Exotic Animal Emergency and Critical Care Medicine

Exotic Animal Emergency and Critical Care Medicine

Edited by

Jennifer E. Graham | DVM, Dipl. ABVP (Avian/Exotic Companion Mammal), Dipl. ACZM
Cummings School of Veterinary Medicine at Tufts University, North Grafton, Massachusetts, USA

Grayson A. Doss | DVM, Dipl. ACZM
School of Veterinary Medicine, University of Wisconsin-Madison, Madison, Wisconsin, USA

Hugues Beaufrère | DVM, PhD, Dipl. ACZM, Dipl. ABVP(Avian), Dipl. ECZM(Avian)
School of Veterinary Medicine, University of California-Davis, Davis, California, USA

WILEY Blackwell

Registered Office
John Wiley & Sons, Inc., 111 River Street, Hoboken, NJ 07030, USA

Editorial Office
111 River Street, Hoboken, NJ 07030, USA

For details of our global editorial offices, customer services, and more information about Wiley products visit us at www.wiley.com.

Wiley also publishes its books in a variety of electronic formats and by print-on-demand. Some content that appears in standard print versions of this book may not be available in other formats.

Library of Congress Cataloging-in-Publication Data

Names: Graham, Jennifer E. (Jennifer Erin), 1974– editor. | Beaufrère, Hugues, 1982– editor. | Doss, Grayson A., 1986– editor.
Title: Exotic animal emergency and critical care medicine / [edited by] Jennifer E. Graham, Hugues Beaufrère, Grayson A. Doss.
Description: Hoboken, NJ : Wiley-Blackwell, [2021] | Includes bibliographical references and index.
Identifiers: LCCN 2020048418 (print) | LCCN 2020048419 (ebook) | ISBN 9781119149231 (cloth) | ISBN 9781119149248 (adobe pdf) | ISBN 9781119149255 (epub)
Subjects: MESH: Animals, Exotic | Emergencies–veterinary | Emergency Treatment–veterinary | Critical Care–methods
Classification: LCC SF997.5.E95 (print) | LCC SF997.5.E95 (ebook) | NLM SF 997.5.E95 | DDC 636.089/025–dc23
LC record available at https://lccn.loc.gov/2020048418
LC ebook record available at https://lccn.loc.gov/2020048419

Cover Design: Wiley
Cover Image: © Grayson Doss, Jennifer E. Graham, Hugues Beaufrère

Set in 9.5/12.5pt STIXTwoText by Straive, Pondicherry, India

SKY10094157_121824

This book is dedicated to those brave souls who are always on high alert, sacrificing sleep and ready to give their all to save a life...and all the feathered, furred, scaled, and amphibious patients they care for.

Contents

List of Contributors

Ali Anwar Bin Ahmad, DVM
Department of Veterinary Services
Singapore Zoological Gardens
Singapore

Hamish Baron, BVSc (Hons), FANZCVS (Avian Medicine and Surgery)
The Unusual Pet Vets
Frankston, Victoria, Australia

Andrew D. Bean, DVM, MPH, Dipl. ABVP (Exotic Companion Mammal Practice)
Avian & Exotic Medicine Service
Animal Emergency and Referral Center of Minnesota
Oakdale, Minnesota, USA

Hugues Beaufrère, Dr.Med.Vet., PhD, Dipl. ACZM, Dipl. ABVP (Avian), Dipl. ECZM (Avian)
Associate Professor
Department of Medicine and Epidemiology
School of Veterinary Medicine
University of California Davis
Davis, California, USA

Diana Binanti, DVM, PhD, Dipl. ECVP
AbLab Veterinary Diagnostic Laboratory
Sarzana, La Spezia, Italy

João Brandão, LMV, MS, Dipl. ECZM (Avian)
Associate Professor, Zoological Medicine
Bell Professorship in Veterinary Clinical Sciences
Zoological Medicine Service
Department of Veterinary Clinical Sciences
College of Veterinary Medicine
Oklahoma State University
Stillwater, Oklahoma, USA

Julie DeCubellis, DVM, MS
Associate Veterinarian
Calgary Avian and Exotic Pet Clinic
Calgary, Alberta, Canada

Marion Desmarchelier, DMV, IPSAV, DES, MSc, Dipl. ACZM, Dipl. ECZM (Zoo Health Management), Dipl. ACVB
Assistant Professor, Department of Clinical Sciences
Faculté de médecine vétérinaire
Université de Montréal
Saint-Hyacinthe, Québec, Canada

Peter M. DiGeronimo, VMD, MSc, Dipl. ACZM,
Veterinarian
Adventure Aquarium
Camden, New Jersey, USA

Nicola Di Girolamo
DMV, MSc (EBHC), PhD, Dipl. ECZM (Herp), Dipl. ACZM
Associate Professor, Zoological Medicine
Exotics and Zoological Service
Department of Veterinary Clinical Sciences
College of Veterinary Medicine
Oklahoma State University
Stillwater, Oklahoma, USA

Grayson A. Doss, DVM, Dipl. ACZM
Clinical Assistant Professor, Zoological Medicine
University of Wisconsin-Madison
Madison, Wisconsin, USA

Constance Fazio, DVM, Dipl. ACVR
Clinical Assistant Professor of Radiology
Department of Small Animal Clinical Sciences
College of Veterinary Medicine
University of Tennessee
Knoxville, Tennessee, USA

Sara Gardhouse, DVM, Dipl. ABVP (Exotic Companion Mammal), Dipl. ACZM
Assistant Professor
Exotic Pet, Wildlife, and Zoological Medicine, Department of Clinical Sciences, College of Veterinary Medicine
Kansas State University
Manhattan, Kansas, USA

Jennifer E. Graham, DVM, Dipl. ABVP (Avian/Exotic Companion Mammal), Dipl. ACZM
Associate Professor of Zoological Companion Animal Medicine
Department of Clinical Sciences
Cummings School of Veterinary Medicine
Tufts University
North Grafton, Massachusetts, USA

Vanessa Grunkemeyer, DVM, MPH, Dipl. ABVP (Avian)
Program Coordinator & Clinical Assistant Professor, UNH Animal Science
Director, UNH Pre-Veterinary Advising
Department of Agriculture, Nutrition, and Food Systems
University of New Hampshire
Durham, New Hampshire, USA

Ruth A. Houseright, DVM, Dipl. ACVP
Yahara Veterinary Research and Diagnostics, LLC
Madison, Wisconsin, USA

Dan H. Johnson, DVM, Dipl. ABVP (Exotic Companion Mammal)
Avian and Exotic Animal Care
Raleigh, North Carolina, USA

Claudia Kabakchiev, DVM
404 Veterinary Emergency and Referral Hospital
Ontario, Canada

Ian Kanda, RVT, VTS (Exotic Companion Animal)
Exotic and Wildlife Technician
Avian, Exotic and Zoological Service
Boren Veterinary Medical Teaching Hospital
College of Veterinary Medicine
Oklahoma State University
Stillwater, Oklahoma, USA

Krista A. Keller, DVM, Dipl. ACZM
Assistant Professor, Department of Veterinary Clinical Medicine
Codirector, Wildlife Epidemiology Laboratory
College of Veterinary Medicine
University of Illinois
Urbana, Illinois, USA

Eric Klaphake, DVM, Dipl. ACZM
Associate Veterinarian
Cheyenne Mountain Zoo
Colorado Springs, Colorado, USA

Carrie Kuzma, DVM, Dipl. ACVR
Clinical Assistant Professor, Diagnostic Imaging
Department of Veterinary Clinical Sciences
College of Veterinary Medicine
Oklahoma State University
Stillwater, Oklahoma, USA

Isabelle Langlois, DMV, Dipl. ABVP (Avian)
Clinical Instructor
Zoological Medicine Service
Department of Clinical Sciences
Faculté de médecine vétérinaire
Université de Montréal
Saint-Hyacinthe, Québec, Canada

Delphine Laniesse, DMV, DVSc, ECZM (Avian), ABVP (Avian)
Evidensia Eläinsairaala
Tammisto, Vantaa
Finland

Rina Maguire, BVSC (Hons 1) Dipl. ABVP Exotic Companion Mammal
Owner and Veterinarian
Beecroft Bird & Exotics Veterinary Clinic
Singapore

Christoph Mans, Dr. med. vet., Dipl. ACZM
Clinical Associate Professor, Zoological Medicine
Department of Surgical Sciences
School of Veterinary Medicine
University of Wisconsin–Madison
Madison, Wisconsin, USA

Anna Martel, DVM
Clinical instructor, Zoological Medicine
Department of Surgical Sciences
School of Veterinary Medicine
University of Wisconsin–Madison
Madison, Wisconsin, USA

Carla Monteiro, LMV
Staff Veterinarian, Zoo Santo Inácio
Exotic/Wild Life Consulting - Clínica Veterinária Atlântida
Porto, Portugal

Helene Pendl, Dr. med. vet.
Pendl Lab
Hematology, Cytology, and Histopathology in Birds and Reptiles
Zug, Switzerland

Sean Michael Perry, DVM, PhD
Associate Veterinarian
Mississippi Aquarium
Gulfport, Mississippi, USA

David N. Phalen, DVM, PhD
Professor
Sydney School of Veterinary Science
University of Sydney
Camden, New South Wales, Australia

David Sanchez-Migallon Guzman, LV, MS, Dipl. ECZM (Avian, Small Mammal), Dipl. ACZM
Professor of Clinical Zoological Companion Animal Medicine and Surgery
Department of Medicine and Epidemiology
School of Veterinary Medicine
University of California–Davis
Davis, California, USA

Rodney Schnellbacher, DVM, Dipl. ACZM
Associate Veterinarian
Zoo Miami
One Zoo Boulevard, Florida, USA

Nico J. Schoemaker, DVM, PhD, Dipl. ECZM (Small Mammal and Avian)
Division of Zoological Medicine
Department of Clinical Sciences
Faculty of Veterinary Medicine
Utrecht University
Utrecht, The Netherlands

Kristin M. Sinclair, DVM, Dipl. ABVP (Avian Practice, Exotic Companion Mammal)
Kensington Bird and Animal Hospital
Kensington, Connecticut, USA

Kurt K. Sladky, MS, DVM, Dipl. ACZM, Dipl. ECZM (Zoo Health Management), Dipl. ECZM (Herpetology)
Clinical Professor, Zoological Medicine
Department of Surgical Sciences
School of Veterinary Medicine
University of Wisconsin–Madison
Madison, Wisconsin, USA

Samantha Swisher, DVM, Dipl. ABVP (Exotic Companion Mammal)
Veterinary Public Health Resident
Department of Veterinary Preventive Medicine
College of Veterinary Medicine
The Ohio State University
Columbus, Ohio, USA

Trent Charles van Zanten, BSc Hons, DVM
Conservation, Research and Veterinary Services
Jurong Bird Park, Wildlife Reserves Singapore
Singapore

Yvonne R.A. van Zeeland, DVM, MVR, PhD, Dipl. ECZM (Avian and Small Mammal), CPBC
Division of Zoological Medicine
Department of Clinical Sciences
Faculty of Veterinary Medicine
Utrecht University
Utrecht, The Netherlands

Claire Vergneau-Grosset, DMV, IPSAV, CES, Dipl. ACZM
Assistant Professor, Zoological Medicine Service
Faculté de médecine vétérinaire
Université de Montréal
Saint-Hyacinthe, Quebec, Canada

Kenneth R. Welle, DVM, Dipl. ABVP, Avian Practice
Clinical Assistant Professor
Zoological Medicine
University of Illinois Veterinary Teaching Hospital
Urbana, Illinois, USA

Peter M. Wencel, DVM
Avian Veterinarian
Al Aseefa Falcon Hospital
Dubai, United Arab Emirates

Stacey L. Wilkinson, DVM, Dipl. ABVP (Reptile & Amphibian)
Owner and Head Veterinarian
Avian and Exotic Animal Hospital of Georgia
Pooler, Georgia, USA

Nicole R. Wyre, DVM, ABVP (Avian), ABVP (Exotic Companion Mammal)
Zodiac Pet and Exotic Hospital
Tin Hau, Hong Kong

Part 1

Exotic Companion Mammals

Section 1

Triage and Stabilization

1

History and Clinical Examination

Nico J. Schoemaker and Yvonne R.A. van Zeeland

Division of Zoological Medicine, Department of Clinical Sciences, Faculty of Veterinary Medicine, Utrecht University, The Netherlands

CONTENTS

Initial Phone Consultation

During the phone call, an initial evaluation of the patient's status needs to be made. Based on the information obtained during the initial phone call, the reception staff or veterinarian can assess whether and when the animal should come. Proper instructions regarding basic first aid procedures and transport instructions to optimize the chances of the patient arriving alive at the clinic should also be relayed during this call.

Is it an Emergency?

Small mammals may present with a variety of emergency signs (see Box 1.1 for an overview). Similar to dogs and cats, emergencies can be broken down into two categories, i.e. "acute" (i.e. resulting from a sudden, recent event, e.g. bite wounds, fall injuries, intoxications) and "chronic" (i.e. resulting from a more chronic, ongoing process, e.g. dental disease, gastritis, vitamin C deficiency in guinea pigs). Especially in small mammal patients, "chronic" emergencies are common due to the animal hiding signs of disease and/or the owner not being experienced enough to recognize signs of illness until the animal is in a severely debilitated condition. As a result, these conditions may be just as life-threatening as "acute" emergencies, thereby warranting a proper assessment to be made during the initial phone call. This emphasizes the importance of having properly trained reception staff, whose primary task is to establish whether the animal can be scheduled for a regular appointment, or whether it needs to come in as an emergency case. If the case classifies as an emergency, it should be determined whether the owner needs to come in immediately (e.g. in case of severe trauma involving blood loss and an open fracture), or whether the appointment can be scheduled later on the same day, but within the next 24 hours (e.g. a rabbit with anorexia for more than 12 hours).

Exotic Animal Emergency and Critical Care Medicine, First Edition. Edited by Jennifer E. Graham, Grayson A. Doss and Hugues Beaufrère.

Box 1.1 Common Emergency Presentations of Small Mammals

Presenting signs noted by the owner that generally warrant immediate attention

Anorexia, decreased appetite
Behavior changes, e.g. hiding, sitting still in a corner, restlessness
Bloated abdomen
Blood loss
Breathing abnormalities, labored breathing
Collapse
Diarrhea, reduced production of droppings (particularly in herbivores)
Dysuria, stranguria
Dystocia (particularly in guinea pigs)
Exophthalmos
Fly strike (particularly in rabbits)
Hematuria
Hypothermia or hyperthermia (including fever, heat stress)
Intoxications (including suspected cases)
Lameness (sudden onset, e.g. due to fractures)
Lethargy, stupor, coma
Lumps, masses (especially in case of sudden onset)
Nasal discharge, sneezing
Neurologic signs, e.g. head tilt, seizures
Paresis/paralysis
Posture changes, e.g. hunched up
Polyuria, altered water intake
Teeth grinding
Traumatic injuries, e.g. bite wounds, fall injuries
Vomiting[a], choking
Weakness
Weight loss

a **Not in herbivorous small mammals, e.g. rabbits, guinea pigs, chinchillas.**

Signalment and (Abbreviated) History

To properly assess the patient's condition over the phone, the information should be obtained regarding the patient's signalment and the presenting problems.

The signalment includes the species, breed, sex, neutering or breeding status, and age of the animal. This information is essential for the initial evaluation of the patient's status. For example, a juvenile that has not eaten for six hours will often be a greater emergency than an adult animal of the same species. Moreover, the information can help to establish an initial differential or tentative diagnosis for the presenting signs.

The owner should also be questioned on the clinical signs that the animal is displaying, including when those signs became apparent. Obvious questions that should be asked are: What is the problem? What signs does the animal show? When did you first notice these signs? Did you notice any changes since then, and if so, what are they?

In cases of trauma, it is helpful to inquire about the nature of the trauma and when it occurred, whether the animal has been unconscious, and if so, for how long. If bleeding was present, the owner should be asked to provide an estimate on the extent of the blood loss. When dealing with or suspicious of an intoxication, the nature of the poison and an estimate of the ingested amount and elapsed time since the ingestion are essential. This preliminary information helps to establish an initial differential or tentative diagnosis, e.g. the sudden onset of severe vomiting in a ferret following ingestion of a foreign body is highly suggestive for an obstruction.

Owner Instructions

The initial phone call should be used to provide the necessary instructions to help stabilize the patient and transport it safely to the clinic. Similarly, instructions can be provided to help calm the animal and minimize its stress during the handling and transport and to ensure that the owner brings along any and all necessary items and/or materials, where applicable.

First Aid at Home

Dependent on the severity and type of emergency, the owner may need to provide basic first aid at home to stabilize the patient and allow the animal to be transported to the clinic safely. Guidelines for first aid in the home environment can be found in Table 1.1.

Transport

The animal should be safely contained during transportation to prevent additional trauma or stress. This is usually best achieved by placing the animal in a suitable carrier (Figure 1.1). Towels can be used to provide a soft bedding. Transportation without a carrier should only be considered if the animal is in shock at which time the animal can be placed on the lap of the co-driver while preferably being wrapped in a blanket. For further guidelines on safe transportation, the reader is referred to Chapter 2.

Materials to Bring Along for the Emergency Visit

Dependent on the presenting signs, the owner can be advised to bring the following along for the visit: feces and urine (when available), vaccination documentation, and photos of the enclosure and living environment. For patients with intermittent clinical signs, videos can be very helpful. When hospitalization may be required, the owner can be asked to bring

Table 1.1 Basic first aid procedures for specific small mammal emergencies.

Type of emergency	Instructions to be provided to the owner
Bleeding (external)	• Apply pressure to stop the bleeding. Hold pressure for at least 3 min before checking if a clot has formed. Alternatively, a bandage may be used for applying pressure to the site • If possible, use a sterile gauze pad to put pressure over the wound. A clean towel, cloth, or handkerchief can be used as an alternative • Do not remove the pad or cloth if it becomes saturated with blood. Instead, apply another one over it and continue applying pressure • If bleeding is severe and, on the legs, a tourniquet (e.g. an elastic band or gauze) can be applied between the wound and the body. To prevent ischemia, the tourniquet can be loosened for 20 s every 15–20 min • If the animal is conscious, some water may be offered for rehydration purposes • In case of an injured claw, styptic powder or flour can be used to stimulate clotting. Several applications may be needed to completely stop the bleeding
Bleeding (internal)	• Symptoms indicating internal bleeding are presence of bleeding from nose, mouth, anus, coughing up blood, blood in urine, pale gums, collapse, and a weak and rapid pulse • If internal bleeding is suspected, the animal should be kept as warm and quiet as possible and transported to the clinic immediately for further treatment
Burns	• Cool the area immediately by immersion or flushing with cool running water or applying a cool compress or cold pack for a minimum of 5–10 min prior to transporting the animal to the clinic • Do not apply any ointments prior to seeking veterinary care • In case of a chemical burn, flush the wound immediately with large quantities of (cool) water • In case of an electric burn (e.g. from biting an electric cord), the animal's mouth may be burnt or lung edema may occur, which may present as labored breathing. In this situation, it is vital to minimize stress and place the animal in a well-ventilated place • While transporting the animal to the clinic, keep it calm by wrapping it in a blanket; avoid overheating or obstructing breathing
Choking, airway obstruction	• If possible, check whether the airway is blocked by the tongue or an object. If this is the case, try to either pull out the tongue or gently remove the object from the oral cavity, e.g. using tweezers or pliers. Care should be taken not to push the object further caudally into the throat and/or waste too much time on trying to get the object out • If the animal is still able to breathe, it is best to try and keep it as calm as possible and transport it to the veterinary clinic immediately • If the airway is not completely obstructed and the animal is able to cough, it may be best to have the animal attempt to cough up the offending particle itself • A (modified) Heimlich maneuver should only be performed if absolutely necessary (i.e. an animal that has collapsed or is in great respiratory distress). For this purpose, a firm (but gentle) upwards press (with the animal placed in sternal recumbency) against the diaphragm is needed to help expel air from the lungs and dislodge objects that are stuck in the trachea. Always ensure that the back and neck are adequately supported during the procedure • Alternative methods include the following: (i) the animal is raised onto its hind legs (or lifted in the air) with the animal's backline against the owner's front, while the arms are placed around the animal just beneath the ribs. The animal is then squeezed firmly in an upward and forward movement for up to four times; (ii) the animal is held upside down by its hind legs and suspended into the air or laid down on its side following which 3–4 firm blows are delivered to the abdomen or side, respectively; and (iii) the animal is held firmly between the forearms whereby the neck and spine are completely immobile, following which the animal is "swung" from a horizontal to a vertical, upside down position. *Note*: This last procedure carries great risk of dropping the animal, potentially leading to severe injuries
Eye injury	• Symptoms indicating eye problems include blepharospasm, pawing, or rubbing the eye, a visible third eyelid that is covering the eye, corneal edema, erythema and/or swelling of the eyelids and/or increased tear production • The animal should be seen by a veterinarian immediately as eye injuries can be extremely painful and can quickly result in blindness if left untreated • Do not apply any medications onto the animal's eye unless these have been advised by a veterinarian

(Continued)

Mammals

Table 1.1 (Continued)

Type of emergency	Instructions to be provided to the owner
Fractures	• Gently place the animal on a flat surface for support • Splinting of a fractured bone is generally not recommended as this may cause further injury • In case of exposed bone, the fracture ends should preferably be covered with sterile gauzes. Alternatively, a freshly laundered (clean) handkerchief or towel can be used to prevent bacterial contamination • Never attempt to push the fractured bone ends back in position • Place the animal in a box or carrier so that it does not try to move around • In case of a leg that is dangling at an odd angle or not moving properly, spinal injury may be present. This requires extra care when moving the animal into a box or carrier
Hypothermia	• Wrap the animal in a thick blanket, jumper, or layer of bubble wrap to prevent further heat loss • If possible, use a heat pack to warm the animal • Reheating is best done slowly. Repeatedly check the animal's body temperature to avoid overheating the animal • If the animal is wet, dry it as quickly as possible to prevent it from cooling down further
Hyperthermia, heat stroke	• If it is not possible to come to the clinic, the animal should be moved into a cooler, shaded area, and out of direct sunlight • Wrap a cool or cold, wet towel around the animal's neck and body. Be careful not to cover the eyes, nose, or mouth. Remove the towel, wring it out, and rewet and wrap it every few minutes • Drizzle water over the animal, concentrating on the head, stomach, ventral neck surface, inner thighs, and footpads. For larger animals, gentle hosing or bathing in cool water can be attempted • Do not apply icepacks to the pet • Cool the animal down slowly. Regularly check the animal's body temperature to avoid hypothermia. Once the temperature has come down to 39 °C (102 °F), cooling down can be stopped following which the animal can be placed in a dry towel
Poisoning, exposure to toxins	• Prevent further exposure, ingestion, or inhalation of the toxic substance • Follow instructions for human exposure to the product, as listed on the label • Bring the product container/packaging along for reference • Collect any material that the animal may have vomited or chewed (wear gloves), place it in a plastic bag and bring the material along for the visit
Seizures	• Clear the area from objects that could lead to injury of the animal • Darken the room and ensure a quiet surrounding • If unconscious, check if the animal is breathing and nothing is obstructing the airway • Do not try to restrain the animal. Wait until the seizuring has stopped before touching or moving the animal • Time how long the seizure lasts • Keep the pet as warm and quiet as possible following the seizure. Reassure the animal if needed • Do not provide any water or food until the animal is fully conscious
Shock	• Keep the animal warm (e.g. using a hot water bottle wrapped in a towel) and minimize stress as much as possible (e.g. placing the animal in a covered box or carrier) • If the animal is conscious, some apple juice or dextrose dissolved in water may be provided for rehydration purposes and provision of extra sugar • If the animal is unconscious, the head needs to be kept level with the rest of the body • The animal should be transported to the veterinarian immediately

Table 1.1 (Continued)

Type of emergency	Instructions to be provided to the owner
Wounds	• Shallow cuts or bite wounds can be cleaned by flushing the wound with iodine solution diluted in warm water to the color of iced tea. If iodine is not available, an antiseptic soap in warm water or a warm saltwater solution (i.e. one teaspoon of salt to one cup of previously boiled water) can be used as an alternative • If a penetrating object is present in the wound, do not attempt to remove it. If possible, reduce the size of the protruding part of the foreign body to 3–4 cm above the skin level. Be careful not to cause damage. If the object has caused a penetrating wound to the chest, restrict the animal's movements and try wrapping the chest and covering the wound with a plastic wrap, without putting further pressure on the penetrating object. Do not attempt to move the object! • Control bleeding, but without putting pressure onto the penetrating object, if present • Any type of breach of the skin carries a risk of (bacterial) infection. A course of antibiotics can help prevent these infections, but only if treated promptly (i.e. within 6–12 hr) • Keep the animal warm and seek help from a veterinarian immediately so that adequate wound care can be provided

Note: Owners should always be made aware that the procedures as mentioned above are only intended to keep the animal alive for transport to the veterinarian and are *never* to be used as a substitute for the provision of veterinary care.

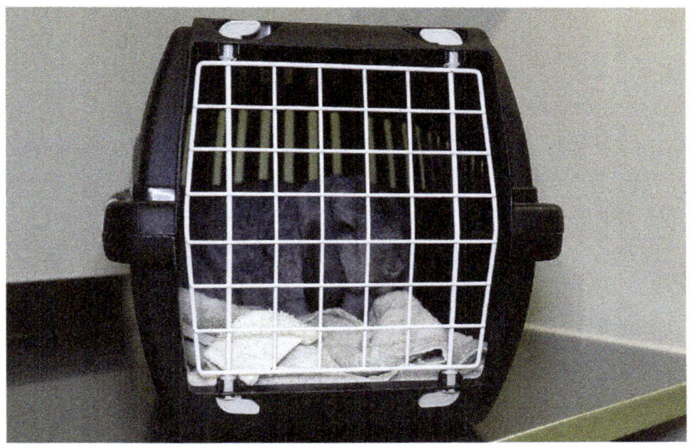

Figure 1.1 A transportation carrier is recommended to allow for safe transportation of any small animal to the veterinary hospital.

along familiar food, bedding, and enrichment to increase patient comfort. In some cases, it may be advised to bring a companion animal as this both helps to reduce stress from hospitalization and prevent problems during reintroduction of the animal to its cage mate(s). When poisoning or toxin exposure is suspected or confirmed, the owner should be instructed to bring along any relevant product packaging, or a photograph or sample of the poison (e.g. plant).

History

If the patient is sufficiently stable, history can be taken prior to examining the animal. Standardized forms ensure that all necessary information is obtained (see Mammal History Form at the end of this chapter and a downloadable form is available at www.wiley.com.). During history taking, the patient may be let out of the cage to acclimatize to the surroundings while simultaneously allowing it to be evaluated from a distance without causing additional stress. If the animal is highly stressed, it can also be left in the carrier. Evaluation from a distance will still be possible if the carrier is strategically placed.

Presenting Signs

Every history starts with a question along the line of "What is the reason for your visit?". In addition to clarifying the nature of the problem for which the owner is seeking veterinary advice, it is important to gather information regarding the time of onset, duration, and clinical course of the presenting signs as well as any treatments that have been attempted prior to the visit (including their effects). Next, questions are asked to obtain an impression of the animal's general condition, including questions pertaining to the food intake, drinking, behavior, respiration, urination, and defecation. Enquiries should be made to find out whether the animal has previously been sick, or whether any contact animals, relatives, or the owner have been experiencing (similar) signs of illness.

Diet and Husbandry

Many of the problems with which small mammals present are the result of a suboptimal diet and/or husbandry. Thus, extra attention should be paid to these topics during the history taking. Dietary questions should not only aim at finding out what food items are being offered, but also at what is actually eaten by the animal and in what quantities. Other relevant aspects in the nutritional history include the ways in which food and water is offered (including how frequently these are refreshed), the source and brand of the provided food, supplements and/or treats (including the frequency and quantities, if applicable), and (recent) changes in the diet provided to the animal.

Husbandry related questions should include questions related to the dimensions and location (e.g. inside or outside, location in the house) of the enclosure, the furnishings and type of bedding, the frequency of cleaning (including the materials used), and climate conditions (e.g. humidity, temperature, drafts).

Other relevant questions include those related to the time spent outside of the enclosure, whether supervision is present during this time and whether potential ingestion of toxins may have taken place. Especially in animals that can roam free unsupervised, claims of the owner with regard to the impossibility of toxin exposure or foreign body ingestion should be interpreted with caution, as these events may have taken place at a time when the owner was not present.

Preventative Treatments

Aside from providing a well-balanced diet and adequate husbandry, different forms of preventive treatments may be provided to exotic small mammals. Dependent on the region, ferrets may be vaccinated against canine distemper virus and rabies; whereas rabbits may be vaccinated against rabies, myxomatosis, and rabbit hemorrhagic disease virus (RHDV and RHDV-2). Rabbits may be given coccidiostatic drugs around the time of weaning to prevent clinical coccidiosis. Other routine preventive treatments provided to small mammals (especially those that have been recently acquired) include antiparasitic treatments for fleas, lice and/or ear, fur, or burrowing mites. Similarly, mammals such as rabbits and guinea pigs may have been preventively treated for dermatophytosis as this is another disease that is commonly seen in (young) rabbits and guinea pigs.

Physical Exam

Primary Survey

General Impression

A general impression of the exotic small mammal patient is obtained through observation of the animal within the cage, carrier, or normal environment of the animal. Preferably, the observations are performed without the animal noticing it to minimally affect its behavior. Asking the owner whether the animal's behavior has changed is important as he/she will most likely be able to provide accurate information on the patient's behavior in its own surroundings.

While observing the animal, attention is paid to the level of consciousness/alertness and behavior, posture and locomotion, body shape and body condition (a Body Condition Score system of either five or nine reference points can be used), condition of the hair coat, and presence of abnormal sounds or other types of noticeable abnormalities. In addition, it is recommended to pay attention to the frequency, type, depth, and regularity of breathing, as respiration will generally be affected following handling. In emergency patients, special attention is paid to the level of consciousness as this helps to determine the level of urgency. When the animal is no longer bright, alert, and/or responsive to its environment, an immediate response is warranted, whereby the ABCDE protocol rather than the standard physical examination protocol should be followed.

ABCDE Protocol

Similar to other companion animals, the ABCDE protocol provides a structured method for evaluation of the small mammal emergency patient. According to this protocol, the following five aspects are subsequently assessed: (i) Airway; (ii) Breathing; (iii) Circulation; (iv) Disability; and (v) Exposure of Environment. If abnormalities are noted, these are first treated before continuing to the next step in the evaluation. Prior to examining the patient, necessary precautions should always be taken so that personal (and patient) safety is ensured.

Airway Examine the airway for signs of obstruction. Signs indicating airway obstruction include paradoxical chest and abdominal movements, increased respiratory effort (particularly during inspiration), cyanosis, and/or presence of abnormal breath sounds or stridor (indicative of an incomplete obstruction or narrowing of the airway). If stridor is present, the type of sound may assist in localizing the obstruction. For example, a sniffing sound is heard in case of a nasal obstruction, whereas a pharyngeal obstruction results in a snoring sound. A typical English "H-," Dutch "G-," or Spanish "J-"sound is indicative for a laryngeal or tracheal obstruction. In case of a nasal obstruction, animals will frequently display open mouth breathing. It is important to realize that rabbits and guinea pigs will only display open mouth breathing in case of severe respiratory distress as their glottis is located on top of their soft palate. In case of airway obstruction, immediate action will be needed to remove the obstruction, e.g. removing mucous or fluids through suction, manually grasping the offending particle, pulling out the tongue, inserting a supraglottic airway device or endotracheal tube and/or performing a tracheostomy. Oxygen should be provided at high concentrations to optimize oxygenation.

Breathing Assess the depth, pattern (type, rhythm), and frequency of the respiratory movements, as well as the presence of accessory respiratory movements (e.g. excessive movement of the nostrils and open mouth breathing) and/or cyanosis. Special attention should be paid to the appearance of the thorax (including any deformities) and the thoracic and abdominal movements. Auscultation will help to evaluate the presence or absence of respiratory sounds, including a decrease or increase in these sounds and the presence of abnormal sounds (e.g. wheezing, whistling). Like dogs and cats, the percussion of the thorax can be performed to identify conditions such as pneumothorax or pleural effusion. However, due to the size of the animal, the procedure is often more difficult to perform and interpret and may be stressful to the patient. As a result, this part of the examination is commonly omitted. In case problems with breathing are identified, similar actions as those described above (i.e. supplementing oxygen and assisted breathing) are indicated.

Circulation The cardiovascular function is evaluated by examining the pulse, mucous membranes, and heart. In many small exotic mammals, the arterial pulse is not easily palpated, but in ferrets, rabbits, and guinea pigs, palpation of the pulse is feasible. If a pulse is present, the rate, quality (i.e. strength, filling, equality), and regularity should be assessed. Inspection of the conjunctival or oral mucosa will provide information on its color and moistness. The capillary refill time (CRT) can be assessed on the unpigmented footpad in many species, except for rabbits as the plantar surface of their feet is covered in thick fur. In rabbits, the unpigmented inside of the pinnae may be used instead. Aside from these parameters, palpation of the temperature of the extremities may also provide additional clues on the quality of the peripheral circulation. The heart can be auscultated for the presence of a heartbeat, and, if a heartbeat is audible, whether the heart sounds are regular and have the expected intensity and whether any murmurs are present. Finally, the examination should focus on identifying the presence of hemorrhage. If hemorrhage is present, adequate action should be taken to control the bleeding. Other actions to be taken will often depend on the specific cause for the cardiovascular collapse but are generally aimed at fluid replacement (except in patients with cardiac failure) and restoration of tissue perfusion.

Disability Assess the patient's mentation (i.e. level of consciousness and responsiveness to the environment) and reflexes, including the cerebral (i.e. corneal and pupillary) and spinal reflexes. It is good to realize that the menace reflex is frequently absent in rabbits and rodents. In addition, the size and symmetry of the pupils can be assessed. Neurological deficits leading to an altered mentation, or absent cerebral reflexes generally indicate a lesion within the cerebrum. Symmetric signs will often have a better prognosis compared to asymmetric signs, as the latter are likely due to focal brain lesions (e.g. neoplasia, infarction, hemorrhage, granuloma) which carry a poor prognosis.

Exposure of Environment During this part of the examination, attention is paid to the influence that the environment may have had on the animal. Aside from checking for the presence of skin lesions, bruises, fractures, or other types of trauma, the animal's body temperature should be taken. Adequate action should be taken to treat and/or prevent hypothermia as well as hyperthermia. In case wounds or fractures are present, these should be treated promptly and appropriately (e.g. cleaning, bandaging).

Secondary Survey

Full Physical Examination

After having gathered the history of the animal and having obtained a general impression of the animal and its enclosure, a complete physical examination of the animal is performed (see Box 1.2 for a checklist of equipment needed for a detailed small mammal physical examination). The structure of the physical examination in the exotic small mammal patient is similar to dogs and cats. However, size and demeanor of the animal may be limiting factors for obtaining accurate information.

Box 1.2 Equipment List for the Detailed Small Mammal Physical Examination

- Infant or pediatric-sized stethoscope
- Ophthalmoscope for oral and ear inspection
- Penlight
- Tape strips and flea comb
- Lubricant and thermometer; distractor treat for ferrets
- Medical ruler (to accurately assess the size of lessons or masses)
- Percussor
- Transparent (acrylic, plastic) box and pipe (to allow visualization of ventral surface area or observe the animal without restraint)

Box 1.3 Focus Areas for a Small Mammal Physical Examination

- Body condition score and/or weight
- Respiratory frequency, depth, type, and rhythm
- Arterial pulse frequency, quality, and rhythm
- Core body temperature
- Coat and skin (including skin turgor)
- Mucous membranes (color, moistness, presence of lesions or hemorrhage, capillary refill time)
- Lymph nodes (shape, size, consistency, painfulness, and mobility)
- Auscultation of the heart and lungs
  - Respiratory rate and sounds
  - Heart rate and sounds
- Abdominal inspection, palpation, and auscultation

The focus areas for the physical examination of a small mammal patient can be found in Box 1.3. As handling and restraint may significantly alter the body temperature, heart/pulse rate, and breathing, these are always evaluated first, whereby breathing is preferably assessed while the animal is still sitting in the carrier. After completing the physical examination, the animal should always be weighed as this will enable accurate drug dosing (if needed) and provide a point of reference for future monitoring purposes (Figure 1.2).

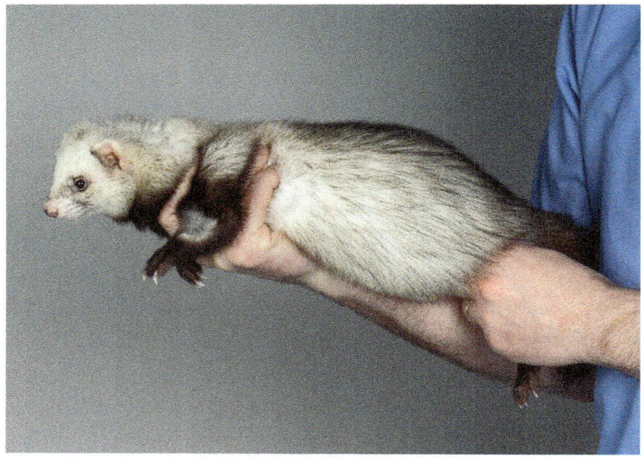

Figure 1.3 Palpation of the pulse in a ferret is often easy to perform with the body of the ferret resting on the arm.

Ferrets

The pulse can be relatively easily assessed at the femoral artery. To facilitate palpation of the pulse, the ferret is preferably placed on the arm rather than on a table (Figure 1.3). Auscultation of the heart is best performed at the level of the 6th to 8th rib. The rectal temperature is preferably measured using a digital thermometer. Ferrets do not tolerate rectal temperature well and a distraction treat may be useful; ideally use something without added sugars to avoid altering blood glucose levels, such as FerreTone™. Reference values for the respiration rate, heart rate, and body temperature can be found in Table 1.2. While taking the temperature, the gender of the ferret can also be assessed (see Section "Gender Determination"). As ferrets may vehemently resist rectal temperature, urination and defecation often occur during this procedure in stressed patients and samples can be opportunistically collected if this happens.

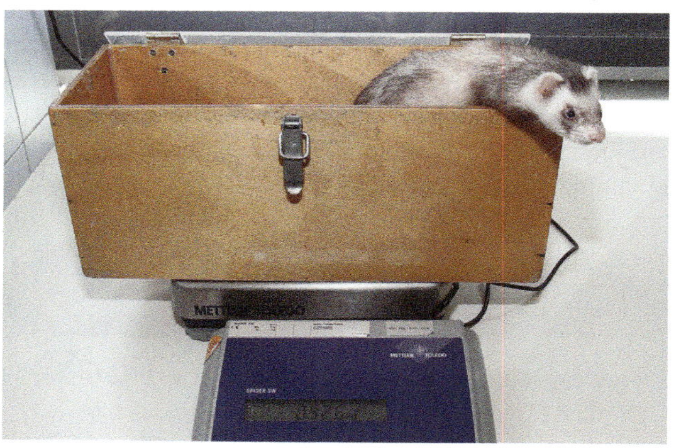

Figure 1.2 Obtaining an accurate weight is extremely important in any small mammal to accurately assess weight changes over time and ensure correct dosing of medication.

The hydration status can be assessed by obtaining the skin turgor of the upper eyelids, evaluating tenting of the skin in the neck or thorax; and evaluating the moistness of the oral mucosa. While checking the oral mucosa, attention should also be paid to the teeth, which should be free from tartar. The CRT can be assessed at an unpigmented footpad, similar to cats.

Since ferrets often have ear mites, special attention should be paid to the external ear canals. The mandibular, axillary, inguinal, and popliteal lymph nodes should be checked. These may appear enlarged in overweight animals. If the lymph nodes also appear firm, a fine needle aspirate should be taken to check for lymphoma as this is a common condition seen in ferrets. A standard physical examination will also include an auscultation of the thorax as well as an abdominal palpation, during which an enlarged spleen will commonly be noted as a coincidental finding.

Table 1.2 Selected biological data and reference ranges of exotic small mammals.

Species	Body weight (g)	Respiratory rate (breaths/min)	Heart rate (beats/min)	Body temperature (°C/°F)	Life expectancy (years)
Ferret	♀ 400–1000 ♂ 600–1500	30–60	180–250	38–40/100–104	5–10
Rabbit	800–7000	30–60	150–300	38–40/100–104	5–10[a]
Guinea pig	700–1200	70–150	220–300	38–39/100–102	4–7
Chinchilla	400–600	40–100	100–300	38–39/100–102	10–15[a]
Rat	225–800	60–120	280–500	38/99–100	2.5–3
Mouse	20–40	80–230	500–725	37.5/99	1–2.5
Syrian hamster	100–200	100–250	280–420	38/99–100	1.5–2
Gerbil	70–130	70–120	260–600	38/99–100	1.5–2.5
Hedgehog	♀ 300–400 ♂ 400–600	25–50	180–280	35.5–37/96–99	4–6
Sugar glider	80–160	16–40	200–300	36/97	10–12

[a] Significant variation reported with some animals living longer.

Rabbits

Although the pulse can be assessed by palpating the femoral artery, the central auricular artery is more commonly used (Figure 1.4). Auscultation of the heart can best be performed at the level of the second to fourth rib. The rabbit's gender is generally assessed while taking the rectal temperature (see Section "Gender Determination"). Reference ranges for vital parameters in the rabbit can be found in Table 1.2.

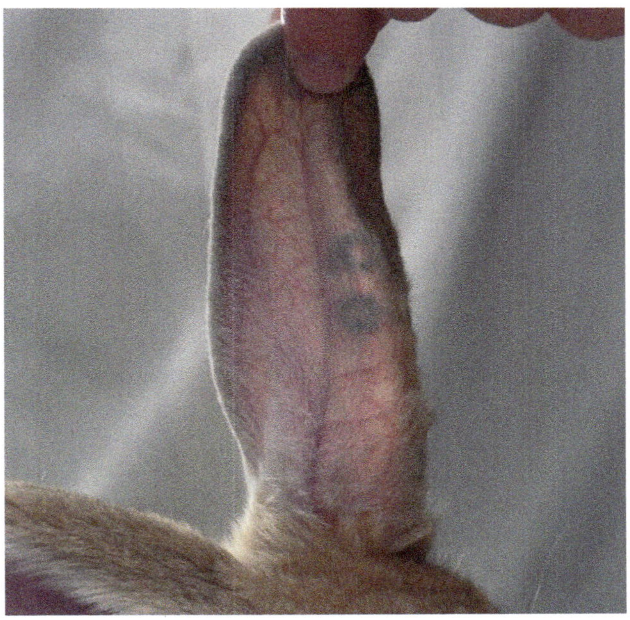

Figure 1.4 The central auricular artery is commonly used for evaluating the pulse of a rabbit.

The hydration status is assessed by evaluating the tenting of the skin over the thorax; and the moistness of the oral mucosa. While checking the oral mucosa, attention should be paid to the position and length of the incisors. As rabbits have dense fur on the plantar surface of their feet, CRT cannot be assessed at the footpads. Instead, CRT is assessed by pressing on the inner surface of the ear pinnae.

Upon examination of the coat and skin, special attention should be paid to the external ear canals and the presence of ear mites. The plantar surface of the hind feet should be inspected to detect (early stages of) pododermatitis, whereas the inner surface of the front paws should be closely inspected for the presence of nasal discharge indicative of (upper) respiratory disease. The mandibular, axillary, inguinal, and popliteal lymph nodes should be evaluated. The mandibular and popliteal lymph nodes may be palpable in healthy animals, dependent on the size of the rabbit. All other lymph nodes will, under normal conditions, be too small to be palpated.

When examining the thorax, palpation of the thorax may help identify the presence of a mass in the cranial mediastinum (i.e. often a thymoma or lymphoma) by caudal displacement of the ictus cordis. In addition, compliance of the thorax may be decreased whereas no breath sounds will be audible upon auscultation of the cranial thorax. Moreover, rabbits with a mediastinal mass will commonly present with bilateral exophthalmos, which can be aggravated upon stressing the animal and/or lifting of the hindquarters (Figure 1.5). Auscultation of the thorax may help detect increased or diminished respiratory sounds, as well as murmurs or irregularities in the heart rhythm.

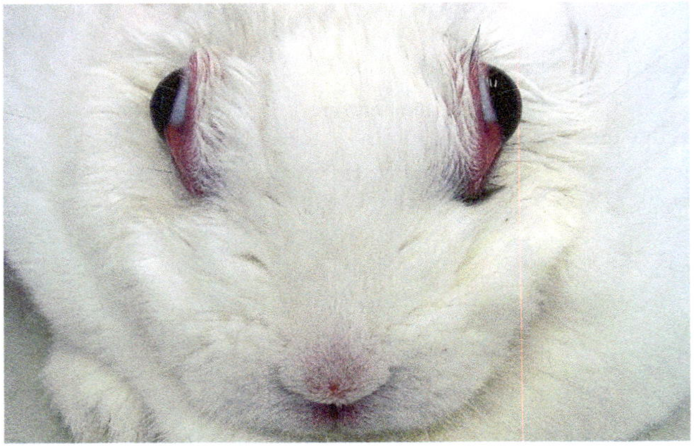

Figure 1.5 Bilateral exophthalmos in a six-year-old male rabbit with a mediastinal mass.

Palpation and auscultation of the abdomen are very important in cases of anorexia to assess the presence of abnormal (gastrointestinal) structures and gastrointestinal motility. In patients suspected of dental problems, an oral examination and palpation of the maxilla and mandible (for the presence of deformities such as abscesses) are recommended. An oral inspection can be performed without sedation using a speculum or otoscope. However, in some patients the procedure can be stressful, thereby warranting sedation or anesthesia to enable the procedure to be performed. In addition, some abnormalities, particularly those in the most caudal portions of the oral cavity, may not be visualized during oral inspection in the awake patient. A more thorough oral inspection while the animal is sedated or anesthetized may therefore be recommended once the patient is stabilized.

Guinea Pigs

Healthy guinea pigs should have an alert demeanor and react to stimuli. When offered greens, they should show interest and (attempt to) eat. On inspection, their eyes should be clear, and their coat should be shining (apart from those with a rex coat).

The physical examination should begin with an assessment of the breathing from a distance, followed by palpation of the pulse at the femoral artery. Due to the size of guinea pigs, a pulse may not always be easily detected, but nevertheless an attempt should be made as this will provide more information than a mere counting of the heart rate. The rectal temperature and gender can subsequently be assessed (see Section "Gender Determination"). Reference values for vital parameters in guinea pigs are found in Table 1.2.

The hydration status can be assessed in a similar fashion as in rabbits, whereby the incisors should also be inspected together with the mucous membranes. Like rabbits, complete inspection of guinea pig's oral cavity should be performed; sedation once the patient is stable to minimize stress can provide a more thorough evaluation or the oral cavity if problems are suspected. The CRT can be assessed by pressing on an unpigmented footpad. A horny overgrowth of the footpads may occasionally be present. Trimming of this hyperkeratotic pad should be done with caution to avoid bleeding.

Just as in rabbits, auscultation of the thorax and abdomen, abdominal palpation and palpation of the jaw are considered part of the standard physical examination.

Chinchillas

When examining a chinchilla, its overall appearance, posture, locomotion, and behavior should be noted. Chinchillas are naturally curious and active animals that carry their tail high if they are healthy. Sick individuals, in contrast, may be lethargic and less responsive to the environment and show signs of weight loss, a hunched posture, abnormal gait, scruffy fur, or labored breathing. Examination in the hand will generally be possible, although sedation may be needed in animals that are not frequently handled. However, it is important to realize that with, but even without sedation, the obtained values will not always reflect the actual values. Results of the physical examination should therefore be interpreted with caution, with the circumstances under which the results were obtained taken into consideration. Reference values for vital parameters in chinchillas can be found in Table 1.2. These are obtained in a similar fashion as in the guinea pig. While determining the gender of the chinchilla (see Section "Gender Determination") special attention should be paid to the penis as it is not uncommon to detect a fur-ring that can lead to phimosis (Figure 1.6); also see Chapter 17.

The hydration status can be assessed in a similar fashion as in the guinea pig. During inspection of the oral mucosa, the incisors can be evaluated. A more thorough inspection of the oral cavity can be performed in a stable, sedated animal, if indicated.

Rats, Mice, Hamsters, and Gerbils

A hands-on physical examination may be challenging to perform in the smaller rodent species. However, inspection of the animal in its cage or on the examination table will reveal valuable information. Aside from assessing the demeanor, posture, gait, and behavior of the animal (including its interest in the environment and interaction with cage mates), the breathing, fur, skin, and body condition can be evaluated. Inspection of the external orifices will provide information on the nature and amount of any discharge that is present. In sick or stressed animals, the area around the eyes and/or nose may stain red due to

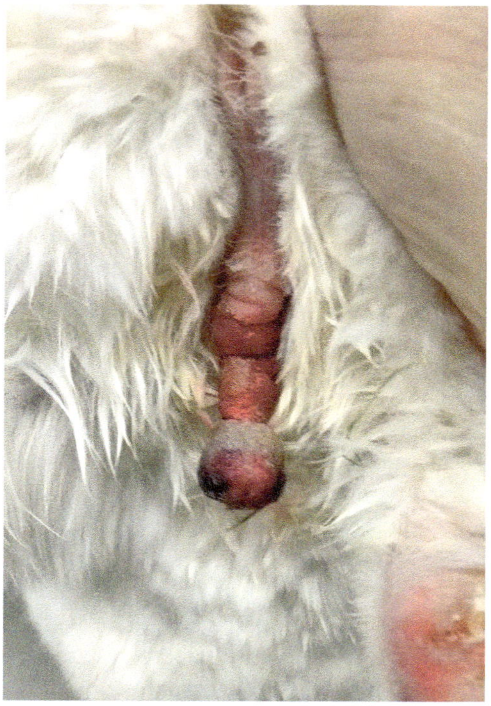

Figure 1.6 In male chinchillas, special attention should be paid to the penis as a fur-ring can be present that can lead to phimosis.

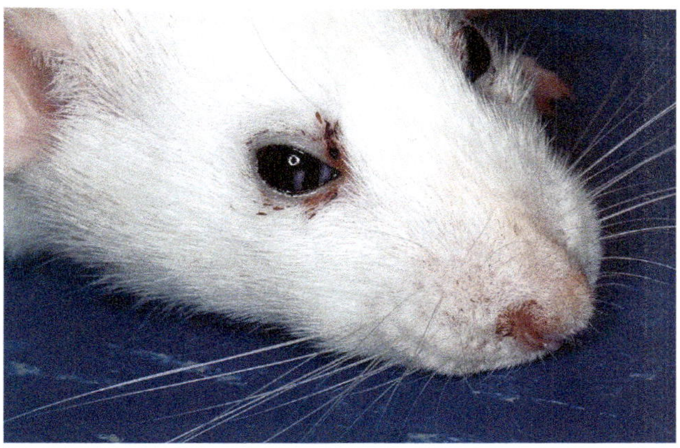

Figure 1.7 Chromodacryorrhea (red tears) is a common finding in ill or stressed rodents.

porphyrin release from the Harderian gland (i.e. chromodacryorrhea; Figure 1.7). One should further be familiar with the location of the scent glands in the different species (e.g. ventral abdominal marking gland in gerbils, paired flank glands in hamsters), as these can easily be mistaken for a lesion if one is not aware of their existence (Figure 1.8).

If the animal's temperament and condition allow it, the physical examination can be continued in the awake animal. Special attention is given to the oral cavity, which should be examined for dentition abnormalities and – in

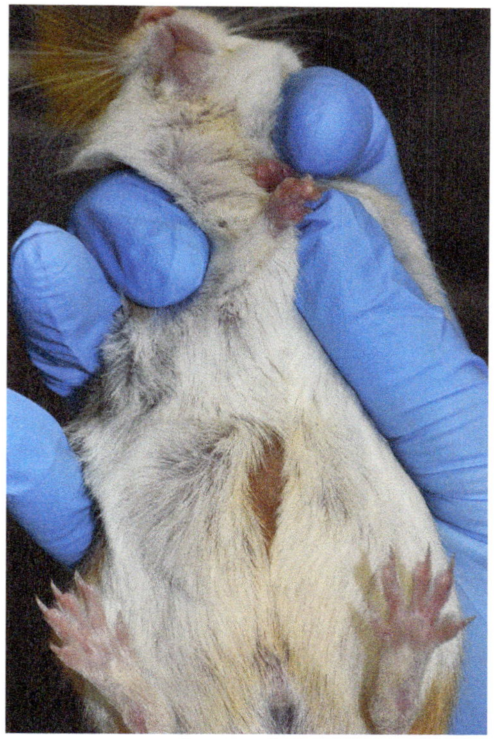

Figure 1.8 Gerbils possess a ventral abdominal scent gland. This hairless area should not be mistaken for a lesion. *Source:* Courtesy of Grayson Doss.

hamsters – for impaction of the cheek pouches. The abdomen is palpated for consistency and the presence of unusual masses. The limbs can also be palpated for tenderness or fractures, whereby special attention is paid to the paws, including the length of the nails and condition of the footpads. Auscultation of the heart and lungs can be attempted using a neonatal/pediatric stethoscope, but the heart and respiration rate will generally be difficult to measure. Abnormal breath sounds, such as "snuffling" in rats and "chattering" in mice, will generally be noticeable without the use of a stethoscope.

Abnormalities that have been noted during inspection (e.g. distended abdomen, labored breathing) should be evaluated further, for which sedation or anesthesia will frequently be needed. Upon handling, many small rodents will produce urine and/or feces, which can be collected for evaluation (see Chapter 11).

Since sedation and handling of the animal can drastically alter the vital parameters (Table 1.2), caution is warranted when interpreting the obtained information. Moreover, one should consider that handling, sedating or anesthetizing a stressed or sick animal can lead to death, thereby warranting the physical examination be performed with extreme caution and as efficiently as possible.

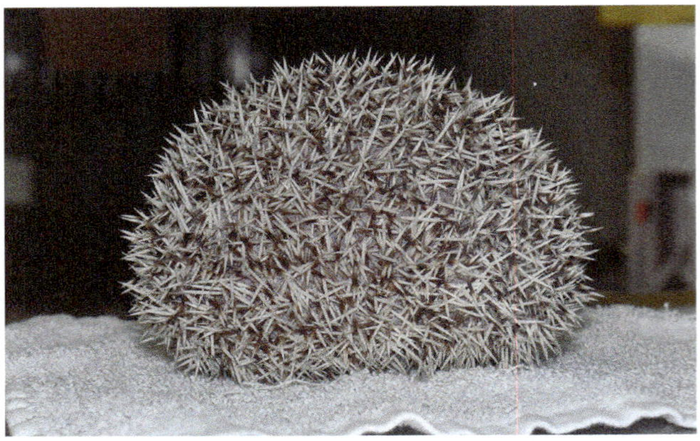

Figure 1.9 A hedgehog rolled up in a defensive posture makes complete physical examination impossible without additional measures allowing unrolling. *Source:* Courtesy of Grayson Doss.

Hedgehogs

Hedgehogs can be challenging to work with as patients. Their ability to roll up into a ball frequently makes it impossible to examine them (Figure 1.9). However, patience and gentle handling, or gentle back stroking of the rump spines will commonly stimulate them to uncurl, allowing for a better visual inspection. Alternatively, the hedgehog can be placed in a shallow pan of water to encourage it to unroll. A healthy, untroubled animal will normally be curious and active and walk with the ventral abdomen raised off the ground (Figure 1.10a,b). The nose should be moist, with no audible respiratory sounds (except if the animal is hissing in defense). The skin in the region of the spines may have a mild dry or flaky appearance but should never be flaking excessively or show signs of erythema, crusts, or quill loss.

For a full physical examination, sedation or anesthesia will commonly be required. Once the animal is sedated, a thorough visual inspection of the eyes, nose, ears, oral cavity, teeth, spines, anal, and urogenital openings can be performed, whereby special attention is paid to the presence of secretions. When inspecting the oral cavity, special attention should be paid to the teeth, gingiva, and tongue, as well as the presence of ulcers, foreign bodies, and/or masses. Hydration status may be assessed by the eyelid turgor. Lymph nodes will normally be difficult to palpate but can become palpable if enlarged, e.g. due to the presence of infection or neoplasia. An abdominal inspection and palpation can be performed to identify the presence of excessive fat, unusual masses, organomegaly, or ascites. Auscultation of the heart and lungs is performed to identify abnormal breath sounds, heart murmurs, or arrhythmias. The femoral pulse should normally be palpable, but obtaining an accurate pulse rate may be difficult. Reference values of biological data of hedgehogs can be found in Table 1.2. Note that the temperature in hedgehogs is approximately 1 °C lower compared to other common small mammals. While taking the temperature, the gender of the hedgehog may be assessed (see Section "Gender Determination"), whereby the prepuce and vulva are carefully checked for the presence of inflammation, discharge, or adherent debris. Toes should also be inspected closely for encircling fibers and overgrown nails.

Sugar Gliders

The physical examination of a sugar glider can best be performed under sedation as animals may be easily stressed and/or bite when handled. More docile animals may be examined while wrapped in a towel and cupped in the palm of the hand. As sugar gliders are nocturnal animals, it is not uncommon for the animal to be asleep during the general inspection. This should thus not be perceived as abnormal, unless the animal is difficult to waken. Once the animal is gently woken, its posture, gait, and demeanor should be

(a) (b)

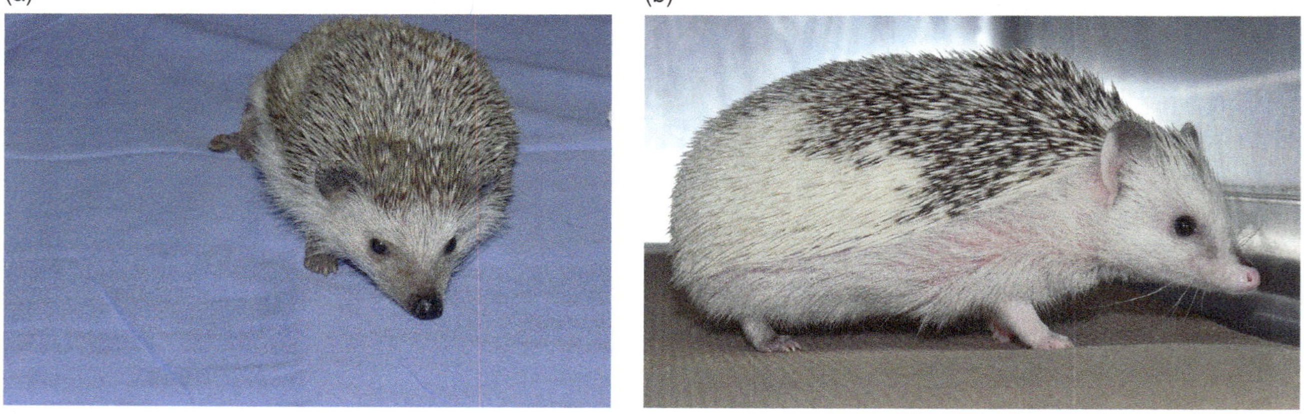

Figure 1.10 (a) Appearance of an ill hedgehog; this animal was dehydrated and unable to ambulate normally. (b) A hedgehog should be curious, active, and walk with the ventral abdomen raised off the ground. *Source:* Courtesy of Grayson Doss.

observed. Following sedation or anesthesia, cloacal temperature, heart rate, and respiration rate can be recorded. Reference values of biological data of sugar gliders can be found in Table 1.2. While taking the temperature, the gender of the sugar glider may be assessed (see Section "Gender Determination"). In addition to assessment of the vital parameters, the heart and lungs should be auscultated using a neonatal/pediatric stethoscope. The fur and skin should be carefully examined for ectoparasites, traumatic injury, fur loss, and hydration status, whereas the oral cavity can be inspected for the presence of fractured teeth, dental abscesses, or tartar. Similarly, the eyes, nose, ears, pouch (in females), and cloacal area (including genitalia) are closely inspected for the presence of abnormalities. The abdomen and major joints should be palpated, and the digits checked for evidence of trauma or overgrown nails.

Gender Determination

Ferrets

The genitalia of ferrets show great resemblance to those of canids (Figure 1.11a,b). Like bitches, jills have a swollen vulva during estrus (Figure 1.11c). In hobs, the J-curved penis is positioned over the abdominal wall with the urethral opening placed just cranial to the pubic bone. Similar to dogs, the penis is supported by a penile bone. In uncastrated males, two marble-sized testicles can be palpated in a furred scrotal sac that is located ventral to the anus. Aside from these characteristics, it is also possible to distinguish males and females based on size as males tend to be bigger and have more body muscle and much larger, wider, and rounder heads than females.

Rabbits

Gender determination in rabbits can be a challenge, especially in young rabbits. This is because the urethral opening can be wide in bucks, thereby resembling the female vaginal opening.

To determine the gender of a rabbit, digital pressure ventral to the urethral opening will result in extrusion of either the penis or the vaginal mucosa. The mucosa will be evenly visible around the penis, while the vaginal mucosa will have the aspect of a droplet whereby the ventral mucosa is easily extruded, while the dorsal mucosa has a tight connection with the skin (Figure 1.12a,b). In contrast to rodents, the penis is located caudal to the testis and lacks a penile bone.

Guinea Pigs

Gender determination in guinea pigs is relatively straightforward and can be done shortly after the animal is born (Figure 1.13a,b). All male rodents have a penile bone which can easily be palpated. Large testes may be found subcutaneously lateral to the anal-genital openings. Placing pressure cranial to the penile bone will result in extrusion of the penis. Female rodents have three external orifices. From cranial to caudal the urethra, vulva and anus can be found. The urethral opening slightly protrudes which

(a) (b) (c)

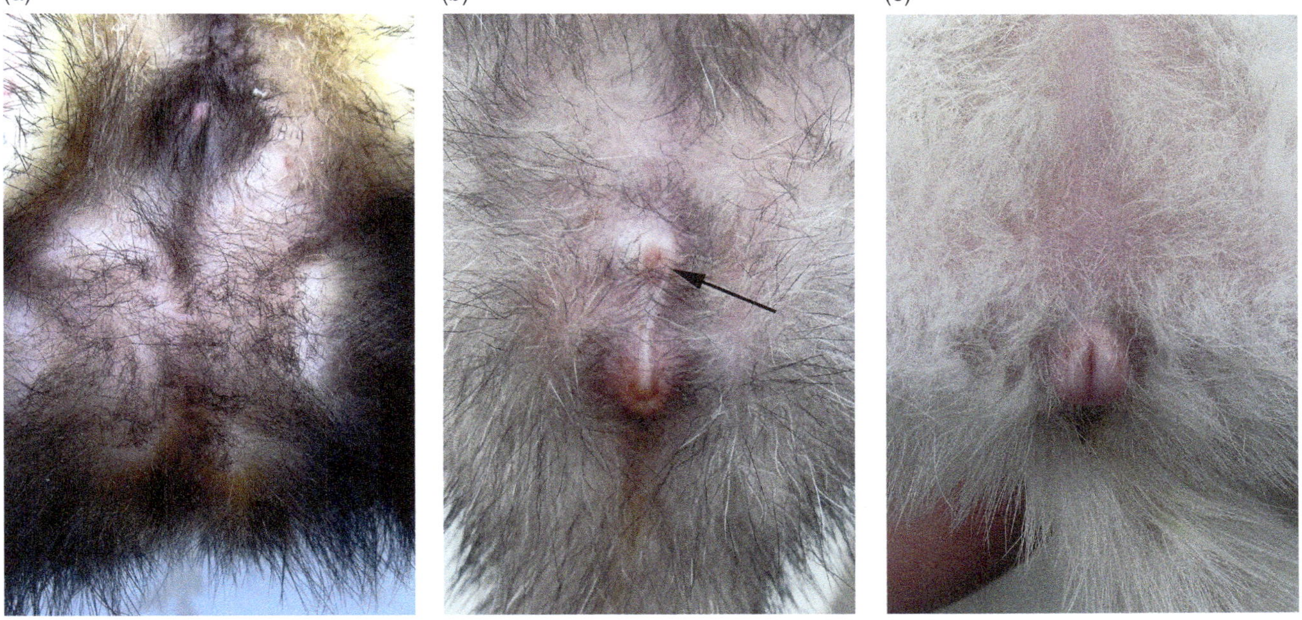

Figure 1.11 Genital openings of the male (a) and female (b) ferret. During estrus, the vulva of the ferret is swollen (c).

(a) (b)

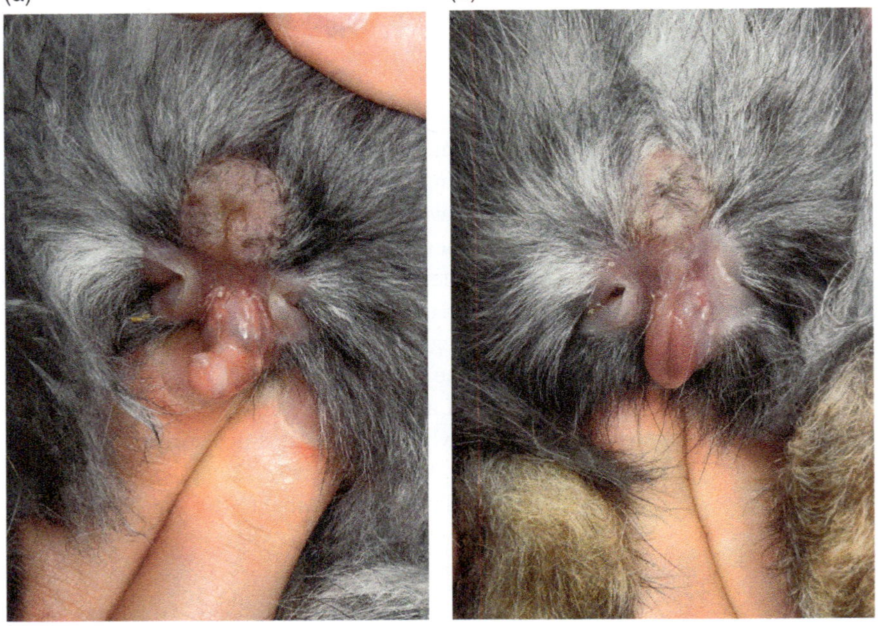

Figure 1.12 Genital openings of the male (a) and female (b) rabbit.

(a) (b)

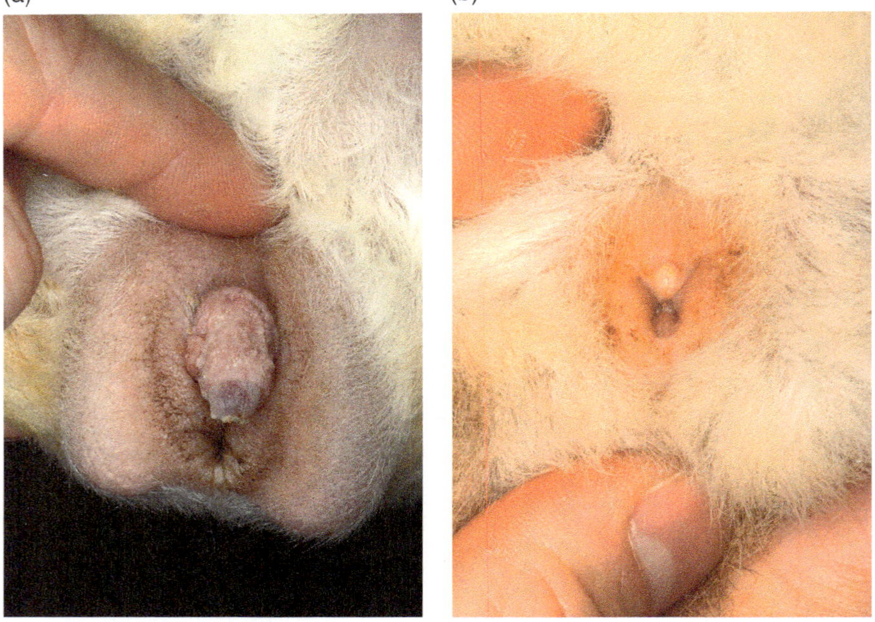

Figure 1.13 Genital openings of the male (a) and female (b) guinea pig.

makes it easy to catheterize. The Y-shaped vulva may be difficult to distinguish due to the presence of a vaginal membrane which is only open for two days around the time of estrus. Both genders have nipples but, in the males, these are generally smaller.

Chinchillas

Although sexing of chinchillas can be done at birth, it is often recommended to recheck the gender at an age of six to eight weeks. When handling a male and female chinchilla simultaneously, the sexes can easily be distinguished (Figure 1.14a,b). For the novice, however, it is easy to mistake the large clitoris in female chinchillas for the penis. Just as in the guinea pig, the penis in chinchillas contains a penile bone which can easily be palpated. In addition, the clitoris is adjacent to the anus, while a small area of skin is present between the anus and penis.

(a) (b)

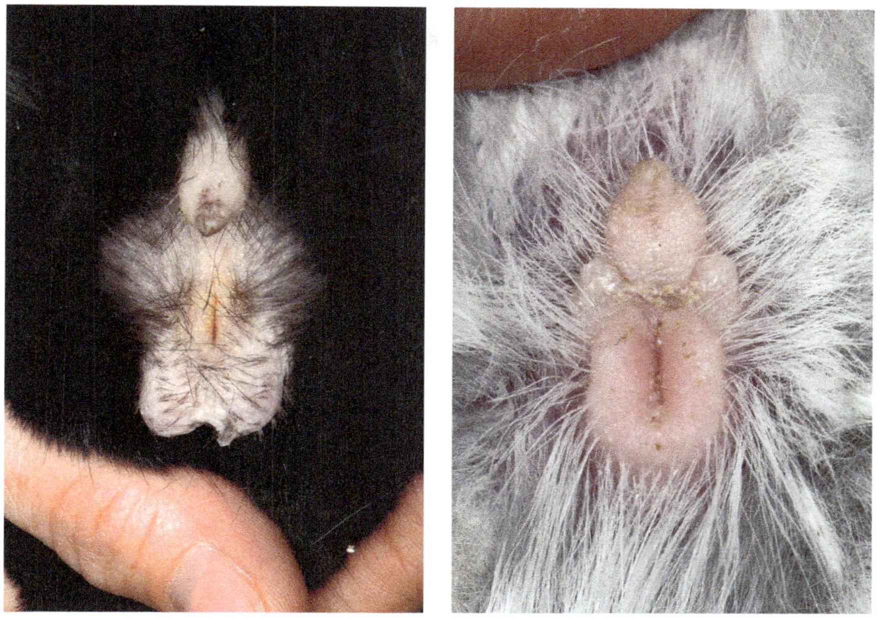

Figure 1.14 Genital openings of the male (a) and female (b) chinchilla.

(a) (b)

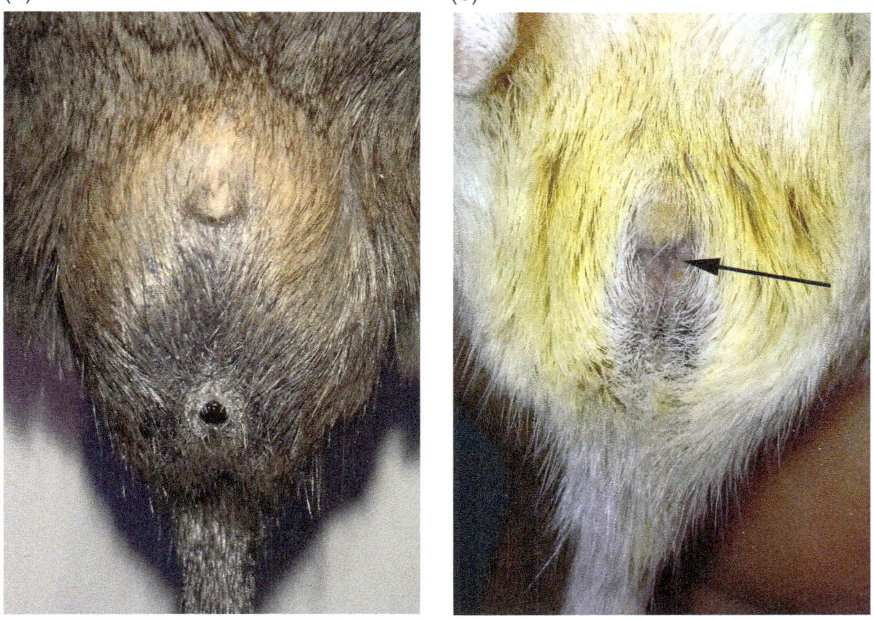

Figure 1.15 Genital openings of the male (a) and female (b) gerbil, exemplifying the gender differences as can be seen in the smaller rodents.

Rats, Mice, Hamsters, and Gerbils

Gender determination in rats, mice, hamsters, and gerbils can be performed in animals of approximately one week old but is easiest to perform in adults. In these rodent species, the distance between the urethral opening and the anus is most frequently used to determine the gender whereby the distance is longest in the male and nearly no distance is present between the openings in the female (Figures 1.15a,b). The presence of nipples in female animals or the obvious large testes of male animals can serve as alternative ways to easily distinguish the two sexes (except for castrated animals or those who have retracted their testes through the open inguinal canals). Female animals are further characterized by the presence of three external orifices. These are especially easy to recognize in gerbils (Figure 1.15b). Female hamsters regularly have a vaginal discharge (after ovulation), which should not be mistaken for a genital infection.

Hedgehogs

Hedgehogs can be sexed as early as two weeks old. Between the genders, obvious differences are present, which are easily spotted unless the hedgehog is rolled up (Figure 1.16A,B). If this happens, consider placing the animal on a glass surface so that the animal can be visualized from below. In the male, the belly button shaped prepuce opening is located halfway down the ventral abdomen whereas the testes are in subcutaneous fat in a para-anal recess and are only palpable during the reproductive season. In females, the urogenital opening is located adjacent to the anus. Females also have five pairs of nipples.

Sugar Gliders

Sugar gliders are easiest to sex when they are sexually mature. To allow gender determination, the animals should be turned over on their backs so that the abdomen can be evaluated. The testicles in the male are located externally in a furry, pendulous scrotum that is located cranially to the prepuce (Figure 1.17a). Under sedation a

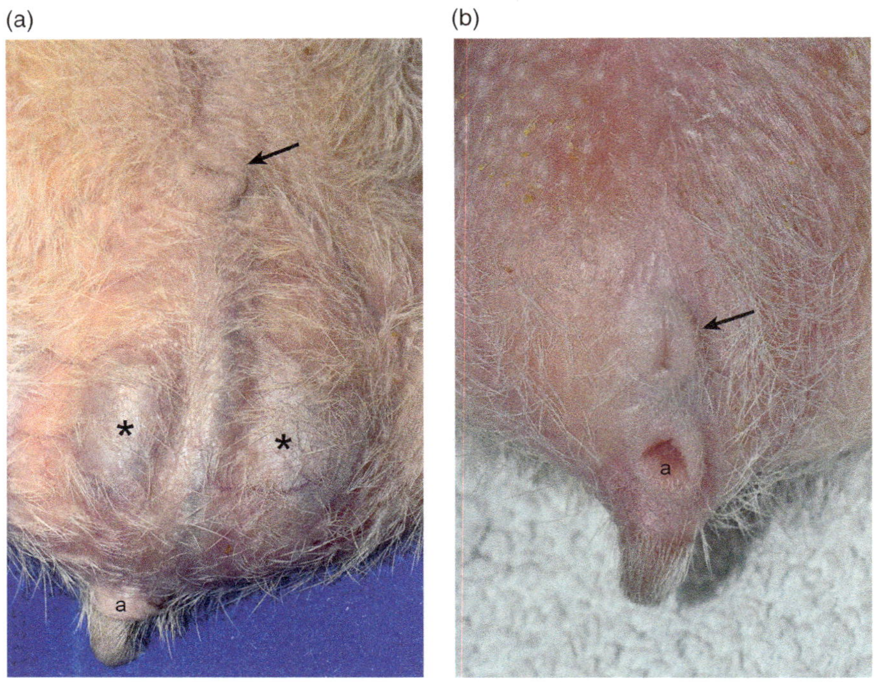

Figure 1.16 Genital openings of the male (a) and female (b) hedgehog. *Source:* Doss and Carpenter [1]. Reproduced with permission from Elsevier.
* = testicles
a = anus
arrow = genital opening

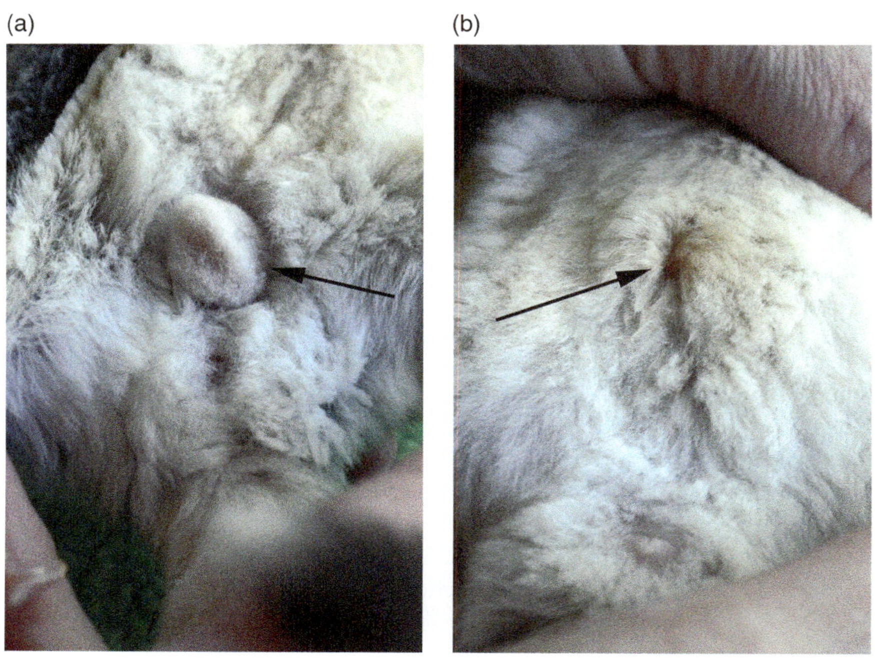

Figure 1.17 Genital openings of the male (a) and female (b) sugar glider.
1.17a = scrotum
1.17b = pouch opening

split penis may be visualized. It is important to realize that the urethral opening is not located at the tip, but at the base of the penis. Male sugar gliders possess scent glands, which are located on the forehead between the eyes and ears (visible as a diamond-shaped bald patch), on the ventral aspect of the throat, and around the cloaca (i.e. paracloacal scent glands). Females typically have a pouch, which is visible as a 1/2″ slit on the ventral abdomen in approximately the same place the testicles are located in the male (Figure 1.17b).

Reference

1 Doss, G.A. and Carpenter, J.W. (2020). African pygmy hedgehogs. In: *Ferrets, Rabbits, and Rodents*, 4e (eds. K.E. Quesenberry, C.J. Orcutt, C. Mans and J.W. Carpenter), 401–415. Saint Louis: Elsevier.

Further Reading

Antinoff, N. (1999). Physical examination and preventive care of rabbits. *Vet. Clin. North Am. Exot. Anim. Pract.* 2 (2): 405–427.

Chitty, J. (2009). Ferrets: physical examination and emergency care. In: *BSAVA Manual of Rodents and Ferrets* (eds. E. Keeble and A. Meredith), 205–218. British Small Animal Veterinary Association.

Daviau, J. (1999). Clinical evaluation of rodents. *Vet. Clin. North Am. Exot. Anim. Pract.* 2 (2): 429–445.

Graham, J. and Mader, D.R. (2012). Basic approach to veterinary care. In: *Ferrets, Rabbits and Rodents: Clinical Medicine and Surgery*, 3e (eds. K.C. Quessenberry and J.W. Carpenter), 157–173. St. Louis: Elsevier Saunders.

Ivey, E. and Morrisey, J. (1999). Ferrets: examination and preventive medicine. *Vet. Clin. North Am. Exot. Anim. Pract.* 2 (2): 471–494.

Lennox, A.M. and Bauck, L. (2012). Basic anatomy, physiology, husbandry, and clinical techniques. In: *Ferrets, Rabbits and Rodents: Clinical Medicine and Surgery*, 3e (eds. K.C. Quessenberry and J.W. Carpenter), 339–353. St. Louis: Elsevier Saunders.

Lichtenberger, M. and Hawkins, M.G. (2009). Rodents: physical examination and emergency care. In: *BSAVA Manual of Rodents and Ferrets* (eds. E. Keeble and A. Meredith), 18–31. British Small Animal Veterinary Association.

Lightfoot, T.L. (1999). Clinical examination of chinchillas, hedgehogs, prairie dogs, and sugar gliders. *Vet. Clin. North Am. Exot. Anim. Pract.* 2 (2): 447–469.

Lumeij, J.T. (2008). Small mammals: rabbit, Guinea pig, chinchilla, golden hamster, mouse, rat, gerbil, ferret, and mink. In: *Medical History and Physical Examination in Companion Animals*, 2e (eds. A. Rijnberk and F.J. van Sluijs), 272–288. Saunders Ltd.

Marini, R.P. (2014). Chapter 11: Physical examination, preventive medicine, and diagnosis in the ferret. In: *Biology and Diseases of the Ferret* (eds. J.G. Fox and R.P. Marini), 235–258. John Wiley & Sons.

Quesenberry, K.E. and Orcutt, C. (2012). Basic approach to veterinary care. In: *Ferrets, Rabbits and Rodents: Clinical Medicine and Surgery*, 3e (eds. K.C. Quessenberry and J.W. Carpenter), 13–26. St. Louis: Elsevier Saunders.

Quesenberry, K.E., Donnelly, T.M., and Mans, C. (2012). Biology, husbandry, and clinical techniques of Guinea pigs and chinchillas. In: *Ferrets, Rabbits and Rodents: Clinical Medicine and Surgery*, 3e (eds. K.C. Quessenberry and J.W. Carpenter), 279–294. St. Louis: Elsevier Saunders.

Richardson, J. and Keeble, E. (2014). Physical examination and clinical techniques. In: *BSAVA Manual of Rabbit Medicine* (eds. A. Meredith and B. Lord), 80–107. British Small Animal Veterinary Association.

Mammal History Form

A detailed history is essential to provide the most appropriate veterinary care for your animal. Please complete this form as accurately as possible. If there is anything you are unsure about, you can discuss it in more depth with the veterinary staff during your appointment.

Animal Details

Name or identification:______________________________

Common or scientific species name: ______________________________

Date of birth: _______ Age: ________ Sex: M/M Neutered/F/F Spayed/Unknown

How long have you had this animal?______________________________

From where did you obtain this animal? ______________________________

Is your animal vaccinated? N/Y

List vaccines and dates given: ______________________________

If applicable, do you have a license (DNR/USDA) to own this animal? N/Y

(Please bring your license with you as a photocopy will be required for the medical record)

Do you have any other pets in the household? N/Y

If so, list the number and the species. ______________________________

When was the last animal added to your household? ______________________________

____

Has your pet had contact with any other animals in the last 30 days?

Do people who have contact with the animal have comparable signs as seen in your animal?

____

Cage Environment

Where is the cage located? Inside/outside Provide details. ______________________________

What percentage of time does you animal spend in the cage? ______________________________

Is your animal supervised when out of the cage? N/Y

What is the cage made of? ______________________________

What are the dimensions of the cage? ______________________________

Have there been any changes in the environment in the last three months? N/Y

Give details. ______________________________

What décor and furnishings are present? ______________________________

Is there ventilation (grills or mesh)? N/Y Please give size/details. ______________________________

What bedding do you use? Please give details. ______________________________

Is your animal litter trained? N/Y

Do you provide any bathing facilities? N/Y Please give details. ______________________________

What is your animal's day and night cycle? ______________________________

Are there any smokers in the house? N /Y Do you use aerosolized substances? N/Y

How often is the cage cleaned? ______________________________

What cleaning/disinfectant agents are used? ______________________________

Diet

How often do you feed your animal? ______________________________

Indicate which foods are eaten, and in what amounts (by weight, or approx. volume)

Pellets brand/amount?__________________ Vegetables type/amount? ________________ Treats type/amount? ________________ Meat or meat products type and amount?_______

Hay type/amount?______________________ Fruits type/amount? __________________ Other details? ____________

____

Do you use any nutritional supplements? N Y, if yes what, how much, and how often: ______________________________

What water supply to you provide? Tap water/bottled water/rain/river water

(Continued)

Mammal History Form *(Continued)*

How is water provided? Bowl/dripper system ____________________
How often is the water changed? ____________________
Do you use any water supplements? N/Y Please give details: ____________________
____

Reason for Presentation Today

What is the primary complaint or what signs you have noticed? ____________________
____

Has this animal received any medication for this primary complaint? If so, what medication has been given, at what dosage and duration? What was the effect of this medication on the primary complaint?
____
____

Has this animal had previous health problems? N/Y Please give details: ____________________
____

Have any other animals or persons in the household had any illness within the last 30 days? ____________________
____
____

Has your animal received any medications in the last three months (i.e. heartworm medication, dewormer, flea treatments)
____
____

General Condition and Functioning

Please provide any changes to the following topics: ____________________
Appetite and food intake: ____________________
Drinking: ____________________
Feces and defecation: ____________________
Urine and urination: ____________________
Behavior, activity, and locomotion: ____________________
Any aspects that need further attention: ____________________

2

Restraint, Handling, and Hospitalization

Nico J. Schoemaker and Yvonne R.A. van Zeeland

Division of Zoological Medicine, Department of Clinical Sciences, Faculty of Veterinary Medicine, Utrecht University, The Netherlands

CONTENTS

Transportation

The ride to the veterinary practice will often be stressful to the animal (and owner) and can aggravate the animal's condition. To minimize the stress during transportation, the following advice can be given to owners:

1) Always use a carrier for transportation, preferably one that the animal is accustomed to. Familiarizing the animal with the carrier is easily achieved by placing the carrier in the living environment of the animal allowing free movement in and out of the carrier. Alternatively, the animal can be placed in the carrier for short durations, while a reward (e.g. a favored toy or food item) is provided.
2) The carrier should provide adequate hiding opportunity so that the animal feels secure (e.g. hay for rabbits and rodents; a sleeping bag for ferrets; or a small [nest]box for hedgehogs and sugar gliders). Placing an additional cloth over the carrier may provide extra seclusion (*Note*: Always make sure that adequate ventilation is maintained). If the journey is long, sufficient food and water should be available in the carrier.
3) Bringing along a familiar cage mate for support can provide comfort for the patient while simultaneously preventing problems with the reintroduction of the animal within the group.
4) Make sure that the ride is as short and smooth as possible and prevent overheating in the car by using the air conditioner.

Exotic Animal Emergency and Critical Care Medicine, First Edition. Edited by Jennifer E. Graham, Grayson A. Doss and Hugues Beaufrère.

5) When an animal is injured, make sure that the injury is stabilized (e.g. by applying bandages) so that it will not worsen during transportation. In severe cases, the animal may benefit from being held on the lap by a passenger.

Handling and Restraint

The safe handling and restraint of exotic companion mammals that present on emergency is essential to quickly triaging and stabilizing these species with minimal stress (see Boxes 2.1 and 2.2). Further specifics on physical exam findings by species is outlined in Chapter 1. Restraint for common venipuncture sites and intravenous (IV) catheter placement is outlined in Chapter 4.

Ferrets

Handling

Most pet ferrets are easy to handle. To pick them up, one hand should be placed around the thorax, while supporting the hind legs with the other hand (Figure 2.1). When being held, ferrets can be extremely active and lively, thereby limiting appropriate examination. The younger the ferret, the more active and more difficult to handle it will be. A distraction can be provided in the form of a favored food item (e.g. liquid diet or paste). In many ferrets, this can distract them sufficiently to allow for the administration of subcutaneous injections (Figure 2.2) or clipping of the nails (Figure 2.3).

Box 2.1 Checklist for Restraint of Small Mammals

Ferrets

- Favored food item (e.g. FerreTone™)
- Towel ("burrito," e.g. for blood collection in the awake animal)
- Leather gloves (uncompliant, aggressive animals)

Rabbits, guinea pigs, chinchillas

- Towel ("burrito")
- Non-slippery mat (especially for rabbits)

Small rodents, hedgehogs, sugar gliders

- Small plastic carrier or box, cup, or acrylic pipe (to allow for visual inspection)
- Sedation or anesthesia (to enable a more thorough examination)
- Gloves or towel (usually only necessary for hedgehogs and sugar gliders)

Box 2.2 Important Tips for Small Mammal Restraint

- Have all necessary items for a procedure ready prior to initiating restraint
- Keep handling time to a minimum
- Especially for rabbits, limit time in the air and place the animal on a sturdy, non-slippery surface to allow for a better grip
- Avoid picking up gerbils by the tail ("tail slip") or chinchillas by the fur ("fur slip")
- Use a cup or small box to pick up and transfer smaller rodents, hedgehogs, and sugar gliders; the box will also allow for an initial visual inspection of the animal and can be used for the induction of anesthesia
- Prevent biting by grasping the animal from dorsal around the neck or shoulders, and placing the thumb and/or fingers right below the mandible while supporting the body with the other hand
- Use a towel ("burrito") if more firm restraint is necessary (e.g. administering drugs)
- Consider scruffing primarily for non-compliant patients (CAVEAT: not in guinea pigs, chinchillas, or hedgehogs)
- Monitor the patient closely during handling and restraint; if the animal becomes dyspneic, stressed, or struggles severely, abort restraint and consider sedation once the patient has recovered
- When a patient is placed on the examination table, keep your eye on it at all times, as they may otherwise fall and injure themselves
- Communicate constantly with restrainer during the examination to prevent injury

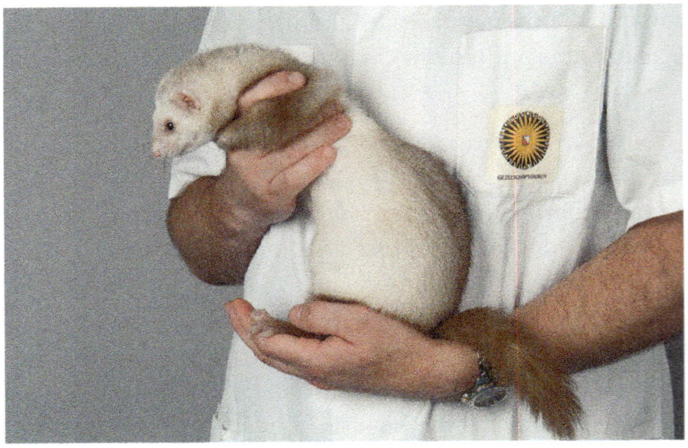

Figure 2.1 Picking up ferrets is frequently accomplished by grabbing them around the thorax while ensuring that the hind legs are supported by the other arm.

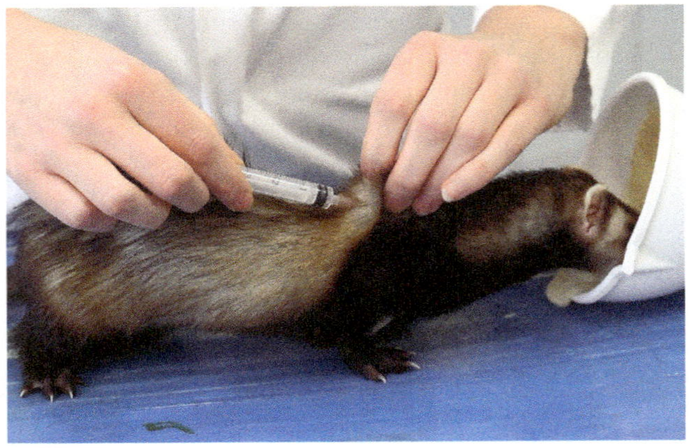

Figure 2.2 Providing the ferret with a favored food item (e.g. FerreTone) will often help to distract them sufficiently to allow for placement of subcutaneous injections, implants, or transponders.

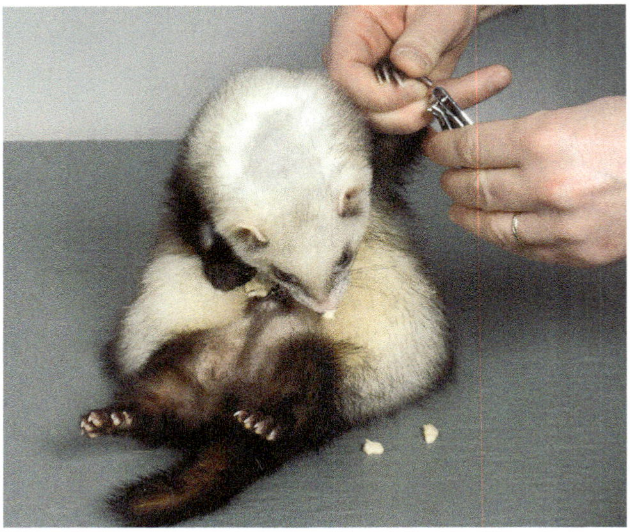

Figure 2.3 By placing a bit of food on the ventral abdomen, the ferret's nails can commonly be clipped without having to resort to further restraint.

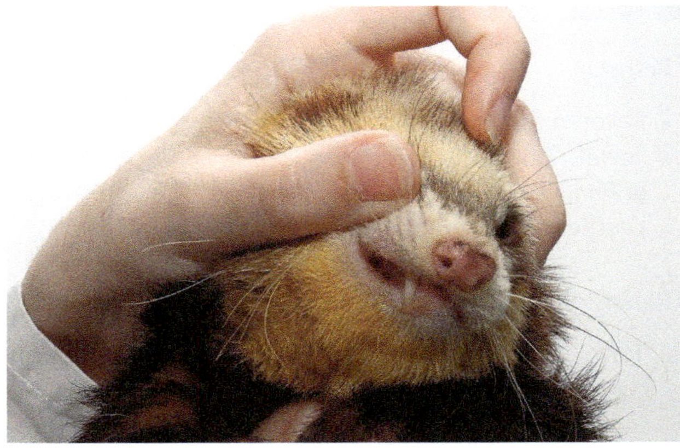

Figure 2.4 Approaching from a caudodorsal direction, placing a hand on top of the head of a ferret and lifting the upper lip with the thumb, the teeth, and gingiva can be inspected.

Restraint

Light restraint will usually suffice to allow a physical examination to be performed. Remember that the tighter the restraint is, the more resistance will be encountered. As ferrets will seldom stand still on a table, it is preferential to have them rest on the lower arm of the examiner with the thorax in the hand and the legs placed on either side of the arm (see Figure 1.3). Using this method, palpation of the femoral pulse and auscultation of the heart and lungs will generally be feasible.

To inspect the teeth and mucous membranes, the ferret's body can be supported with one hand while the other hand is placed over the head of the ferret from dorsal and behind, to allow the upper lip to be lifted with the thumb (Figure 2.4).

Abdominal palpation is often easiest to perform when the ferret is placed on the table and held at the front end. In case of a less friendly ferret which tends to bite, or when performing a painful procedure (e.g. placement of an intramuscular injection), the ferret may be scruffed by the neck (Figure 2.5), or, alternatively, restrained by placing the hand dorsally around the head and neck, just beneath the base of the skull. This will frequently result in the ferret opening its mouth and allowing for an oral inspection to be performed without having to sedate the animal. To facilitate the administering of an injection, a hind leg of the ferret may be held above the knee while stretching the body by holding the neck with the other hand (Figure 2.6). This position will also facilitate taking the ferret's temperature, especially if it is otherwise struggling too much.

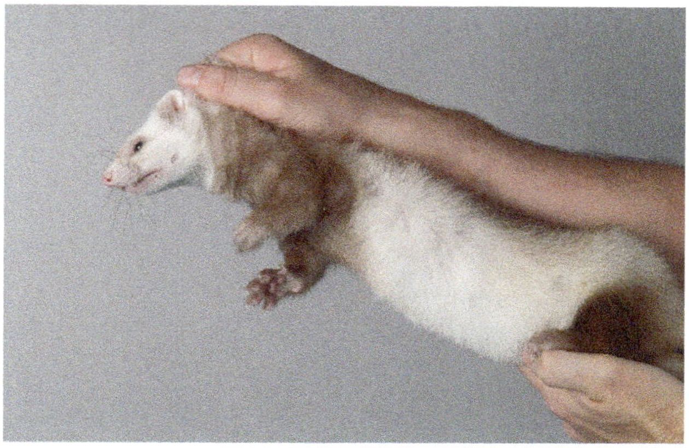

Figure 2.5 Scruffing of a ferret. Many ferret owners are accustomed to scruff their ferret and will often voluntarily use this technique to allow for further examination of their animal.

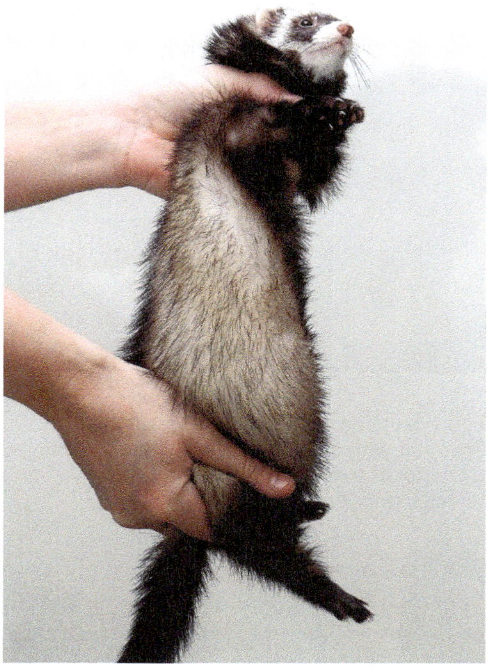

Figure 2.6 Administering an injection to a ferret can easily be accomplished by having the body of the ferret rest against the lower arm of the handler while restraining the hind legs just above the knee.

Risks

The risk of being bitten by a ferret is no greater than with a cat or dog. Young (intact) ferrets which have not been handled frequently (yet), however, have a slightly higher tendency to bite. Luckily, most owners will be able to provide reliable information on the likelihood that their ferret(s) will bite. When ferrets bite, they may not let go easily. To stimulate the ferret to let go, it may be needed to hold it under a running faucet as this usually results in an instant release of the grip.

Rabbits

Handling

Proper handling of rabbits is necessary to prevent fractures of the spine and hind legs. As rabbits have very powerful hind legs, it is essential to continuously support the hindquarters during handling. Some veterinarians prefer to hold one hand under the thorax while picking up the rabbit, whereas others like to grasp a skinfold over the thorax (Figure 2.7). As many animals start to struggle upon being picked up, the handling time in the air should be kept as short as possible. Rabbits should be placed back in a carrier or cage with the rear end first to prevent them from jumping into their cage with too much force.

(a)

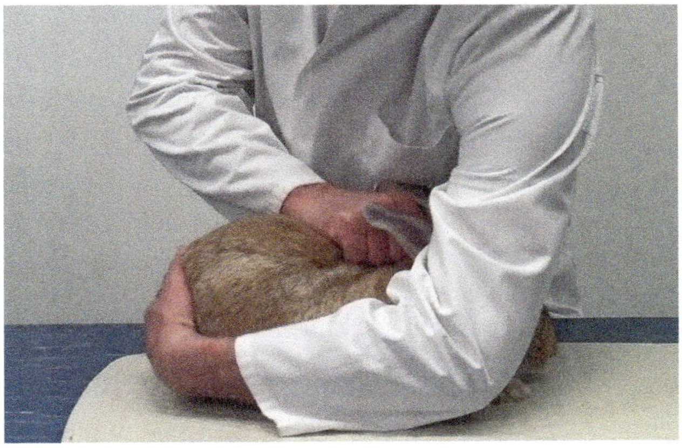

(b)

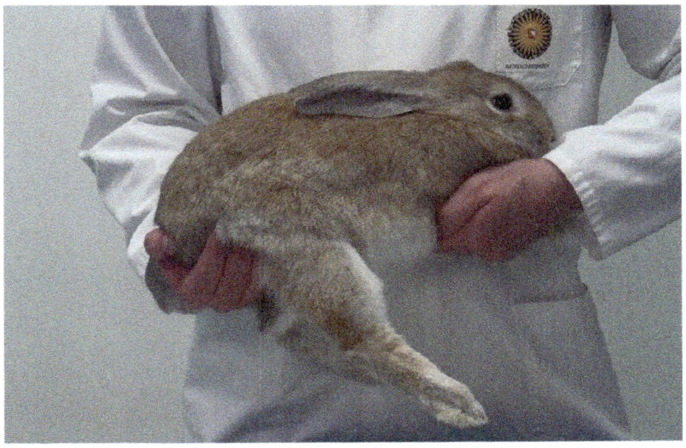

Figure 2.7 Common techniques used for handling rabbits: the animal is held by either grasping a skinfold over the thorax (a) or supporting the thorax with the hand (b). The hind legs should always be supported to prevent the animal from being able to deliver a powerful kick with the hind legs and injuring its spine.

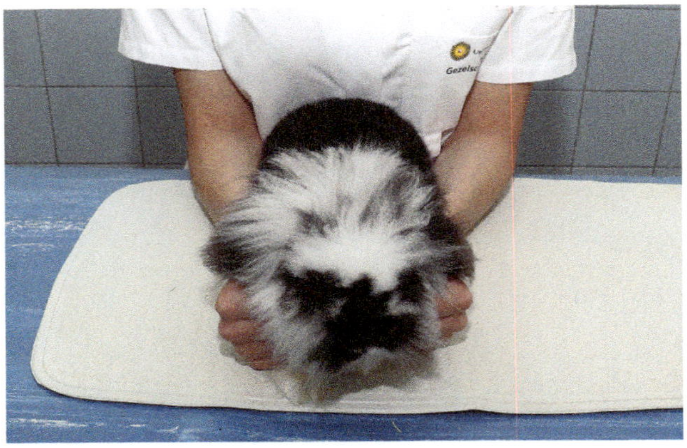

Figure 2.8 When examining a rabbit, the authors prefer to stand behind the rabbit with both arms beside the rabbit to provide optimal control of the rabbit and prevent it from jumping, unexpectedly from the table.

When examining the rabbit on a table, it is recommended to use a non-slippery surface (e.g. bathmat) to create stability and prevent the feet from sliding out underneath the rabbit. During the exam, care should be taken not to lose control of the rabbit as it may easily jump off the table and injure itself. The authors prefer to stand behind the rabbit while examining it on the table while having both arms next to the rabbit so that it cannot unexpectedly jump to the side (Figure 2.8).

Restraint

Wrapping a rabbit in a towel (also called a "bunny burrito") will help prevent it from struggling and injuring itself (Figure 2.9). However, this does not mean that the procedure is not stressful or detrimental to the rabbit. Holding the rabbit restrained in a towel for a prolonged time may result in the rabbit overheating. In highly stressed rabbits, placing a hand over their eyes can help to calm them down.

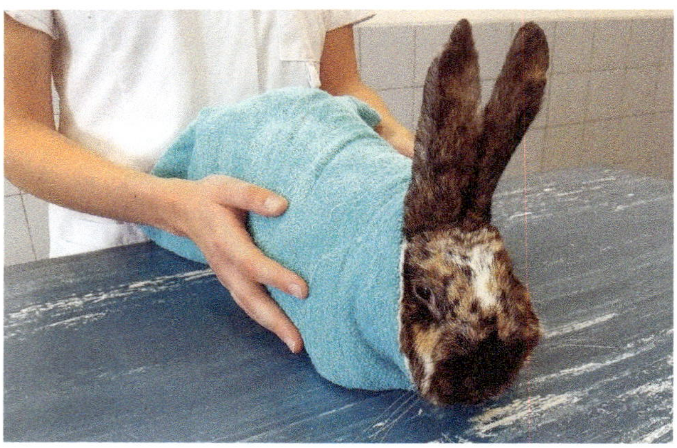

Figure 2.9 A "bunny burrito" is a commonly used method for restraining a rabbit to administer medication. By wrapping a towel around the animal, the rabbit can be prevented from struggling and injuring itself.

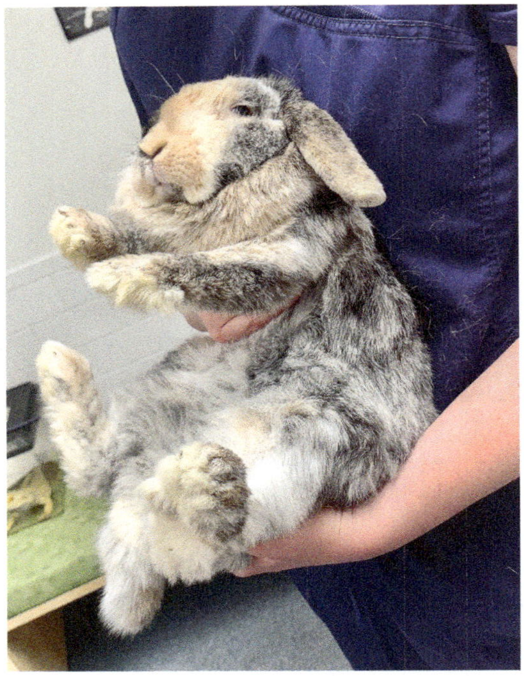

Figure 2.10 C-shape hold of a rabbit allows for inspection of the rabbit's underside and is a helpful position to facilitate obtaining rectal body temperature and performing a nail trim. *Source*: Courtesy of Jennifer Graham.

Although rabbits become calm when placed on their backs, it is important to realize that this so-called state of "hypnosis" or "tonic immobility" is associated with an (initial) increase in blood pressure as well as increases in plasma concentrations of adrenocorticotropic hormone (ACTH), corticosterone, and norepinephrine. These physiological responses indicate that the procedure induces stress rather than calms the animal. Caution is therefore warranted when applying this technique. Briefly, restraining a rabbit in this position may facilitate obtaining a rectal temperature and examining the perineal region but a "C-shape" hold is preferred (Figure 2.10).

Risks

The handling and restraint of rabbits usually carries little risks for the handler, as rabbits rarely bite or scratch. However, incorrect handling can pose serious consequences as rabbits are more vulnerable to spinal fractures and (sub)luxations and subsequent paresis or paralysis of the hind legs due to the fragility of their skeleton (see Chapter 15). Some studies suggest that rabbits have a lower skeletal density than other species, such as cats. While ovariectomy/ovariohysterectomy is recommended in rabbits, this can have a negative influence on bone density and as such might represent an additional explanation for the presence of osteoporosis in rabbits.

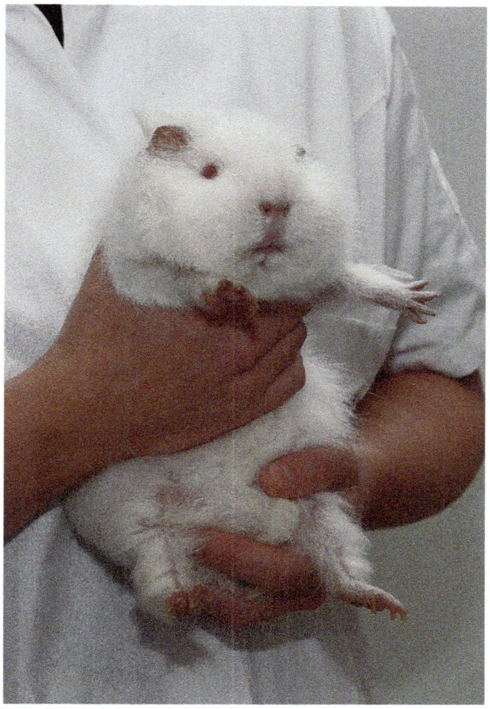

Figure 2.11 To handle a guinea pig, one hand is held under the thorax while the other hand is placed under the animal's rear for additional support of the hind legs.

Guinea Pigs

Handling

Guinea pigs are gentle animals that seldom bite. Getting them out of their cage can be challenging as they will often try to escape from being picked up. Guinea pigs can best be picked up by cupping the hands and scooping the animal, rather than grabbing over the dorsum. Once scooped up, the guinea pig will generally sit quietly and let itself be examined. When holding a guinea pig, one hand is held under the thorax while the other supports the guinea pig's hind legs, without restraining them (Figure 2.11). Like rabbits, the guinea pig should be placed onto a flat surface as soon as possible following which its head or back may be covered by the hands of the owner or technician to keep it calm and prevent it from walking away.

Restraint

Actual restraint is seldom needed as guinea pigs will rarely fiercely resist handling. Gently scooping one's non-dominant hand under their chin and across the front of their shoulders and forelimbs while standing behind the guinea pig often enables a physical exam to be performed with the other hand. Guinea pigs cannot be scruffed as they have little subcutaneous space over their neck and/or back. In case restraint is necessary (e.g. to administer medication), the guinea pig may be wrapped in a towel (i.e. a guinea pig burrito), similar to rabbits (Figure 2.12).

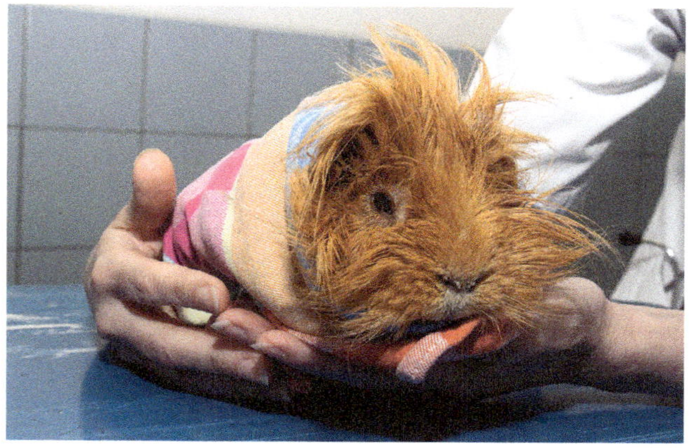

Figure 2.12 Similar to rabbits, guinea pigs may be wrapped in a towel (guinea pig burrito) to prevent it from struggling, and providing comfort during medicating and force feeding.

Risks

The risk associated with handling guinea pigs is minimal for both the handler (i.e. the animals will rarely bite) and animal itself, although in obese guinea pigs with concurrent hepatic lipidosis liver ruptures have been reported. Pet guinea pigs (particularly young ones or those that were recently acquired) do carry a potential zoonotic risk for handlers, as they may carry dermatophytes.

Chinchillas

Handling

Chinchillas will seldom bite when they are used to being handled. However, it is important to approach them as gently and calmly as possible.

The chinchilla's body weight is too high to lift them by their tail without providing support to the body. The preferred technique for handling chinchillas is to encircle the thorax with one hand while the other is used to hold the tail to direct it into the desired location (Figure 2.13). Particularly, calm chinchillas may also have their hindquarters cupped in one hand while the other hand encircles the thorax. As chinchillas have very short nails, there is little risk of the chinchilla being able to resist being picking up by grabbing hold of objects or the cage bars.

Restraint

Firm restraint is rarely needed in chinchillas. Scruffing is not desired as their fur easily epilates when pulled ("fur slip"). If restraint is needed, wrapping the chinchilla into a towel (i.e. a chinchilla burrito) can prove helpful.

Risks

As mentioned under restraint, the natural defense mechanism of chinchillas to escape from the grip of a predator is the so-called "fur slip." When the fur lets loose, this will usually not

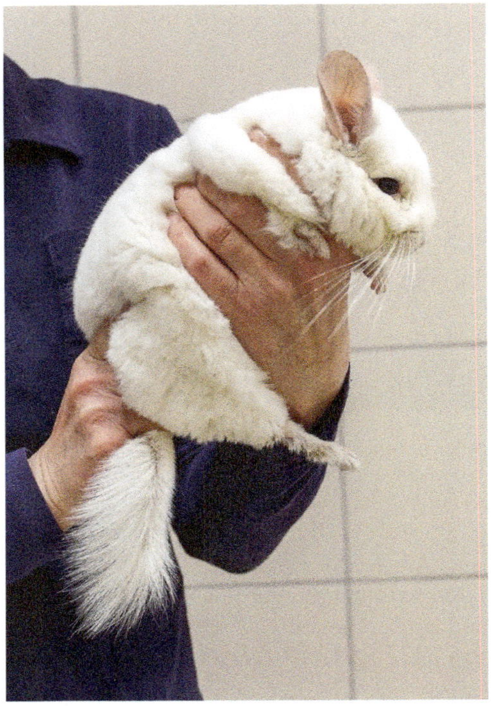

Figure 2.13 Chinchillas are easily handled by encircling their thorax with one hand while holding the tail with the other hand.

result in large areas of fur loss, unless a large amount of fur is held. It may take a considerable time for the fur to fully regrow, whereby the regrown fur may have a different shade. Chinchillas should therefore not be held by the fur.

Chinchillas will rarely bite, even if handled incorrectly. The major zoonotic risk from chinchillas is the potential transmission of *Giardia*, as chinchillas are frequently reported as carriers.

Rats, Mice, and Gerbils

Handling

Of the smaller rodent species, rats are most accustomed to being handled and frequently appear to enjoy being picked up and petted. In general, rats can be handled in a similar manner as chinchillas, whereby the animal is picked up by supporting the thorax and cupping the hindquarters or likewise the tail can be used to direct it to a certain location.

Mice and gerbils are much less tolerant of being handled than rats unless they are scooped up with an open hand. As a result, it is important to determine in advance what needs to be done so that the handling time can be kept as short as possible. Moreover, the handling of the animal will alter most of the physical parameters so that obtained values must be interpreted with great caution. The authors, therefore, recommend trying to obtain as much information

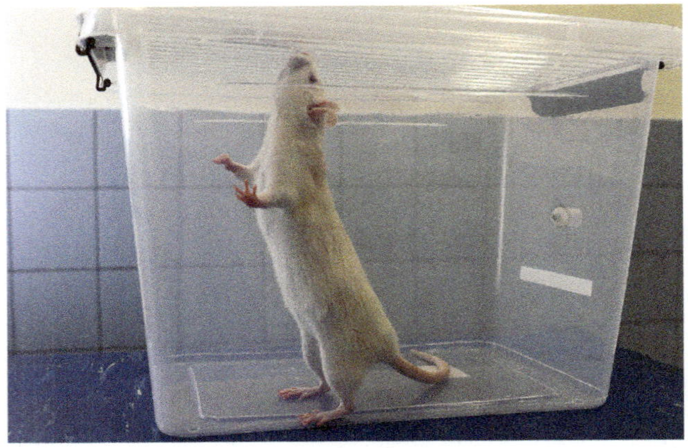

Figure 2.14 Placing a rat in a plastic carrier will not only allow inspection of the exterior of the rat, but also its explorative behavior.

from the visual inspection of the animal before attempting to handle it. Small clear plastic pet carriers are often very useful for facilitating a visual exam (Figure 2.14). When the animal needs to be picked up, take into consideration that many of the small rodents may be more accustomed to being handled by their owners than by an unfamiliar person. As such, it may be advisable to request the owner to pick up the animal from its cage instead of trying to catch it yourself. An alternative to grabbing the animal with the open hand is a small box or container used to scoop the animal out of its cage.

Restraint

It has for long been common practice to pick up mice and gerbils that are not accustomed to handling, by grabbing them at the base of their tail, followed by scruffing them. It has been shown, however, that this method is perceived as extremely stressful. Restraint should therefore preferably be achieved by handling them with a (paper) towel (Figure 2.15), or by letting them walk into a pipe/tunnel (Figure 2.16).

Rats can either be restrained by holding them in a towel or by encircling their neck and applying pressure to both elbows (Figure 2.17). Using this method, the front legs will be crossed across the body and prevent the rat from bending or turning the head and biting the handler. Just as mice, rats do not appreciate being scruffed. These animals will likely bite the handler during a subsequent attempt to pick up the animal.

Sedation or anesthesia may facilitate examination in a less stressful manner in rats, mice, and gerbils, although induction may be perceived as stressful as well.

Risks

Rats that are accustomed to handling usually do not bite. However, when distressed or handled inappropriately, they can bite hard. A potential complication of such a bite

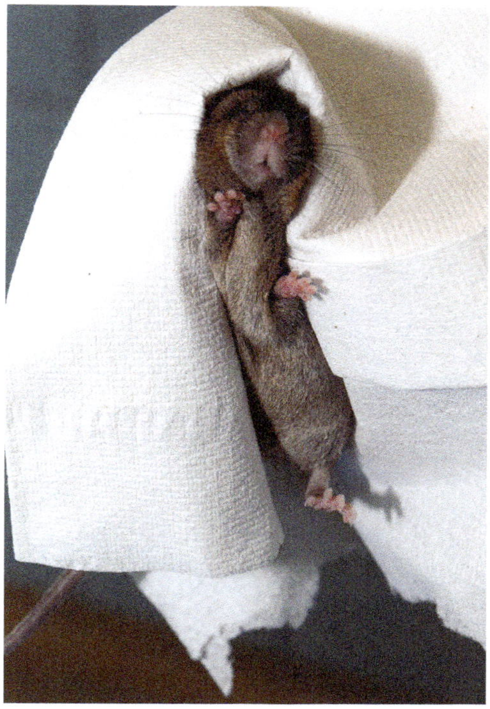

Figure 2.15 Instead of scruffing a mouse, which has been proven to be stressful to the animal, these animals can be held in a paper towel.

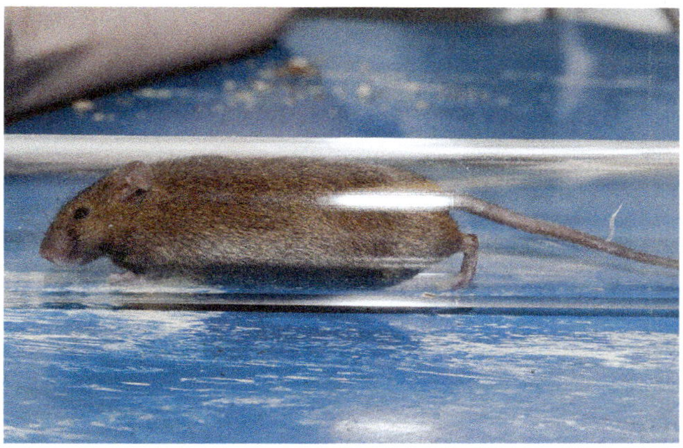

Figure 2.16 A technique advocated in laboratory animal medicine is to let mice walk into transparent tubes to transport them from one location to the other, instead of picking them up by the tail.

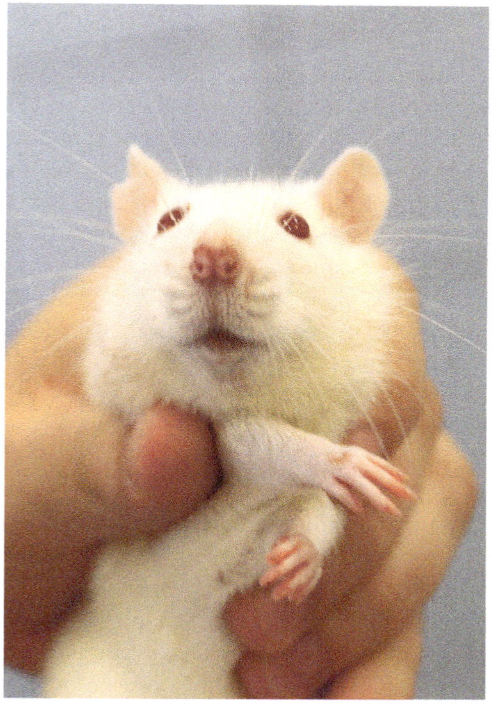

Figure 2.17 A good way to restrain rats is to encircle their neck and cross their front legs across their chest by applying pressure to both elbows. This will help to prevent the animal from being able to turn or bend its head to bite.

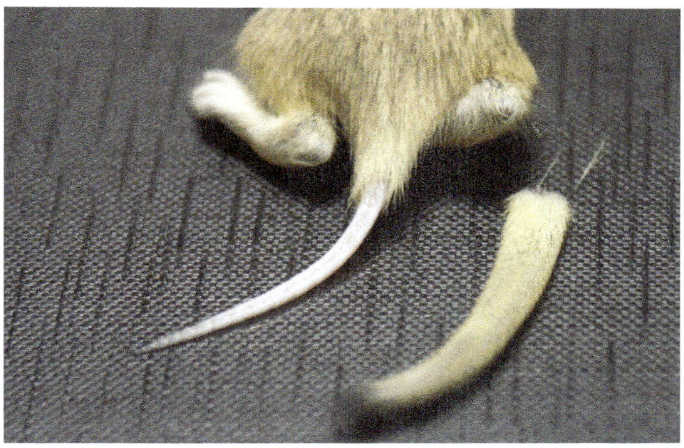

Figure 2.18 When the tail of a gerbil (or mouse) is handled too far caudally, there is a considerable risk for "tail slip" whereby the skin of the tail is stripped from the vertebrae. *Source*: Courtesy of Katleen Hermans, Ghent University, Belgium.

wound is "rat-bite fever." This condition is caused by an infection with *Streptobacillus moniliformis* and/or *Spirillum minus*. Clinical signs will generally appear 6–10 days following infection and may comprise recurrent fever, vomiting, muscle ache, and enlarged lymph nodes.

It is not uncommon for rodents to be injured due to a fall or being dropped to the floor. Similarly, placing a rodent on the table may pose a risk of the animal falling off the table, although most small rodents are able to distinguish heights and will not unexpectedly fall.

Inappropriate handling of gerbils (and mice), whereby they are picked up too far caudally at the tail, also carries a considerable risk for "tail slip" (Figure 2.18). This condition is a well-known defense mechanism of rodents, whereby the skin is sloughed from the tail to enable the rodent to escape from its predator. Following the injury, the exposed part of the tail will eventually become necrotic and fall off. To prevent this from occurring, it is recommended to amputate the tail at the level where the skin ends.

Rats and mice may be carriers of lymphocytic choriomeningitis virus (LCMV), a virus predominantly carried by wild rodents, that may be transmitted to people. Symptoms may occur in two out of three infected people, between 2- and 21 days post-infection. Although most symptoms are mild, they may progress to meningitis, especially in prenatal and immunocompromised people. LCMV is spread via contact with rodent urine, feces, saliva, or blood. Fortunately, outbreaks are rare.

Hamsters

Handling

As Syrian hamsters are solitary and nocturnal creatures, most of them do not appreciate being handled. To prevent aggression, it is advised to wake the hamster prior to approaching it. Some hamsters can be scooped up in the hand (Figure 2.19). For those that are less accustomed to being handled, a small cup or container can be used to scoop up the animal and transfer it from one area to another. Transferring the hamster to a clear plastic pet carrier will facilitate a visual exam.

Restraint

Restraint of hamsters is best achieved by picking them up with a towel and then encircling the neck, similar to what is done in rats (Figure 2.20).

Risks

Hamsters may deliver a fierce bite when approached suddenly without warning or waking them up. Similarly, they can bite when restrained inappropriately.

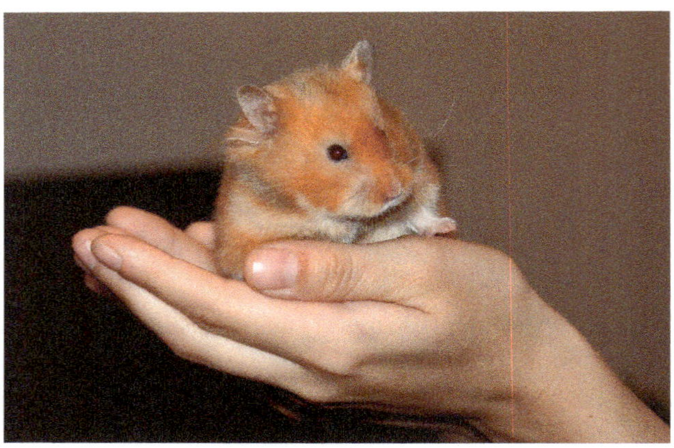

Figure 2.19 Although hamsters are known to easily bite their handler, some will allow being picked up by cupped hands and sit on the open palm.

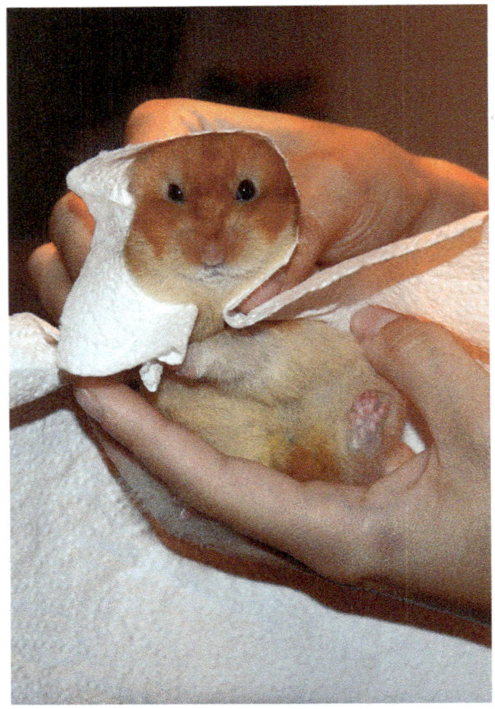

Figure 2.20 Just as in mice and gerbils, handling hamsters by their scruff is stressful, especially since they have very loose, elastic skin in which they can easily maneuver necessitating an even firmer grip. Handling a hamster in a paper towel and holding the hamster behind the mandibles will prevent the handler being bitten.

Just as mice and rats, Syrian hamsters may be carriers of LCMV.

Hedgehogs

Handling

Handling hedgehogs can be challenging, not because they tend to bite (as they seldom will), but because they will frequently roll up into a ball, thereby preventing further inspection or examination (Figure 2.21). There are several methods described that can be used to unroll a hedgehog, of which some may work in one animal, but fail in another. These methods include the following:

1) In docile hedgehogs and those that are used to being handled, a little bit of time and patience is all that is needed for the animal to unroll and allow further inspection without additional force.
2) Some hedgehogs will unfold when stroked in a backward motion over the spines.
3) Some hedgehogs unroll after placing them in an upright position and gently rocking them up and down.

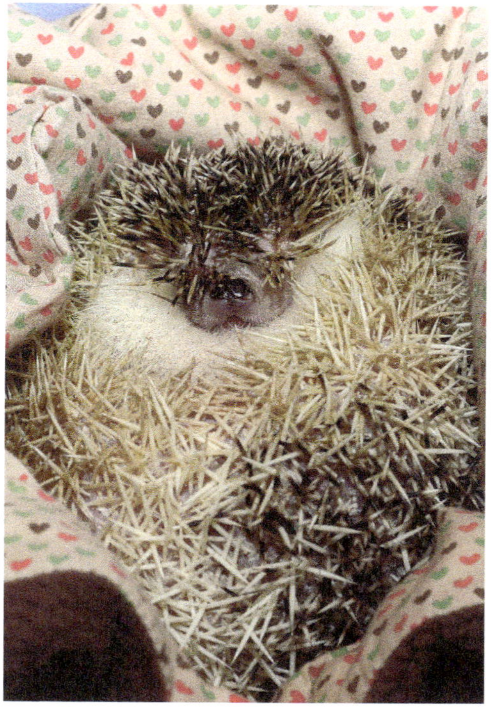

Figure 2.21 Hedgehogs will frequently roll up into a ball when handled or touched, thereby preventing further examination of the animal. As unrolling them can be challenging, chemical restraint is often used to enable the clinician to further inspect and examine the animal.

4) The hedgehog's hind legs can be lifted, following which the animal will stretch itself out to try and place its front legs on the table for support.
5) When the hedgehog is slightly unrolled, a thumb may be placed on the back of the head following which pressure can be applied to the back of the animal (a towel is placed over the spines to prevent the handler from being pricked) to further unroll the hedgehog. This method is considered more forceful.
6) The hedgehog can be placed in a shallow pan of water, while ensuring the animal's nose and mouth are above the water. This will generally stimulate the animal to unroll.
7) By grasping the muscular ventral ring, which is responsible for the animal's ability to roll up, and then gently stretching the muscle outward, the animal can be unrolled. To be able to perform this procedure, the handler will need to wear gloves to protect him/herself against the spines.

Only in animals that are accustomed to being handled will a physical examination be possible without sedation.

Restraint

In many cases, transferring hedgehogs to a clear plastic pet carrier will facilitate a visual exam often allowing gait assessment, visualization of the ventrum, and an initial inspection of the face and head (Figure 2.22). The spines of a hedgehog prevent manual restraint in animals that refuse to unroll. Chemical restraint (induction with isoflurane or sevoflurane) is typically necessary if further investigations have to take place.

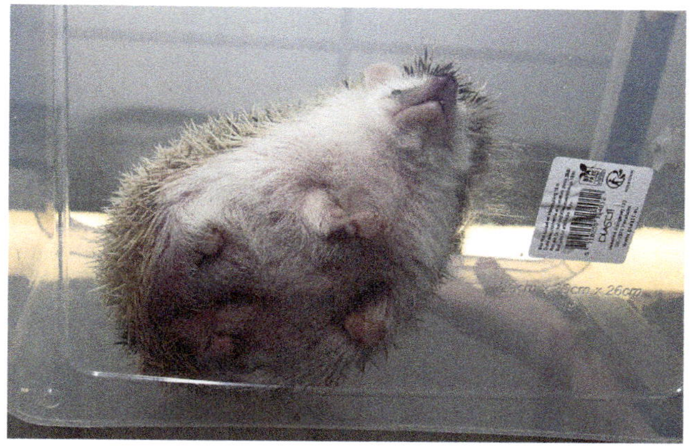

Figure 2.22 Placing a hedgehog in a plastic container may allow it to relax and unroll. This will allow inspection from all sides. These containers may also be used as an induction box by letting sevoflurane flow into them.

Risks

When handling a hedgehog, the spines may prick and lead to some degree of discomfort. In some cases, allergic reactions (urticaria) have been noted following the handling of a hedgehog. This may be prevented by wearing protective gloves or using a towel. Aside from rolling up in a ball, huffing, and puffing are defensive mechanisms indicating distress to the animal. Hedgehogs will rarely, if ever, bite.

Sugar Gliders

Handling

When sugar gliders are handled frequently, they will usually allow handling in the clinic. Those that are less accustomed to being handled will likely try to bite an approaching hand. When startled, a sugar glider may easily escape from the hand. As sugar gliders are nocturnal animals, it is recommended to schedule consultations in the morning, at a time when they are less active and thus easier to handle.

Like hamsters, transportation from one enclosure to the other may best be accomplished using a nest box with a hinge. Once in the clinic, the nest box can be taken out of the transportation cage, allowing the sugar glider to be taken out of the box more easily. A cotton glove, cloth, or cotton bag can be used to protect the

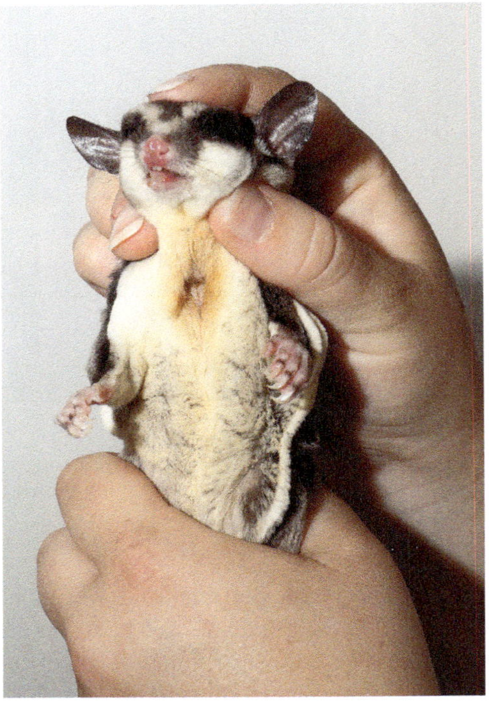

Figure 2.23 Handling of sugar gliders can be achieved by placing the head in between the thumb and middle finger, whereby the index finger can be placed on top of the head for further control. The rest of the hand is used to support the remainder of the body.

handler from being bitten. Once the sugar glider is captured, the head is carefully located and held between the thumb and middle finger. For further control, the index finger can be placed on top of the head while the remainder of the body is supported in the rest of the hand (Figure 2.23). The cloth can subsequently be pulled back from the head and ventral side of the body, allowing for examination of the sugar glider. In more docile sugar gliders, the animal may be lifted by the tail to allow for inspection (and palpation) of the abdomen, including the pouch.

Restraint

The difference between handling and restraint is minimal. Chemical restraint will often be needed to allow for a more thorough examination to be performed.

Risks

Improper handling of sugar gliders carries a great risk of being bitten. With their sharp teeth, they can easily break the skin. However, gentle handling and proper socialization of the animal will help to avoid biting and scratching by the animal.

Hospitalization

Ward Considerations

As most small mammals are prey species, it is advised to hospitalize them separately from predatory species such as dogs, cats, and ferrets. For ferrets, this separation is not essential.

It is recommended to have specialized cages available for the provision of supplemental oxygen and heat. Incubators are ideal for most small mammal patients. It is also important to ensure an optimal temperature in the ward. For rabbits, the ambient temperature should preferably not exceed 22 °C/71.6 °F as rabbits tolerate heat poorly and higher temperatures will result in reduced food intake.

In each ward, a table should preferably be present which can be used to examine and treat the patients. Cupboards are useful to store the different types of food, food and water bowls, towels, syringes, needles, etc. A counter with a sink and faucet is recommended for refreshing the water and preparing syringe feeding formulas. From a hygiene perspective, cleaning of the cages should not be performed in the same sink.

Once an animal is discharged, the cage and all other materials and equipment that have been used during the animal's stay should be disinfected. Different types of disinfectants can be used, of which dilute sodium hypochlorite (bleach) is one that can be used in most circumstances. As legislation differs per country, the reader is referred to the national guidelines on the selection and use of sanitizers and disinfectants.

Cage Requirements

Ferrets

When hospitalizing a ferret, the cage must be escape proof, as ferrets are notorious escape artists. Be aware that many ferrets can squeeze through tight spaces and will either get caught while trying to escape or succeed and start roaming around the ward.

Suitable housing for a ferret is big enough to accommodate an area for sleeping, eating, and a litter box (Figure 2.24). All items that are placed into the cage should be sturdy and/or tightly secured; otherwise, the ferret will tip these over and soil the rest of the cage. The litter box should be placed as far away from the feeding station as possible. A box or hammock can provide a suitable sleeping area.

The cage bottom should preferably consist of easy-to-clean, solid material. Cloths, towels, or old T-shirts can be used for bedding material.

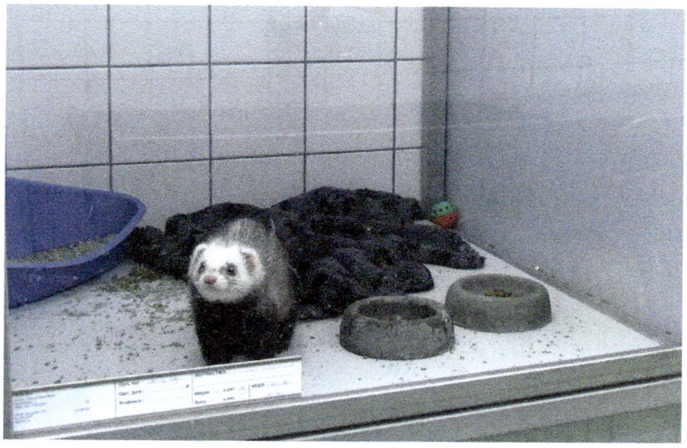

Figure 2.24 Ferrets are notorious escape artists and can easily squeeze through tiny spaces. In this case, the cage does not have any bars so that escape is impossible.

Rabbits

A rabbit's cage should be provided with sufficient bedding so that the rabbit has a soft surface to lay on, and urine is adequately absorbed. A layer of newspaper covered by a layer of (preferably dust-free) bedding (e.g. paper pulp, softwood shavings) will generally work well. Following surgery, rabbits can best be housed on towels or absorbent paper. A litter box may be provided to rabbits that are accustomed to using this. In case excrements need to be collected, the bedding may temporarily be removed. It is essential to document the nature of any droppings in the cage to assess for changes that might suggest the onset of gastrointestinal (GI) disturbance.

In addition, plenty of hay should be provided as this serves both as bedding and roughage that is needed for proper gastrointestinal motility. It is preferred to provide rabbits with their regular diet during the hospitalization period. This not only applies to the type of pellet provided, but also to the type of vegetables the rabbit prefers to eat. Also, ask the owner how the rabbit is used to receiving the drinking water, as some rabbits may not be accustomed to drinking out of a water bottle versus a bowl.

As rabbits are social animals, concurrently hospitalizing a regular cage mate for additional support and companionship can be considered, although this is less ideal if the rabbit will be receiving IV fluids, as this increases the incidence of having the IV lines chewed. The presence of a hiding box is important to provide the rabbit with additional security and seclusion. Moreover, the housing should be high enough to enable the rabbit to stand upright on its hind legs to assess its surroundings. If feasible, the owner can bring along any toys or items that the animal plays with at home as this can help the animal to feel more "at home."

Guinea Pigs

Requirements for guinea pig housing do not differ greatly from those for a rabbit. Although guinea pigs will not jump out of their cage, it is advisable to cover the cage to provide them with an additional sense of security. The provision of hiding opportunities (e.g. a cardboard box) is also advised for guinea pigs to enable them to retreat if desired (Figure 2.25). Like ferrets, guinea pigs tend to tip over their food and water bowls. Bowls should be sturdy enough and/or secured tightly to prevent them from being tipped over.

Chinchillas

In the home environment, chinchillas will often be provided with a cage that has multiple levels, ladders, and platforms as these animals love elevations. However, in a hospital situation, a multi-level cage is not recommended, as a debilitated chinchilla may easily fall and injure itself. Multi-level cages can also make it difficult to catch the animal.

A hiding box is highly recommended, as is a solid bottom, which prevents their legs from getting caught between the bars. (Paper) towels are ideal bedding material in a hospital situation. Hay should be provided to chinchillas, as this offers them opportunities to hide, and comprises an essential part of their diet. If the practice does not have the regular food of the chinchilla available, ask the owner to bring the animal's regular food.

If chinchillas need to be hospitalized for longer periods, it is ideal to provide the chinchilla with a (weekly) dust bath to maintain a good coat quality. For short hospital visits, these baths are generally not required. Co-housing with a cage mate will not only provide the animal with highly needed social support but at the same time also helps avoid problems with reintroduction.

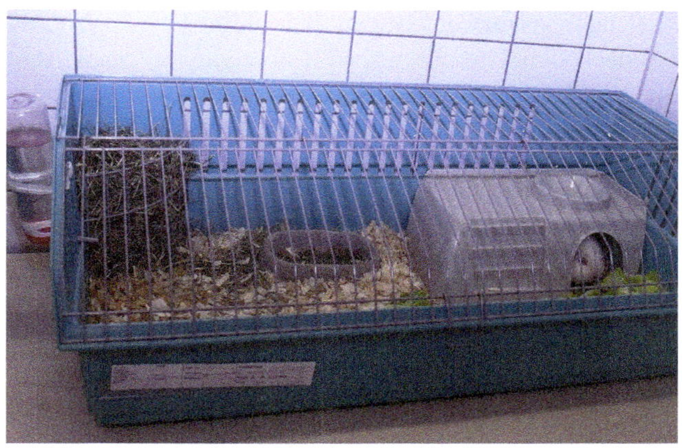

Figure 2.25 The cage of a guinea pig has sufficient padding, a layer of newspaper covered by a layer of bedding. Plenty of hay should be provided. The presence of a hiding box is important to provide the guinea pig with additional security and seclusion. Guinea pigs should have food and water bowls that are sturdy enough to prevent them from being tipped over.

Rats, Mice, Hamsters, and Gerbils

The housing of smaller rodents (i.e. rat, mouse, hamster, and gerbil) largely follows similar guidelines for all species. The housing should contain a solid floor that will allow for the provision of deep enough bedding material for the animal to hide. Many different types of bedding materials are available for these species, of which aspen wood shavings and paper or / corncob by-products are the most frequently recommended. Pine and cedar wood shavings may contain toxins and are therefore discouraged to be used. In animals with respiratory disease, paper towels or shredded cardboard are preferred to limit upper airway irritation from dust. Other types of dust-free bedding (e.g. cotton, hemp fiber) can also be used.

Water bottles are preferred as a water source, as smaller rodents will frequently fill a water bowl with bedding, resulting in no water access. It is important to check the water bottles regularly to ensure that the sipper is not occluded. Also, beware that bottles may leak, especially when bedding is pushed against the sipper.

Hedgehogs

Hedgehogs should be housed in an enclosure with a smooth surface and smooth sides to prevent them from climbing the walls and injuring themselves when falling from a height. Newspapers, shavings, and hay can function as bedding. Some hedgehogs are accustomed to using a litter box and are preferably provided with one if this is the case.

Compared to other small companion mammals, the optimum ambient temperature for hedgehogs is much higher and ranges from 24 to 29 °C/75.2 to 84.2 °F. To provide additional heat, an infrared lamp or heating mat (placed underneath the cage to prevent the animal from burning itself) may be used. A hiding box (e.g. cardboard box or flower pot) is essential for hedgehogs as they are nocturnal. As hedgehogs may defecate in their hiding box, this should be checked daily and replaced if necessary, to ensure that their (sleeping) environment is kept clean.

Sugar Gliders

Sugar gliders are nocturnal animals with an arboreal lifestyle. Like chinchillas, it is best to keep them in a cage that is not too high and allows for easy capture of the animal when hospitalized. To prevent the animals from escaping, the maximum space between the cage bars should be 6 mm. Since sugar gliders do not like to move around on the ground, branches, or perches should be provided in the cage for climbing. A newspaper placed on the bottom of the cage will be suitable to serve as bedding. A nest box of approximately 25 × 10 × 15 cm with a hinged top and a circular opening of at least 5 cm is ideal for the sugar glider to sleep in and allows for easy capture of the animal (see Section "Handling and Restraint"). A piece of cloth can serve as nest material. Like hedgehogs, sugar gliders should be kept in slightly higher temperature ranges (24–27 °C/75.2–80.6 °F is optimal) than other small mammals.

Daily Monitoring

Daily monitoring of all hospitalized patients is essential. This involves obtaining a general impression of the animal's activity, mentation, and appetite as well as an evaluation of the animal's excreta. A physical examination should be performed in those animals requiring extra care and attention. In any patient that has undergone surgery or has any type of injury, the bandage and/or injury should be carefully checked.

Records should always be kept to allow evaluation of the course of the disease over time. These should minimally include the following: physical examination findings; body weight; water and food consumed; the amount, color, and consistency of the urine and droppings; any medication, food, fluids, or other types of treatment provided to the animal (including dosages, frequency, and route of administration). A common mistake is to compare daily findings rather than evaluating them in relation to the whole hospitalization period. Writing findings such as the weight, body temperature, respiration, and/or heart rate down in a chart, will help to provide an overview and facilitate visualization of a (gradual) progress or decline in the animal's condition. Ideally, add which vital parameters should be monitored and how frequently by species (i.e. monitoring of fecal output in rabbits, guinea pigs, and chinchillas; food intake monitoring in all species; activity and respiratory monitoring are more practical in small rodents than measuring heart rate to minimize the stress of handling).

Further Reading

Ballard, B. and Rockett, J. (2009). *Restraint & Handling for Veterinary Technicians & Assistants*. Cengage Learning.

Bradbury, A.G. and Dickens, G.J.E. (2016). Appropriate handling of pet rabbits: a literature review. *J. Small Anim. Pract.* 57 (10): 503–509.

Cao, T., Cao, T., and Shirota, T. (2001). Bone mineral density in mandibles of ovariectomized rabbits. *Clin. Oral Implants Res.* 12 (6): 604–608.

Carli, G. (1974). Blood pressure and heart rate in the rabbit during animal hypnosis. *Electroencephalogr. Clin. Neurophysiol.* 37 (3): 231–237.

Carli, G., Farabollini, F., and Di Prisco, C.L. (1979). Plasma corticosterone and its relation to susceptibility to animal hypnosis in rabbits. *Neurosci. Lett.* 11 (3): 271–274.

Chitty, J. (2009). Ferrets: biology and husbandry. In: *BSAVA Manual of Rodents and Ferrets* (eds. E. Keeble and A. Meredith), 193–204. British Small Animal Veterinary Association.

Drescher, B. and Loeffler, K. (1991). The effects of different housing systems on the structure of long bones in Chinchilla and New Zealand White rabbits. Part 2. *Tierarztliche Umschau* 46 (12): 736–738.

Dúcs, A., Bilkó, Á., and Altbäcker, V. (2009). Physical contact while handling is not necessary to reduce fearfulness in the rabbit. *Appl. Anim. Behav. Sci.* 121 (1): 51–54.

Dyer, S.M. and Cervasio, E.L. (2008). An overview of restraint and blood collection techniques in exotic pet practice. *Vet. Clin. North Am. Exot. Anim. Pract.* 11 (3): 423–443.

Ewell, A.H., Cullen, J.M., and Woodruff, M.L. (1981). Tonic immobility as a predator-defense in the rabbit (*Oryctolagus cuniculus*). *Behav. Neural Biol.* 31 (4): 483–489.

Farabollini, F., Facchinetti, F., Lupo, C., and Carli, G. (1990). Time-course of opioid and pituitary-adrenal hormone modifications during the immobility reaction in rabbits. *Physiol. Behav.* 47 (2): 337–341.

Fisher, P.G. (2005). Equipping the exotic mammal practice. *Vet. Clin. North Am. Exot. Anim. Pract.* 8 (3): 405–426.

Fisher, P.G. (2010). Standards of care in the 21st century: the rabbit. *J. Exot. Pet Med.* 19 (1): 22–35.

Grand, T.I. (1977). Body weight: its relation to tissue composition, segment distribution, and motor function. I. Interspecific comparisons. *Am. J. Phys. Anthropol.* 47 (2): 211–239.

Johnson-Delaney, C.A. (2005). Safety issues in the exotic pet practice. *Vet. Clin. North Am. Exot. Anim. Pract.* 8 (3): 515–524.

Johnson-Delaney, C.A. (2006). Common procedures in hedgehogs, prairie dogs, exotic rodents, and companion marsupials. *Vet. Clin. North Am. Exot. Anim. Pract.* 9 (2): 415–435.

Keeble, E. (2009). Rodents: biology and husbandry. In: *BSAVA Manual of Rodents and Ferrets* (eds. E. Keeble and A. Meredith), 1–17. British Small Animal Veterinary Association.

Mader, D.R. (2004). Basic approach to veterinary care. In: *Ferrets, Rabbits, and Rodents: Clinical Medicine and Surgery*, 2e (eds. K.E. Quesenberry and J.W. Carpenter), 147–154. St. Louis: WB Saunders.

Malley, D. (2007). Safe handling and restraint of pet rabbits. *Practice* 29 (7): 378–386.

McBride, E.A., Day, S., McAdie, T.M. et al. (2006). Trancing rabbits: relaxed hypnosis or a state of fear? In: *Proceedings of the VDWE International Congress on Companion Animal Behaviour and Welfare*, 135–137. Flemish Veterinary Association.

Meredith, A. and Johnson-Delaney, C. (2010). *BSAVA Manual of Exotic Pets*, 5e. British Small Animal Veterinary Association.

Mitchell, M.A. and Tully, T.N. (2004). Zoonotic diseases. In: *Ferrets, Rabbits and Rodents: Clinical Medicine and Surgery*, 2e (eds. K.E. Quesenberry and J.W. Carpenter), 429–434. St Louis: WB Saunders.

Richardson, V.C. (2008). *Diseases of Small Domestic Rodents*. Wiley.

Saunders, R. (2014). Husbandry. In: *BSAVA Manual of Rabbit Medicine* (eds. A. Meredith and B. Lord), 13–26. British Small Animal Veterinary Association.

Sheldon, C.C., Sonsthagen, T.F., and Topel, J. (2006). *Animal Restraint for Veterinary Professionals*. Mosby Elsevier.

Tamura, Y. (2010). Current approach to rodents as patients. *J Exot. Pet Med.* 19 (1): 36–55.

Zaffarano, B. (2010). Ferrets: examination and standards of care. *J. Exot. Pet Med.* 19 (1): 73–81.

3

Oxygen Therapy

Sara Gardhouse

Department of Clinical Sciences, College of Veterinary Medicine, Kansas State University, Manhattan, USA

CONTENTS

Indications for Oxygen Therapy in Exotic Companion Mammals

Oxygen therapy is critical in the ill exotic companion mammal (ECM), often as a life-saving measure. The importance of oxygen therapy is in part due to the high metabolism of ECMs and also due to their high oxygen consumption rates, both associated with their small size [1]. As a result, ECMs are very susceptible to even short periods of hypoxemia [1]. In humans, interruption of pulmonary gas exchange for greater than five minutes can result in irreversible damage to the vital organs, particularly the brain [2]. In comparison, rodents can develop irreversible brain injury within 30 seconds of respiratory arrest [1].

Oxygen is the most commonly used drug in emergency medicine, with obvious benefits to hypoxemic patients. Hypoxemia is defined as inadequate oxygenation of arterial blood (PaO_2 <80 mmHg, sea level) [3]. Hypoxia is defined as an inadequate amount of oxygen to meet the metabolic needs of the tissue's cells [4]. Hypoxemia results in a reduced arterial oxygen content (CaO_2), which in turn can result in tissue hypoxia [3].

The oxygen content of arterial blood is dependent on the concentration of hemoglobin and the binding affinity or degree of oxygen saturation (SaO_2) of the hemoglobin present [3]. Delivery of arterial oxygen to the tissues is usually in a form that is bound to hemoglobin, with only a small amount delivered unbound in the plasma [3]. The general purpose of oxygen therapy is to improve the arterial oxygen content (CaO_2) which resultantly acts to decrease the risk of tissue hypoxia [3]. Provision of supplemental oxygen to hypoxic patients increases the arterial oxygen content through two mechanisms: increasing hemoglobin saturation (SaO_2) and increasing dissolved plasma oxygen levels [3].

Oxygen therapy is an essential part of patient resuscitation and stabilization in times of critical illness [5]. In cases of suspected hypoxemia or patients at risk of tissue hypoxia, non-invasive oxygen supplementation will provide benefit to the ECM before handling for a physical examination, diagnostics, and treatments [3]. For patients that have ongoing respiratory distress despite oxygen therapy, supplemental oxygen should be provided via a face mask during the brief, limited physical examination. Many ECMs

Exotic Animal Emergency and Critical Care Medicine, First Edition. Edited by Jennifer E. Graham, Grayson A. Doss and Hugues Beaufrère.

Table 3.1 Normal respiratory rates by species.

Species	Respiratory rate (breaths/min)
Rabbits [8]	32–60
Ferrets [9]	33–36
Guinea pigs [10]	42–104
Chinchillas [11]	45–80
Rats [12]	115
Mice [13]	60–220
Hamster [14]	33–127
Hedgehog [15]	25–50
Sugar glider [15]	16–40

are obligate nasal breathers, and therefore, all ECMs should be quickly evaluated for nasal discharge or crusting of the nose that could be cleared and provide significant relief prior to placement in oxygen [6, 7].

In all animals, airway resistance is inversely related to the radius of the airways [1]. As a result, even slight changes in the overall lower airway diameter due to edema or accumulation of secretions can have a dramatic effect on the work of breathing in small ECMs [1]. A compounding factor in obligate nasal breathers is the presence of secretions or mucus occluding the nares or oral cavity that can contribute to severe hypoxemia [6, 7].

Clinical signs of respiratory distress in ECMs include tachypnea, dyspnea, open-mouth breathing (often agonal in obligate nasal breathers), a marked abdominal component to respirations, extended head and neck postures and, in severe cases, presence of cyanosis (Table 3.1) [16].

One of the key factors in treatment of respiratory disease is early recognition of hypoxemia. Hypoxemia results in a decrease in the oxygen content of arterial blood which can in turn cause a severe tissue hypoxia [3]. In the face of tissue hypoxia with normal hemoglobin levels (>5 g/dl), visible cyanosis can occur [17]. The delivery of oxygen to tissues (tissue oxygen delivery, DO_2) depends on two factors: (i) arterial oxygen content (CaO_2) and (ii) cardiac output (CO). This means that increasing CO has the potential to limit tissue hypoxia in some hypoxemic patients [3]. There are different types of hypoxemia that can occur including those as a result of ventilation–perfusion (V/Q) mismatch, intrapulmonary shunts, diffusion impairments, hypoventilation, and a decreased fraction of inspired oxygen [18].

The recognition of hypoxemia in ECMs is extremely limited due to the difficulties that are associated with collection of arterial blood gas samples. It is possible in rabbits to obtain a sample from the auricular artery to look at PaO_2 levels, but this is not commonly done in the awake rabbit [19]. In dogs and cats, a PaO_2 value of less than 80 mmHg is consistent with hypoxemia, and when values drop below 60 mmHg, severe hypoxemia is considered to be present [3]. Arterial blood hemoglobin saturation (SaO_2 or SpO_2) values that are less than 95% are considered representative of hypoxemia in dogs and values less than 90% are associated with life-threatening hypoxemia [18]. In dogs, arterial oxygen saturation greater than 95% typically corresponds with a PaO_2 of greater 80 mmHg, while an SpO_2 less than 90% typically corresponds with a PaO_2 less than 60 mmHg in patients breathing room air [18].

Since arterial samples can rarely be obtained in ECMs, the use of pulse oximeters is common to estimate the approximate hemoglobin oxygen saturation level ($SpO_2 \approx SaO_2$). The use of pulse oximetry allows for a non-invasive technique to measure oxygen saturation. SaO_2 and PaO_2 are affected by the same pulmonary processes, and SpO_2 and SaO_2 are often used as surrogate markers of PaO_2 [18].

In an emergent setting, pulse oximetry is a readily available, inexpensive, user friendly tool that can be rapidly used to detect the presence of hypoxemia [20]. Pulse oximetry measures oxygen saturation of the blood through illumination of the skin and detection of changes in light absorption between oxygenated blood (oxyhemoglobin) and deoxygenated blood (reduced hemoglobin) [20]. The pulse oximeter then looks at the ratio of absorbance between these wavelengths with calibration against direct measurements of arterial oxygen saturation (SaO_2) to determine the measurement of arterial saturation (SpO_2) by the pulse oximeter [20]. In humans, the difference between SpO_2 and SaO_2 is less than 2% when the SaO_2 value is above 90%; however, the precision of the reading worsens when the SaO_2 is lower than 90% [20]. Similarly, in ferrets, values obtained by pulse oximetry have been demonstrated to closely relate to oxygen saturation, when measured by blood gas analysis, with the most precise measurements being noted when oxygen saturation was between 90% and 100% [21]. In addition to ferrets, the use of pulse oximetry has been validated in rabbits, with accuracy at hemoglobin saturation values greater than 85% and rats, with variability demonstrated at anywhere from 60% to 75% saturation [22–24]. Depending on the species, the pulse oximeter can be placed in various locations (Table 3.2).

In ECMs, differences exist in the oxygen–hemoglobin dissociation curve compared to companion mammals such as dogs and cats. It is well known that specific environmental adaptations to a low oxygen tension (high altitude) result in a shift of the curve to the left [25]. Metabolic need for oxygen appears to shift the curve in the other direction [25]. This means, ECMs, being very small mammals tend to have dissociation curves that are markedly shifted to the right in comparison with larger mammals like dogs due to an increased metabolic need for oxygen [25]. The reason for this is that the oxygen consumption per gram of tissue is significantly higher

Table 3.2 Pulse oximeter probe placement by species.

	Tail	Toes/legs	Rectum	Scrotum/vulva	Pinna	Tongue
Rabbits		C	F	C	C	C
Ferrets		C	F	C		C
Rodents	C (some species)	C	F	C		C

F, flat reflectance (rectal probe); C, clip probe.

in smaller animals compared to larger animals, which resultantly means that at the cellular level, the diffusion gradient also must be higher in smaller animals [25]. As a result, the oxygen–hemoglobin dissociation curve is in favor of off-loading oxygen to the tissues in order to allow for appropriate tissue support at higher metabolic rates, at the expense of hemoglobin with an overall decreased oxygen affinity [25]. It is also important to keep in mind the fact that many of these species are obligate nasal breathers, and with significant upper airway disease, severe hypoxemia can occur [6, 7].

Oxygen Toxicity

As mentioned previously, oxygen is the most commonly prescribed drug in medicine [5]. With this information in mind, however, it should be of note that oxygen should be prescribed, administered, and monitored by trained staff [5]. There is a common belief that oxygen is safe in all situations, and many are unaware of the dangers associated with inappropriate oxygen therapy, resulting in hyperoxemia [5]. It is important to note that there is no evidence of the benefits of oxygen therapy in patients that are normoxemic or very mildly hypoxemic [26, 27]. The toxicity is associated with damage to the pulmonary epithelium [3]. The degree of damage to the pulmonary epithelium depends on two main factors: (i) fraction of inspired oxygen and (ii) duration of therapy [3]. The onset of toxicity varies with the atmospheric pressure, with higher atmospheric pressures demonstrating earlier onset of toxicity [28]. In humans, exposure to 100% oxygen at sea level for 24–48 hours can be tolerated, but longer exposure produces definite tissue injury [28]. At higher atmospheric pressure, characteristic pulmonary lesions occur within 3–6 hours of exposure with severe signs at 10 hours [28]. There have been no known detrimental effects in humans with less than 12 hours of 100% oxygen exposure, and though no definitive studies exist in small mammals, a similar rule could be assumed [28]. Susceptibility to oxygen exposure and toxicity is very variable, depending on the age, species, and strain of animal [29]. Given the knowledge that this variability exists, it is prudent to maintain FiO_2 levels at less than 50% when patients are going to require prolonged oxygen therapy to manage hypoxemia associated with respiratory disease.

Oxygen Administration Techniques

Non-invasive Administration Methods

Flow-By Oxygen

Flow-by oxygen is a simple and easy method of administration, especially in an emergent situation; however, it does come with limitations [30]. The oxygen tubing must be held adjacent to or within 2 cm of the patient's nostril in order to be effective [3]. An FiO_2 of 25–40% can be achieved when a flow rate of 2–3 L/min is used [3]. This administration method is typically well tolerated by patients during the initial triage stages, but is wasteful and inappropriate for use long-term [3]. It is important to keep in mind that ECMs are easily stressed with handling, so this administration technique should be a short-term solution to oxygen therapy [31].

Face Mask

A face mask can be utilized to provide oxygen therapy in an emergent situation (Figure 3.1). This should only be considered as a temporary method of administration as handling an ECM in respiratory distress can be very stressful and further exacerbate the respiratory distress. The mask should be loose, but well-fitted to the patient; the mask should not be a tight fit in order to allow for carbon dioxide and heat to escape [32]. Oxygen flow rates greater than

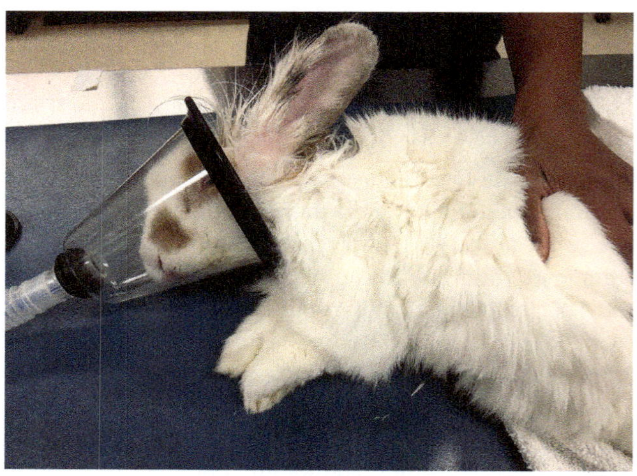

Figure 3.1 Oxygen therapy via face mask in a rabbit.

100 ml/kg/min are needed with a mask that is well-fit to the patient [32]. If the mask is large and poorly fitted, higher oxygen flow rates (300 ml/kg/min) may be needed [32]. Short-term use of face masks provides a higher FiO_2 than do other modalities such as an oxygen chamber [30]. Oxygen therapy delivered using a face mask has also been demonstrated to be more effective at increasing the partial pressure of arterial oxygen than oxygen flow by supplementation [30]. Face mask oxygen therapy can also be useful to allow for a brief hands-on physical examination of the ECM patient in respiratory distress.

Oxygen Chamber or Cage

The oxygen chamber or cage provides the easiest and least stressful route of oxygen therapy to ECMs since they provide a hands-off approach to the patient [30]. These oxygen cages are available commercially and have specific control of oxygen concentration, humidity, temperature, and the ability to monitor carbon dioxide levels [33]. Often times, these cages are large enough, that the entire travel carrier of the ECM can be placed directly into the chamber, minimizing handling, and thus minimizing stress that could exacerbate the respiratory distress. The fraction of inspired oxygen in these cages typically can reach 40% [31]. These cages are vented to decrease buildup of the expired carbon dioxide [33]. The use of oxygen analyzer devices can be useful to determine what FiO_2 is being supplied and allow for appropriate adjustment of oxygen levels [34]. An example of an oxygen analyzer is the MiniOX® [35]. It is very important to keep in mind the humidity and temperature of these enclosures, as excessively humid or warm enclosures can contribute to respiratory distress in these patients. The ideal temperature for each patient will vary depending on the species, with the ultimate goal of maintaining the temperature range within the ideal thermoneutral zone for the patient [36]. Species of special note that are particularly intolerant of excess heat are the chinchilla and guinea pig, due to natural histories that involve adaptations to higher elevations and mountain environments [37]. Although oxygen chambers are extraordinarily useful, they do come with inherent disadvantages including lack of direct access to the patient, loss of FiO_2 levels on immediate opening of the door of the cage, higher risk of hyperthermia, high cost of commercial units, and large amounts of oxygen usage [30, 38].

Other methods of oxygen administration have been described including transport cages wrapped in plastic wrap with oxygen tubing inserted through the bars. As a temporary measure, this can be effective, but it should be kept in mind there is no control of temperature and humidity and no control over the allowance for escape of carbon dioxide [30].

Invasive Administration Methods

Nasal Oxygen Prongs and Catheters

While nasal oxygen prongs and catheters are commonly employed in small animal medicine as an effective means of providing supplemental oxygen, they are not commonly used in ECMs. There are a multitude of reasons for this: Nasal prongs are easily dislodged; nasal prongs provide an unknown concentration of FiO_2, and the large diameter of the neonatal nasal prongs (3 mm) precludes their use in most ECMs [30]. Additionally, many ECMs are obligate nasal breathers, so the placement of a large diameter tube in one of their nostrils can be incredibly stressful [6, 7]. Another difficulty that may be encountered with nasal oxygen catheters in ECMs is the potential for maxillary tooth elongation into the nasal cavity, making passage of the nasal oxygen catheter impossible [39].

Nasotracheal Intubation

Nasotracheal intubation is a useful method in an emergent situation to provide high levels of oxygen to a patient [40]. The technique is performed by advancing the nasal oxygen catheter into the trachea [41]. The tube should be directed ventrally and medially into the ventral nasal meatus [42]. Previously, there has been significant concern with this technique, due to concerns for introduction of pathogens into the lungs, and necessity for high oxygen flow rates; however, in a study of New Zealand white rabbits, high oxygen flow rates were unnecessary, and no evidence of lung disease was noted in the rabbits [42]. Nasotracheal intubation takes advantage of the fact that the rabbits are an obligate nasal breather [42]. In a normal rabbit, the epiglottis is entrapped on the dorsal surface of the soft palate, and thus, this facilitates the direct passage of air from the nasopharynx into the larynx and trachea [42]. Resultantly, a tube passed nasally should traverse this natural pathway from the nasopharynx to the larynx to the trachea [42]. The flipped soft palate is one of the described difficulties with orotracheal intubation and is actually a benefit of nasotracheal intubation [42]. A common indication for the use of nasotracheal intubation is cases where the oral cavity is the primary area of interest [41]. Contraindications for the use of nasotracheal intubation include the presence of upper respiratory disease, pre-existing edema of the nasal passages, and pre-existing narrowing of the nasal passages, such as from apical elongation from the teeth [42, 43]. Complications of this technique are usually associated with traumatic nasotracheal intubation where repeated attempts result in damage to the soft tissue structures and nasal turbinates which can result in swelling and nasal passageway obstruction [41]. Although mentioned previously that there is little evidence to support introduction of

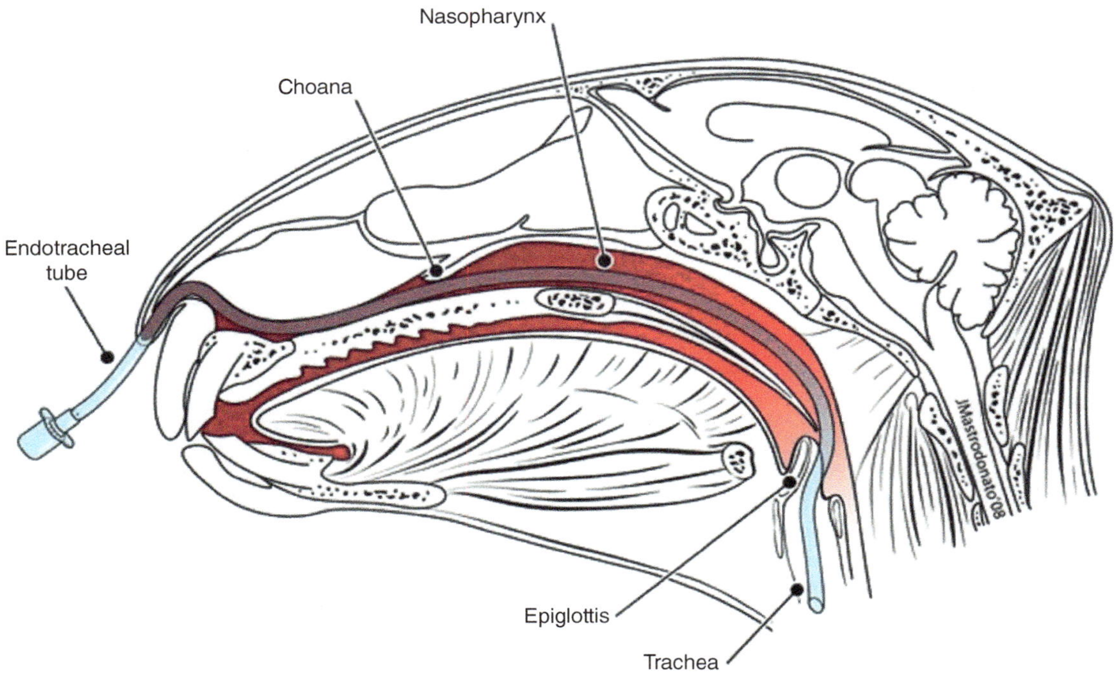

Figure 3.2 Illustration schematic of nasotracheal intubation in a rabbit. The pathway of the endotracheal tube follows the external nares and then passes through the ventral nasal meatus, choana, and nasal pharynx, at which point it reaches the trachea. *Source:* From Devalle [42]. © 2009, American Association for Laboratory Animal Science.

bacteria into the lungs, in cases of known upper respiratory infection, it may be prudent to avoid the use of nasotracheal intubation [42, 43].

To place a nasotracheal tube, the first step is an anesthetic plan that produces appropriate muscle relaxation. Supplemental oxygen via face mask or flow by should be provided to the patient throughout the procedure. A 2% lidocaine solution at a dose of 1–2 mg/kg can be instilled into the nasal passages with a syringe. Following lidocaine administration, wait 60 seconds for the lidocaine to take effect, while providing ongoing oxygen supplementation. The correct position is critical for success. The rabbit should be positioned in sternal recumbency with hyperextension of the head and neck. This position allows for optimal alignment of the nasopharynx with the trachea, allowing the endotracheal tube to pass smoothly into the trachea. The diameter of the nasal passage of rabbits, even large ones, is quite small, and therefore, it is usually not possible to pass a tube any larger than 2.0–2.5 mm. Conservative application of sterile lubricant should be placed on the end of the tube prior to placement. Too much lubricant can result in obstruction of the tube. The bevel of the endotracheal tube is then inserted into the ventral nasal canal and directed in a ventromedial direction. A small degree of resistance is normal due to the normal nasal passageway, but significant resistance or a "crunching" sound likely indicate the tube is too large, or the tube is passing through the nasal turbinates and the tube should be redirected [43]. The rabbit often coughs when the tube enters into the trachea [43] (Figure 3.2).

Oral Endotracheal Intubation

Oral endotracheal intubation is the most common method of securing an airway in ECMs, though with the smaller rodents presents significant challenges. In an emergency setting, indications for orotracheal intubation include signs of imminent respiratory arrest [44]. Once intubated, positive pressure ventilation can be used [44].

In ferrets, endotracheal intubation is commonly compared to the cat and is easy to perform, even in an emergency situation [45]. Ferrets weighing less than 800 g can usually accommodate a 2.0–2.5 mm uncuffed endotracheal tube, and ferrets weighing greater than 1 kg can usually accommodate a 3.0 cuffed endotracheal tube or 3.5 uncuffed endotracheal tube [46] (Figures 3.3 and 3.4 [47]).

In rabbits, orotracheal intubation can be challenging due to the narrow oral cavity lined by cheek teeth on both sides, long tongue with a large base, decreased jaw opening, and potential for laryngospasm [48]. Many different techniques have been described for the intubation of rabbits including the blind method, the modified blind method, videoendoscopic methods, and direct visualization [48]. Complications

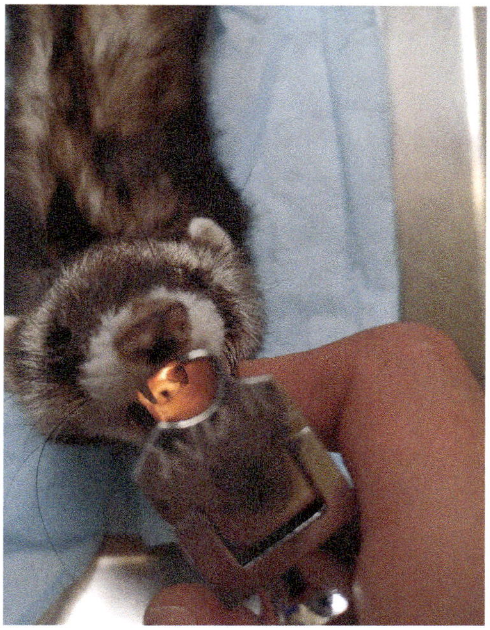

Figure 3.3 Oral endotracheal intubation in a ferret demonstrating visualization of the glottis. *Source:* Courtesy of Sarah Birch, RVT.

with orotracheal intubation include difficult placement, trauma to the oropharyngeal soft tissue, laryngospasm, tube dislodgement, and postintubation oropharyngeal swelling after intubation [48]. For intubation using the blind technique, visualization of air flow through the endotracheal tube, listening for patient respiration, or monitoring of end-tidal carbon dioxide followed by careful manipulation of the tube is needed [48]. This technique is not useful in cases of respiratory arrest due to absence of airflow [48]. With inexperience, this technique can result in significant laryngospasm and laryngeal trauma [48]. Another method of intubation in rabbits is with the use of the laryngoscope and direct visualization of the larynx; however, this technique presents significant challenges, as often the laryngoscope blade is wider than the narrow oral cavity and cheek teeth preventing appropriate visualization [48]. Other intubation options in rabbits include the use of a fiberoptic laryngoscope that allows for easy insertion of the endotracheal tube by using a laryngoscope placed inside the tube, allowing direct visualization of the trachea [48]. Similarly, an endoscope can be used to visualize the larynx and guide placement of the endotracheal tube (see Figures 7.7 and 7.8) [48]. The most common endotracheal tube sizes in rabbits range from 2.0 to 3.5 mm depending on the size of the rabbit [45]

Currently, three main types of endoscopes are commonly utilized for endotracheal intubation in exotic small mammals: (i) the 2.7 mm 30° Hopkins rod-lens telescope (Karl Storz Veterinary Endoscopy America); (ii) the 1.9 mm semi-rigid fiber optic endoscope (MDS Incorporated); and (iii) the 1.0 mm semi-rigid fiber optic endoscope (Karl Storz and MDS) [49]. The 2.7 mm telescope can accommodate endotracheal tubes with an internal diameter of 3.0 mm or greater [49]. The 30° angle of the rigid scope is beneficial to get a clear view of the glottis, but the rigid nature of the scope limits visualization in patients with a difficult airway or positioning [49]. The 0° angle of the 1.9 and 1.0 mm scopes may result in more difficult visualization of the glottis, and more difficult entry through the laryngeal folds due to the flat surface, compared to the angled surface of the 30° scope that helps to open the laryngeal folds on entry [49]. The 1.9 mm semi-rigid scope can accommodate tubes with an internal diameter of 2.0 mm, and the 1.0 mm semi-rigid scope can accommodate tubes with an internal diameter of 1.5 mm [49]. Varying light sources ranging from a handheld table top unit, to cameras and video monitors can be utilized for visualization [49].

Intubation in guinea pigs, chinchillas, and degus carries its own set of challenges due to their unique oropharyngeal anatomy and is unlikely to be feasible in an emergency setting [49]. In guinea pigs, and chinchillas, and degus the caudal aspect of the tongue is continuous with their soft palate with a very small opening, referred to as the palatal ostium [49]. The palatal ostium is formed by the soft palate, the palatoglossal arches on either side, and the tongue [49]. The folds of soft palate that surround the palatal ostium are very vascular, and significant trauma and hemorrhage can occur if this area is damaged during attempts at intubation [50]. Additionally, guinea pigs almost always have a large amount of food in their mouth, which impedes visualization and complicates ability to intubate them. In addition to these complicating factors, both species have a small laryngeal opening [49]. Endoscopic techniques with the use of a guide and elevation of the patient on a dental board can help to facilitate successful intubation [49]. In guinea pigs and chinchillas, an 8-Fr urinary catheter or 2.0–2.5 mm endotracheal tube is generally a good fit [49].

Hedgehogs and sugar gliders can be intubated with 1.0–1.5 mm silicone tubes [49]. Endoscope assistance can be utilized for their intubation [49].

Rats and other small mammals can be challenging but possible with the use of a small laryngoscope and direct visualization or endoscopic guidance [49]. The size of the tube for intubation typically ranges from 1.0 to 1.5 mm or a 14–16-gauge intravenous (IV) catheter (Table 3.3) [49].

Prairie dogs, though uncommon pets, are seen in clinical practice. Techniques utilized in rabbits can also be employed in prairie dogs, though they tend to be more challenging [49]. The soft palate of prairie dogs is longer than rabbits, often obscures the glottis, and they have a

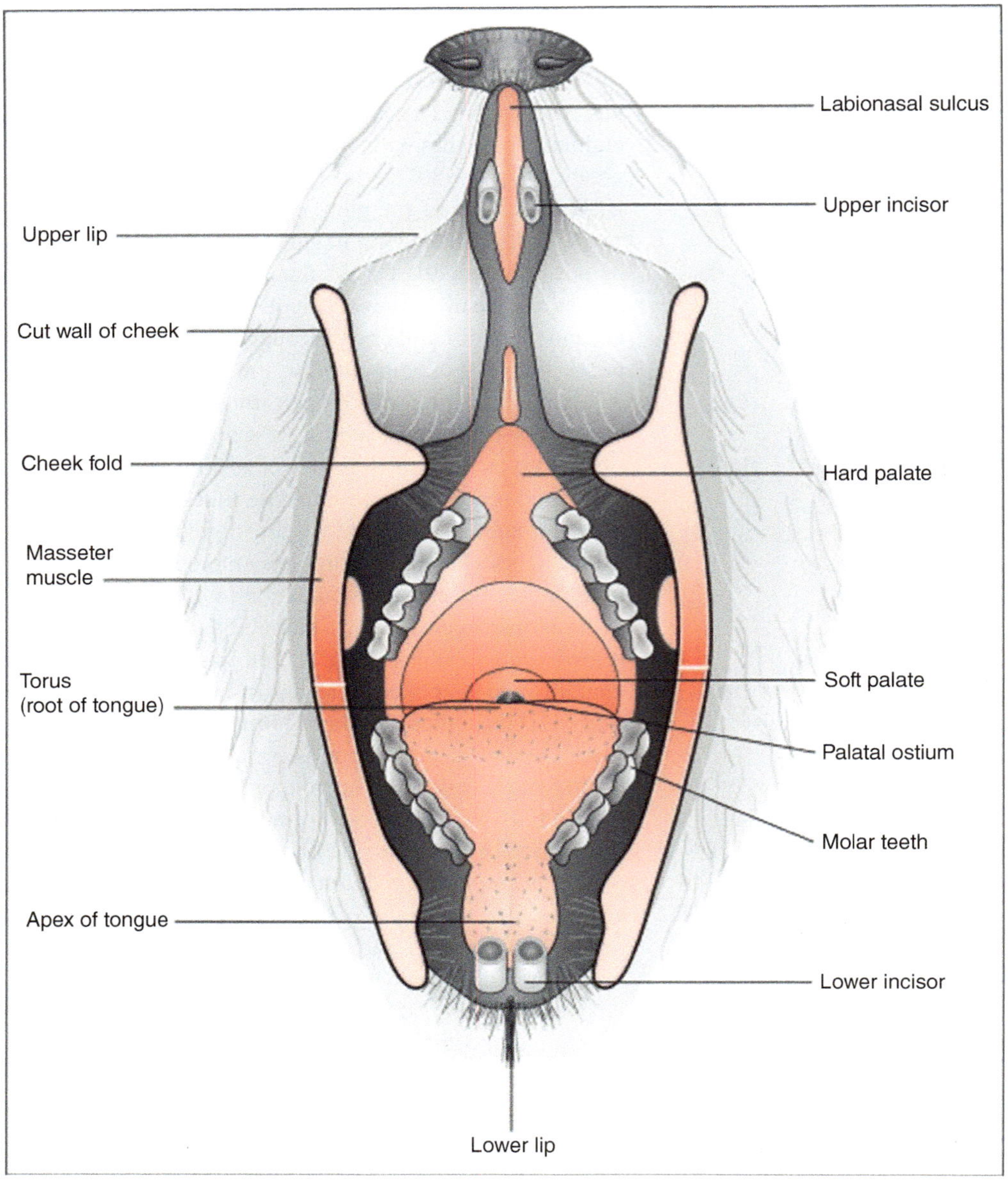

Figure 3.4 Oral anatomy of the ferret. *Source:* From O'Malley [47]. © 2005, Elsevier.

smaller glottal opening than rabbits [49]. Typically, a 2.0–2.5 mm endotracheal tube can be placed [49].

It is important to keep in mind that with small diameter tubes, risk of occlusion of the tube with saliva, lubricant, or occlusion from kinking of the tube are significant risks and require close monitoring [49]. Use of an end-tidal CO_2 monitor on the patient can be useful to help detect endotracheal tube complications [49].

Confirmation of tube placement is similar to other species [49]. The patient may cough as the tube is passed, condensation may be seen on the inside of the endotracheal tube, or condensation may be seen on a glass slide placed at the end of the tube, air movement can be detected by listening for breath sounds, or movement of the chest can be detected when a breath is provided with the rebreathing bag [49]. If endoscopic guidance is used, direct visualization of tube placement can be confirmed [49].

Laryngeal Mask Airway (LMA) Devices and Supraglottic Airway Devices (SGAD)

The laryngeal mask airway (LMA) is a supraglottic airway device (SGAD) that was initially developed by a human anesthesiologist as an alternative to mask ventilation [51]. It is

Table 3.3 Normal endotracheal tube sizes by species [49].

Species	Tube size
Rabbit	2.0–3.5 mm ID
Ferret	2.0–2.5 mm ID
Prairie dog	2.0–2.5 mm ID
Guinea pig	8F
	2.0–2.5 mm ID
Chinchilla	8F
	2.0–2.5 mm ID
Hedgehog	1.5 mm ID
Sugar glider	1.5 mm ID
Rat	1.0–1.5 mm ID
	14–16 gauge

ID, internal diameter.
Source: Adapted from Johnson [49].

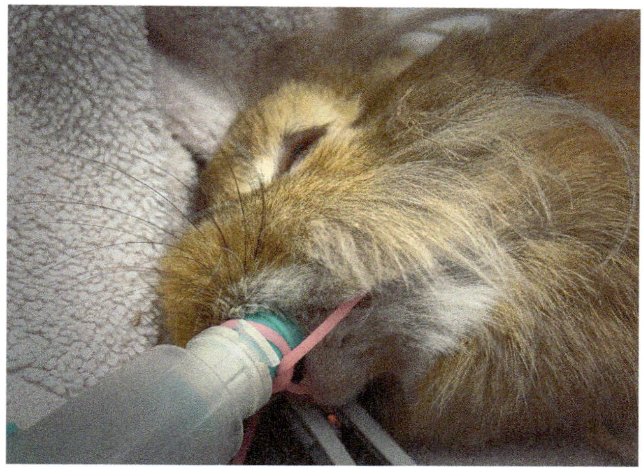

Figure 3.6 Adult rabbit with v-gel Advanced Rabbit Supraglottic Airway Device in place. *Source:* Courtesy of DocsInnovent Ltd.

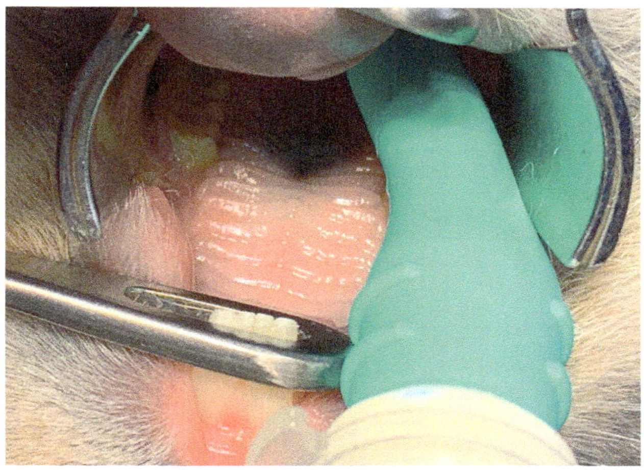

Figure 3.7 Adult rabbit with v-gel Advanced Rabbit Supraglottic Airway Device in place. *Source:* Courtesy of DocsInnovent Ltd.

commonly also used in humans in an emergency setting to manage difficult airways [51]. The pediatric LMA has been used in rabbits as an alternative to endotracheal tube placement and results in easier placement than an endotracheal tube, especially in the emergency setting [52]. It has also been noted, however, that the LMA submits more isoflurane waste than when the rabbit is intubated [52]. Of important note, since pediatric human devices are not specifically designed for rabbits, complications including lingual cyanosis, gastric tympany, and an incomplete airway seal have been demonstrated with these devices in rabbits [52–54].

More recently, a SGAD specific to rabbits (v-gel® ADVANCED) has been created which allows for rapid management of the rabbit's airway and administration of positive pressure ventilation with proper placement (Figure 3.5) [55]. The v-gel has the benefit of ease of placement by a novice clinician using end-tidal CO_2 guidance, combined with minimal to no airway trauma (Figures 3.6 and 3.7) [55]. Placement time for the SGAD in rabbits is short, ranging from 14 to 38 seconds [55]. In one study comparing the placement of a v-gel to oral endotracheal intubation, consistency in the time taken to secure an airway was demonstrated with the v-gel with the longest time being 38 seconds with the v-gel compared to 171 seconds with an endotracheal tube [55]. The difference in time to placement of oral endotracheal tubes was magnified in this study when failed intubation is considered [55]. An advantage of the v-gel over the human pediatric LMA is that the rabbit v-gel is specifically shaped to mirror the pharyngeal airway anatomical structures of the rabbit (Figure 3.8) [54, 55]. The combination of the unique shape with the soft gel-like material allows for creation of a strong seal with minimal airway trauma [55]. Additionally, it is suggested by the manufacturer that the v-gel does not

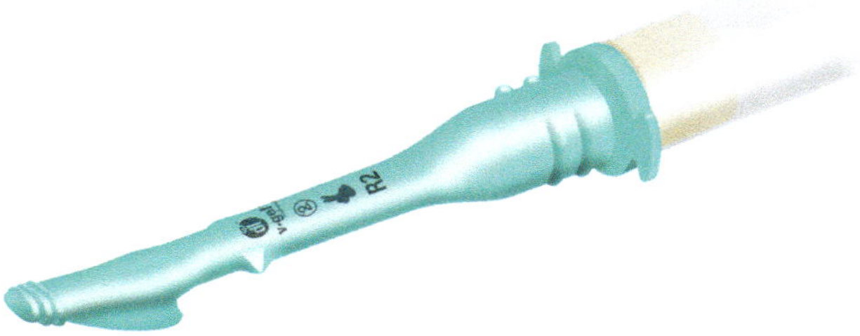

Figure 3.5 v-gel Advanced Rabbit Supraglottic Airway Device (https://docsinnovent.com/products/v-gel-rabbit). *Source:* Courtesy of DocsInnovent Ltd.

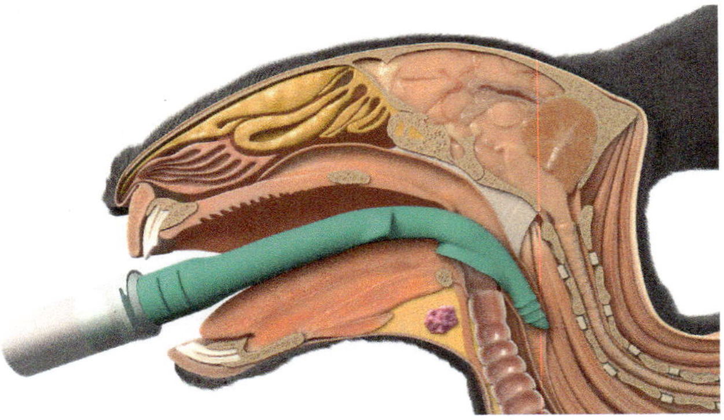

Figure 3.8 Model of adult rabbit showing anatomic location of appropriate placement of v-gel Advanced Rabbit Supraglottic Airway Device (https://docsinnovent.com/products/v-gel-rabbit). *Source:* Courtesy of DocsInnovent Ltd.

RABBIT v-gel® sizing guide		
Size	Ideal body weight of rabbit	Product code
R1	0.6–1.5 kg (1.3–3.5 lb)	D30001
R2	1–2 kg (2–4.5 lb)	D30002
R3	1.8–3.5 kg (4–8 lb)	D30003
R4	2.5–4 kg (5–9 lb)	D30004
R5	3.5–5 kg (8–11 lb)	D30005
R6	4.5 kg+ (10 lb+)	D30006

Figure 3.9 v-gel Advanced Rabbit Supraglottic Airway Device sizing guide (https://docsinnovent.com/products/v-gel-rabbit). *Source:* Courtesy of DocsInnovent Ltd.

result in airway narrowing as does placement of an endotracheal tube, which may resultantly decrease work of breathing [56]. The rabbit v-gel is available in a wide variety of sizes for rabbits ranging from rabbits weight 0.6 kg to 4.5+ kg (Figure 3.9) [56].

In a recent study on rabbit airway devices, a comparison was made between the rabbit v-gel SGAD, to a human infant SGAD, a pediatric LMA and standard endotracheal intubation during assisted ventilation (AV) or controlled ventilation (CV) in anesthetized rabbits [57]. The results of this study demonstrated that the rabbit v-gel SGAD was easily placed in the shortest time to successful placement when compared to endotracheal tubes and other perilaryngeal airway devices [57].

Preliminary studies demonstrate that the use of the R1 v-gel may be of benefit in hedgehogs in place of a face mask

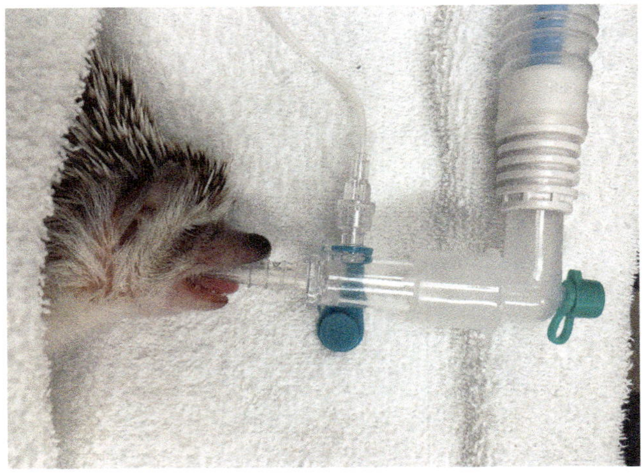

Figure 3.10 Appropriate placement of a v-gel in an African pygmy hedgehog. *Source:* Courtesy of Grayson Doss.

(Figure 3.10). Development of similar devices for guinea pigs [58] and chinchillas is underway.

Percutaneous Emergency Airway Access

Percutaneous emergency airway access is rarely utilized in ECMs, but in cases where the animal is not able to be intubated and a life-threatening situation with need for oxygen supplementation is required, it can be a life-saving technique [3]. In small animal patients (dogs and cats), percutaneous emergency airway access is achieved through transtracheal oxygen catheters or a tracheotomy [3]. The placement of transtracheal oxygen catheters in ECM is similar to other companion animals, with exceptions in intact female rabbits that have large dewlaps that may impede access. Transtracheal oxygen catheters provide a means of administering oxygen rapidly, with potential for manual ventilation, especially in cases of respiratory arrest when intubation is not possible [3]. In species such as guinea pigs, chinchillas, and small rodents where emergency oral endotracheal intubation is not possible, the use of a transtracheal oxygen catheter may provide a more reliable and rapid means of airway access. This technique is, however, invasive and may not be desirable by some owners.

Alternatively, a recent study examining cardiopulmonary resuscitation (CPR) techniques in rabbits demonstrated that tight-fitting face masks can provide effective respiratory support in rabbits during CPR when intubation is not possible [59]. Since in many cases, intubation is too challenging and time-consuming to undertake in an emergency situation, forced mask ventilation is an attractive alternative [60]. If face mask ventilation is elected in an emergent situation, it is important to clear the oral cavity of food and secretions and ensure that the mask is a tight fit with a strong seal [60]. Use of 20–30 breaths per minute with visualization of thoracic excursions is appropriate in the respiratory arrest situation [60]. This technique can result in rapid filling of the stomach with air, and this should be monitored throughout the CPR process.

Tracheostomy

Tracheostomy is a technique well described in dogs and cats as a method of emergency airway access [61]. Although this technique does appear to be well tolerated in dogs, there is very limited experience with this technique in ECM and it is questionable whether this technique would be well tolerated in patients that survive.

Common Respiratory Diseases of Exotic Small Mammals

Respiratory disease is common in ECMs and can be caused by a large number of underlying etiologies, with infectious being a common cause. Since rabbits and rodents are obligate nasal breathers, upper respiratory tract disease can be as concerning as lower respiratory tract disease [6, 7].

Rabbits

Infectious Etiologies

Respiratory disease in rabbits has been historically referred to as pasteurellosis or snuffles, with *Pasteurella multocida* implicated as the underlying cause; however, many other bacterial agents such as *Bordetella bronchiseptica*, *Staphylococcus* sp., and *Pseudomonas* sp., as well as anaerobes can be involved [6]. Rhinitis and sinusitis are the most common forms of pasteurellosis with evidence of mucopurulent discharge from the eyes and nares [6]. As a result of grooming, crusting of the forearms is often noted [6]. Chronic infection with extension to the lower respiratory tract is not uncommon [6]. Viral diseases associated with primary respiratory disease in rabbits have not been identified [6].

Non-infectious Etiologies

Any space occupying mass in the respiratory tract or extra-respiratory tract mass can also result in significant respiratory distress. Given that rabbits are obligate nasal breathers, any signs of open-mouth breathing are significant and representative of serious respiratory compromise [6]. Non-infectious etiologies of respiratory distress include neoplasia of the nasal turbinates, most commonly adenocarcinoma, primary lung tumors, and secondary lung metastases [6]. Thymomas are a common presentation in adult rabbits, with the presence of respiratory signs occurring as a result of a space occupying cranial mediastinal mass [6]. A common clinical sign of thymoma in rabbits is bilateral exophthalmos, as a result of compromised return of blood to the heart [6]. Allergens have also been reported as a cause of rhinitis and chronic bronchitis in rabbits [6]. In any rabbit with upper respiratory clinical signs, a thorough oral examination in combination with diagnostic imaging (dental radiographs, skull computed tomography) should always be undertaken, as the signs can be a result of apical elongation or abscessation of the teeth [6].

Rodents

Guinea Pigs

There are many factors that are involved in the development and progression of respiratory disorders in guinea pigs, including overcrowding, improper nutrition, and issues related to the housing environment (inadequate ventilation, changes in humidity and temperature, extreme weather [hot or cold], excessive dust) [62].

Infectious Etiologies Many different pathogens can result in respiratory disease in guinea pigs, including bacterial, viral, and fungal [62]. Bacterial pneumonia can present as a significant respiratory disease in guinea pigs, with common etiologic agents including *B. bronchiseptica* and *Streptococcus pneumoniae* [62]. Common sources of infection include rabbits and dogs, who can be asymptomatic carriers of the infection [62]. Both infections result in lower respiratory tract signs [62]. Clinical signs of bacterial pneumonia include anorexia, ocular and nasal discharge, abnormal respiratory sounds, lethargy, and sneezing, which can progress to tachypnea and dyspnea [62]. Chlamydiosis caused by *Chlamydia caviae* and *Chlamydia psittaci* have also been reported in guinea pigs which may initially present as conjunctivitis and rhinitis, but progress to bronchitis and pneumonia [62]. Bronchopneumonia in association with an adenovirus has been reported in guinea pigs [62].

Non-infectious Etiologies Bronchogenic papillary adenoma, bronchogenic, and alveologenic adenocarcinoma, as well as lymphosarcoma and leukemia linked to a type C retrovirus resulting in mediastinal lymphadenopathy and dyspnea, have all been reported in guinea pigs [62]. Guinea pigs are susceptible to heat stroke because they are a species native to cooler regions of South America [62]. Other non-infectious etiologies of respiratory distress in guinea pigs to consider include cardiovascular disease and toxins [62].

Chinchillas

There are many factors that are involved in the development and progression of respiratory disorders in chinchillas, including overcrowding, improper nutrition, and issues related to the housing environment (inadequate ventilation, changes in humidity, and temperature, extreme weather [hot or cold], excessive dust) [62].

Infectious Etiologies Although *S. pneumoniae*, *Pseudomonas*, and *Pasteurella pneumotropica* are normal inhabitants of the respiratory tract of chinchillas, pneumonia can occur under stressful conditions with invasion of *S. pneumoniae* and *B. bronchiseptica* [62].

Non-infectious Etiologies Chinchillas are susceptible to heat stroke because they are a species native to cooler regions of South America [62]. Other non-infectious etiologies of respiratory distress in chinchillas to consider include cardiovascular disease and toxins [62].

Prairie Dogs

Respiratory disease is a common presentation in prairie dogs [63]. In many cases, poor husbandry is an underlying factor, including factors such as high levels of dust, humidity, or poor ventilation, and resolution of signs can be seen when the husbandry is corrected [63]. Infectious respiratory disease has also been reported in prairie dogs [63]. Another very common etiology of respiratory distress in prairie dogs is obstructive respiratory disease associated with pseudo-odontomas [64].

Rats

Respiratory disease is an extremely common presentation of the pet rat [65]. Infectious causes are common with frequent etiologic agents being *Mycoplasma pulmonis*, *Streptococcus pneumonia*, and *Corynebacterium kutscheri* [65]. Viruses can also be implicated in disease but are less common [65]. The resultant disease in rats is often referred to as chronic respiratory disease (CRD) [65]. Disease often involves both the upper and lower respiratory tract [65]. Neoplasia, both primary and secondary to metastasis, have also been reported to cause respiratory disease in rats [65].

General

Clinical signs consistent with upper airway disease can be caused by dental malocclusion in rabbits and rodents. The incisors of all rabbits and rodents are aradicular (open-rooted), hypsodont (high-crowned), and elodont (continuously growing) [66]. These features when combined with trauma, inappropriate diet, or disease can result in abnormal growth of these teeth, which subsequently results in dental malocclusion [66]. Inflammation, abnormal growth, and bony reaction surrounding the apex of these teeth can result in impingement of the surrounding soft tissue structures, including the nasal passages [66]. Prairie dogs specifically develop pseudo-odontoma formation from trauma [64] with impingement of the nasal passages.

References

1. Heard, D. (2014). Rodents. In: *Zoo Animal and Wildlife Immobilization and Anesthesia*, 2e (eds. G. West, D. Heard and N. Caulkett), 893–903. Ames, IA: Wiley-Blackwell.
2. MSD (2017). Overview of Respiratory Arrest – Critical Care Medicine. MSD Manual Professional Edition.
3. Mazzaferro, E.M. (2015). Oxygen therapy. In: *Small Animal Critical Care Medicine*, 2e (eds. D.C. Silverstein and K. Hopper), 77–80. Saunders.
4. Williams, P., Pageau, R., Whalen, C.-A. et al. (2013). *Oxygen Therapy Clinical Best Practice Guidelines*, 1–44. College of Respiratory Therapists of Ontario.
5. Kane, B., Decalmer, S., and O'Driscoll, B.R. (2013). Emergency oxygen therapy: from guideline to implementation. *Breathe* 9: 247–254.
6. Johnson-Delaney, C.A. and Orosz, S.E. (2011). Rabbit respiratory system: clinical anatomy, physiology and disease. *Vet. Clin. North Am. Exot. Anim. Pract.* 14: 257–266.
7. Longley, L. (2008). Mammal anaesthesia. In: *Anaesthesia of Exotic Pets* (ed. L.A. Longley), 27–35. Elsevier.
8. Nowland, M.H., Brammer, D.W., Garcia, A. et al. (2015). Biology and diseases of rabbits. In: *Laboratory Animal Medicine*, 3e (eds. J.G. Fox, L.C. Anderson, G.M. Otto, et al.), 411–461. https://doi.org/10.1016/B978-0-12-409527-4.00010-9.
9. Mayer, J., Marini, R.P., and Fox, J.G. (2015). Biology and diseases of ferrets. In: *Laboratory Animal Medicine*, 3e (eds. J.G. Fox, L.C. Anderson, G.M. Otto, et al.), 577–622. https://doi.org/10.1016/B978-0-12-409527-4.00014-6.
10. Shomer, N.H., Holcombe, H., and Harkness, J.E. (2015). Biology and diseases of guinea pigs. In: *Laboratory Animal Medicine*, 3e (eds. J.G. Fox, L.C. Anderson, G.M. Otto, et al.), 247–283. https://doi.org/10.1016/B978-0-12-409527-4.00006-7.
11. Hsu, C.C., Chan, M.M., and Wheler, C.L. (2015). Biology and diseases of chinchillas. In: *Laboratory Animal*

Medicine, 3e (eds. J.G. Fox, L.C. Anderson, G.M. Otto, et al.), 387–409. https://doi.org/10.1016/B978-0-12-409527-4.00009-2.

12 Otto, G.M., Franklin, C.L., and Clifford, C.B. (2015). Biology and diseases of rats. In: *Laboratory Animal Medicine*, 3e (eds. J.G. Fox, L.C. Anderson, G.M. Otto, et al.), 151–207. Academic Press. https://www.sciencedirect.com/science/article/pii/B9780124095274000043 (accessed 4 May 2019).

13 Whary, M.T., Baumgarth, N., Fox, J.G. et al. (2015). Biology and diseases of mice. In: *Laboratory Animal Medicine*, 3rde (eds. J.G. Fox, L.C. Anderson, G.M. Otto, et al.), 43–149. Academic Press.

14 Miedel, E.L. and Hankenson, F.C. (2015). Biology and diseases of hamsters. In: *Laboratory Animal Medicine*, 3e (eds. J.G. Fox, L.C. Anderson, G.M. Otto, et al.), 209–245. Academic Press.

15 Johnson, D.H. (2011). Hedgehogs and sugar gliders: respiratory anatomy, physiology, and disease. *Vet. Clin. North Am. Exot. Anim. Pract.* 14: 267–285.

16 Lennox, A.M. (2012). Respiratory disease and Pasteurellosis. In: *Ferrets, Rabbits and Rodents – Clinical Medicine and Surgery*, 3e (eds. K.E. Quesenberry and J.W. Carpenter), 205–216. St. Louis, MO: Elsevier, Inc.

17 Kyavar, M. and Sadeghpour, A. (2014). Cyanosis. In: *Comprehensive Approach to Adult Congenital Heart Disease* (eds. A. Sadeghpour, M. Kyavar and A. Alizadehasl), 37–43.

18 Haskins, S. (2014). Hypoxemia. In: *Small Animal Critical Care Medicine*, 2e (eds. D. Silverstein and K. Hopper), 81–86. St. Louis, MO: Saunders.

19 Fick, T.E. and Schalm, S.W. (1986). A procedure for arterial blood sampling in the rabbit. *Lab. Anim.* 20: 138–139.

20 Jubran, A. (2015). Pulse oximetry: review. *Crit. Care* 19: 272.

21 Olin, J.M., Smith, T.J., and Talcott, M.R. (1997). Evaluation of noninvasive monitoring techniques in domestic ferrets (*Mustela putorius furo*). *Am. J. Vet. Res.* 58: 1065–1069.

22 Vegfords, M., Sjöberg, F., Lindberg, L.G. et al. (1991). Basic studies of pulse oximetry in a rabbit model. *Acta Anaesthesiol. Scand.* 35: 596–599.

23 Bernard, S.L., An, D., and Glenny, R.W. (2004). Validation of the Nonin 8600V Pulse Oximeter for heart rate and oxygen saturation measurements in rats. *Contemp. Top. Lab. Anim. Sci.* 43: 43–45.

24 Decker, M.J., Conrad, K.P., and Strohl, K.P. Noninvasive oximetry in the rat. *Biomed. Instrum. Technol.* 23: 222–228.

25 Schmidt-Neilsen, K. and Larimer, J.L. (1958). Oxygen dissociation curves of mammalian blood in relation to body size. *Am. J. Phys.* 195: 424–428.

26 Abernethy, A.P., McDonald, C.F., Frith, P.A. et al. (2010). Effect of palliative oxygen versus room air in relief of breathlessness in patients with refractory dyspnoea: a double-blind, randomised controlled trial. *Lancet* 376: 784–793.

27 O'Driscoll, B.R. (2008). Short burst oxygen therapy in patients with COPD. *Monaldi Arch. Chest Dis.* 69: 70–74.

28 Chawla, A. and Lavania, A.K. (2001). Oxygen toxicity. *Med. J.* 57: 131–133.

29 Capellier, G., Maupoil, V., Boussat, S. et al. (1999). Oxygen toxicity and tolerance. *Minerva Anestesiol.* 65: 388–392.

30 Samal, P., Jena, D., and Gupta, A. (2018). Oxygen therapy in small animals: a review. *Int. J. Livest. Res.* 8 (2): 1.

31 Lee-Fowler, T. (2018). Feline lower airway disease. In: *Textbook of Small Animal Emergency Medicine* (eds. K.J. Drobatz, K. Hopper, E. Rozanski and D.C. Silverstein), 220–224. Hoboken, NJ, USA: Wiley https://doi.org/10.1002/9781119028994.ch34.

32 Boysen, S.R. and Mathews, K.A. (2017). Respiratory emergencies. In: *Veterinary Emergency and Critical Care Manual*, 3e (ed. K.A. Mathews), 37–84. Guelph, ON: Lifelearn, Inc.

33 Anon (2020). Intensive Care Units (ICU) – Snyder Manufacturing. https://www.snydermfg.com/products/intensive-care-units-icu (accessed 9 November 2019).

34 Wilding, L.A., Hampel, J.A., Khoury, B.M. et al. (2017). Benefits of 21% oxygen compared with 100% oxygen for delivery of isoflurane to mice (*Mus musculus*) and rats (*Rattus norvegicus*). *J. Am. Assoc. Lab. Anim. Sci.* 56: 148–154.

35 Anon (2020). MiniOx I Oxygen Analyzer – Respicare Inc. http://respicare.ph/product/mini-ox (accessed 9 November 2019).

36 Walsberg, G.E. (2020, 2000). Small mammals in hot deserts: some generalizations revisited. *Bioscience* 50: 109.

37 DeCubellis, J. (2016). Common emergencies in rabbits, guinea pigs, and chinchillas. *Vet. Clin. North Am. Exot. Anim. Pract.* 19: 411–429.

38 Drobatz, K.J. and Macintire, D.K. (2012). Respiratory emergencies. In: *Manual of Small Animal Emergency and Critical Care Medicine*, 2e (eds. D.K. Macintire, K.J. Drobatz and S.C. Haskins). Chichester, UK: Wiley-Blackwell.

39 Capello, V. (2008). Diagnosis and treatment of dental disease in pet rodents. *J. Exot. Pet. Med.* 17: 114–123.

40 Roppolo, L.P., Vilke, G.M., Chan, T.C. et al. (1999). Nasotracheal intubation in the emergency department, revisited. *J. Emerg. Med.* 17: 791–799.

41 Prasanna, D. and Bhat, S. (2014). Nasotracheal intubation: an overview. *J. Maxillofac. Oral Surg.* 13: 366–372.

42 Devalle, J.M.S. (2009). Successful management of rabbit anesthesia through the use of nasotracheal intubation. *J. Am. Assoc. Lab. Anim. Sci.* 48: 166–170.

43 Varga, M. (2017). Airway management in the rabbit. *J. Exot. Pet. Med.* 26: 29–35.

44 Hopper, K. Basic mechanical ventilation. In: *Small Animal Critical Care Medicine*, 2e (eds. D. Silverstein and K. Hopper), 161–166. St. Louis, MO: Elsevier Inc.

45 Dehn, S. (2009). Intubation of select exotic species for the veterinary technician. In: *NAVC Conference*, 36. Orlando, FL.

46 Johnson-Delaney, C.A. (2005). Ferret cardiopulmonary resuscitation. *Semin. Avian Exot. Pet Med.* 14: 135–142.

47 O'Malley, B. (2005). *Clinical Anatomy and Physiology of Exotic Species: Structure and Function of Mammals, Birds, Reptiles, and Amphibians.* Saunders, Ltd.

48 Thompson, K.L., Meier, T.R., and Scholz, J.A. (2017). Endotracheal intubation of rabbits using a polypropylene guide catheter. *J. Vis. Exp.* 2017: 1–8.

49 Johnson, D.H. (2010). Endoscopic intubation of exotic companion mammals. *Vet. Clin. North Am. Exot. Anim. Pract.* 13: 273–289.

50 Turner, M.A., Thomas, P., and Sheridan, D.J. (1992). An improved method for direct laryngeal intubation in the guinea pig. *Lab. Anim.* 26: 25–28.

51 Verghese, C., Mena, G., Ferson, D.Z. et al. (2013). Laryngeal mask airway. In: *Benumof and Hagberg's Airway Management*, 4e (ed. C.A. Hagberg), 443–465. Philadelphia, PA: Elsevier.

52 Smith, J.C., Robertson, L.D., Auhll, A. et al. (2004). Endotracheal tubes versus laryngeal mask airways in rabbit inhalation anesthesia: ease of use and waste gas emissions. *Contemp. Top. Lab. Anim. Sci.* 43: 22–25.

53 Bateman, L., Ludders, J.W., Gleed, R.D. et al. (2005). Comparison between facemask and laryngeal mask airway in rabbits during isoflurane anesthesia. *Vet. Anaesth. Analg.* 32: 280–288.

54 Kazakos, G.M., Anagnostou, T., Savvas, I. et al. (2007). Use of the laryngeal mask airway in rabbits: placement and efficacy. *Lab. Anim.* 36: 29–34.

55 Engbers, S., Larkin, A., Rousset, N. et al. (2017). Comparison of a supraglottic airway device (v-gel®) with blind orotracheal intubation in rabbits. *Front. Vet. Sci.* 4: 49.

56 Anon. Docsinnovent. https://docsinnovent.com/products/product/rabbit-v-gel (accessed 16 November 2019).

57 Uzun, M., Kiraz, H.A., Ovali, M.A. et al. (2015). The investigation of airway management capacity of v-gel and cobra-PLA in anaesthetised rabbits. *Acta Cir. Bras.* 30: 80–86.

58 van Zeeland, Y., Schoemaker, N., and Crotaz, I. (2018). Development and use of a supraglottic airway device in guinea pigs. In: *Exoticscon Proceedings*, 779–780. Atlanta, GA.

59 Buckley, G.J., DeCubellis, J., Sharp, C.R. et al. (2011). Cardiopulmonary resuscitation in hospitalized rabbits: 15 cases. *J. Exot. Pet. Med.* 20: 46–50.

60 Lichtenberger, M. and Lennox, A.M. (2012). Critical care of the exotic companion mammal (with a focus on herbivorous species): the first twenty-four hours. *J. Exot. Pet. Med.* 21: 284–292.

61 Nicholson, I. and Baines, S. (2012). Complications associated with temporary tracheostomy tubes in 42 dogs (1998 to 2007). *J. Small Anim. Pract.* 53: 108–114.

62 Yarto-Jaramillo, E. (2011). Respiratory system anatomy, physiology, and disease: guinea pigs and chinchillas. *Vet. Clin. North Am. Exot. Anim. Pract.* 14: 339–355.

63 Thas, I., Wagner, R.A., and Thas, O. (2019). Clinical diseases in pet black-tailed prairie dogs (*Cynomys ludovicianus*): a retrospective study in 206 animals. *J. Small Anim. Pract.* 60: 153–160.

64 Phalen, D.N., Antinoff, N., and Fricke, M.E. (2000). Obstructive respiratory disease in prairie dogs with odontomas. *Vet. Clin. North Am. Exot. Anim. Pract.* 3: 513–517.

65 Kling, M.A. (2011). A review of respiratory system anatomy, physiology, and disease in the mouse, rat, hamster, and gerbil. *Vet. Clin. North Am. Exot. Anim. Pract.* 14: 287–337.

66 Verstraete, F.J.M. (2003). Advances in diagnosis and treatment of small exotic mammal dental disease. *Semin. Avian Exot. Pet Med.* 12: 37–48.

4

Catheterization and Venipuncture

Yvonne R.A. van Zeeland and Nico J. Schoemaker

Division of Zoological Medicine, Department of Clinical Sciences, Faculty of Veterinary Medicine, Utrecht University, The Netherlands

CONTENTS

Blood Sample Collection

Venipuncture

Equipment/Materials

It is important to determine beforehand which parameters need to be measured and what samples need to be collected so that all necessary materials can be gathered (Box 4.1; Figure 4.1). Because the blood volumes that can be collected will usually be small, miniature container tubes (e.g. Microtainer tubes, Becton–Dickson) are considered ideal (Figure 4.1). Alternatively, pre-heparinized syringes can be used to omit the step of blood transfer, thereby minimizing sample loss and preventing the blood to clot. Particularly in rabbits and rodents, which have rapid clotting times and small peripheral veins that prevent rapid blood collection, this is highly beneficial. Pre-heparinized syringes are commercially available in 1- and 2-ml variants (e.g. PICO syringes, Radiometer; RAPIDlyte, Siemens; Figure 4.1), but can also be self-made by coating the inside of the needle and syringe with heparin through drawing up and expelling heparin.

When less than 0.1 ml is needed, a heparinized microhematocrit tube can be inserted into the hub of a needle to collect the blood through capillary action. Simultaneously, a blood smear can be prepared using the “slide-to-slide” technique, preferably using blood that has not been in contact with an anticoagulant to prevent alterations to the blood cells.

Small needles (i.e. 22-gauge or smaller; Figure 4.1) and 1 – 3 ml syringes are preferred for blood sampling in small mammals to limit the risk of post-puncture hemorrhage or collapse of the vessel. However, the contents should be carefully transferred from the syringe as expelling it with too

Exotic Animal Emergency and Critical Care Medicine, First Edition. Edited by Jennifer E. Graham, Grayson A. Doss and Hugues Beaufrère.

Box 4.1 Equipment Needed for Blood Collection in Small Mammals

- Needles (20- to 31-gauge, dependent on the species involved; 26-gauge is a size that will work for most species while minimizing the risk of hemorrhage)
- Syringes (1–3 ml)
- Microtainer tubes
- Microhematocrit tubes
- Microscopic slides
- Self-made or commercial pre-heparinized syringes can be used as an alternative to avoid having to transfer the blood to a container or tube
- Alcohol, to be used sparingly. Preferably a small piece of cotton is used to apply alcohol to the skin to prevent soaking and hypothermia of the animal
- Scissors (if hair needs to be clipped)
- Midazolam/isoflurane or sevoflurane (if sedation or anesthesia is needed)

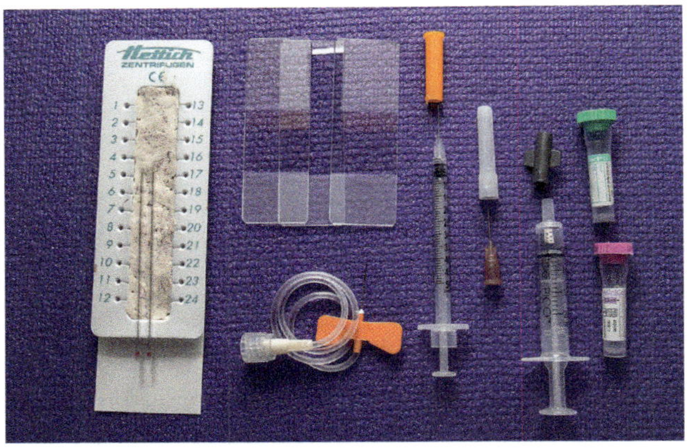

Figure 4.1 Materials that can be used during blood collection in small mammals include from left to right, microhematocrit tubes (including clay), microscope slides to make blood smears, a 25-gauge butterfly needle, an insulin syringe, or a pre-heparinized syringe, 26-gauge needles, and microtainer tubes.

much force may lead to hemolysis. For delicate procedures (e.g. collection of blood in mice), 0.3–0.5 ml insulin syringes are recommended (Figure 4.1). Alternatively, the needle may be used separately to puncture or lance the blood vessel to allow blood to flow freely into the collection tube. Usually, the amount that can be collected through this method will suffice for a basic panel (i.e. packed cell volume [PCV], estimated total and differential white blood cell count, total protein, glucose, and blood urea nitrogen). Petroleum jelly or silicone grease can be applied to the puncture site beforehand to prevent the blood from spreading into the fur.

Dependent on the species, age, temperament, and health status of the patient, blood collection can be performed in an awake (restrained) or sedated animal. In many patients, the authors prefer the use of a (mild) sedative (e.g. midazolam) or anesthetic agent (e.g. [dex]medetomidine, isoflurane, or sevoflurane) to facilitate blood collection and avoid unnecessary stress. However, most rabbits tolerate blood to be collected awake with minimal restraint.

Restraint, sedation, and anesthesia can significantly alter blood parameters. Similarly, fasting (which is generally recommended for four to six hours in ferrets and for one to two hours in other small mammals to enable safe sedation or anesthesia) can affect blood values.

A topical anesthetic (e.g. EMLA cream, AstraZeneca) can be applied to the venipuncture site to increase compliance of non-sedated patients or allow for a lighter plane of sedation to be used. Prior shaving will be necessary, and following application the area should be covered loosely with a bandage to allow the cream to take effect (~30 minutes), while preventing environmental contamination or ingestion by the patient during grooming. Care should be taken not to exceed the toxic threshold, especially in the smaller species. Similarly, alcohol, used to disinfect and direct the hairs away from the puncture site, should be used sparingly to prevent vasoconstriction (which impedes blood collection) and prevent cooling of the patient.

Moderate warming of the patient through placing it in a warm incubator (39 °C or 102 °F), under a heat lamp or onto a warm heating pad for 5–10 minutes before the procedure can help to improve access by inducing peripheral vasodilatation. However, continuous monitoring is necessary to prevent overheating and distress, especially in chinchillas. Alternatively, the body part that needs to be sampled (e.g. tail or extremity) can be placed in a warm water bath (35–40 °C or 95–104 °F) for 5–10 seconds for dilation of the vessels to occur.

Sample Size

Generally, a maximum of 1% of the animal's lean body weight (BW) or 10% of its total blood volume (which in most species comprises 6–8% of the body weight) can be safely collected from healthy small mammals. An overview of blood sample sizes to be collected in commonly seen small mammal patients is found in Table 4.1. In elderly, obese or severely debilitated, hypoproteinemic or anemic patients, sampled volumes should be lowered to 0.5% of the lean body

Table 4.1 Common maximum blood sample sizes and collection sites in adult small mammals.

Species	BW (g)[a]	Maximum sample size (ml)[b]	Sample sites – typical order of approach	Pitfalls
Necessary sample size				
Cell blood count (CBC)/ Chem – outside lab		**1**		
Vetscan[c]; i-STAT[d]		**0.1**		
CBC – in house		**0.01–0.1**		
General rule		**1 ml/100 g**		
Ferret	♂ 900–1800	7.2–12.6	CVC, jugular, lateral saphenous, cephalic	
	♀ 600–1200	4.2–8.4		
Rabbit	800–6000	4.8–36	Lateral saphenous, auricular, jugular, cephalic	—
Guinea pig	750–1200	6–10	CVC, jugular, cephalic, lateral saphenous	Cephalic and saphenous are small
Chinchilla	400–700	2.8–4.9	CVC, jugular	All other veins are too small
Rat	♂ 450–520	3–3.6	Lateral and dorsal tail, lateral saphenous	Small size
	♀ 250–300	1.5–2.1		
Mouse	20–40	0.2–0.3		Small size
Gerbil	50–130	0.35–0.9		Small size
Hamster	80–150	0.5–1.0		Small size
Hedgehog	♂ 400–600	2–6	Jugular, CVC, lateral saphenous, cephalic	Lateral saphenous, cephalic very small
	♀ 300–400	1.5–4.0		
Sugar glider	80–160	0.5–1.0	CVC, jugular	Small size

CVC, cranial *Vena cava*.
[a] Body weights vary by individual, age, gender, and season.
[b] Only take the minimum amount of blood necessary for diagnostics or blood donation.
[c] Point of care analyzer Abaxis Vetscan VS2 (Abaxis, Union City, CA, USA 94587).
[d] Point of care analyzer VetScan i-STAT1 (Abaxis, Union City, CA, USA 94587).

mass, or 0.8% over a period of 14 days. This rule also applies to the smaller-sized animals because of the risk of post-puncture hemorrhage, cardiovascular collapse, and death upon exceeding a loss of 20–25% of the blood volume. Fortunately, many point-of-care analyzers (e.g. VetScan, Abaxis) can analyze samples as small as 100 μl, thereby rarely necessitating the collection of such amounts. Should large sample volumes be anticipated or inadvertently have been collected, double the amount of replacement fluids should be given immediately through the intravenous (IV), intraosseous (IO), intraperitoneal, or subcutaneous (SQ) route (see also Chapter 8).

Venipuncture Sites

The vascular anatomy of small mammals resembles that of the larger companion animals, thereby allowing for similar approaches to be used. However, difficulties may be encountered due to the animal's size or anatomic features (e.g. short neck in guinea pigs). Restoration of blood volume will occur within 24 hours following venipuncture, whereas restoration of hemoglobin, hematocrit, and total red blood cell count may take up to two weeks. Since blood loss greater than 20–25% can lead to hypovolemic shock and death if not treated promptly, pressure should always be applied to the venipuncture site to prevent hematoma formation. In patients with suspected coagulopathies, the cephalic or saphenous veins are preferred over the larger vessels (e.g. cranial vena cava, jugular vein) as a bandage can be placed to ensure adequate hemostasis.

Ferrets

The jugular vein and cranial vena cava are preferred for obtaining larger samples, whereas the cephalic and lateral saphenous veins may be used if smaller volumes are required. Fasting for three to six hours is recommended for safe anesthesia and correct interpretation of the results.

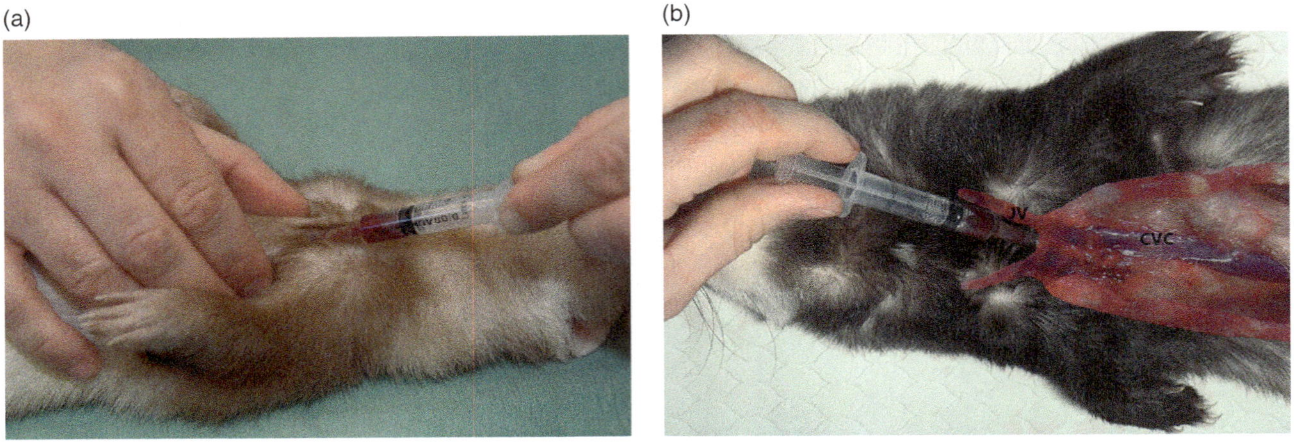

Figure 4.2 In ferrets, large volumes of blood can easily be collected from the cranial vena cava. The ferret is placed in dorsal recumbence, and the needle (26-gauge) is inserted on the left side of the manubrium in the junction with the first rib in a 30° angle to the body in the direction of the contralateral hindleg (a). The anatomy layover image (b) demonstrates that the cranial vena cava slightly deviates to the right explaining why the needle is best inserted on the left side of the manubrium. It also demonstrates that the heart and lungs are located far away from the injection site.

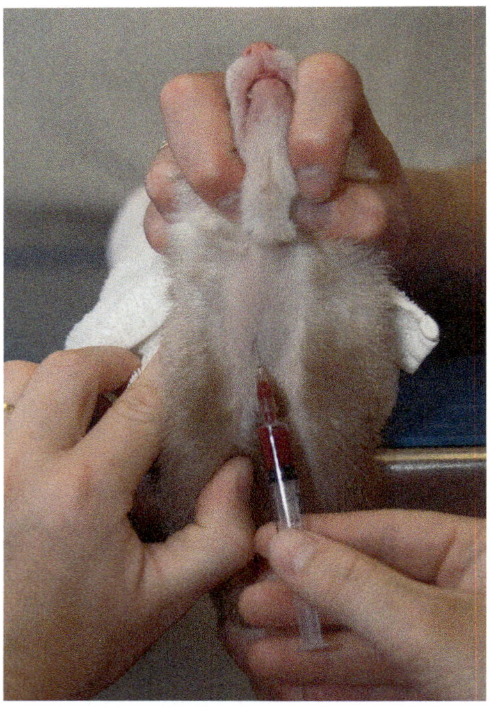

Figure 4.3 Blood collection from the jugular vein in ferrets is performed in a similar fashion as in cats. Restraint can be more challenging and using a towel wrapped around the body and hindlegs may be helpful.

Cranial Vena Cava The cranial vena cava is the authors' preferred location for blood collection, as this site allows greater volumes of blood to be obtained with relative ease and minimal risk (i.e. the relatively long thorax minimizes the risk of puncturing the heart or lungs). Sedation or anesthesia will often be required to facilitate collection and prevent injury due to sudden movement. As anesthesia can alter blood parameters (e.g. hematocrit, white blood cell count), blood should be collected quickly following induction.

Phlebotomy is usually performed using a 25- to 27-gauge needle and 3–10 ml[1] syringe. The ferret should be placed in dorsal recumbency with the head and neck extended and the front legs placed along the chest. The needle is subsequently inserted into the thoracic inlet in the junction of the left first rib and the manubrium sterni, at a 30° angle into the body, whereby the needle is directed toward the opposite hind leg (Figure 4.2). Following full insertion of the needle, the plunger is pulled back while the needle is slowly withdrawn until the syringe fills with blood. Alternatively, negative pressure can be applied once the needle has penetrated the skin following which the needle is slowly advanced until blood begins to appear.

Jugular Vein Blood collection from the jugular vein is performed in the awake or sedated animal using a similar technique as in the cat. Dependent on the size of the ferret, a 20- to 25-gauge needle can be used, which can be bent at a 30° angle to facilitate collection. Restraint is accomplished by wrapping the ferret in a towel or placing it in sternal recumbency with the front legs pulled down over the edge of the table, and the head and neck extended upward (Figure 4.3). Visibility of the vessel, which is located slightly more lateral than in cats, can be enhanced by shaving and applying pressure at the thoracic inlet. Blood

1 For blood transfusion.

should flow easily into the syringe; if this is not the case, the head may be overextended and can be moved up and down to facilitate blood flowing into the syringe.

Cephalic Vein The cephalic vein is located on the dorsal aspect of the front leg and can be used for the collection of small blood samples (e.g. for measuring glucose) using the technique as used in dogs and cats. To prevent collapse of the vein during venipuncture, a 25- to 29-gauge needle on an insulin or 1 ml syringe is used. Restraint is accomplished by wrapping the ferret in a towel or by scruffing it, whereby it is held in a vertical position. To increase the visibility of the vein, a tourniquet may be placed just proximal to the elbow. A topical anesthetic cream (e.g. EMLA) can be applied 30 minutes before venipuncture to increase patient compliance.

Lateral Saphenous Vein The lateral saphenous vein is located on the lateral side of the hind leg, just cranial to the hock joint. This vessel is mostly used if small amounts of blood are needed. To engorge the vessel, the rear leg is grasped at the level of the stifle while the ferret is placed in lateral (or ventral) recumbency. A 25- to 29-gauge needle and insulin or 1 ml syringe is subsequently used to draw blood with minimal risk of vessel collapse. Shaving may be necessary to increase visibility of the vein.

Rabbits

In rabbits, blood may be drawn from the lateral saphenous vein, marginal ear vein, jugular vein, and cephalic vein. As rabbit blood vessels are fragile, blood samples need to be taken cautiously to prevent hematoma formation. Moreover, rabbit blood quickly clots at room temperature, necessitating the use of a pre-heparinized syringe. Rabbits usually allow blood collection without anesthesia but are prone to catecholamine-related cardiac arrest when severely stressed and debilitated. As a result, close monitoring with minimal restraint or sedation is recommended.

Lateral Saphenous Vein The lateral saphenous vein runs from medial to lateral, diagonally across the lateral aspect of the tibia, and can usually be accessed with relative ease and minimal stress for the rabbit. It therefore is the preferred vessel for venipuncture by the authors. To restrain the rabbit, it is placed in sternal recumbency at the edge of the table with its head situated between the restrainer's elbow and body. By grabbing the hind leg at the crux of the stifle, the hind leg can be extended while simultaneously occluding venous return (Figure 4.4). The vein can be located by palpation following which alcohol can be applied to enable visualization of the vein. As the vein is prone to collapse and lies very superficial, the use of a 25- to 27-gauge needle bent at a 30° angle or a pre-heparinized 25-gauge butterfly catheter attached to a 1–3 ml syringe is preferred. As hematomas are easily formed, the vein should be held off well to ensure adequate hemostasis.

Marginal Ear Vein The marginal ear vein runs laterally on the ear and will usually allow for small samples to be obtained with minimal restraint and stress to the rabbit. Shaving or plucking can enhance its visibility, but care should be taken not to tear or damage the delicate skin. Warming of the ears (e.g. using a plastic glove filled with warm water) induces vasodilatation, thereby facilitating blood collection. The handler can engorge the vessel by compressing it at the base of the ear, following which a 25- to 27-gauge needle (bent at a 30° angle) is inserted into the vein. As many rabbits react with head shaking which may lead to laceration of the vein, application of a topical anesthetic cream 30 minutes before sample collection should be considered. Thrombosis and consequential sloughing of the pinna are a rare complication, but may occur in dwarf breeds or following injection of toxic or irritating substances.

Jugular Vein The jugular vein can be accessed using the method as described in the ferret. However, the authors prefer other methods as the animal's breathing can be severely compromised due to dislodging of the glottis from the soft palate, necessitating the rabbit to breathe through its mouth. Respiration should thus be monitored closely and sedation is considered to reduce stress.

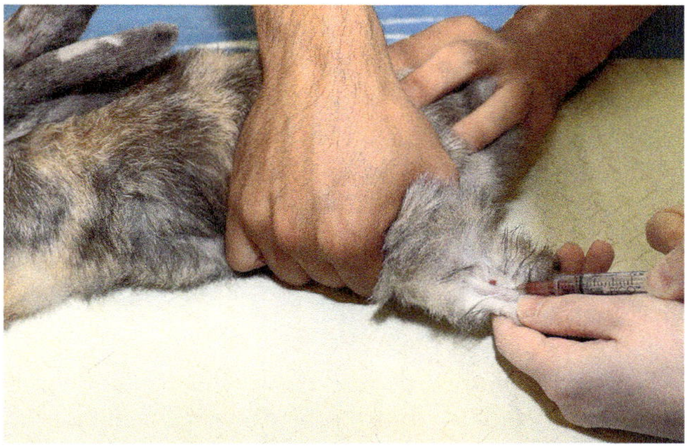

Figure 4.4 The most ideal location for collection of blood in rabbits is from the lateral saphenous vein. One person will firmly hold the hind leg above the knee, thereby also extending the hindleg. As the vein lies very superficial, it is recommended to slightly bend the needle to prevent puncturing through the vein.

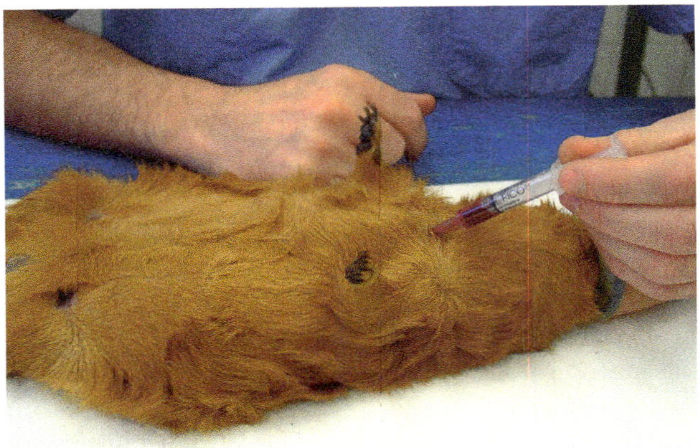

Figure 4.5 Cranial vena cava venipuncture in a guinea pig. The technique and landmarks used for puncturing the cranial vena cava are largely similar to those in ferrets. However, rather than directing the needle toward the contralateral hind leg, it is directed toward the contralateral front leg, resulting in a steeper angle of insertion.

Cephalic Vein The cephalic vein is located and accessed in a similar manner as described in the ferret.

Guinea Pigs

Blood collection in guinea pigs is considered challenging because of their relatively small-sized vessels and their build (i.e. short neck and legs, and compact body). The lateral saphenous and cephalic veins are readily accessible but will only allow collection of small quantities of blood. When larger amounts of blood are needed, (blind) puncturing of the jugular vein or cranial vena cava is recommended, for which the animal needs to be sedated or anesthetized. As guinea pigs have longer prothrombin times than e.g. rabbits, rats, or hamsters, their blood will take longer to clot.

Cranial Vena Cava The technique and landmarks used for puncturing the cranial vena cava are largely similar to those in ferrets. However, rather than directing the needle toward the contralateral hind leg, it is directed toward the contralateral front leg, resulting in a steeper angle of insertion (Figure 4.5). This, together with the use of small, short (1/2–5/8 in.) needles, minimizes the risk of puncturing the heart. Like ferrets, guinea pigs should be anesthetized for the procedure.

Jugular Vein Guinea pigs have short, thick necks which render blood collection from the jugular vein difficult. As the procedure is similarly stressful as in rabbits, sedation or anesthesia is highly recommended. Following induction, the guinea pig is placed on its rear end, with the legs placed alongside the thorax, and the neck and head extended in an upward direction. Shaving may aid in visualization, but often a blind approach is needed for which the rami of the mandible and the thoracic inlet are located with the thumb and fingers to indicate the direction in which the jugular vein should run.

Cephalic Vein The technique used to access the cephalic vein is like that described in the rabbit and ferret.

Lateral Saphenous Vein The lateral saphenous vein runs dorsally and then laterally across the tarsus. Shaving will often be needed to visualize the vessel. Pressure is placed on the thigh to extend the leg and engorge the vessel, as described for the rabbit. Samples are collected using a 25- to 27-gauge needle and 1 ml syringe, or directly from the needle hub following puncturing of the vessel.

Femoral Vein To collect blood from the femoral vein, which runs on the medial side of the thigh, the guinea pig should be anesthetized and placed in dorsal recumbency with the leg abducted so that the femur lies in an approximately 90° angle to the long axis of the body. The femoral pulse is palpated to localize the femoral artery and adjacently running vein. The needle should be directed perpendicular to the skin or at a 45° angle to the long axis of the femur and inserted about 6 mm deep at the location where the body wall meets the upper thigh, just behind the inguinal nipple and midway along the upper thigh. If accidentally puncturing the artery, pressure should be applied for at least two minutes to promote hemostasis.

Chinchillas

Potential venipuncture sites used in chinchillas include the cranial vena cava and the jugular, cephalic, femoral, and lateral saphenous veins. Sedation is generally preferred as chinchillas are highly sensitive to stress. Techniques are largely similar to those described in the guinea pig, apart from the jugular vein being located superficial and prone to laceration and hemorrhage.

Rats, Mice, Gerbils, and Hamsters

Many of the smaller rodents have veins that are too small to bleed with a needle and syringe. It may therefore be necessary to punch or lance the vein or perform a "blind stick" to puncture the larger vessels. Many of the bleeding sites used in laboratory animals are not considered ethically acceptable for use in pets (e.g. cardiac puncture or sampling of the retro-orbital venous sinus or sublingual veins). The lateral tail veins, cranial vena cava, and the lateral saphenous, femoral and jugular veins are accessible in pet rodents. Usually, some form of restraint (e.g. sedation, anesthesia, or commercially available restraint tube) will be necessary. The use of a topical anesthetic cream may reduce discomfort for the awake animal. Size of the needle used will largely depend on the type and size of the animal involved.

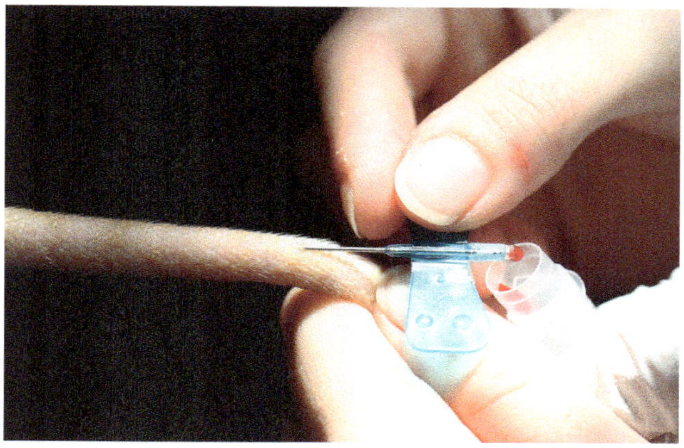

Figure 4.6 The dorsal tail vein can be used to collect blood from rats. After vasodilation has been induced, a small gauge needle can be used to puncture the vein to let blood flow into a microhematocrit or microtainer tube. *Source:* Courtesy of Katleen Hermans.

Lateral and Dorsal Tail Veins The dorsal[2] or lateral tail veins can be used in mice and rats. Vasodilation can be induced by placing the patient in a warm incubator or placing the tail in a warm water bath, following which a 21- to 25-gauge needle can be used to puncture the vein (Figure 4.6). To facilitate access to the deeper veins, a rubber band may be used as a tourniquet. In gerbils, venipuncture of the tail is discouraged because of the possibility of inducing "tail slip."

Lateral Saphenous Vein The lateral saphenous vein can often be punctured without anesthesia. Following clipping of the hair, the animal is placed in a modified 50 ml syringe case that serves as a restraint tube. Next, the hind leg is extended, and the vein occluded by placing a tourniquet or grasping the skin above the stifle. The vein can subsequently be punctured using a 20- to 25-gauge needle held at a 90° angle to the skin to allow blood to flow into a microhematocrit tube. Hemostasis is achieved by releasing the pressure on the leg. Removal of the clot or scab from the punctured area will usually suffice to obtain further material.

Submandibular Veins In (anesthetized) mice, the submandibular veins can be accessed by puncturing the skin with an 18- to 23-gauge needle or lancet at a 90° angle, just caudal to the mandibular joint, at the location where the orbital and submandibular veins join to form the jugular vein. The scab or clot can be removed if additional samples are needed. Potential risks associated with this technique include laceration of the skin, damage to the surrounding tissues, and bleeding into the mouth or ear canal.

2 Only in rats.

Jugular Veins To collect blood from the jugular vein, the animal needs to be anesthetized and placed in dorsal recumbency, with the head and neck hyperextended (*Note*: A strip of gauze or piece of string tied around the upper incisors can help with achieving this hyperextension). The needle (23–26G, connected to a 1–3 ml syringe) is subsequently inserted through the pectoral muscles, just cranial to where the external jugular vein passes between the clavicle and pectoral muscle.

Cranial Vena Cava General anesthesia is mandatory to minimize complications (including hemorrhage and puncture or laceration of the heart or trachea). The animal should be placed in dorsal recumbency with the forelegs placed alongside the thorax to allow the needle (25–27G, on a 1–2 ml syringe) to be inserted lateral to the manubrium and just cranial to the first rib, in the direction of the opposite femoral head at a 30° downward angle. To collect the sample, the needle may need to be advanced anywhere from 2 to 10 mm. Pressure is applied to the collection site for up to 30 seconds to ensure proper hemostasis.

Cephalic Vein The approach to the cephalic vein is like that in the other companion animals, although the needle is generally inserted without a syringe attached. A tourniquet can be used to occlude the vein and allow for better visualization of the vessel. General anesthesia will usually be required.

Hedgehogs

General anesthesia is usually needed to collect blood from hedgehogs, as they have a tendency to curl up into a ball and raise their spines when awake. Veins that are accessible for venipuncture include the jugular vein, cranial vena cava, and the cephalic, lateral saphenous, and femoral veins. As these last three vessels are very small and collapse easily, these are only suitable for collection of small volumes. As recently published by G. Doss, the preferred site to collect larger volumes of blood in the hedgehog is the jugular vein. The venipuncture site is at the thoracic inlet, where the internal and external jugular veins split into separate branches just cranial to the medial portion of the clavicle. The area of the manubrium is palpated to identify the clavicle and a finger is used to locate the bilateral indentation formed between the base of the ventral neck and the attachment of the clavicle to the manubrium. The needle and syringe should be positioned as close to 90° to the table as possible during entry and the entry point location can be verified by examining the location of the papillae of the paired cervical mammary glands present in both male and female hedgehogs; the skin entry point should fall a couple of millimeters cranial to an imaginary line drawn between the two papillae (Figure 4.7). Sampling from the cranial vena cava and femoral vein require extra

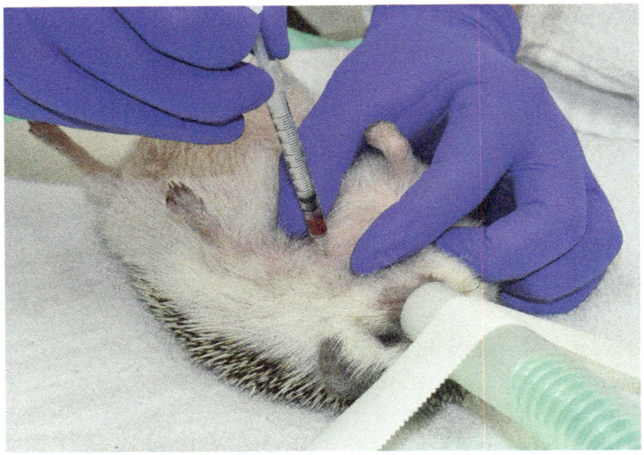

Figure 4.7 The jugular vein is the preferred site for blood collection in hedgehogs. The venipuncture site is at the thoracic inlet, where the internal and external jugular veins split into separate branches just cranial to the medial portion of the clavicle. *Source:* Courtesy of Grayson Doss.

care to prevent laceration of the vessel or damage to surrounding structures as this can lead to significant morbidity and mortality.

Sugar Gliders

Because of the small size of the peripheral vessels, blood collection in sugar gliders is usually achieved from the jugular vein and cranial vena cava, which allow samples of up to 1 ml to be collected. The approach to these vessels is largely similar to the guinea pig (cranial vena cava) and other rodents (jugular vein). In case smaller volumes (0.1–0.25 ml) are needed, the lateral saphenous, cephalic, femoral, and ventral tail veins can be accessed using the technique as described for rodents. Anesthesia will be needed to safely perform the procedure.

Jugular Vein The jugular vein is difficult to visualize in sugar gliders but can be punctured by inserting a 25- to 27-gauge needle connected to a 1 ml syringe midway between the point of the shoulder and the mandibular ramus.

Cranial Vena Cava The cranial vena cava should be approached using a similar technique as described for the guinea pig, using a needle and syringe size as described for the jugular vein. Similar to rodents and hedgehogs, this technique poses a risk for accidental cardiocentesis and damage to the vein or surrounding thoracic structures.

Arterial Sampling

Arterial blood samples are indicated for blood gas analysis. However, arterial sampling is challenging due to the size of the peripheral arteries, and carries a risk of significant hemorrhage, thereby leading to further compromise of an already debilitated patient. As a result, it is infrequently performed in small mammals. Following puncture of the artery, pressure should be applied for a minimum of one to three minutes to achieve hemostasis.

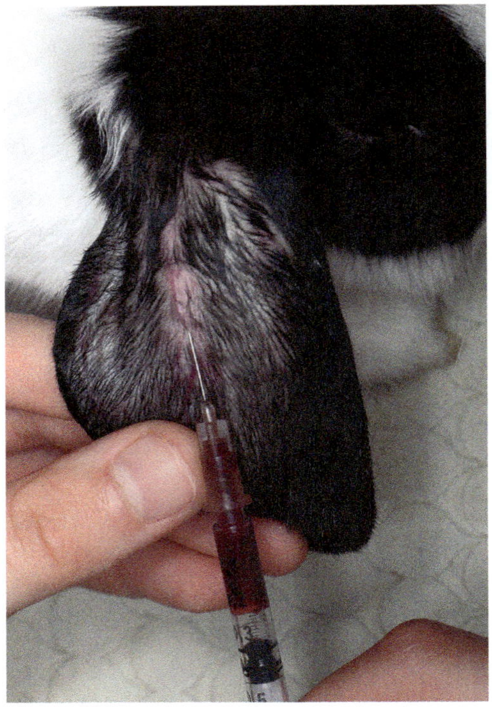

Figure 4.8 Blood collection from the central auricular artery in a rabbit. After blood collection, the injection site should be held off longer than when blood is collected from a vein.

Central Ear Artery

In rabbits, the central ear artery (Figure 4.8) is readily accessible for arterial blood sampling and can be punctured using a 21- or 22-gauge needle that is inserted parallel to and then directed into the vessel, aiming it toward the base of the ear. Thrombosis and sloughing of the pinna may occur as sequela to arterial sampling.

Ventral or Caudal Tail Artery

In rats, mice, and ferrets, the ventral or caudal tail artery can be used. As the procedure can be painful, general anesthesia is recommended, whereby the animal is placed in dorsal recumbency. Prior warming of the tail (e.g. using a warm compress or warm water bath) ensures vasodilation to promote easier access to the vessel. In ferrets, a 20- to 21-gauge needle on a 1- to 3-ml syringe should be inserted into the groove on the ventral midline of the tail at approximately 1–2 in. (2–5 cm) away from the base of the tail, with the needle pointing in a 45° angle toward the body. In rats and mice, a 19- to 27-gauge needle with (rat) or without (mouse) a plunger-less syringe attached can be used. The needle should be inserted in the ventral midline of the tail at approximately one-third of the distance from the tail base, using a 30° angle. Following correct insertion into the artery a "pop" should be felt, and blood will start filling the syringe or microtainer tube without negative pressure needed.

Dorsal Tail Artery

In rats, the dorsal tail artery can be used for obtaining arterial blood samples. In the ventral recumbent patient, the needle is inserted at the dorsal midline at an angle of 30°, and advanced until a characteristic "pop" is felt, and the hub of the needle begins to fill with blood.

Medial Tibial Artery

In sugar gliders, arterial blood sampling can be attempted from the medial tibial artery. This vessel can be visualized relatively easily, but tends to roll, thereby making it difficult to puncture.

Collection from Blood Donors

Fresh whole blood from a donor is most commonly used for blood donations in small mammals due to the limited donor pool and difficulties associated with storing and banking. Blood transfusions can generally be accomplished easily in most small mammals provided an adequate donor is available and intravenous (Figure 4.9) or intraosseous access can be achieved in the recipient (see Section "Catheterization").

Donor Selection

Blood collected should only take place from young to middle aged, healthy donors that ideally have a normal complete blood count (with a hematocrit of at least 40%), biochemistry profile, and are tested negative for species-specific infectious agents that can potentially be transmitted via blood (e.g. Aleutian disease virus in ferrets, *Encephalitozoon cuniculi* in rabbits). Moreover, a donor that is of a similar size or larger than the recipient is preferred. This is most important to consider in rabbits, rats and ferrets, in which large size differences exist between breeds or genders. In ferrets, donor animals should have been vaccinated against distemper and rabies, and – in countries where heartworm disease is prevalent – have been tested negative for microfilaria, whereas donor rabbits should have been vaccinated against myxomatosis or rabbit hemorrhagic disease virus (RHDV and RHDV2), if these diseases are prevalent in the country or region of residence.

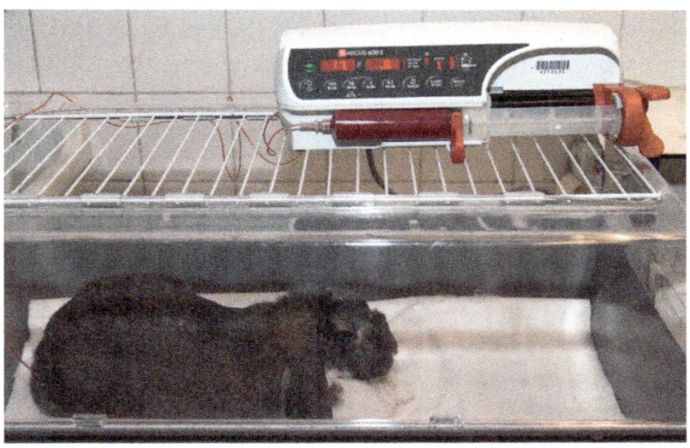

Figure 4.9 Blood transfusions can be performed in small mammals, whereby the rabbit and ferret will be the most common species that will be presented for this type of treatment.

Donor Testing/Typing

When performing a blood transfusion, antibodies present in the serum of the recipient may react to the presence of red-blood-cell-antigen from the donor cells, thereby resulting in acute hemolysis and transfusion reactions. In ferrets, blood groups have not been identified, minimizing the risk for acute transfusion reactions and enabling provision of multiple transfusions, even from the same donor, without prior cross-matching. In other species, information is lacking on the existence of blood groups. In rabbits (and rodents, if enough blood is available), a simple cross-matching test is therefore recommended to assess donor-recipient compatibility and minimize the risk for complications. For this purpose, the following procedures are carried out:

1) Collect blood in an ethylenediamine tetraacetic acid (EDTA) tube from both the patient and donor animal.
2) Mix two drops of plasma from the recipient with one drop of blood from the donor on a microscopic slide at room temperature and observe for the presence of agglutination (i.e. major cross-match).
3) Repeat the procedure with two drops of plasma from the donor and one drop of blood from the patient (i.e. minor cross-match).
4) If agglutination is observed (particularly during the major cross-match) blood from the selected donor should *not* be transfused into the patient.

Technique and Storage

Blood transfusions in small mammals are performed using similar equipment to dogs and cats (Box 4.2). However, needle sizes will vary according to the patient size and species involved. Prior to the procedure, the PCV of the patient and donor should be checked to calculate the amount to be transfused using the following formula:

Box 4.2 Equipment Needed to Perform Blood Transfusions in Small Mammals

Materials required for blood collection from the donor

- Sterile surgical gloves
- Butterfly needles of appropriate size
- Collection syringe of appropriate size filled with suitable anticoagulant (i.e. citrate, heparin)
- Scissors (if hair needs to be clipped from the venipuncture site)
- Alcohol
- Sedative and/or anesthetic agent

Materials required for administration of blood to the recipient

- Intravenous catheter (see Box 4.3 for further information)
- Collection syringe filled with the donor's blood mixed with anticoagulant
- Transfusion set attached to a filter
- Syringe pump/driver

Note: Regardless of the species, the procedure should be performed aseptically in both donor and recipient. Sedation or anesthesia of the donor animal is required to enable safe collection of the needed blood volume.

$$\text{Required anticoagulated blood volume}(\text{ml}) = \text{Patient's body weight}(\text{BW, in kg}) \times 70 \times (\text{PCV}_{\text{desired}} - \text{PCV}_{\text{patient}}) / \text{PCV}_{\text{donor}}$$

The target PCV (i.e. $\text{PCV}_{\text{desired}}$) will generally lie between 25% and 30%, especially for ongoing blood loss. As a rule of thumb, a rise in PCV of 1% and 10% can be accomplished by administering a volume of respectively 2–3 and 20 ml/kg. Care should be taken not to exceed the maximum collectable amount, as this may lead to vascular compromise and collapse of the donor. To compensate for the volume lost, replacement fluids should be provided (see Chapter 8).

Blood collection may be accomplished in a sedated or anesthetized animal. Agents that can cause vasoconstriction (e.g. medetomidine) or hypotension (e.g. acepromazine) should be avoided. In ferrets, isoflurane may significantly decrease hematocrit at 15 minutes post induction due to uptake of red blood cells by the spleen. As a result, some veterinarians prefer propofol or alfaxalone as this induces a rapid induction and recovery without affecting the hematocrit.

To prevent clotting and maintain cell viability (especially if storage is required), an anticoagulant preservative should be used. The following anticoagulants are considered suitable for transfusion purposes:

- Citrate-phosphate-dextrose-adenine (CPDA-1), used in a ratio of 1 ml of anticoagulant to 7–9 ml of whole blood. This anticoagulant allows blood to be stored in the refrigerator for up to 35 days;
- Citrate-phosphate-dextrose (CPD), used in a ratio of 1 : 7;
- Acid-citrate-dextrose (ACD) used in a ratio of 1 : 7;
- Heparin, used in a ratio of 5–10 units per 1 ml of blood. Since the action of heparin is slowly reversed, blood should be used within 48 hours to prevent clotting.

Usually, one of the larger vessels (e.g. jugular vein, cranial vena cava) is used, although in rodents, the lateral saphenous or lateral tail veins may also be considered. Techniques are largely similar to regular venipuncture, but slightly larger needles (e.g. 20- to 22-gauge) are required to minimize the risk of erythrocyte damage. A butterfly needle is often preferred as the needle can be held steadily while blood is being aspirated. Throughout and following blood collection, the syringe should be gently rocked to ensure adequate mixing of blood with the anticoagulant.

Catheterization

Intravenous

Intravenous (IV) catheters can be placed to administer fluids, medications, induce anesthesia, and deliver (emergency) drugs, and anesthetic and/or analgesic agents. Popular sites include the cephalic vein, lateral saphenous vein, and, in rabbits, the marginal ear vein. If the patient is too small to access the peripheral veins, the use of a central vessel (e.g. jugular vein), placement of an intraosseous catheter (see Section "Intraosseous"), or a vascular cutdown technique (as a final resort) should be considered. All required materials (see Box 4.3) need to be laid out prior to removing the patient from its cage. In addition, sedation or anesthesia should be considered to facilitate placement and minimize stress.

Cephalic Vein

To place a catheter in the cephalic vein, the patient should be placed in sternal recumbency. A non-slip surface is preferred to prevent the animal's feet from sliding away underneath its body. Restraint can be accomplished by placing one arm around the animal's body and pulling the body toward the side, following which the vessel can be held off using the thumb and index finger. Alternatively, an elastic band or similar material can be used as a tourniquet (Figure 4.10). Following shaving and aseptic preparation of

Box 4.3 Equipment Needed for Placement of Intravenous Catheters in Small Mammal Patients

- Clippers or razor
- *Optional:* Tourniquet (e.g. elastic band)
- Chlorhexidine scrub
- Isopropyl alcohol
- Gauze sponges
- *Optional:* 20- to 25-gauge hypodermic needle
- Sterile, heparinized saline
- One to two milliliter syringe for flushing
- Indwelling catheters of appropriate size (i.e. 20- to 26-gauge, dependent on the species)
- Pediatric T-port or intermittent infusion plug
- White porous tape
- Roll gauze (0.5 in./1.3 cm)
- Elastic wrap (0.5 in./1.3 cm)
- Fluid pump or burette (Figure 4.9)
- *Optional:* Topical anesthetic cream (e.g. EMLA cream [AstraZeneca])

(a) (b)

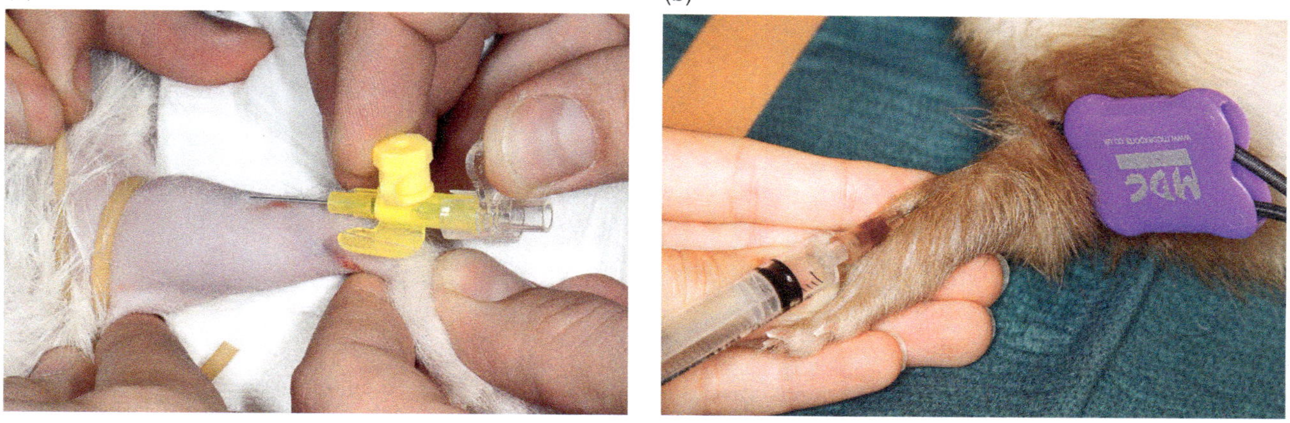

Figure 4.10 Holding off the cephalic vein can be achieved by using a rubber band (a), or specifically developed tourniquet devices (b) that can be placed proximally to the blood collection site.

the venipuncture site, the catheter is placed using a similar technique as described for dogs and cats. However, the skin in ferrets and some rabbits can be tough and difficult to penetrate, in which case a relief hole may be created to help facilitate placement. In rabbits (and many rodents), due to the fragility of their veins, it may help to have an assistant gently thread the catheter in. Once the catheter is in place, an intermittent infusion plug, or pediatric T-port can be placed onto the hub of the catheter. Next, the catheter is flushed with a small amount of saline and secured in a similar manner as in dogs and cats. Too much tape may cause a catheter to slide out; the authors therefore recommend placing one or two needle caps (cut to the correct size) on either size of the catheter to help stabilize its position and prevent the leg from bending (and the vessel from occluding). A small piece of roll gauze and elastic can be used to stabilize and cover the catheter.

Lateral Saphenous Vein

Catheterization of the lateral saphenous vein takes place with the animal in sternal recumbency, whereby the body of the animal is restrained against the body of the assistant. The assistant can subsequently place his/her hand around the hind limb, just proximal to the stifle, to hold off the vessel. A similar method is used to place the catheter as described for the cephalic vein. However, due to the different anatomy of the hind limb, taping the catheter correctly into place is somewhat more challenging.

Marginal Ear Vein

Due to the possible risk of (chemical) phlebitis, thrombosis, and sloughing of the pinna, the marginal ear vein should only be used for the administration of fluids and non-irritating substances. Catheter placement can be facilitated through placing a hand around the base of the pinna to stabilize the ear, whereby the ear vein is held off with either the thumb or index finger. Once the needle is inserted and advanced into the vessel, a roll of gauze or syringe case is placed on the inner side of the pinna to provide a suitable base to secure the catheter (Figure 4.11).

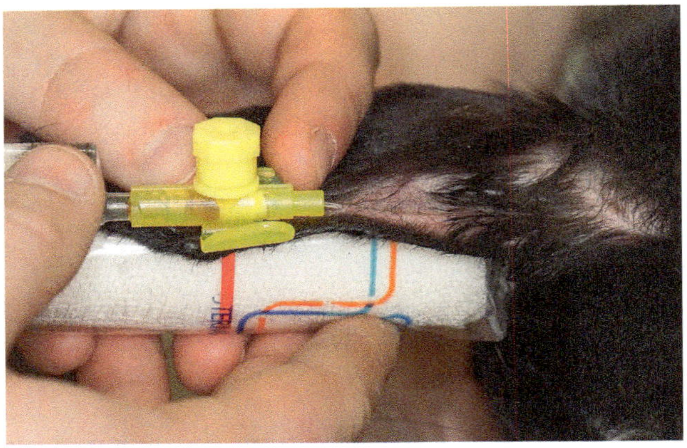

Figure 4.11 The marginal ear vein is commonly used to place IV catheters in rabbits. To prevent occlusion of the vein by bending of the pinna, a role of gauze is placed under the pinna, after which it is held in place by using tape.

Catheter Maintenance

If not removed immediately (e.g. following surgery), catheters should be cared for at least once daily. Bandages should be removed and the area around the catheter gently cleaned and observed for signs of inflammation. The catheter should be pulled if signs of redness or swelling are present, or if the site is painful or warm to the touch.

Vascular Cutdown Techniques

Because of the high risk of introducing bacteria into the bloodstream, vascular cut-down techniques should only be attempted in emergency situations where immediate vascular access is required (i.e. significant cardiovascular collapse), and other alternatives (i.e. percutaneous or intraosseous catheters) have failed or are contraindicated (e.g. patients with metabolic bone disease). Contraindications include the presence of cellulitis, overlying skin disease, coagulopathies, or vein thrombosis.

Vessels to be used include the external jugular vein, cephalic vein, or the lateral saphenous vein (see Box 4.4 for an overview of the necessary equipment). In conscious patients, the use of a local anesthetic (e.g. lidocaine) is highly recommended. Following location of the vein, clipping of the fur, and aseptic preparation of the skin, a full-thickness transverse skin incision is made over the site. Next, the subcutaneous tissue is bluntly dissected to the level of the vein. Once the vessel is freed from the surrounding fascia, suture loops or a hemostat placed proximal and distal under the vein can help to stabilize and raise the vessel parallel to the skin surface (Figure 4.12). Next, the largest catheter possible is placed in the vessel and secured using the proximal tie, whereas the distal loops are gently tied to occlude the vessel at the distal end to prevent hemorrhage. Intravenous tubing can be attached to the catheter, following which the skin is sutured and a bandage is placed. Maintenance follows guidelines similar to those for percutaneous catheters.

Potential complications include the failure to cannulate the vessel, hemorrhage, air embolism, thrombosis, infection, and transection of a nerve or artery.

Arterial

Arterial catheter placement is indicated for blood pressure measurement and monitoring, or to enable (repeated) arterial blood sampling for blood gas analysis or evaluation of acid-base status. In clinical practice, arterial catheter placement will only be feasible in rabbits as in most other species (even ferrets), the peripheral arterial vessels are too small to allow for catheter placement. The central auricular artery is most commonly used, although catheterization of the femoral artery (only in an anesthetized animal) or

Box 4.4 Equipment Required for Vascular Cut-Down in Small Mammals

- Clippers or razor
- Surgical scrub
- Sterile gloves
- Small surgical drape or towels
- Sterile gauze pads
- *Optional:* Tourniquet
- Syringe of appropriate size (e.g. 5 ml)
- Needle of appropriate size (e.g. 25-gauge)
- Scalpel blade (No. 10 or 11)
- Metzenbaum scissors
- Thumb forceps
- Curved mosquito hemostats
- Needle holders
- Absorbable suture material (size 3–0 or 4–0)
- Appropriately sized intravenous catheter(s); intravenous tubing
- Pediatric T-port, intermittent infusion plug, or catheter cap
- Sterile, heparinized saline
- White tape (0.5–1.0 in./1.3–2.6 cm)
- Bandage material (roll gauze, elastic wrap)
- *Optional:* Local anesthetic (e.g. lidocaine); if not using general anesthesia

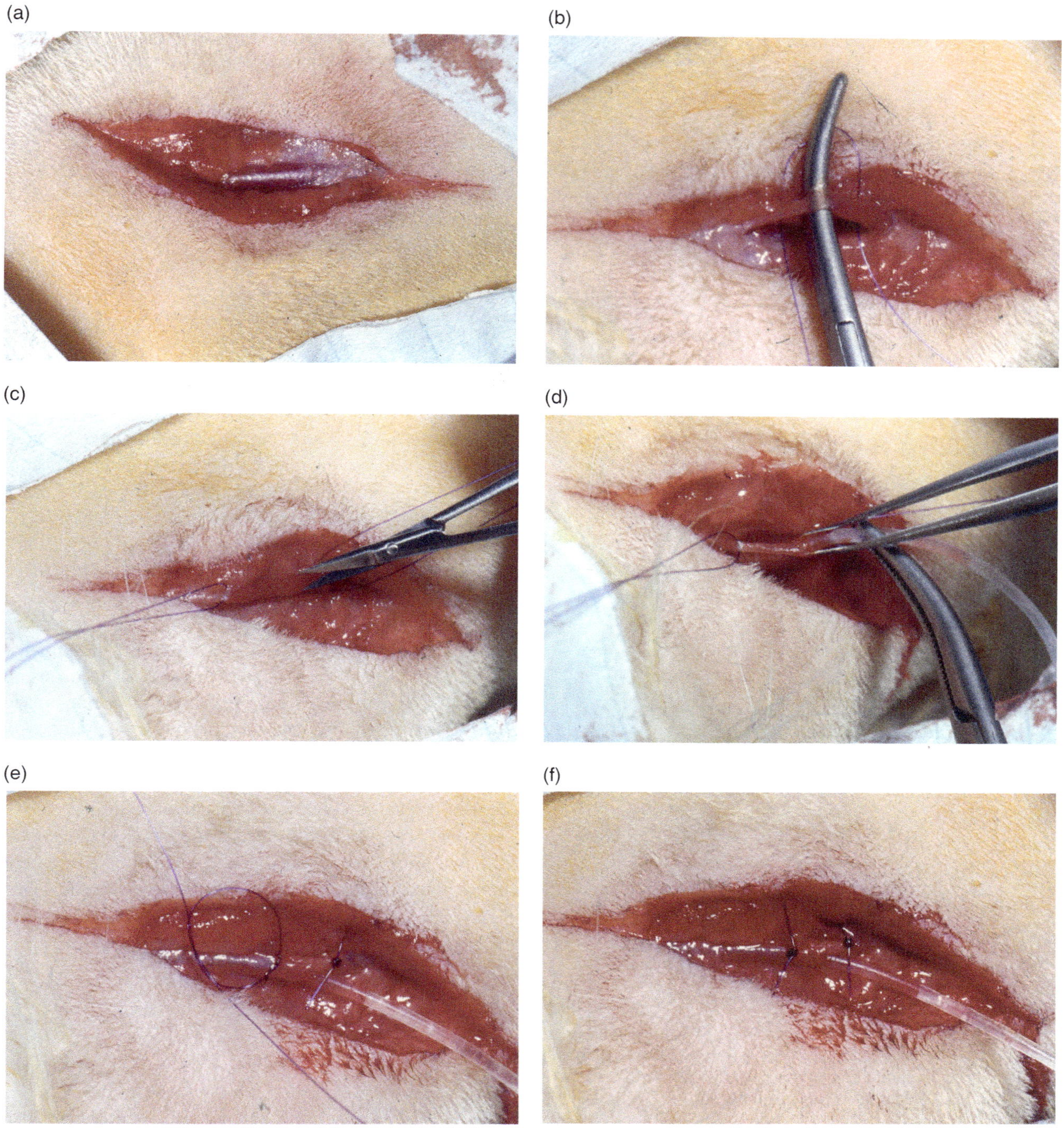

Figure 4.12 To be able to place a catheter in the jugular vein in ferrets, this vein needs to be approached surgically. A longitudinal incision is made just sagittal to the vein, and the subcutaneous (SC) tissue is carefully dissected away from the vein (a). The vein is then freed from the surrounding SC tissue (b). Suture material is placed proximal and distal to the intended location for placement of the catheter (c). After opening the vein, a silicone tube/catheter can be inserted into the vein (d). The proximal portion of the vein is occluded, while a circumferential suture is placed around the vein and catheter (e, f).

medial saphenous artery can also be attempted. In a conscious rabbit, topical anesthetics (e.g. EMLA cream) are highly recommended. The technique is similar to that for intravenous catheter placement, with the exception that the artery may be slightly harder to puncture due to its thick, elastic wall. Ischemic necrosis and sloughing of the ears can occur following catheterization of the central ear artery. Since chemical irritation of the artery (e.g. by drugs)

Box 4.5 Equipment Needed for Intraosseous Catheter Placement in Small Mammals

- Clippers
- Sterile gloves
- Surgical blade (No. 11 or 15)
- Local anesthetic (e.g. lidocaine)
- Spinal or hypodermic needle of appropriate size (18- to 25 gauge).
  A suitable needle should be long enough to extend one-third to one-half of the length of the medullary cavity and wide enough to occupy between one-third and two-thirds of the medullary cavity at its thinnest portion
- Cerclage wire or stainless-steel suture (can serve as a stylet for hypodermic needles)
- Sterile, heparinized saline
- Catheter cap or infusion plug
- Needle holders
- Non-absorbable suture material (size 3-0 to 4-0)
- Porous white tape
- Bandage material

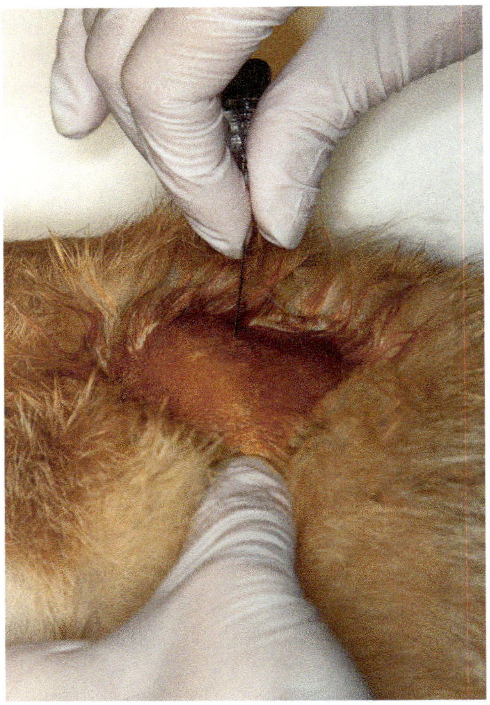

Figure 4.13 The authors prefer placement of intraosseous catheters in the proximal femur as there is minimal-to-no risk of insertion into a joint, and the animal has the least amount of discomfort after the catheter has been placed.

greatly increases this risk, intra-arterial administration of fluids or medications should best be avoided.

Intraosseous

Intraosseous (IO) catheters are indicated when intravascular access is difficult or impossible to achieve. Equipment needed for placement of an IO catheter can be found in Box 4.5. Appropriately sized injection or spinal needles will serve as suitable IO catheters for most small mammal patients. Preferably, the needle should occupy between one- to two-thirds of the marrow cavity at the thinnest portion and extend one-third to one-half of the marrow length

Sites that are considered suitable for IO catheter placement in small mammals include the proximal humerus, proximal tibia, and proximal femur (Figure 4.13). Appropriate analgesia (e.g. local infusion of lidocaine at a maximum dose of 1 mg/kg) and/or heavy sedation or general anesthesia are generally recommended. Confirmation of correct placement usually requires two-directional radiography as no other method (e.g. firm seating, appearance of blood in the hub, checking for patency through injection of fluids) will be 100% reliable (Figure 4.14). Larger catheters (up to 22-gauge) may be connected to a low-volume pediatric infusion pump, but for smaller catheters, fluid administration will only be accomplished by bolus infusion through a

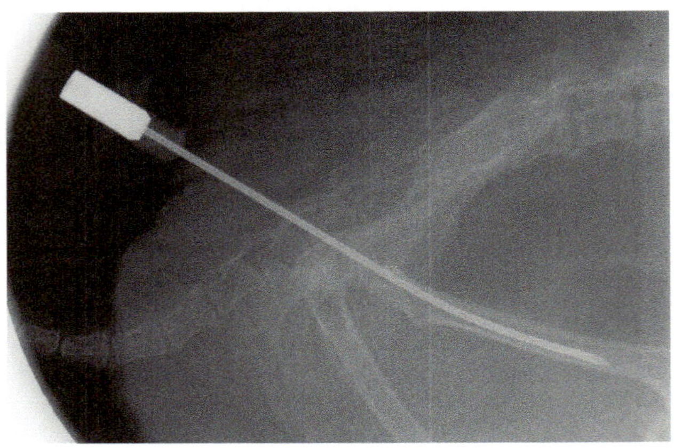

Figure 4.14 Lateral radiograph of an intraosseous catheter placed in the proximal femur of a hedgehog. Anterior–posterior radiographs should also be taken as the needle may have been inserted parallel to the femur.

syringe. Care should be taken to avoid excessive pressure, as fluids may leak into the adjacent tissues. Pain management (see Chapter 7) is also important to consider for any patient with an IO catheter.

Proximal Femur

Intraosseous catheterization of the femur is accomplished with the animal in lateral recumbency and the femur slightly adducted, following which the greater trochanter, the trochanteric fossa, and the body of the femur are identified as landmarks. Insertion is accomplished through the top of the greater trochanter (in rabbits) or trochanteric fossa (in ferrets, rodents – identifiable as a depression medial to the greater trochanter; *Note*: This can be challenging due to the extensive amount of muscle covering the area). Following aseptic preparation of the insertion site and infusion of the local anesthetic into the periosteum and overlying tissues, a stab incision is made over the insertion site. Using a firm twisting motion, the needle is then drilled into the proximal cortex as if placing an intramedullary pin. Once the cortex is passed, the needle should easily advance into the medullary cavity. Upon removal of the stylet, immediate but gentle flushing with heparinized saline will prevent clotting and minimize the risk of fat or bone marrow emboli formation. The catheter can then be fitted with standard IV injection caps and secured into place using butterfly tape and simple interrupted or horizontal mattress sutures. Additional tape may be applied to the catheter in a crisscross fashion, if needed.

Proximal Tibia

To place a catheter in the proximal tibia, the animal should be placed in lateral recumbency, following which the stifle is flexed and the tibia grasped firmly. The catheter is introduced at the tibial crest at the insertion of the patellar ligament, thereby avoiding penetration of the knee joint. Dependent on the size of the patient and shape of the tibia, the angle at which the needle needs to be inserted will differ slightly from species to species. During insertion, the needle should be gently rotated and kept as straight as possible to prevent creating a larger entrance hole through which fluids may leak out. Once the catheter passes the cortex, it can be advanced further until resistance is encountered, indicating that the opposite cortex has been reached.

Humerus

Intraosseous catheter placement into the proximal humerus requires the animal be placed in lateral recumbency with the shoulder flexed. The greater tubercle serves as a landmark for entry for the needle, which can be placed and secured in a similar manner as described for the proximal tibia and femur.

Catheter Maintenance

Intraosseous catheters may be left in place for up to 72 hours following placement. The catheter site should be inspected at least daily to evaluate correct placement and possible infection. Potential complications include extravasation of fluids from the catheter site, infection, formation of fat or bone marrow emboli, catheter occlusion, or – rarely – fractures, cellulitis, abscess formation, or tissue necrosis (e.g. due to extravasation of irritating substances).

Urinary

Urinary catheterization may be performed to treat a urinary obstruction, perform therapeutic flushing or contrast radiography of the urinary tract, or when requiring an

Box 4.6 Equipment Needed for Urethral Catheterization of Small Mammals

- Urinary catheter or intravenous catheter (with needle removed), appropriate for the size of the animal
- 24-gauge IV catheter (used to dilate the urethral opening in male ferrets)
- Sterile gloves
- Sterile gauze sponges
- Small sterile drapes or towels
- Dilute chlorhexidine solution
- Sterile water-soluble lubricant
- Sterile saline
- Sterile empty IV bag with administration set, to use as a closed urinary system
- Syringes of appropriate size to collect a sterile urine sample
- Needle holders
- Non-absorbable suture material (size 3–0 or 4–0)
- White tape
- Bandage material
- +/− Elizabethan or soft collar
- Vaginal speculum (female ferrets, rabbits)
- Sedation or anesthesia is usually required to enable catheterization. The use of a local anesthetic (e.g. lidocaine) can be considered but make sure not to exceed toxic levels (i.e. 1 mg/kg)

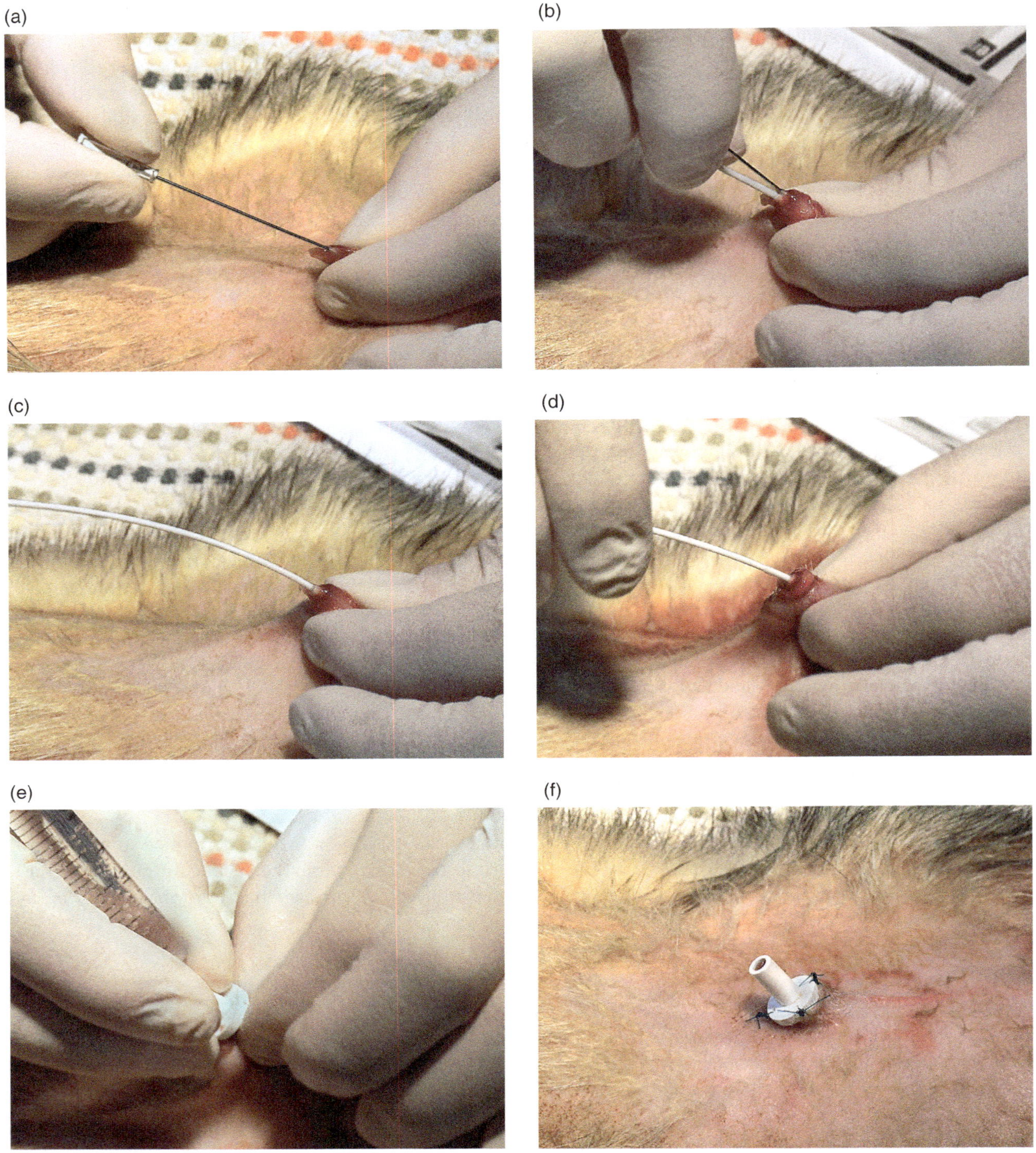

Figure 4.15 Urethral catheterization in a ferret following aseptic preparation of the preputial region. A 22-gauge blunt needle is used to dilate the urethral opening (a). With the blunt needle used as a guide, a polyurethane urinary catheter is inserted into the urethra (b, c). If resistance is felt at the pelvic flexure (d), repeated gentle flushing and lubrication can assist catheter passage (e). If a urethral catheter is used, the catheter hub can be sutured to the prepuce (f). *Source:* Courtesy of Angela Lennox.

uncontaminated urine sample (e.g. for bacterial culture). Equipment needed to perform a urinary catheterization in small mammals is listed in Box 4.6. Complications include urethral tear or rupture secondary to rough or repeated attempts at catheterization, rupture of the bladder due to overextension or over-insertion, dysuria due to mucosal swelling and/or urinary tract infection, and – if significant damage is present – urethral stricture formation.

Ferrets

Urethral obstruction is common in hobs due to the presence of urinary calculi or prostatomegaly secondary to adrenocortical disease. To enable urine to pass, catheterization is warranted, but can be challenging due to the animal's size and J-shaped penile bone (Figure 4.15). Otherwise, the catheter placement and maintenance are like that of the tomcat. A 3.0–3.5 French tomcat catheter (i.e. Slippery Sam™ Tomcat Urethral Catheter) or red rubber tube that is frozen prior to insertion will usually suffice. General anesthesia is recommended to achieve adequate muscle relaxation. Following induction and with the ferret in dorsal recumbency, the penis is extruded by applying digital pressure to the craniodorsal surface of the prepuce. Following exposure of the J-shaped *os penis*, the penis can be prevented from slipping back by grabbing the prepuce at the mucocutaneous junction using a gauze sponge. Dilute chlorhexidine and saline can be used to clean the penis, after which a lubricated catheter is gently inserted into the small, slit-like urethral opening located on the ventral surface of the penis, in between the two osseous projections of the penis. To facilitate placement, the urethral opening can be dilated by placing a 24-gauge IV catheter (without needle) into the tip of the urethra and then flushing with saline. Resistance can be encountered when passing the pelvic flexure, necessitating repeated flushing and relubrication to allow the catheter to advance. Once in place, the catheter can be secured with butterfly tape strips at the penile entry and at another point located approximately 3–5 cm away, and sutured to the skin, if needed. Additionally, a body wrap can be placed around the ferret's torso to secure the line.

Catheterizing jills can be difficult, but, fortunately, this is rarely needed. Sedation or anesthesia is generally required, following which the animal is placed in ventral recumbency with the hind legs elevated (e.g. using a towel or cloth placed underneath). Following aseptic preparation of the vulva, a vaginal speculum is used to locate the urethral opening in the floor of the urethral vestibule, approximately 1 cm cranial to the clitoral fossa. A 3.5 French urinary catheter with wire stylet can subsequently be introduced into the urethral opening and advanced into the bladder following which it can be secured by placing butterfly tape strips at the level of the vulva and the tail (3–5 cm from the vulva) and suturing these to the skin, if needed.

In both hobs and jills, a urine collection device can be attached to allow urine to flow freely and measure urine production. If the animal attempts to remove the catheter, placement of an E-collar should be considered.

Rabbits

Rabbits are preferably sedated or anesthetized for urinary catheterization. The perineal area should be thoroughly washed with dilute disinfectant, rinsed, and dried. Dependent on the size of the rabbit, a 4- to 9-French sterile feline urinary catheter with stylet can be used.

Bucks are best placed in dorsal or lateral recumbency, or, if not anesthetized, in a seated position. The prepuce is retracted to expose the penis following which the catheter can be introduced. Some resistance may be palpated when passing the pelvic rim. When entering the bladder, urine will usually flow from the catheter, following which the catheter can be sutured in place, if needed.

Catheterization of the vesicular gland is a risk in male rabbits, and can be prevented using a modified "digital pressure" catheterization technique; slowly thread the catheter into the urethra using one hand, while the index fingertip of the other hand is placed immediately caudal to the pubic symphyses, helping to divert the catheter from entering the vesicular gland. A retrospective study on 45 rabbits showed this technique to be successful in over 95% of rabbits, whereas regular catheterization resulted in failure in over one-third of rabbits.

Does are best placed in sternal recumbency, whereby the hindquarters can be slightly elevated using sandbags, towels, or foam pads. Following proper cleaning of the perineal area, the vulva is pulled slightly caudal, following which the urinary catheter is introduced in the vagina and

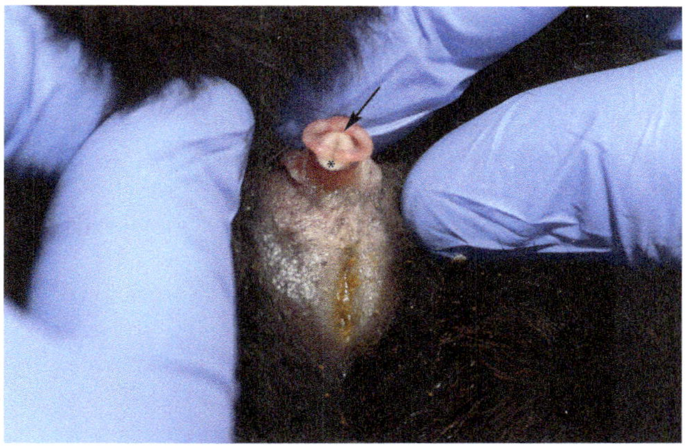

Figure 4.16 The penis of a guinea pig can be held in a gloved hand to allow insertion of a urine catheter. It is important to distinguish the intromittent sac (*) from the urethral opening (arrow).

directed ventrally along the floor of the vagina into the urethral opening. If resistance is felt, the catheter can best be retracted and rotated slightly before re-advancing. Additionally, if an obstruction is suspected, a small volume of bodily-warm, sterile water or saline can be introduced to try and flush the obstruction back into the bladder. Urine flow confirms correct placement, following which the catheter can be sutured into place, if needed.

Guinea Pigs

To insert a urethral catheter in the male guinea pig, sedation or anesthesia is highly recommended. Following induction, the animal is placed in dorsal recumbency, with the hind legs directed toward the person performing the procedure. Using gentle manipulation, the glans penis[3] is everted from the preputial sac and flushed with sterile saline to remove gross debris. Fixing the glans penis between the thumb and index finger (Figure 4.16) will facilitate localization of the external urethral opening dorsal of the glans. A soft, flexible, 3- to 5-French catheter can be introduced into the urethral opening, while avoiding the intromittent sac, which is located just ventral to the urethral orifice. The catheter can then be advanced in a craniodorsal direction until reaching the first curve of the S-shaped penis. At this point, the penis should be extended further in a caudal direction to help guide the catheter past this point. Following gentle manipulation and after passing the second curvature, the catheter will pass into the bladder, allowing urine to flow freely. Alternatively, retrograde flushing and aspiration with sterile saline can be used to confirm correct positioning, following which the catheter can be sutured in place, if needed.

Urethral catheter placement in the female is relatively easy to accomplish and is associated with fewer complications than catheterization of male guinea pigs. Once sedated or anesthetized, the animal is placed in ventral recumbency, with the hind limbs positioned toward the person carrying out the procedure. A sterile, lubricated 3- to 5-French catheter is inserted along the ventral wall of the urethral opening and readily advanced into the bladder.

3 In guinea pigs, the glans penis has a rounded tip and is covered with saw-toothed white scales or spurs that represent a unique feature of the hystricomorph rodent family to which guinea pigs and chinchillas belong.

Rodents

Urinary tract catheterization is rarely performed in small rodents and may be difficult to perform in males, whereas in females the procedure is relatively easy to perform as the external urinary orifice is readily visualized. Sedation or anesthesia is usually required, following which the animal can be placed in ventral recumbency with the tail bent upwards and backward over the body to gain access to the urethral papilla, which is located anterior to the vaginal opening. Dependent on the size of the animal, a 24-gauge IV catheter (without stylet, in mice) or 3.5-French catheter (in rats) can be used. For short-term placement, the catheter can be taped to the tail.

Catheter Maintenance

It is generally recommended to maintain urinary catheters for no more than one to three days to avoid the development of a urinary infection. Treatment with antibiotics (e.g. TMP/S) may be initiated for prevention. Catheters should be checked daily to ensure correct placement and patency of the catheter. In addition, the bladder size should be evaluated frequently to confirm that it is empty. It is recommended to repeat urinalysis and urine culture one week after removal of the catheter.

Further Reading

Briscoe, J.A. and Syring, R. (2004). Techniques for emergency airway and vascular access in special species. *J. Exot. Pet Med.* 13 (3): 118–131.

Brown, C. (2006). Blood collection from the cranial vena cava of the ferret. *Lab Anim.* 35 (9): 23–24.

Brown, C. and Mans, C. (2007). Urethral catheterization of the male Guinea pig (*Cavia porcellus*). *Lab Anim.* 36 (7): 20–21.

Brown, C. (2011). Urethral catheterization in the female Guinea pig (*Cavia porcellus*). *Lab Anim.* 40 (2): 42–43.

Brown, S.A. (1997). Clinical techniques in domestic ferrets. *Semin. Avian Exot. Pet Med.* 6 (2): 75–85.

Clair, M.B., Sowers, A.L., Davis, J.A., and Rhodes, A.L. (1999). Urinary bladder catheterization of female mice and rats. *J. Am. Assoc. Lab. Anim. Sci.* 38 (3): 78–79.

Doss, G. (2020). Proximal jugular venipuncture in African pygmy hedgehogs (*Atelerix albiventris*). *J. Exot. Pet Med.* 35 (3): 94–96.

Dyer, S.M. and Cervasio, E.L. (2008). An overview of restraint and blood collection techniques in exotic pet practice. *Vet. Clin. North Am. Exot. Anim. Pract.* 11 (3): 423–443.

Feldman, B.F. and Kristensen, A.T. (1995). Modern veterinary blood banking practices and their applications in companion animal practice. *Vet. Clin. North Am. Exot. Anim. Pract.* 25 (6): 1231–1243.

Hohenhaus, A.E. (2004). Importance of blood groups and blood group antibodies in companion animals. *Transfus. Med. Rev.* 18 (2): 117–126.

Joslin, J.O. (2009). Blood collection techniques in exotic small mammals. *J. Exot. Pet Med.* 18 (2): 117–139.

Kristensen, A.T. and Feldman, B.F. (1995). General principles of small animal blood component administration. *Vet. Clin. North Am. Exot. Anim. Pract.* 25 (6): 1277–1290.

Lanevschi, A. and Wardrop, K.J. (2001). Principles of transfusion medicine in small animals. *Can. Vet. J.* 42 (6): 447.

Lennox, A.M. (2007). Emergency and critical care procedures in sugar gliders (*Petaurus breviceps*), African hedgehogs (*Atelerix albiventris*), and prairie dogs (*Cynomys* spp.). *Vet. Clin. North Am. Exot. Anim. Pract.* 10 (2): 533–555.

Lennox, A.M. (2008). Intraosseous catheterization of exotic animals. *J. Exot. Pet Med.* 17 (4): 300–306.

Lichtenberger, M. (2004). Transfusion medicine in exotic pets. *Clin. Tech. Small Anim. Pract.* 19 (2): 88–95.

Manning, D.D. and Bell, J.A. (1990). Lack of detectable blood groups in domestic ferrets: implications for transfusion. *J. Am. Vet. Med. Assoc.* 197 (1): 84–86.

Mitchell, S. (2011). Venipuncture techniques in pet rodent species. *J. Exot. Pet Med.* 20 (4): 284–293.

Ness, R.D. (1999). Clinical pathology and sample collection of exotic small mammals. *Vet. Clin. North Am. Exot. Anim. Pract.* 2 (3): 591–620.

Parasuraman, S., Raveendran, R., and Kesavan, R. (2010). Blood sample collection in small laboratory animals. *J. Pharmacol. Pharmacother.* 1 (2): 87–93.

Perry-Clark, L.M. and Meunier, L.D. (1991). Vascular access ports for chronic serial infusion and blood sampling in New Zealand white rabbits. *Lab. Anim. Sci.* 41 (5): 495–497.

Uthamanthil, R.K., Hachem, R.Y., Gagea, M. et al. (2013). Urinary catheterization of male rabbits: a new technique and a review of urogenital anatomy. *J. Am. Assoc. Lab. Anim. Sci.* 52 (2): 180–185.

5

Wound Care and Bandaging Techniques

Nico J. Schoemaker and Yvonne R.A. van Zeeland

Division of Zoological Medicine, Department of Clinical Sciences, Faculty of Veterinary Medicine, Utrecht University, The Netherlands

CONTENTS

Principles of Wound Healing

Stages of Wound Healing

Following injury, the wound healing process ensures that tissue continuity is restored, either through restoring of the tissue itself, or by replacing the tissue by collagen thereby forming a scar. Wound healing starts directly after injury has taken place. Four phases can be distinguished, i.e. inflammation, debridement, repair, and maturation, which may run concurrent to each other.

Inflammatory Phase

This phase is initiated immediately following the traumatic insult and is characterized by the onset of vasoconstriction of the smaller vessels to limit hemorrhage, followed 5–10 minutes later by vasodilatation which results in the leakage of fibrinogen and coagulation factors. These will stimulate a clot to be formed which acts as a barrier protecting the wound against infections and providing the basis for further wound repair. At this stage, an increased vascular permeability is seen, which allows for release of cytokines and growth factors, and an influx of inflammatory cells (i.e. macrophages, neutrophils, lymphocytes, and fibroblasts) into the injured tissue. This results in the typical signs associated with inflammation: redness, swelling, heat, and pain.

Debridement Phase

During the debridement phase, exudate is formed consisting of degenerated white blood cells, dead tissue, and wound fluid. Neutrophils and monocytes first appear at the wound site 6 and 12 hours following the injury, respectively. Neutrophils contribute to wound debridement and prevention of infections by phagocytosis of bacteria and cellular debris. They also release enzymes and growth factors that facilitate the breakdown of necrotic material and stimulate

Exotic Animal Emergency and Critical Care Medicine, First Edition. Edited by Jennifer E. Graham, Grayson A. Doss and Hugues Beaufrère.

the monocytes to transform into macrophages. Like neutrophils, macrophages help remove necrotic tissue, bacteria, and foreign material. They secrete chemotactic and growth factors that recruit mesenchymal cells, stimulate angiogenesis, and modulate matrix formation, thereby leading to the formation of granulation tissue.

Repair Phase

The repair phase starts three to five days after the injury. In this phase, fibroblasts, originating from undifferentiated mesenchymal cells, play an important role. They migrate into the wound along the fibrin strands and deposit collagen, elastin, and proteoglycans. At the same time, new capillaries are formed out of capillary buds that invade the area. The endothelial cells of these capillaries release plasminogen activator that is fibrinolytic and clears the path for the new granulation bed. Red coloring indicates healthy granulation tissue that is highly resistant to infection, whereas unhealthy granulation tissue has a whitish appearance due to the high fiber content and lack of capillaries.

Granulation tissue helps to provide a surface for the epithelium to migrate across (*Note:* Epithelialization does not occur over non-viable tissue). Aside from playing a role in epithelialization, the granulation tissue plays an important role in wound contraction. Wound contraction is usually noticeable five to nine days following the injury and takes place under influence of myofibroblasts that are located on the wound edges.

Maturation Phase

Once enough collagen has been deposited, the maturation phase of wound healing starts (i.e. approximately 2.5–3 weeks after the initial trauma). During this phase, which may continue for several years, remodeling takes place whereby the collagen fibers become oriented along the direction in which stress is placed on the wound. Original strength of the tissue will never be regained, but over time up to 80% of the original strength can be regained. Clinically, a flattening and softening of the scar can be noted.

Factors Affecting Wound Healing

To stimulate wound healing, the wound should be kept moist (to stimulate epithelialization) and warm (to allow cells to migrate quicker into the wound).

Factors that negatively affect wound healing include wound infections and a (sterile) inflammation caused by presence of foreign objects in the wound (e.g. dirt, sutures, and implants), seroma formation (accumulation of fluids in a dead space inhibits migration of fibroblasts into the injured area), and abundant use of antiseptics in and around wounds (due to suppressing the effects of local inflammatory mediators). Caution is therefore warranted when applying the latter solutions on or near wounds.

Other factors affecting wound healing include the following:

- Impaired blood supply (e.g. due to infections, trauma, and tight bandages) negatively affects wound healing as adequacy of circulation is essential for delivery of nutrients and oxygen to the area. If ischemia is present, hyperbaric oxygen therapy may be attempted to help promote recirculation
- Type of wound or wound repair technique (e.g. incisions created with a scalpel blade heal faster than those created with scissors or lasers as the latter instruments will usually result in more wound margin necrosis)
- Body condition and age of the patient, i.e. malnourished and/or elderly animals, are likely to have delayed wound healing
- Concurrent (systemic) illness, including shock, hypotension, blood loss, electrolyte imbalances, and sepsis, can negatively affect the wound healing process. Since these conditions frequently accompany wounds, it is vital that they are appropriately addressed. Similarly, liver disease (resulting in decreased production of clotting factors and proteins that are needed for regeneration) and – particularly in guinea pigs – vitamin C deficiency (resulting in impaired collagen formation) may delay wound healing
- Stress and pain can result in endogenous corticosteroid release which suppresses the rate of wound contraction and predisposes to infections. Iatrogenic administration of anti-inflammatory steroids may also negatively affect wound healing. These effects may be reversed using vitamin A and/or anabolic steroids
- Radiation and chemotherapy are also known to suppress wound healing. It is therefore advised to delay the use of these treatment options for at least two weeks following surgery

Pre-treatment Considerations

Prior to treating any wound, the patient needs to be assessed to identify the presence of any life-threatening injury, systemic illness, or other conditions that may first need to be addressed (see Chapter 1). If active bleeding is present, this should be stopped first, either by applying pressure to the wound or by placing a tourniquet or ligature proximal to the lesion. Similarly, the patient may require fluids and/or oxygen to treat concurrent shock and/or hypotension. Once the patient is deemed stable, wound management takes place by following the six steps outlined below:

- Prevent further wound contamination
- Debride dead and dying tissue

- Remove foreign debris and contaminants
- Provide adequate wound drainage
- Establish a viable vascular bed
- Select the appropriate method of closure

If the patient is deemed unstable, and proper wound management needs to be delayed, the wound should be moistened with 0.9% saline and covered with sterile bandaging materials to protect it from further damage. Further assessment, cleaning, and debridement of the wound then may be performed at a later stage.

Wound Assessment

To protect the clinician and patient against infection, examination gloves should be worn during assessment of the wound. In addition, the temperament of the animal may necessitate sedation or anesthesia.

For a traumatically induced open wound, the extent and type of damage, and the potential presence of contamination need to be assessed. In addition, the size and location of the wound; presence of necrotic debris, foreign substances, and/or purulent material; extent or damage of any underlying tissues; potential damage of blood supply and innervation; and potential demarcation of vital tissues should be taken into consideration.

If a wound infection is suspected, swabs should be taken from the deepest area of the wound and submitted for culture and sensitivity testing. Samples can also be collected for in-house cytology and/or Gram stain to help determine the type of culture that should be requested (i.e. aerobic, anaerobic, or both) and guide preliminary antibiosis. Tissue biopsies or other diagnostic tests (e.g. radiographs) should be considered in case of chronic or unresponsive wounds to exclude concomitant arthritis, osteomyelitis, or neoplastic processes.

Clipping of hairs, which is preferred to shaving to reduce risk of infection, will facilitate inspection of the wound. For traumatic wounds, clipping is preferably also avoided to prevent wound infection. If hair must be removed, it is best to cover the wound with a (sterile) ointment (e.g. a honey containing ointment) to prevent the clipped hairs from contaminating the wound.

Wound Classification

There are several methods for wound classification, each using its own set of criteria, including the nature/etiology (e.g. abrasion, avulsion, incision, laceration, puncture, contusion, bruise, or burn wound), skin disruption (open vs. closed), duration, and degree of wound contamination. The most widely used system is descriptive in nature and uses four classifications based on the degree of wound contamination (i.e. clean, clean-contaminated, contaminated, and dirty; Box 5.1.). Another, perhaps more practical method for classification of wounds is primarily based on the wound duration, which at the same time also provides an indication of the level of wound contamination. In this classification system, three classes can be distinguished (i.e. Class I, II, and III; Box 5.2).

Classification systems help to make decisions regarding the method of wound closure as well as necessity to initiate antibiotic therapy. However, a recent study found that the

Box 5.1 Wound Classification System According to the Degree of Wound Contamination

Classification	Definition
Clean	Wounds that are surgically created under aseptic conditions
Clean-contaminated	Wounds with minimal contamination that can be effectively removed
Contaminated	Wounds in which gross contamination with (foreign) debris is present
Infected or dirty	Wounds in which thick, viscous exudate is present, indicative for an infection
	Number of bacterial organisms that is present exceeds 10^5 organisms per gram of tissue

Box 5.2 Wound Classification System According to the Wound Duration and Degree of Contamination

Classification	Definition
Class I	Minimally contaminated wounds; less than 6 h old
Class II	Wounds with significant contamination; between 6 and 12 h old
Class III	Wounds which are grossly contaminated and exist for more than 12 h

chance of wound infection did not significantly differ in patients in which wounds were closed prior to or after 12 hours from the time they occurred, indicating that the distinction based on time frame may not necessarily be reliable for predicting the outcome of a wound. See Mickelson et al. [1] for more information on wound classification in exotic pets.

Wound Management

Wound Debridement, Cleansing, and Decontamination

After assessing the wound, it should be cleaned, starting with (manual) removal of the visible debris. Provision of analgesia is highly recommended (see also Chapter 7) prior to handling of the wound. Local application of lidocaine (e.g. infiltration or splash block) has been found highly effective without affecting the wound healing process. Epinephrine, in contrast, does affect wound healing, so care should be taken to avoid using a product containing this drug in the wound.

Wound cleaning continues with copious flushing of the wound with bodily warm sterile saline or any other isotonic solution. A 20–60 ml syringe combined with an 18- or 19-gauge needle builds up sufficient pressure (7–8 psi) to effectively flush the wound. Placing the patient on a grate with a collecting container underneath helps prevent the animal from becoming soaked with lavage fluid, which in turn can lead to severe heat loss and hypothermia.

Scrubbing of wounds should be avoided as this damages the tissue and promotes infection. Similarly, antiseptic agents should mainly be used to clean the area around the wound and preferably not be flushed onto the wound as their cytotoxic effects may delay wound healing. Chlorhexidine (0.05% solution) least affects the wound healing process and possesses significantly higher bactericidal activity with long residual effects, and is therefore preferred over the use of povidone-iodine (1%) as an antiseptic for wound lavage. In rabbits, guinea pigs, and rodents, the use of a trypsin-containing spray has been reported to aid in the digestion of necrotic tissue and also proven beneficial in case of myiasis.

During wound lavage, debris should never be flushed into inaccessible areas of the wound as this may lead to edema and potentially infection. Magnifying loupes may be used to assure that all debris has been removed from the visible surface and wound edges. In addition, radiographs or an ultrasonographic evaluation may assist in assuring that no contaminants are present in the deeper parts of the wound.

Debridement of the wound is subsequently performed to remove heavily contaminated and devitalized tissues and promote wound healing. For this purpose, surgical (i.e. using sharp scissors or a scalpel blade), enzymatic (e.g. trypsin and Castor oil), and/or mechanical (e.g. adherent bandages, polyurethane sponges, or calcium alginate) techniques can be used. Determining whether the tissue is still viable may not always be easy. Dependent on the type of tissue, demarcation may take anywhere from 24 hours to up to five days. Criteria that can be used to determine viability of the tissue include color, consistency of the tissue, and presence of contraction and circulation (blood flow). Until delineation between viable and non-viable tissue is clear, surgical debridement should be performed conservatively to avoid removing excessive amounts of potentially viable tissue.

The use of drains should be considered in any (infected) wound with deeper areas to provide an outlet for tissue fluids that may otherwise easily accumulate, leading to pocket formation or abscesses. However, in rabbit wounds, drains will usually not work due to the nature of their pus (i.e. thick and caseous).

Closure Techniques

Dependent on the type of wound that is present, wounds can be allowed to heal by primary closure, delayed primary closure, secondary closure, or by second intent. When surgically closing a wound, the use of an absorbable monofilament suture material (e.g. polydioxanone [PDS], poliglecaprone [Monocryl]) in the smallest size possible (e.g. 4-0 to 6-0) is recommended. In addition, the amount of suture material that is placed in the wound should be kept to a minimum. Where possible, placement of skin sutures should be avoided in rabbits, guinea pigs, and other rodent species due to their propensity to chew and lick sutures through their normal grooming behavior. Instead, a subcuticular pattern with a buried knot can be used. Sutures should also never be too tight when closing the wound, as this can lead to discomfort and increase the risk of the animal starting to chew the sutures or surgical site. For small wounds, tissue adhesive can be used to achieve closure.

Primary Closure

Primary wound closure takes place directly following the initial presentation and is indicated when the wound is clean, less than six hours old and closure can be achieved without tension or creation of a dead space. Various techniques (e.g. undermining, tension-relieving techniques, or skin flaps) are available to relieve tension and help oppose the skin edges to close the wound for unimpeded wound healing. Primary closure should *not* be attempted in wounds that have been contaminated by feces, saliva, soil, or purulent exudate.

Delayed Primary Closure

Delayed primary closure can be considered if the wound is older than eight hours and/or minimal contamination or tissue trauma is present. Cleaning and some debridement will generally be needed for these wounds. Prior to closure, which takes place prior to the initiation of the granulation phase (i.e. within one to five days after the injury), a bandage should be placed to protect the wound. Once the wound is considered clean and free of infection, closure can be attempted in a similar fashion as during a primary closure.

Closure by Second Intent

When a wound is contaminated and/or considerable tissue loss is present, the wound is managed as an open wound. Adequate treatment comprises flushing and debridement of the wound, following which bandages can be placed to protect the wound while healing. Granulation will take place followed by contraction and epithelization (see Section "Principles of Wound Healing"). For wounds that are under constant tension, the wound may not heal completely by second intent. In those cases, surgical intervention by secondary closure is advised.

Secondary Closure

Secondary closure is performed on wounds that do not close by second intent and takes place after granulation tissues have been formed. Prior to closing the wound the granulation tissue is resected and fresh skin margins are created. Following apposition of the wound edges, closure can take place. After closure, it is advisable to apply an absorbent bandage to protect the wound and absorb any exudate that may be produced.

Factors Affecting the Decision on the Closure Technique to be Used

Several factors need to be taken into consideration when deciding the preferred technique for wound closure (see Box 5.3). If an infection is present, the wound cannot be closed immediately, and bandaging will be needed. In case of severe trauma and/or large wounds, primary closure will not be possible either as demarcation is needed to distinguish vital from non-vital tissues. Following demarcation, delayed primary closure or secondary closure may be possible, during which surgical flaps or other tension-relieving surgical techniques can be applied to help close the defect. Wounds that are left to heal by second intent can close completely resulting in normal-appearing skin. However, second intent healing also carries significant disadvantages such as contracture with disfigurement, scarring, and/or incomplete healing, particularly in areas where a lot of movement and tension is present (e.g. around joints and other moving parts of the body). In those cases, secondary closure is advised.

Topical Medication

Many different topical medications for wound care are available. Scientific information to support their efficacy, however, is extremely scarce. A small selection of wound treatment options will be discussed here.

Topical Antibiotics The use of antibiotic creams and ointments is controversial. Reported advantages of using topical antimicrobials for infected wounds include achievement of high tissue concentrations of the antimicrobial drug at the site of interest; the limited amount of antimicrobial needed; and the omission of parenteral administration which limits the risk of potential systemic side effects occurring. The latter is especially valuable in the small mammal species with a sensitive gastrointestinal (GI)-system (e.g. guinea pigs, rabbits, and chinchillas). A topical treatment induces minimal pain and/or stress for the patient and is in many cases easier to administer. Disadvantages of the use of topical medication, however, include the potential interference with wound healing; lack of evidence on the drug's effectiveness in case of topical application; and potential risk of ingestion (e.g. during grooming) or absorption through the skin, which may potentially lead to side effects (especially in case of oral ingestion in herbivorous small mammals). In a position paper on antimicrobial stewardship in wound care, it was reported that antibiotic therapy is only indicated in clinically infected wounds. Preferably, the antibiotic is chosen based on the results of a culture and sensitivity of the bacteria infecting the wound. Pending the results, treatment may be initiated. A common ointment to use for this purpose is silver sulfadiazine. This medication has good antimicrobial effectivity, and bacterial resistance to this drug is rarely seen.

Aloe Vera Of all the available plant extracts, aloe vera is probably the one that is best known. Acemannan is a component of aloe vera extract which has been shown to promote wound healing by increasing fibroblast proliferation and epidermal growth. In a comparative study in which full-thickness burn wounds were induced in guinea pigs and then treated with either a placebo, an aloe vera extract, silver sulfadiazine, or a salicylic acid cream, the aloe vera extract was the only topical treatment which significantly decreased healing time by approximately 40%. Similar results have been published in rats. Nevertheless, scientific evidence on the effectivity of aloe vera is still questioned in a Cochrane systemic review.

Honey Like aloe vera, honey has been used in wound healing for thousands of years and is used with increasing frequency in veterinary medicine. It has a broad-spectrum antibacterial effect, and may also stimulate the immune response, reduce inflammation, and enhance the autolytic debridement process.

Box 5.3 Factors Affecting the Decision on the Wound Closure Technique to be Used

1) Amount of time that has elapsed since the injury. Wounds that are less than 6 h old can be closed primarily; wounds older than 6–8 h are best treated with bandages and closed later, once they are clean and free of infection
2) Degree of contamination. Clean wounds can be closed immediately, whereas delayed closure will be needed in case of contamination. Severe contamination and infection of a wound will require extensive lavage and bandaging prior to attempting closure
3) Amount of tissue damage that is present. The larger the wound, the more difficult it will be to close without tension. Thus, large wounds are preferably left to heal by secondary intent (while using protective bandaging). Following granulation, epithelialization, and contraction of the initial wound, secondary closure may be attempted, if the wound is clean and free of infection to speed up the healing process
4) Completeness of the wound debridement. Closure should only be attempted once debridement is complete; partially debrided wounds or those that require further bandaging are best left to heal by secondary intent, which may be followed by secondary closure if complete debridement can be achieved
5) Status of wound vascularization. In case blood supply to the wound is questionable, closure should not be attempted until it has been adequately determined whether the tissue is viable or not
6) Overall health status of the patient. Debilitated patients or patients that are in shock or have a systemic illness may have an increased anesthetic risk, thereby limiting the options for surgical closure and necessitating the wound to be treated initially using bandages
7) Amount of tension on the wound edges and/or degree of dead space present following closure of the wound. If it is expected that closure of the wound will either result in a large amount of tension or a large amount of dead space, the risk for complications (e.g. seroma formation, infection, wound dehiscence) is greater. In those cases, bandaging of the wound is preferred over primary closure
8) Location of the wound. Particularly if the wound is located on the head or extremities, primary closure will be difficult as there is little loose skin in these regions thereby necessitating the use of skin flaps or healing by second intent
9) Temperament of the patient. In case of highly stressed or aggressive animals, options for regular (e.g. daily) replacement of bandages may be limited and may require the use of a sedative or anesthetic to complete the procedure. In these patients, wound closure is preferably achieved as soon as possible
10) Financial constraints for the owner. Healing by second intent is cheapest compared to other techniques for wound closure and can be considered for those owners that do not have the financial means to allow primary or secondary closure of the wound

Source: Adapted from MacPhail [2].

Bandages and Dressings

Bandages serve various purposes that help to promote wound healing. They can be applied to hold plain and medicated dressings in place; support or immobilize a body part; apply pressure to control hemorrhage; obliterate dead space or cavities; and protect a wound from external trauma, contamination, and desiccation.

A commonly heard complaint in practice is that many of the small mammalian species (particularly rabbits and rodents) will chew their bandage, thereby prohibiting these from being applied, or necessitating the use of an Elizabethan collar to prevent the animal from chewing the bandage. However, as chewing may also indicate discomfort, it is important to verify that the bandage is well placed before assuming the chewing is a nuisance behavior that needs to be addressed by placing a collar.

Bandages are usually comprised of three basic layers, i.e. the primary layer (or contact dressing); the secondary or intermediate (absorbent) layer; and the tertiary or outer (protective) layer.

Primary Layer

The primary layer or dressing refers to the material that is directly applied to the surface of the wound and may serve different functions depending on the stage of wound healing. The choice for the type of dressing is based on the type of wound. Dressings may be divided in the following categories (with overlapping functions): adherent, non-adherent, absorptive, semi-occlusive, occlusive, and moisture-retaining. Adherent dressings, such as those used in wet-to-dry and dry-to-dry bandages, are used to clean wounds, absorb produced fluids, and help debride necrotic tissue. Non-adherent (or – more appropriately – low-adherent) dressings, on the other hand, are primarily used for healthy wounds in which granulation tissue has formed. These usually consist of mesh containing paraffin (or similar product) and serve a main purpose to retain the wound moisture to encourage epithelialization, while simultaneously allowing excess fluid to be drained from the wound, thereby preventing tissue maceration. Two subtypes can be distinguished, i.e. semi-occlusive and occlusive dressings. Semi-occlusive dressings allow air to penetrate and exudate to leave the wound, whereas occlusive dressings have a moisture containing inner side, and an outer side that is impermeable to air and prevents penetration of contaminants, thereby rendering these ideal to use for non-exudative wounds.

Secondary Layer

The secondary layer of a bandage serves to hold the primary layer in place and functions as an absorbent, particularly in exudate-producing wounds. The secondary layer provides uniform compression, improved stability, and reduces the risk of applying the bandage too tightly, thereby preventing circulatory compromise. Gauze pads, cotton, and cast padding can all be used as secondary layer. In exudate-producing wounds, the secondary layer may initially be thick to ensure proper absorption of wound fluids, but its thickness may gradually decrease during treatment once the amount of exudate produced declines.

Tertiary Layer

The primary function of the tertiary layer is to keep the bandage in place and serves as a protective layer for the primary and secondary layer. It may also provide extra stability to the bandage and/or provide the necessary pressure to control hemorrhaging. Many of the materials used for the tertiary layer (e.g. Elastoplast [Smith and Nephew], Vetrap [3 M Animal care products]) are self-adherent which make them easy to use. Especially when using elastic bandages, care must be taken to not wrap the layer too tightly as this may result in circulatory compromise.

Bandaging Techniques

Types of Bandages

Wet-to-Dry Bandages

Wet-to-dry bandages are indicated for exudate-producing wounds that are not clean. The primary layer consists of sterile gauze that is moistened with sterile saline and applied directly to the wound. This adherent layer is then covered with dry sterile gauze, which will allow the dry gauze to absorb the fluid from the wet gauze. Consequently, necrotic tissue and debris from the wound will adhere to the drying gauze. Following removal of the bandage, the adhered materials will consequently also be removed, thereby explaining the cleaning action of this type of bandage. To facilitate bandage removal (and decrease patient discomfort), it is advised to moisten the bandage with sterile saline prior to its removal. However, saline should be used sparingly as it may negatively influence the cleaning effect of this type of bandage (and may lead to hypothermia if the animal gets soaked with water). Wet-to-dry bandages need to be replaced at least daily, but more frequent changes are commonly needed in case of extremely dirty wounds. Since adjacent tissues may be traumatized by this type of bandage, it is recommended that they are applied for no more than five days.

Dry-to-Dry Bandages

A dry-to-dry bandage is similar to a wet-to-dry bandage with the exception of the moist primary layer being replaced by a dry gauze. The function of both is, however, similar (i.e. remove debris from the wound). Dry-to-dry bandages are often recommended for highly exudative wounds as these allow for a better absorption of fluids than the wet-to-dry bandages.

Stabilizing Bandages (Including Splints)

Stabilizing bandages are most commonly used in case of fractures but may also be used to deter tension forces from sutured wounds (e.g. tendon repair, etc.). In a Robert Jones bandage, secondary and tertiary layers are alternated to create extra stability. When greater stability is needed, splints may be used. Dependent on the size of the animal, materials such as lighting matches (e.g. in mice), or pieces of tongue depressors (e.g. in ferrets) can be used. Aluminum finger splints may also serve as a suitable splint or cast for many of the small mammals, as these are pliable, lightweight, and may be easily cut to the proper size.

Bandaging Techniques for Different Locations

Bandaging techniques in small mammals do not differ from those used in other companion animals. However, applying the bandages may be more challenging due to the size of the patient. Bandage materials often need to be trimmed down to allow proper placement. A bandage should always be applied smoothly and evenly to prevent a tourniquet effect and eliminate ridges or bulking that can cause discomfort or skin necrosis. The owner should furthermore be taught to monitor their pet's behavior and the bandage for signs of swelling, odor, or discomfort to allow for complications to be detected early. It is essential to keep the bandage dry and clean, e.g. by placing auto-adhesive plastic wraps on the plantar surface of leg or foot bandages.

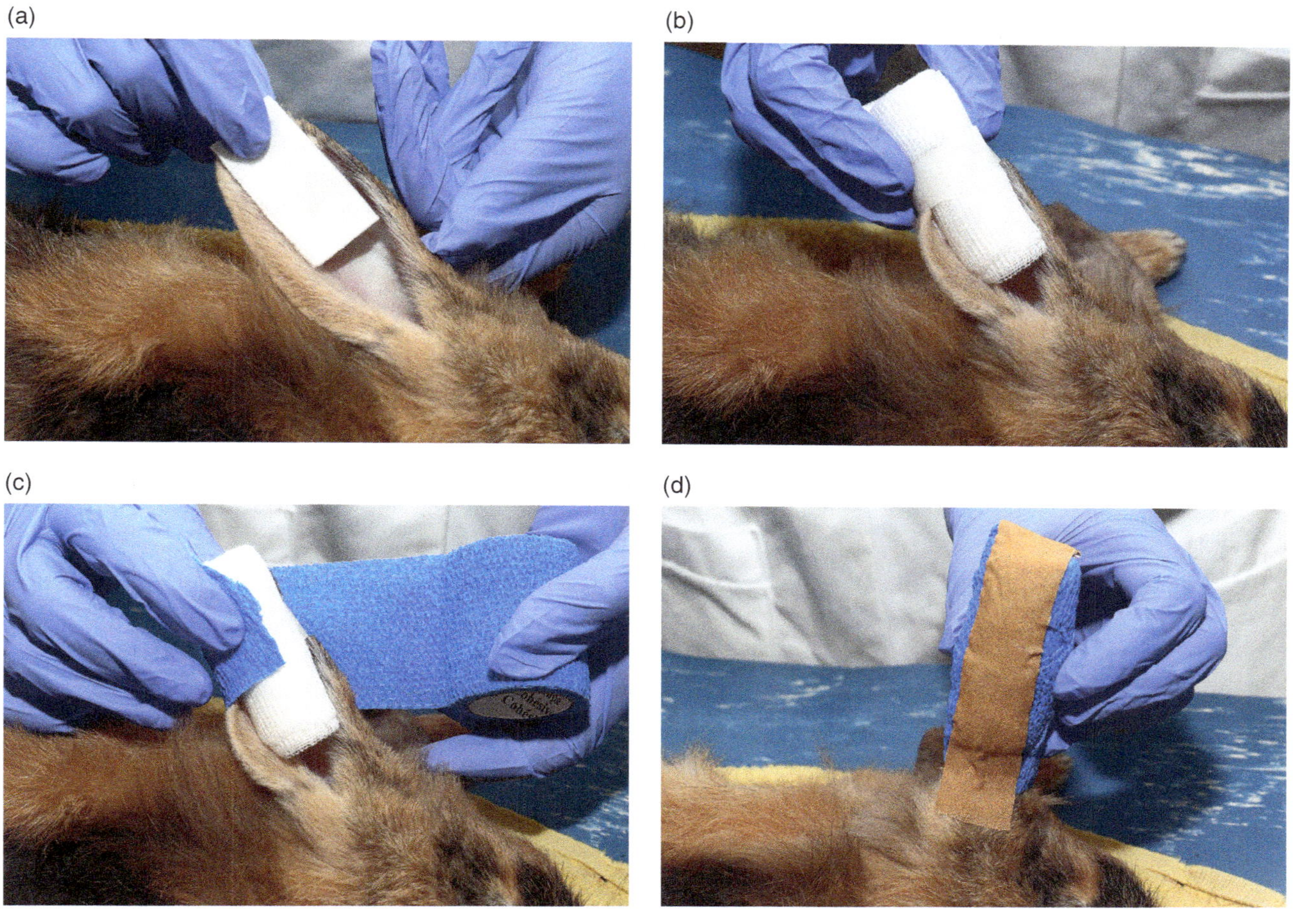

Figure 5.1 To provide support to the pinnae when placing an ear bandage in rabbits, the pinnae are not placed against the head, as is done in dogs, but a roll of gauze is placed within the ear (b) after having applied a piece of gauze as primary layer (a). Vetwrap (3 M Animal care products) is used as tertiary layer to hold the bandage in place (c). An adhesive tape is placed over the bandage and adjacent hairs to ensure that the bandage stays in place (d).

Ear and Head Bandages In most small animals, except for rabbits, the ear will be too small to allow for any type of bandage to be placed, whereas in rabbits, the cartilage in their ears prohibits these from being folded over the head, as performed in dogs. As an alternative, a roll of bandage can be placed inside the ear for support while bandaging the rest of the ear (Figure 5.1). Keeping the bandage in place by incorporating the head can be a challenge as the bandage will easily cover the laterally placed eyes. Suturing the bandage to the base of the ear may prevent it from sliding off.

Tie-Over Bandage In areas where it is difficult to keep the bandage in place (e.g. the torso), a tie-over bandage may be used. These bandages can be particularly helpful to use in smaller rodents, including guinea pigs, as they allow bandaging of the affected area (e.g. head, shoulder, back, and hip) with a limited amount of material, rendering the animal more comfortable and more accepting of the bandage. The principle behind tie-over bandages is to hold the primary and secondary layers of the bandage in place using non-absorbable suture loops that are placed around the wound. Both layers can either be held in place by attaching them to the suture loops themselves or be held in place by lacing gauze or tape through the loops, following which an adhesive tertiary layer (e.g. Tegaderm) can be applied locally. Alternatively, the padding or secondary layer can be wrapped around the torso and abdomen firmly, but without causing constriction. Each layer should overlap the underlying one over one third to one half of the padding's width. By wrapping the secondary and tertiary layers between the front legs and over the shoulders in a crisscross fashion, slippage can be prevented. Similarly, adhering one fourth to one half inch of tape to the hair, or

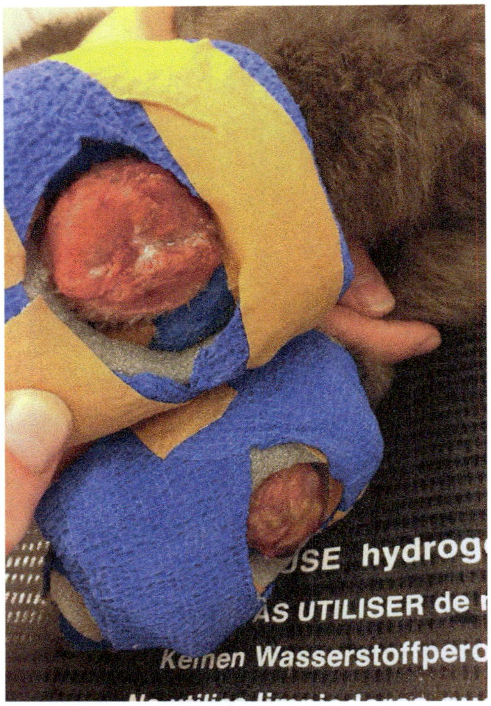

Figure 5.2 Pododermatitis can present in many different stages. In this rabbit, bilateral, proliferative lesions were present. By cutting a hole in a foam insulation pipe, pressure on the lesion is released and helps allow the wound to heal and enable daily inspection of the lesions.

placement of a stockinette, can help to maintain the bandage in place.

Foot and Leg Bandages The most common indications for placing foot and leg bandages include fractures (whereby incorporation of splints is frequently indicated) and pododermatitis. Sedation or anesthesia is often required to ensure proper placement. In case of leg bandages, porous tape stirrups, long enough to reach the tarsus can be applied to the primary layer to prevent it from slipping. The intermediate and outer layer are then applied starting distally with one half to two thirds overlapping, whereby the last two layers are wrapped around the hips (or shoulder) and the bandaged leg in a crisscross fashion to prevent the bandage from slipping. Adhering one fourth to one half inch of tape to the hairs will often be helpful for this purpose, too. In the smaller rodent species (e.g. mice, hamsters), it is recommended to include the toes in the bandage to prevent the animals from auto-mutilating them. Alternatively, easy-to-remove tape can be used to cover and protect the toes while allowing the owner to assess them on a regular basis.

In animals with pododermatitis, the bandage serves a vital role in reducing pressure load to the wound, thereby acting as a pressure relief bandage. Pressure relief can best be achieved by applying a soft ring around the wound which will then bear the weight (i.e. a doughnut bandage). Due to the long metatarsi of rabbits, a piece of insulation pipe that is cut in half and placed under the metatarsi often provides an ideal "shoe" for the foot. A hole cut in the insulation material over the area where the wound is located will help to alleviate pressure on the plantar surface (Figure 5.2). The insulation material is then incorporated in the bandage in a similar fashion as would be done with a splint.

Tail Bandages A tail bandage is applied in a similar fashion as in dogs and cats. The greatest challenge with these bandages is to prevent them from sliding off. The most common technique to help prevent this is to use a tape stirrup of which the one half is taped to the end of the tail and the other half extends further from the end of the tail. After applying the secondary layer to the tail, the extended part of the tape stirrup is twisted around and taped to the bandage, following which an adhesive bandage is used as a tertiary layer to cover the other layers. Alternative techniques to prevent the bandage from sliding off include suturing the bandage to the base of the tail or incorporating the hairs of the tail in the secondary layer with every turn of the padding (*Note:* This will only be feasible in animals with a furred tail).

References

1 Mickelson, M.A., Mans, C., and Colopy, S.A. (2016). Principles of wound management and wound healing in exotic pets. *Vet. Clin. North Am. Exot. Anim. Pract.* 19 (1): 33–53.

2 MacPhail, C.M. (2012). Surgery of the integumentary system. In: *Small Animal Surgery Textbook*, 4e (ed. W.T. Fossum), 190–288. Philadelphia, PA, USA: Elsevier Health Sciences.

Further Reading

Akhoondinasab, M.R., Akhoondinasab, M., and Saberi, M. (2014). Comparison of healing effect of aloe vera extract and silver sulfadiazine in burn injuries in experimental rat model. *World J. Plast. Surg.* 3 (1): 29–34.

Dat, A.D., Poon, F., Pham, K.B., and Doust, J. (2012). Aloe vera for treating acute and chronic wounds. *Cochrane Database Syst. Rev.* (2): CD008762. https://doi.org/10.1002/14651858.CD008762.pub2.

Edlich, R.F., Rodeheaver, G.T., Thacker, J.G. et al. (2010a). Revolutionary advances in the management of traumatic wounds in the emergency department during the last 40 years: part I. *J. Emerg. Med.* 38 (1): 40–50.

Edlich, R.F., Rodeheaver, G.T., Thacker, J.G. et al. (2010b). Revolutionary advances in the management of traumatic wounds in the emergency department during the last 40 years: part II. *J. Emerg. Med.* 38 (2): 201–207.

Garzotto, C.K. (2008). Wound management. In: *Small Animal Critical Care Medicine* (eds. D. Silverstein and K. Hopper), 676–682. Philadelphia, PA, USA: Elsevier Health Sciences.

Graham, J.E. (2004). Rabbit wound management. *Vet. Clin. North Am. Exot. Anim. Pract.* 7 (1): 37–55.

Hernandez-Divers, S.M. (2004). Principles of wound management of small mammals: hedgehogs, prairie dogs, and sugar gliders. *Vet. Clin. North Am. Exot. Anim. Pract.* 7 (1): 1–18.

Hess, L. and Tater, K. (2004). Dermatologic diseases. In: *Ferrets, Rabbits and Rodents: Clinical Medicine and Surgery* (eds. K.E. Quesenberry and J.W. Carpenter), 194–202. St. Louis, MO, USA: Elsevier Health Sciences.

Jacobsen, S. (2016). Topical wound treatments and wound-care products. In: *Equine Wound Management*, 3e (eds. C. Theoret and J. Schumcher), 75–99. Ames, IA, USA: Wiley.

Langlois, I. (2004). Wound management in rodents. *Vet. Clin. North Am. Exot. Anim. Pract.* 7 (1): 141–167.

Lipsky, B.A. and Hoey, C. (2009). Topical antimicrobial therapy for treating chronic wounds. *Clin. Infect. Dis.* 49 (10): 1541–1549.

Lipsky, B.A., Dryden, M., Gottrup, F. et al. (2016). Antimicrobial stewardship in wound care: a position paper from the British Society for Antimicrobial Chemotherapy and European Wound Management Association. *J. Antimicrob. Chemother.* 71 (11): 3026–3035.

Manning, P.J., Wagner, J.E., and Harkness, J.E. (1984). Biology and disease of guinea pigs. In: *Laboratory Animal Medicine* (eds. J.G. Fox, B.J. Cohen and F.M. Loew), 149–181. Orlando, FL, USA: Academic Press.

Molan, P.C. and Rhodes, T. (2015). Honey: a biologic wound dressing. *Wounds* 27 (6): 141–151.

Pavletic, M.M. (2011). *Atlas of Small Animal Wound Management and Reconstructive Surgery*. Ames, IA, USA: Wiley.

Pilny, A.A. and Hess, L. (2004). Ferrets: wound healing and therapy. *Vet. Clin. North Am. Exot. Anim. Pract.* 7 (1): 105–121.

Prevaldi, C., Paolillo, C., Locatelli, C. et al. (2016). Management of traumatic wounds in the emergency department: a secondary publication. *Emerg. Care J.* 12 (2): 31–34.

Quinn, J.V., Polevoi, S.K., and Kohn, M.A. (2014). Traumatic lacerations: what are the risks for infection and has the 'golden period' of laceration care disappeared? *Emerg. Med. J.* 31: 96–100.

Rodriguez-Bigas, M., Cruz, N.I., and Suarez, A. (1988). A comparative evaluation of aloe vera in the management of burn wounds in guinea pigs. *Plast. Reconstr. Surg.* 81 (3): 386–389.

Waldron, D.R. and Trevor, P. (1993). Management of superficial skin wounds. In: *Textbook of Small Animal Surgery*, 2e (ed. D. Slatter), 269–280. Philadelphia, PA, USA: WB Saunders.

6

CPR and Euthanasia

Yvonne R.A. van Zeeland and Nico J. Schoemaker

Division of Zoological Medicine, Department of Clinical Sciences, Faculty of Veterinary Medicine, Utrecht University, The Netherlands

CONTENTS

Cardiopulmonary Resuscitation (CPR)

Cardiopulmonary resuscitation or CPR is an emergency procedure that combines the use of basic and advanced life support (ALS) measures to revive patients with cardiac and/or respiratory arrest. The primary goal of any CPR procedure is to preserve the function of the brain and other vital organs while attempting to restore spontaneous blood circulation and breathing. As the preservation of neurologic function comprises an essential component of successful resuscitation, the term cardiopulmonary cerebral resuscitation (CPCR) is nowadays preferred.

Indications

CPCR is indicated in patients with cardiopulmonary arrest (CPA). Typically, patients will be unconscious and unresponsive with non-functional ventilation and/or ineffective circulation. Dependent on the cause, patients may present with absent or abnormal respirations (e.g. agonal breathing pattern) and/or have a non-functional perfusion (e.g. resulting from ventricular fibrillation or asystole). Because successful revival and survival are related directly to the underlying condition, the primary disease process should be taken into consideration. In many hospitals, the patient's condition, prognosis, and costs of CPCR are discussed with the owner so that the team can act accordingly if the patient collapses. The owner is commonly offered three options, i.e. (i) Code red – do not resuscitate (DNR); (ii) Code yellow – permission to intubate, ventilate, medicate, and use external chest compressions to resuscitate the animal (i.e. external CPCR); or (iii) Code green – permission for full resuscitation with internal cardiac massage, if deemed appropriate.

Out-of-Hospital Arrest

Out-of-hospital cardiopulmonary arrest (OHCPA) is defined as the cessation of breathing and/or cardiac activity that occurs outside of the hospital setting (usually the owner's home). Under these conditions, chances for successful patient revival are generally slim. Nevertheless, an attempt can be made to administer CPCR to the patient. For this purpose, it is vital to provide appropriate instructions to the

Exotic Animal Emergency and Critical Care Medicine, First Edition. Edited by Jennifer E. Graham, Grayson A. Doss and Hugues Beaufrère.

owner on how to check their pet's vital functions and provide emergency care. Guidelines for proper at-home CPCR include the following:

1) *Danger:* Ensure that the owner can safely approach the pet;
2) *Response:* Instruct the owner to evaluate consciousness by observing for signs of movement and evaluating the animal's response to a call of its name. Ask the owner to gently touch the animal and attempt to wake the animal up;
3) *Send for help:* Instruct the owner to get a second person (if not present) that can take over the call while the owner assists the pet;
4) *Airway:* If the animal is unconscious, provide appropriate instructions for checking the airway (i.e. pulling out the tongue, looking for any obstructions, and removing these);
5) *Breathing:* Have the owner watch the chest to see if it is rising and falling; if the animal is not breathing, instruct the owner how to perform rescue breathing (see Section "Basic Life Support");
6) *Circulation:* Have the owner check the pulse, gums, and/or heartbeat. If no circulation is present, instruct how to perform chest compressions (see Section "Basic Life Support").

Owners should be notified to try and get the animal to the veterinary clinic as soon as possible and continue CPCR for as long as they can until they have reached the clinic (where a professional team can take over) or until the animal has a palpable pulse or heartbeat that is strong and regular again. Even when resuscitation at home is successful, transportation to the clinic should take place immediately for further examination and care.

In Hospital Arrest

A CPA is classified as an "in-hospital" cardiopulmonary arrest (IHCPA) if it occurs in a hospitalized patient who had a pulse at the time of admission and when it is unrelated to an anesthetic event. Most patients suffering from in-hospital arrest are found to have pre-existing morbidities and/or display clinical abnormalities in the 24 hours prior to the arrest, with the commonest reasons being cardiac arrhythmias, acute respiratory insufficiency, and hypotension. In rabbits, IHCPAs are predominantly related to handling, which may lead to acute myocardial stunning (i.e. Takotsubo cardiomyopathy) because of stress-induced catecholamine release. In ferrets, vaccine reactions and acute traumatic incidents have been reported as causes for IHCPA, but no studies have thus far investigated causes for in-hospital arrest in small mammalian species.

Compared to OHCPA, survival-to-discharge rates and changes for a favorable outcome are likely higher in IHCPA patients as veterinary staff is better equipped to respond timely and adequately to CPA. To facilitate recognition of patients at risk, and ensure adequate monitoring and intervention, cage-side rounds during shift changes have been recommended. The mnemonic "H's and T's" is commonly used to identify patients at risk for CPA or assess specific etiologies during CPCR (see Table 6.1). In addition, rapid response systems, such as present in human hospitals, may be applied in the veterinary practice.

Table 6.1 Overview of (reversible) etiologies for CPA.

6 H's	5 T's
Hypovolemia or hemorrhage	Toxins or tablets
Hypoxia or hypoventilation	Tension pneumothorax
Hydrogen ions (acidosis)	Tamponade (pericardial effusion)
Hyper- or hypo-electrolytes (Na^+, K^+, Ca^{2+}, Mg^{2+})	Thrombosis or thromboembolism
Hypoglycemia	Trauma
Hypo- or hyperthermia	

Anesthesia-Related Arrest

Anesthesia-related CPA is defined as a cessation of respiratory and/or cardiac activity that can be attributed to an anesthetic event, from induction until the patient is fully awake.

Small mammal patients are prone to anesthesia-related CPA. A study investigating the risk for perioperative morbidity and mortality demonstrated that, compared to dogs and cats, the risk for anesthetic-related death in most small mammals is often 10-fold greater (see also Table 6.2). Factors rendering these species at greater risk for anesthesia-related complications include the following:

- a relative high surface-area-to-volume ratio and higher metabolic rates that predispose to (perioperative) hypothermia and hypoglycemia;
- a higher sensitivity to stress (e.g. from handling during induction of anesthesia);
- limited accessibility of veins for intravenous (IV) catheterization;
- technical difficulties experienced upon endotracheal intubation (preventing adequate ventilation and/or predisposing to complications due to incorrect intubation);
- higher predilection for (undetected) preoperative morbidities (e.g. respiratory, digestive, and/or fluid balance disorders);
- relative inexperience of veterinarians with anesthesia of these patients.

Nonetheless, compared to other forms of CPA, anesthesia-related arrest represents one of the more treatable causes of CPA in veterinary patients. Close patient monitoring facilitates early detection of an impending arrest. Moreover, identifying high-risk patients and/or situations (e.g. patients with pre-existent morbidities and/or

Table 6.2 Risk of anesthesia-related death in companion animals.

Species	Number of anesthesia/sedation-related deaths	Number of sedated/anesthetized animals	Risk of anesthetic-related mortality (95% CI)
Dogs	163	98 036	0.17% (0.14–0.19%)
Cats	189	79 178	0.24% (0.20–0.27%)
Ferret	4	600	0.67% (0.18–1.70%)
Rabbit	114	8209	1.39% (1.14–1.64%)
Guinea pig	49	1288	3.80% (2.76–4.85%)
Chinchilla	11	334	3.29% (1.38–5.21%)
Hamster	12	246	4.88% (2.19–7.57%)
Rat	8	398	2.01% (0.87–3.92%)
Other small mammals	7	232	3.02% (1.22–6.12%)

Source: Brodbelt [1]and Brodbelt et al. [2].

undergoing specific surgical procedures, specific events such as intubation, extubation, or repositioning of the patient) allows for anticipation of potential complications (see also Chapter 7). Vigilant monitoring should also continue throughout the recovery period as >50% of anesthetic-related CPA events have been found to occur in this phase (particularly within the first three hours post-operation).

General Principles

CPCR can be complicated in small mammals due to their size, anatomic, and physiologic diversity, and lack of evidence on treatment efficacy. Nonetheless, the CPCR principles and techniques in small mammals roughly follow similar guidelines as those established for humans and other companion animals.

First, the patient should be evaluated using the ABCDE approach (airway, breathing, circulation, disability, and environment, see also Chapter 1) following which basic life support (BLS) can be provided to promote oxygenation, ventilation, and circulation. In addition, ALS can be provided which consists of electrocardiographic evaluation of the cardiac rhythm, administration of drugs and fluids, defibrillation, monitoring during CPCR, and post-resuscitation care. Installment of a crash cart or specifically designated area where the necessary supplies (see Box 6.1) are readily available is also highly recommended to maximize the chances of a successful outcome.

Evidence-Based Literature

In human medicine, the science behind the CPCR technique is periodically reviewed by the International Liaison Committee on Resuscitation (ILCOR), which comprises a consortium of emergency and critical care scientists. Joint efforts of this consortium and the American Heart Association resulted in the development of the first International CPR Guidelines in 2000, which have been continuously updated ever since (for the latest guidelines, see https://eccguidelines.heart.org/circulation/cpr-ecc-guidelines). In 2012, the American College of Veterinary Emergency Critical Care (ACVECC) started a similar initiative called the Reassessment Campaign on Veterinary Resuscitation (RECOVER) with the intention to draft a set of evidence-based clinical guidelines for veterinary CPCR (see www.acvecc-recover.org and www.veccs.org). Although these consensus guidelines have been primarily designed for CPCR in dogs and cats, most of the information can be extrapolated for use in small mammals. However, evidence to support the use of these CPCR guidelines in small mammals is scarce, being mainly derived from expert opinion and few case reports. A study reviewing the outcomes of CPCR in 15 rabbits with CPA determined that return of spontaneous circulation (ROSC) occurred in approximately 45% of patients (similar to reports in other species) following the use of conventional CPCR techniques. Based on these findings, the authors concluded conventional techniques for other species to be similarly effective in rabbits.

Resuscitation Protocol

Resuscitation protocols follow similar guidelines that include the universal "ABCD" algorithm, representing the major components of CPCR (i.e. airway, breathing, circulation, and drugs). Guidelines further divide the components of this algorithm into two major categories, i.e. basic life support (BLS) and advanced life support (ALS), which are often applied simultaneously. A flowchart for small mammal resuscitation, based on extrapolation of the current guidelines for dogs and cats, can be found in Box 6.2.

Box 6.1 Emergency Equipment for Small Mammal CPCR

Equipment that needs to be readily available in case of a small mammal emergency

- Dosage sheet for commonly used emergency drugs
- Calculator
- Notepad and pen
- Emergency drugs (e.g. atropine, epinephrine/adrenaline, doxapram, antidotes)
- Endotracheal tubes (ETTs) of appropriate sizes for small mammals (e.g. 2.0–3.5); *Note:* In smaller mammals, intravenous catheters (without needle) can be used for endotracheal intubation
- Stylet pre-adjusted to fit the above-mentioned ETTs
- Supraglottic airway device (SGAD, for rabbits)
- Laryngoscope with #1 straight blade
- Face masks of appropriate sizes for small mammals
- Pediatric ambu bag
- Oxygen delivery system
- Gauze bandages for opening the mouth, holding the tongue and/or tying the ETT or SGAD in place
- Syringes of various sizes (i.e. 1 ml, 3–10 ml, 20–50 ml)
- Needles of various sizes (e.g. 22- to 28 gauge)
- Intravenous catheters of appropriate sizes (e.g. 22- to 29 gauge)
- Butterfly infusion catheters or appropriate size for subcutaneous and/or intraperitoneal fluid administration (e.g. 19- to 27 gauge)
- Spinal or hypodermic needles appropriate for intraosseous catheterization
- Catheter injection plugs and intravenous lines
- Infusion pump
- Sterile fluids (e.g. saline)
- Rubber band tourniquet (or similar material) and hemostat
- Stomach tubes of appropriate size (e.g. 3–14 French)
- Stethoscope
- ECG monitor
- Audio Doppler unit with appropriate cuffs
- Pulse oximeter
- Capnograph
- Thermometer
- Heating pad or heating source
- Clippers
- Cotton or gauze pads
- Alcohol
- Lubricating gel (e.g. electrode or ultrasound gel)
- Tape
- Vetrap or other bandage materials

Basic Life Support

Basic Life Support should be initiated immediately following recognition of an (impending) CPA to promote blood flow to the heart and brain, and limit injury to these organs until spontaneous circulation has been restored. Despite the CAB approach (i.e. circulation, airway, and breathing) being advocated for people in recent years, the ABC approach (i.e. airway, breathing, and circulation; see also Box 6.3) is still considered more appropriate in veterinary patients as, in contrast to human medicine, CPAs are not commonly associated with primary cardiac disease. Dependent on the abnormalities observed, ventilatory support and/or chest compressions may begin. If the patient with the (impending) arrest is anesthetized, anesthesia should be stopped immediately by turning off the inhalant anesthetic vaporizer and/or administering reversal agents. At this stage, if possible, a search for potentially reversible causes (e.g. hypoxemia,

Box 6.2 Flowchart for Provision of CPCR to Small Mammals

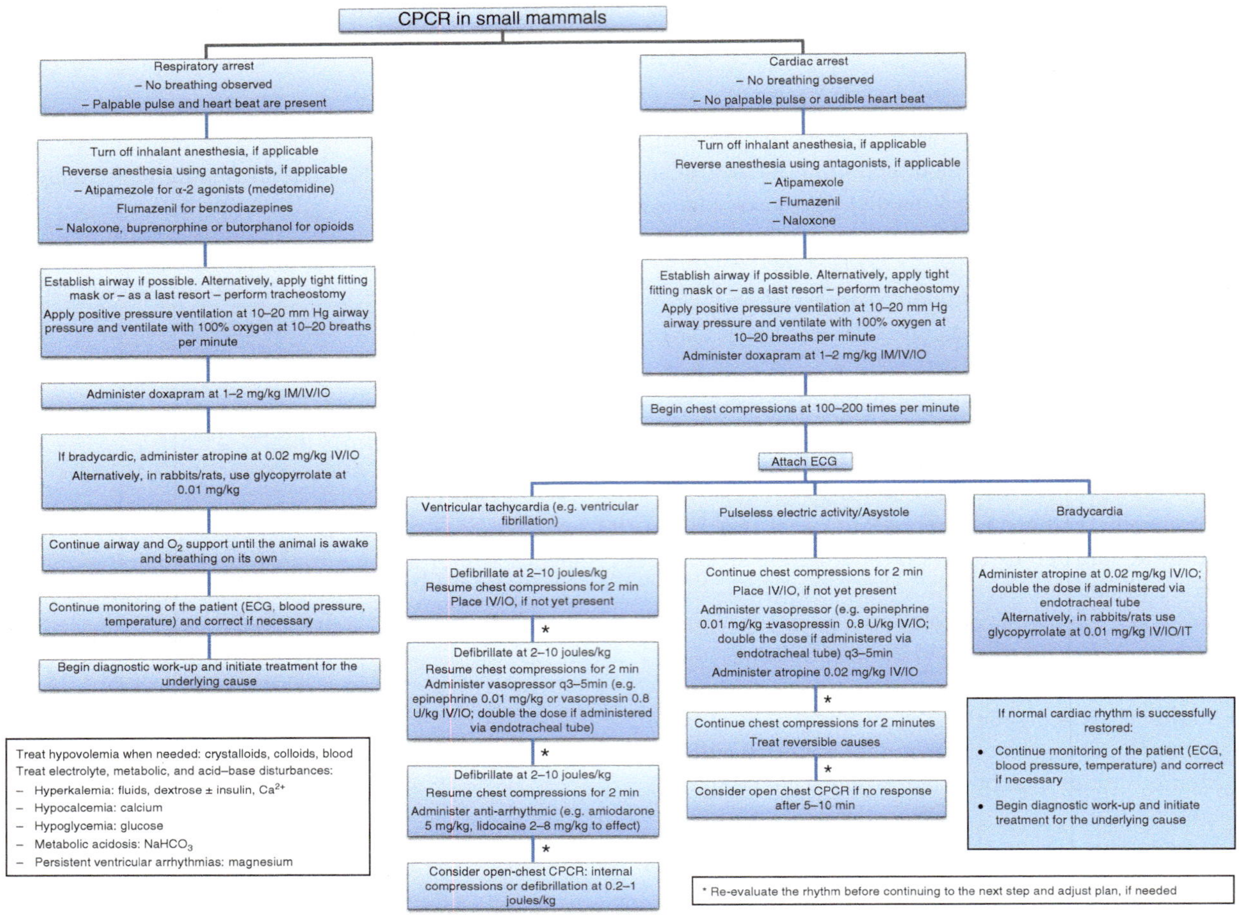

hypercarbia, hypovolemia, hypothermia, electrolyte, metabolic, or acid–base disturbances) should be initiated, while the other team members assemble to start the CPCR, draw up the emergency drugs, and gather any other supplies that are necessary for ALS.

Ventilatory Support

In patients with respiratory arrest, the following protocol needs to be followed:

1) Check the airway and remove any visible obstructions in the oral cavity.
2) Secure airway access through one of the following routes:
   a. Endotracheal intubation: This may be challenging in many small mammals given their narrow oral cavity and even more so in rabbits and rodents since many of these species are obligate or dependent nasal breathers. In ferrets, use a 2.0 or 2.5 uncuffed ETT (technique similar to the cat); in rabbits and larger guinea pigs, use an endoscope-guided technique (see Chapter 7).
   b. In rabbits, place a species-specific supraglottic airway device (see Chapter 7). The smallest size (R1) has been used to successfully intubate hedgehogs.
   c. Place a tight-fitting face mask over the mouth and nose to deliver forced high-flow ventilation (Figure 6.1). *Note*: This may lead to significant gastric bloat due to leakage of air into the esophagus, which can subsequently hinder the proper movement of the diaphragm.
   d. Perform an emergency tracheostomy using a similar technique as described in the dog and cat (Figure 6.2). Due to the invasiveness of the procedure and potential risk of post-surgical stricture formation, this technique should only be considered as a last resort.
3) Evaluate correct placement of the ETT or supraglottic airway device by evaluating for chest movement, listening for lung sounds, capnography, and/or direct visualization of the larynx.

4) Turn off any anesthetic gases and flush the circuit.
5) Initiate positive pressure ventilation (e.g. using an ambu bag, demand valve, or anesthetic machine) using 100% oxygen:
   a. Administer breaths at a rate of 10–20 breaths per minute,[1] and using a tidal volume of 10 ml/kg.
   b. Keep airway pressure between 10 and 20 mmHg.
   c. Inspiratory time of approximately one second.

   Note: In patients with respiratory arrest occurring shortly after induction or during anesthesia, a few breaths and addressing the precipitating cause (e.g. decreasing anesthetic concentration) may be all that is needed to promote return to normal breathing.
6) Monitor end-tidal carbon dioxide (ETCO2) with a capnograph connected to the breathing circuit, if possible. Adjust the tidal volume, inspiratory time, and respiratory rate to prevent hypercapnia (<45 mmHg; see Section "Monitoring").
7) Administer doxapram as a respiratory stimulant (see Section "Drugs"); side effects can be significant (e.g. cardiac arrhythmias, muscle fasciculation, and seizures); therefore, its use should be limited to patients that cannot be intubated or otherwise allow control of ventilation.
8) In absence of adequate materials to support ventilation, administer mouth-to-mouth, or mouth-to-nose breathing by cupping the hands around the animal's muzzle, placing the mouth over it, and blowing air into the mouth or nose until the chest expands. *Note:* Consider the potential for transmission of zoonotic diseases prior to initiating mouth-to-mouth or mouth-to-nose breathing!
   a) During the first 60 seconds, administer breaths every 3–5 seconds.
   b) Reassess breathing and circulation.
   c) If necessary, resume mouth-to-nose breathing at a slower pace (i.e. every six seconds).

Chest Compressions

In small mammals, due to their high metabolic rate, the time frame between the onset of CPA and the development of severe neurologic damage is short. The following protocol is recommended to regain cardiovascular function and limit the risk of permanent damage:

1) Upon identifying cardiac arrest, commence chest compressions immediately.
   a) Administer chest compressions at a rate of 100 times per minute using one of the following methods:
      i) Place fingers and thumb on opposite sides of the chest;
      ii) Use a two-hand technique with the fingers of each hand on opposite sides of the chest. *Note:* When using this technique, care should be taken to avoid compression using only the tips of the fingers.

Compressions should encompass approximately half of the total compression-release cycle to ensure that sufficient time is available for complete recoiling of the chest.
   b) Continue chest compressions throughout the provision of ventilatory support and for at least two minutes. Should alternate rescue breaths and chest compressions be considered, a cardiac compression-to-ventilation ratio of 15:1 or 30:2 is recommended.
   c) Re-evaluate the patient's status and identify whether a palpable pulse is present. If needed, change between compressors before resuming chest compressions.
   d) Resume chest compressions with greater force if the previous session has not resulted in a palpable pulse.
2) Monitor cardiac activity with a stethoscope and electrocardiography (ECG) and the effectiveness of compressions with a Doppler probe.
   a) ECG allows for evaluation of the cardiac rhythm and determines in large part the subsequent steps that need to be taken (see Section "Advanced Life Support"). Leads are placed in similar locations as in dogs and cats. Hypodermic needles provide a good alternative to pads which commonly fail to result in a signal.
   b) A Doppler probe can be positioned over the heart or across the jugular or peripheral arteries of the legs or tail to identify a pulse. A cuff can be placed around the legs or tail to monitor blood pressure (Figure 6.3).
3) Placement of an intraosseous (IO) or intravenous catheter should be considered to allow fluids or medication to be administered (see Section "Vascular Access").
4) In dogs and cats, internal cardiac massage is recommended if efforts are ineffective after two to five minutes of external compressions or if a disease process would limit the effectiveness of closed thorax compressions. In small mammals, unless in surgery, this is not commonly performed.

1 Research has indicated that hyperventilation as well as high peak inspiratory pressure can be harmful and should be avoided to prevent compromise of venous return. As a result, current guidelines recommend lower respiratory rates, i.e. between 10 and 20 breaths per minute for small mammals.

Box 6.3 ABC Approach in Patients Suspected of CPA

A = Airway	Listen for the presence of stridor indicative of upper airway obstruction and check whether the oral cavity is clear by opening the mouth and pulling out the tongue. Any foreign objects or excess mucous present should be removed
B = Breathing	Evaluate the color of the mucus membranes for the presence of cyanosis and assess the animal's breathing for abnormalities in rate, rhythm, depth, and type. Initiate ventilatory support in patients with absent or highly abnormal respirations
C = Circulation	Evaluate the animal's pulse (i.e. frequency, quality, and rhythm), heart rate, mucous membranes, and capillary refill time. Initiate circulatory support, including cardiac compressions, in patients with no effective circulation (i.e. absence of a palpable pulse)

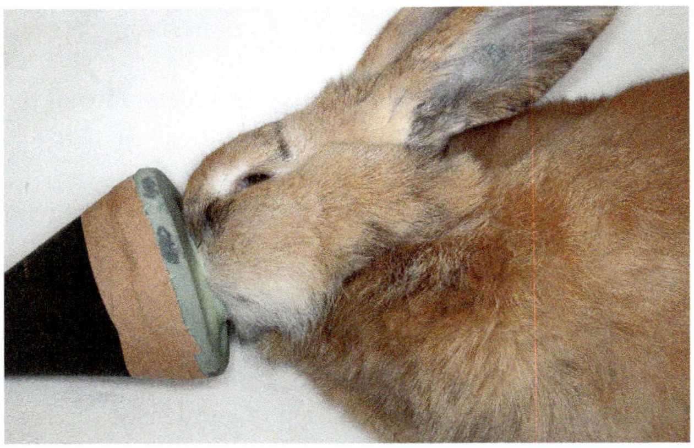

Figure 6.1 A tight-fitting face mask may be used to attempt to ventilate a rabbit in respiratory arrest.

Advanced Life Support

The primary purpose of ALS is to restore the electrical and mechanical activity of the heart. During ALS, an electrocardiographic evaluation of the arrest rhythm is made, followed by drug and fluid administration and/or defibrillation, as indicated. Regardless of initiating ALS, BLS procedures should be continued.

Electrocardiography

The major rhythms associated with arrest include asystole, sinus bradycardia, pulseless electrical activity (PEA, i.e. presence of normal to slow electrical activity without the mechanical activity of the myocardium), and ventricular tachycardia (i.e. ventricular fibrillation [VF] or flutter). Dependent on the arrhythmia that is present, specific treatment can be administered (Table 6.3). For further information on placement of the ECG electrodes see Chapter 7.

Vascular Access

Potential routes for delivery of fluids and drugs include the intravenous, intraosseous, intratracheal, or intracardial route. The latter is no longer recommended because of the risk of myocardial damage and/or arrhythmias. The intratracheal route can be used for various drugs (i.e. naloxone, atropine, epinephrine, doxapram, lidocaine, and vasopressin), especially if the intravenous or intraosseous route is not readily available. Doubling the dose is recommended. In addition, dilution with sterile saline or water to a volume of 2–4 ml may help to facilitate absorption. To administer the drugs, a red rubber tube of appropriate diameter can be passed down the ETT to the level of the bifurcation. Next, two positive pressure breaths should be given to promote the distribution of the drugs across the tracheobronchial tree.

Vascular access should be obtained as soon as possible (but without interfering with resuscitation!). More information on the placement of intravenous or intraosseous catheters and fluid therapy can be found in Chapters 4 and 8.

Drugs

See Table 6.4 for an overview of the most commonly used emergency drugs for CPCR, including their indications, dosages, and routes of administration.

Defibrillation

Electrical defibrillation is recommended in the case of ventricular fibrillation or flutter. In all other types of arrest arrhythmias, defibrillation is contraindicated as it can cause severe myocardial damage. Moreover, many standard handheld defibrillators do not provide low enough energy levels for small mammal patients and often have paddles that are too large. However, newer defibrillators have adhesive patch electrodes and lower energy ranges which may be more suitable to use in smaller patients. The first attempt should include one countershock, using an energy level of 2–5 joules/kg, following which the energy is increased to 5–10 joules/kg. In addition, epinephrine may be administered to help convert the rhythm. Chest compressions should recommence immediately following administering the shock and can be interrupted shortly after two minutes to re-evaluate the rhythm to decide on the next step to take.

Monitoring

Monitoring is vital during any CPCR procedure. Similar to anesthetic procedures, monitoring can take place by the clinical evaluation of the patient as well as by the use of monitoring aids (see also Chapter 7). However, some clinical signs and monitoring aids may not provide reliable information during CPCR. Of all the parameters to be measured,

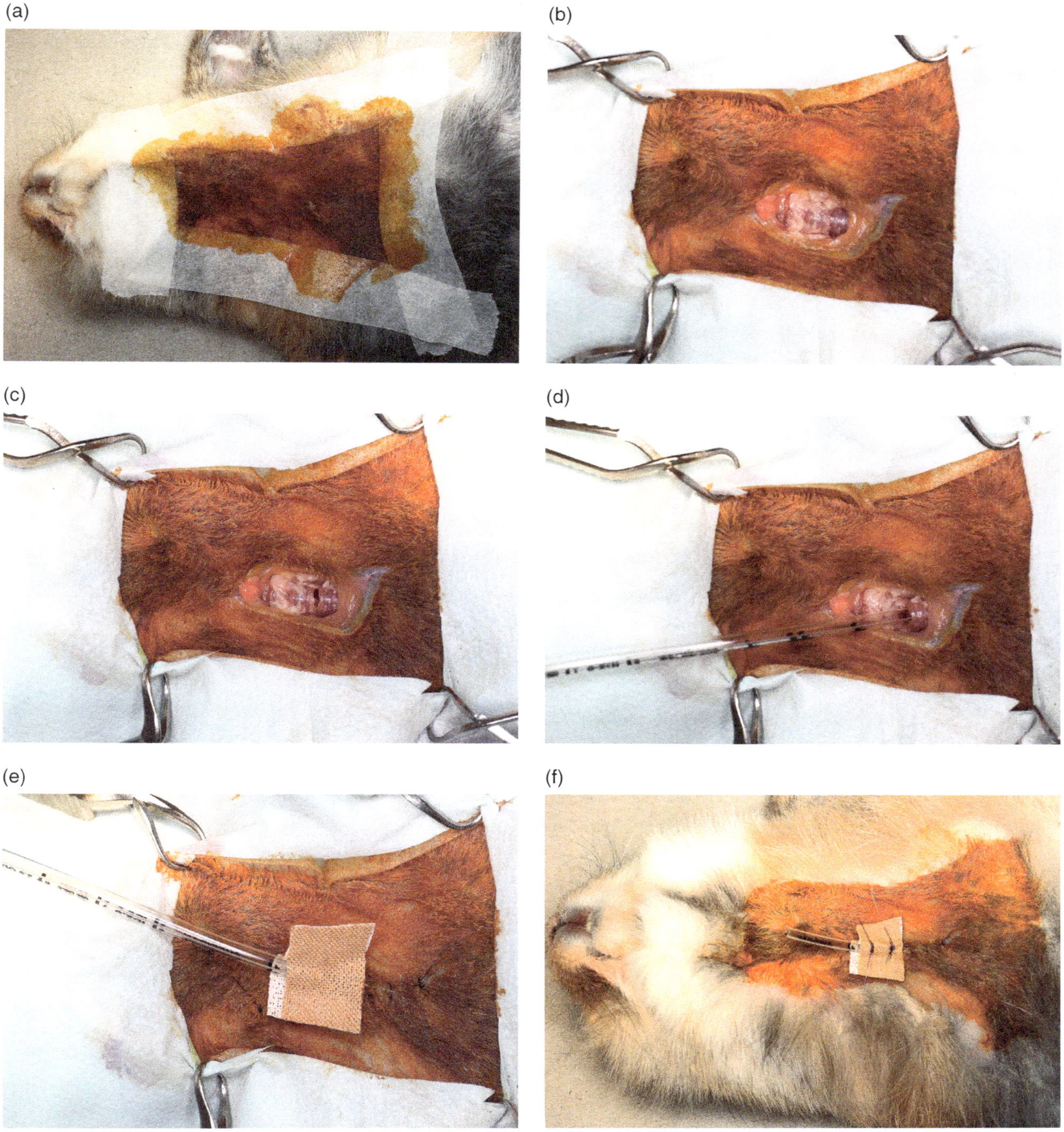

Figure 6.2 The ventral surface is shaved and disinfected prior to performing a tracheostomy (a). A ventral midline skin incision is made, parallel to trachea and just below the larynx, after which the trachea is isolated by bluntly dissecting through the SC fat, fascia, and the sternohyoid and sternothyroid muscles (b). The trachea is incised transversely between the trachea rings, taking care not to exceed 50% of the tracheal circumference (c). An endotracheal tube of appropriate size is inserted into the trachea (d). After the closure of the incision, the tube is secured to the skin by using adhesive tape around the tube (e) and sutures through the skin and the tape (f).

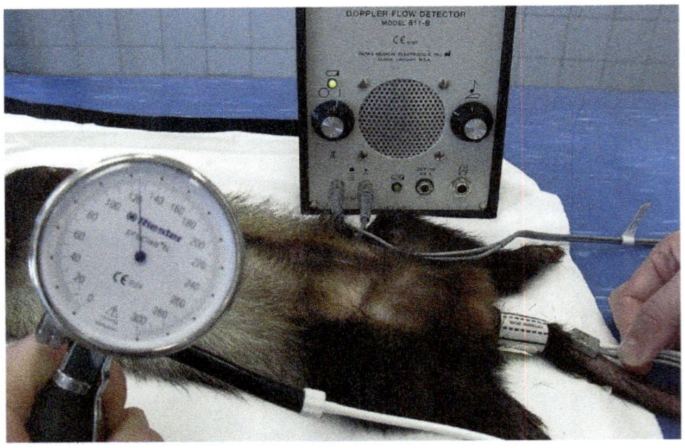

Figure 6.3 Blood pressure can either be measured through an automated blood measure monitor or by using a Doppler and an oscillometer.

$ETCO_2$ is considered the best indirect indicator of cardiac output and pulmonary blood flow as both parameters are directly proportional to each other if ventilation is kept constant. As such, this should be measured in any patient that is intubated. Upon improvement of the flow during effective CPCR, the $ETCO_2$ will also steadily increase. In fact, in humans, $ETCO_2$ is one of the best indicators of successful ROSC. In general, the following guidelines should be considered for $ETCO_2$ readings in patients with CPA:

- **$ETCO_2$ <10 mmHg (<1.3%):** incorrect intubation, ineffective CPCR technique, or hyperventilation (if adequate perfusion is established). If present for more than 15–20 minutes following initiation of CPCR, a successful outcome becomes highly unlikely
- **$ETCO_2$ 12–18 mmHg (1.6–2.4%):** ROSC
- **ETCO2 > 45 mmHg (>6%):** hypoventilation or increased CO_2 delivery to the lungs after ROSC

Table 6.3 Major arrest rhythms and their treatment.

Heart rhythm	Treatment
Asystole (flat line; complete absence of electrical heart activity)	- Start chest compressions - If hyperkalemia suspected or present: o Calcium gluconate 50 mg/kg o Insulin 0.2 U/kg o Glucose or dextrose 25% diluted 1:4; 0.25–1 ml/kg over 5 min o Sodium bicarbonate: mEq = BW (kg) × 0.3 × deficit (give ½ dose initially and re-evaluate) - Epinephrine (0.01 mg/kg) or vasopressin (0.8 U/kg) - ±Atropine (0.02 mg/kg) - Consider open chest cardiac massage if no response is obtained within 5–10 min - *Note:* Fine ventricular fibrillation may resemble asystole on ECG!
Pulseless electrical activity (PEA) (presence of a normal ECG trace or arrhythmia, but no muscular activity present – no audible heart sounds or palpable pulse)	- Start chest compressions - Administer atropine (0.02 mg/kg) and epinephrine (0.01 mg/kg) or vasopressin (0.8 U/kg) - Defibrillation may be attempted with pulseless ventricular tachycardia (see ventricular fibrillation) - Address the underlying cause - Consider open chest cardiac massage if normal rhythm and circulation have not been successfully restored within 5–10 min
Sinus bradycardia (normal P, QRS, and T waves, but occurring in slower rate)	- Address the underlying cause (e.g. increased vagal tone due to GI, urinary, or thoracic disease; hyperkalemia due to urinary obstruction or rupture) - Administer atropine at 0.02 mg/kg
Ventricular fibrillation (indicates lack of coordinated mechanical activity)	- External defibrillation at 2–10 joules/kg for 3× with 2-min intervals; re-evaluate the rhythm following each cycle - Continue chest compressions in the meantime - From the second cycle onward, add epinephrine (0.01 mg/kg) or vasopressin (0.8 U/kg) to the treatment protocol q3–5 min - Following the third defibrillation, an anti-arrhythmic (e.g. lidocaine 2–8 mg/kg, amiodarone 5 mg/kg) may be administered
Ventricular flutter (prefibrillatory rhythm)	- Lidocaine (2–8 mg/kg) IV/IO - If ineffective following two boluses and no perfusion is present, defibrillation may be attempted (see ventricular fibrillation)

Table 6.4 Common emergency drugs, including their indications, dosages, and routes of administration in small mammals.

Drug	Indication(s)	Dosage and route of administration[a]
Aminophylline	Bronchodilator; treatment of airway obstruction from e.g. asthma. Do not use concurrently with doxapram	4 mg/kg PO,IV
Amiodarone	Mixed class anti-arrhythmic with actions on sodium, potassium, and calcium channels as well as α- and β- adrenergic effects; recommended in case of ventricular fibrillation or ventricular tachycardia refractory to repeated electrical conversion	5 mg/kg IV,IO (slowly, if possible)
Atipamezole	α2 adrenergic antagonist. Reversal of dexmedetomidine or medetomidine anesthesia	Same volume as medetomidine. SC,IM
Atropine	Muscarinic receptor (M2) antagonist with anticholinergic effects; increased automaticity of the sinus node and improved conduction at the atrioventricular node, resulting in increased heart rate. Recommended for patients with symptomatic bradycardia and patients with anesthesia-related CPA *Note 1:* Also causes mydriasis, thereby rendering pupillary responses unreliable for post-resuscitative monitoring *Note 2:* May be less effective in rabbits due to presence of atropinesterase in the blood – glycopyrrolate may be considered as an alternative	During CPR: 0.02–0.04 mg/kg IV,IO,IT Non-emergency situations: 0.05–0.2 mg/kg SC,IM
Buprenorphine	Partial μ-opioid agonist and κ-opioid antagonist; used to partially reverse the effects of opioid medications such as fentanyl and morphine. Also frequently used to provide analgesia	0.02–0.04 mg/kg SC,IM
Butorphanol	Mixed κ-opioid agonist μ-opioid antagonist; used to partially reverse the effects of opioid medications such as fentanyl and morphine. Also frequently used to premedicate due to its sedative and analgesic properties	0.2–0.4 mg/kg SC,IM
Calcium gluconate	Mineral supplement; used during CPCR in cases of pre-existing hypocalcemia, calcium channel blocker toxicity, and/or temporary amelioration of hyperkalemia	50 mg/kg SC,IM
Dexamethasone	Glucocorticoid with anti-inflammatory properties, gluconeogenetic, and membrane-stabilizing effect. Has not been found to result in improved neurologic recovery or have other positive effects on post-arrest outcome. Thus, its use is not recommended, except in ferrets with collapse due to (suspected) insulinoma. May also be used to treat anaphylactic shock	0.5–2 mg/kg SC,IM,IV,IP
Diphenhydramine	Antihistaminergic drug; used to treat and/or prevent anaphylactic shock (consider using prior to e.g. vaccinations)	1–2 mg/kg PO,IM,IV,IO
Dobutamine	Sympathomimetic drug with primary actions on β1-receptors; used to treat hypotension due to poor cardiac contractility	1–15 μg/kg/min IV,IO
Dopamine	Sympathomimetic drug; used to treat hypotension due to poor cardiac contractility or vasodilatation	1–10 μg/kg/min IV,IO
Doxapram	Respiratory stimulant; stimulates ventilation by direct stimulation of carotid chemoreceptors and non-selective stimulation of CNS neurons. Particularly used in patients with respiratory arrest. Side effects can be significant (e.g. cardiac arrhythmias, muscle fasciculation, seizures), therefore its use should be limited to patients that cannot be intubated or otherwise allow control of ventilation	2–10 mg/kg IV,IO,IT,IC or sublingual
Dextrose	See glucose	PO
Epinephrine	α- and β-adrenergic agonist; peripheral vasoconstriction, increased aortic diastolic pressure. Use in case of ventricular fibrillation, asystole, and pulseless electrical activity (PEA); Initial resuscitation efforts should include a low dose of epinephrine to be administered; a high dose may be considered if continued resuscitation efforts are unsuccessful Effects may be diminished in hypoxic or acidotic patients	Low dose: 0.01–0.02 mg/kg SC,IM,IV, IO,IT,IC q3–5min High dose: 0.1–0.2 mg/kg SC,IM,IV,IO,IT,IC CRI: 0.05–5 μg/kg/min IV,IO

(Continued)

Mammals

Table 6.4 (Continued)

Drug	Indication(s)	Dosage and route of administration[a]
Fluids	Colloids, crystalloids, blood etc. Can be used alone or in combination to treat hypovolemia and shock **Crystalloids (isotonic, saline):** primarily used to restore blood volume and promote perfusion **Crystalloids (hypertonic):** treatment and/or prevention of cerebral edema; induces hypernatremia, with subsequent expansion of plasma volume due to passive movement of fluids into the vascular system **Colloids (e.g. hetastarch, dextran 70):** promote the rapid expansion of intravascular volume (smaller volumes needed compared to crystalloids) **Blood or blood products:** primarily used to treat (severe) anemia *Note 1:* Overzealous fluid administration should be avoided as this can result in fulminant, life-threatening pulmonary edema, and decreased myocardial perfusion. Fluids should be used conservatively in euvolemic patients. In addition, regular blood pressure monitoring is highly recommended *Note 2:* Hypertonic fluids should be used with caution to avoid cellular swelling and hypomyelinosis	Crystalloids, isotonic: max 10 ml/kg IV,IO in normovolemic patients Crystalloids, hypertonic: 2–4 ml/kg IV,IO Colloids: 2–5 ml/kg IV,IO
Flumazenil	Benzodiazepine antagonist; used to reverse the effects of benzodiazepines such as midazolam and diazepam	0.01–0.2 mg/kg IV,IO
Furosemide	Loop diuretic; may be used to treat pulmonary edema	1–4 mg/kg SC,IM,IV,IO
Glucose	Used in patients with hypoglycemia and/or hyperkalemia *Note:* Caution is warranted when administering glucose as hyperglycemia has been associated with increased risk for post-ischemic brain damage and decreased neurologic recovery. Preferably reserved for patients highly suspected of or diagnosed with hypoglycemia	50% diluted 1:1 with saline: 0.25–1 ml/kg IV,IO In patients with suspected hypoglycemia, sublingual administration of a few drops of 50% dextrose may also be considered
Glycopyrrolate	Muscarinic receptor (M3) antagonist with anticholinergic effects; can be used to decrease bronchial secretions and increase heart rate (particularly in rabbits with atropinesterase activity – onset of action is seen following 30–45 seconds)	0.01–0.02 mg/kg SC,IM,IV,IO
Lidocaine	Local anesthetic and (class 1b) anti-arrhythmic drug; prevents the influx of sodium into the cell, thereby functioning as a membrane stabilizer and blocking the generation or conduction of action potentials. Used primarily to treat post-resuscitation ventricular arrhythmias if amiodarone is unavailable *Note 1:* Increases the defibrillation threshold and should therefore be avoided if defibrillation is possible *Note 2:* Overdose results in CNS effects including excitement, tremors, and collapse	2–8 mg/kg (preferably use lower dose) SC,IM,IV,IO,IT
Magnesium sulfate	Mineral supplement; may be useful in refractory ventricular tachycardia and/or in the treatment of patients with concurrent hypomagnesemia and hypocalcemia	0.2 mEq/kg SC,IM,IV,IO

Table 6.4 (Continued)

Drug	Indication(s)	Dosage and route of administration[a]
Mannitol	Highly potent osmotic diuretic; induces reflex vasoconstriction in cerebral vessels and improves blood viscosity; used primarily in the treatment and/or prevention of cerebral edema or patients with increased intracranial pressure (particularly in patients with neurologic deficits in post-resuscitation phase). Osmotic effects can be observed approximately 15–20 min following administration *Note 1:* Intermittent administration is preferred over continuous administration to avoid increased permeability of the blood–brain barrier *Note 2:* Regular monitoring of serum osmolality is recommended as increased osmolality may increase the risk for acute renal failure	0.5–1.5 g/kg IV,IO over 20 min q8h
Naloxone	Opiate antagonist; used to reverse the effects of opioid medications such as fentanyl and morphine	0.02–0.05 mg/kg SC,IM,IV,IO,IT
Prednisolone	Glucocorticoid with anti-inflammatory properties, gluconeogenic, and membrane-stabilizing effect. Has not been found to result in improved neurologic recovery or have other positive effects on post-arrest outcome. As a result, its use is not recommended, except in ferrets with collapse due to (suspected) insulinoma. May also be used to treat anaphylactic shock	1–2 mg/kg PO,SC,IM 10–20 mg/kg IV (for treatment of anaphylactic shock)
Potassium chloride	Mineral supplement; used in the treatment of hypokalemia (e.g. in patients with diuretic therapy, diarrhea and/or alkalosis) *Note:* Avoid administration rates > 0.5 mEq/kg/min (separate infusion may be needed in patients which require rapid fluid administration). ECG monitoring during administration is highly recommended to prevent overdosing	<0.5 mEq/kg/min IV,IO
Sodium bicarbonate ($NaHCO_3$)	Crystalline salt; its use can be considered in patients with severe pre-existing metabolic acidosis, extreme hyperkalemia, calcium channel blocker overdose, prolonged CPCR (>10 min), and/or in case of significant bicarbonate loss (e.g. via kidney or GI tract). *Note:* Patients suffering from lactic acidosis secondary to lack of perfusion are best treated by the restoration of blood flow. If possible, acid–base status should be evaluated prior to utilizing $NaHCO_3$	0.5–1 mEq/kg IV,IO q10min Calculation of exact amount: mEq = BW (kg) × 0.3 × deficit; provide ½ deficit initially and re-evaluate
Vasopressin	Non-adrenergic vasopressor. Induces pronounced vasoconstriction through direct stimulation of vasopressin (V1) receptors. Use in case of ventricular fibrillation, asystole, or PEA. Preferred option for patients with metabolic acidosis or hypoxia. May be followed by administration of epinephrine	0.1–0.8 U/kg IV,IO,IT q3–5min CRI: 0.01–0.04 U/kg/min IV,IO
Yohimbine	α2-adrenergic antagonist. Reversal of xylazine anesthesia	0.2 mg/kg SC,IM

IC, intracardiac; IM, intramuscular; IO, intraosseous; IP, intraperitoneal; IT, intratracheal; IV, intravenous; PO, per os; SC, subcutaneous; CRI, constant rate infusion; CNS, Central nervous system.

[a] When using the intratracheal route, doubling of the dose is recommended.

Aside from $ETCO_2$ measurements, continued monitoring of the patient's ECG is essential as this enables the identification and treatment of the different arrest rhythms (see Section "Electrocardiography"). Moreover, blood gas analysis can provide information on peripheral circulation. During CPCR, the use of venous blood gases is recommended over the use of arterial blood gases, as these will reveal the presence of metabolic acidosis during CPCR, thereby providing a better representation of the oxygenation and acid–base status of peripheral tissues. Blood from the jugular vein may be used as an indicator of cerebral oxygenation and extraction. Collected blood can also be used to evaluate other biochemical parameters (e.g. glucose, potassium, and calcium) which may help to guide further therapy.

Effective CPCR strives to achieve the following goals:

- $ETCO_2 \geq 30$–40 mmHg (≥ 4–5.3%) and normoxia
- Mean (direct) arterial blood pressure ≥ 50 mmHg (*Note:* In small mammals, measurements will mostly be feasible in rabbits)
- Normal acid–base status
- Normal glucose and electrolytes (K^+, Na^+, and Ca^{2+})

Failure to achieve these goals within a reasonable time frame (i.e. 15–20 minutes) will indicate a poor prognosis for recovery in humans, dogs, and cats. Moreover, a coma that lasts for more than four hours carries a poor prognosis for full neurologic recovery (whereas this is not necessarily the case if the animal fails to regain consciousness within the first few hours following ROSC). In patients that do not regain consciousness after CPCR, brain stem reflexes, including the pupillary light reflex (PLR),[2] corneal reflex, withdrawal response to pain and motor responses, are considered to provide important prognostic information. Should these (and in particular the PLR) responses be absent for more than 24 hours following ROSC, chances of successful neurologic recovery will be slim.

Post-arrest Care

Patients that have sustained CPA are at increased risk for recurrence of CPA, particularly if the primary cause has not been identified. Post-resuscitative care is initially directed to stabilize the patient, followed by therapy to treat or prevent complications and/or the underlying disease. Close monitoring of the patient is essential, particularly during the first 24–48 hours. This includes both regular assessments of the patient's clinical parameters as well as monitoring of parameters such as ECG, blood pressure, pulse oximetry, $ETCO_2$, and venous blood gases (if possible). Diagnostic work-up is aimed at identifying (and treating) the potential underlying causes for the arrest to help prevent re-arrest as well as establish a prognosis and proper treatment regimen for the patient.

Depending on the abnormalities found, specific treatments may be initiated. For example, the use of dopamine, dobutamine, vasopressin, or epinephrine may be warranted in case of (suspected) poor cardiac output, whereas mannitol (±furosemide) is the preferred treatment in case of cerebral edema. Drug therapy is also warranted in case of cardiac arrhythmias (e.g. lidocaine or amiodarone for persistent ventricular tachycardia; atropine for bradycardia). In addition, ventilatory support (including supplemental oxygen) or active warming should be considered in patients with respiratory depression or hypothermia, respectively. Particularly in the small mammal patients, the provision of adequate nutritional support is essential to a good recovery (see Chapter 8).

Euthanasia

Euthanasia (derived from the Greek terms "eu" [i.e. good] and "thanatos" [i.e. death]) is the common term used to describe the ending of a life in such a way that pain and distress are minimized. According to AVMA guidelines on euthanasia, the primary duties of a veterinarian in this process are to the following:

1) induce death when it is a matter of welfare and/or in the animal's best interest; and
2) use humane techniques that result in as fast, painless, and distress-free induction of death as possible.

Indications

In accordance with recommendations for other companion animals, the decision to euthanize any patient should primarily be based on the (long-term) expectations regarding the animal's welfare and quality of life. Insurmountable suffering is likely occurring in animals suffering from a chronically debilitating disease, such as chronic renal or respiratory disease, cardiomyopathies, (progressive) neurologic disease, or neoplastic conditions. Euthanasia may also be considered in animals suffering from diseases that will result in recurrent pain and/or distress (e.g. dental disease in species with hypsodont teeth and molars such as rabbits, guinea pigs, chinchillas, and degus) and/or acute diseases that induce great pain and/or severe discomfort to the animal (e.g. severe trauma, spinal injuries).

Technique

Euthanasia methods are comparable to those in the other companion animals. If an IV or IO catheter is in place/can be placed (see Chapter 4), this route may be elected for administering the euthanasia solution, as well as the anesthetic agents to induce sedation or general anesthesia prior to euthanasia.

In case vascular access is not achievable, the intracardiac, intrathoracic, intrarenal, intrahepatic, and/or intraperitoneal routes may be elected. Of these, the intraperitoneal

2 PLR can be transiently lost and reappear during the first six hours post-ROSC. Thus, caution is warranted when interpreting results from this test. In addition, resuscitation drugs such as atropine and epinephrine can affect the pupillary diameter (although this does not have to interfere with PLR).

Table 6.5 Common euthanasia drugs in small mammals.

Drug	Dosage
Pentobarbitone	0.2–1 ml/kg or 150 mg/kg IV, IO, IC; 2–3× recommended dose when using the IP or intrathoracic route
Potassium chloride	1–2 mmol/kg IV, IO, or IC; general anesthesia required prior to administration
Propofol	Given to effect, IV or IO
T61 (a mixture of embutramide, mebezonium iodine, tetracaine hydrochloride)	0.3 ml/kg IV, IO, IP, IC, intrathoracic, intrarenal, or intrahepatic following sedation or anesthesia
Thiopentone	Given to effect, IV or IO

IC, intracardiac; IO, intraosseous; IP, intraperitoneal; IV, intravenous.

route will usually take longer to take effect. For any of these routes, the patient should be adequately sedated or anesthetized to minimize stress, pain, and discomfort.

Drugs

Any of the available euthanasia solutions that are used for euthanasia of companion animals are usable in small mammal patients as well. Dependent on national legislation, commonly used euthanasia agents include those containing pentobarbitone, potassium chloride or a mixture of embutramide, mebezonium iodide, and tetracaine hydrochloride (e.g. T61). Dosages are similar to those described in other species (see Table 6.5).

Necropsy

The post-mortem examination procedure in small mammals is like that of other species and consists of a gross post-mortem examination followed by a cytological and histopathological examination and – dependent on the findings – other diagnostic tests such as bacteriologic culture, parasitology, virology, and/or polymerase chain reaction (PCR) for specific pathogens. Having a pre-printed checklist of findings is useful to ensure that all necessary information is collected. Moreover, any unusual findings or abnormalities can be photographed for additional documentation.

References

1 Brodbelt, D.C. (2006). The confidential enquiry into perioperative small animal fatalities. Doctoral dissertation. Royal Veterinary College, University of London.

2 Brodbelt, D.C., Blissitt, K.J., Hammond, R.A. et al. (2008). The risk of death: the confidential enquiry into perioperative small animal fatalities. *Vet. Anaesth. Analg.* 35 (5): 365–373.

Further Reading

Adams, J.G. (2014). Cardiopulmonary cerebral resuscitation (CPCR). In: Veterinary Anaesthesia, 11e. Elsevier Health Sciences (eds. K.W. Clarke and C.M. Trim), 645–669. St. Louis, MO: Elsevier.

Boller, M., Kellett-Gregory, L., Shofer, F.S., and Rishniw, M. (2010). The clinical practice of CPCR in small animals: an internet-based survey. *J. Vet. Emerg. Crit. Care* 20 (6): 558–570.

Boller, M. and Fletcher, D.J. (2012). RECOVER evidence and knowledge gap analysis on veterinary CPR. Part 1: evidence analysis and consensus process: collaborative path toward small animal CPR guidelines. *J. Vet. Emerg. Crit. Care* 22 (s1): S4–S12.

Brainard, B.M., Boller, M., and Fletcher, D.J. (2012a). RECOVER evidence and knowledge gap analysis on veterinary CPR. Part 5: Monitoring. *J. Vet. Emerg. Crit. Care* 22 (s1): S65–S84.

Brainard, B.M., Haskins, S.C., Hopper, K. et al. (2012b). RECOVER evidence and knowledge gap analysis on veterinary CPR. Part 7: Clinical guidelines. *J. Vet. Emerg. Crit. Care* 22 (s1): S102–S131.

Briscoe, J.A. and Syring, R. (2004). Techniques for emergency airway and vascular access in special species. *Semin. Avian Exot. Pet Med.* 13 (3): 118–131.

Brodbelt, D.C. (2009). Perioperative mortality in small animal anaesthesia. *Vet. J.* 182 (2): 152–161.

Buckley, G.J., DeCubellis, J., Sharp, C.R., and Rozanski, E.A. (2011). Cardiopulmonary resuscitation in hospitalized rabbits: 15 cases. *J. Exot. Pet Med.* 20 (1): 46–50.

Cole, S.G., Otto, C.M., and Hughes, D. (2002). Cardiopulmonary cerebral resuscitation in small animals–a clinical practice review. Part 1. *J. Vet. Emerg. Crit. Care* 12 (4): 261–267.

Cole, S.G., Otto, C.M., and Hughes, D. (2003). Cardiopulmonary cerebral resuscitation in small animals – a clinical practice review. Part II. *J. Vet. Emerg. Crit. Care* 13 (1): 13–23.

Costello, M.F. (2004). Principles of cardiopulmonary cerebral resuscitation in special species. *Semin. Avian Exot. Pet Med.* 13 (3): 132–141.

Di Girolamo, N., Toth, G., and Selleri, P. (2016). Prognostic value of rectal temperature at hospital admission in client-owned rabbits. *J. Am. Vet. Med. Assoc.* 248 (3): 288–297.

Feldman, D.B. and Seely, J.C. (1988). Necropsy Guide: Rodents and the Rabbit. CRC Press.

Fernandez, C.M., Peyton, J.L., Miller, M. et al. (2013). Successful cardiopulmonary resuscitation following cardiopulmonary arrest in a geriatric chinchilla. *J. Vet. Emerg. Crit. Care* 23 (6): 657–662.

Hildreth, C.D. (2016). Preparing the small animal hospital for avian and exotic animal emergencies. *Vet. Clin. North Am. Exot. Anim. Pract.* 19 (2): 325–345.

Hofmeister, E.H., Brainard, B.M., Egger, C.M., and Kang, S. (2009). Prognostic indicators for dogs and cats with cardiopulmonary arrest treated by cardiopulmonary cerebral resuscitation at a university teaching hospital. *J. Am. Vet. Med. Assoc.* 235 (1): 50–57.

Hopper, K., Epstein, S.E., Fletcher, D.J., and Boller, M. (2012). RECOVER evidence and knowledge gap analysis on veterinary CPR. Part 3: Basic life support. *J. Vet. Emerg. Crit. Care* 22 (s1): S26–S43.

Huynh, M., Boyeaux, A., and Pignon, C. (2016). Assessment and care of the critically ill rabbit. *Vet. Clin. North Am. Exot. Anim. Pract.* 19 (2): 379–409.

Johnson-Delaney, C.A. (2005). Ferret cardiopulmonary resuscitation. *Semin. Avian Exot. Pet Med.* 14 (2): 135–142.

Leary, S., Underwood, W., Anthony, R. et al. (2013). AVMA Guidelines for the Euthanasia of Animals: 2013 Edition. American Veterinary Medical Association.

Lee, S.K., Vaagenes, P., Safar, P. et al. (1989). Effect of cardiac arrest time on cortical cerebral blood flow during subsequent standard external cardiopulmonary resuscitation in rabbits. *Resuscitation* 17 (2): 105–117.

Lichtenberger, M. (2007). Shock and cardiopulmonary-cerebral resuscitation in small mammals and birds. *Vet. Clin. North Am. Exot. Anim. Pract.* 10 (2): 275–291.

Lichtenberger, M. and Ko, J. (2007). Critical care monitoring. *Vet. Clin. North Am. Exot. Anim. Pract.* 10 (2): 317–344.

Lichtenberger, M. and Lennox, A.M. (2012). Critical care of the exotic companion mammal (with a focus on herbivorous species): the first twenty-four hours. *J. Exot. Pet Med.* 21 (4): 284–292.

Lyon, A.R., Rees, P.S., Prasad, S. et al. (2008). Stress (Takotsubo) cardiomyopathy – a novel pathophysiological hypothesis to explain catecholamine-induced acute myocardial stunning. *Nat. Clin. Pract. Cardiovasc. Med.* 5 (1): 22–29.

McIntyre, R.L., Hopper, K., and Epstein, S.E. (2014). Assessment of cardiopulmonary resuscitation in 121 dogs and 30 cats at a university teaching hospital (2009–2012). *J. Vet. Emerg. Crit. Care* 24 (6): 693–704.

McLaughlin, A. and Strunk, A. (2016). Common emergencies in small rodents, hedgehogs, and sugar gliders. *Vet. Clin. North Am. Exot. Anim. Pract.* 19 (2): 465–499.

McMichael, M., Herring, J., Fletcher, D.J., and Boller, M. (2012). RECOVER evidence and knowledge gap analysis on veterinary CPR. Part 2: preparedness and prevention. *J. Vet. Emerg. Crit. Care* 22 (s1): S13–S25.

Onuma, M., Ono, S., Ishida, T. et al. (2009). Mortality rate related to anesthesia-associated complications in 111 ferrets. *Jpn. J. Vet. Anesth. Surg.* 40 (4): 85–88.

Peberdy, M.A., Kaye, W., Ornato, J.P. et al. (2003). Cardiopulmonary resuscitation of adults in the hospital: a report of 14 720 cardiac arrests from the National Registry of Cardiopulmonary Resuscitation. *Resuscitation* 58 (3): 297–308.

Plunkett, S.J. and McMichael, M. (2008). Cardiopulmonary resuscitation in small animal medicine: an update. *J. Vet. Intern. Med.* 22 (1): 9–25.

Rozanski, E.A., Rush, J.E., Buckley, G.J. et al. (2012). RECOVER evidence and knowledge gap analysis on veterinary CPR. Part 4: advanced life support. *J. Vet. Emerg. Crit. Care* 22 (s1): S44–S64.

Sandroni, C., Nolan, J., Cavallaro, F., and Antonelli, M. (2007). In-hospital cardiac arrest: incidence, prognosis and possible measures to improve survival. *Intensive Care Med.* 33 (2): 237–245.

Smarick, S.D., Haskins, S.C., Boller, M., and Fletcher, D.J. (2012). RECOVER evidence and knowledge gap analysis on veterinary CPR. Part 6: post-cardiac arrest care. *J. Vet. Emerg. Crit. Care* 22 (s1): S85–S101.

Varga, M. (2014). Post-mortem examination of rabbits. In: Textbook of Rabbit Medicine, 2e, 472–482. St Louis, MO: Elsevier.

Waldrop, J.E., Rozanski, E.A., Swanke, E.D. et al. (2004). Causes of cardiopulmonary arrest, resuscitation management, and functional outcome in dogs and cats surviving cardiopulmonary arrest. *J. Vet. Emerg. Crit. Care* 14 (1): 22–29.

7

Analgesia, Anesthesia, and Monitoring

Yvonne R.A. van Zeeland and Nico J. Schoemaker

Division of Zoological Medicine, Department of Clinical Sciences, Faculty of Veterinary Medicine, Utrecht University, The Netherlands

CONTENTS

Injection Sites

The injection sites and techniques in small mammals are identical to those in other mammals. Administration of drugs by the intramuscular (IM), intraperitoneal (IP), or subcutaneous (SC) route is relatively straightforward to accomplish in most species. Dependent on the route selected, however, the rate of drug absorption, and thereby the effect, may vary. The subcutaneous and intramuscular routes are generally preferred, as the intraperitoneal route has a relatively high failure rate.

Subcutaneous

The loose skin located on the dorsum of rabbits, guinea pigs, chinchillas, and ferrets is most ideal to be used for subcutaneous (SC) injections (Figure 7.1). As ferrets may react painfully to these injections, distracting them with a (small amount of) preferred liquid food should be attempted. However, adequate restraint may be needed to prevent it from attempting to bite. In ferrets, the neck area is best avoided as the skin in this region is at least twice as thick compared to that of the dorsum. In small rodents, SC injections can be placed from cranial to caudal in the scruff (Figure 7.2).

Intramuscular

Intramuscular (IM) injections can be administered into the large lumbar muscles on either side of the spine, just cranial to the pelvis (Figure 7.3). Alternatively, the quadriceps muscles may be used. To prevent damage to the sciatic nerve that runs

1 Analgesia, amnesia, muscle relaxation, and abolition of autonomic reflexes with maintenance of homeostasis.

2 Lower doses can mainly be achieved when adding analgesic and/or other injectable or inhalant anesthetics to the protocol (i.e. balanced anesthesia).

Exotic Animal Emergency and Critical Care Medicine, First Edition. Edited by Jennifer E. Graham, Grayson A. Doss and Hugues Beaufrère.

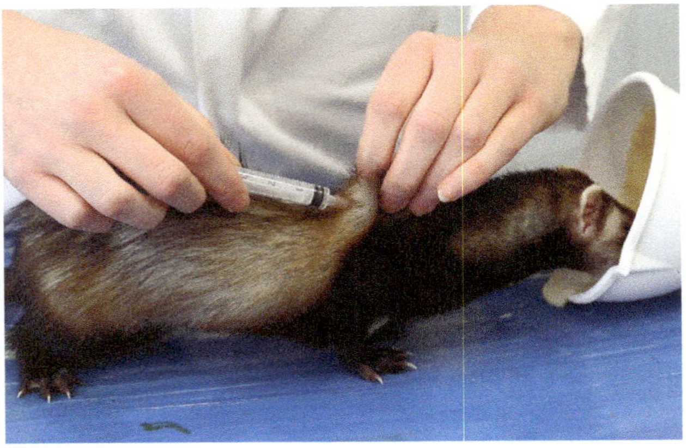

Figure 7.1 (Same figure as Figure 2.2) Placement of a subcutaneous injection in ferrets is best performed over the thorax as they have ample subcutaneous space and the skin is much thinner compared to that of the neck.

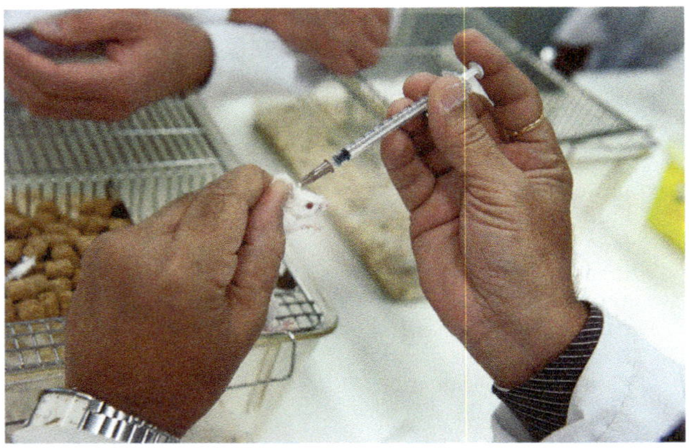

Figure 7.2 Subcutaneous injections in mice are placed from cranial to caudal in the scruff. *Source:* Courtesy Thomas Dobber, UMC Utrecht, the Netherlands.

along the caudal portion of the leg, the injection is best placed into the cranial aspect of the hind leg. Intramuscular injections may be painful, potentially even more so in small rodents due to the relatively small size of their muscles. In rabbits, IM administration of ketamine-xylazine combinations for anesthesia can result in myonecrosis, vasculitis, myositis, and sciatic neuronal degeneration. Moreover, IM administration of ketamine–medetomidine combinations were found to provide little benefit over SC administration (i.e. onset of anesthesia was only two minutes delayed when using the SC route, but markedly less resistance was encountered). As such, the authors highly recommended the use of the SC over the IM route.

Intraperitoneal

Intraperitoneal (IP) injections are given in the left caudal quadrant of the abdomen. Preferably, the animal is held head down to decrease the risk of puncturing a vital organ.

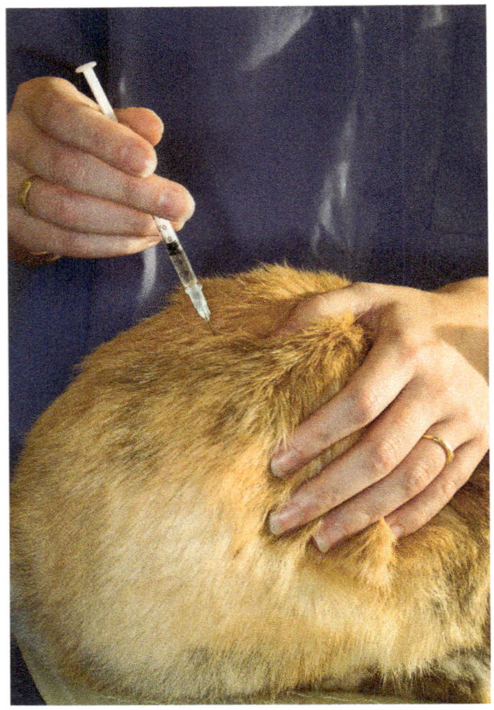

Figure 7.3 In rabbits, an intramuscular injection can be administered into the lumbar muscle just cranial to the pelvis.

In laboratory small rodents, the IP route is frequently used. However, accidental injections into the viscera, fat or other tissues may occur, leading to unreliable results or side-effects due to under- or overdosing, without the possibility to adjust the dose accordingly. It is therefore recommended to only use the IP route for drugs that carry a wide safety margin. In the larger small mammals, IP injections are rarely given.

Analgesia

Recognizing Pain/Indications

Assessing pain is difficult as individuals experience and express pain in a different manner. In prey species, such as rabbits and rodents, assessment of pain is often challenging as these species tend to hide pain to avoid predation. Lack of activity, burrow building, and decreased food and/or water consumption are nonspecific signs that may indicate pain. In addition, animals may sit in a hunched position or lay flat on the floor, hide in the back of the cage (facing away from the observer), show signs of aggression upon being approached, display less grooming activity, and/or salivate excessively. Animals may also vocalize when in pain, especially when being handled.

Since the early 1990s, facial expression has been used for the assessment of pain in people and animals. Mice were the first species in which facial expressions in response to pain were assessed, leading to the development of a so-called facial grimace scale. This scale assesses pain by evaluating five facial features, i.e. orbital tightening, cheek flattening, nose bulging (including downwards movement of the nose tip), whisker change (i.e. positioned backward against the cheeks), and rotation and flattening of the ears against the head. A grimace scale based on similar characteristics later followed for rats, rabbits, and ferrets (see References for further information).

Principles of Analgesia

Different classes of analgesics can be used to prevent, reduce or eliminate the sensation of pain at different stages. This principle lies at the basis of multimodal pain management. The advantage of this approach is the combined use of analgesic drugs results in an additive and/or synergistic effect, while the risk for adverse side-effects is reduced as lower doses of the individual drugs are needed. Where possible, preemptive analgesia, i.e. administering pain medication before the occurrence of pain, should be considered to increase the efficacy of analgesic therapy.

Drug Classes

Different classes of analgesics exist, each exerting their own action on the peripheral and central nervous systems. The most commonly used analgesics include non-steroidal anti-inflammatory drugs (NSAIDs), opioids, and local anesthetics.

Non-steroidal Anti-Inflammatory Drugs

NSAIDs exert an inhibitory action on cyclo-oxygenase 1 and 2 (COX-1 and COX-2), the enzymes responsible for prostaglandin production which cause the pyrexia and pain associated with inflammation. However, prostaglandins also regulate renal and gastrointestinal mucosal perfusion. As a result, caution is warranted when using NSAIDs, particularly long term, as the reduced perfusion that results from lowered prostaglandin synthesis may increase the risk for renal or gastrointestinal disorders (i.e. renal papillary necrosis, gastric ulcers). Nevertheless, rather than avoiding the use of NSAIDs out of fear of potential side effects, additional therapies addressing the potential side effects should be considered, as chronic pain can negatively influence both the recovery and welfare of the patient. Additional therapies may include the use of supplemental fluid therapy to ensure adequate hydration as well as the use of proton-pump inhibitors/antacids (e.g. ranitidine, omeprazole) or gastric protectants (e.g. sucralfate) to help protect the gastrointestinal mucosa.

Meloxicam and carprofen, both potent COX-2 inhibitors, are the most frequently used NSAIDs in small mammals. Since these drugs supposedly have less effect on the gastrointestinal mucosa and kidney function, they are generally considered safer to use than flunixin-meglumine or ketoprofen. Dosages for commonly used NSAIDs can be found in Table 7.1.

Opioids

Opioids are used for the management of moderate to severe visceral pain and exert their analgesic effects by binding to μ-, κ-, and/or δ-opioid receptors. Side effects include sedation, respiratory depression, and reduced gastrointestinal motility. The latter has not been seen when using buprenorphine in rabbits, therefore allowing this drug to be used safely in animals with gastric stasis. Moreover, side-effects as seen following opioid use can also occur as a sequela to pain itself, therefore warranting a carefully weighed decision and patient evaluation prior to deciding to withhold opioids.

Buprenorphine is a potent μ-opioid receptor agonist, but reportedly has fewer side effects than some of the other opioids. Profound sedation can be seen following doses greater than 20 μg/kg, particularly in ferrets. Duration of action will generally vary between 6 and 12 hours. For optimal functionality, the analgesic and sedative effects need to be balanced carefully, which requires regular patient assessment and according dose adjustment. In rodents, higher dosages (0.2 mg/kg) are deemed necessary (Table 7.2). Sustained-release formulations can be

Table 7.1 Dosages, routes of administration, and dose intervals of NSAIDs in small mammals.

	Dose (mg/kg), Route, Interval			
Drug	**Rabbit**	**Ferret**	**Guinea pig**	**Rodents**
Carprofen	2–4 mg/kg PO, SC q12–24h	1–4 mg/kg PO, SC q12–24h	4 mg/kg PO, SC q12–24h	5–10 mg/kg PO, SC q12–24h
Meloxicam	0.3–1.5 mg/kg SC, PO, IV q24h	0.1–0.2 mg/kg SC, PO, IV q12–24h	1–2 mg/kg SC, PO, IV q24h	1–5 mg/kg SC, PO, IV q12–24h
Ketoprofen		1–5 mg/kg SC, IM, IV q24h		

Table 7.2 Dosages, routes of administration, and dose intervals of opioids in small mammals.

	Dose (mg/kg), Route, Interval			
Drug	**Rabbit**	**Ferret**	**Guinea pig**	**Rodents**
Buprenorphine	0.02–0.1 mg/kg SC, IM, IV q6–12h	0.01–0.05 mg/kg SC, IM, IV q6–12h	0.2 mg/kg SC, IM, IV q8–12h	0.2 mg/kg SC, IM, IV q12h
Butorphanol	0.1–0.5 mg/kg SC, IM, IV q2h	0.05–0.5 mg/kg SC, IM, IV q 2–12h	1–2 mg/kg SC, IM, IV q4h	1–2 mg/kg SC, IM, IV q4h
Fentanyl – fluanisone (Hypnorm: 0.315 and 10 mg/ml, respectively)	0.5 ml/kg		1 ml/kg	0.3–0.4 ml/kg
Hydromorphone		0.1–0.2 mg/kg SC, IM, IV		
Oxymorphone	0.1–0.3 mg/kg SC, IM, IV q3-4h	0.05–0.2 mg/kg SC, IM, IV q6-8h	0.2–0.5 mg/kg SC, IM, IV	0.2–0.5 mg/kg SC, IM, IV
Morphine	2–5 mg/kg SC, IM q3-4h	0.05–5 mg/kg SC, IM q2-6h	2–5 mg/kg SC, IM q4h	2–5 mg/kg SC, IM q4h
Tramadol	> 10 mg/kg PO q12–24h	10 mg/kg PO q24h		5–80 mg/kg PO

considered, which have shown effectiveness for up to 12 hours and three days in mice and rats, respectively.

Butorphanol is assumed to have agonistic effects on μ-, δ-, and κ-opioid receptors, with the highest affinity for the κ-opioid receptor. Although its analgesic effects are similar to buprenorphine, it has greater sedative effects and potentially induces more respiratory depression. Moreover, its analgesic effects last shorter than those of buprenorphine. Nevertheless, in rodent species, it should be considered as many species (including rats, mice, and guinea pigs) have been found to possess a high number of κ-opioid receptors in their brain.

Morphine, a μ-opioid receptor agonist, may result in nausea and vomiting in ferrets when administering a dose within the therapeutic range. The systemic use should therefore be done with caution in ferrets. Similarly, parenteral use of morphine should be avoided in rabbits, as morphine (10 mg/kg IM) significantly decreases GI-transit times. Epidural injections (0.1 mg/kg), on the other hand, can result in effective analgesia with limited systemic side effects. This route may thus be considered and will provide effective perioperative analgesia in rabbits or ferrets for up to 12–24 hours.

Hydromorphone and oxymorphone, both μ-opioid receptor agonists, have been used in rabbits and ferrets and have fewer side effects compared to morphine. Anecdotally, doses similar or slightly higher than those recommended for dogs and cats seemingly are effective and well-tolerated in small mammals.

Fentanyl, a short-acting and highly potent μ-opioid receptor agonist, provides excellent analgesia, and is often combined with other anesthetic agents for balanced, multi-modal anesthesia. The combination with fluanisone (commercially available as Hypnorm®) is probably the most well-known and has been widely recommended for use in mice, rats, guinea pigs, and rabbits. Respiratory depression is a potential but serious side effect, thereby warranting frequent assessment of the patient's ventilatory status and recommending against its use if no manual or mechanically assisted ventilation can be achieved. Fentanyl is also well-known for use as constant rate infusion (CRI) in rabbits and ferrets, both peri- and post-operatively, and can also be used topically, similar to dogs and cats. In rabbits, for example, application of a 25 mg/h fentanyl patch resulted in plasma concentrations within the therapeutic range for people for at least 72 hours. However, hair regrowth quickly impeded absorption of the drug.

Tramadol is a synthetic 4-phenyl-piperidine analog of codeine that exerts effects on the μ-opioid receptor as well as the serotoninergic, catecholaminergic, and GABA-systems. It is frequently used to treat mild to moderate pain in humans, dogs, and cats. In small mammals, its use is controversial, with little to no existent information on its pharmacokinetic properties or palatability. In rabbits, effective analgesia has anecdotally been reported using dosages of 6–12 mg/kg q12–24h. However, doses of 11 mg/kg did not result in plasma concentrations within the analgesic range for humans. In addition, palatability has been found to be problematic. In ferrets, doses of 5 and 10 mg/kg resulted in excitatory reactions with no reduction or abolishment of responses to a toe pinch. In chinchillas, dosages up to 20 mg/kg were not found to exert any analgesic effect, whereas higher dosages (40 mg/kg) resulted in severe, transient neurologic side effects (i.e. epileptic seizures). In rats,

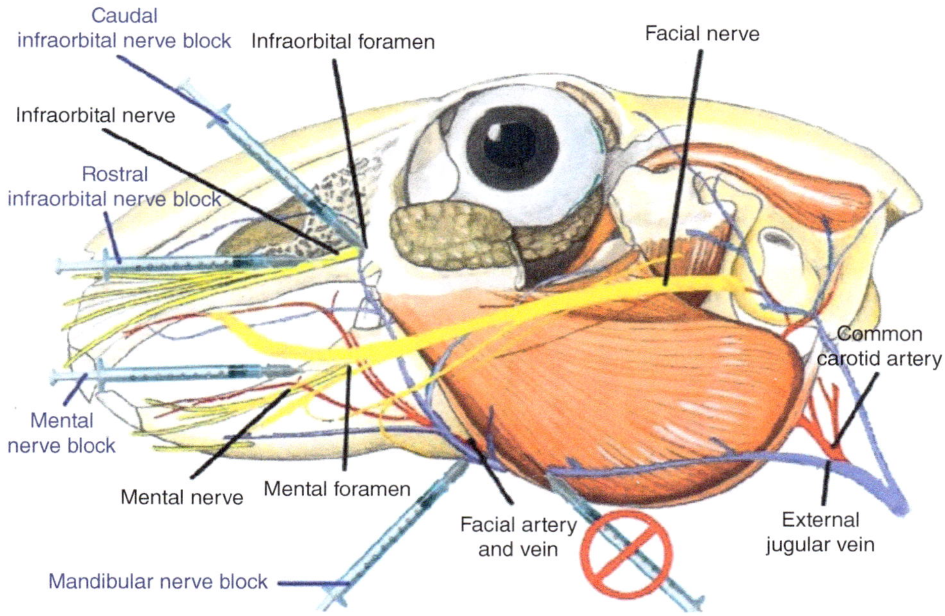

Figure 7.4 Injection sites for placement of dental blocks in rabbits. *Source:* Lennox [2]. © 2008, Elsevier.

an obvious gender difference in efficacy has been observed, with dosages of 40 mg/kg inducing an analgesic effect similar to that of buprenorphine (30 µg/kg) in male rats, whereas, in the female rats, the same effect could be achieved following dosages of 30 mg/kg. In mice, this gender difference was also observed, with dosages of 80 mg/kg resulting in adequate post-operative analgesia in female mice, but lacking effect in the male individuals.

Local Anesthetics (Local Blocks)

Local anesthetics, which reversibly block transmission of nociceptive signals from nerve endings to the central nerve system, can provide a valuable addition to any multimodal anesthetic protocol. Bupivacaine and lidocaine are most commonly used, with lidocaine exerting a faster onset of action (i.e. within three minutes following administration), but of much shorter duration than that of bupivacaine (of which effects may last for up to five hours). Moreover, bupivacaine has twice the potency of lidocaine. The drugs' effects are highly predictable and minimally affect the animal's systemic physiology, if given in the proper dose. Exceeding the maximum dose (i.e. 1–2 mg/kg) can lead to severe systemic complications, including fatal cardiac arrest.

Local anesthetics can be administered through the topical, intra-articular, intravenous, and epidural route to provide local or regional anesthesia. Other options include local infiltration into the skin and subcutis, and incisional line, ring, or splash blocks. Following administration, it is advised to wait at least five minutes for the local anesthetic to be fully effective.

In rabbits and rodents, local anesthetics are particularly useful for dental procedures and five different nerve blocks have been described, i.e. infraorbital, mental, mandibular, maxillary, and palatine nerve block (Figure 7.4; see also Lichtenberger and Ko [1]). Intra-testicular blocks can be used during orchiectomy. However, the authors highly recommend sedating the animal prior to injecting anything in a testicle.

Sciatic and femoral nerve blocks with lidocaine (1 mg/kg) and bupivacaine (0.5 mg/kg) have been successfully used during femoral fracture repair in rabbits and guinea pigs, whereas lumbosacral epidural blocks with lidocaine (4 mg/kg) or bupivacaine (1 mg/kg) can be considered in rabbits or ferrets to accomplish a sensory and motor block of the hindquarters for up to 40 minutes. Techniques are similar to those described for other companion animals.

Other Drugs

Alpha-2 adrenergic antagonists (e.g. medetomidine and dexmedetomidine) possess analgesic properties. However, as these drugs can severely impact the cardiovascular system, they are deemed unsuitable for severely ill and/or debilitated patients. Similarly, caution is warranted in elderly patients and those with cardiac compromise, despite the suggestion that heart rate and cardiac output will not be affected by low doses, such as those used during CRI.

Ketamine, a NMDA (*N*-methyl-D-aspartate) receptor antagonist, has profound sedative effects, and can therefore not be used as a stand-alone analgesic, but may have added value during anesthesia (e.g. combined with fentanyl for CRI) due to its anesthetic sparing effects. Ketamine CRI can also be considered as adjunct analgesia during the postoperative period, during which it can be combined with opioids or other analgesics.

Sedation

Indications

Many of the procedures performed by veterinarians (e.g. blood or urine sampling, fine needle aspiration, diagnostic imaging, nail clipping, or grooming) may be stressful for the smaller mammals. Previously, manual restraint (e.g. scruffing, towel restraint, or so-called "hypnosis") was common practice to enable these procedures. However, as studies have shown that excessive amounts of glucocorticoids may be released during such restraint, sedation has nowadays replaced many of these techniques.

Commonly Used Sedatives and Tranquilizers

Benzodiazepines (e.g. diazepam, midazolam) are the most commonly used sedatives in small mammals. Midazolam in particular has gained tremendous popularity, because of its efficacy and limited risk of cardiorespiratory side effects, making this drug relatively safe to use, even in critically ill animals. In patients with severe respiratory distress, midazolam aids in alleviating hypoxia-induced anxiety, leading to deeper and slower breaths and increased respiratory efficiency. Dependent on the dose, midazolam (0.2–1 mg/kg) will induce mild to moderate sedation in rabbits, rodents, and ferrets that lasts up to one hour, which is sufficient for most non-invasive procedures. Midazolam is also frequently used in combination with butorphanol, which potentiates its sedative effects and provides additional analgesia. Due to their synergistic effects, lower dosages are needed (0.1–0.3 mg/kg, each).

Other drugs that can be used to sedate or tranquilize small mammals include phenothiazine derivatives (e.g. acepromazine, chlorpromazine) and α2-adrenergic agonists (xylazine, medetomidine, dexmedetomidine, to be used in lower doses). Phenothiazine derivatives should not be used in critical small mammal patients due to their vasodilatory effects. Detomidine gel has been used as a sedative in ferrets, with doses of $3\,mg/m^2$ (~0.3 mg/kg) enabling blood collection to be performed in one out of two animals.

Finally, alfaxalone is a neuroactive steroid that can be used for sedation, induction of anesthesia, and for total intravenous anesthesia. Respiratory depression/apnea can occur, particularly if given rapidly IV; therefore, SC and IM adminstration may be preferable. Using a lower dose in conjunction with other premedication drugs can help smooth patient recovery.

Risks and Benefits

Side effects of benzodiazepines, especially midazolam, pose little risk and are generally considered safe to use, even in critically ill small mammal patients. In case of overdosing, flumazenil may be used to antagonize the effects, but in the authors' opinion, this is rarely needed.

Medetomidine and dexmedetomidine can produce significant cardiovascular and respiratory depression. Close monitoring of the patient is therefore warranted. Atipamezole can be administered to reverse the actions of these drugs.

Anesthesia

Principles of Balanced Anesthesia

The term balanced anesthesia was introduced by Lundy in 1926, who suggested that a mixture of drugs and techniques (i.e. injectable and inhalant anesthetics; local and systemic analgesics) should be used to produce the different components of general anesthesia, to maximize effect but minimize the risk of adverse effects as dosages of the individual drugs can be lowered.

Indications

Anesthesia is indicated for any (surgical or other) procedure that can induce pain. In high-risk patients, sedation combined with local anesthesia can be considered for minor surgical procedures.

Pre-anesthetic Considerations

Patient Evaluation

To select the most appropriate form of anesthesia, an extensive history and physical examination should be performed to assess the patient's clinical condition (see Chapter 1). During the examination, special attention is given to commonly occurring, but frequently undetected, changes to the respiratory system. Especially in elderly ferrets, extra attention should be paid to the cardiac system. Moreover, the animal's weight should be obtained to allow for accurate dosing of drugs and fluids. Additional diagnostic work-up can be performed, if necessary.

Based on the findings from aforementioned exams and similar to dogs and cats, the patient is classified into one of five ASA-categories (i.e. ASA-I to ASA-V; Table 7.3) to help determine the risks associated with the procedure and establish whether and which stabilizing procedures and anesthetic protocol should be implemented.

Nutritional Status and Fasting

Withholding food and water for longer periods prior to anesthesia is not needed in rabbits and rodents as they are unable to vomit. However, in rabbits, guinea pigs, and chinchillas, removal of food for one hour prior to anesthesia will reduce the amount of food that is retained in their oral cavity. In guinea pigs, the authors also find it helpful to flush the

Table 7.3 ASA classification system based on clinical findings.

ASA class	Description
I	Normal, healthy patient
II	Patient with mild systemic disease, without functional limitations
III	Patient with moderate systemic disease, with functional limitations
IV	Patient with severe systemic disease that poses a constant threat to life
V	A moribund patient who is, with or without intervention, not expected to survive anesthesia and will likely die within 24 hours

oral cavity with water just prior to induction. A cotton swab can subsequently be used to remove any remaining food particles and ascertain that the oral cavity is clean.

In ferrets, fasting for approximately three to four hours is usually recommended to prevent hypoglycemic episodes in animals with an insulinoma. However, this may not lead to complete gastric emptying. Hence, longer fasting periods may be considered when an insulinoma is not suspected or diagnosed.

Preoxygenation

In all small mammals, especially those with (suspected) cardiac and/or respiratory disease, preoxygenation is recommended to improve oxygen saturation prior to surgery. Preoxygenation can usually be achieved by placing the animal in an infant incubator or oxygen cage while oxygen flows continuously. Alternatively, the cage or carrier can act as an oxygen cage by covering it in plastic in which small holes are made, and allowing oxygen to run freely into the carrier/cage. Sedation may also be considered, following which oxygen can be delivered through a face mask or tube held in front of the nose and mouth; ideally at no more than 2 cm from the nostrils (Figure 7.5).

Induction of Anesthesia

Premedication

As the pungent odors of gas anesthetics (isoflurane > sevoflurane) can be stressful to small mammal patients, mask induction without the use of additional premedication is no longer recommended. Aside from midazolam-butorphanol combinations (see Sedatives), the combination of fentanyl and fluanisone can be used, if available. The latter combination is primarily advantageous to use because of its vasodilatory effect which facilitates placement of the IV catheter. (Dex)medetomidine and ketamine combinations

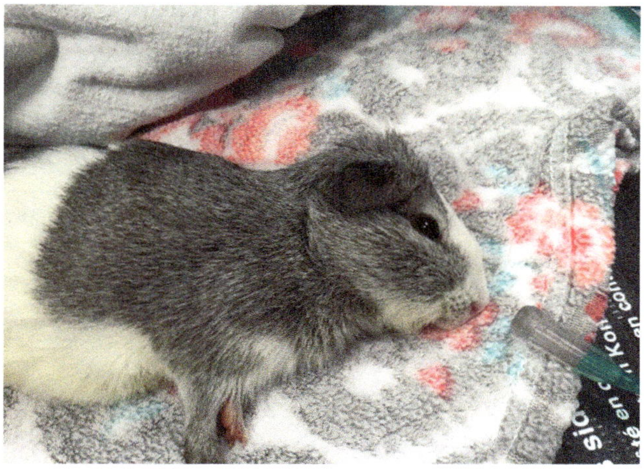

Figure 7.5 Flow by O_2 in a guinea pig provided by a tube at the recommended distance of 2 cm distance from the nostrils. *Source:* Courtesy of Cummings School of Veterinary Medicine at Tufts University.

can also be used to induce anesthesia, but should only be used in patients which are considered cardiovascularly stable. Alfaxalone in combination with other drugs (benzodiazepines, opiods, α2-adrenergic agonists) are also commonly used in premedication protocols.

Table 7.4 contains a selection of agents that are used during premedication of laboratory animals. The authors recommend using the lower ends of the dose ranges as a starting point.

Anticholinergic drugs (i.e. atropine, glycopyrrolate) can be added to the anesthetic protocol to reduce bronchial secretions that may obstruct the airway. However, as salivary viscosity may increase, thereby posing a similar risk for airway obstruction, the decision to use anticholinergics should always be made after carefully weighing the benefits and pitfalls. Because of their vagolytic effect, anticholinergics are indicated if (profound) bradycardia is present. In rabbits, glycopyrrolate (0.01 mg/kg IV) is preferred over atropine (0.02 mg/kg IV) to treat bradycardia because atropinesterase (present in the blood of many rabbits) can quickly inactivate the administered atropine.

Intubation

Intubation of small mammals (particularly rabbits and rodents) is generally considered challenging due to the narrowness of the oral cavity, with the large tongue, cheek teeth, and long soft palate obscuring visualization of the epiglottis and laryngeal opening. As a result, facemasks are frequently used as an alternative, but these will not allow adequate ventilation to be provided when inadequate breathing or apnea is present. With some practice, endotracheal intubation can be accomplished blind in (larger) rabbits. Following placement

Table 7.4 A selection of premedication agents and suggested doses commonly used in small mammals.

	Dose (mg/kg)						
Drug	**Rabbit**	**Ferret**	**Guinea pig**	**Rat**	**Mouse**	**Hamster**	**Gerbil**
Fentanyl and fluanisone (0.315 mg and 10 mg/ml)[a]	0.2–0.5	0.5	1	0.2–0.6	0.1–0.3	0.2–0.6	0.5–1
Medetomidine	0.1–0.5	0.01–0.08	0.5	0.03–0.1	0.03–0.1	0.03–0.1	0.1–0.2
Dexmedetominde	0.05–0.25	0.005–0.04	0.25	0.015–0.05	0.015–0.05	0.015–0.05	0.05–0.1
Ketamine	3–10	10–20	22–44	25–40	22–44	20–40	40–60
Midazolam	0.5–2	0.25–0.5	2–5	2–5	2–5	2–5	2–5
Alfaxalone	1–5	1–5	2–5	2–20	5–20		

Note: combination of drugs allows for lower dosages to be used.
[a] The dose of fentanyl and fluanisone is given in ml/kg.

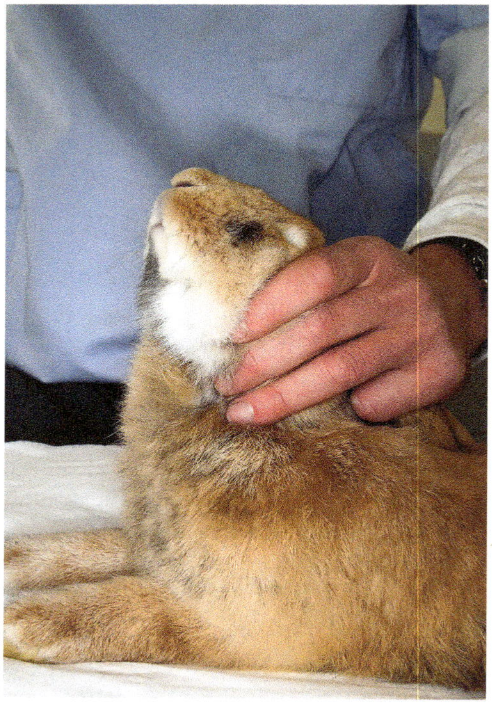

Figure 7.6 To allow tracheal intubation the nose of the rabbit needs to be directed dorsally to align the oropharynx with the larynx and trachea.

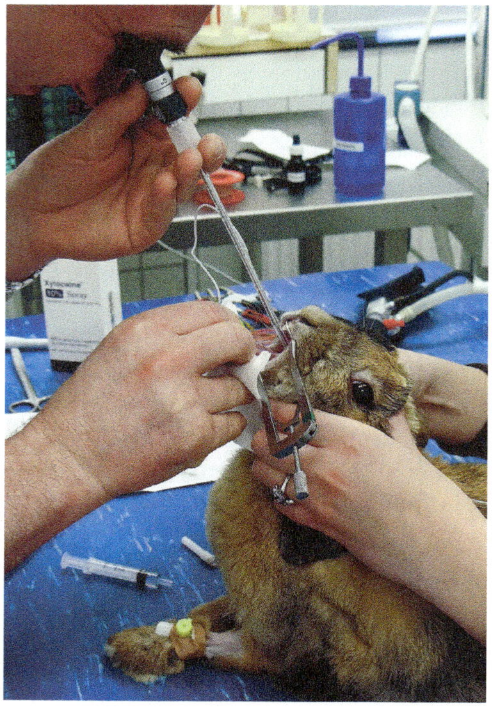

Figure 7.7 By inserting an endoscope in the endotracheal tube and directing the endoscope into the trachea, visual placement of the tube into the trachea is accomplished.

in ventral recumbency, the rabbit's head is extended as far backward as possible (i.e. [almost] perpendicular to the body; Figure 7.6). The tube is then inserted in between the molars toward the larynx and while listening to ensure that breath sounds are always audible (or CO_2 trace visible, if using capnography to assist with intubation), the tube can be further advanced into the larynx. Endoscopy greatly aids in intubation as it allows visualization of the larynx, thereby decreasing the risk of (laryngeal) trauma and enabling successful intubation of animals as small as rats and sugar gliders (Figures 7.7 and 7.8).

Supraglottic airway devices (SGADs) provide a practical alternative to endotracheal intubation. In rabbits, devices specifically adapted to the rabbit's oropharyngeal anatomy have been developed (Figure 7.9); see Chapter 3 for more information. Rather than being inserted into the trachea, SGADs rest on top of the larynx to ensure an open airway (Figure 7.10). As a result, these are generally quicker and easier to place, with less risk for traumatizing the upper airway mucosa but otherwise similar benefits to endotracheal intubation (i.e. proper airway seal resulting in less

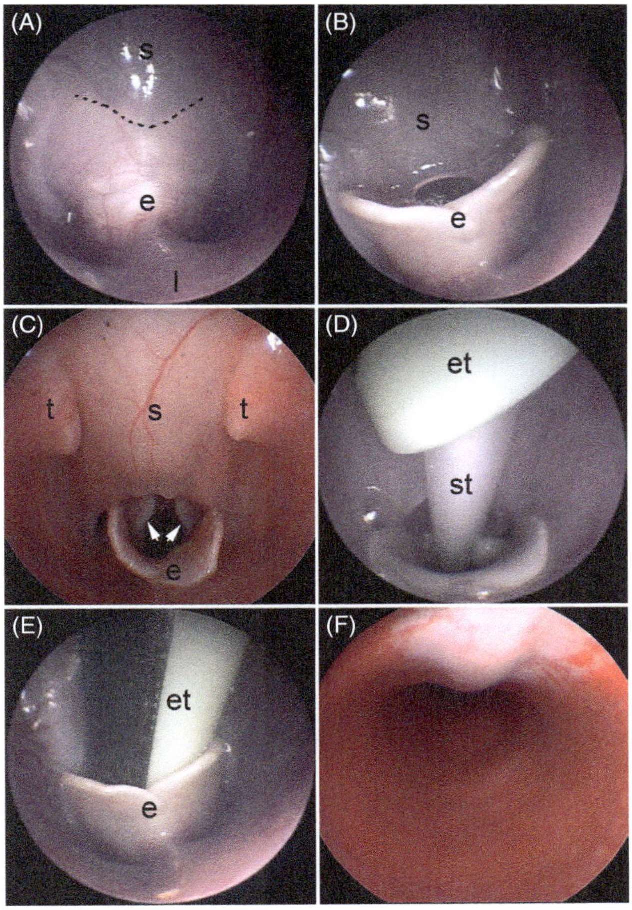

Figure 7.8 Rabbit laryngotracheoscopy and intubation. (A) View of the normal larynx in the nasal breathing rabbit. Note that the epiglottis (e) at the base of the tongue (l) is buttoned over the caudal edge of the soft palate (s). The cranial edge of the epiglottis can be seen through the semitransparent caudal soft palate (dotted line). (B) By placing gentle dorsal pressure on the anesthetized rabbit, it is easy to disengage the cranial edge of the epiglottis (e) from the soft palate (s). If the rabbit is semi-conscious then swallowing quickly re-engages the epiglottis and soft palate. (C) View of the larynx in an anesthetized rabbit, after dorsal displacement on the caudal soft palate has disengaged the epiglottis. The freed epiglottis (e), arytenoid cartilages (arrows), caudal soft palate (s) and tonsils (t) are visible. (D) Intubation in a rabbit using side by side endoscopic guidance. An endotracheal tube (et) and stylet (st) have been introduced into the caudal buccal cavity. The stylet is first directed through the glottis under endoscopic (or laryngoscopic) to act as a guide for the endotracheal tube. (E) Intubation in a rabbit using side by side endoscopic guidance. The endotracheal tube (et) is then advanced along the stylet, over the epiglottis (e) and into the trachea. (F) Intubation in a rabbit using over the endoscope technique. The endotracheal tube is slid up the endoscope, before the endoscope is passed through the glottis and into the anterior trachea. Once a clear view of the trachea has been obtained, as shown, then the endotracheal tube is advanced off the endoscope and into the trachea, as the endoscope is withdrawn. *Source:* Reprinted with permission (C) Stephen J. Divers, University of Georgia, Athens, GA, USA.

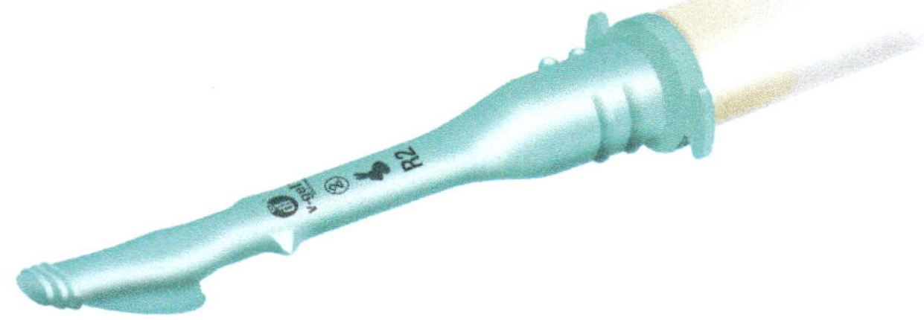

Figure 7.9 (same figure as Figure 3.5) v-gel® Advanced Rabbit Supraglottic Airway Device (https://docsinnovent.com/products/v-gel-rabbit). The largest device is for rabbits ⩾4.5 kg while the smallest device is suitable for rabbits 0.6 kg and up. *Source:* Courtesy of DocsInnovent Ltd.

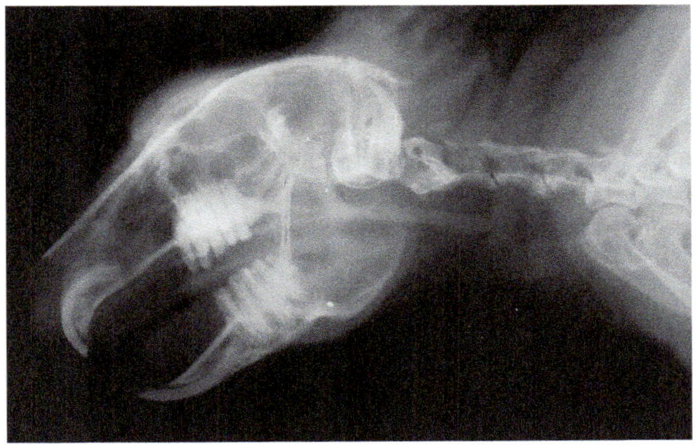

Figure 7.10 A radiograph of the head of a rabbit with a supraglottic airway device in place. The opening of the device is placed over the glottis.

isoflurane leakage and enabling assisted ventilation, if needed). Thus, in rabbits, their use has been highly advocated. Limitations include difficulty to work in the mouth easily with the device in place (i.e. dental work), potential of malposition resulting from patient movement (which is less commonly seen with newer models), and the necessity of continuous capnography to verify correct positioning. For other small mammals (i.e. guinea pigs, rats, mice), similar devices, adapted to the animal's unique anatomy, are currently under development.

Catheterization

Placement of an intravenous catheter is highly recommended in any patient that is anesthetized as it will enable (anesthetic and emergency) drugs and fluids to be administered quickly. The cephalic or saphenous vein are preferred locations for catheter placement in most small mammals, although the marginal ear vein can also be used in rabbits. If intravenous access is not feasible (e.g. small veins), placement of an intraosseous catheter should be

Table 7.5 A selection of injectable anesthetic agents and suggested doses commonly used in small mammals.

	Dose (mg/kg)						
Drug	**Rabbit**	**Ferret**	**Guinea pig**	**Rat**	**Mouse**	**Hamster**	**Gerbil**
Fentanyl/fluanisone and midazolam[a]			8	2.7	10	4	8
Ketamine/ Medetomidine	5–15/0.25	4–8/0.05–0.1	40/0.5	75/0.5	75/1	100/0.25	75/0.5
Ketamine/ Dexmedetomidine	5/0.02/0.01 (F)[b]	5/0.03	3–5/0.05	75/0.5	75/0.5		
Alfaxalone/ medetomidine/ butorphanol					40–80/0.3/5		

[a] Mix 1 ml fentanyl/fluanisone with 2 ml water for injection. Then add 1 ml midazolam (5 mg/ml). Dose is given in ml/kg.
[b] (F) = fentanyl.

considered. More information on catheter placement and maintenance is found in Chapter 4.

Injectable Agents

The injectable agents that are used to sedate and/or premedicate small mammals can also be used for injectable anesthesia (Table 7.5). The most frequently used combination is (dex)medetomidine with ketamine. Many publications mention relatively high doses of ketamine (ranging from 15 to 75 mg/kg), but since ketamine cannot be reversed and skeletal muscle tone can be increased for a considerable time, use of the lowest possible dose is advised. In rabbits and ferrets, the authors frequently use doses as low as 3, up to 10 mg/kg, for sedation and induction of anesthesia.

In some countries, fentanyl/fluanisone is frequently combined with midazolam. This combination provides stable anesthesia for approximately 20–40 minutes and can partially be reversed using butorphanol, which simultaneously provides some post-operative analgesia.

Propofol (<10 mg/kg IV) and alfaxalone (<12 mg/kg SC, IM or IV) are induction agents which are frequently mentioned as anesthetic agents. However, as these do not possess analgesic properties, additional analgesia is required for painful/surgical procedures. Both propofol and – to a lesser extent – alfaxalone may induce apnea, warranting the need for airway access to be achieved quickly.

Antidotes: For many injectable anesthetics, antidotes are available, which increases the safety of their use. Exceptions are propofol and alfaxalone, which have a relatively short duration of action (<15 min), and ketamine. For α2-adrenergic agonists, atipamezole (same volume as [dex] medetomidine used) or – the less commonly used – yohimbine (0.2–1 mg/kg) are available. Flumazenil (0.05–0.1 mg/kg) is used to reverse midazolam, although this is only required if very high doses were given. Buprenorphine or butorphanol can be used to antagonize opioid effects, and are usually preferred as they also provide post-anesthetic analgesia. Naloxone (0.01–0.1 mg/kg) can be used if severe side effects are present.

Inhalant Anesthesia

Isoflurane and sevoflurane are the most commonly used inhalant anesthetics. Both produce a rapid induction and recovery and facilitate quick adjustments to the depth of anesthesia. Although induction and recovery with sevoflurane may be quicker compared to isoflurane, the clinical relevance of this difference is debatable. Nevertheless, sevoflurane has a less pungent odor than isoflurane and will pose a lesser risk for breath-holding, particularly in rabbits and guinea pigs. Sevoflurane furthermore appears to provide a more stable heart rate and less hypotension compared to isoflurane, rendering it slightly safer to use in patients (especially those with cardiovascular disease).

Monitoring

Peri-anesthetic Monitoring (and Supportive Care)

Depth of Anesthesia

Depth of anesthesia is monitored through assessment of reflexes, including the righting, palpebral, corneal, toe pinch – leg withdrawal, and pinna reflex. The righting reflex is the first reflex to be lost and is not suitable to determine surgical depth of anesthesia as painful stimuli may still elicit a response from the animal. Similarly, the palpebral reflex is lost at a light plane of anesthesia in most species.

However, in rabbits, this reflex – like the corneal reflex – is only lost at a dangerously deep level of anesthesia. The toe pinch – leg withdrawal reflex is generally considered the method of choice to reliably assess anesthetic depth in small mammals. In rabbits, this reflex is lost sooner in the hind leg than in the front leg. However, as research has shown that the front leg reflex does not have to disappear in order for surgery to take place, evaluating the reflex of the hindleg will suffice. As the toe pinch – withdrawal reflex may be difficult to perform in rodents, the tail pinch – withdrawal reflex is commonly used as an alternative. Similarly, pinching the ear is a reliable indicator of anesthetic depth, with lack of response indicating a surgical plane of anesthesia.

Additional parameters used to indicate the depth of anesthesia include the (loss of) muscle and jaw tone; presence or absence of vocalizations and/or gross purposeful movements; and changes in the rate, depth, and pattern of respiration and/or heart rate.

Cardiovascular Function

Cardiovascular function can be assessed in a similar manner as during a physical exam (i.e. evaluate mucous membranes, pulse frequency, and heart). However, accessibility may be a challenge when the patient is draped for surgery. The use of monitoring equipment allows for continued evaluation of the patient's vital parameters, but these will never fully replace a qualified assistant that is alert to the patient's clinical condition. Thus, whenever a monitor fails, or displays aberrant values, focus should be placed on evaluating the patient first.

Electrocardiography (ECG) allows for adequate monitoring of the heart rate and rhythm in small mammals. However, this does not necessarily equate to adequate myocardial function and contractility! As many monitors are not capable of accurately determining the animal's heart rate, manual calculation may be needed. In small mammals, the feet's plantar surface is generally too small to properly place sticker electrodes, hence requiring the use of crocodile clips or hypodermic needles to obtain a signal (Figure 7.11). Electrode gel or alcohol can help to improve contact.

Pulse oximetry is used to measure oxygen saturation and can be used to determine pulse rate and rhythm if an audible sound is produced. The tongue is usually considered the best site for placement but may not be accessible in all patients. In such cases, it can be attempted to obtain a satisfactory signal from the ear, digit, or tail. Information obtained with a pulse oximeter may be unreliable in patients with decreased blood pressure and/or vasoconstriction as pulsations are inadequate to allow an accurate signal to be obtained.

Doppler ultrasonic flow probes are a commonly used monitoring tool in small mammals. By placing the Doppler probe directly over a peripheral artery (e.g. central auricular or femoral artery) or the heart, blood flow can be detected, thereby enabling the pulse (or heart) rate and rhythm to be monitored.

Blood pressure measurement can be performed directly by cannulation of an (peripheral) artery, or indirectly using a non-invasive blood pressuring device. Size is a limiting factor for direct blood pressure measurement in small mammals, with the exception of rabbits in which the central auricular artery can be cannulated (see Chapter 4). In other species, blood pressure measurement is only feasible using non-invasive techniques, of which the Doppler technique is the most commonly used. After placing the occlusive cuff just proximal to the elbow or knee, or – in ferrets – at the base of the tail (Figure 7.12), the Doppler probe is placed

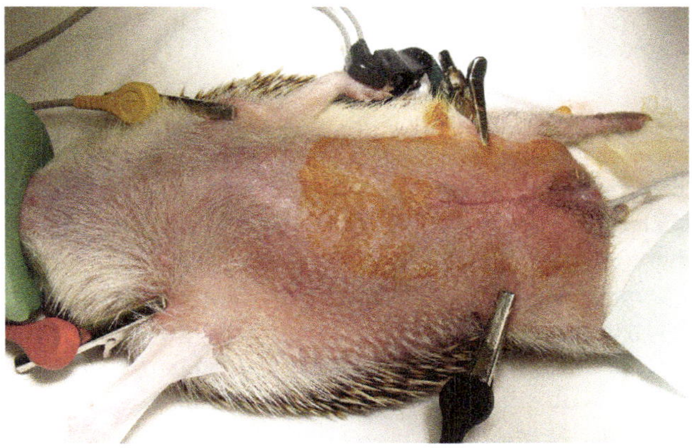

Figure 7.11 Alligator clips were placed on this hedgehog to monitor electrical activity of the heart during pyometra surgery.

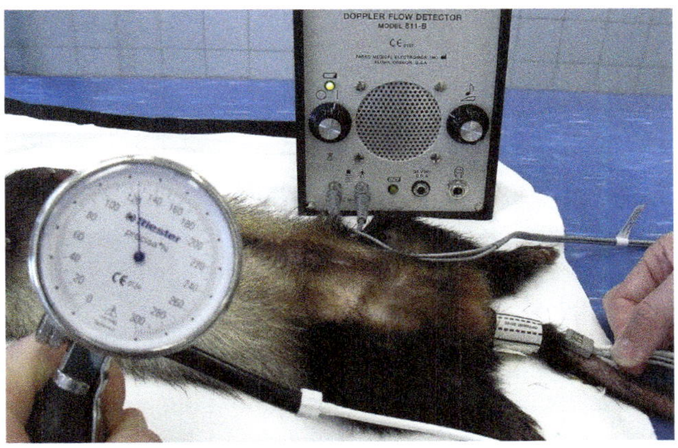

Figure 7.12 (same figure as Figure 6.4). Blood pressure can either be measured through an automated blood measure monitor or by using Doppler and an oscillometer. After placing the occlusive cuff at the base of the tail in ferrets, the Doppler probe is placed distal from the cuff to identify at what cuff pressure a signal is lost or found again.

distal from the cuff to identify at what cuff pressure a signal is lost or found again. The forelimb (or tail in ferrets) usually provides the best results, whereby a cuff width to limb circumference ratio of approximately 40% is recommended. Although values obtained using this technique should not be considered as absolute, repeated measurements are useful to observe trends in blood pressure over time, and evaluate whether pressures remain above 90 mmHg.

Cardiovascular support: Intravenous, or intraosseous access (see Chapter 4) are recommended for any surgical procedure, as many of the anesthetic agents will result in hypotension. During surgical procedures, fluid therapy is usually recommended at a rate of 10 ml/kg/h. In case of bradycardia or cardiac arrest, anesthesia should always be discontinued immediately and/or reversed by the use of an antagonist, if possible. The use of atropine should be considered for bradycardia, whereas adrenaline is recommended in patients with cardiac arrest (see Chapter 6).

Respiration

The respiratory function can be assessed through the evaluation of the mucous membrane color and respiration rate. However, visualization of respiration may be challenging in draped patients, especially if the patient is small. To adequately monitor respiratory function, capnography is therefore highly recommended.

Capnography allows measurement of carbon dioxide (CO_2) concentrations in the expired air. With the obtained end-tidal CO_2 tension ($ETCO_2$), the arterial partial pressure of carbon dioxide ($PaCO_2$) can be estimated. $ETCO_2$, therefore, provides information on both alveolar ventilation as well as cardiac output. In small mammals, capnography may be accomplished using either a side-stream or an in-line sampling method, whereby the latter provides the most accurate results, but also increases the resistance to the anesthetic circuit.

Respiratory support: Intubation is pivotal for adequate respiratory support, including assisted ventilation through intermittent positive pressure ventilation (IPPV). If IPPV is used, the ventilator is usually set to a tidal volume of 10–15 ml/kg, with a respiration rate of 20–40 breaths per minute and pressures of approximately 15–20 mmHg.

Should apnea or hypoventilation be encountered, anesthesia should immediately be discontinued and/or reversed. Moreover, intubation should be attempted, if airway access has not yet been achieved. Re-insertion or suction of the endotracheal tube may be necessary in patients with suspected tube blockage. If intubation is unsuccessful or not feasible, gentle compression of the thorax may provide some ventilation of the lungs. Doxapram may be administered to stimulate ventilation, although this has largely gone out of favor.

Temperature

The small size and relatively large body surface to body volume ratio of small mammals renders them especially sensitive to anesthesia-related hypothermia. However, in animals with thick fur (e.g. rabbits), hyperthermia can also occur, especially during the hot summer days. Monitoring the patient's core-body temperature throughout the procedure is therefore essential and can be accomplished using a regular (digital) thermometer, or – preferably – using an esophageal or rectal probe to allow for continuous measurement.

Maintenance of normothermia (or rather: prevention of heat loss) can be achieved through the use of active warming devices such as water blankets, a Bair hugger™, or a Hot dog® warming system. Heat loss can be reduced by minimizing the area that is shaved, limiting the use of antiseptic solutions, and covering the patient with an insulating blanket. In addition, the inspired air can be humidified and fluids warmed to body temperature prior to administration.

Hypothermia can be treated through increasing the temperature of the warming device, or use of an additional heating device. Placing a heat lamp over the surgery site or increasing the environmental temperature may also help. Under all circumstances, if applicable, the body cavity should be closed as quickly as possible, so the patient can be woken up to recover in a warm incubator. At this time, frequent temperature monitoring is imperative as hyperthermia can easily occur.

Hyperthermia can occur in animals with thick fur, with rabbits being particularly sensitive to overheating (especially if shaving is not necessary). To cool the patient down, turn off any active heating device, spray alcohol on the footpads and exposed skin, and provide cool intravenous fluids. Temperature monitoring is warranted as cooling the patient too quickly may inadvertently result in hypothermia.

Post-Anesthetic Considerations

As almost two-thirds of the anesthetic related mortalities occur in the post-anesthetic period, close monitoring of the patient during the first hours after anesthesia is recommended. During this period, the heart rate, respiration rate, and temperature should be monitored regularly. The IV catheter should be maintained, if possible, to enable quick administration of fluids, glucose, or CPR medications, if needed. As small mammals tend to rapidly develop hypoglycemia if they do not eat, food should be provided as quickly as possible after anesthesia. Ferrets will frequently accept a liquid diet, even when they are not yet fully awake. Rabbits and other herbivorous small mammals may be provided with fresh leafy green vegetables directly after anesthesia to stimulate eating and should be fed a critical care formula if food intake stays behind in the first 6–12 hours after an anesthetic procedure. Fecal output should also be evaluated in combination with auscultation of GI-tract motility as this may frequently be suppressed during the post-anesthetic period. (*Note: this is of particular importance in the herbivorous species, which heavily rely on an adequate gastrointestinal motility for the digestion of food.*) Prokinetic drugs (e.g. cisapride, metoclopramide) can be considered if intestinal sounds are not audible. Adequate pain management is essential in the first days of post-surgery, as pain may significantly suppress the recovery of any small mammal patient.

References

1 Lichtenberger, M. and Ko, J. (2007). Anesthesia and analgesia for small mammals and birds. *Vet. Clinics North Am. Exot. Anim. Pract.* 10 (2): 293–315.

2 Lennox, A.M. (2008). Clinical technique: small exotic companion mammal dentistry – anesthetic considerations. *J. Exot. Pet Med.* 17 (2): 102–106.

Further Reading

Aguiar, J., Mogridge, G., and Hall, J. (2014). Femoral fracture repair and sciatic and femoral nerve blocks in a Guinea pig. *J. Small Anim. Pract.* 55 (12): 635–639.

Barter, L.S. (2011). Rabbit analgesia. *Vet. Clinics North Am. Exot. Anim. Pract.* 14 (1): 93–104.

Beyers, T.M., Richardson, J.A., and Prince, M.D. (1991). Axonal degeneration and self-mutilation as a complication of the intramuscular use of ketamine and xylazine in rabbits. *Lab. Anim. Sci.* 41 (5): 519–520.

Brodbelt, D.C., Blissitt, K.J., Hammond, R.A. et al. (2008). The risk of death: the confidential enquiry into perioperative small animal fatalities. *Vet. Anaesth. Analg.* 35 (5): 365–373.

Carli, G., Farabollini, F., and Di Prisco, C.L. (1979). Plasma corticosterone and its relation to susceptibility to animal hypnosis in rabbits. *Neurosci. Lett.* 11 (3): 271–274.

Das, R.G. and North, D. (2007). Implications of experimental technique for analysis and interpretation of data from animal experiments: outliers and increased variability resulting from failure of intraperitoneal injection procedures. *Lab. Anim.* 41 (3): 312–320.

Deflers, H., Bolen, G., Gandar, F. et al. (2013). Influence of Buprenorphine on the European Rabbit's (*Oryctolagus cuniculus*) gastro-intestinal motility. In: *Proceedings of the First International Conference on Avian, Reptile, and Exotic Medicine*, Wiesbaden, Germany, 200.

Deflers, H., Bolen, G., Gandar, F., Bréthaut, E., Farnir, F., Marlier, D. (2014) Influence of morphine on the rabbit gastrointestinal tract. *Proceedings Association of Exotic Mammal Veterinarians Conference* Orlando, FL, October 18–24 2014.

d'Ovidio, D., Rota, S., Noviello, E. et al. (2014). Nerve stimulator-guided sciatic-femoral block in pet rabbits (*Oryctolagus cuniculus*) undergoing hind limb surgery: a case series. *J. Exot. Pet Med.* 23 (1): 91–95.

Ebert, T.J., Harkin, C.P., and Muzi, M. (1995). Cardiovascular responses to sevoflurane: a review. *Anesth. Analg.* 81 (6S): 11S–22S.

Flecknell, P.A. (2015). *Laboratory Animal Anaesthesia*, 4e. London: Academic Press.

Flecknell, P.A. and Mitchell, M. (1984). Midazolam and fentanyl-fluanisone: assessment of anaesthetic effects in laboratory rodents and rabbits. *Lab. Anim.* 18 (2): 143–146.

Flecknell, P.A., Lofgren, J.L.S., Dyson, M.S. et al. (2015). Preanesthesia, anesthesia, analgesia, and euthanasia. In: *Laboratory Animal Medicine*, 3e (eds. J.G. Fox, L.C. Anderson, G. Otto, et al.), 1136–1201. St. Louis, MO: Elsevier.

Foley, P.L., Henderson, A.L., Bissonette, E.A. et al. (2001). Evaluation of fentanyl transdermal patches in rabbits: blood concentrations and physiologic response. *Comp. Med.* 51 (3): 239–244.

Foley, P.L., Liang, H., and Crichlow, A.R. (2011). Evaluation of a sustained-release formulation of buprenorphine for analgesia in rats. *J. Am. Assoc. Lab. Anim. Sci.* 50 (2): 198–204.

Giral, M., García-Olmo, D.C., Gómez-Juárez, M., and Gómez de Segura, I.A. (2014). Anaesthetic effects in the ferret of alfaxalone alone and in combination with medetomidine or tramadol: a pilot study. *Lab. Anim.* 48 (4): 313–320.

Graham, J. and Mader, D.R. (2012). Basic approach to veterinary care. In: *Ferrets, Rabbits and Rodents: Clinical Medicine and Surgery* (eds. K.E. Quesenberry and J.W. Carpenter), 174–182. St. Louis, MO: Elsevier.

Hawkins, M.C. and Pascoe, P.J. (2012). Anesthesia, analgesia, and sedation of small mammals. In: *Ferrets, Rabbits and Rodents: Clinical Medicine and Surgery* (eds. K.E. Quesenberry and J.W. Carpenter), 429–451. St. Louis, MO: Elsevier.

Johnson, D.H. (2010). Endoscopic intubation of exotic companion mammals. *Vet. Clinics North Am. Exot. Anim. Pract.* 13 (2): 273–289.

Keating, S.C., Thomas, A.A., Flecknell, P.A., and Leach, M.C. (2012). Evaluation of EMLA cream for preventing pain during tattooing of rabbits: changes in physiological, behavioural and facial expression responses. *PLoS One* 7 (9): e44437. https://doi.org/10.1371/journal.pone.0044437.

Langford, D.J., Bailey, A.L., Chanda, M.L. et al. (2010). Coding of facial expressions of pain in the laboratory mouse. *Nat. Methods* 7 (6): 447–449. https://doi.org/10.1038/nmeth.1455.

Lennox, A.M. (2014). Safe sedation and immobilization of unusual exotic species encountered in practice. *J. Exot. Pet Med.* 23 (4): 363–368.

Lichtenberger, M. and Ko, J. (2007). Critical care monitoring. *Vet. Clinics North Am. Exot. Anim. Pract.* 10 (2): 317–344.

Mans, C. and Evenson, E. (2016). Analgesic efficacy and safety of hydromorphone and tramadol in Chinchillas *(Chinchilla lanigera)*. In: *Proceedings ExoticsCon 2016*, Portland, OR, August 27–September 1 2016, 409.

Miller, A.L. and Richardson, C.A. (2011). Rodent analgesia. *Vet. Clinics North Am. Exot. Anim. Pract.* 14 (1): 81–92.

van Oostrom, H., Schoemaker, N.J., and Uilenreef, J.J. (2011). Pain management in ferrets. *Vet. Clinics North Am. Exot. Anim. Pract.* 14 (1): 105–116.

Phillips, B.E., Harms, C.A., and Messenger, K.M. (2015). Oral transmucosal detomidine gel for the sedation of the domestic ferret (*Mustela putorius furo*). *J. Exot. Pet Med.* 24 (4): 446–454.

Quesenberry, K.E. and Orcutt, C. (2012). Basic approach to veterinary care. In: *Ferrets, Rabbits and Rodents: Clinical Medicine and Surgery* (eds. K.E. Quesenberry and J.W. Carpenter), 13–26. St. Louis, MO: Elsevier.

Reijgwart, M.L., Schoemaker, N.J., Pascuzzo, R. et al. (2017). The composition and initial evaluation of a grimace scale in ferrets after surgical implantation of a telemetry probe. *PLoS One* 12 (11): e0187986. https://doi.org/10.1371/journal.pone.0187986.

Richardson, D.A. (2015). Comparison of the V-gel® supraglottic airway device and non-cuffed endotracheal tube in the time to first capnograph trace during anaesthetic induction in rabbits. *Vet. Nurse* 6: 426–432.

Schoemaker, N.J., Mol, J.A., Lumeij, J.T. et al. (2003). Effects of anaesthesia and manual restraint on the plasma concentrations of pituitary and adrenocortical hormones in ferrets. *Vet. Rec.* 152 (19): 591–594.

Sladky, K.K., Horne, W.A., Goodrowe, K.L. et al. (2000). Evaluation of epidural morphine for postoperative analgesia in ferrets (*Mustela putorius furo*). *J. Am. Assoc. Lab. Anim. Sci.* 39 (6): 33–38.

Sotocinal, S.G., Sorge, R.E., Zaloum, A. et al. (2011). The rat grimace scale: a partially automated method for quantifying pain in the laboratory rat via facial expressions. *Mol. Pain* 7 (1): 1. https://doi.org/10.1186/1744-8069-7-55.

Souza, M.J., Greenacre, C.B., and Cox, S.K. (2008). Pharmacokinetics of orally administered tramadol in domestic rabbits. *Am. J. Vet. Res.* 69 (8): 979–982.

Spivey, W.H., McNamara, R.M., MacKenzie, R.S. et al. (1987). A clinical comparison of lidocaine and bupivacaine. *Ann. Emergency Med.* 16 (7): 752–757.

Swisher, S. and Lennox, A. (2015). Analgesia in small exotic mammals: a review. *Adv. Small Anim. Med. Surg.* 28 (11): 1–3.

Taylor, B.F., Ramirez, H.E., Battles, A.H. et al. (2016). Analgesic activity of tramadol and buprenorphine after voluntary ingestion by rats (*Rattus norvegicus*). *J. Am. Assoc. Lab. Anim. Sci.* 55 (1): 74–82.

Wenger, S. (2012). Anesthesia and analgesia in rabbits and rodents. *J. Exot. Pet Med.* 21 (1): 7–16.

Williams, A.M. and Wyatt, J.D. (2007). Comparison of subcutaneous and intramuscular ketamine–medetomidine with and without reversal by atipamezole in Dutch belted rabbits (*Oryctolagus cuniculus*). *J. Am. Assoc. Lab. Anim. Sci.* 46 (6): 16–20.

Wolfe, A.M., Kennedy, L.H., Na, J.J., and Nemzek-Hamlin, J.A. (2015). Efficacy of tramadol as a sole analgesic for postoperative pain in male and female mice. *J. Am. Assoc. Lab. Anim. Sci.* 54 (4): 411–419.

van Zeeland, Y.R.A. and Schoemaker, N.J. (2014). Current anaesthetic considerations and techniques in rabbits - Part I: Pre-anaesthetic considerations and commonly used analgesics and anaesthetics. *Eur. J. Companion Anim. Pract.* 24 (4): 19–30.

van Zeeland, Y.R.A. and Schoemaker, N.J. (2014). Current anaesthetic considerations and techniques in rabbits - Part II: Induction, maintenance and the post-anaesthetic period. *Eur. J. Companion Anim. Pract.* 24 (4): 31–45.

van Zeeland, Y.R.A., Meuwissen, A., Hoytink, I. et al. (2016). Risk assessment of different delivery methods for isoflurane anesthesia in rabbits. In: *Proceedings ExoticsCon 2016*, Portland, OR, August 27–September 1 2016, 499–500.

8

Nutrition and Fluid Therapy

Yvonne R.A. van Zeeland and Nico J. Schoemaker

Division of Zoological Medicine, Department of Clinical Sciences, Faculty of Veterinary Medicine, Utrecht University, The Netherlands

CONTENTS

Nutrition

Indications

Nutritional support is warranted in most small mammal patients presenting with decreased food intake. Due to the animals' high metabolic rate, anorexia will quickly result in depletion of the already limited glycogen stores and hypoglycemia. In addition, the negative energy balance resulting from decreased food intake combined with increased energy requirements during disease will result in a breakdown of fat and muscle and subsequent cachexia. Mobilization of free fatty acids may lead to (life-threatening) hepatic lipidosis and ketoacidosis, especially in obese patients and hindgut fermenters such as rabbits, guinea pigs, and chinchillas.

Adequate food intake is paramount to proper digestive function. Lack of food intake poses a risk for malnutrition and development of nutritional deficiencies (e.g. vitamin C deficiency in the guinea pig[1]), which can affect both normal physiological processes and those responsible for inflammation and tissue repair. Inadequate food intake poses a risk for breakdown of tight junctions and loss of the epithelial barrier in the gastrointestinal tract, followed by bacterial translocation and sepsis. Provision of adequate nutritional support, along with fluid therapy, is therefore key to prevent and/or treat these potentially lethal conditions.

Nutritional support strategies aim to prevent and/or correct (obvious) nutritional deficiencies and imbalances, minimize metabolic derangements and catabolism of lean body tissue, and return the animal's appetite and subsequent food intake to adequate amounts. Repletion of body weight during hospitalization is *not* an immediate goal per se as this will only occur following resolution of the primary underlying disease process. Nevertheless, ongoing weight loss should be prevented and addressed appropriately.

Nutritional Requirements

Proper nutritional support of the critical care patient comprises the provision of adequate amounts of nutrients and energy to

1 Guinea pigs lack L-gulonolactone oxidase and are therefore not able to synthesize vitamin C.

Exotic Animal Emergency and Critical Care Medicine, First Edition. Edited by Jennifer E. Graham, Grayson A. Doss and Hugues Beaufrère.

Table 8.1 Recommended percentages of protein, fat, carbohydrates, and fiber in the diets of small mammals.

	Rabbit	Guinea pig	Chinchilla	Rat/mouse/gerbil	Ferret	Hedgehog	Sugar glider
Protein (%)	12–16	16–20	16–20	14–20	35	30–50	19–25
Fat (%)	1.5–2	?		5	20–30	10–20	6–14
Carbohydrate (%)	<15				<30		
Fiber (%)	16–25	12–20	15–35	<20	Low	3–27	

support critical physiologic processes and meet the additional demands of the inflammatory response and tissue repair.

Nutrient requirements for common small mammal species can be found in Table 8.1. However, dependent on the underlying disease process, nutrient requirements may be altered. For example, protein requirements will often be increased in patients with inflammatory processes and/or wounds or other types of tissue trauma. Most of the commercially available critical care and recovery diets (see next paragraph) will meet these requirements.

Like other animals, the basal metabolic rate (BMR, i.e. metabolic rate at complete rest) is used to calculate the minimum daily caloric requirements. In small mammals, BMR is calculated using the formula $BMR = 70 \times W^{0.75}$ (kcal/kg/d). Maintenance energy requirement (MER, i.e. metabolic rate based on activity) can subsequently be determined by correcting the BMR for the animal's health status and activity pattern (i.e. 1.2–1.5×BMR for convalescing animals; 2× BMR for growing, or sick and/or debilitated animals). Next, the amount of food to be fed can be calculated based on energy content and divided over the day's feeding sessions (i.e. 10–20 ml/kg at a time for up to two to four times a day). *Note: As many variables may affect the animal's energy requirements* (e.g. *age, neutering status, physical activity, environmental temperatures*), *and food is commonly spilled during feeding, the calculated amounts should be considered a starting point rather than an absolute number.*

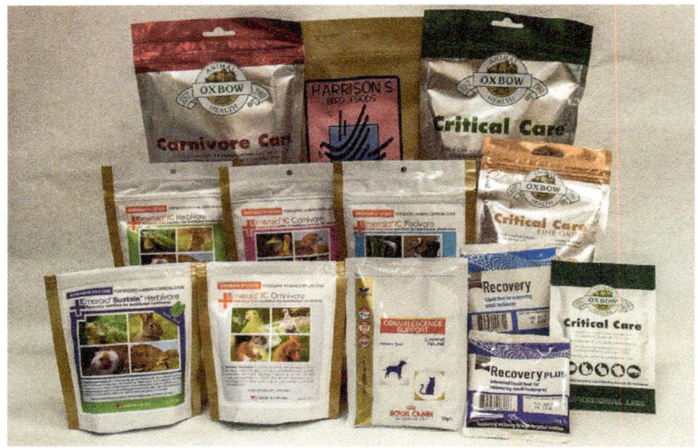

Figure 8.1 A wide variety of nutritional support diets are commercially available tailored to the specific needs of the different species.

Table 8.2 Recommended composition (diet: water ratio) of Emeraid Critical Care formula for common small mammal patients.

	Omnivore	Carnivore	Herbivore	Water
Rabbit/ chinchilla/ guinea pig/ degu			4	4
Sugar glider/ mouse	6			4
Rat/gerbil	4.5		1	4
Hamster	3		2	4
Hedgehog	1.5	1.5		4
Ferret		2		4

Nutritional Diets/Feeding Formulas

A wide variety of feeding formulas has become available in the past decade(s) (Figure 8.1), and new/updated products are brought to the market on a regular basis. In alphabetical order, the following companies produce feeding formulas specifically tailored to small mammal patients: Lafeber Company (Cornell, IL, USA); Oxbow Animal Health (Murdock, NE, USA); and Supreme Pet Foods (Suffolk, United Kingdom).

The Lafeber Company produces Emeraid® IC intensive care nutrition that is specifically intended for debilitated/cachectic herbivores, omnivores, carnivores, and piscivores, and animals with digestive disorders that benefit from receiving easily digestible nutrients (including those suffering from hypoalbuminemia). The diets contain high levels of glutamine and arginine, hydrolyzed proteins, and a highly digestible blend of fats (including a balanced amount of omega 3 and 6 polyunsaturated fatty acids) and simple carbohydrates for energy. Additional benefits include the consistency (i.e. the formula is liquid enough to pass through any size of feeding tube), shelf life (i.e. the formula can be stored in the refrigerator for up to 24 hours after preparation), and ability to use the products in combination to create a mix that is adapted to the species' specific needs (see Table 8.2). However, as the fiber content in the herbivore IC diet is limited, it should not be used for more than three weeks. Instead, the animal should be switched to Emeraid Sustain™ for herbivores which functions as a maintenance diet for the later stages of recovery.

Oxbow Animal Health produces Critical Care® for herbivores and carnivores (i.e. Critical Care for Herbivores [in apple-banana or anise flavor], Carnivore Care™). Both diets are complete maintenance diets that can be fed to sick or convalescing animals and is readily accepted by the animal when syringe-fed. The formula for herbivores contains a high percentage of non-digestible fiber and is (relatively) low in fat and carbohydrates to ensure adequate gastrointestinal motility and digestion. Due to the high-fiber content, the formula will easily clog a 5-8 Fr tube (even when blenderized), thereby rendering it unsuitable for nasogastric tube feeding. A specific formula (i.e. Critical Care Fine grind®) was therefore designed to enable nasogastric tube feeding using a 5 Fr nasogastric tube. An Omnivore Care diet has recently been added to the company's product line.

Supreme Pet Foods produces a Recovery and RecoveryPlus diet for the small herbivorous patient. In addition to a higher level of fibers (25% instead of 19%), the RecoveryPlus diet also contains pre- and probiotics that anecdotally support gastrointestinal function and restoration of the normal bacterial gut flora.

For ferrets and other carnivores, high-quality liquid support diets for dogs and cats (e.g. Convalescence Support Instant Diet, Royal Canin, Aimargues, France) are frequently used and found highly effective by the authors. Similarly, diluted canned support diets for dogs and cats (e.g. Hill's® prescription diet™ a/d®, Topeka, KS, USA) may be used. For omnivorous species (e.g. rats, mice, hamsters), parrot hand-feeding formulas (e.g. Harrison Juvenile, Harrison's Bird Foods, Brentwood, TN, USA) or baby foods can be used. The latter products can also be used in herbivorous patients as a short-term alternative in case the owner is unable to book an appointment. Alternatively, the owner can be advised to soak the regular pellets and feed these as a mash to animal.

Routes

Factors such as the underlying disease, patient compliance, and clinical condition of the animal are important determinants to select the appropriate route for nutritional support. Whenever possible, the oral or enteral route should be used. Not only is it the safest, simplest, and least expensive, but also the most physiologic route of administration. Enteral feeding can be accomplished by one of several techniques: appetite stimulation, force feeding using a syringe, and/or tube feeding using an orogastric, nasogastric, or esophageal tube. If enteral feedings are not tolerated or the gastrointestinal tract should be bypassed for longer than five days (e.g. in case of severe, acute pancreatitis or paralytic ileus), parenteral feeding should be considered.

Regardless of the route chosen, food should remain available for voluntary consumption (unless enteral food intake is contra-indicated). Provision of favored treats and food items, and, in herbivorous species, provision of fresh grass, greens (e.g. dandelion greens, cilantro, endive) and hay, can help to stimulate the animal's appetite.

Syringe Feeding

Many small mammals will readily tolerate hand feeding by a syringe, sometimes eating food voluntarily out of a syringe without the necessity to restrain the animal. Anorectic ferrets will also commonly eat liquid force-feeding formulas readily out of a bowl (Figure 8.2).

In rabbits and rodents, syringe feeding can be accomplished by placing the tip of the syringe in the diastema (Figure 8.3). To facilitate administering the formula, the animal can be wrapped in a towel (see Chapter 2 – Restraint and Handling). Syringe feeding in carnivores is accom-

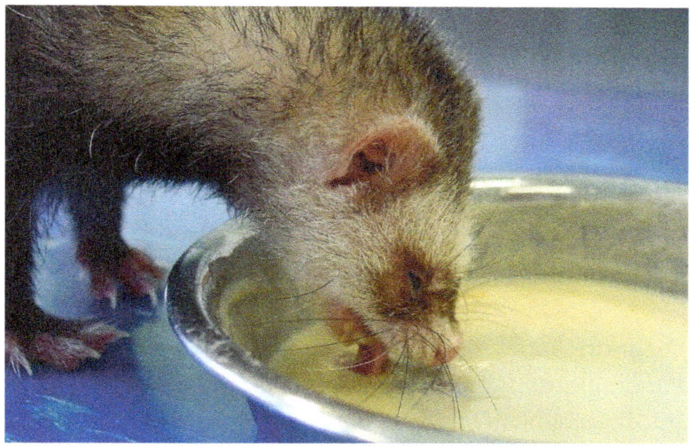

Figure 8.2 Many ferrets will eat the liquid feeding formulas readily out of a dish or bowl.

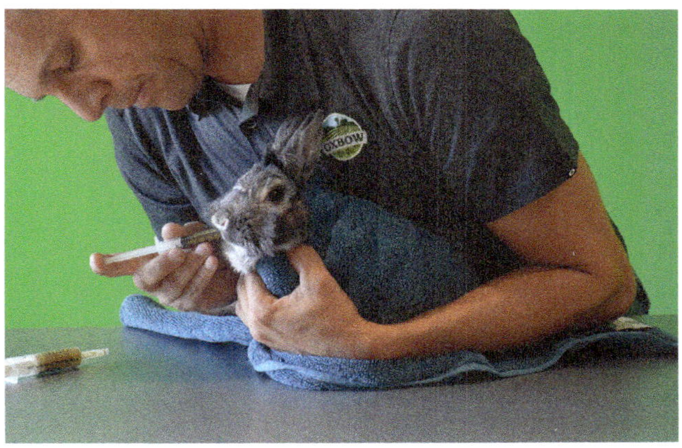

Figure 8.3 Syringe feeding in a rabbit. The syringe is best placed in the diastema of the mouth (just behind the incisors). *Source:* Courtesy of Oxbow Animal Health.

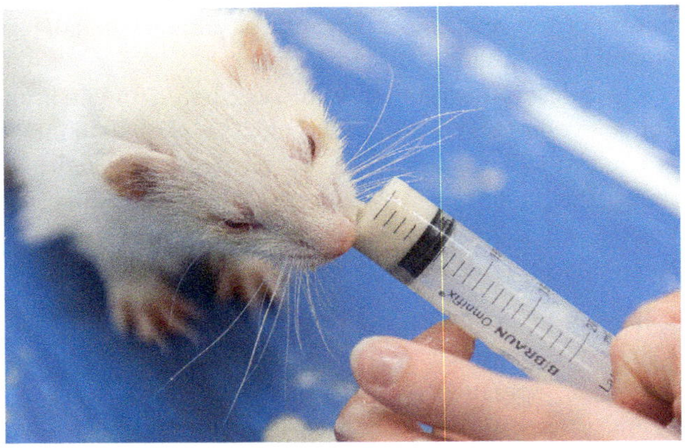

Figure 8.4 Carnivores, such as this ferret, can best be fed by placing the syringe in the corner of the mouth.

plished by placing the syringe tip in the corner of the mouth (Figure 8.4). To prevent aspiration, syringe feeding should be done slowly with sufficient breaks in between to allow the animal to swallow. Although some producers of herbivore diets provide specific syringes with wider tips, these could pose a risk for food aspiration, as the animal may unintentionally be made to swallow large volumes of food too quickly. The authors therefore prefer to use 1 ml syringes to ensure delivery of smaller volumes (i.e. 0.05–0.1 ml for smaller rodents and sugar gliders; 0.25 ml for hedgehogs, chinchillas and guinea pigs; up to 1 ml for rabbits and ferrets). When feeding high-fiber diets, the tip of the syringe can be removed to prevent clogging.

Orogastric Tube

An orogastric tube can be used to administer food directly into the stomach (Figure 8.5a). The authors only recommend this technique for single dosing, e.g. to provide instant nutrition to a severely debilitated animal in which placement of a nasogastric or esophagostomy tube is not feasible. For chronic use, the technique is deemed unsuitable, as placement can be extremely stressful for the animal thereby negatively influencing it's recovery. Consequently, the authors also recommend sedation when attempting this technique in any of the small mammals (Note: this may negatively affect the animal's ability to swallow, thereby increasing the risk of accidental insertion in the trachea). A mouth gag or speculum can be used to prevent the animal from biting the tube and swallowing the severed portion.

For orogastric feeding, a flexible, round-tipped rubber catheter of an appropriate diameter (e.g. 8-Fr in guinea pigs, 10-Fr in ferrets, 18- to 22-Fr in rabbits) should be used (Figure 8.5b). In the smaller rodents, commercially available feeding needles (13-22G) may be used. The length of insertion should be premeasured by determining the distance from the mouth to the last rib and marking this distance on the tube or needle. Following lubrication, the tube is inserted through the mouth gag or speculum following which the animal is allowed to swallow the tube. In rabbits, the neck can be slightly flexed to facilitate placement. Next, the tube is gently but rapidly passed through the esophagus into the stomach. Correct placement may be confirmed by observing the patient for signs of choking or coughing, aspirating gastric contents, or auscultating the cranial abdomen while injecting 5–10 ml of air into the tube[2] and

2 If the tube is placed into the stomach, characteristic bubbling noises of turbulent air flow should be audible, whereas coughing and/or condensation in the lumen of the tube can be noted if the tube is placed into the trachea. In case of gastric dilatation, fluid and gas may start flowing from the tube once it passes the cardia.

(a) (b)

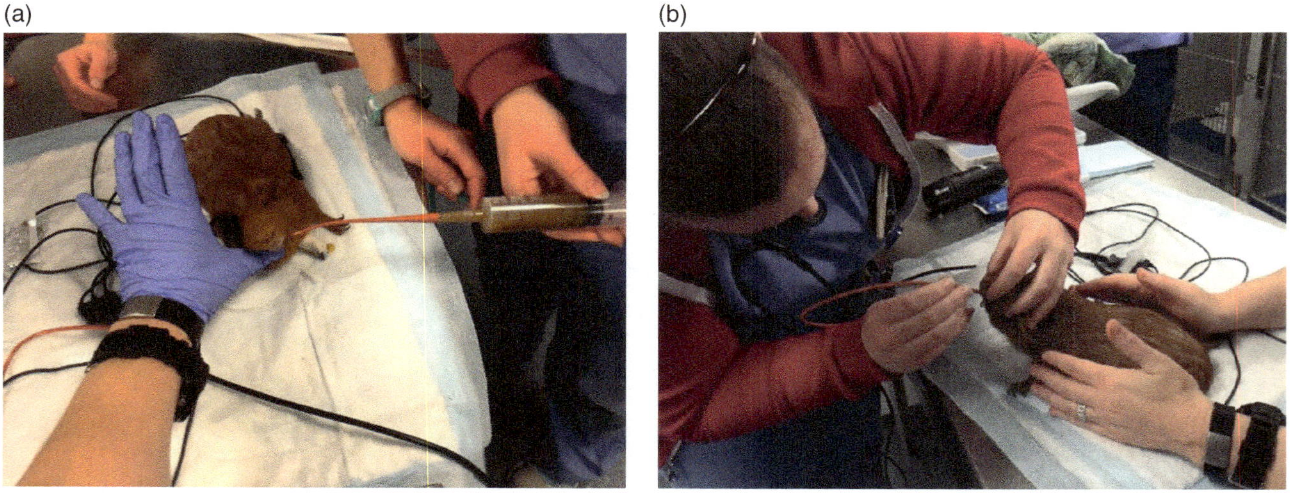

Figure 8.5 (a) Orogastric tube in a guinea pig. In this case, material is being suctioned from the stomach to reduce bloat. (b) Initial placement of the orogastric tube in the patient. (a). *Source:* Courtesy of Cummings School of Veterinary Medicine at Tufts University.

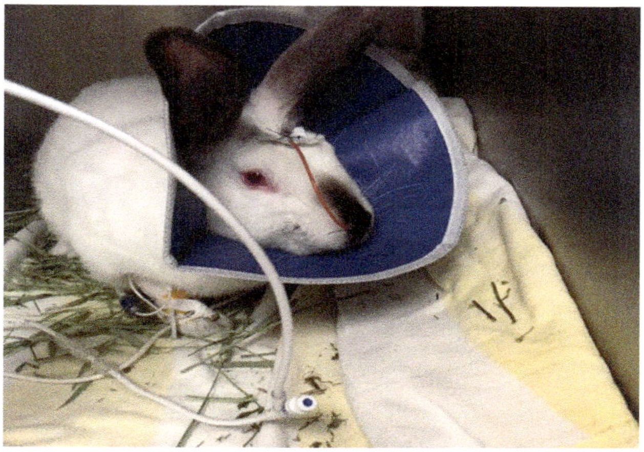

Figure 8.6 Nasogastric tube in a rabbit. This rabbit was also receiving intravenous lipid therapy for witnessed ingestion of ibuprofen by the owner. *Source:* Courtesy of Cummings School of Veterinary Medicine at Tufts University.

checking for negative pressure when the tube is pulled backed into the esophagus. In addition, small quantities of water may be passed down the tube prior to administering the food. Following feeding, the tube is immediately withdrawn while leaving the syringe attached or crimping the tube to prevent leakage and possible aspiration.

Nasogastric Tube

Placement of a nasogastric tube is recommended in anorectic rabbits and guinea pigs that are too weak or nauseous to swallow syringe-fed food (Figure 8.6). To enable passing of the nasal cavity, 5- to 8-Fr flexible feeding tubes should be used in rabbits, whereas 3.5-Fr tubes are considered appropriate for guinea pigs. As the small diameter precludes administration of high-fiber diets, nasogastric tube feeding can only be executed using specific formulas such as Oxbow Critical Care Fine grind or Emeraid Herbivore IC.

Similar to orogastric tubes, the length of insertion (distance between tip of the nose and last rib) needs to be premeasured and marked on the tube. Next, a local anesthetic (e.g. 2% lidocaine gel) is administered into the animal's nostril and allowed 5–10 minutes to take effect.

Proper restraint or sedation is necessary to place the nasogastric tube. In rabbits, the head should be flexed ventrally to prevent the tube from entering the trachea. The tube should be inserted ventromedial in the ventral nasal meatus and gently advanced until the mark on the tube has reached the nostril. Correct placement can be verified through radiographs or one of the methods described for the orogastric tube. The tube is then sutured (or glued) to the laterodorsal nasal surface and to the dorsal surface of the head, following which the remainder of the tube can be coiled over the body and wrapped under a bandage. Feeding formula can be delivered via a syringe every six hours, followed by a small amount of water to ensure patency. Most patients will readily accept a nasogastric tube, allowing it to remain in place until the animal starts eating on its own. However, in some patients, the tube may lead to irritation and nasal discharge, warranting early removal and initiation of antibiotic therapy.

Esophagostomy Tube

Esophagostomy tubes allow feeding (and administering medication) to be performed with relative ease without adverse reaction of the patient or interfering with normal feeding. Esophagostomy tubes are frequently placed in ferrets, but can be placed in other small mammals, including rabbits and hedgehogs, as well. In rabbits, placement is more difficult due to the narrow oral cavity and thus not routinely performed. However, if long-term nutritional support is required (e.g. in case of jaw fractures or trauma or surgery to the mouth or pharynx), placement of an esophagostomy tube should be considered.

In ferrets, an 8-Fr flexible, enteric feeding tube may be used. The animal should be properly anesthetized (see Chapter 7 – Analgesia, Anesthesia and Monitoring) as this is a surgical procedure. Placement is performed on the left side of the neck using a similar technique as described in the cat (Figure 8.7a–d). After shaving, aseptic preparation, and marking of the feeding tube (distance from entry site to the last rib), a curved mosquito forceps is inserted through the mouth into the esophagus with the tip pointing laterally to allow a stab incision to be made over the tip through the skin, subcutis, and esophageal wall to allow it to exit through the skin. Using the mosquito forceps, the feeding tube is then pulled through the incision back into the oral cavity, turned 180°, and directed back into the oral cavity and esophagus. Once at the incision site, the tube is retracted gently to allow the tube to pass and advance further down the esophagus until it reaches the stomach (as indicated by the mark). Sutures are placed proximal to the incision site to fix the tube into position, following which a bandage is placed loosely around the neck to prevent the ferret from pulling the tube. Food should be withheld the first few hours, but once the animal has recovered fully from the anesthesia, liquid (carnivore) diet may be administered through the tube at a dose of 10–15 ml/kg q6h.[3] Prior to each feeding session, the oral cavity should be inspected for presence of a regurgitated tube and water (approx. 1–1.5 ml) flushed down the tube to ensure its patency. Once food

3 Frequency of feeding may be adjusted according to the animal's body weight.

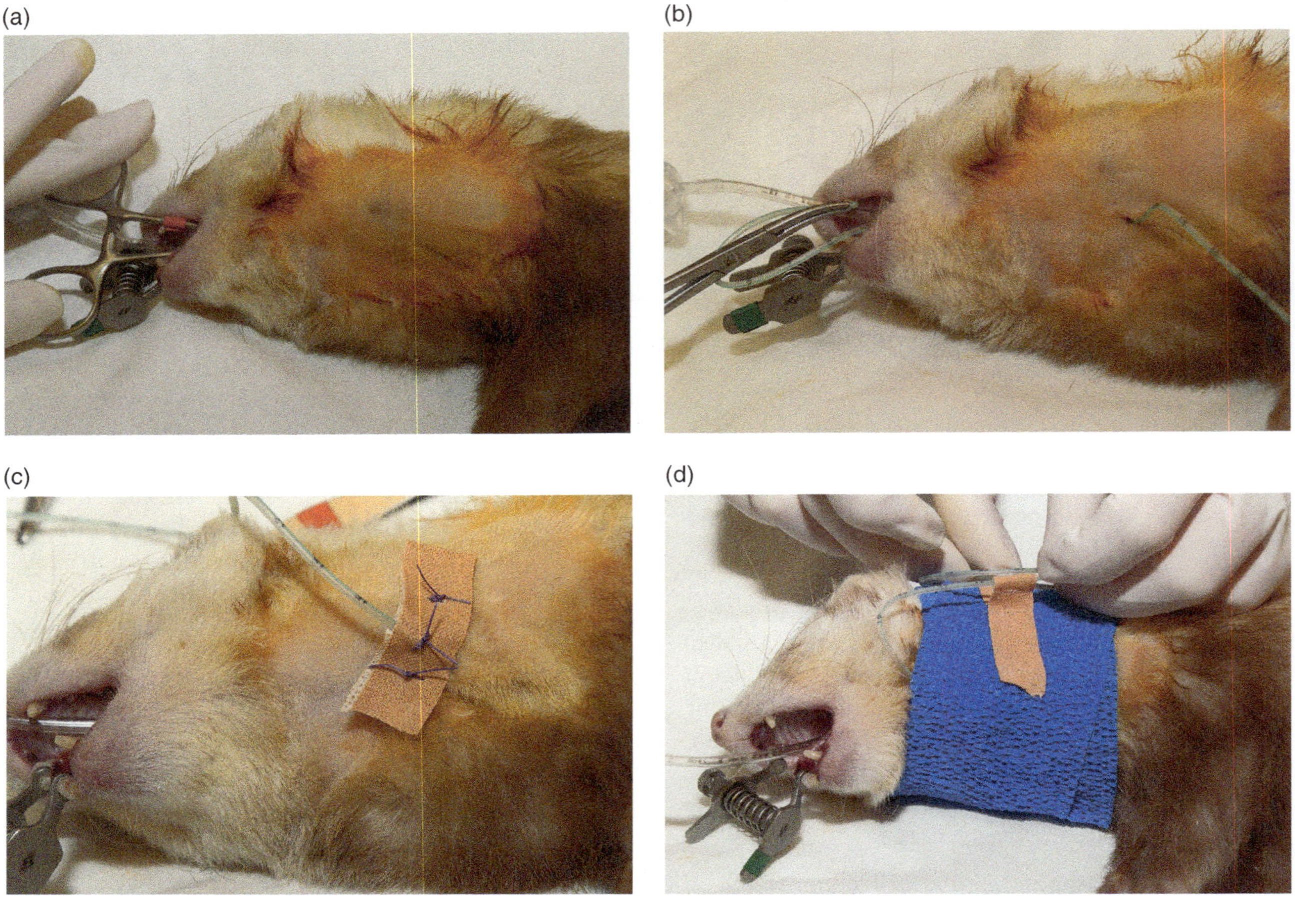

Figure 8.7 (a) Placement of an esophageal feeding tube in a ferret cadaver. After shaving, aseptic preparation, and marking of the feeding tube (distance from entry site to the last rib), a curved mosquito forceps is inserted through the mouth into the esophagus with the tip pointing laterally to allow a stab incision to be made over the tip through the skin, subcutis, and esophageal wall to allow it to exit through the skin. (b) Using the mosquito forceps, the feeding tube is then pulled through the incision back into the oral cavity, turned 180°, and directed back into the oral cavity and esophagus. (c) Sutures are placed proximal to the incision site to fix the tube into position. (d) A bandage is placed loosely around the neck to prevent the ferret from pulling the tube.

(and medication) is administered, the tube should be flushed once more to prevent clogging. Should this inadvertently occur, gentle flushing with a small amount of cola may help to resolve the obstruction. Esophageal tubes can usually be left in place up to six weeks or until the animal's appetite returns. After pulling the tube, the insertion site is allowed to heal by second intent.

Complications associated with placement of esophagostomy tubes in companion animals include necrosis, infection, and abscess formation at the tube entrance site, spontaneous tube removal by the patient, hemorrhage, vomiting, and kinking of the tube during placement.

Parenteral

Parenteral nutrition can be given to ferrets and rabbits in a similar fashion as is done in dogs and cats (see Tables 8.3 and 8.4; Remillard [1]). Primary indications for parenteral nutrition include prolonged periods of vomiting, acute pancreatitis, severe malabsorptive disorders, and severe ileus. Two major types of parenteral nutrition are as follows:

- Total parenteral nutrition (TPN), which is typically delivered via a central venous catheter and provides the total energy requirement of the patient;
- Partial parenteral nutrition (PPN), which is intended for short-term use in a non-debilitated patient with average nutritional requirement and delivers only a portion (i.e. 40–70%) of the animal's energy requirements, thereby lowering the osmolarity of the solution and allowing it to be administered through a large peripheral vein (e.g. lateral saphenous or femoral vein).

Table 8.3 Total nutrient admixture formula for a 1 kg ferret.

	Rate of administration	PN composition
Body weight	1.0 kg (= 293 × kgBW$^{0.75}$)	
Resting energy requirement	293 kJ	
Central catheter	550 or greater mOsm/l	
Nutritional component		
Percent Kcal from glucose	20% = 59 kJ	8 ml of 50% dextrose
Percent Kcal from lipid	80% = 235 kJ	28 ml of 20% lipid solution
Protein–calorie ratio	4 g/418 kJ = 2.8 g protein	33 ml of 8.5% AA solution
B vitamins	1 ml/418 kJ	1 ml
MultiTrace	1 ml/418 kJ	1 ml
		71 ml total
Fluid and electrolyte component		
Volume of crystalloid (norm R)	100 ml/kg BW = 100	100–71 from above = 29 ml
Phosphorous supplementation	10 nM/l × 0.11 = 1 nM	1.0–1.0 from above = 0 ml KPO_4
Potassium supplementation	30 mEq/l × 0.11 = 0.3 mEq	3.0–2.4 from above = 0.6 mEq = 0.3 ml KCl

Final volume = 112 ml with a 717 mOsm/l with a final electrolyte concentration.

Sodium	71.66 mEq/l	Calcium	0.0 mEq/l
Potassium	29.9 mEq/l	Zinc	6.25 µg/ml
Magnesium	4.1 mEq/l	Copper	2.5 µg/ml
Phosphate	9.8 mM/l	Manganese	0.63 µg/ml
Chloride	56.3 mEq/l	Chromium	25.0 ng/ml

Administration orders: TNA solution IV at 4.2 ml/h for 24 h via central catheter.

Source: From Remillard [1]. Reproduced with permission of Elsevier.

Central, peripheral, intraosseous, and/or intraperitoneal catheters may be used to administer parenteral nutrition with an osmolarity of less than 550 mOsm/l, whereas those with an osmolarity greater than 550 mOsm/l may only be administered into a central vein. The latter is commonly needed in ferrets as they have relatively high protein requirements, making it likely that the osmolarity exceeds 600 mOsm/l. In this species, the central catheter can be placed in the medial saphenous vein and then advanced into the caudal vena cava. As phlebitis is a common complication, silicone and polyurethane catheters are the only catheters to be considered when parenteral nutrition must be given for more than three days.

Parenteral nutrition always requires a dedicated catheter that is placed aseptically to minimize the risk for infection. Multi-lumen catheters are generally recommended as these can remain in place for longer periods while simultaneously providing other ports, e.g. for blood sampling and administering other fluids and medications. Formulation of TPN and PPN solutions is often adjusted to the individual patient, with most solutions comprising a carbohydrate source (dextrose), a protein source (amino acids), and a fat source (lipids). Vitamins and trace minerals can be added, if needed. Care should be taken never to exceed the animal's resting energy requirement (RER) as this may lead to metabolic complications (e.g. hyper- or hypoglycemia, hyperlipidemia, refeeding syndrome, acid-base disturbances).

Although technically feasible, clinical use of TPN has not been reported in small mammals, likely because of the lack of knowledge regarding exact nutrient requirements

Table 8.4 Total nutrient admixture formula for a 2.3 kg rabbit.

	Rate of administration	PN composition
Body weight	2.3 kg (= 293 × kgBW$^{0.75}$)	
Resting energy requirement	547 kJ	
Peripheral catheter	550 or less mOsm/l	
Nutritional component		
Percent Kcal from glucose	20% = 109 kJ	15 ml of 50% dextrose
Percent Kcal from lipid	80% = 438 kJ	52 ml of 20% lipid solution
Protein–calorie ratio	2 g/418 kJ = 2.6 g protein	30 ml of 8.5% AA solution
B vitamins	1 ml/418 kJ	1.3 ml
MultiTrace	1 ml/418 kJ	1.3 ml
		99.6 ml total
Fluid and electrolyte component		
Volume of crystalloid (norm R)	100 ml/kg BW = 230	230–99 from above = 131 ml
Phosphorous supplementation	10 nM/l × 0.23 l = 2.3 nM	2.3–0.9 from above = 1.4 nM = 0.5 ml KPO_4
Potassium supplementation	30 mEq/l × 0.11 l = 0.3 mEq	6.9–4.1 from above = 2.8 mEq = 1.4 ml KCl

Final volume = 230 ml with a 534 mOsm/l with a final electrolyte concentration.

Sodium	92.25 mEq/l	Calcium	0.0 mEq/l
Potassium	30.07 mEq/l	Zinc	5.1 μg/ml
Magnesium	3.0 mEq/l	Copper	2.1 μg/ml
Phosphate	9.8 mMl	Manganese	0.5 μg/ml
Chloride	67.1 mEq/l	Chromium	20.4 ng/ml

Administration orders: TNA solution IV at 9.5 ml/h for 24 h via peripheral catheter.

Source: From Remillard [1]. Reproduced with permission of Elsevier.

and the high costs involved. In rabbits in which TPN was experimentally applied, hepatocellular degeneration and portal tract inflammation were apparent in most animals as early as one week following the start of parenteral feeding. Some changes resolved after refeeding the animals, but in some animals, changes were permanent (i.e. portal fibrosis, functional cholestasis). In addition, complete colonic stasis occurred, indicating that parenteral feeding should be avoided if enteral feeding is an option.

Monitoring

In any patient receiving nutritional support, the body weight, fecal production (amount, consistency), and potential ongoing losses (e.g. due to diarrhea, vomiting, exudative wounds) should be monitored. Physical examination findings such as a decrease in subcutaneous fat stores, muscle wasting, and presence of edema or ascites will help to determine whether adjustments to the nutritional protocol are necessary. Although changes in body weight are often the primary parameter for evaluating adequate nutritional intake, weight changes should always be considered in relation to the animal's body condition as shifts in fluid dynamics can easily mask weight loss and/or be mistaken for weight gain. Thus, weight changes can only serve as a reliable parameter when fluid balance, urination, and fecal production are in order.

Especially in the herbivorous mammals, gastrointestinal hypomotility is a frequent sequela to inadequate fiber intake, resulting in decreased fecal pellet production and diminished gut sounds. Thus, these parameters deserve special attention during the physical exam.

Table 8.5 Guidelines for assessing hydration status in companion animals.

% Dehydration	Eyeball position	Skin tenting (seconds)	Mucous membranes
Normal	Normal	<1	Moist
1–5	Normal	1–4	Moist
6–8	Slightly sunken	5–10	Tacky
9–10	Gap between eyeball and surrounding tissues	11–15	Tacky to dry
>10[a]	Large gap and very sunken	16–45	Dry

[a] Often accompanied by signs of hypovolemic shock.

In patients with nasogastric or esophageal tubes, daily monitoring of the insertion site and patency of the tube is required. In addition, patients should be monitored for gastrointestinal signs (e.g. regurgitation, vomiting, cramping, bloating, diarrhea) and/or signs of volume overload or aspiration pneumonia. Serum electrolytes, glucose and liver values, and urinary ketones may be evaluated to detect metabolic changes (e.g. hypo- or hyperglycemia, electrolyte disturbances, hepatic lipidosis).

In patients receiving parenteral nutrition, sepsis, thrombophlebitis, and metabolic disturbances (e.g. hyperglycemia, electrolyte imbalances, hyperlipidemia) may occur. Frequent monitoring of vital signs, catheter exit sites, and routine biochemistry panels may help to detect and treat these potential complications in an early stage.

Fluid Therapy

Indications

The purpose of fluid therapy is to increase tissue perfusion; correct acid-base, electrolyte imbalances, fluid deficits and hypotension; supply daily fluid needs; and replace ongoing fluid losses. Thus, fluid therapy is a key element in the treatment of any sick, debilitated, or recovering small mammal. In patients with anemia, fluid therapy may be provided in the form of a blood transfusion or blood product.

Due to their small size and high metabolism, small mammals' daily fluid requirements are relatively high (50–100 ml/kg/day) when compared to that of dogs and cats. Dehydration and shock may therefore easily occur following a decrease in food and fluid intake. Clinical signs observed in small mammals with shock include altered mentation, prolonged capillary refill time (CRT), pale mucous membranes, a weak and thready pulse, hypotension, bradycardia/tachycardia, tachypnea, weakness, hypothermia, cold extremities, and reduced urine output. Dehydrated animals, in contrast, will commonly present with sunken eyes, prolonged skin tenting, and tacky to dry mucous membranes (see Table 8.5). In hindgut fermenters, hydration status is not always readily assessed as they initially will withdraw fluids from their large intestinal tract, hindering accurate estimation of fluid losses. As a result, decreased fecal production and gastrointestinal hypomotility will be the first clinical sign of dehydration in these species.

Fluid Types

Fluids given to small mammal patients can be divided into four groups, i.e. crystalloids, colloids, hemoglobin-based oxygen carriers, and blood. Fluids should preferably be administered bodily warm (i.e. 38–39 °C; 100.4–102.3 °F) to prevent cooling of the patient, except in hyperthermic patients. To ensure that the fluids are at an optimal temperature for administration, these can best be kept in fluid incubators set at the appropriate temperature.

Crystalloids

Isotonic crystalloids are the most commonly used fluids in critically ill patients and ideal to use during both the rehydration and maintenance phases of fluid therapy (see the paragraphs under *Fluid requirements* for the recommended doses). In addition, crystalloids can serve as a basis for intravenous administered drugs and/or to supplement the patient with minerals such as potassium, dextrose, calcium chloride, calcium gluconate, sodium bicarbonate, and water-soluble B vitamins. As fluid therapy frequently results in dilution of plasma potassium and subsequent hypokalemia, routine supplementation with potassium is recommended, for which the following correction formula can be used to calculate the amount to supplement: $(5-[K]) \times BW\ (kg) \times 0.6\ =\ \_\_$ mmol correction

(*Note: 5 represents the desired plasma concentration; [K] the actual plasma concentration*). For example, the amount of potassium needed for correction in an 800-g ferret with a plasma potassium concentration of 3.4 mmol/l will be: $(5-3.4)\times 0.8\times 0.6 = 0.77$ mmol, whereby the maximum amount administered should not exceed 0.5 mmol/kg/h (indicating this amount should be given over at least two hours). Alternatively, potassium may be orally supplemented. A formula for adding bicarbonate to crystalloids can be found in Table 6.4.

Hypertonic crystalloids (e.g. 7.5% saline) are used predominantly for resuscitation of hypovolemia and can be administered in small volumes (i.e. 3–5 ml/kg) over 10 minutes. The high osmolarity of the fluid draws fluids from the interstitial and intracellular spaces into the intravascular space, thereby resulting in rapid expansion of the intravascular volume. Due to this effect, the use of hypertonic saline should be avoided in dehydrated patients, as they already have a volume-depleted extravascular fluid compartment.

Colloids

Colloids are fluids that contain large molecular weight substances and include products such as plasma, dextrans, hydroxyethyl starch (hetastarch), and hemoglobin-based oxygen carriers (HBOC). When the vascular endothelium is intact, these substances (except plasma) remain within the plasma compartment, thereby aiding in rapid correction of hypotension with a minimal risk of developing edema. A specific HBOC fluid historically used in small mammal medicine was Oxyglobin®. This product contains purified, polymerized bovine hemoglobin and may be used in patients with anemia if donor blood is not available or cross-matching is not possible. Unfortunately, to the author's knowledge, the product is currently not available.

Colloids can be administered as boluses in doses of up to 5 ml/kg IV or IO over a period of 10–20 minutes until blood pressure and heart rate have normalized. Daily doses should not exceed 20 ml/kg. Dosages for Oxyglobin are lower compared to the other colloids (i.e. 2 ml/kg over 10–15 minutes, or continuous rate infusion [CRI] at 0.2–0.4 ml/kg/h).

Blood Products

Indications for blood transfusions include an increased need for albumin, coagulation factors, and/or red blood cells. Although thrombocytopenia is sometimes mentioned as an indication for blood transfusion, platelets are usually lost during the collection process as they tend to aggregate against the plastic of the collection syringe. Aside from the need for blood transfusions in animals with acute trauma, rabbits are most commonly presented with chronic blood loss due to uterine pathology (e.g. venous aneurysm, cystic endometrial hyperplasia, or endometrial carcinoma). In ferrets, pancytopenia is seen in jills with hyperestrogenism due to persistent estrus. Chronic blood loss may also occur due to *Helicobacter*-associated gastric ulcers. Criteria for donor selection, testing and typing, as well as storage of blood are found in *Chapter 4 – Catheterization and Venipuncture*.

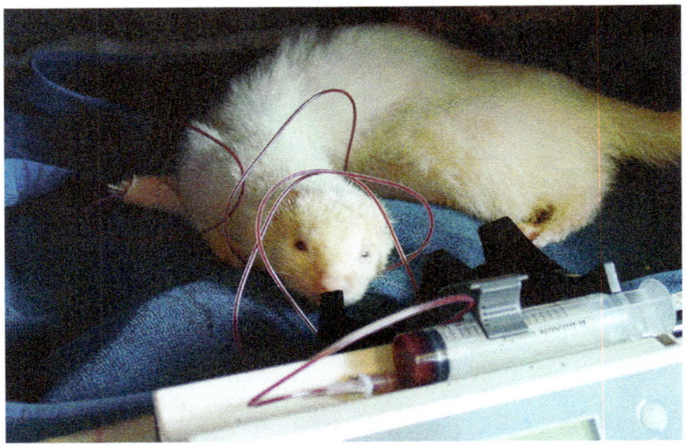

Figure 8.8 Blood transfusions in ferrets are relatively easy, as ferrets do not have blood groups and most owners have multiple ferrets. The cephalic vein is most commonly used to provide the blood.

The most common route for administering blood or blood products is the intravenous route (Figure 8.8), although the intraosseous route can be used as well. To minimize the risk of bacterial growth in blood that is stored at room temperature, blood transfusions should be completed within four hours. Prewarming of the blood to approximately 42 °C (107.6 °F) is recommended to prevent development of hypothermia. An 18-mm filter system attached to intravenous tubing should be used to remove blood clots and debris that may predispose to embolism. The recommended rate of administration during the first 20 minutes of the transfusion is 1.5 ml/kg/h, following which the rate may gradually be increased up to 12 ml/kg/h if no transfusion reactions are observed. Once all the blood has been administered, fluid therapy can be continued with crystalloids. The packed cell volume (PCV) can be remeasured after one to two hours to evaluate the effect.

As a last resort, it has recently been found that a xenotransfusion with feline red blood cells can be given to ferrets and rabbits when species specific blood is not available.

Transfusion Reactions Transfusion reactions have not been reported in small mammals, but may nevertheless occur. Establishing a base line[4] prior to the start of the transfusion and rechecking these parameters at least every 30 minutes will aid in early detection of possible transfusion reactions. Acute hemolytic transfusion reactions will most likely occur in case of a mismatch between the blood of the donor and that of the recipient. Clinical signs include signs of disseminated intravascular coagulation, bronchospasm, and vascular collapse. Should these signs be observed, the transfusion should be stopped immediately and administration of corticosteroids, fluids, and bronchodilators be initiated.

The "febrile non-hemolytic reaction" is another type of transfusion reaction characterized by hyperthermia. If this occurs, the transfusion should be stopped for 15 minutes and restarted at a slower rate, with more frequent monitoring (e.g. every 5–10 minutes). If no hemolysis is seen, the transfusion may be continued.

Fluid Requirements

The amount of fluids required varies according to the condition of the patient. Fluid requirements are highest in patients in shock, which require rapid administration of large amounts of fluids over a short period to replace the intravascular volume and restore tissue perfusion and oxygenation (i.e. the resuscitation phase of fluid therapy). Once the patient has been stabilized, the rehydration phase of fluid therapy is initiated where the focus lies with correction of interstitial fluid deficits and rehydrating the patient. Patients that are stable, but do not drink themselves, will need to be given enough fluids to maintain the fluid balance (i.e. maintenance phase).

Shock Fluids

In patients with hypovolemic shock, the major goal of fluid therapy is to restore normotension as quickly as possible. This can best be achieved by administering fluids IV or IO. As peripheral circulation is severely diminished, the common perception is that, during hypotension, subcutaneous (SC) fluids will hardly be absorbed. However, providing SC fluids is always preferred to providing no fluids at all.

Resuscitation can generally be safely accomplished using a combination of crystalloids, colloids, and rewarming procedures:

1) In severely hypovolemic patients (i.e. systolic blood pressure below 40 mmHg), hypertonic saline (7.2–7.5%) can be given in a bolus at 3 ml/kg over a period of 10 minutes, followed by administration of colloids at a similar dose and rate. Continued blood pressure measurement is indicated to monitor the effects.
2) Once blood pressure is above 40 mmHg, the hypertonic saline can be replaced by a bolus infusion of isotonic crystalloids at 10–15 ml/kg combined with a bolus of colloids at 5 ml/kg given over 5–10 minutes. This procedure needs to be repeated four times per hour until the systolic blood pressure is above 90 mmHg.
3) Once normotension (>90 mmHg) is achieved, administration of colloids is stopped, and further replacement fluid therapy is given with crystalloids, and the rehydration phase may be initiated. Alternatively, colloids can be continued at a CRI of 0.8 ml/kg/h until the blood pressure, heart rate, CRT, and mucous membrane color have normalized.

Simultaneous with fluid resuscitation, rewarming should take place over one to two hours using warm water bottles, forced air heating blankets, warming of intravenous fluids, and/or placing the patient in a preheated incubator. Regularly temperature rechecks are required to prevent hyperthermia.

Patients with non-responsive shock should be evaluated and treated for potential underlying causes (e.g. excessive vasodilation or vasoconstriction, hypoglycemia, electrolyte imbalances or acid-base disturbances, hypoxemia, cardiac dysfunction). If the condition perseveres despite correction of the underlying causes, treatment for non-responsive shock is continued by bolus or CRI administration of Oxyglobin (2 ml/kg over 10–15 minutes or 0.2–0.4 ml/kg/h; not currently commercially available) or colloids (5 ml/kg over 10 minutes). In addition, the use of vasopressors, such as dopamine (5–10 μg/kg/min), can be considered to treat refractory hypotension.

Replacement/Losses

During the rehydration phase of fluid therapy, fluids are provided to correct for the interstitial fluid losses and dehydration. Interstitial fluid deficits are typically associated with a decrease in skin turgor (Figure 8.9), sunken eyes, and tacky to dry mucous membranes (see Table 8.3). As parameters can be affected by decreased body fat and increased age, caution is warranted with too strict interpretation of the guidelines for estimating fluid deficits.

Rehydration of the interstitial compartment is best accomplished using isotonic replacement fluids as these can easily diffuse to the different body fluid compartments. The amount of fluid that needs to be given to replace the

4 Baseline to include the demeanor, core body temperature, pulse, respiratory rate, mucous membrane color, and capillary refill time.

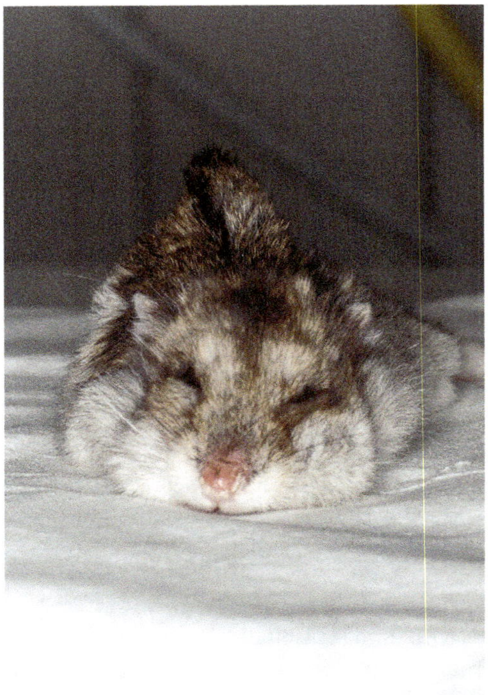

Figure 8.9 Severely prolonged skin turgor in a debilitated Campbell's dwarf hamster. After tenting the skin did not return to its original position.

deficit needs to be calculated based on the estimated dehydration status. Fluid deficits are usually replaced over a period of 4–24 hours,[5] dependent on the rate of fluid losses as well as the patient's clinical status. The formula used to calculate the fluid requirement to correct the fluid deficit is: % dehydration × kg × 1000 ml/l.

Example: A ferret of 1.2 kg has an estimated dehydration of 7%. This ferret will have a fluid deficit of 0.07 × 1.2 × 1000 = 84 ml.

The calculated amount of fluid to correct for dehydration should be added to the maintenance fluid requirements and requirements to compensate for ongoing fluid losses to replenish the total fluid losses.

Maintenance

During the maintenance phase, fluids, and electrolytes are provided to replace ongoing losses, meet metabolic demands, and restore intracellular water balance until the patient is eating and drinking on its own. Due to the higher metabolism and body surface to bodyweight ratio, small mammals are assumed to have higher maintenance requirements (i.e. 50–100 ml/kg/day) compared to dogs and cats. As overhydration through IV or IO administration may result in lung edema and potentially death, it is important to monitor the fluid balance (fluid intake versus loss). Enteral feeding can be used to supply part of the animal's maintenance requirements and should be considered when calculating the required fluid volumes and rates.

5 In patients with interstitial fluid losses that are cardiovascularly stable, fluid losses may be replaced over a period of 12–24 hours. If fluid losses are more rapid, replacement of fluid deficits may be accomplished over a period of four to six hours.

Routes

Oral

Oral rehydration is only advised when dehydration is estimated to be less than 5% as uptake is postulated to be slow. The patient should be able to swallow and show no signs of gastrointestinal compromise. In rabbits, the percentage of total body water in the digestive tract can be as high as 12%, compared to 3% in dogs. As a result, providing oral fluids to rehydrate the GI tract is therefore advised in hindgut fermenters. However, parenteral fluids will also be required to ensure adequate provision of fluids for the rest of the body.

Rectal

The intrarectal administration of fluids has been described in rabbits, whereby warmed isotonic fluids are administered in the rectum over a period of 15 minutes to aid in the recovery of hypovolemic shock.

Subcutaneous

Subcutaneous fluids should primarily be given to patients that are considered stable and less than 5% dehydrated. However, the risks of catheter placement may outweigh its benefits in some patients with shock. In these patients, the administration of subcutaneous fluids may be considered until the patient is stable enough for placement of the catheter. Only isotonic fluids may be given subcutaneously, as hypertonic solutions will cause a shift of fluids into the interstitial space and worsen electrolyte imbalances.

Volumes of up to 100–150 ml/kg/day can be provided through the subcutaneous route and are usually divided over two to four times per day. Although large amounts (i.e. up to 40–50 ml/kg) can be given in one location, some authors recommend not to give more than 20 ml/kg in the same location at once to minimize the risk for (avascular) skin necrosis.

Subcutaneous fluid boluses, consisting of 0.18% NaCl combined with 4% dextrose (10–15 ml/kg), may be administered preoperatively to conveniently replace intra-operative water losses and anticipated postoperative deficits. Once administered, this fluid will be slowly absorbed, hence limiting its value in treating cardiovascular failure.

Intraperitoneal

Especially in small rodents, the intraperitoneal route allows for easy and effective administration of fluids which are readily absorbed due to the large surface of the peritoneum. Overhydration is reported, but in animals with normal functioning kidneys risks are considered limited as osmotic pressure will prevent overloading the vascular system. In hindgut fermenters, the peritoneal space is less ideal to be used as a route for fluid administration as the cecum can potentially be punctured during placement of a peritoneal catheter. However, in rabbits, peritoneal dialysis has experimentally been performed following percutaneous placement of a commercial 15-Fr peritoneal catheter. However, surgical placement may be considered to avoid accidental perforation of the cecum. Complications of the procedure include peritonitis, pain, infection of the catheter site, protein loss, and overhydration, thereby rarely resulting in a successful outcome. Moreover, the technique is labor-intensive and time-consuming, thereby rendering it a technique that should only be used as a last resort in pet rabbits with oliguric or anuric renal failure.

Intravenous/Intraosseous

The intravenous (IV) route is considered the preferred route of fluid therapy for resuscitation and rehydration. As discussed in Chapter 4, the intraosseous (IO) route is equally effective in terms of fluid administration rates and therapeutic agent dosing. Since placement of an IO catheter requires anesthesia, the IV route is preferred whenever possible. Catheters should be removed within three days following placement to prevent infections at the insertion site.

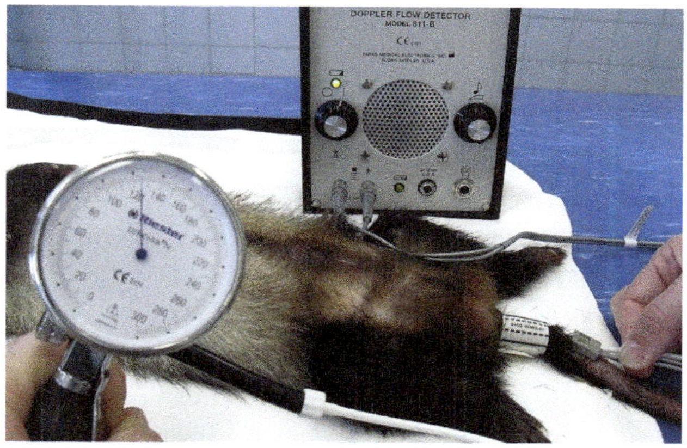

Figure 8.10 (Same as Figure 6.3) Indirect blood pressure measurement can most easily and, accurately, be measured at the tail in ferrets.

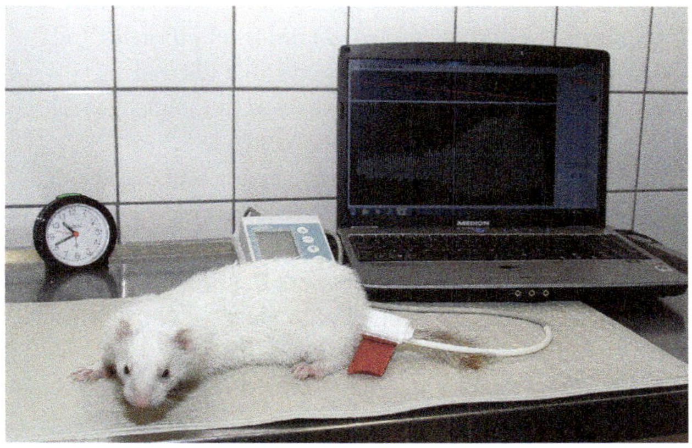

Figure 8.11 Blood pressure measurement in a ferret with an HDO monitor in a research setting. On the laptop, the normal curve of the blood pressure wave is seen to check whether the measurement was performed correctly.

Monitoring

The effect of fluid therapy can be monitored using clinical parameters such as the animal's general demeanor, skin turgor, CRT, moistness and color of mucous membranes, respiratory rate, pulse quality and frequency, body temperature, and temperature of the extremities. In addition, the patient's weight should be monitored carefully as large, rapid increases provide a good indication of rehydration. Urinary output should be measured concurrently as the absence of urinary production combined with great weight increases suggest potential overhydration of a patient with anuric or oliguric renal failure. Other signs indicating overhydration include the onset of breathing difficulties combined with crackles heard upon auscultation of the lungs. The latter indicates the presence of lung edema which warrants immediate discontinuation of IV or IO fluid therapy as well as the provision of supplemental oxygen therapy and (IV or IO) administration of diuretics (e.g. furosemide 1–4 mg/kg q8h).

Blood pressure measurements also allow monitoring of fluid therapy effects. As previously mentioned, the goal is to increase systolic blood pressure to above 90 mmHg. Accurate blood pressure measurement will require the use of an intra-arterial catheter for direct arterial blood pressure measurement. However, this will seldom be possible in small mammals other than rabbits. Indirect blood pressure measurements, in contrast, are generally easier to obtain, whereby the front leg and tail are considered the preferred locations for cuff placement. While the combination of a sphygmomanometer and an ultrasonic Doppler device is most commonly used in small mammals (Figure 8.10), the use of high definition oscillometry (HDO) is gaining interest (Figure 8.11). As indirect blood pressure measurements seldom provide accurate measurements, trends are more important to monitor than actual values.

As fluid therapy is also given to correct acid-base and electrolyte imbalances and may influence many plasma parameters (e.g. PCV, total protein, albumin, urea, creatinine, Ca, P, Na, K), daily collection of blood should be considered for monitoring purposes. In the smaller-sized mammals, this may not be feasible due to their limited blood volume, but in the larger mammalian this should be considered to adjust and optimize the therapeutic plan.

Reference

1 Remillard, R.L. (2006). Parenteral nutrition support in rabbits and ferrets. *J. Exot. Pet Med.* 15 (4): 248–254.

Further Reading

Adamovicz, L., Bullen, L., Saker, K., and Grunkemeyer, V. (2016). Use of an esophagostomy tube for management of traumatic subtotal glossectomy in an African pygmy hedgehog (*Atelerix albiventris*). *J. Exot. Pet Med.* 25 (3): 231–236.

DiBartola, S.P. and Bateman, S. (2012). Introduction to fluid therapy. In: *Fluid Therapy in Small Animal Practice* (ed. S.P. DiBartola), 265–280. St. Louis, MO: Elsevier.

Graham, J. (2006). Common procedures in rabbits. *Vet. Clin. North Am. Exot. Anim. Pract.* 9 (2): 367–388.

Hohenhaus, A.E. (2012). Blood transfusion and blood substitutes. In: *Fluid Therapy in Small Animal Practice* (ed. S.P. DiBartola), 585–604. St. Louis, MO: Elsevier.

Huynh, M., Boyeaux, A., and Pignon, C. (2016). Assessment and care of the critically ill rabbit. *Vet. Clin. North Am. Exot. Anim. Pract.* 19 (2): 379–409.

Lennox, A.M. (2007). Emergency and critical care procedures in sugar gliders (*Petaurus breviceps*), African hedgehogs (*Atelerix albiventris*), and prairie dogs (*Cynomys spp*). *Vet. Clin. North Am. Exot. Anim. Pract.* 10 (2): 533–555.

Lichtenberger, M. (2004). Principles of shock and fluid therapy in special species. *Semin. Avian Exot. Pet Med.* 13 (3): 142–153.

Lichtenberger, M. and Lennox, A.M. (2012). Emergency and critical care of small mammals. In: *Ferrets, Rabbits and Rodents: Clinical Medicine and Surgery*, 3e (eds. K.E. Quesenberry and J.W. Carpenter), 532–544. St Louis, MO: Elsevier.

Lichtenberger, M. and Lennox, A.M. (2012). Critical care of the exotic companion mammal (with a focus on herbivorous species): the first twenty-four hours. *J. Exot. Pet Med.* 21 (4): 284–292.

de Matos, R.E.C. and Morrisey, J.K. (2006). Common procedures in the pet ferret. *Vet. Clin. North Am. Exot. Anim. Pract.* 9 (2): 347–365.

McLaughlin, A. and Strunk, A. (2016). Common emergencies in small rodents, hedgehogs, and sugar gliders. *Vet. Clin. North Am. Exot. Anim. Pract.* 19 (2): 465–499.

Proença, L.M. and Mayer, J. (2014). Prescription diets for rabbits. *Vet. Clin. North Am. Exot. Anim. Pract.* 17 (3): 485–502.

Section 2

Diagnostics

9

STAT Diagnostics in Exotic Companion Mammals

Sara Gardhouse

Department of Clinical Sciences, College of Veterinary Medicine, Kansas State University, Manhattan, USA

CONTENTS

Exotic mammal emergencies should be triaged and handled in a similar manner to other mammals. However, it is important to keep in mind that the natural history, physiology, and behavior of many exotic animals warrants special handling techniques due to their easily stressed nature and propensity to destabilize rapidly [1].

Point-of-Care Testing (POCT)

Point-of-care testing (POCT) refers to the use of pathology laboratory tests that are performed near the patient, without the use of a traditional laboratory [2]. The use of POCT is critical to the emergency evaluation of any patient [2]. It enables rapid clinical decision making in the process of diagnosing a patient, either ruling in or out specific disease processes, treatment decisions, essential patient monitoring tools, and resource utilization [2]. It is always important, however, to keep in mind that the rapid results afforded by POCT do not always result in improved patient care if the test performance is questionable due to quality of the test, failure of the test, or lack of operator training [2]. POCT should be used with a specific clinical question in mind to help aid in a patient's diagnosis and should not be used as a replacement for main laboratory testing, and rather as a complement to it [2].

Point-of-Care Blood Sampling

As with any emergency patient, aside from a good history and physical examination, evaluation of the blood is a very important component of the initial evaluation of a critical exotic mammal patient [3]. Though this is extraordinarily useful and important information, a unique challenge faced with exotic mammals may be the difficulties associated with blood collection and the stability of the patient and necessary restraint (i.e. sedation or anesthesia) that is required to acquire such a sample [3]. Various studies in laboratory small mammals have been undertaken that

Exotic Animal Emergency and Critical Care Medicine, First Edition. Edited by Jennifer E. Graham, Grayson A. Doss and Hugues Beaufrère.

generally demonstrate that 1% of body weight can be safely removed from healthy individuals [4]. However, it is important to keep in mind that the animals that present as an emergency are typically not healthy, may be anemic or hypovolemic, and the sampling volume may need to be adjusted accordingly [3]. An ideal minimum database should include a packed cell volume, total protein, blood glucose, and a blood smear that should be evaluated [5].

Packed Cell Volume (PCV) and Total Protein (TP)

Both a packed cell volume (PCV) and total protein (TP) can be easily obtained and evaluated from a microhematocrit capillary tube. PCV evaluates the percentage of the red blood cells in circulating blood [6]. TP is measured with a refractometer which measures the angle of refraction between air and an aqueous solution. The TS is measured with the use of a refractometer and is evaluated based on the refraction angle that is produced [7]. The angle of refraction that is created by a plasma sample is a result of the combined concentration of all solutes, which is the total solids (TS) [7]. The refractometer measures total solids and then approximates this value to a total plasma protein value on the scale of the refractometer (reticle scale) [7]. The plasma total solids concentration that is provided by the refractometer is approximately 15–20 g/l greater than the total protein concentration, due to the contributions that come from glucose, urea, and cholesterol [7]. As a result of this, total solids will increase in animals with increased glucose, and increased cholesterol, and would be expected to occur in samples with gross lipemia or hemolysis [7]. Given these challenges associated with total solids measurement and the contribution from nonprotein solids, refractometric tests overall have reduced sensitivity compared to laboratory chemistry profiles [7]. As a consequence of this, total solids are often incorrectly referred to as total protein, but it is important to keep in mind that they are not the same. In normal samples, the non-protein solids account for a small contribution and are assumed to be normal and unchanged; however, in samples that contain a large amount of non-protein solids, the refractometer will give a falsely high total protein reading. This stresses the importance of critical evaluation of a biochemistry profile. It is also of important note to consider the difference between plasma total protein and serum total protein, as plasma total protein may be slightly higher due to the inclusion of plasma fibrinogen [8].

Indications

PCV should be evaluated in all emergent patients, but particularly those where there is a suspicion of anemia, due to blood loss, red blood cell destruction, or failure of bone marrow production. PCV is also useful in cases where an increased number of red blood cells (erythrocytosis) is suspected either due to dehydration or an abnormal increase in red blood cell production. TP should be evaluated in any emergent patients as well, but particularly patients with a concern for protein loss such as blood loss, protein-losing enteropathy, protein-losing nephropathy, or malnutrition. Increased TP is usually indicative of dehydration but can also be seen with chronic disease.

Normal PCV and TP reference ranges for commonly seen exotic small mammals are provided in Table 9.1. Evaluation of the PCV and TP together can already help in the formulation of differential diagnoses for the patient, as well as guide therapeutics (Table 9.2).

Table 9.1 Normal PCV and TP reference ranges for common exotic small mammals.

Species	PCV (%)	TP (g/dl)
Rabbits [9]	34–43	5.0–7.5
Ferrets [10]	47–59	5.0–6.8
Guinea pigs [11]	43 ± 12	4.5–5.9
Chinchillas [12]	37 (35–40)	5.6 (5.3–6.0)
Mice [13]	34–50	4.6–6.9
Rats [13]	33–47	5.6–7.4
Hedgehogs [14]	36 ± 7	5.8 ± 0.7
Sugar Gliders [15]	45–53	5.1–6.1
Hamsters [13]	45–52	5.2–7.0
Gerbils [13]	41–52	5.6 (4.6–6.3)

Table 9.2 Interpretation of PCV and TP.

Packed cell volume (%)	Total protein (g/dl)	Differential diagnoses
Increased	Increased	Dehydration – verify with urine specific gravity
Increased	Normal	Dehydration, protein loss
Increased	Decreased	Acute blood loss
Normal	Increased	Anemia, dehydration
Normal	Normal	Normal
Normal	Decreased	Protein loss
Decreased	Increased	Anemia, dehydration
Decreased	Normal	Red blood cell destruction
Decreased	Decreased	Whole blood loss

Source: Based on Fielding et al. [16].

Other Uses for a Hematocrit Tube Sample

It is also very important to examine the hematocrit tube when it is removed from the centrifuge to evaluate the buffy coat which can give a general idea of the white blood cell count of the animal [17]. The buffy coat is present between the layer of red blood cells and the plasma and should normally be less than 1 % [18]. If a large buffy coat is noted, it can represent an elevation in the white blood cell count [18].

It is also very important to examine the plasma layer of the hematocrit tube for evidence of lipemia, hemolysis, or icterus [19]. When lipemia is present, the plasma will appear cloudy or white in color [20]. When hemolysis is present, the plasma will often have a pink color [20]. If hemolysis is present, factors such as toxins such as heavy metal or aflatoxin, sepsis, or errors in sample collection should all be considered [20].

Blood Glucose (BG)

Blood glucose (BG) is easily evaluated with a plasma, serum, or whole blood sample. The most common analyzers utilized in a point of care (POC) setting for assessment of blood glucose include a glucometer, blood gas analyzer, or POC biochemistry analyzer.

Glucometers

The use of human or veterinary glucometers often demonstrate significant differences in blood glucose values when compared to laboratory biochemistry profiles [21–23]. However, in some species, glucometers may be useful to evaluate for trends or significant concerns in an exotic small mammal patient. In general, in exotic small mammals, veterinary glucometers have been demonstrated to overestimate the BG value, and human glucometers have been demonstrated to underestimate the BG value (Table 9.3) [21–23].

Normal blood glucose values measured by standard laboratory analyzers vary by exotic small mammal species (Table 9.4).

There are several conditions and situations in exotic small mammals that warrant the evaluation of a BG immediately upon presentation.

Ferrets that present on emergency should always have a blood glucose value assessed immediately [22]. Hypoglycemia in ferrets is a very common presentation, often secondary to pancreatic islet β-cell tumors, more commonly referred to as insulinomas [22]. Other differentials for hypoglycemia in this species include septicemia, severe hepatic insufficiency, hypoadrenocorticism, or starvation, though are much less common [24].

Guinea pigs have also been reported with insulinomas, and therefore, lethargic or weak guinea pigs should also have blood glucose values evaluated [25–27].

Blood glucose has also been utilized as a prognostic indicator in rabbits [28]. A significant relationship between blood glucose and food intake, signs of stress, and severity of clinical disease has been demonstrated in rabbits [28]. Stressed rabbits demonstrate a higher blood glucose than rabbits with no signs of stress [28]. Rabbits with complete anorexia demonstrate higher blood glucose values than those with normal food intake or hyporexia [28]. Severe hyperglycemia (>20 mmol/l, 360 mg/dl) has been demonstrated to be associated with conditions with a poor prognosis [28]. In cases of confirmed intestinal obstruction, the mean blood glucose value was demonstrated to be 24.7 mmol/l (444.6 mg/dl) compared to rabbits presenting with non-obstructive gastrointestinal stasis with a mean blood glucose of 8.5 mmol/l (153 mg/dl) [28]. Overall, the use of BG in rabbits is useful as both an indicator of the severity of a rabbit's condition on presentation and also to help with differentiation of gastrointestinal stasis versus intestinal obstruction [28].

Table 9.4 Normal blood glucose values for exotic companion mammals.

Species	Blood glucose (mg/dl)
Rabbits [9]	74–148
Ferrets [10]	99–135
Guinea pigs [11]	80–110
Chinchillas [12]	180 (163–197)
Mice [13]	90–193
Rats [13]	50–135
Hamsters [13]	84.0 ± 18.5 (M), 100.0 ± 16.6 (F)
Sugar gliders [15]	130–183
Hedgehogs [14]	89 ± 30

Table 9.3 Utility of handheld glucometers in exotic companion mammals.

Species	Veterinary glucometer: Canine	Veterinary glucometer: Feline	Human glucometer	Recommendation
Black-tailed prairie dogs (*Cynomys ludovicianus*) [21]	Overestimates BG	Overestimates BG	Underestimates BG	None of the measurement methods were consistently accurate
Ferrets (*Mustela putorius furo*) [22]	Overestimates BG	Overestimates BG	Underestimates BG	Veterinary glucometer on canine setting most accurate
Rabbits (*Oryctolagus cuniculus*) [23]	Overestimates BG	Overestimates BG	Underestimates BG	Human glucometer most accurate

Lactate

Lactate is produced by the enzyme lactate dehydrogenase as the end product of pyruvate metabolism during both aerobic and anaerobic glucose metabolism [29, 30]. Lactate is produced during times of tissue hypoperfusion when decreased oxygen delivery to the tissues results in a change to anaerobic glycolysis, leading to provision of energy through the conversion of pyruvate to lactate [29]. The end result of this process is an elevation in lactate values on bloodwork. Common causes of elevated lactate values include shock, low cardiac output states, acute liver failure, severe sepsis, neoplasia, seizures, poisoning, and drug therapy [31]. The measurement of lactate in an emergency setting can be performed with the use a blood gas/electrolyte panel, or a point-of-care lactate meter.

Lactate exists as a pair of stereoisomers (more specifically enantiomers), L-lactate, and D-lactate [30, 31]. L-lactate is measured by POC analyzers, and it is used to detect local and systemic hypoperfusion, as well as a monitoring tool for response to treatment [30]. L-lactate values have been frequently used as a prognostic indicator in human medicine, with increasing levels of hyperlactatemia being associated with an increased mortality rate [29, 32]. This has also been demonstrated in veterinary medicine, where L-lactate has been demonstrated to have both diagnostic and prognostic value with shock [33, 34]. D-lactate is produced through metabolism of glucose and carbohydrates by gastrointestinal bacteria [31]. Although this value may have some clinical use, it is not commonly measured.

Reference ranges for lactate in many exotic small mammal species are lacking (Table 9.5); however, L- and D-lactate values have been described for rabbits, with D-lactate values being similar to other mammals, and L-lactate values being higher in healthy rabbits compared with other mammals [30]. It was also demonstrated in this study that the agreement between blood gas analyzers and portable analyzers with laboratory results demonstrated a significant difference in lactate values [30]. A single value on arrival at an emergency hospital has been demonstrated to have poor diagnostic or prognostic value, but serial monitoring of L-lactate concentrations can provide important information [38]. If a sudden increase in L-lactate concentration is noted in conjunction with evidence of a metabolic acidosis, this can be an indicator of metabolic distress in the patient [38]. In critically ill rabbits, L-lactate values were demonstrated to be persistently low with minimal fluctuations, compared with rabbits that had a good prognosis, where lactate values were seen to be increased [38].

Table 9.5 Lactate values for exotic companion mammals.

Species	Blood L-lactate (mmol/l)
Rabbits [30]	6.9 ± 2.7 (portable analyzer)
	7.1 ± 1.6 (blood gas analyzer)
Ferrets [35] (reference interval)	0.3–1.5 (portable analyzer)
Guinea Pigs [36] (min-max)	
Short hair English guinea pigs	0.11–0.56 (blood gas analyzer)
Duncan-Hartley guinea pigs	0.003–0.73 (blood gas analyzer)
Rats [37] (reference interval)	
Male Wistar rats	1.9–5.61 (blood gas analyzer)
Female Wistar rats	1.15–5.42 (blood gas analyzer)
Mice [37] (reference interval)	
Male C57/BL6 mice	0.04–1.09 (blood gas analyzer)
Female C57/BL6 mice	0.04–0.8 (blood gas analyzer)

Blood Smear Evaluation

Evaluation of the blood smear is an invaluable tool in the assessment of a critical patient. Examination of the monolayer of a well-prepared and properly stained blood smear will allow for evaluation of the morphology of the cells, allow cellular counts and estimates to be obtained, and allow for evaluation of other features on the blood smear [39]. Morphology of the erythrocytes (RBC=red blood cell), leukocytes (WBC=white blood cell), and platelets can be examined on the blood smear [39]. Changes in the orientation, size, shape, and the color of the cells on the blood smear can be useful indicators of disorders such as anemia, neoplasia, infection, inflammation, myeloproliferative disorders, and defects in the bone marrow [39]. These changes may be missed if only an automated analyzer is used; hence, reiterating the importance of looking at a blood smear [39]. Not only can the blood smear be used for evaluation of the morphology of cells, the blood smear can also be used to assess cellular counts and estimates [39]. Evaluation of the blood smear can provide an assessment of both the relative and absolute values of segmented neutrophils (or heterophils), band neutrophils (or heterophils), lymphocytes, monocytes, eosinophils, and basophils [39]. These values are useful to help evaluate for the presence of infection and inflammation [39]. The slide is also useful to evaluate for the presence of other changes such as immature cells, inclusions, parasites, cellular clumping, and toxic changes [39].

Coagulation Testing

There is minimal information regarding coagulation testing in small mammals [40, 41]. Prothrombin time (PT) and activated partial thromboplastin time (aPTT) are the most commonly performed blood coagulation tests [42]. A prolonged PT is indicative of a deficiency or inhibition of the extrinsic pathway, compared to a prolonged aPTT which is indicative of a deficiency or inhibition of the intrinsic pathway [42]. When both parameters are prolonged, it may be suggestive of a deficiency or inhibition of the common pathway [42]. Results of aPTT testing have been questioned as many testing modalities use an aPTT reagent that contains soy phosphates and rabbit brain phosphatides [42]. PT has also been performed with rabbit brain reagent as well [43]. This makes the utility of these tests, particularly in rabbits, questionable.

Blood Gas and Acid-Base Evaluation

Blood gas evaluation is a critical tool in the assessment of a patient and can provide valuable information on the severity of the illness or injury, to assist in diagnosis, to determine fluid therapy needs, and to assist in determination for other treatment needs of the patient [44]. Ideally, arterial samples are utilized for blood gas analysis, but often venous samples are used due to ease of sample collection. If a venous sample is used, assessment of blood oxygenation and lung efficiency is not possible, but venous samples do provide a better reflection of the metabolic status of the body [44]. The vast majority of the values differ only by a small amount when comparing venous and arterial samples, except for the PO_2, which is significantly lower in the venous sample [44]. Abnormalities of the metabolic component are more common in veterinary medicine than those of the respiratory component [44].

Proper sample collection is critical to ensure accurate results and should be done with collection into an airtight heparinized syringe [45]. Sample storage will affect results, with changes in the PO_2 noted after only 12 minutes [46]. There are many different radiometers available for sample analysis, some with more extensive analyte panels (ABL800 FLEX, Radiometer Medical, Bronshoj, Denmark), and some with more limited panels (I-STAT, Abbott Laboratories, Princeton, USA). Direct measurement of pH, partial pressure of oxygen (PO_2), partial pressure of carbon dioxide (PCO_2), electrolytes, and metabolites is performed and used to calculate parameters such as bicarbonate (HCO_3), total CO_2 (TCO_2), O_2 saturation, anion gap (AnGap), or base excess (BE) [47]. It is important to keep in mind that the formulas or nomograms that are used to calculate the calculated values are validated for human plasma but are not validated for veterinary species, and thus, should always be examined critically when interpreting them [47].

The first step in interpreting a blood gas analysis is to determine whether or not the patient is normal, and if not normal, determining the primary disturbance [44]. This step is carried out by evaluating the pH of the blood and determining if the patient is acidemic (low blood pH) or alkalemic (high blood pH) or eudremic (neutral pH). In dogs and humans, eudremia is considered to be 7.4, and the reference point in rabbits appears to be similar [47–49]. The availability of reference ranges for exotic small mammals is limited, although some do exist [47]. If reference ranges are not available, it is best to interpret the values compared to other known mammalian references ranges, such as dogs and cats.

The pH is then evaluated in conjunction with the PCO_2 and [HCO_3^-] [44]. Evidence of an elevated pH with a low PCO_2 provides evidence of a respiratory alkalosis [44]. Evidence of a low pH with a high PCO_2 is indicative of a respiratory acidosis [44]. If the patient has a low base excess and a low pH, a metabolic acidosis exists [44]. Conversely, if the patient has a high base excess with an elevated pH, a metabolic alkalosis exists [44].

To determine the primary disturbance on the blood gas profile, it is important to evaluate the pH, PCO_2, and HCO_3^- in concert [48]. If the disorder is respiratory in origin, the pH will change in the opposite direction of the PCO_2 and the HCO_3^- [48]. Conversely, if the disorder is metabolic in origin, the pH will change in the same direction as the PCO_2 and the HCO_3^- [48].

Following the initial evaluation, it is also important to evaluate for a compensatory response [47]. As a whole, the respiratory system attempts to compensate for metabolic acid–base disorders and the metabolic system attempts to compensate for respiratory acid–base disorders [47]. This compensation occurs in parallel with the primary disorder to try to keep the pH stable [47]. If the compensatory response appears to be adequate, it can help to rule out disorders of the compensatory system. However, in many cases, multiple systems are dysfunctional and compensation may be inadequate or absent, leading to a diagnosis of a complex or mixed acid–base disturbance [47].

Once the type of acid–base disorder is identified, additional information about the condition of the patient, and the cause of the acidemia or alkalemia can be obtained by calculating the strong ion difference (SID), anion gap (AG), and base excess (BE) [50].

$$\text{SID}(\text{simplified}) = \text{Na}^+ - \text{Cl}^-$$

or

$$\text{SID} = \left(\text{Na}^+ + \text{K}^+ + \text{Ca}^{2+}\right) - \left(\text{Cl}^- + \text{lactate}\right)$$

The simplified SID is a rapid and efficient way to determine the underlying electrolyte changes associated with acid–base disorders that need to be corrected [51]. A high

SID means that chloride ions are lost in comparison with sodium ions, which can be an indicator of vomiting, gastrointestinal obstruction, or that other causes of hypernatremia are present, such as diabetes insipidus [52]. A low SID means that chloride ions are increased in comparison to sodium ions which creates a hyperchloremic metabolic acidosis or that sodium levels are decreased comparatively to chloride in situations such as diarrhea [52].

The normal anion gap in dog ranges from approximately 12–24, and 13–27 mmol/l in cats, and is useful to further characterize metabolic acidosis [53]. It represents the disparity between the major measured plasma cations (sodium and potassium) and the anions (chloride and bicarbonate) [54]. An elevated anion gap in the face of metabolic acidosis coincides with an increase in lactate, ketones, or renal acids, most commonly seen in starvation and uremia [55]. When the anion gap is normal in the face of metabolic acidosis, diarrhea or urinary loss of bicarbonate is suspected as the underlying cause [56].

$$AG = \left(Na^{+} + K^{+}\right) - \left(Cl^{-} + HCO_3^{-}\right)$$

The base excess is a calculated quantity that ranges from −4 to 4 in most mammals [50]. The base excess represents the metabolic component of the acid–base balance and is calculated from the blood pH and $PaCO_2$. In cases of metabolic alkalosis, the base excess increases, and in cases of metabolic acidosis, the base excess decreases. There is some question of the utility of the base excess because it does not take into account the appropriateness of the response for any given disorder.

Electrolytes (Na/Cl, K, Ca, Phos)

Point-of-care blood-gas analyzers and point-of-care biochemistry analyzers provide electrolyte values that can be useful when trying to determine more information about a patient's acid–base status (for example, the SID and AG) and to provide information that may benefit from correction with fluid therapy.

POC analyzers also provide information about calcium status (either total or ionized) and phosphorus, which can also aid in determining the next diagnostic and treatment steps for the patient. Of important note, the calcium metabolism of rabbits is unique, and ionized calcium values higher than seen in other species are normal in this group of animals [57]. In cases of ionized hypercalcemia, differentials include hypervitaminosis D, nutritional secondary hyperparathyroidism, osteolytic lesions, rodenticides, and artifactual causes (ex. lipemia) [58–60]. In the face of hypocalcemia, differentials such as low dietary calcium or vitamin D_3, hypoparathyroidism, terminal chronic renal failure, and sepsis should be considered [58, 60]. Phosphorus levels are linked in close association with calcium and can be directly affected by changes in both vitamin D and parathyroid hormone [60]. Differentials for hyperphosphatemia include renal disease, hypervitaminosis D, nutritional secondary hyperparathyroidism, or as an artifact with hemolysis [60]. Hypophosphatemia is seen with dietary deficiency of phosphorus, hypovitaminosis D (together with hypocalcemia), diabetic ketoacidosis, or chronic glucocorticoid therapy [60, 61].

Biochemistry (Point-of-Care)

Biochemical profiles that are comprehensive are critical in the workup of emergent small mammal patients; however, submission to a reference laboratory is often required, prolonging obtaining the results and thus, diagnosis and treatment are delayed. When available, veterinary point of care analyzers such as the Vetscan (Abaxis, Union City, CA, USA) should be utilized for immediate evaluation, if total sample volume permits. If the patient is very small, and only a small sample can be obtained, it may be more appropriate to submit the entirety of the blood sample to the reference laboratory to gain the most benefit from the sample submission.

Evaluation of Temperature

Measurement of body temperature is critical in exotic small mammals for evaluation of health status, and in some species, has been associated with prognosis. In rabbits, a significant association between the presence of hypothermia at the time of admission or during hospitalization and mortality has been demonstrated [62]. It is of important note, that hypothermia in rabbits is ultimately linked to an increased risk of death, but is not the underlying cause of death [62]. Timing of temperature evaluation is also critical, demonstrated by a study in chinchillas, where manual restraint for greater than three minutes resulted in a significant increase in rectal temperature [63]. Rectal thermometer insertion depth is also a critical component to the value obtained on the digital thermometer [63]. At this time, it is not known if aggressive or passive rewarming is the preferred rewarming method in rabbits [64].

Body temperature in marsupials (i.e. sugar gliders) is lower than that of eutherian mammals [15]. Since marsupials have a cloaca, often what is measured is the cloacal temperature, which is lower than the actual body temperature [15]. The true rectal temperature of a marsupial can be

Table 9.6 Normal body temperatures of common exotic small mammals.

Species	Temperature (°C(°F))
Rabbits [9]	38.5–39.5 (101.3–103.1)
Ferrets [10]	37.8–40.0 (100.0–104.0)
Guinea pigs [11]	37.2–39.5 (99.0–103.1)
Chinchillas	37–38 (98.6–100.4)
Sugar gliders [15]	36.4 (97.3)
Hedgehogs [14]	35.4–37.0 (95.7–98.6)
Mice [65]	37–37.2 (98.8–99.3)
Rats [66]	37.5 (99.5)
Hamsters [67]	36.2–37.5 (97.2–99.5)
Gerbils [13]	38.2 (100.8)

obtained by directing the thermometer dorsally into the rectum [15]. Body temperature in hedgehogs also tends to be lower than that of most mammals [14].

Normal body temperatures of common exotic small mammals are provided in Table 9.6.

Cardiovascular Assessment

Evaluation of the cardiovascular system is critical in the assessment of the small mammal patient. The biggest difficulties encountered when evaluating the cardiovascular system of the small mammal patient are small patient size and lack of standardized reference ranges. Information about cardiovascular monitoring equipment can be found in "Chapter 28: Analgesia, Anesthesia and Monitoring."

Clinical Assessment

Cardiovascular disease has been reported in most exotic small mammals, and common histories given by owners include lethargy, weakness, decreased appetite, exercise intolerance, and increased respiratory effort [68–70]. Thoracic auscultation should be performed in all emergency small mammal patients to allow for evaluation of the heart rate, rhythm, and presence of abnormal cardiac sounds. Normal heart rates should be known for the species being evaluated and are provided in Table 9.7. The normal anatomy of the heart, including the difference from common domestic species, has been well described for most small mammal species [68, 70, 73]. It can be difficult to evaluate a pulse in some of the smaller exotic mammals; however, in the larger mammals such as rabbits and ferrets, the femoral artery is most easily palpated [74]. Other potential locations to palpate a pulse include the dorsal pedal artery, auricular artery (particularly in rabbits), and the caudal (tail) artery [75]. Mucous membrane color and capillary refill time should be assessed as part of a thorough evaluation of the cardiovascular system [5]. Pale pink, white, or injected mucous membranes with a capillary refill time of greater than two seconds can be consistent with shock [5]. Skin turgor is also a useful tool in the assessment of the cardiovascular system [76].

Table 9.7 Normal heart rates and respiratory rates for exotic small mammal species.

Species	Heart rate (beats/min)	Respiratory rate (breaths/min)
Rabbits [9]	200–300	32–60
Ferrets [71]	200–400	33–36
Guinea pigs [11]	230–380	42–104
Chinchillas [72]	200–350	45–80
Rats [66]	250–500	115
Mice [65]	310–840	60–220
Hamster [67]	280–412	33–127
Hedgehogs [14]	180–280	25–50
Sugar gliders [15]	200–300	16–40

Doppler evaluation of the cardiovascular system is extremely useful to evaluate the rate and rhythm of the heart [74]. The Doppler transducer can be placed directly over the heart in very small patients or can be placed on a superficial artery such as the carotid, carpal, or femoral artery [75].

Blood pressure measurement in exotic small mammals can be challenging. Arterial blood pressure is evaluated as a function of heart rate, blood volume, stroke volume, and arterial compliance [77]. The evaluation of blood pressure should be used in conjunction with other diagnostics as part of the cardiovascular assessment and evaluation of tissue perfusion. A low blood pressure can be indicative of reduced blood flow and impaired oxygenation of major organs [78]. Blood pressure can be measured directly or indirectly [74]. Direct arterial blood pressure monitoring is uncommon in most exotic small mammals, although can be highly reliable and accurate in rabbits when an over-the-needle catheter is placed in the central ear artery [79]. The coccygeal artery may be utilized in larger ferrets [80]. However, in small patients, less than 2 kg, the placement of the catheter may change the pressure wave formation, making interpretation challenging [81]. Additionally, in very small patients, the vessel is also at increased risk of thromboembolism [81].

Indirect blood pressure measurement is more common and is a less invasive approach [74]. There are two main methods of indirect blood pressure including oscillometry and Doppler ultrasonic sphygmomanometry [74]. Although mean arterial pressure (MAP) is the most clinically important measurement, it is not known what is measured by these methods in exotic small mammals. In other species, systolic arterial pressure is measured by the Doppler technique, although there is evidence that Doppler blood pressure may be more reflective of MAP in cats [82]. In either case, the cuff width to limb circumference ratio should be 30–40% [83]. The smallest cuff size is a #1 blood pressure cuff. This cuff size is theoretically too large for many exotic small mammals but can be used for trending purposes. Typically, Doppler is recommended over oscillometric monitoring in exotic small mammals, for a number of reasons. Oscillometric techniques can fail due to the inability to obtain measurements with rapid heart rates (>200 bpm), small patient size, and hypothermia [79, 84]. In most exotic small mammals, the Doppler probe is placed on the medial aspect of the forelimb, targeting the radial carpal artery, or the dorsal aspect of the hind limb, targeting the dorsal pedal or femoral arteries [79, 84–86]. The coccygeal artery can also be used for Doppler probe placement in ferrets [80].

Table 9.8 Electrocardiographic values for 52 clinically normal ferrets.[a]

Parameter	Mean, or Mean ± SD (range) (n = 25)	Value (n = 27)
Age (months)	10–20	5.2
Male/female ratio	All male	1.25
Body weight (kg)	1.4 ± 0.2	Not available
Rhythm		
Normal sinus	Not available	67%
Sinus arrhythmia	Not available	33%
Heart rate (beats/min)	196 ± 26 (140–240)	233 ± 22
Mean electrical axis, frontal plane (degrees)	+86.1 ± 2.5 (79.6–90.0)	+77.2 ± 12.0
Lead II measurements		
P amplitude (mV)	Not available	0.122 ± 0.007
P duration (s)	Not available	0.024 ± 0.004
PR interval (s)	0.056 ± 0.0086 (0.04–0.08)	0.047 ± 0.003
QRS duration (s)	0.044 ± 0.008 (0.035–0.06)	0.043 ± 0.003
R amplitude (mV)	2.21 ± 0.42 (1.4–3.0)	1.46 ± 0.84
QT interval (s)	0.11 ± 0.02 (0.08–0.14)	0.12 ± 0.04

[a] All ferrets were sedated with ketamine–xylazine. *Source:* Morrisey and Kraus [89]. © 2012, Elsevier.

Electrocardiograms

Cardiac muscle cells produce electrical activity, and this can be monitored with the use of an electrocardiogram (ECG) tracing [75]. The ECG tracing is composed of three primary complexes which includes the P wave, QRS complex, and T wave [87]. ECG evaluation is a useful tool when detection of arrhythmias occurs, which is common with acid–base and electrolyte abnormalities. Given that exotic companion mammals (ECM) are small with rapid heart rates, the ECG must be able to measure this, which is best done with low-voltage machines and fast recording speeds (up to 100 mm/s) [86, 88]. Many ECMs have very delicate skin, and the standard alligator clips can tear the skin. Instead, the clips can be attached to small-gauge hypodermic needs placed through the skin. The adhesive pads can also be utilized but may also tear the skin on removal.

In ferrets, a pronounced sinus arrhythmia is common and normal [89]. Additionally, first- and second-degree atrioventricular block are a common incidental finding in ferrets [89]. High-grade second-degree atrioventricular (AV) block or third-degree AV block warrant further investigation in the ferret [89]. Abnormal ECG findings in ferrets include tachycardia, and premature complexes, either atrial or ventricular in origin, that occur secondary to cardiac disease [89]. In ferrets diagnosed with insulinomas, sinus bradycardia may be seen [89]. Reference values for ECGs in ferrets have been published (Table 9.8) [90, 91]. Most ferrets do not like alcohol, and use of ECG coupling gel is recommended [89]. Right lateral positioning is recommended [89].

In rabbits, the most common cardiovascular concerns are related to thymomas, valvular disease, and congestive heart failure [92]. Rabbits should have a normal sinus rhythm which does not include a respiratory sinus arrhythmia [92]. Reference values for ECGs in rabbits have been published (Table 9.9) [70, 93].

Respiratory Assessment

Assessment of the respiratory system should be done in conjunction with assessment of the cardiovascular system. If the patient displays signs of respiratory distress, oxygen supplementation should be initiated prior to handling. Additionally, flow by oxygen therapy can be provided by face mask throughout the examination process. For animals with signs of respiratory distress, the examination process should be kept brief, with rest periods in oxygen in between.

Table 9.9 Electrocardiographic values in clinically normal pet rabbits.

ECG parameter	Values	Values
Heart rate	198–330 (mean 264) beats/minute	240 beats/minute (mean)
Measurements (lead II)		
P wave		
Amplitude (height)	0.04–0.12 mV	0.04–0.07 mV
Duration (width)	0.01–0.05 s	0.02–0.04 s
P-R interval		
Duration	0.04–0.08 s	0.05–0.07 s
QRS complex		
R-wave amplitude	0.03–0.039 mV	0.12–0.2 mV
Duration	0.02–0.06 s	0.03–0.04 s
Q-T interval		
Duration	0.08–0.16 s	—
T wave		
Amplitude	0.05–0.17 mV	—
Electrical axis (frontal plane)	43–80°	—
Body weight	1.1–7.9 (mean 2.57) kg	—

Source: From Morrisey and Kraus [89]. © 2012, Elsevier.

Respiratory rate and effort should be evaluated for every small mammal presenting on emergency. Respiratory distress in exotic small mammals is a common emergency presenting complaint. Since rabbits and rodents are obligate nasal breathers, upper respiratory tract disease can be as concerning as lower respiratory tract disease [71, 72].

In rabbits, respiratory distress can be associated with disease of both the upper and lower respiratory tract, as well as the pleural space [94]. Dyspneic rabbits are critical patients that must be approached with extreme caution, patience, and quiet. Many of the rabbit patients that present with respiratory signs are unstable and may require time in a dark, quiet room with oxygen therapy prior to handling. Given that rabbits are obligate nasal breathers, open-mouth breathing is a poor prognostic indicator when it is noted in these species [71, 94]. Once stable, a thorough physical examination to localize the respiratory issue, along with bloodwork, imaging, cytology, and culture should be considered for diagnostic purposes.

Infectious respiratory disease in rabbits has been historically referred to as pasteurellosis or snuffles, with *Pasteurella multocida* implicated as the underlying cause; however, many other bacterial agents such as *Bordetella bronchiseptica*, *Staphylococcus* sp., and *Pseudomonas* sp., as well as anaerobes can be involved [71]. Rhinitis and sinusitis are the most common forms of pasteurellosis with evidence of mucopurulent discharge from the eyes and nares [71]. As a result of grooming, crusting of the forearms is often noted [71]. Chronic infection with extension to the lower respiratory tract is not uncommon [71]. Viral diseases associated with primary respiratory disease in rabbits have not been identified [71].

Any space-occupying mass in the respiratory tract or extra-respiratory tract mass can also result in significant respiratory distress. Given that rabbits are obligate nasal breathers, any signs of open mouth breathing are significant and representative of serious respiratory compromise [71]. Noninfectious etiologies of respiratory distress include neoplasia of the nasal turbinates, most commonly adenocarcinoma, primary lung tumors, and secondary lung metastases [71, 94]. Neoplasias that result in metastasis to the lungs include uterine adenocarcinoma, osteosarcoma, lymphoma, and mammary carcinoma [94–98].

Thymomas and thymic lymphomas are not an uncommon presentation of adult rabbits, with the presence of respiratory signs occurring as a result of a space occupying cranial mediastinal mass [71, 94]. A common clinical sign of thymoma in rabbits is bilateral exophthalmos, as a result of compromised return of blood to the heart [71]. Allergens have also been reported as a cause of rhinitis and chronic bronchitis in rabbits [71]. In any rabbit with upper respiratory clinical signs, a thorough oral examination in combination with diagnostic imaging (dental radiographs, skull computed tomography) should always be undertaken, as the signs can be a result of apical elongation or abscessation of the teeth [71].

In rats, most cases of infectious respiratory disease are multifactorial, although *Mycoplasma pulmonis* is the most significant and serious bacterial pathogen [99]. Other infectious agents that are commonly implicated include *Streptococcus pneumoniae*, *Corynebacterium kutscheri*, Sendai virus, pneumonia virus of mice, rat respiratory virus, cilia-associated respiratory bacillus, and *Haemophilus* species [99]. In the immediate term, stabilization of the patient with oxygen supplementation, nebulization, and injectable antibiotics are key [99]. Once stabilized, additional diagnostics such as bloodwork, radiographs, and/or a computed tomography scan of the chest can be considered [99]. Differentials such as neoplasia should also be considered in cases of rat respiratory distress [99].

Respiratory distress is also not an uncommon presentation in the ferret, although there are few causes of primary respiratory disease in captive ferrets [100]. The presence of clinical signs, such as dyspnea, tachypnea, and coughing can occur with diseases such as canine distemper virus, influenza virus, Aleutian disease, heartworm disease, congestive heart failure, lymphoma, trauma, anemia, heatstroke, anaphylactic reactions, fungal disease, and metabolic disturbances [100]. Just like other small mammals, the initial management of a dyspneic ferret should be focused on stabilizing the patient in the form of oxygen therapy. Once stabilized, additional diagnostics such as bloodwork, radiographs, and/or a computed tomography scan of the chest can be considered.

Pulse Oximeter

Pulse oximetry is commonly used in small mammal patients but with limited information about the accuracy. Pulse oximetry measures oxygen saturation of the blood through illumination of the skin and detection of changes in light absorption between oxygenated blood (oxyhemoglobin) and deoxygenated blood (reduced hemoglobin) [101]. The pulse oximeter then looks at the ratio of absorbance between these wavelengths with calibration against direct measurements of arterial oxygen saturation (SaO_2) to determine the measurement of arterial saturation (SpO_2) by the pulse oximeter [101]. In humans, the difference between SpO_2 and SaO_2 is less than 2% when the SaO_2 value is above 90%; however, the precision of the reading worsens when the SaO_2 is lower than 90% [101]. Similarly, in ferrets, values obtained by pulse oximetry have been demonstrated to closely relate to oxygen saturation, when measured by blood gas analysis, with the most precise measurements being noted when oxygen saturation was between 90% and 100% [102]. In addition to ferrets, the use of pulse oximetry has been validated in rabbits, with accuracy at hemoglobin saturation values greater than 85% and rats, with variability demonstrated at anywhere from 60% to 75% saturation [103–105]. Depending on the species, the pulse oximeter can be placed in various locations, working most effectively on unpigmented regions of the skin (example the feet) (Table 9.10). Pulse oximeters may also provide valuable information on heart rate.

Capnography

Capnography is a useful tool in anesthetized patients or obtunded patients that are intubated [106]. Capnometry measures the maximum value of carbon dioxide that is measured at the end of expiration, which in turn is a reflection of the amount of CO_2 that is present in the alveolar gas [106]. Measurement of the end-tidal carbon dioxide concentration ($EtCO_2$) has demonstrated utility in determining the arterial concentration of carbon dioxide ($PaCO_2$) [106]. Normocapnia in mammals is associated with an $EtCO_2$ of 35–45 mmHg [107]. Patients with $ETCO_2$ values less than 35 mmHg are considered to be hypocapnic, and values from 65 to 75 mmHg are considered to be hypercapnic [107]. Both hypoventilation and hypercapnia are concerns for obtunded patients or patients that are under general anesthesia [106]. The capnograph wave is useful for assessing the adequacy of ventilation and perfusion to the lungs as it has been well correlated with arterial CO_2 [106]. Capnography has been demonstrated to provide useful estimations of the $PaCO_2$ in rabbits and ferrets [102, 108].

Evaluation of Defecation

The fecal and urine output of any exotic companion mammal should always be evaluated closely to determine if

Table 9.10 Pulse oximeter probe placement by species.

	Tail	Toes/legs	Rectum	Scrotum/Vulva	Pinna	Tongue
Rabbits		C	F	C	C	C
Ferrets		C	F	C		C
Rodents	C (some species)	C	F	C		C

F = flat reflectance (rectal probe); C = clip probe.

there are concerns with the digestive or urinary tracts. Evaluation of the feces and urine are fast, and easy diagnostic tests that can help to dictate the diagnostic and therapeutic plan for a patient.

Rabbits and Rodents

In rabbits and rodents, reduction in fecal output is a common presenting complaint, often falling under the umbrella of gastrointestinal stasis [109]. When normal, rabbits and rodents should always pass enough feces that by the time they present to you, there are fecal balls present in their carrier [109]. Abnormal fecal presentations in these species can include smaller fecal balls, lower volume of fecal balls, or absence of fecal balls entirely [109]. Gastrointestinal stasis is often caused by a multitude of factors including low fiber in the diet, inappropriate diet (usually too high in carbohydrates), stress, dehydration, and any other causes of illness [109]. In rabbits and rodents with gastrointestinal stasis, the goal is to determine the underlying cause of the stasis, followed by aggressive supportive care with analgesia, fluid therapy, and enteral feedings [109]. A common conundrum in rabbits is determining if a true gastric obstruction is present [109]. Usually, the obstructions in rabbits are created by dehydrated masses of ingesta and hair that with appropriate therapy will resolve without the use of surgery [109]. Aside from gastric outflow obstructions, the duodenum and the ileocecal junction are the most common sites of impaction [109]. The decision to take a rabbit or rodent to surgery for an obstruction of the gastrointestinal tract is not one that is taken lightly and all diagnostic tests should point to this being the appropriate decision. Blood gas analysis demonstrating a hypochloremic metabolic alkalosis, abdominal radiographs, and abdominal ultrasound can all help to point in the direction of a diagnosis of gastrointestinal obstruction [109, 110].

True diarrhea in rabbits and rodents is also an emergency presentation that can have a high mortality rate if not managed appropriately [109]. In very young rabbits, diarrhea is often secondary to coccidiosis caused by *Eimeria* species [109]. Other common causes of diarrhea in rabbits include inappropriate diets resulting in an imbalance of bacteria leading to overgrowth of *Escherichia coli* and *Clostridium* species that produce toxins [109].

Cecal dysbiosis can also occur in rabbits when the diet is inappropriate and too high in sugars and other simple carbohydrates that change the bacterial flora balance and also result in yeast overgrowth [109]. The result of cecal dysbiosis is production of abnormal cecotrophs which owners often refer to as diarrhea [109]. The cecotrophs are often large, pasty, foul-smelling, soft cecotrophs [109]. Supportive care is indicated in these cases with strict diet changes [109].

Ferrets

Diseases of the gastrointestinal tract are a common emergency presentation in ferrets, and it is important to be able to differentiate the potential differential diagnoses based on the clinical presentation of the ferret [111]. Given the short gastrointestinal tract and rapid gastrointestinal transit time, any gastrointestinal disturbances in ferrets appear quickly, including common emergent presentations such as diarrhea and anorexia [111]. Clinical signs of gastrointestinal upset in ferrets are typically nonspecific and include collapse, lethargy, anorexia, dehydration, nausea, bruxism, ptyalism, pawing at the mouth, frequent swallowing, gagging, diarrhea, and vomiting [112]. Diarrhea can result in rapid dehydration in the ferret with such a short transit time, and it can be difficult to distinguish between large and small bowel diarrhea in this species [112].

Gastrointestinal emergencies in ferrets often differ by age group with young ferrets commonly presenting with gastrointestinal foreign bodies [111]. Occasionally, coccidia and giardia are seen in young ferrets [111]. Historically, proliferative bowel disease was seen in young ferrets, with only rare cases reported in North America today [111]. In adult ferrets, inflammatory bowel disease, eosinophilic enteritis, lymphoplasmacytic enteritis, *Helicobacter mustelidae*, epizootic catarrhal enteritis (coronavirus), and neoplasia of the gastrointestinal tract are more common presentations [111].

Initial stabilization to correct dehydration and electrolyte imbalances is critical in the early stages of presentation, followed by pursuit of diagnostics to determine the underlying cause of gastrointestinal signs [112]. Aside from routine bloodwork (complete blood count, biochemistry profile), imaging including radiographs, ultrasound, computed tomography, and potential endoscopy should be considered [112]. In cases of febrile ferrets, a fecal culture should be pursued to evaluate for *Campylobacter jejuni* and *Salmonella* spp. [113].

Other Tests

A fecal floatation can be performed if looking specifically for parasitic infections. A fecal occult blood test is recommended in any patient that demonstrates concerns for melena, weight loss, anorexia, or evidence of gastroenteritis. Melena can be seen as dark tarry feces in all mammals and is an indicator of upper gastrointestinal tract hemorrhage. A fecal occult blood test is beneficial in confirming the presence of blood; however, a complete dietary evaluation with the owner is important, as certain foods can cause false positives with this test [114]. Understanding how the fecal occult blood test works is important to interpretation of the test results. The Guaiac-based fecal occult blood tests are based on detection of the activity of peroxidase in heme/hemoglobin [114]. This means that when substances containing peroxidase are ingested, they can result in a false-positive test result [114]. Foods that are high in peroxidase include broccoli, cauliflower, radishes, turnips, and some melons [114]. Animal food products high in heme contents such as beef, lamb, and processed foods containing these meats can also result in false-positive test results [114]. The false-positive effects of peroxidase containing foods can be mitigated by delaying time to evaluation after smearing [115].

Evaluation of the Urinary System

Rabbits and Rodents

Disorders of the urinary system are common in rabbits and rodents [116].

Common renal presentations in rabbits include renal insufficiency, acute renal failure, and chronic renal failure, as well as urolithiasis [116]. The most common clinical signs of urinary disease in rabbits include polyuria, polydipsia, incontinence, inappropriate elimination behavior, perineal urine scalding, hematuria, stranguria, and pollakiuria [116]. Rabbits have a unique calcium metabolism, having evolved to maximize absorption of dietary calcium, with any extra being excreted in the urine as calcium carbonate [116]. In most mammals, intestinal absorption of calcium is linked to vitamin D_3, but in rabbits, intestinal absorption is independent of vitamin D_3 levels, meaning that an increase in dietary calcium directly results in an increase in urinary calcium excretion [117, 118]. Resultantly, urolithiasis, and hypercalciuria in the rabbit is common, with suspected predisposing factors to include decreased exercise, and a diet consisting of free-choice pellets, and alfalfa hay [116]. Diagnosis is standard and urinalysis may reveal crystalluria with calcium oxalate, ammonium phosphate, calcium carbonate, and monohydrate crystals all being reported, in addition to proteinuria and hematuria [116]. Treatment depends on the location of the urolith, but typically involves surgical removal [116]. Prevention involves, diet changes, increased exercise, in addition to examination of the water source.

Both acute and chronic renal failure have been reported in rabbits, more commonly older rabbits [116]. Diagnosis and treatment are similar to other species, with common biochemistry abnormalities including azotemia, hypercalcemia, and hyperphosphatemia [116].

A unique and important cause of renal disease in rabbits to consider is infection with the microsporidian, obligate, intracellular protozoan *Encephalitozoon cuniculi* [116]. Disease typically results in nonsuppurative, granulomatous nephritis that can progress to interstitial fibrosis [116]. Disease is usually chronic and subclinical but can result in renal failure [116].

Urolithiasis is a common problem in guinea pigs, with the high mineral content and alkaline nature of guinea pig urine suspected to favor the formation of crystals and precipitation of stones [119]. Calcium carbonate is the most common stone composition found in guinea pigs, though historically, it was reported as calcium oxalate [119, 120]. Clinical signs depend on the size and location of the calculi, with common reports of hematuria, stranguria, dysuria, as well as nonspecific signs of generalized illness [119]. Diagnosis and treatment are similar to other mammalian species, with urinary calculi typically being radiopaque [119]. Urinalysis data from guinea pigs with urinary calculi have been reported and found the mean $\pm$ SD urine specific gravity was 1.015 ± 0.008 (range 1.004–1.046) and urine pH was 8.4 ± 0.5 (range 6.5 to >9) [120]. The most commonly reported abnormality on urine sediment was hematuria, followed by the presence of mucous and lipid droplets [120]. Various crystals, including calcium carbonate, calcium oxalate, and struvite are common, but similar to other animals, are not predictive of the type of mineral found in the calculi [120]. Urine culture should be performed as deemed necessary [119].

Other urinary presentations of guinea pigs include cystitis and urinary tract infections, as well as chronic renal failure [119].

Male chinchillas can develop urinary calculi and obstructive urolithiasis, with the most common underlying stone composition being calcium carbonate [121, 122]. The most common clinical presentations include hematuria, stranguria, pollakiuria, and anuria [121, 122]. Diagnosis and treatment are similar to other mammalian species [121]. Recurrence of uroliths is common in chinchillas, with a better prognosis reported for cystic uroliths compared to urethral uroliths [121].

Red, orange, or brown urine in rabbits and rodents is a common presenting complaint and is most commonly caused by porphyrinuria or hematuria [116]. Pigmented urine in the rabbit and rodent can occur as a result of diet, uterine disease, renal disease, and stress [116]. In order to distinguish porphyrin pigments from hemoglobin, a Wood's lamp can be used to demonstrate fluorescence of porphyrin but not hemoglobin [116]. True hematuria can be determined on examination of the sediment with the presence of five or more red blood cells per high power field [116]. A urine dipstick that demonstrates a positive reaction for blood can indicate hematuria or hemoglobinuria [116].

Ferrets

Urinary emergencies in ferrets are usually a result of two causes. The first cause is a result of prostatic cysts or prostatic enlargement due to underlying adrenal gland disease [123]. The second cause is a result of stones, with struvite, calcium oxalate, and cystine being reported [123]. Both diseases can result in acute renal failure (ARF) if obstruction ensues [123]. Other, less common causes of ARF include toxin exposure [123]. Ibuprofen, and less commonly acetaminophen, can result in ARF, with neurologic and gastrointestinal signs being seen in addition to ARF with ibuprofen toxicity [123]. ARF in ferrets can present with polyuria, polydipsia, oral ulcers, and nonspecific signs of illness [123]. Abnormal bloodwork results include hyperphosphatemia, hyperkalemia, reduced total carbon dioxide levels, and azotemia [123]. Imaging is an important diagnostic step in these cases [123]. Treatment should be aimed at the underlying cause of failure, which may include leuprolide acetate injections or deslorelin implants for adrenal gland disease, and relief of obstruction with surgical removal for urolithiasis [123]. In addition to treatment of the underlying cause, supportive therapy including fluid therapy, and appropriate nutritional support should be provided to the ferret [123]. A detailed review of adrenal gland disease and ferret urolithiasis is beyond the scope of this chapter but can be found in the relevant literature and Chapter 14 [24, 123].

Chronic renal failure (CRF) is a common disease in older ferrets and presents similar to other mammals [123].

Other causes of renal disease in ferrets include Aleutian disease, pyelonephritis, renal neoplasia, cystitis, bladder tumors, and prostatic tumors [123].

Normal urinalysis results for ferrets have been reported [124]. The overall urine specific gravity range for ferrets is reported as 1.026–1.070, though differences in male and female ferrets have been reported [124]. Trace protein is a common finding in the urine of ferrets, with it being more commonly reported in male versus female ferrets on urine dipstick [124]. Urine is acidic, as is typical for a carnivore, ranging from 5.0 to 7.5 [124].

Urine sediment evaluation is useful for detection of cells, crystals, and casts [125].

Point-of-Care Ultrasound (POCUS)

Point-of-care ultrasound (POCUS) in exotic small mammal patients has the potential to provide information that assists in the diagnostic analysis of the patient, narrow differential diagnoses and help to guide clinical therapy. Portable ultrasound machines are typically used for POC assessment and are often of lower quality and resolution than standard ultrasound machines; therefore, in most cases, a follow-up, thorough ultrasound should be performed once the patient has been stabilized.

Indications

The indications to perform POCUS in exotic small mammals are similar to the indications to perform POCUS in other mammals, including detection of free fluid in the peritoneal, pleural, and pericardial spaces, evaluation of trauma patients for evidence of pneumothorax, penetrating injury patients, as well as any abnormalities such as palpation of an abdominal mass on physical examination [126]. Both the thorax (T-FAST) and abdomen (A-FAST) can be evaluated with the ultrasound [127]. FAST ultrasound examinations are useful to diagnosis effusion and can be relied upon to rule in and out the presence of free fluid [127]. Some soft tissue diagnoses are more user-dependent and should trigger the need for confirmatory imaging [127].

Limitations

Ultrasonography in exotic small mammals is similar to other mammalian species but can be limited by the small size of the patient, and understanding unique anatomical features of exotic companion mammals. In some cases, more advanced imaging such as radiographs, and computed tomography may be indicated [127].

References

1 Paul-Murphy, J. (2007). Critical care of the rabbit. *Vet. Clin. North Am. Exot. Anim. Pract.* 10: 437–461.

2 Nichols, J.H. (2013). Point-of-care testing. In: *Immunoassay Handbook* (ed. D. Wild), 455–463. Elsevier.

3 Ott, J.J. (2009). Blood collection techniques in exotic small mammals. *J. Exot. Pet Med.* 18: 117–139.

4 Diehl, K.H., Hull, R., Morton, D. et al. (2001). A good practice guide to the administration of substances and removal of blood, including routes and volumes. *J. Appl. Toxicol.* 21: 15–23.

5 Reineke, E.L. (2014). *Evaluation and Triage of the Critically Ill Patient*, 2e. Elsevier Inc.

6 Whitbread TJ. Laboratory tests routinely performed in veterinary medicine. https://www.merckvetmanual.com/special-pet-topics/diagnostic-tests-and-imaging/laboratory-tests-routinely-performed-in-veterinary-medicine (accessed 19 November 2019).

7 Hayes, G.M., Mathews, K., Floras, A. et al. (2011). Refractometric total plasma protein measurement as a cage-side indicator of hypoalbuminemia and hypoproteinemia in hospitalized dogs. *J. Vet. Emerg. Crit. Care* 21: 356–362.

8 Lumeij, J.T. and De Bruijne, J.J. (1985). Evaluation of the refractometric method for the determination of total protein in avian plasma or serum. *Avian Pathol.* 14: 441–444.

9 Nowland, M.H., Brammer, D.W., Garcia, A. et al. (2015). Biology and diseases of rabbits. In: *Laboratory Animal Medicine*, 3e (eds. J.G. Fox, L.C. Anderson, G.M. Otto, et al.), 411–461. https://doi.org/10.1016/B978-0-12-409527-4.00010-9.

10 Mayer, J., Marini, R.P., and Fox, J.G. (2015). Biology and diseases of ferrets. In: *Laboratory Animal Medicine*, 3e (eds. J.G. Fox, L.C. Anderson, G.M. Otto, et al.), 577–622. https://doi.org/10.1016/B978-0-12-409527-4.00014-6.

11 Shomer, N.H., Holcombe, H., and Harkness, J.E. (2015). Biology and diseases of guinea pigs. In: *Laboratory Animal Medicine*, 3e (eds. J.G. Fox, L.C. Anderson, G.M. Otto, et al.), 247–283. https://doi.org/10.1016/B978-0-12-409527-4.00006-7.

12 Quesenberry, K.E., Donnelly, T.M., and Mans, C. (2012). Biology, husbandry, and clinical techniques of guinea pigs and chinchillas. In: *Ferrets, Rabbits and Rodents – Clinical Medicine and Surgery*, 3e (eds. K.E. Quesenberry and J.W. Carpenter), 279–294. St. Louis, MO: Elsevier Inc.

13 Lennox, A.M. and Bauck, L. (2012). Small rodents basic anatomy, physiology, husbandry, and clinical techniques. In: *Ferrets, Rabbits and Rodents – Clinical Medicine and Surgery*, 3e (eds. K.E. Quesenberry and J.W. Carpenter), 339–353. St. Louis, MO: Elsevier Inc.

14 Ivey, E. and Carpenter, J.W. (2012). African hedgehogs. In: *Ferrets, Rabbits and Rodents – Clinical Medicine and Surgery*, 3e (eds. K.E. Quesenberry and J.W. Carpenter), 411–427. St. Louis, MO: Elsevier Inc.

15 Ness, R.D. and Johnson-Delaney, C.A. (2012). Sugar gliders. In: *Ferrets, Rabbits and Rodents – Clinical Medicine and Surgery*, 3e (eds. K.E. Quesenberry and J.W. Carpenter), 393–410. St. Louis, MO: Elsevier Inc.

16 Fielding, L.C. and Magdesian, G.K. (2011). Review of packed cell volume and total protein for use in equine practice. *AAEP Proc.* 57: 318–321.

17 Coppen, M.J., Noble, C.J., and Aubrey, C. (1981). Evaluation of buffy-coat microscopy for the early diagnosis of bacteraemia. *J. Clin. Pathol.* 34: 1375–1377.

18 Dhurat, R. and Sukesh, M. (2014). Principles and methods of preparation of platelet-rich plasma: a review and author's perspective. *J. Cutan. Aesthet. Surg.* 7: 189.

19 Salvagno, G.L., Lippi, G., Gelati, M. et al. (2012). Hemolysis, lipaemia and icterus in specimens for arterial blood gas analysis. *Clin. Biochem.* 45: 372–373.

20 Martínez-Subiela, S. and Cerón, J.J. (2005). Effects of hemolysis, lipemia, hyperbilirrubinemia, and anticoagulants in canine C-reactive protein, serum amyloid a, and ceruloplasmin assays. *Can. Vet. J.* 46: 625–629.

21 Higbie, C.T., Eshar, D., and Bello, N.M. (2015). Evaluation of three point-of-care meters and a portable veterinary chemistry analyzer for measurement of blood glucose concentrations in black-tailed prairie dogs (*Cynomys ludovicianus*). *Am. J. Vet. Res.* 76: 532–539.

22 Petritz, O.A., Antinoff, N., Chen, S. et al. (2013). Evaluation of portable blood glucose meters for measurement of blood glucose concentration in ferrets (*Mustela putorius furo*). *J. Am. Vet. Med. Assoc.* 242: 350–354.

23 Selleri, P., Di Girolamo, N., and Novari, G. (2014). Performance of two portable meters and a benchtop analyzer for blood glucose concentration measurement in rabbits. *J. Am. Vet. Med. Assoc.* 245: 87–98.

24 Rosenthal, K.L. and Wyre, N.R. (2012). Endocrine diseases. In: *Ferrets, Rabbits and Rodents – Clinical Medicine and Surgery*, 3e (eds. K.E. Quesenberry and J.W. Carpenter), 86–102. St. Louis, MO: Elsevier Inc.

25 Künzel, F. and Mayer, J. (2015). Endocrine tumours in the guinea pig. *Vet. J.* 206: 268–274.

26 Vannevel, J.Y. and Wilcock, B. (2005). Insulinoma in 2 guinea pigs (*Cavia porcellus*). *Can. Vet. J.* 46: 339–341.

27 Hess, L.R., Ravich, M.L., and Reavill, D.R. (2013). Diagnosis and treatment of an insulinoma in a guinea pig (*Cavia porcellus*). *J. Am. Vet. Med. Assoc.* 242: 522–526.

28 Harcourt-Brown, F.M. and Harcourt-Brown, S. (2012). Clinical value of blood glucose measurement in pet rabbits. *Vet. Rec.* 170: 674.

29 Bou Chebl, R., El Khuri, C., Shami, A. et al. (2017). Serum lactate is an independent predictor of hospital mortality in critically ill patients in the emergency department: a retrospective study. *Scand. J. Trauma Resusc. Emerg. Med.* 25: 1–7.

30 Langlois, I., Planché, A., Boysen, S.R. et al. (2014). Blood concentrations of D- and L-lactate in healthy rabbits. *J. Small Anim. Pract.* 55: 451–456.

31 Pang, D. and Boysen, S. (2007). Lactate in veterinary critical care: pathophysiology and management. *J. Am. Anim. Hosp. Assoc.* 43: 270–279.

32 Widgren B, Ekhardt M (2012). Blood lactate: a useful analysis in emergency: 1–7. https://acutecaretesting.org/-/media/acutecaretesting/files/pdf/blood-lactate--a-useful-analysis-in-emergency-care.pdf.

33 Delesalle, C., Dewulf, J., Lefebvre, R.A. et al. (2007). Determination of lactate concentrations in blood plasma and peritoneal fluid in horses with colic by an Accusport analyzer. *J. Vet. Intern. Med.* 21: 293–301.

34 de Papp, E., Drobatz, K.J., and Hughes, D. (1999). Plasma lactate concentration as a predictor of gastric necrosis and survival among dogs with gastric dilatation-volvulus: 102 cases (1995-1998). *J. Am. Vet. Med. Assoc.* 215: 49–52.

35 Yuschenkoff D, Graham JE, Sharkey L, et al. (2020). Reference Interval Determination of Blood Gas Parameters in Healthy Ferrets. Press

36 Scnchez-Aparicio, P., Mota-Rojas, D., Verduzco-Mendoza, A. et al. (2009). Reference values for blood gas analysis, electrolytes and critical biochemical variables for short-hair-English and Duncan–Hartley guinea pigs anaesthetized with xylazine-ketamine. *J. Anim. Vet. Adv.* 8: 1893–1899.

37 Hartmann, M., Tran, N., Zacharowski, K. et al. (2007). Clinical chemistry reference database for Wistar rats and C57/BL6 mice. *Biol. Chem.* 388: 547–554.

38 Ardiaca, M., Dias, S., Montesinos, A. et al. (2016). Plasmatic L-lactate in pet rabbits: association with morbidity and mortality at 14 days. *Vet. Clin. Pathol.* 45: 116–123.

39 Adewoyin, A.S. and Nwogoh, B. (2014). Peripheral blood film – a review. *Ann. Ibadan Postgrad. Med.* 12: 71–79.

40 Pikula, J., Adam, V., Bandouchova, H. et al. (2007). Blood coagulation times in the European brown hare (*Lepus europaeus*). *Vet. Clin. Pathol.* 36: 361–363.

41 Meier, P. and Gygax, P. (1990). A comparison of different reagents for the activated partial thromboplastin time in rabbit and rat plasma. *Thromb. Res.* 59: 883–886.

42 Lin, C.-H., Liu, C.-Y., Shih, C.-H. et al. (2014). A sample-to-result system for blood coagulation tests on a microfluidic disk analyzer. *Biomicrofluidics* 8: 052105.

43 Jagadeeswaran, P. and Sheehan, J.P. (1999). Analysis of blood coagulation in the zebrafish. *Blood Cells Mol. Dis.* 25: 239–249.

44 Mathews, K.A. and Bosch, L. (2017). Acid-base assessment. In: *Veterinary Emergency and Critical Care*, 3e (ed. K.A. Mathews), 579–588. Guelph, ON: Lifelearn, Inc.

45 Davis, M.D., Walsh, B.K., Sittig, S.E. et al. (2013). AARC clinical practice guideline: blood gas analysis and hemoximetry: 2013. *Respir. Care* 58: 1694–1703.

46 Haskins, S.C. (1977). Sampling and storage of blood for pH and blood gas analysis. *J. Am. Vet. Med. Assoc.* 170: 429–433.

47 Ardiaca, M., Bonvehí, C., and Montesinos, A. (2013). Point-of-care blood gas and electrolyte analysis in rabbits. *Vet. Clin. North Am. Exot. Anim. Pract.* 16: 175–195.

48 Bateman, S.W. (2008). Making sense of blood gas results. *Vet. Clin. North Am. - Small Anim. Pract.* 38: 543–557.

49 de Morais, H.S.A. and DiBartola, S.P. (1991). Ventilatory and metabolic compensation in dogs with acid-base disturbances. *J. Vet. Emerg. Crit. Care* 1: 39–49.

50 Durward, A. and Murdoch, I. (2003). Understanding acid-base balance. *Curr. Paediatr.* 13: 513–519.

51 Stockham, S.L. and Scott, M.A. Blood gases, blood pH, and strong ion difference. In: *Fundamentals of Veterinary Clinical Pathology*, 2e (eds. S.L. Stockham and M.A. Scott), 559–592. Ames, IA: Blackwell Publishing.

52 Boyle, M. and Baldwin, I. (2002). Introduction to an alternate view of acid/base balance: the strong ion difference or Stewart approach. *Aust. Crit. Care* 15: 14–20.

53 DiBartola, S.P. (2012). Electrolyte and acid-base disorders. In: *Small Animal Clinical Diagnosis by Laboratory Methods*, 5e (eds. M.D. Willard and H. Tvedten), 112–125. St. Louis, MO: Elsevier Inc.

54 Ford, R.B. and Mazzafero, E.M. (2012). Laboratory diagnosis and test protocols. In: *Kirk and Bistner's Handbook of Veterinary Procedures and Emergency Treatment*, 9e (eds. R.B. Ford and E.M. Mazzaferro), 551–634. St. Louis, MO: Elsevier Inc.

55 Reddi, A.S. and Reddi, A.S. (2018). High anion gap metabolic acidosis. In: *Fluid, Electrolyte and Acid-Base Disorders* (ed. A.S. Reddi), 339–365. Springer International Publishing.

56 Kraut, J.A. and Madias, N.E. (2012). Differential diagnosis of nongap metabolic acidosis: value of a systematic approach. *Clin. J. Am. Soc. Nephrol.* 7: 671–679.

57 Eckermann-Ross, C. (2008). Hormonal regulation and calcium metabolism in the rabbit. *Vet. Clin. North Am. Exot. Anim. Pract.* 11: 139–152.

58 Sirault, B. (2016). Hypo and hypercalcemia: from diagnosis to treatment. *Rev. Med. Brux.* 37: 334–339.

59 Zagzag, J., Hu, M.I., Fisher, S.B. et al. (2018). Hypercalcemia and cancer: differential diagnosis and treatment. *CA Cancer J. Clin.* 68: 377–386.

60 Stockham, S.L. and Scott, M.A. (2008). Calcium, phosphorus, magnesium, and their regulatory hormones. In: *Fundamentals of Veterinary Clinical Pathology*, 2e (eds. S.L. Stockham and M.A. Scott), 593–638. Ames, IA: Blackwell Publishing.

61 Felsenfeld, A.J. and Levine, B.S. (2012). Approach to treatment of hypophosphatemia. *Am. J. Kidney Dis.* 60: 655–661.

62 Di Girolamo, N., Toth, G., and Selleri, P. (2016). Prognostic value of rectal temperature at hospital admission in client-owned rabbits. *J. Am. Vet. Med. Assoc.* 248: 288–297.

63 Ozawa, S., Mans, C., and Beaufrère, H. (2017). Comparison of rectal and tympanic thermometry in chinchillas (*Chinchilla lanigera*). *J. Am. Vet. Med. Assoc.* 251: 552–558.

64 Vassal, T., Benoit-Gonin, B., Carrat, F. et al. (2001). Severe accidental hypothermia treated in an ICU: prognosis and outcome. *Chest* 120: 1998–2003.

65 Whary, M.T., Baumgarth, N., Fox, J.G. et al. (2015). Biology and diseases of mice. In: *Laboratory Animal Medicine*, 3e, 43–149. Academic Press.

66 Otto, G.M., Franklin, C.L., and Clifford, C.B. (2015). Biology and diseases of rats. In: *Laboratory Animal Medicine*, 3e, 151–207. Academic Press. Available at: https://www.sciencedirect.com/science/article/pii/B9780124095274000043. Accessed May 4, 2019.

67 Miedel, E.L. and Hankenson, F.C. (2015). Biology and diseases of hamsters. In: *Laboratory Animal Medicine*, 3e, 209–245. Academic Press.

68 Heatley, J.J. (2009). Cardiovascular anatomy, physiology, and disease of rodents and small exotic mammals. *Vet. Clin. North Am. Exot. Anim. Pract.* 12: 99–113.

69 Wagner, R.A. (2009). Ferret cardiology. *Vet. Clin. North Am. Exot. Anim. Pract.* 12: 115–134.

70 Pariaut, R. (2009). Cardiovascular physiology and diseases of the rabbit. *Vet. Clin. North Am. Exot. Anim. Pract.* 12: 135–144.

71 Johnson-Delaney, C.A. and Orosz, S.E. (2011). Rabbit respiratory system: clinical anatomy, physiology and disease. *Vet. Clin. North Am. Exot. Anim. Pract.* 14: 257–266.

72 Longley, L. (2008). Mammal anaesthesia. In: *Anaesthesia of Exotic Pets*, 27–35. Elsevier.

73 Truex, R.C., Belej, R., Ginsberg, L.M. et al. (1974). Anatomy of the ferret heart: an animal model for cardiac research. *Anat. Rec.* 179: 411–422.

74 Flecknell, P. (2015). Managing and monitoring anaesthesia. In: *Laboratory Animal Anaesthesia*, 4e (ed. P. Flecknell), 77–108. Boston: Elsevier.

75 Ozeki, L. and Caulkett, N. (2015). Monitoring. In: *Zoo Animal and Wildlife Immobilization and Anesthesia*, 2e (eds. G. West, D. Heard and N. Caulkett), 149–165. Ames, IA: Wiley-Blackwell.

76 Matchett, C.A., Marr, R., Berard, F.M. et al. (2012). Veterinary care. In: *The Laboratory Ferret* (eds. C.A. Matchett, R. Marr, F.M. Berard, et al.), 29–61. Boca Raton, FL: CRC Press.

77 Shahoud JS, Aeddula NR. Physiology, arterial pressure regulation.; 2019.

78 Cooper, E. (2015). Hypotension. In: *Small Animal Critical Care Medicine*, 2e (eds. D.C. Silverstein and K. Hopper), 46–50. Elsevier Health Sciences.

79 Ypsilantis, P., Didilis, V.N., Politou, M. et al. (2005). A comparative study of invasive and oscillometric methods of arterial blood pressure measurement in the anesthetized rabbit. *Res. Vet. Sci.* 78: 269–275.

80 van Zeeland, Y.R.A., Wilde, A., Bosman, I.H. et al. (2017). Non-invasive blood pressure measurement in ferrets (*Mustela putorius furo*) using high definition oscillometry. *Vet. J.* 228: 53–62.

81 Heard, D. (2016). Anesthesia. In: *Current Therapy in Avian Medicine and Surgery* (ed. B. Speer), 612. St. Louis, MO: Elsevier Inc.

82 Caulkett, N.A., Cantwell, S.L., and Houston, D.M. (1998). A comparison of indirect blood pressure monitoring techniques in the anesthetized cat. *Vet. Surg.* 27: 370–377.

83 Acierno, M.J., Brown, S., Coleman, A.E. et al. (2018). ACVIM consensus statement: guidelines for the identification, evaluation, and management of systemic hypertension in dogs and cats. *J. Vet. Intern. Med.* 32: 1803–1822.

84 Harvey, L., Knowles, T., and Murison, P.J. (2012). Comparison of direct and Doppler arterial blood pressure measurements in rabbits during isoflurane anaesthesia. *Vet. Anaesth. Analg.* 39: 174–184.

85 Kuwahara, M., Yagi, Y., Birumachi, J.I. et al. (1996). Non-invasive measurement of systemic arterial pressure in guinea pigs by an automatic oscillometric device. *Blood Press. Monit.* 1: 433–437.

86 Heard, D. (2015). Lagomorphs (rabbits, hares, and pikas). In: *Zoo Animal and Wildlife Immobilization and Anesthesia*, 2e (eds. G. West, D. Heard and N. Caulkett), 1558–1559. Ames, IA: Wiley-Blackwell.

87 Hancock, E.W., Deal, B.J., Mirvis, D.M. et al. (2009). AHA/ACCF/HRS recommendations for the standardization and interpretation of the electrocardiogram. Part V: electrocardiogram changes associated with cardiac chamber hypertrophy a scientific statement from the American Heart Association electrocardiography. *J. Am. Coll. Cardiol.* 53: 992–1002.

88 Heard, D. (2014). Rodents. In: *Zoo Animal and Wildlife Immobilization and Anesthesia*, 2e (eds. G. West, D. Heard and N. Caulkett), 893–903. Ames, IA: Wiley-Blackwell.

89 Morrisey, J. and Kraus, M. (2012). Cardiovascular and other diseases. In: *Ferrets, Rabbits and Rodents – Clinical Medicine and Surgery* (eds. K.E. Quesenberry and J.W. Carpenter), 62–77. St. Louis, MO: Elsevier Inc.

90 Bone, L., Battles, A.H., Goldfarb, R.D. et al. (1988). Electrocardiographic values from clinically normal, anesthetized ferrets (*Mustela putorius furo*). *Am. J. Vet. Res.* 49: 1884–1887.

91 Smith, S.H. and Bishop, S.P. (1985). The electrocardiogram of normal ferrets and ferrets with right ventricular hypertrophy. *Lab. Anim. Sci.* 35: 268–271.

92 Huston, S.M., Ming-Show Lee, P., Quesenberry, K.E. et al. (2012). Cardiovascular disease, lymphoproliferative disorders, and thymomas. In: *Ferrets, Rabbits and Rodents*

– *Clinical Medicine and Surgery* (eds. K.E. Quesenberry and J.W. Carpenter), 257–268. St. Louis, MO: Elsevier Inc.

93 Lord, B., Boswood, A., and Petrie, A. (2010). Electrocardiography of the normal domestic pet rabbit. *Vet. Rec.* 167: 961–965.

94 Lennox, A.M. (2012). Respiratory disease and pasteurellosis. In: *Ferrets, Rabbits and Rodents – Clinical Medicine and Surgery*, 3e (eds. K.E. Quesenberry and J.W. Carpenter), 205–216. St. Louis, MO: Elsevier, Inc.

95 Sharma, R., Parimoo, H., and Sharma, B. (2013). Histopathology of metastatic uterine adenocarcinoma in a rabbit. *Indian J. Vet. Pathol.* 37: 210–212. Available at: https://www.researchgate.net/publication/262182080_Histopathology_of_metastatic_uterine_adenocarcinoma_in_a_rabbit (accessed 20 November 2019).

96 White, S.D., Campbell, T., Logan, A. et al. (2000). Lymphoma with cutaneous involvement in three domestic rabbits (*Oryctolagus cuniculus*). *Vet. Dermatol.* 11: 61–67.

97 Ishikawa, M., Kondo, H., Onuma, M. et al. (2012). Osteoblastic osteosarcoma in a rabbit. *Comp. Med.* 62: 124–126.

98 Schöniger, S., Horn, L.C., and Schoon, H.A. (2014). Tumors and tumor-like lesions in the mammary gland of 24 pet rabbits: a histomorphological and immunohistochemical characterization. *Vet. Pathol.* 51: 569–580.

99 Brown, C. and Donnelly, T.M. (2012). Disease problems of small rodents. In: *Ferrets, Rabbits and Rodents – Clinical Medicine and Surgery* (eds. K.E. Quesenberry and J.W. Carpenter), 354–372. St. Louis, MO: Elsevier Inc.

100 Barron, H.W. and Rosenthal, K.L. (2012). Respiratory diseases. In: *Ferrets, Rabbits and Rodents – Clinical Medicine and Surgery*, 3e (eds. K.E. Quesenberry and J.W. Carpenter), 78–85. St. Louis, MO: Elsevier Inc.

101 Jubran, A. (2015). Pulse oximetry: review. *Crit. Care* 19: 272.

102 Olin, J.M., Smith, T.J., and Talcott, M.R. (1997). Evaluation of noninvasive monitoring techniques in domestic ferrets (*Mustela putorius furo*). *Am. J. Vet. Res.* 58: 1065–1069.

103 Vegfords, M., Sjöberg, F., Lindberg, L.G. et al. (1991). Basic studies of pulse oximetry in a rabbit model. *Acta Anaesthesiol. Scand.* 35: 596–599. Available at: http://www.ncbi.nlm.nih.gov/pubmed/1785236. (accessed 6 November 2019).

104 Bernard, S.L., An, D., and Glenny, R.W. (2004). Validation of the Nonin 8600V Pulse Oximeter for heart rate and oxygen saturation measurements in rats. *Contemp. Top. Lab. Anim. Sci.* 43: 43–45.

105 Decker, M.J., Conrad, K.P., and Strohl, K.P. Noninvasive oximetry in the rat. *Biomed. Instrum. Technol.* 23: 222–228. Available at: http://www.ncbi.nlm.nih.gov/pubmed/2752232. (accessed 6 November 2019).

106 Stanford, M. (2004). Practical use of capnography in exotic animal anesthesia. *Exotic DVM* 6: 57–60.

107 Beck, C., Barthel, F., Hahn, A.M. et al. (2014). Evaluation of a new side-stream, low dead space, end-tidal carbon dioxide monitoring system in rats. *Lab. Anim.* 48: 1–5.

108 Evans, J.M., Hogg, M.I.J., and Rosen, M. (1977). Correlation of alveolar PCO_2 estimated by infra-red analysis and arterial PCO_2 in the human neonate and the rabbit. *Br. J. Anaesth.* 49: 761–764.

109 Oglesbee, B.L. and Jenkins, J.R. (2012). Gastrointestinal diseases. In: *Ferrets, Rabbits and Rodents – Clinical Medicine and Surgery*, 3e, 193–204. St. Louis, MO: Elsevier Inc.

110 Whitlock, R.H., Tasker, J.B., and Tenant, B.C. (1975). Hypochloremic metabolic alkalosis and hypokalemia in cattle with upper-gastrointestinal obstruction. *Am. J. Dig. Dis.* 20: 595–596.

111 Hoefer, H.L., Fox, J.G., and Bell, J.A. (2012). Gastrointestinal diseases. In: *Ferrets, Rabbits and Rodents – Clinical Medicine and Surgery*, 3e (eds. K.E. Quesenberry and J.W. Carpenter), 27–45. St. Louis, MO: Elsevier Inc.

112 Orcutt, C.J. (1998). Emergency and critical care of ferrets. *Vet. Clin. North Am. Exot. Anim. Pract.* 1: 99–126.

113 Stanke, N.J., Graham, J.E., Orcutt, C.J. et al. (2011). Successful outcome of hepatectomy as treatment for liver lobe torsion in four domestic rabbits. *J. Am. Vet. Med. Assoc.* 238: 1176–1183.

114 Sinatra, M.A., St. John, D.J.B., and Young, G.P. (1999). Interference of plant peroxidases with Guaiac-based fecal occult blood tests is avoidable. *Clin. Chem.* 45: 123–126.

115 Young, G.P., Sinatra, M.A., and St. John, D.J.B. (1996). Influence of delay in stool sampling on fecal occult blood test sensitivity. *Clin. Chem.* 42: 1107–1108.

116 Klaphake, E. and Paul-Murphy, J. (2012). Disorders of the reproductive and urinary systems. In: *Ferrets, Rabbits and Rodents – Clinical Medicine and Surgery* (eds. K.E. Quesenberry and J.W. Carpenter), 217–231. St. Louis, MO: Elsevier Inc.

117 Buss, S.L. and Bourdeau, J.E. (1984). Calcium balance in laboratory rabbits. *Miner. Electrolyte Metab.* 10: 127–132.

118 Cheeke, P.R. and Amberg, J.W. (1973). Comparative calcium excretion by rats and rabbits. *J. Anim. Sci.* 37: 450–454.

119 Hawkins, M.G. and Bishop, C.R. (2012). Disease problems of guinea pigs. In: *Ferrets, Rabbits and*

Rodents – Clinical Medicine and Surgery (eds. K.E. Quesenberry and J.W. Carpenter), 295–310. St. Louis, MO: Elsevier Inc.

120 Hawkins, M.G., Ruby, A.L., Drazenovich, T.L. et al. (2009). Composition and characteristics of urinary calculi from guinea pigs. *J. Am. Vet. Med. Assoc.* 234: 214–220.

121 Martel-Arquette, A. and Mans, C. (2016). Urolithiasis in chinchillas: 15 cases (2007 to 2011). *J. Small Anim. Pract.* 57: 260–264.

122 Mans, C. and Donnelly, T.M. (2012). Disease problems of chinchillas. In: *Ferrets, Rabbits and Rodents – Clinical Medicine and Surgery* (eds. K.E. Quesenberry and J.W. Carpenter), 311–325. St. Louis, MO: Elsevier Inc.

123 Pollock, C.G. (2012). Disorders of the urinary and reproductive systems. In: *Ferrets, Rabbits and Rodents – Clinical Medicine and Surgery*, 3e (eds. K.E. Quesenberry and J.W. Carpenter), 46–61. St. Louis, MO: Elsevier Inc.

124 Eshar, D., Wyre, N.R., and Brown, D.C. (2012). Urine specific gravity values in clinically healthy young pet ferrets (*Mustela furo*). *J. Small Anim. Pract.* 53: 115–119.

125 Roxe, D.M. (1990). Urinalysis. In: *Clinical Methods: The History, Physical, and Laboratory Examinations*, 3e (eds. H.K. Walker, W.D. Hall and J.W. Hurst), 868–871. Boston: Butterworths.

126 Boysen, S.R. and Lisciandro, G.R. (2013). The use of ultrasound for dogs and cats in the emergency room AFAST and TFAST. *Vet. Clin. North Am. - Small Anim. Pract.* 43: 773–797.

127 Smith, Z.A., Postma, N., and Wood, D. (2010). FAST scanning in the developing world emergency department. *S. Afr. Med. J.* 100: 105–108.

10

Diagnostic Imaging

João Brandão[1], Peter M. DiGeronimo[2], and Carrie Kuzma[1]

[1] Department of Veterinary Clinical Sciences, College of Veterinary Medicine, Oklahoma State University, Oklahoma, USA
[2] Adventure Aquarium Camden, New Jersey, USA

CONTENTS

Introduction – Indications for Diagnostic Imaging

The advent of diagnostic imaging techniques has revolutionized both human and veterinary medicine and surgery. Since W.C. Roentgen discovered X-rays in 1895, various imaging modalities have been developed including radionuclide imaging, ultrasonography (US), computed tomography (CT), magnetic resonance imaging (MRI), and digital radiography [1]. Most of these are currently available to exotic animal clinicians.

Diagnostic imaging allows for noninvasive evaluation of internal structures assisting the clinician to achieve a definitive diagnosis, to provide an accurate prognosis, and to determine the most appropriate therapy.

Some imaging modalities, such as radiographs and CT, may expose the personnel involved to harmful radiation. Radiation safety should be followed as described for small animals [2].

Image Acquisition and Normal Anatomy

Radiographs

Positioning (By Species, Sedated vs. Anesthesia)

Patient malpositioning during radiographic exposure is the most common reason for nondiagnostic radiographs or misdiagnosis, especially for practitioners less experienced in exotic animal practice [3]. Physical restraint is necessary to achieve proper positioning and chemical restraint, that is sedation or general anesthesia, may be beneficial. In emergency cases, chemical restraint may not be ideal in unstable patients. Positioning for diagnostic imaging is often uncomfortable and physical restraint alone may cause additional stress and struggling thus making it contraindicated in painful, respiratory, or cardiovascularly compromised patients. There is limited research of the effects of sedation and general anesthesia on the quality and interpretation of exotic mammal radiographs. However, chemical restraint can improve radiographic quality by reducing

Exotic Animal Emergency and Critical Care Medicine, First Edition. Edited by Jennifer E. Graham, Grayson A. Doss and Hugues Beaufrère.

motion artifacts and allowing for more precise positioning and increasing the safety of the patient and technical staff [3]. See Chapter 7 for more information on sedation and general anesthesia in exotic mammal emergencies.

Orthogonal views yield more diagnostic information than single views. Typical orthogonal views include ventrodorsal and right and/or left lateral projections. To acquire ventrodorsal images, the patient is positioned in dorsal recumbency and the limbs are extended cranially and caudally (Figures 10.1 and 10.2). To minimize radiation exposure to personnel performing patient restraint, tape or rolled gauze can be applied to the limbs and used to position the animal. The midline sternum should overlap the spine. For lateral projections, the contralateral shoulder and the hip joints should overlap (Figure 10.3). Quality of positioning should be confirmed once the images are available, and the radiographs repeated if necessary. Similar to other small animals, foam wedges, troughs, and small sandbags can be helpful positioning aids for some patients. In some species, it may be helpful to use some unusual devices, such as tape or chip clips in hedgehogs or a "hanging ferret." In emergency cases, proper positioning may not be possible for unstable patients and the time and effort associated with repeating radiographs may preclude obtaining ideally positioned images. In these cases, even poorly positioned radiographs should be critically evaluated for information that may be clinically valuable.

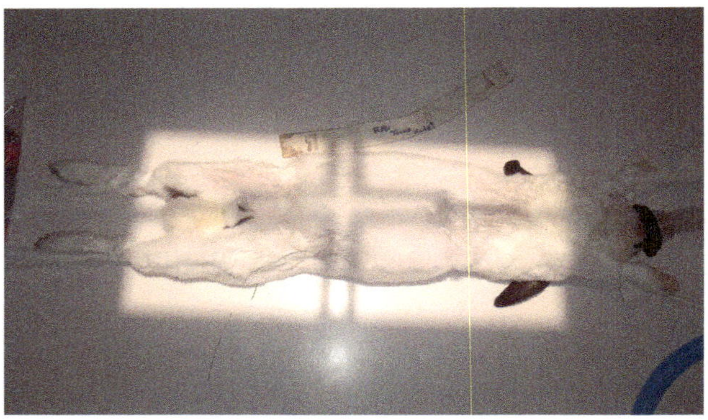

Figure 10.1 Positioning of a rabbit under general anesthesia for ventro-dorsal whole-body radiographs.

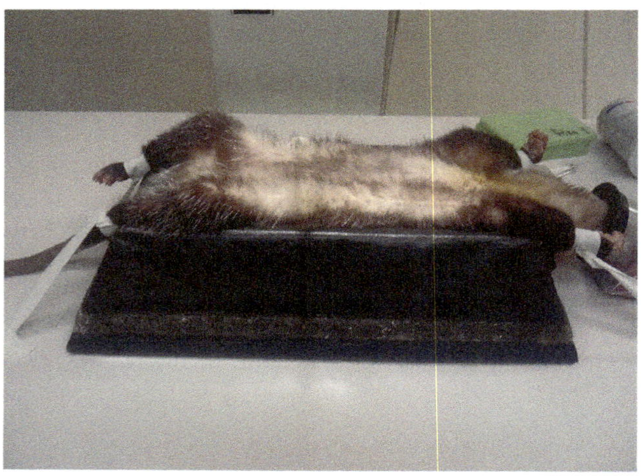

Figure 10.2 Positioning of a Virginia opossum (*Didelphis virginiana*) under general anesthesia for ventro-dorsal whole-body radiographs.

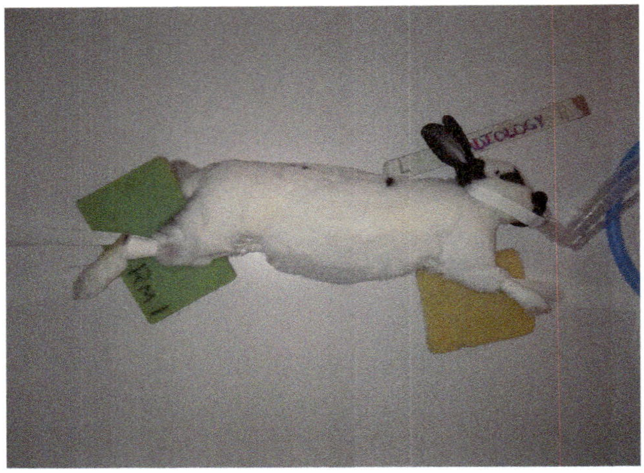

Figure 10.3 Positioning of a rabbit under general anesthesia for left lateral whole-body radiographs.

(a) (b)

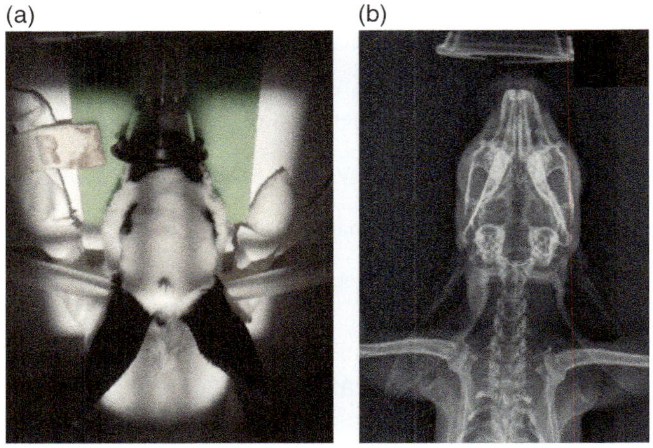

Figure 10.4 Positioning of a presumptively healthy rabbit under general anesthesia for dorso-ventral skull projection and associated radiographic image.

Skull radiographic evaluation can be very useful for assessment of dental and ear disease. Although CT may provide more detail for these conditions, radiography is commonly available and it may provide enough information to make a diagnosis. Nevertheless, skull radiographs may not be essential of the emergency management of a patient. Skull radiographs should include the following projections: dorsoventral (Figure 10.4) and/or ventrodorsal, lateral (Figure 10.5), left and right oblique views (Figure 10.6). Craniocaudal "skyline" skull view may also be useful. For the oblique views, markers should be placed in a standardize manner so the appropriate identification

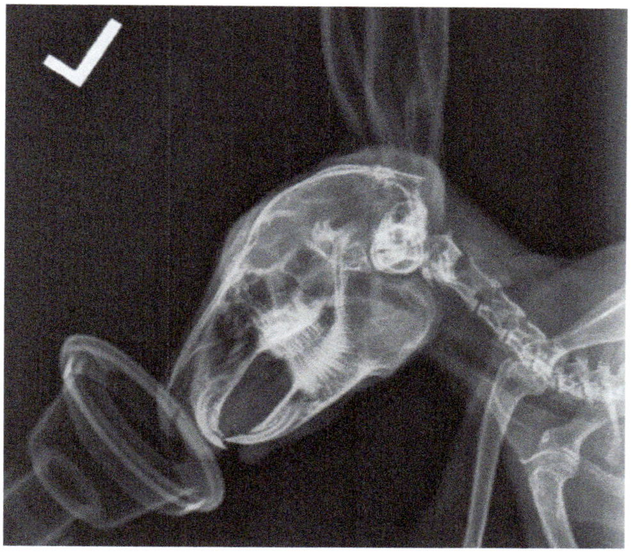

Figure 10.5 Left lateral skull radiographic image of a presumptively healthy rabbit under general anesthesia.

of the structures can be made. If the area of interest is the ear, the positioning of the skull may have to be more oblique, in comparison for the assessment of the mandible and maxilla.

Complications/Contraindications

The decision to take radiographs must be made on a case by case basis as patients may decompensate due to physical or chemical restraint associated with positioning. This is especially important for dyspneic patients. If radiographs may provide diagnostic or prognostic information that will influence case management, then the benefit may outweigh the risk. No diagnostics should be performed if the results will not affect management of the case.

Contrast Studies

Gastrointestinal and urogenital contrast studies can be performed using positive (e.g. barium, iohexol) or negative (e.g. gas) contrast agents or a combination of the two along with standard radiographic or fluoroscopic techniques. Intravenous contrast can be administered for cardiovascular assessment. Myelography relies on the injection of a contrast agent into the subarachnoid space to evaluate the spinal cord and nerve roots for suspected compression.

Contrast studies may be useful to identify potential obstruction, stenosis, and foreign bodies, but may not be commonly performed as an emergency procedure. There is limited information regarding normal contrast studies and contrast transit times in exotic mammals.

Positive and/or negative contrast injected retrograde into the urinary tract may improve the assessment of the mucosa, wall thickness, and luminal content of the urinary bladder [4].

Gastrointestinal contrast studies can be achieved by administration of 5 ml/kg air (pneumogastrography) or 3–10 ml/kg positive contrast. Double-contrast studies are useful for delineating foreign bodies and wall lesions, like ulcers and tumors [4]. In rabbits, the cecum contained 32% of a liquid contrast agent (^{14}C-labeled polyethylene glycol and ^{51}Cr-labeled ethylenediaminetetraacetic-acid) given via gastric fistula within one hour [5]. Anesthesia may decrease intestinal motility. Such has been shown in rats with brief (<6 minutes exposure) isoflurane anesthesia [6].

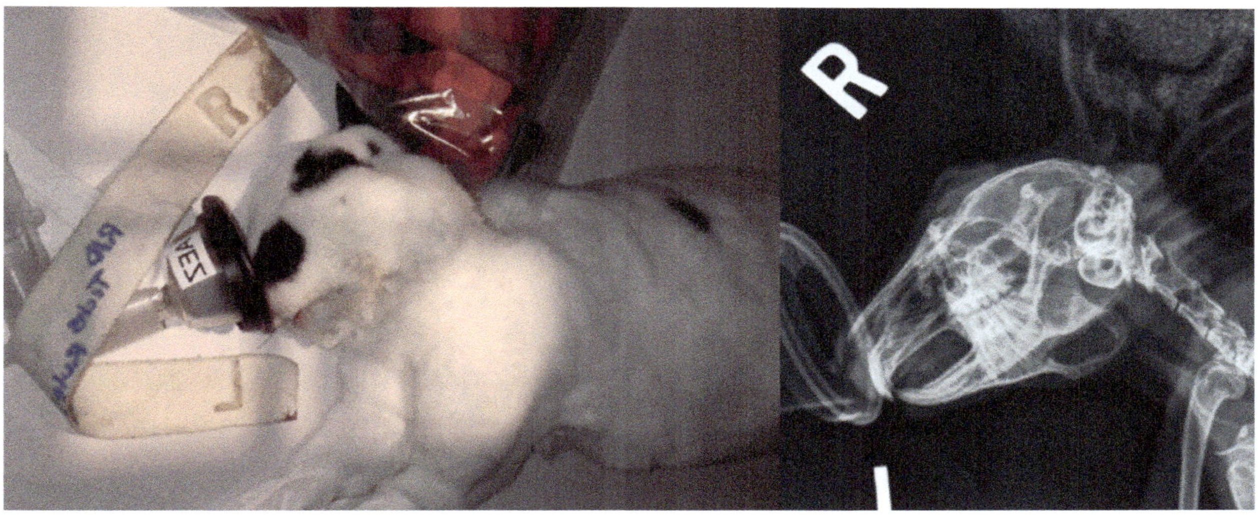

Figure 10.6 Positioning of a presumptively healthy rabbit under general anesthesia for right oblique skull projection and associated radiographic image. The rabbit is placed in right lateral recumbency and the radiographic projection is dorsal 30° lateral – ventrolateral oblique.

Normals (Lateral and DV or VD Views by Species)

Radiography is the most commonly available diagnostic imaging modality. Species-specific anatomical variation, however, makes its interpretation challenging and dependent on the skill, experience, and knowledge of the clinician. Radiographs of presumed healthy animals can be found on the following images; rabbit (Figures 10.7–10.9), ferret (Figure 10.10), and guinea pig (Figure 10.11). Radiographs of selected diseases in small mammals can be found on the following images; cardiomegaly in a ferret (Figures 10.12 and 10.13), ferret with pleural and peritoneal effusion (Figures 10.14 and 10.15), guinea pig with dyspnea secondary to suspected bacterial pneumonia (Figures 10.16 and 10.17), and guinea pig with ovarian cysts (Figure 10.18). There are a number of studies that describe the radiographic findings that correlate with normal anatomical structures of small mammals including rabbits [7–17], guinea pigs [9, 10], chinchillas [9, 10, 18], ferrets [19–22], rats [23], African hedgehogs (*Atelerix albiventris*) [24], black-rumped agoutis (*Dasyprocta prymnolopha*) [25], and common marmosets (*Callithrix jacchus*) [26].

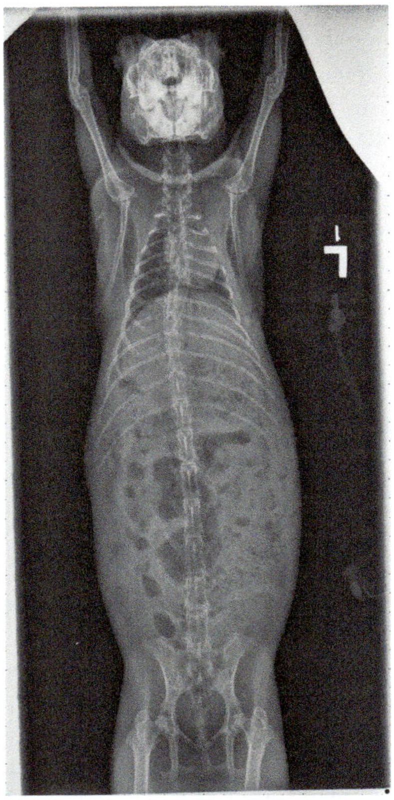

Figure 10.7 Full body ventro-dorsal projection of a domestic rabbit. This projection includes rostrocaudal projection of the skull ("skyline view") that may be useful to evaluate for dental disease.

Because the mammalian skeleton is typically bilaterally symmetrical, interpretation of radiographs to assess for orthopedic disease can be facilitated by comparison of affected sites

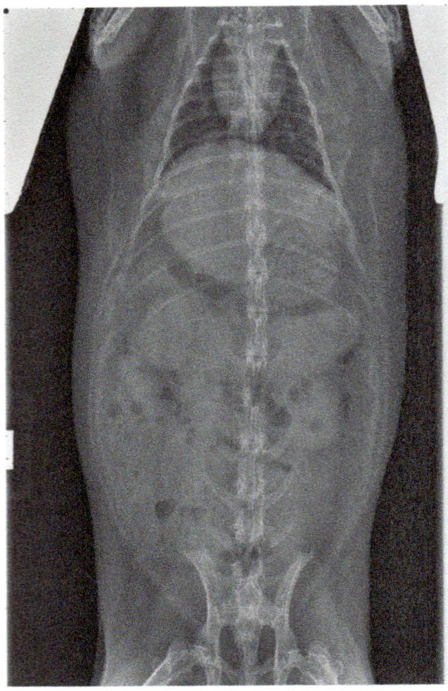

Figure 10.8 Ventro-dorsal projection of a domestic rabbit.

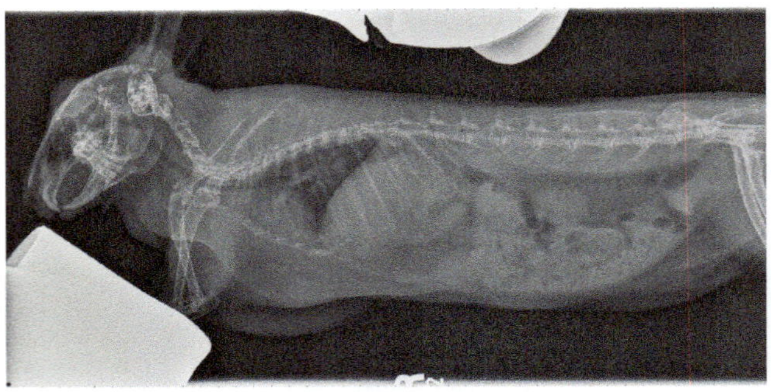

Figure 10.9 Right lateral projection of a domestic rabbit.

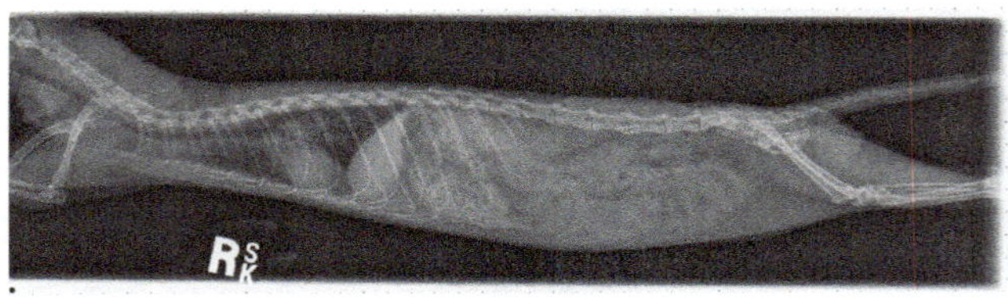

Figure 10.10 Right lateral projection of a normal female ferret. Note ingesta within stomach. Gastrointestinal foreign body should be considered as in small animal (dog and cat) practice. Splenomegaly is common finding in domestic ferrets and is not necessarily indicative of pathology.

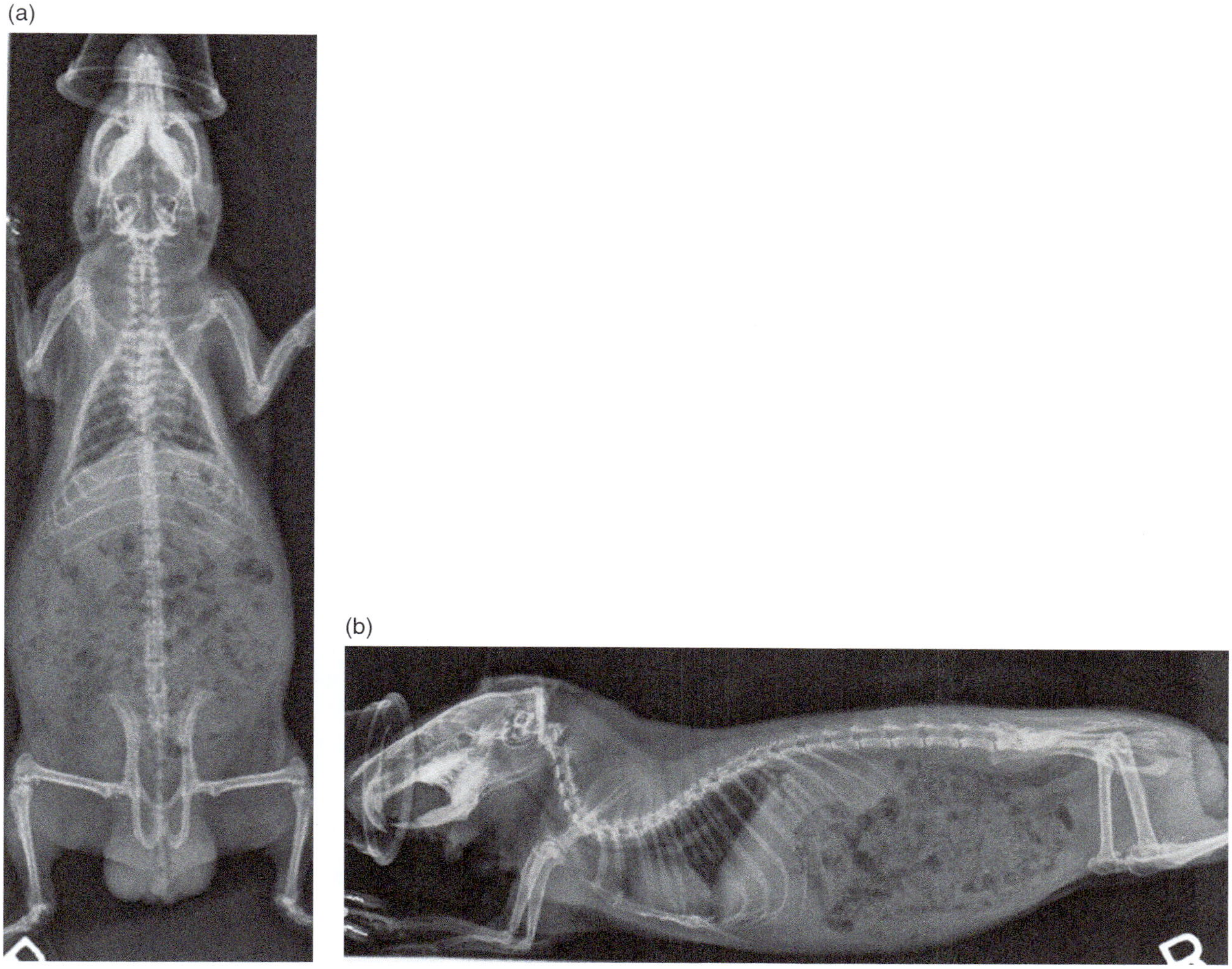

Figure 10.11 Whole body VD (a) and right lateral (b) of a presumed healthy guinea pig. *Source:* Images courtesy of Samantha Loeber, University of Wisconsin–Madison.

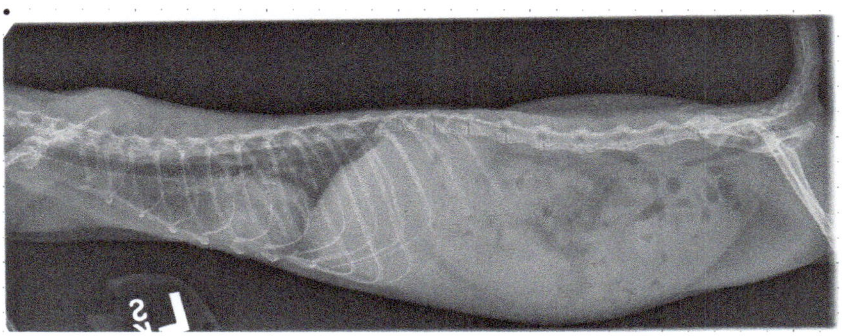

Figure 10.12 Left lateral projection of a ferret with cardiac disease. The cardiac silhouette is enlarged with a pulmonary bronchiolar pattern. Moderate peritoneal effusion indicated by the decreased abdominal serosal margin detail. Subcutaneous emphysema is dorsal to the thorax from fluid administration. Splenomegaly also suspected.

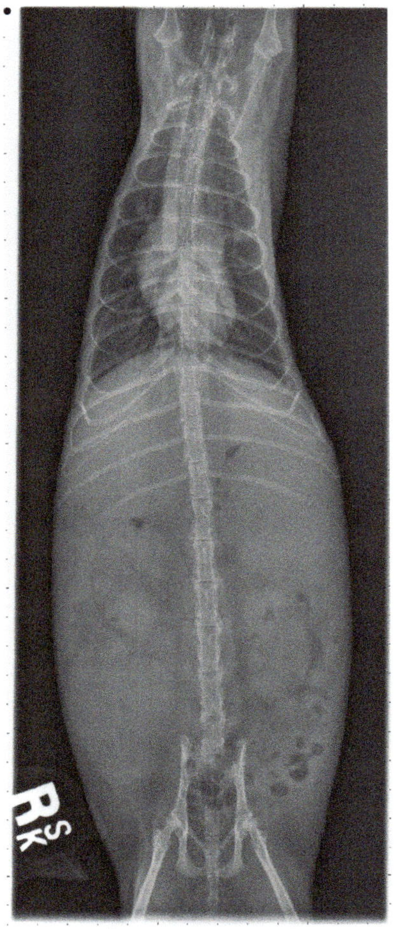

Figure 10.13 Ventro-dorsal projection of a ferret with cardiac disease. Cardiac silhouette is enlarged and there is vascular distention consistent with cardiac disease and likely hypertension. There is abaxial deviation of the caudal principal bronchi, suggestion of left atrial enlargement. Moderate peritoneal effusion indicated by the decreased abdominal serosal margin detail. Subcutaneous emphysema is adjacent to the left scapula from fluid administration. Mild widening of the pleural fissure lines which are indicative of pleural effusion.

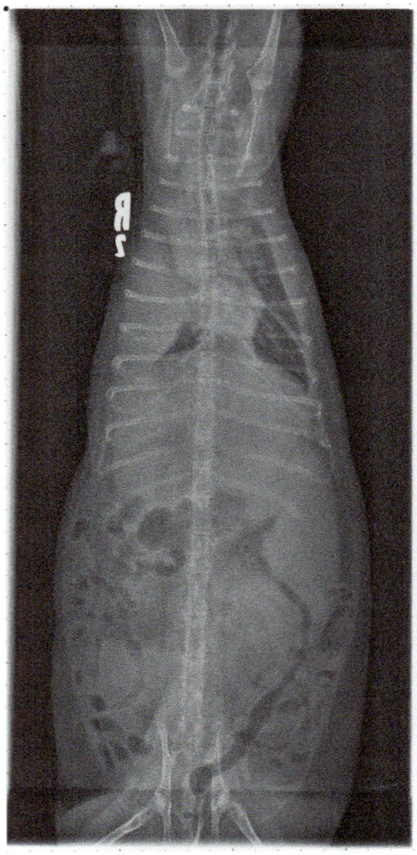

Figure 10.14 Ventro-dorsal projection of a ferret with pleural and peritoneal effusions. Splenomegaly is also suspected.

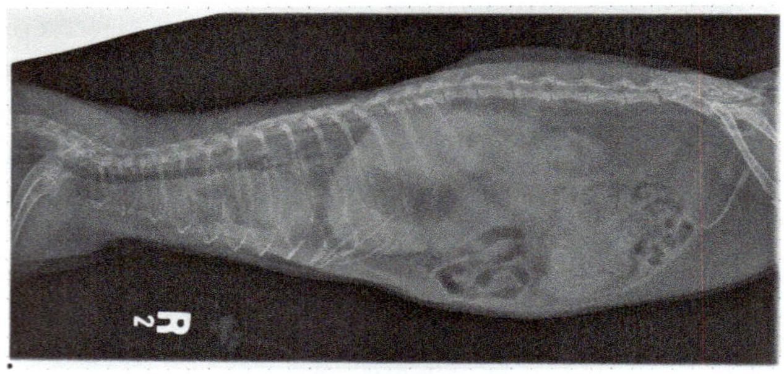

Figure 10.15 Right lateral projection of a ferret with pleural and peritoneal effusions. Mild gastric distension is present.

with the unaffected contralateral structure even without prior knowledge of the species-specific anatomy [3].

Ultrasound

Indications

On emergency presentation, ultrasound (US) can be useful for quick patient assessment. Depending on the structures of interest, this modality can require minimal physical restraint. Chemical restraint may be indicated for sample collection by aspiration or centesis.

Ultrasonography is commonly performed to assess the thorax (e.g. pleura, heart) and abdomen and, to a lesser extent, certain skull structures (e.g. eye, ear). Ultrasonographic examination is warranted for patients with suspected renal, liver, or reproductive disease, pregnancy or pregnancy toxemia, gastrointestinal (e.g. diarrhea, vomiting) or urinary signs (e.g. stranguria, hematuria), and in cases of trauma [27].

General Information

Ultrasound allows for noninvasive imaging of internal structure without harmful biological effects [28] and allows

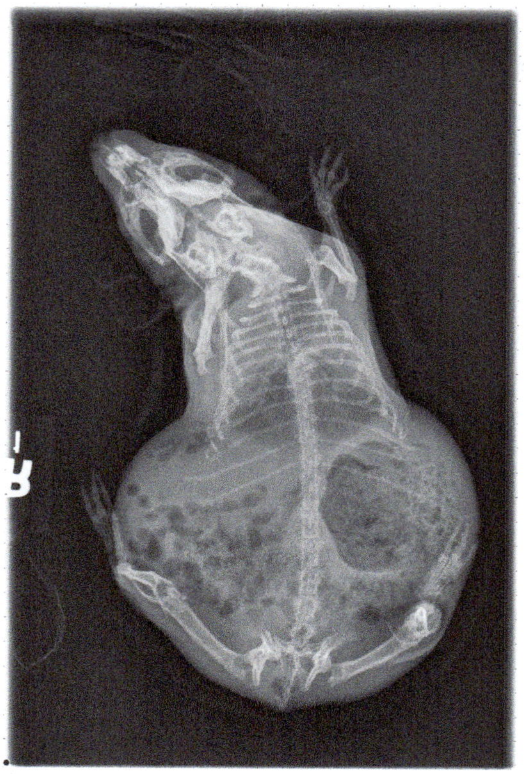

Figure 10.16 Standing dorsoventral projection of a guinea pig presented for dyspnea. Cranial lung lobes are homogeneously soft tissue opaque; the caudal lung lobes are gas filled with an unstructured interstitial pulmonary pattern. Gas in the stomach and intestines may be secondary to aerophagia in cases of severe dyspnea.

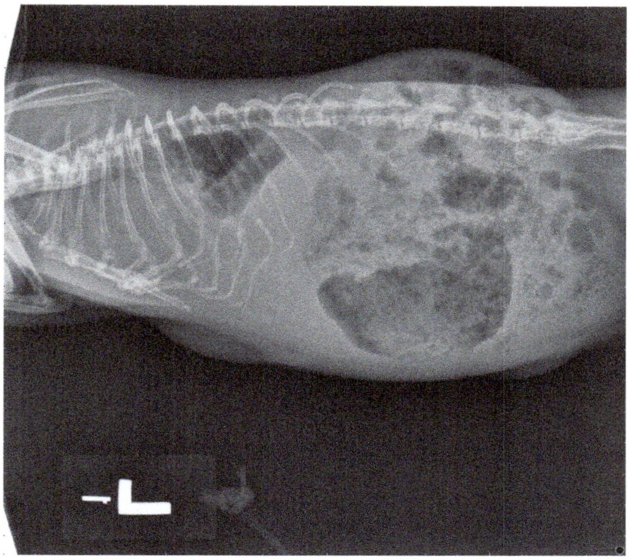

Figure 10.17 Left lateral projection of the same guinea pig from Figure 10.16. Soft tissue opacity of the cranial lung has completely obscured the cardiac silhouette and border efface the ventral diaphragm.

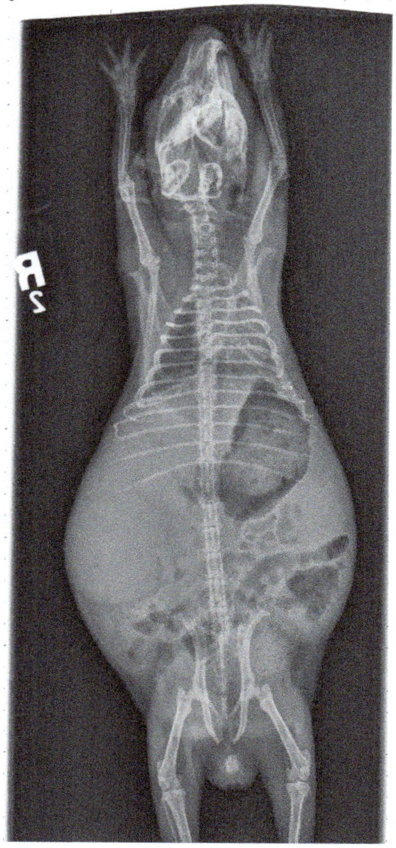

Figure 10.18 Ventro-dorsal projection of a sedated female guinea pig. Large, round soft tissue opacities are present bilaterally in the cranial to mid-abdomen consistent with ovarian cysts. Although typically benign, they may cause clinical signs such as hyporexia or gastrointestinal ileus due to a space-occupying mass effect.

for the use of color and power Doppler, pulse wave, and M mode capabilities. Small size, high definition transducers (e.g. 10–5 MHz 25 mm linear array transducer) may be beneficial for smaller patients. Due to the large range of patient sizes, multiple probes of different shapes (e.g. linear and curve) ranging from 3.5 to 20 MHz may be necessary [4].

Conduction of ultrasound is enhanced by fluids and hampered by gas [29]. Gas in the gastrointestinal tract of herbivorous small mammals, especially species like rabbits and guinea pigs that have well-developed ceca, will obstruct the image. Ultrasound can still yield diagnostic information and may be indicated nonetheless. Image quality is improved by clipping the fur and/or applying alcohol or acoustic coupling gel. Care must be taken when clipping the fur of species with sensitive or thin skin such as rabbits. Excessive clipping or alcohol use can precipitate hypothermia, an important consideration for small animals with high metabolic rates. Ideally, coupling gel should be warmed prior to application. Ferrets may become intractable if alcohol is used as they have well-developed olfactory systems and often find alcohol extremely obnoxious. In chinchillas, clipping the fur may be avoided if sufficient gel is applied [4].

Species Specific Information

Abdominal Ultrasound

Liver torsion is a common emergency presentation of rabbits that may present with clinical signs similar to those associated with gastrointestinal ileus. While hematology and biochemistry may suggest liver torsion, definitive diagnosis may be made by ultrasonographic evaluation. Common findings may include hepatomegaly or an abnormally large liver lobe, rounded lobar margins, mixed hepatic parenchymal echogenicity, hyperechoic perihepatic mesentery, and free peritoneal fluid (Figures 10.19 and 10.20) [30]. Color flow Doppler may reveal a lack of or decreased blood flow in the affected liver lobe(s) [30]. In exotic mammals, hepatic lipidosis can be a sequela of anorexia and may result in diffuse and homogenous hyperechogenic hepatic parenchyma on ultrasonography [27].

Reproductive disease is common in intact female rabbits over four years of age [31]. Clinical signs, such as vulvar bleeding or discharge, are often non-specific to any one reproductive disease and can be confounded with urinary tract disease. Ultrasound may help differentiate reproductive from urinary disease and may identify neoplasia of the reproductive tract (e.g. uterine or ovarian adenoma or adenocarcinoma), endometritis, pyometra, or mummified fetuses. Ovarian cysts are commonly diagnosed in guinea pigs. Ultrasonographically, cysts have thin walls, contain variable amounts of anechoic fluid, are contiguous with the ovaries, and may be visualized dorsal to the kidney [32]. Cysts are often multilocular, although unilocular cysts or neoplastic cysts have also been described [32]. Ultrasound has also been used to detect intra-abdominal abscesses in guinea pigs [33]. Ultrasonography can also be used to diagnose pregnancy and identify viable fetuses [34].

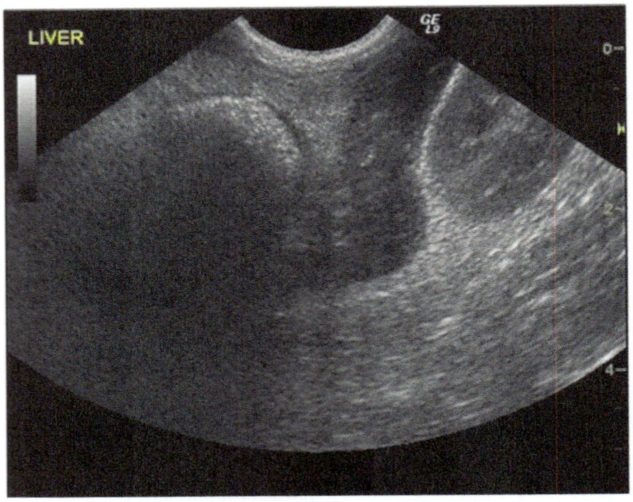

Figure 10.20 Ultrasonographic examination of cranial abdomen of a rabbit that was presented for decreased appetite and cranial abdominal pain. Torsion of the right caudate liver lobe appeared as a hypoechoic, oblong mass-like structure with mildly irregular and rounded margins in the right dorsal abdomen near the right kidney. Vascular structures were observed within the lobe but no blood flow was detected with Doppler. The rabbit appeared painful when imaging this region. *Source:* Courtesy of Jennifer Reetz.

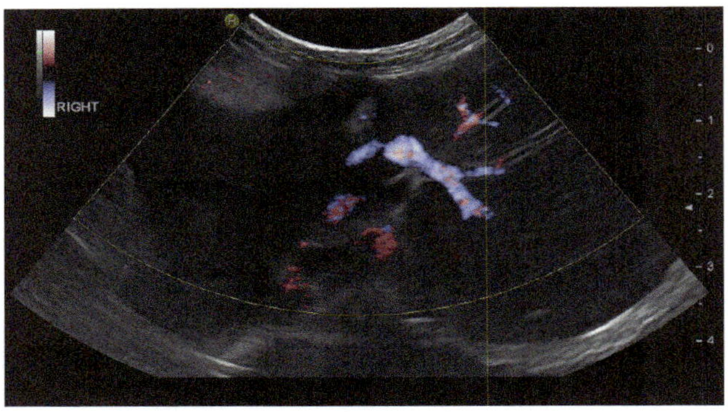

Figure 10.19 Transverse image of the liver of a rabbit at the level of the porta hepatis. The right liver is heterogeneously hypoechoic and mildly irregularly marginated, and lacks Doppler signal on Power Doppler evaluation, when compared to the left. A torsion of the caudate hepatic lobe was confirmed surgically in this patient. Note the surrounding hyperechoic mesentery, consistent with focal peritonitis. *Source:* Courtesy of Alexandre Le Roux.

Abdominal ultrasound is indicated when urinary tract disease, especially obstruction, is suspected (Figure 10.21). Ultrasound-guided cystocentesis is preferred in hind gut fermenters, such as rabbits, guinea pigs, and chinchillas, to minimize risk of accidental damage to the large cecum. Uroliths may be diagnosed by detecting the associated acoustic shadowing [27]. Ultrasound has been used to diagnose a ureterolith and an adrenal tumor in a guinea pig [35]. Ultrasound-guided percutaneous antegrade hydropropulsion has also been reported to relieve a ureteral obstruction in a pet guinea pig [36]. Male ferrets may present with signs of urinary obstruction due to prostatomegaly secondary to hyperadrenocorticism or to urolithiasis [37]. Urolithiasis is more prevalent in males, usually affects the lower urinary tract (bladder and urethra), and is most commonly cysteine [38]. Some species (e.g. guinea pig, chinchilla, ferret) have an os penis that should not be confused with a urolith [27].

Hyperadrenocorticism can be presumptively diagnosed in ferrets based on the identification of unilaterally or bilaterally abnormal adrenal glands evaluated with ultrasound.

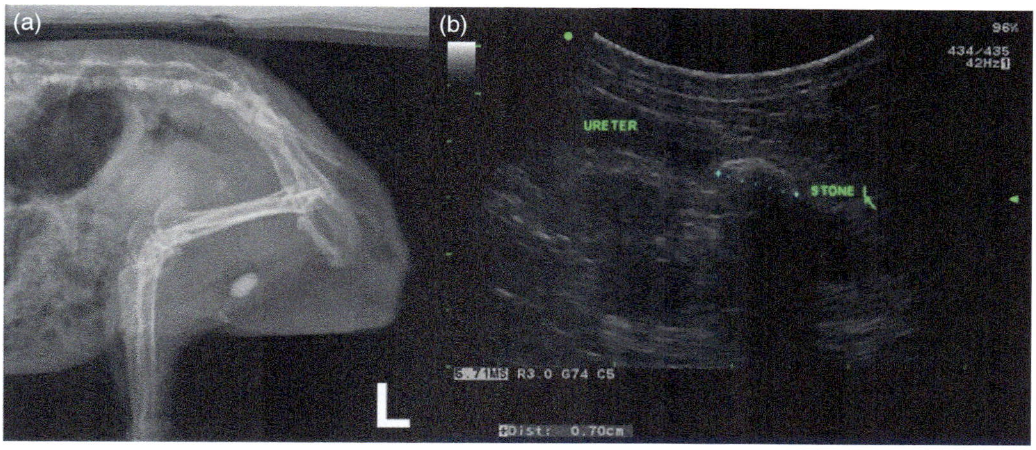

Figure 10.21 (a) Lateral abdominal radiograph of a four-year-old intact male guinea pig presented for suspected blood in the urine. An ovoid urethral calculus can be seen caudal to the pelvic limbs and a small ovoid calculus present dorsal to the femurs and superimposed with the urinary bladder (ultimately diagnosed as a ureterolith on ultrasound). Also note the periarticular degenerative changes of the stifles. The urethral calculus was removed by urethrotomy but no surgical treatment was pursued for the second calculus (b) Ultrasound of the same patient at three months. A ureteral calculus is present within the ureter. Imaging diagnosis: ureterolith, urethrolith, and stifle osteoarthritis.

Affected adrenal glands often have a rounded appearance, an increased cranial-caudal pole length (>3.9 mm), a heterogeneous structure, increased echogenicity, and/or signs of mineralization [39].

Thoracic Ultrasound

Thoracic ultrasound for the assessment of structures other than the heart may be indicated in certain cases. Ultrasound can be used to quickly and safely assess for pleural effusion, such as chylothorax [40, 41], hemothorax, or pneumothorax, even in debilitated patients undergoing triage and stabilization [42]. Air in the lungs renders thoracic ultrasonography challenging. Thymoma or thymic lymphoma are common diagnoses in rabbits that may be suggested by thoracic ultrasound. Common clinical signs include dyspnea and tachypnea due to a space-occupying thoracic mass or secondary pleural effusion, and bilateral exophthalmos secondary to pooling of blood in the retrobulbar venous plexus as a consequence of cranial vena cava compression [43]. Although CT may provide higher quality diagnostic images, ultrasound can be used to directly image the mediastinum and to obtain ultrasound-guided aspirates for cytology [43].

Ultrasonography is not ideal as a single imaging modality of the thorax since air will interfere with imaging. It may help to guide aspiration of pleural effusion (thoracocentesis) [42] or of pulmonary nodules identified on radiographs. The practicality of fine-needle aspiration depends on the location of the lesion and potential risks associated with damaging other structures.

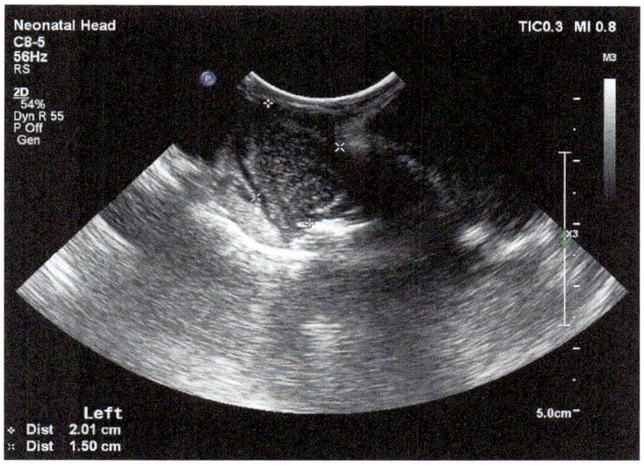

Figure 10.22 Ultrasound of the retrobulbar region of the right eye of a three-year-old rabbit that presented with left-sided exophthalmos. Caudal to the left globe, a heterogeneous well-encapsulated mass was present. Purulent material was obtained from an ultrasound guided aspirate. Imaging diagnosis: retrobulbar abscess.

Skull Ultrasonography

Ocular and periocular ultrasonography may allow the identification of intra- and peri-ocular abscesses and neoplasia [27]. These patients may present exophthalmic or buphthalmic due to retrobulbar abscesses (Figure 10.22), commonly associated with dental abscesses in animals with elodont dentition [44]. Ultrasound has been used to assess exophthalmos in a rabbit with a *Taenia serialis* cyst [45].

Otitis media and/or interna are common findings among several species of exotic companion mammals and are usually due to bacterial infections [46]. Otitis media is associated with respiratory disease in rabbits, as infection can spread via the Eustachian tube to the tympanic bulla and middle and inner ears [47]. Clinical signs associated with otitis include nystagmus, varying degrees of head tilt, loss of balance, and other neurological deficits. Although clinical signs can be severe, they are not pathognomonic. Differential diagnoses include *Encephalitozoon cuniculi* in rabbits and pituitary neoplasia in rats. It has been shown that US can be used for the assessment of the auditory system in domestic animals such as dogs [48], cats [49], and cows [50]. This technique has also been described in rabbits and rats. In rabbits, the anatomy of the ear has been described using US. A 12 MHz linear transducer was found to be most appropriate [51]. From a lateral approach, the external ear canal could be visualized to the level of the external acoustic meatus while the tympanic bullae itself could only be visualized from a ventral approach [51]. Rats can be assessed using a ventral approach to the caudal aspect of the skull [52]. A study compared the value of CT, radiograph, and US for the diagnosis of induced otitis (tympanic bullae filled with water-based gel) in rabbit cadavers [16]. CT was the most accurate diagnostic method, but US produced better results than radiography [16].

Normals

References for some normal anatomical structures imaged by abdominal ultrasonography have been reported for rabbits [53], rat [23, 54], guinea pigs [55], chinchilla [56], African hedgehog [57], and ring-tailed coati (*Nasua nasua*) [58]. Thoracic ultrasonographic references have not been reported in small mammals. Ultrasonographic evaluation of the auditory bullae has been reported in rabbits [16].

Advanced Diagnostic Imaging (Brief)

Echocardiography

On an emergency presentation, a brief echocardiogram can be performed to investigate the presence of emergent condition such as pericardial effusion which may require aspiration. Complete cardiac assessment should be performed after stabilization. Selected normal echocardiographic values for certain small mammal species can be found in Table 10.1.

Fluoroscopy

Fluoroscopy is not a common procedure performed on emergency; however, it may be useful to assess the functionality and/or motility of certain organs such as the gastrointestinal tract including the esophagus, trachea and tracheal collapse, among others. Clinically, relevant information on small mammal fluoroscopy applicable to emergency presentations appears to be underreported.

Computed Tomography (CT)

CT uses X-rays and computer calculations to produce two-dimensional images as a "slice" of the patient which can be digitally reconstructed to produce three-dimensional

Table 10.1 Selected normal echocardiographic values for small mammals.

	Ferret	Rabbit	Guinea pig	Chinchilla	Hedgehog
N	30	52	12	17	13
IVSd (mm)	2.2–5	1.3–2.8	1.1–2.4	1.2–2.4	1.3–1.7
IVSs (mm)	2.6–7	2.2–4	1.6–3		1.8–2.6
LVIDd (mm)	5.8–11.8	11.4–17.4	6.1–7.6	5.4–7.4	6.4–8.4
LVIDs (mm)	2.9–8.9	7.6–12.5	4–4.7	2.8–4.8	5.2–6.4
LVFWd (mm)	2–6.4	1.7–2.7	1.5–3.1	2.2–3	1.4–1.8
LVFWs (mm)	3.7–7.8	2.4–4.6	1.6–4		1.9–2.7
FS (%)	5–61	24.2–36.1	30.4–40.9	30–50	16.5–26.5
EF (%)	31–100	52–70.6	64.9–76.9		
Ao (mm)	3.3–7.3	6.7–9.8	4.2–5.2	2.6–4.6	3.2–4
LA (mm)	3.5–10.7	7.4–12	4.3–5.6	3.7–6.1	4.8–6.4

N, sample size; IVSd, interventricular septum end diastole; IVSs, interventricular septum end systole; LVIDd, left ventricular internal diameter end diastole; LVIDs, left ventricular internal diameter end systole; LVFWd, left ventricular free wall end diastole; LVFWs, left ventricular free wall end systole; FS, fractional shortening; EF, ejection fraction; Ao, Aorta; LA, left atrium. *Source:* From Beaufrere et al. [59]. © 2016, Elsevier.

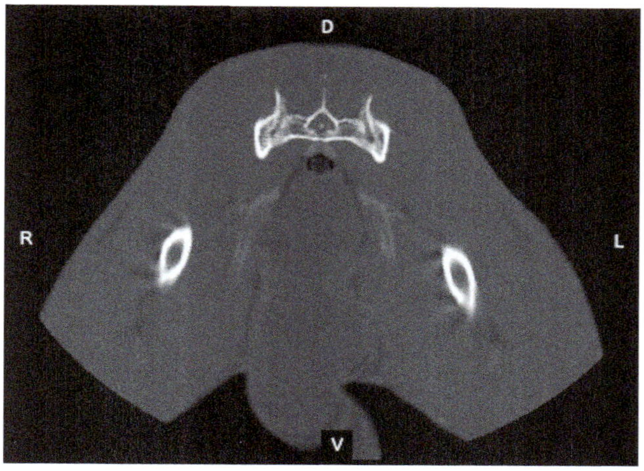

Figure 10.23 Transverse CT image of the caudal abdomen of a six-year-old intact male rabbit presented for a fluid filled mass within the right scrotum. At the caudal aspect of the abdomen at the level of the sacrum, ventral herniation of the urinary bladder can be seen. The herniation was more prominent to the right-sided and associated with the right testicle. Imaging diagnosis: urinary bladder herniation.

images of internal anatomy without interference from adjacent and overlying structures [4, 60]. It is particularly useful to assess bony structures and, to a lesser extent, soft tissue. Three-dimensional reconstructions are helpful to plan surgical procedures (Figure 10.23). Assessment of soft tissue can be enhanced by the use of intravenous iodine-based contrast agents. CT requires complete immobilization which necessitates general anesthesia, although newer generation units require less time per scan, allowing diagnostic imaging to be achieved in some cases with heavy sedation alone. Although this technology may not be commonly available, it has gained significant popularity in recent years. For particularly small patients, micro-CT units have been used in research, but this technology is not currently readily available in clinical practice.

CT is particularly useful for the assessment of respiratory tract, skull (to evaluate the reserve crowns of animals with elodont dentition, nasal cavity [Figure 10.24], and inner ear [Figure 10.25]), and patients with neoplasia and potential metastasis.

Normal computed tomographic anatomy has been described in rabbits [7, 16, 61–64], guinea pigs [62], and chinchillas [62, 65]. MicroCT has been reported in rabbits [63, 66], guinea pigs [67], and rats [68].

Magnetic Resonance Imaging (MRI)

MRI uses computer generation of images by measuring the hydrogen content of tissues [4]. This method does not

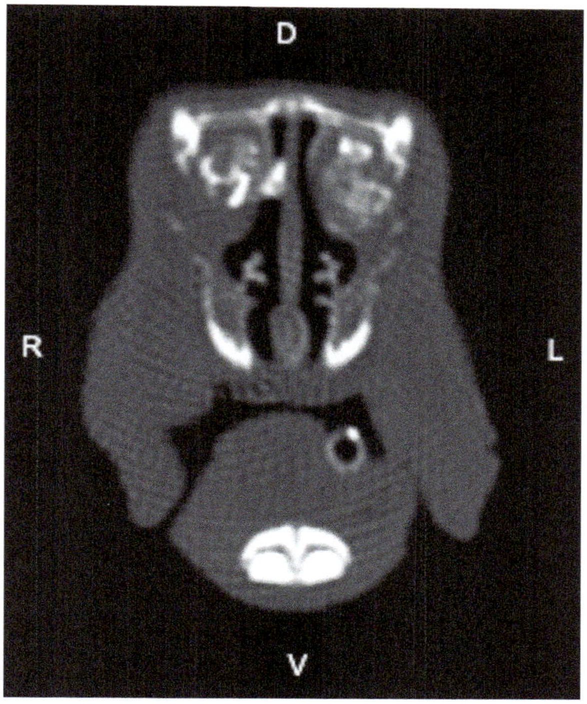

Figure 10.24 Transverse CT image of the skull of a seven-year-old neutered male rabbit which presented with chronic nasal discharge. Bilateral heterogeneous soft tissue and mineral attenuation at the cranial dorsal aspect of the maxillary sinuses. Imaging diagnosis: rostral maxillary sinusitis and rhinitis.

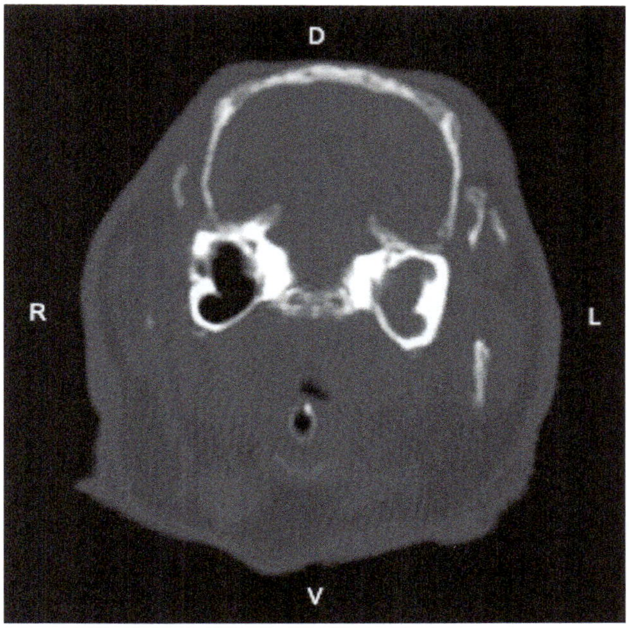

Figure 10.25 Transverse CT image of the skull of a three-year-old spayed female rabbit which presented with left-sided head tilt. On CT, fluid attenuating material within the left tympanic bulla was identified. Imaging diagnosis: left-sided otitis media.

produce radiation and spatial resolution and soft-tissue contrast is higher with this technique than with CT [4]. MRI is relatively expensive, not widely available in primary care or even referral practices, and requires more time for image acquisition than any other modality necessitating prolonged anesthesia. Nevertheless, MRI is the diagnostic test of choice for intracranial and spinal cord lesions, although there is a limited information regarding the application and interpretation of MRI in exotic mammals (rabbits [69, 70]).

Clinical Presentations Requiring Emergent Imaging

Investigations of:

GI Disease/FB

Gastrointestinal disease and foreign bodies, especially trichobezoars, are common findings in hindgut fermenters. Trichobezoars are challenging to diagnose by imaging because they are difficult to distinguish from normal ingesta. Radiographs may be useful to assess for gastric distension or gas in the gastric antrum or pylorus, suggestive of an obstructive gastric foreign body, such as a trichobezoar. Ultrasound may be useful, but gas in the stomach or cecum may impair or limit imaging acquisition. Other foreign bodies, particularly metal, are readily identified on radiographs.

Gastrointestinal dilation and volvulus (GDV) have been reported in guinea pigs (Figure 10.26) [71–73]. Clinical signs of GDV in guinea pigs include abdominal distension and tympany, abdominal pain, lack of intestinal sounds on abdominal auscultation, short sharp shallow breaths, and cardiovascular signs [72]. Interestingly, GDV has not been reported in rabbits although other torsions have been reported; mesenteric root and cecal torsion [74], and intestinal torsion [75]. Gastric dilation with and without torsion has been rarely reported in black-footed ferrets (*Mustela nigripes*) [76] and domestic ferrets [77].

Gastrointestinal foreign bodies are commonly reported in ferrets. The inquisitive behavior of ferrets may be predisposing these species to this condition. Ferrets typically present with a history of vomiting and/or diarrhea. Diagnostic imaging (radiography and/or ultrasonography) typically allow clinical diagnosis (Figure 10.27).

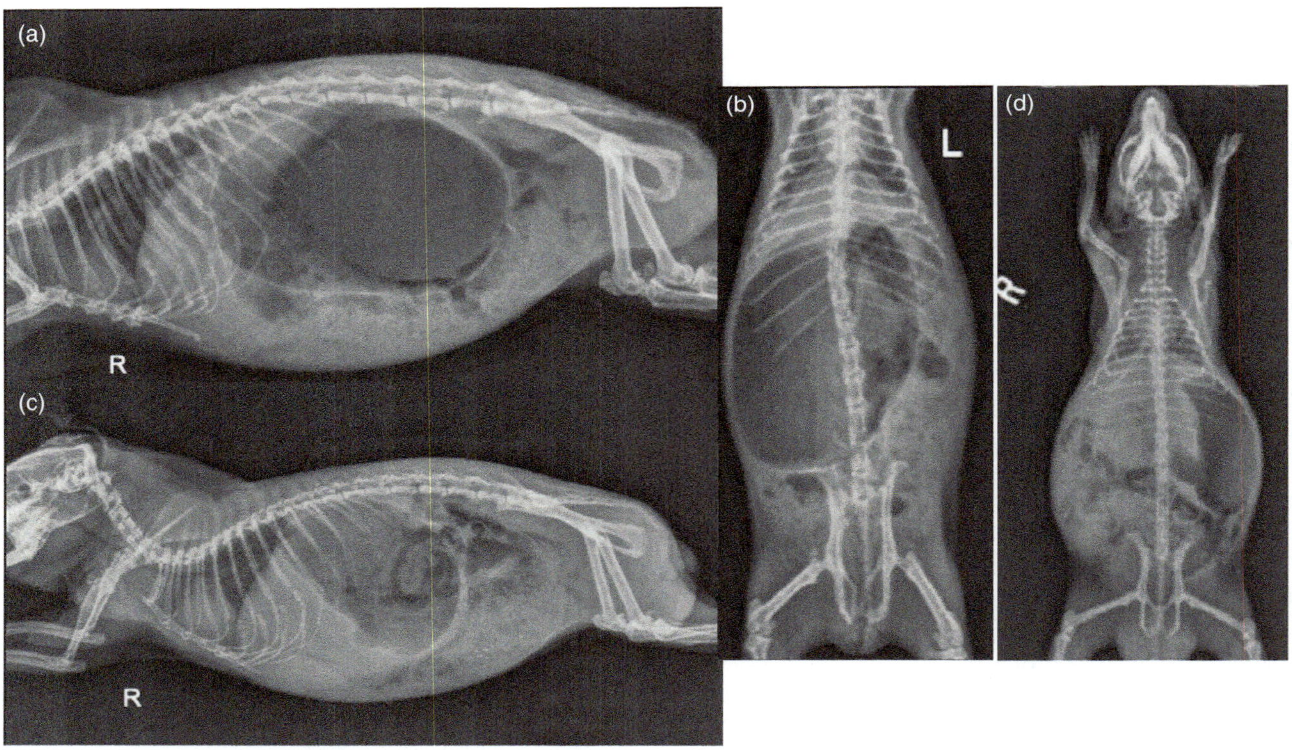

Figure 10.26 (a) and (b) Whole-body VD and right lateral radiographs of an adult guinea pig that presented for dry heaving and gagging. The stomach is markedly gas distended and displaces part of the cecum caudally and to the left. The small intestines are displaced craniodorsally to the left cranial aspect of the abdomen. Imaging diagnosis: Gastric dilatation and volvulus. (c) and (d) Whole-body VD and right lateral radiographs of an adult guinea pig that presented for lethargy and abdominal distention. Moderate gastric distention and caudal displacement of the gastric axis from hepatomegaly on the lateral projection. Moderate gastric distention with a gas filled pylorus which is positioned to midline by hepatomegaly. Flattening of the lesser curvature is noted from the hepatomegaly as well.

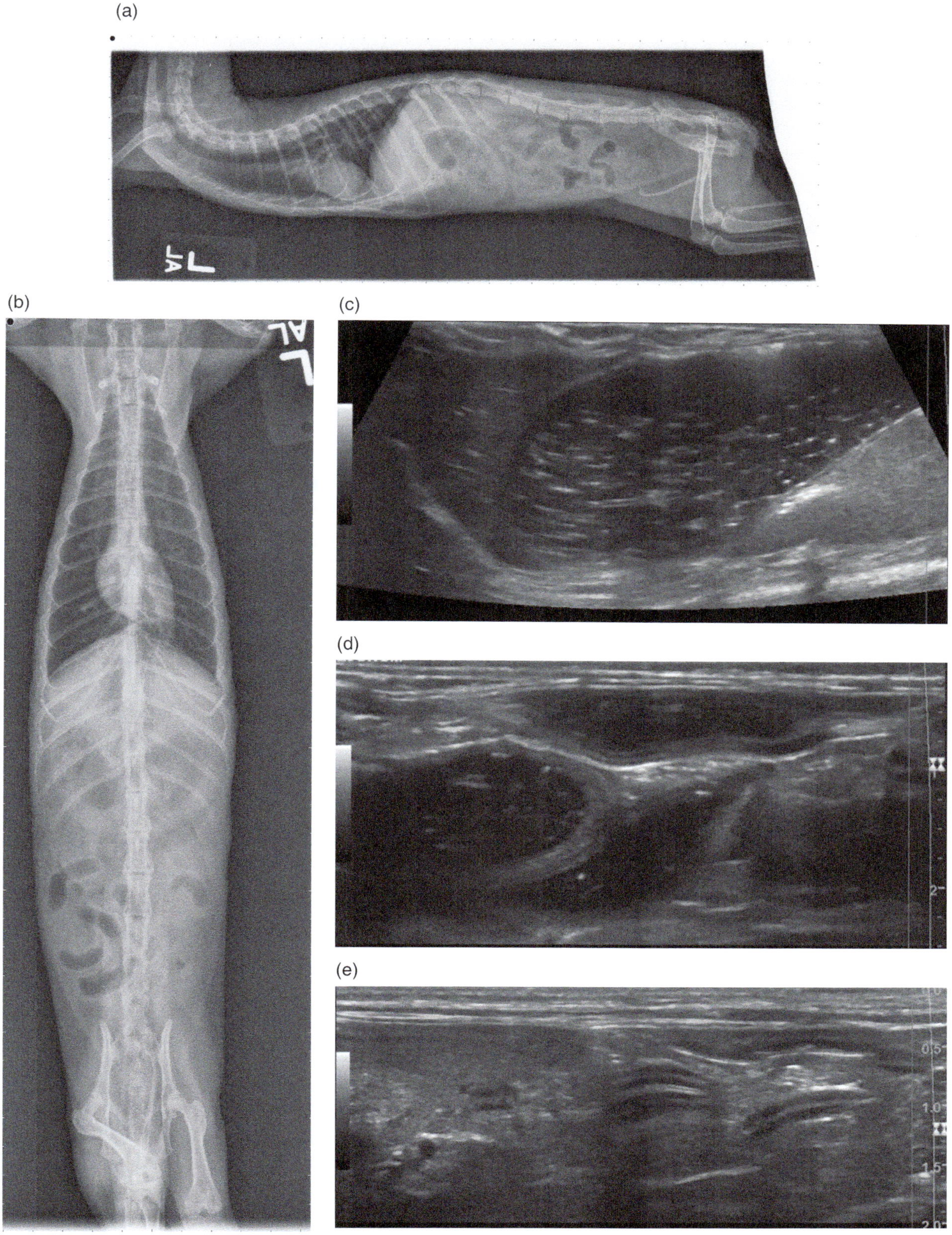

Figure 10.27 Whole body VD (a) and left lateral (b) radiograph of a ferret with a gastrointestinal foreign body. The stomach is distended and numerous small intestinal loops are gas filled and dilated. Smaller diameter intestinal loops are noted just caudal to the stomach indicating two populations and a small intestinal mechanical obstruction. Abdominal ultrasound images of selected gastrointestinal sections (stomach (c), and jejunum (d, e)) of a ferret with a gastrointestinal foreign body. Note the fluid filled stomach with suspended hyperechoic foci. Similar findings are within multiple small intestinal loops in image (d). In image (e), the normal empty small intestinal loops correspond to the radiographic two population pattern of small intestine. *Source:* Images courtesy of Samantha Loeber, University of Wisconsin–Madison.

Dyspnea

Dyspnea can result from respiratory or extra-respiratory disease. Pneumonia can be diagnosed by radiography and/or CT. Diagnostic imaging may reveal nodules consistent with pulmonary abscesses, especially in species that produce caseous pus (e.g. lagomorphs and rodents). Depending on the location of the lesions, ultrasound may be used to further assess and collect samples by fine-needle aspiration for cytology and/or bacterial/fungal cultures and/or molecular testing. Infectious (e.g. bacterial with or without an underlying viral component, and fungal) and non-infectious causes (e.g. endogenous lipid deposition) should be considered in cases of pneumonia in small mammals [78–82]. Rabbits may develop respiratory infections (with or without pneumonia) secondary to bacterial infection such as *Pasteurella multocida*, *Staphylococcus* sp., and *Mycobacterium* sp. [79] Rodents such as guinea pigs and rats, may develop respiratory infections (with or without pneumonia) secondary to bacterial infection such as *Bordetella bronchiseptica*, *Chlamydia* spp., cilia-associated respiratory bacillus, *Corynebacterium kutscheri*, *Haemophilus* spp., *Klebsiella pneumoniae*, *Mycobacterium* sp., *Mycoplasma* spp., among others [81]. Murine respiratory mycoplasmosis (also known as chronic respiratory disease) in rodent species is caused by *Mycoplasma pulmonis*. This chronic and progressive disease is very common in pet rats [83]. Fungal pneumonias should be considered in ferrets. Ferrets can also develop bacterial pneumonia and an underlying viral component (e.g. distemper and influenza) should be considered [84–86]. Extra-respiratory causes of dyspnea include mediastinal masses, such as thymomas in rabbits. Thymic lymphomas are also possible but appear less common [87]. Rabbits with thymomas typically present with dyspnea, exercise intolerance, and bilateral exophthalmos [87]. These masses will likely displace the trachea dorsally which should be noticeable on radiographs and on CT. For suspected mediastinal masses, CT is the imaging modality of choice, although US may also be performed. CT and US can also be useful for the collection of samples for cytology. Although not commonly reported, pneumothorax can occur in exotic mammals. This may be caused by trauma and iatrogenic causes such as pulmonary overinflation, or pulmonary and systemic disease (Figure 10.28) [88, 89].

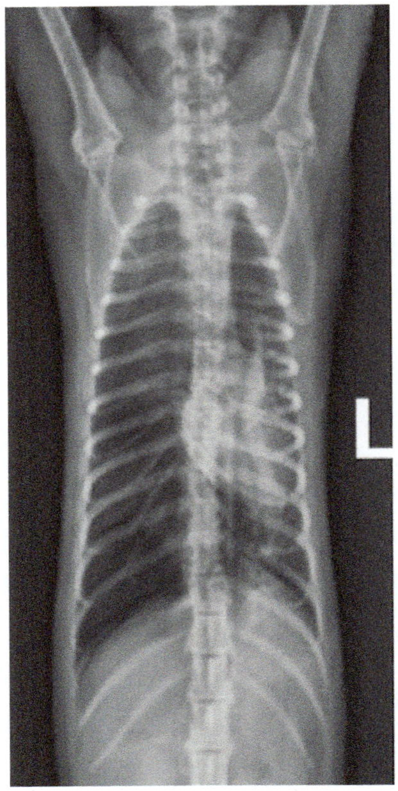

Figure 10.28 Ventro-dorsal thoracic radiograph of a five-year-old intact male kinkajou (*Potus favus*) presented with severe dyspnea. There is a mediastinal shift to the left. A pneumothorax, more severe within the right hemithorax can be seen. Imaging diagnosis: pneumothorax with pulmonary atelectasis.

Trauma

Focused assessment with sonography for trauma, triage and tracking (FAST) has been described and used in small animal emergency medicine for the evaluation of the thorax (T-FAST) and abdomen (A-FAST) [90]. FAST increases the sensitivity of US examination and expedites decision making to improve outcomes. T-FAST and A-FAST are particularly useful in cases of blunt force trauma and to screen for abdominal, pleural and pericardial effusions, and pneumothorax. Ultrasound-guidance also improves recovery of fluid samples by abdominocentesis compared to blind centeses [91]. Although adaptation of FAST US to the unique anatomy of exotic small mammals has not been described, clinicians with access to US should be familiar with FAST techniques to assist in triaging emergencies. A-FAST is performed in right and left lateral recumbencies and systematically scans four-points: diaphragmato-hepatic, spleno-renal, hepato-renal, and cysto-colic (Figure 10.29) [90]. The presence, contour, and wall of the gall bladder and urinary bladder should be evaluated. An abdominal fluid score (0–4; where 0 = no effusion at any point and 4 = effusion seen at each point) should be assigned. T-FAST is performed in right and left lateral or sternal recumbencies and systematically scans five-points: stationary bilateral chest tube sites (dorso-lateral thorax), bilateral pericardium sites moving along short and long axes of the heart, and the diaphragmato-hepatic site [90]. At the chest tube site, the glide sign excludes pneumothorax, lung rockets indicate interstitial lung fluid (e.g. edema, hemorrhage), and the step sign indicates thoracic wall trauma or pleural space disease. Pericardial and diaphragmato-hepatic sites can be used to identify pleural or pericardial effusion and cardiac tamponade.

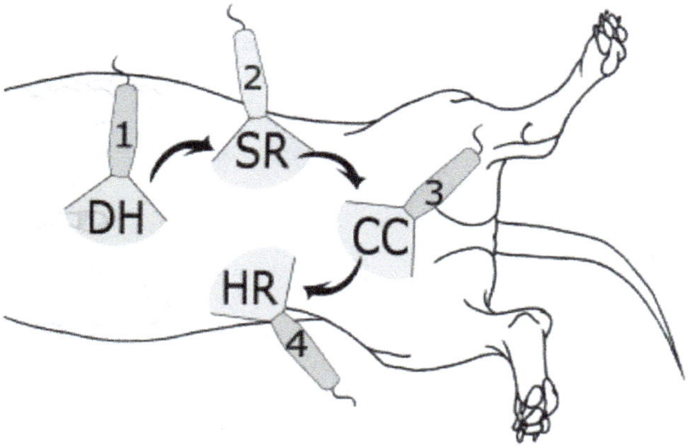

Figure 10.29 Depiction of the 4-point abdominal focused assessment with sonography for trauma, triage and tracking (AFAST), protocol performed in right lateral recumbency beginning at the diaphragmatico-hepatic (DH) view, followed by the spleno-renal view (SR), the cysto-colic view (CC), and completed at the hepato-renal view (HR). Direction (arrows) and order of AFAST exam (numbered ultrasound probes) are illustrated. *Source:* From Lisciandro and Gregory [90]. © 2011, John Wiley & Sons.

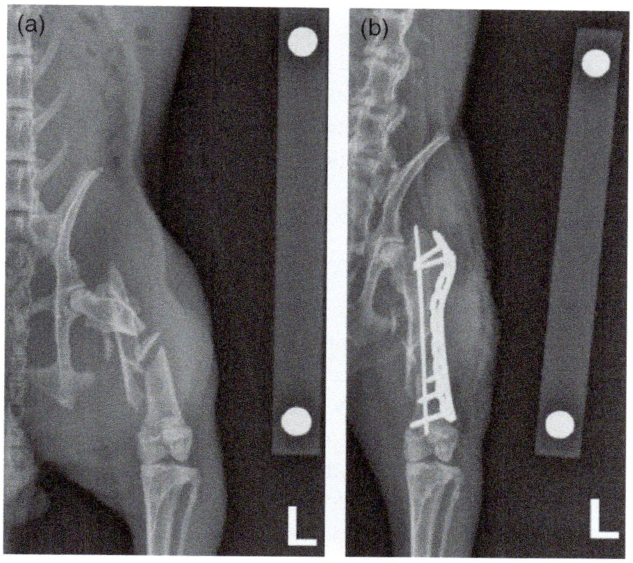

Figure 10.30 Left pelvic limb craniocaudal radiograph of a 6-month-old intact rabbit presented after a traumatic incident. (a) Comminuted fracture with sharp margins on the left femur, with the largest fragment moderately craniodorsally displaced and increased soft tissue swelling around the fracture. (b) Left femoral fracture reduced and stabilize. An intramedullary pin with an orthopedic plate and five orthopedic screws are present on the dorsal aspect of the femur. Imaging diagnosis: comminuted femoral fracture and subsequent surgical repair.

Lameness

Diagnostic imaging can be used in exotic small mammals for the evaluation of lameness as it is applied in small animal medicine. Radiographs taken with appropriate technique can be used to evaluate for trauma or fracture of long bones (Figures 10.30 and 10.31) and trauma or effusion of joints. Signs of degenerative joint disease and osteoarthritis are similar as in other mammals.

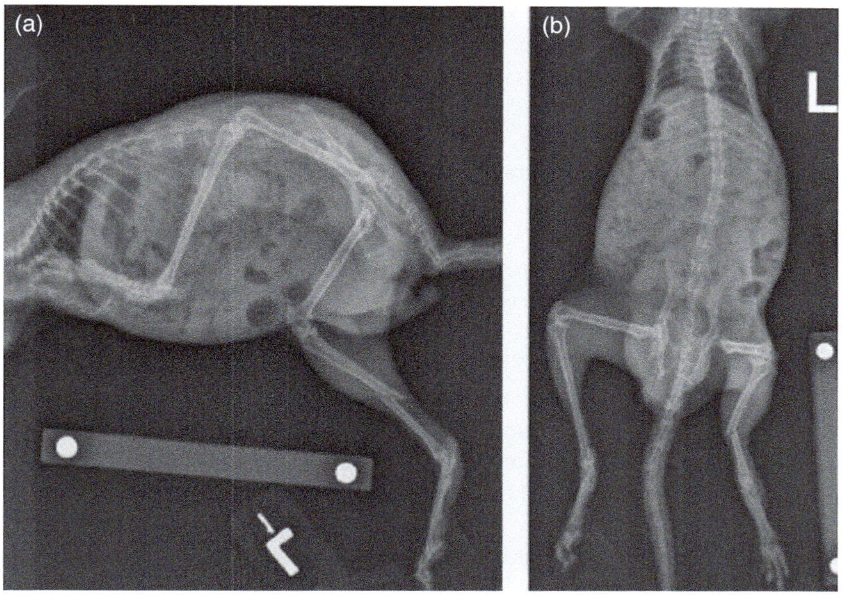

Figure 10.31 Left lateral (a) and ventro-dorsal (b) projections of whole-body radiographs of a chinchilla that was presented for acute onset lameness of <2 days duration. Positioning was facilitated by general anesthesia and the use of tape stirrups around metacarpi and metatarsi. There are short, oblique mid-diaphyseal fractures of the left tibia and fibula that are displaced proximally, cranially, and laterally with associated soft tissue swelling. Imaging diagnosis: tibial and fibular fracture. *Source:* Images courtesy of Emily Elser and Jantra Suran.

Prolapses/Reproductive Complications

For reproductive emergencies, radiographs may be used to count fetuses and identify obstetrical obstructions. Ultrasonography may be used to determine the viability of fetuses by identifying fetal heartbeats. Diagnostic imaging can be used to screen for neoplasia and pyometra as in small animal medicine. Prolapses associated with reproductive complications are uncommon. Nevertheless, uterine prolapse can be associated with dystocia or other reproductive diseases. Imaging may be useful to determine the cause of the prolapse.

References

1 Doi, K. (2006). Diagnostic imaging over the last 50 years: research and development in medical imaging science and technology. *Phys. Med. Biol.* 51: R5–R27.

2 Thrall, D. and Widmer, W. (2013). Radiation protection and physics of diagnostic radiology. In: Textbook of Veterinary Diagnostic Radiology (ed. D. Thrall), 2–21. St. Louis, MO: Elsevier Health Sciences.

3 Williams, J. (2002). Orthopedic radiography in exotic animal practice. *Vet. Clin. North Am. Exot. Anim. Pract.* 5: 1–22.

4 Redrobe, S. (2001). Imaging techniques in small mammals. *Semin. Avian Exot. Pet. Med.*: 187–197.

5 Pickard, D. and Stevens, C. (1972). Digesta flow through the rabbit large intestine. *Am. J. Physiol.-Leg. Conte.* 222: 1161–1166.

6 Torjman, M.C., Joseph, J.I., Munsick, C. et al. (2005). Effects of isoflurane on gastrointestinal motility after brief exposure in rats. *Int. J. Pharm.* 294: 65–71.

7 Van Caelenberg, A.I., De Rycke, L.M., Hermans, K. et al. (2011). Comparison of radiography and CT to identify changes in the skulls of four rabbits with dental disease. *J. Vet. Dent.* 28: 172–181.

8 Hammond, G., Sullivan, M., Posthumus, J. et al. (2010). Assessment of three radiographic projections for detection of fluid in the rabbit tympanic bulla. *Vet. Radiol. Ultrasound* 51: 48–51.

9 Boehmer, E. and Crossley, D. (2009). Objective interpretation of dental disease in rabbits, guinea pigs and chinchillas. *Tierarztl. Prax. Ausg. K Klientiere Heimtiere* 37: 250–260.

10 Gracis, M. (2008). Clinical technique: normal dental radiography of rabbits, guinea pigs, and chinchillas. *J. Exot. Pet Med.* 17: 78–86.

11 Dorotea, S., Banzato, T., Bellini, L. et al. (2016). Radiographic anatomy of dwarf rabbit abdomen with normal measurements. *Bulg. J. Vet. Med.* 19: 96–107.

12 Gibbs, C. and Hinton, M.H. (1981). Radiological examination of the rabbit. The head, thorax and vertebral column. *J. Small Anim. Pract.* 22: 687–703.

13 Hinton, M. and Gibbs, C. (1982). Radiological examination of the rabbit: II. The abdomen. *J. Small Anim. Pract.* 23: 687–696.

14 King, A.M., Cranfield, F., Hall, J. et al. (2010). Radiographic anatomy of the rabbit skull with particular reference to the tympanic bulla and temporomandibular joint: part 1: lateral and long axis rotational angles. *Vet. J.* 186: 232–243.

15 King, A.M., Cranfield, F., Hall, J. et al. (2010). Radiographic anatomy of the rabbit skull, with particular reference to the tympanic bulla and temporomandibular joint. Part 2: ventral and dorsal rotational angles. *Vet. J.* 186: 244–251.

16 King, A.M., Posthumus, J., Hammond, G. et al. (2012). Comparison of ultrasonography, radiography and a single computed tomography slice for the identification of fluid within the tympanic bulla of rabbit cadavers. *Vet. J.* 193: 493–497.

17 Onuma, M., Ono, S., Ishida, T. et al. (2010). Radiographic measurement of cardiac size in 27 rabbits. *J. Vet. Med. Sci.* 72: 529–531.

18 Brenner, S.Z., Hawkins, M.G., Tell, L.A. et al. (2005). Clinical anatomy, radiography, and computed tomography of the chinchilla skull. *Compendium* 27: 933–944.

19 Eshar, D., Briscoe, J.A., and Mai, W. (2013). Radiographic kidney measurements in North American pet ferrets (*Mustela furo*). *J. Small Anim. Pract.* 54: 15–19.

20 Proks, P., Stehlik, L., Paninarova, M. et al. (2015). Congenital abnormalities of the vertebral column in ferrets. *Vet. Radiol. Ultrasound* 56: 117–123.

21 Onuma, M., Kondo, H., Ono, S. et al. (2009). Radiographic measurement of cardiac size in 64 ferrets. *J. Vet. Med. Sci.* 71: 355–358.

22 Stepien, R.L., Benson, K.G., and Forrest, L.J. (1999). Radiographic measurement of cardiac size in normal ferrets. *Vet. Radiol. Ultrasound* 40: 606–610.

23 Dorotea, S.B., Banzato, T., Bellini, L. et al. (2016). Kidney measures in the domestic rat: a radiographic study and a comparison to ultrasonographic reference values. *J. Exot. Pet Med.* 25: 157–162.

24 Black, P.A., Marshall, C., Seyfried, A.W. et al. (2011). Cardiac assessment of African hedgehogs (*Atelerix albiventris*). *J. Zoo Wildl. Med.* 42: 49–53.

25 de Moura, C.R., das Neves Diniz, A., da Silva Moura, L. et al. (2015). Cardiothoracic ratio and vertebral heart scale in clinically normal Black-rumped agoutis (*Dasyprocta prymnolopha*, Wagler 1831). *J. Zoo Wildl. Med.* 46: 314–319.

26 Wagner, W.M. and Kirberger, R.M. (2005). Radiographic anatomy of the thorax and abdomen of the common marmoset (*Callithrix jacchus*). *Vet. Radiol. Ultrasound* 46: 217–224.

27 Redrobe, S. (2006). Ultrasound of exotic species. In: Diagnostic Ultrasound in Small Animal Practice (ed. P. Mannion), 301–331. Ames, IO: Blackwell Publishing.

28 King, A.M. (2006). Development, advances and applications of diagnostic ultrasound in animals. *Vet. J.* 171: 408–420.

29 Capello, V. and Lennox, A.M. (2011). Diagnostic imaging of the respiratory system in exotic companion mammals. *Vet. Clin. North Am. Exot. Anim. Pract.* 14: 369–389. vii.

30 Graham, J. and Basseches, J. (2014). Liver lobe torsion in pet rabbits: clinical consequences, diagnosis, and treatment. *Vet. Clin. North Am. Exot. Anim. Pract.* 17: 195–202.

31 Saito, K., Nakanishi, M., and Hasegawa, A. (2002). Uterine disorders diagnosed by ventrotomy in 47 rabbits. *J. Vet. Med. Sci.* 64: 495–497.

32 Bean, A.D. (2013). Ovarian cysts in the guinea pig (*Cavia porcellus*). *Vet. Clin. North Am. Exot. Anim. Pract.* 16: 757–776.

33 Zorn, S., Molnár, V., Bíró, F. et al. (2000). Ultrasonographic detection of abdominal abscess in two guinea pigs. *Acta Vet. Hung.* 48: 271–276.

34 Griffin, P.C., Bienen, L., Gillin, C.M. et al. (2003). Estimating pregnancy rates and litter size in snowshoe hares using ultrasound. *Wildl. Soc. Bull.*: 1066–1072.

35 Gaschen, L., Ketz, C., Lang, J. et al. (1998). Ultrasonographic detection of adrenal gland tumor and ureterolithiasis in a guinea pig. *Vet. Radiol. Ultrasound* 39: 43–46.

36 Eshar, D., Lee-Chow, B., and Chalmers, H.J. (2013). Ultrasound-guided percutaneous antegrade hydropropulsion to relieve ureteral obstruction in a pet guinea pig (*Cavia porcellus*). *Can. Vet. J.* 54: 1142–1145.

37 Chen, S. (2010). Advanced diagnostic approaches and current medical management of insulinomas and adrenocortical disease in ferrets (*Mustela putorius* furo). *Vet. Clin. North Am. Exot. Anim. Pract.* 13: 439–452.

38 Nwaokorie, E.E., Osborne, C.A., Lulich, J.P. et al. (2013). Epidemiological evaluation of cystine urolithiasis in domestic ferrets (*Mustela putorius* furo): 70 cases (1992–2009). *J. Am. Vet. Med. Assoc.* 242: 1099–1103.

39 Kuijten, A.M., Schoemaker, N.J., and Voorhout, G. (2007). Ultrasonographic visualization of the adrenal glands of healthy ferrets and ferrets with hyperadrenocorticism. *J. Am. Anim. Hosp. Assoc.* 43: 78–84.

40 Pilny, A.A. and Reavill, D. (2008). Chylothorax and thymic lymphoma in a pet rabbit (*Oryctolagus cuniculus*). *J. Exot. Pet Med.* 17: 295–299.

41 Levshin, S., Eshar, D., and Naor, A. (2016). Idiopathic chylothorax in a pet rabbit (*Oryctolagus cuniculus*). *Compan. Ani.* 21: 534–537.

42 Johnson, D.H. (2012). Emergency presentations of the exotic small mammalian herbivore trauma patient. *J. Exot. Pet Med.* 21: 300–315.

43 Andres, K.M., Kent, M., Siedlecki, C.T. et al. (2012). The use of megavoltage radiation therapy in the treatment of thymomas in rabbits: 19 cases. *Vet. Comp. Oncol.* 10: 82–94.

44 Wagner, F. and Fehr, M. (2007). Common ophthalmic problems in pet rabbits. *J. Exot. Pet Med.* 16: 158–167.

45 O'Reilly, A., McCowan, C., Hardman, C. et al. (2002). *Taenia serialis* causing exophthalmos in a pet rabbit. *Vet. Ophthalmol.* 5: 227–230.

46 Daniel, H.J., Means, L.W., Dressel, M.E. et al. (1973). Otitis media in laboratory rats. *Physiol. Psychol.* 1: 7–8.

47 Lennox, A. (2012). Respiratory disease and Pasteurellosis. In: Ferrets, Rabbits, and Rodents: Clinical Medicine and Surgery, 3e (eds. K. Quesenberry and J. Carpenter), 205–216. St. Louis, Mo: Elsevier/Saunders.

48 Dickie, A.M., Doust, R., Cromarty, L. et al. (2003). Comparison of ultrasonography, radiography and a single computed tomography slice for the identification of fluid within the canine tympanic bulla. *Res. Vet. Sci.* 75: 209–216.

49 King, A.M., Weinrauch, S.A., Doust, R. et al. (2007). Comparison of ultrasonography, radiography and a single computed tomography slice for fluid identification within the feline tympanic bulla. *Vet. J.* 173: 638–644.

50 Bernier Gosselin, V., Babkine, M., Gains, M.J. et al. (2014). Validation of an ultrasound imaging technique of the tympanic bullae for the diagnosis of otitis media in calves. *J. Vet. Intern. Med.* 28: 1594–1601.

51 King, A.M., Hall, J., Cranfield, F. et al. (2007). Anatomy and ultrasonographic appearance of the tympanic bulla and associated structures in the rabbit. *Vet. J.* 173: 512–521.

52 Robertson J, Sippel K, Breshears M, et al. 2016 Feasibility of ultrasonography for the assessment of the tympanic bullae and pituitary gland in cadaveric rats (*Rattus norvegicus*). *Exotics Con 2016 Main Conference Proceedings, Portland, August 27 – September 1 2016.* 655–656.

53 Banzato, T., Bellini, L., Contiero, B. et al. (2015). Abdominal ultrasound features and reference values in 21 healthy rabbits. *Vet. Rec.* 176: 101.

54 Banzato, T., Bellini, L., Contiero, B. et al. (2014). Abdominal anatomic features and reference values determined by use of ultrasonography in healthy common rats (*Rattus norvegicus*). *Am. J. Vet. Res.* 75: 67–76.

55 Beregi, A., Molnar, V., Zorn, S. et al. (2000). Abdominal ultrasonography in pet guinea pigs. *Acta Vet. Hung.* 48: 261–269.

56 Ferrari, M., da Silva, W.A.C., and Monteiro, R.V. (2013). Ultrasonographic features of the chinchilla (*Chinchilla lanigera*) kidney. *J. Exot. Pet Med.* 22: 393–395.

57 Chang Lanata P. Caracterización ecográfica del sistema excretor del erizo de tierra africano. *Facultad de Ciencias Veterinarias y Pecuaria Santiago*. Chile: Unversidad de Chile 2014:11.

58 Ribeiro, R.G., Costa, A.P., Bragato, N. et al. (2013). Normal sonographic anatomy of the abdomen of coatis (Nasua nasua Linnaeus 1766). *BMC Vet. Res.* 9: 124.

59 Beaufrere, H., Schilliger, L., and Pariaut, R. (2016). Cardiovascular system. In: Current Therapy in Exotic Pet Practice (eds. M. Mitchell and T.N. Tully), 151–220. St. Louis, MO: Elsevier Health Sciences.

60 Mackey, E.B., Hernandez-Divers, S.J., Holland, M. et al. (2008). Clinical technique: application of computed tomography in zoological medicine. *J. Exot. Pet Med.* 17: 198–209.

61 Van Caelenberg, A.I., De Rycke, L.M., Hermans, K. et al. (2010). Computed tomography and cross-sectional anatomy of the head in healthy rabbits. *Am. J. Vet. Res.* 71: 293–303.

62 Capello, V. and Cauduro, A. (2008). Clinical technique: application of computed tomography for diagnosis of dental disease in the rabbit, guinea pig, and chinchilla. *J. Exot. Pet Med.* 17: 93–101.

63 De Rycke, L.M., Boone, M.N., Van Caelenberg, A.I. et al. (2012). Micro-computed tomography of the head and dentition in cadavers of clinically normal rabbits. *Am. J. Vet. Res.* 73: 227–232.

64 Zotti, A., Banzato, T., and Cozzi, B. (2009). Cross-sectional anatomy of the rabbit neck and trunk: comparison of computed tomography and cadaver anatomy. *Res. Vet. Sci.* 87: 171–176.

65 Crossley, D., Jackson, A., Yates, J. et al. (1998). Use of computed tomography to investigate cheek tooth abnormalities in chinchillas (*Chinchilla laniger*). *J. Small Anim. Pract.* 39: 385–389.

66 Sasai, H., Iwai, H., Fujita, D. et al. (2014). The use of micro-computed tomography in the diagnosis of dental and oral disease in rabbits. *BMC Vet. Res.* 10: 1–8.

67 Souza, M.J., Greenacre, C.B., Avenell, J.S. et al. (2006). Diagnosing a tooth root abscess in a guinea pig (*Cavia porcellus*) using micro computed tomography imaging. *J. Exot. Pet Med.* 15: 274–277.

68 Clark, D.P. and Badea, C.T. (2014). Micro-CT of rodents: state-of-the-art and future perspectives. *Phys. Med.* 30: 619–634.

69 Van Caelenberg, A.I., De Rycke, L.M., Hermans, K. et al. (2011). Low-field magnetic resonance imaging and cross-sectional anatomy of the rabbit head. *Vet. J.* 188: 83–91.

70 Müllhaupt, D., Augsburger, H., Schwarz, A. et al. (2015). Magnetic resonance imaging anatomy of the rabbit brain at 3 T. *Acta Vet. Scand.* 57: 47.

71 Mitchell, E.B., Hawkins, M.G., Gaffney, P.M. et al. (2010). Gastric dilatation-volvulus in a guinea pig (*Cavia porcellus*). *J. Am. Anim. Hosp. Assoc.* 46: 174–180.

72 Nógrádi, A.L., Cope, I., Balogh, M. et al. (2017). Review of gastric torsion in eight guinea pigs (*Cavia porcellus*). *Acta Vet. Hung.* 65: 487–499.

73 Dudley, E.S. and Boivin, G.P. (2011). Gastric volvulus in guinea pigs: comparison with other species. *J. Am. Assoc. Lab. Anim. Sci.* 50: 526–530.

74 Gleeson, M., Chen, S., Fabiani, M. et al. (2019). Mesenteric root and cecal torsion in a domestic rabbit (*Oryctolagus cuniculus*). *J. Exot. Pet Med.* 28: 76–81.

75 Maksimović, A., Spahija, N., Čamo, D. et al. (2020). A unique case of spontaneous intestinal volvulus in a pet rabbit. *Veterinaria* 69: 65–68.

76 Hinton, J.D., Aitken-Palmer, C., Joyner, P.H. et al. (2016). Fatal gastric dilation in two adult black-footed ferrets (*Mustela nigripes*). *J. Zoo Wildl. Med.* 47: 367–369.

77 Geyer, N.E. and Reichle, J.K. (2012). What is your diagnosis? *J. Am. Vet. Med. Assoc.* 241: 45–47.

78 Perpiñán, D. and Ramis, A. (2011). Endogenous lipid pneumonia in a ferret (*Mustela putorius* furo). *J. Exot. Pet Med.* 20: 51–55.

79 Johnson-Delaney, C.A. and Orosz, S.E. (2011). Rabbit respiratory system: clinical anatomy, physiology and disease. *Vet. Clin. North Am. Exot. Anim. Pract.* 14: 257–266.

80 Johnson, D.H. (2011). Hedgehogs and sugar gliders: respiratory anatomy, physiology, and disease. *Vet. Clin. North Am. Exot. Anim. Pract.* 14: 267–285. vi.

81 Kling, M.A. (2011). A review of respiratory system anatomy, physiology, and disease in the mouse, rat, hamster, and gerbil. *Vet. Clin. North Am. Exot. Anim. Pract.* 14: 287–337. vi.

82 Yarto-Jaramillo, E. (2011). Respiratory system anatomy, physiology, and disease: guinea pigs and chinchillas. *Vet. Clin. North Am. Exot. Anim. Pract.* 14: 339–355. vi.

83 Graham, J.E. and Schoeb, T.R. (2011). *Mycoplasma pulmonis* in rats. *J. Exot. Pet Med.* 20: 270–276.

84 Darrow, B., Mans, C., Drees, R. et al. (2014). Pulmonary blastomycosis in a domestic ferret (*Mustela putorius* furo). *J. Exot. Pet Med.* 23: 158–164.

85 Eshar, D., Mayer, J., Parry, N.M. et al. (2010). Disseminated, histologically confirmed *Cryptococcus* spp. infection in a domestic ferret. *J. Am. Vet. Med. Assoc.* 236: 770–774.

86 Johnson-Delaney, C.A. and Orosz, S.E. (2011). Ferret respiratory system: clinical anatomy, physiology, and disease. *Vet. Clin. North Am. Exot. Anim. Pract.* 14: 357–367. vii.

87 Kunzel, F., Hittmair, K.M., Hassan, J. et al. (2012). Thymomas in rabbits: clinical evaluation, diagnosis, and treatment. *J. Am. Anim. Hosp. Assoc.* 48: 97–104.

88 Reuter, J.D., Fowles, K.J., Terwilliger, G.A. et al. (2005). Iatrogenic tension pneumothorax in a rabbit (*Oryctolagus cuniculus*). *Contemp. Top. Lab. Anim. Sci.* 44: 22–25.

89 Glassman, A., Ramachandran, A., Lyon, S. et al. (2020). Streptococcal toxic shock syndrome in a captive kinkajou (*Potos flavus*). *J. Exot. Pet Med.* 33.

90 Lisciandro, G.R. (2011). Abdominal and thoracic focused assessment with sonography for trauma, triage, and monitoring in small animals. *J. Vet. Emerg. Crit. Care (San Antonio)* 21: 104–122.

91 Crowe, D. (1984). Diagnostic abdominal parentesis techniques – clinical evaluation in 129 dogs and cats. *J. Am. Anim. Hosp. Assoc.* 20: 223–230.

11

Clinical Pathology

Carla Monteiro[1] and João Brandão[2]

[1] Exotic/Wild Life Consulting – Clínica Veterinária Atlântida, Porto, Portugal
[2] Department of Veterinary Clinical Sciences, College of Veterinary Medicine, Oklahoma State University, Oklahoma, USA

CONTENTS

Hematology

Complete Blood Cell Count

RBC Assessment

Like small animals, exotic mammals do not have nucleated red blood cells (RBCs), therefore, automated cell counters can be used. This is particularly useful in emergency conditions because results of the hematologic evaluation may be available more rapidly. Nevertheless, if no in-house hematology analyzer is available, blood smears are useful as well as other blood parameters (packed cell volume [PCV] and total solids [TS]). Although these methods are more time consuming, with practice, a quick assessment of the blood components can be readily performed (Table 11.1).

The blood volume of the rat is reported to vary from 5.0 to 7.1 ml per 100 g of body weight, and it is possible to collect approximately 5.5 ml/kg of blood during a single collection without risk [6]. The blood volume of the Syrian hamster varies between 65 and 80 ml per kilogram of body weight, and 1 ml can be safely collected during a single withdrawal [6]. Erythrocytes are relatively short-lived (45–68 days); therefore, the presence of a greater degree of polychromasia (1–18% in healthy rats and mice) and anisocytosis on a blood smear is expected [1]. The presence of a low number of Howell–Jolly bodies, basophilic stippling, and nucleated RBCs are also common in rodents [1].

In the adult guinea pig, the blood volume is approximately 69–75 ml per kilogram of body weight, and 8–10% of the blood volume can be safely collected in a single aspiration [6]. Polychromasia is commonly observed with higher rates (4.5%) in juveniles versus adults (1.5%) [1].

The estimated total blood volume in rabbits is approximately 57–78 ml/kg of body weight [3]. New Zealand white rabbits have been safely bled at rates of 6–8 ml/kg/wk [3]. Estimated life span is 50 days, therefore, polychromasia (2–5%) is also common (Figure 11.1) [3]. Poikilocytosis can be observed in rabbits. In one study, fragmentation and

Exotic Animal Emergency and Critical Care Medicine, First Edition. Edited by Jennifer E. Graham, Grayson A. Doss and Hugues Beaufrère.

Table 11.1 Selected hematological parameters in exotic mammals.

Blood parameter	Rat [1]	Mice [1]	Gerbils [1]	Hamster [1]	Guinea pig [1, 2]	Rabbit [1, 3]	Ferret [1, 4, 5]
Hematocrit (%)	38–51	35–52	35–50	36–55	37–50	33–35	Albino 42–61 Fitch 36–51
Hemoglobin (g/dl)	12–16	10–17	10–17	10–16	11.4–17.2	10–17.4	Albino 14.8–18.2 Fitch 12–17.4
Mean corpuscular volume (fl)	55–62	45–55	46–60	65–78	23.1–27.2	58–66.5	Fitch 42.6–51
Mean corpuscular hemoglobin concentration (g/dl)	30–34	30–38	30–33	28–37	28.2–38.9	29–37	Fitch 30.3–34.9
Red blood cell diameter (μm)	5–7	5–7	5–7	5–7	6.6–7.9	6.5–7.5	5.94 (males) and 6.32 (females)

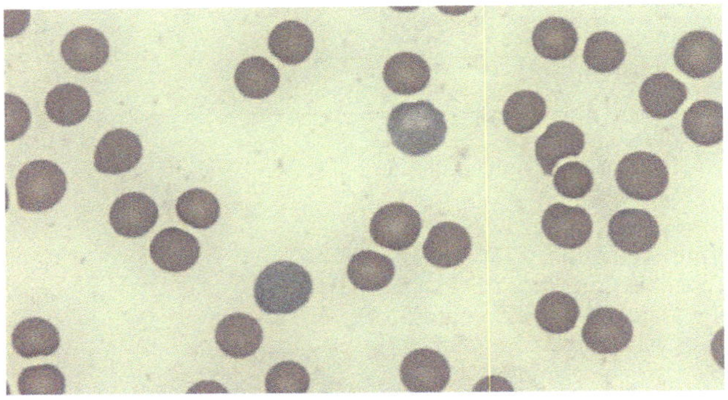

Figure 11.1 Normal red blood cells (Wright's stain) from a rabbit. Note the presence of polychromasia. *Source:* Images courtesy of Ian Kanda.

acanthocytosis were higher in rabbits with inflammatory disease and malignant neoplasia [7]. The percentage of fragmented cells correlated with percentage of polychromasia, RBC distribution width, and heterophil, monocyte, globulins, and fibrinogen concentrations [7]. Echinocytosis was significantly associated with renal failure, azotemia, and acid-base/electrolyte abnormalities [7].

The hematology of ferrets resembles that of domestic carnivores, one of the exceptions is the hematocrit values and total RBC counts, tending to be higher [1]. Under sevoflurane and isoflurane anesthesia, the ferret can experience a significant decrease in the PCV. Under isoflurane, a decrease of approximately 38 ± 9% has been observed, while sevoflurane caused 43 ± 12% decrease [4, 8]. In another study, PCV decreased by approximately 36%, with the maximum effects occurring at 15 minutes after induction, but returned to their original state 45 minutes after anesthesia [9].

Hematocrit and PCV are used to measure RBC mass. Although commonly used interchangeably, hematocrit is a calculated value produced by automated hematology analyzers while PCV is the value directly measured from centrifugated blood in a microhematocrit tube. PCV is an easy, fast, inexpensive, and accurate way to evaluate the fraction of the blood volume which is occupied by erythrocytes, expressed as a percentage or decimal fraction [10]. The increase in the PCV can be classified as relative or absolute [10]. A common cause of increased relative PCV is dehydration (by reducing the water in the plasma content, the fraction of PCV in the total volume is relativity increased), so, to improve the diagnostic value, a PCV increase must always be evaluated in correlation with TS [10]. Another cause of relative increase of PCV is splenic contraction [10]. Absolute increase of the PCV is a consequence of a genuine increase of the RBCs, polycythemia. It can be of primary origin – *polycythemia vera* – or secondary, like high altitude hypoxia, neoplasia, or another organ pathology [10, 11]. Polycythemia vera in a ferret has been reported once and the patient was managed with a combination of phlebotomy and hydroxyurea, and remained stable for 12 months at which time it died of acute venous infarction of the small and large intestine [12]. Polycythemia was also reported in a ferret with tetralogy of Fallot [13]. Most of the causes of PCV decrease are similar to other animals and may include hyperestrogenism (secondary to intact female ferrets, or neutered with ovarian remnant), hyperadrenocorticism, chronic inflammation, uterine adenocarcinoma, endometrial aneurysm, and lead toxicosis [1, 3, 14–16]. Rabbit PCV can be altered by external factors, e.g. environmental temperature. Rabbits kept for one to three hours at 28 °C (82 °F) showed elevated PCV [15] (Table 11.2).

WBC Assessment

A simple blood smear can give immediate information with a small drop of blood: white blood cell (WBC) count estimate and differential, WBC morphologic abnormalities or toxic changes, identification of hemoparasites, and platelet estimates. When estimating the WBC, the number of leukocytes per 40× objective from at least five fields is counted.

Table 11.2 Concomitant interpretation of hematocrit (HCT) and total plasma protein (TPP) concentration.

HCT	Low TPP	Normal TPP	High TPP
Normal	Gastrointestinal protein loss, proteinuria, severe liver disease, vasculitis	Normal	Increased globulin synthesis, dehydration-masked anemia
High	A combination of splenic contraction and a source of protein loss	Splenic contraction, primary or secondary erythrocytosis, dehydration-masked hypoproteinemia	Dehydration
Low	Substantial ongoing or recent blood loss, overhydration	Increased erythrocyte destruction, decreased erythrocyte production, chronic blood loss	Anemia of inflammatory disease, neoplasia (multiple myeloma), lymphoproliferative diseases

The average number is then multiplied by 1000 to estimate the total WBC [6]. In ferrets, the WBC tends to be lower compared to other domestic carnivores and it can be decreased under anesthesia with isoflurane [4]. Leukopenia is observed in cases of hyperestrogenism (in a later stage), hyperadrenocorticism, viral diseases (influenza, canine distemper virus), and some cases of lymphoma although leukocytosis is a more common presentation [5]. Leukocytosis is evident in initial cases of hyperestrogenism, lymphoma, and bacterial and parasitic infections [5]. Ferrets rarely develop a marked leukocytosis (concentrations greater than 20000/μl) with inflammatory disease, other than in cases of disseminated idiopathic myositis (DIM), and a left shift is rare [1].

Lymphocytes are the most common WBC in the rabbit peripheral blood smear. The second most common is the heterophil. Neutrophils in rabbits and many rodents are commonly called heterophils or pseudoeosinophils, because they contain small pink acidophilic granules in an almost colorless cytoplasm. The eosinophils are larger than the heterophils, making it possible to distinguish between both cells [17]. The percentage of basophils and eosinophils can vary between different rabbit breeds [3, 15]. In the rabbit, the WBC differential count is very important in the evaluation of the blood smear. Leukocytosis is not the common inflammatory response to an infectious disease, but a shift from lymphocyte-predominant to heterophil-predominant counts [15]. This alteration in the lymphocyte/heterophil ratio can also appear in stressful situations, that may persist for up to 48 hours [18]. Leukocytosis can be present in cases of lymphosarcoma [18] but also in situations of prolonged heat stress [15]. Leukopenia is often present in acute infections (with a normal differential count), chronic stress, or chronic infection [15]. In rodents, a variety of factors can influence total and differential WBC count, such as circadian rhythm, breed, and gender. Guinea pigs, chinchillas, mice, and rats are normally lymphocytic; therefore, early inflammation often reveals an increase in heterophils and decrease in lymphocytes with either a normal leukocyte count or leukopenia [1, 2, 19]. Guinea pigs have unique large mononuclear cells called Foa-Kurloff cells, that contain a single, large cytoplasmic inclusion, and are referred to as the Kurloff body (Figure 11.2). The exact function of these cells is not known, but many speculate they might function as killer cells. Apparently influenced by sex hormones, and appear in reduced number in immature male guinea pigs [1] (Table 11.3).

Platelet Assessment (Thrombocytes)

Platelets are defined as cytoplasmic fragments that arise from megakaryocytes within the bone marrow and participate in hemostasis [3]. Mammalian platelets originate from the bone marrow and are involved in hemostasis. Normal platelets are smaller than RBC and are shaped like flat disks. They tend to be round but can vary slightly in shape and size. Guinea pig platelets appear as 2–3 mm irregular oval cytoplasmic fragments with concentric dark inner and lighter outer staining regions [2]. Large platelets, the so-called macroplatelets or shift platelets, can present and

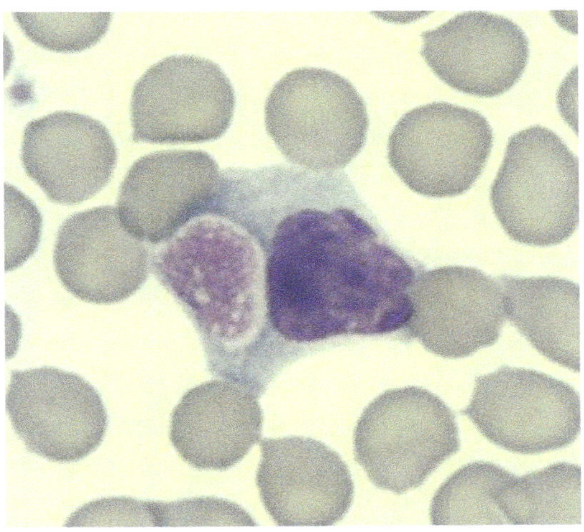

Figure 11.2 Kurloff body in a guinea pig lymphocyte (Wright's stain). *Source:* Image courtesy of Ian Kanda.

Table 11.3 General and some species-specific characteristics of leukocytes.

Cell type	General characteristics	Species-specific characteristics
Heterophils/ Neutrophils	• Contain numerous small granules that vary from colorless to pale-staining to dark-staining	
Eosinophils	• Large cytoplasmic granules become increasingly eosinophilic in color as the cell matures	• Trapezoidal pattern in guinea pig and other rodents • Needle-shaped pattern in rabbits
Basophils	• Species-specific variations in the color and ultrastructural appearance of the granules	• Guinea pig often stain reddish-purple to black • Rabbit have granules with coiled threaded pattern • Other rodents have a homogeneous pattern
Monocytes	• Generally, the largest leukocytes in peripheral blood • Do not vary grossly in appearance with species	
Lymphocytes	• Varies depending upon the species, lymphocyte type, and degree of activation, varying in size, color of cytoplasm (light to dark blue), and degree of nuclear chromatin condensation	

For additional species-specific information see Figures 11.3–11.6.

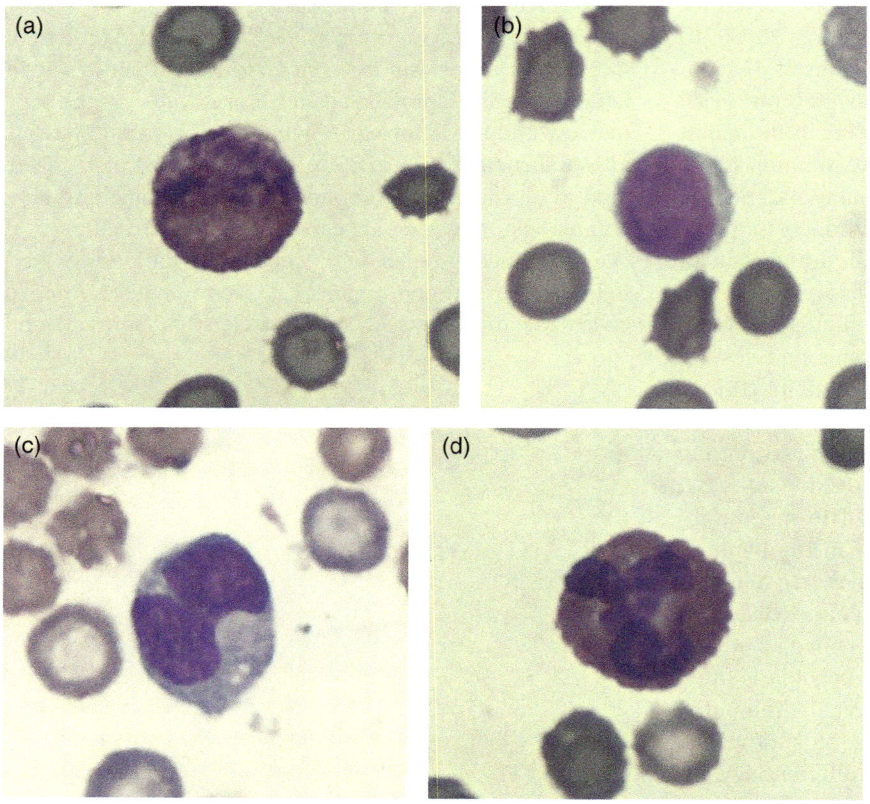

Figure 11.3 Normal white blood cells from rabbits. (a) neutrophil (Diff Quick stain); (b) lymphocyte (Diff Quick stain); (c) monocyte (Diff Quick stain); (d) eosinophil (Diff Quick stain). *Source:* Images courtesy of Ian Kanda.

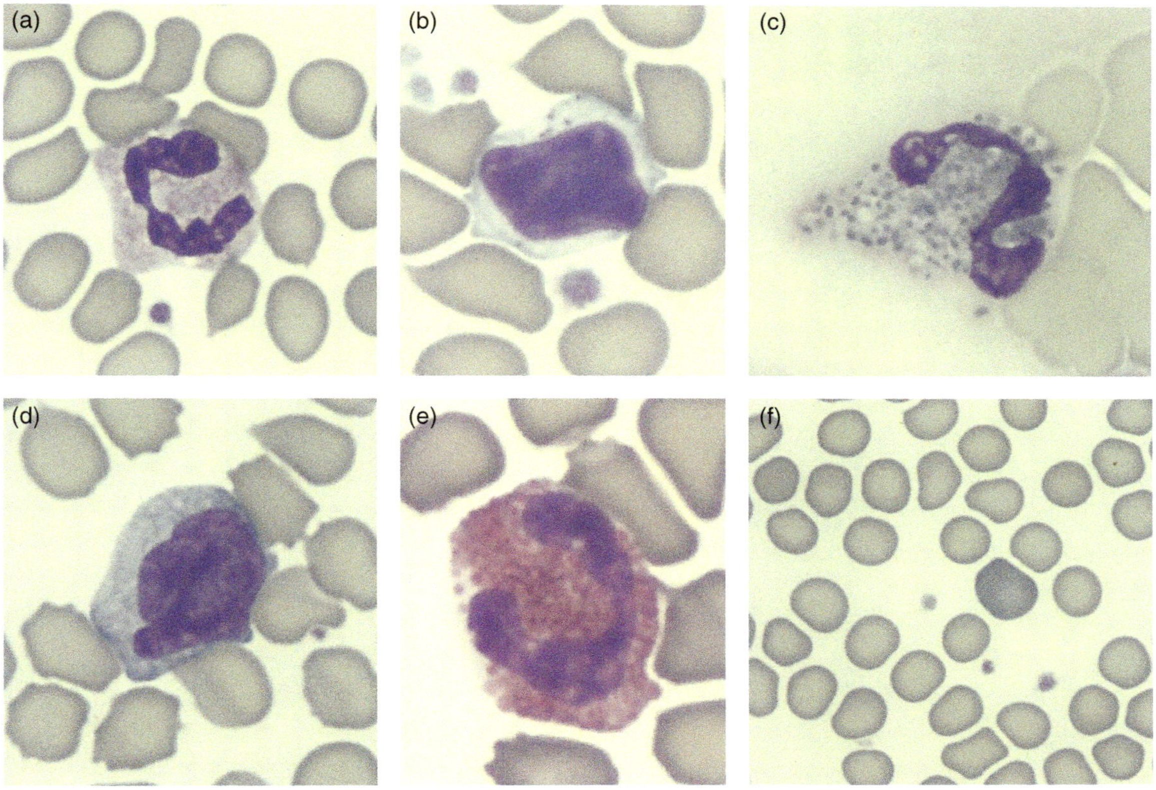

Figure 11.4 Normal blood cells from guinea pigs: (a) heterophil (Wright's stain); (b) lymphocyte (Wrights stain); (c) basophil (Wright's stain); (d) monocyte (Wright's stain); (e) eosinophil (Diff Quick stain); (f) red blood cells with polychromasia (Wright's stain). *Source:* Images courtesy of Ian Kanda.

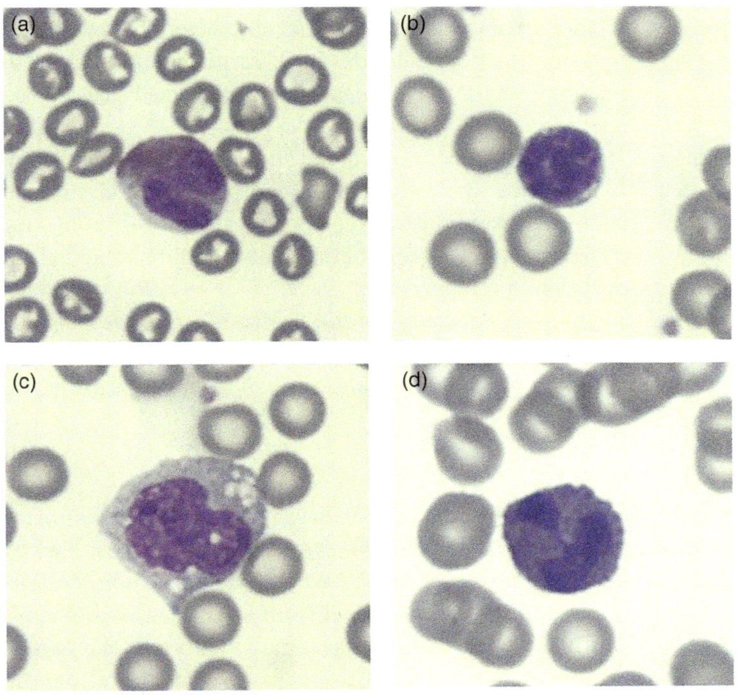

Figure 11.5 Normal white blood cells from chinchillas: (a) heterophil (Wright's stain); (b) lymphocyte (Wright's stain); (c) monocyte (Wright's stain); (d) eosinophil (Wright's stain). *Source:* From Fisher [20]. © 2006, Elsevier.

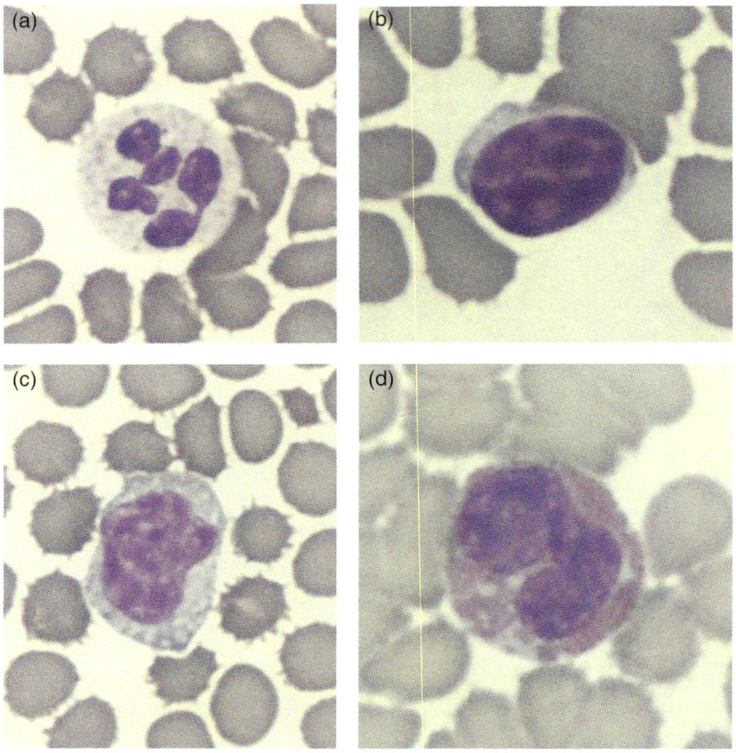

Figure 11.6 Normal white blood cells from ferrets: (a) neutrophil (Diff Quick stain); (b) lymphocyte (Diff Quick stain); (c) monocyte (Diff Quick stain); (d) eosinophil (Wright's stain). *Source:* Images courtesy of Ian Kanda.

their presence may be suggestive of accelerated thrombocytopoiesis with an early release of immature forms into the circulating blood [1]. It is common to have clumps of platelets on the blood smear and this can decrease the overall number of platelets on the slide.

To estimate the platelet count from a blood film, obtain the average number of platelets in ten 100× (oil-immersion) fields and multiply that number by 15000 resulting in a platelet count/μl. It is possible also to assess whether or not there is an adequate number of platelets on a blood film by obtaining the average number of platelets per oil-immersion field; there should be at least five platelets per oil-immersion field, to consider the number of platelets is adequate [1]. Normal platelet concentrations for most mammals are greater than 100000/ml of blood, although higher platelet concentration in rodents is common [1]. A total platelet count decrease can occur in hibernating hamsters [1]. The occurrence of increase in the total platelet count (>1000000/μl), without changes in total WBC, is considered to be an important marker of inflammation in guinea pigs as well as other small mammals [1].

Blood Smear

With the advent of automated analyzers, hematology in mammalian species is not commonly performed solely on blood smear estimates. Nevertheless, blood smears are of great help to the clinician. This is a fast and inexpensive method that complements the automated hematological results. Also, if an automated analyzer is not available, estimation from the blood smear can be performed as described above.

The major benefit of a blood smear interpretation is that it allows the assessment of the morphology of circulating cells. Furthermore, it can also allow the clinician/technician to identify structures that should not be present in the circulating blood.

Anemia is caused by loss, destruction, or lack of production of RBCs. In cases of anemia, blood smear assessment will provide information regarding the regenerative response of the body or lack thereof. If hematopoiesis is increased, it is likely that there will be a higher rate of polychromasia. As stated above, because exotic mammal erythrocytes have a shorter lifespan than dog and cat erythrocytes, it is common to have an increased rate of polychromasia, independent of a regenerative response. If an anemic animal has no significant polychromasia, it may mean that the regeneration has not started to occur, or that there may be an abnormality with the bone marrow. In the latter case, bone marrow aspirates may be indicated.

Interpretation of regeneration should be complemented with the hematology results. Macrocytosis usually correlates with a regenerative anemia. Most regenerative anemias have an increased MCV and a decreased MCHC. Hypochromasia is determined by the presence of pale-staining erythrocytes with an increased area of central pallor [1]. Hypochromatic erythrocytes are suggestive of iron deficiency [1]. In adults, hypochromatic erythrocytes are a consequence of pathologies like parasitosis, gastrointestinal ulcers, inflammatory bowel disease, or neoplasms (chronic blood loss), while in juveniles is usually diet-related (e.g. reduce iron intake) [1].

In cases of severe inflammation or infection, it is common to find indications in the WBC evaluating the blood smear. A term that is commonly used is "left shift." "Left shift" indicates that there is a high number of young, immature WBCs in circulation. It is said that in ferrets, a left shift is rare [1]. Toxic changes of the WBC are related to changes in granulocyte cells (Figure 11.7). These changes are commonly found in patients with sepsis. Toxic granulations are dark coarse granules found in granulocytes, particularly neutrophils or heterophils.

Although uncommon, it is occasionally possible to see bacteria in the circulating blood cells (Figure 11.8). This is highly suggestive of severe bacteremia and the prognosis in these cases is poor. Blood culture should be performed and the patient should receive intensive care, including intravenous antibiotics.

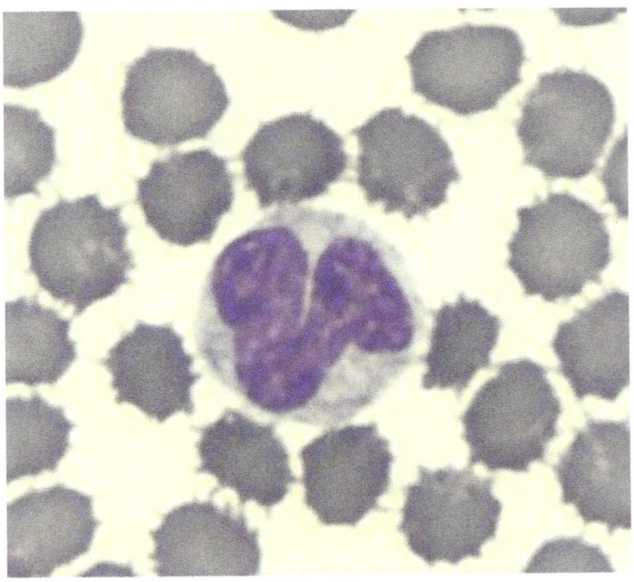

Figure 11.7 Band neutrophil in a ferret (Diff Quick stain). *Source:* Image courtesy of Ian Kanda.

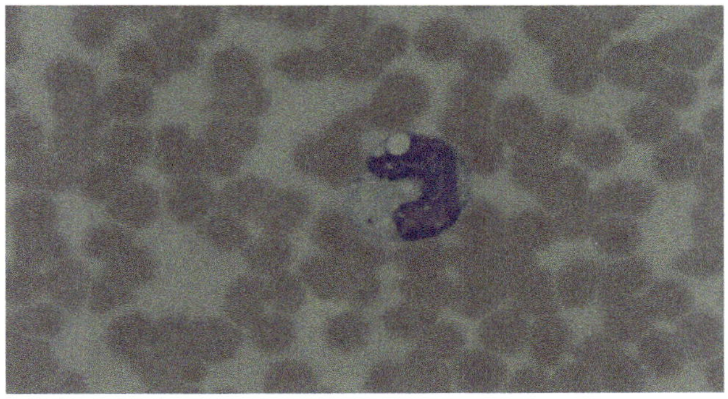

Figure 11.8 Bacteria in a circulating neutrophil from a kinkajou (*Potos flavus*).

Biochemical Evaluation

Protein Characterization

Total Protein, Albumin, Globulin

It is common to use the term total protein and TS interchangeably; however, TS are measured with a refractometer which measures the refractive index. This can be used as an estimate for total protein (which are the constituents of plasma that have the most effect on the refractive index). This assessment is done on plasma (which contains fibrinogen), so values are usually higher than that seen on chemistry panels run on serum (which lacks fibrinogen). This is a simple intuitive method that allows the estimation of the concentration of TS that has a constant correlation with total protein in the plasma [21]. The gold standard for the quantification of protein and its portions is protein electrophoresis.

Plasma appearance is related to color and transparency. The normal plasma should be clear and colorless to light yellow, depending on the carotenoid pigment and bilirubin concentrations [22]. An increase in yellow coloration may be associated with increased bilirubin concentration (fasting, liver failure), while red discoloration is associated with hemoglobinemia (intravascular hemolysis or inappropriate collection techniques, and prolonged storage). White opaque plasma (lipemia) may be associated with a recent meal (postprandial lipemia), pregnancy, lactation, metabolic, or systemic diseases (anorexia, hyperadrenocorticism, diabetes mellitus, pancreatitis, cholestasis, hepatic lipidosis) [22].

Plasma total protein includes albumin and globulins. The liver is the sole site of albumin synthesis and hypoalbuminemia is a hallmark of advanced liver disease in all species [23]. In rabbits, hypoalbuminemia is most likely to be associated with nutritional factors such as inadequate cecotrophy, inappropriate diet, starvation or malnutrition associated with dental disease, primary or secondary hepatic neoplasia, and hepatic coccidiosis [23]. A hyperalbuminemia is not an indication of any specific disease, although an increased albumin level in conjunction with a raised PCV is indicative of dehydration [23]. Ferrets with cystic renal disorders had hypoalbuminemia, presumably the result of enhanced renal loss or inappetance [5]. Hypoalbuminemia also occurs in ferrets with excessive dietary iron, Aleutian disease, epizootic catarrhal enteritis, hepatic coccidiosis, and *Cryptococcus* sp. [5] Plasma globulins are made up of a range of proteins including carrier proteins and immunoglobulins or antibodies. The types of globulin can be separated into fractions by electrophoresis. The globulin fraction is made up of α1, α2, β, and γ globulins. Protein electrophoresis can be used to assess the presence of inflammatory conditions in rabbits [24]. Infection is often reflected as a decrease in the A/G ratio attributable to increases in concentrations of globulins, including the γ-globulin fraction that contains IgG [24]. Rabbits suspected of having an *Encephalitozoon cuniculi* infection or other clinical abnormalities had a higher concentration of γ-globulins and decreased A/G ratio when compared to clinically normal rabbits [24].

Fibrinogen (Species-specific)

Fibrinogen is a large protein synthesized by the liver that constitutes about 5% of the total plasma protein, and its concentration can be estimated from the difference in protein content before and after heat treatment of plasma [25, 26]. Fibrinogen is included in the beta portion of globulins, which consists of several proteins classified as "acute-phase" proteins [18]. Fibrinogen is more consistently increased during inflammation in horses and cattle than it is in dogs and cats [25].

In addition, fibrinogen (factor I) is a major component of blood clots [26]. Fibrinogen is the final substrate in the coagulation cascade as it is converted to fibrin by thrombin [5]. Low plasma fibrinogen concentrations are therefore associated with an increased risk of bleeding due to impaired primary and secondary hemostasis [27]. It also plays an important role in platelet aggregation by linking activated platelets [26].

Overall, there are limited reports of the use of fibrinogen for the health assessment of exotic mammals, both in terms of inflammation or coagulopathies. It is said that fibrinogen correlates with inflammation in rabbits, although the correlation is not as evident as in other species [18]. Experimental infection of rabbits with *Escherichia coli* and *Staphylococcus aureus* induced increased fibrinogen levels [28, 29]. It is said that the fibrinogen level in ferret plasma is two times higher than that in rats [30]; however, other studies do not seem to support this finding (Table 11.4). Nevertheless, fibrinogen in ferrets can be elevated due to infectious and other inflammatory diseases, pregnancy, and myeloproliferative disorder [5].

Table 11.4 Normal values of fibrinogen.

Species	Fibrinogen (mg/dl)	References
Rabbit	Male 318.8 ± 48.5^a and 258.7 ± 28.7^b Female 288.2 ± 31.6^a and 238.6 ± 13.6^b	[26]
Rat	Male 239.9 ± 32.8^a and 190.3 ± 15.2^b Female 199.6 ± 26.5^a and 158.2 ± 10.3^b	[26]
Ferret	107.4 ± 19.8^c	[31]
Prairie dogs	$224–626^d$	[32]

[a] Prothrombin-time–derived fibrinogen assay.
[b] Clauss assay.
[c] Turbidimetric method.
[d] STA Compact USB hemostasis analyzer.

Renal Values

BUN, CREA

Blood urea nitrogen (BUN) and creatinine are commonly used to assess renal function in mammals. Urea is the main end product of protein catabolism in the liver of mammals [33]. Urea is passively reabsorbed by carrier-mediated diffusion in the distal convoluted tubule, which also contributes to the concentration gradient, and electrolytes are continually reabsorbed in the distal convoluted tubule as well [34]. Urea reabsorption accounts for approximately 25–40% of the filtered urea [35]. The BUN concentration is inversely proportional to the GFR, but it is not produced and excreted at a constant rate [35]. Serum levels are influenced by protein levels in the diet, liver function, intestinal absorption of nitrogen, and the state of hydration [35]. Rabbit BUN has a diurnal fluctuation, peaking in the late afternoon and early evening, which is thought to be correlated to the ingestion of cecotrophs [33, 36]. Laboratory rodent diet protein levels may vary from 12% to 24%, resulting in significant changes in BUN in healthy animals [37]. A decrease in BUN may be caused by anabolic steroids, diminished protein intake, and severe hepatic insufficiency [33]. Elevated BUN can be used to quantify levels of dehydration or decreased renal excretion, possibly due to renal dysfunction in mammalian patients [34]. Renal increase of BUN results from loss of 50–70% nephrons [33]. Because the BUN may be influenced by nonrenal factors, creatinine generally serves as a better indicator of renal function [20].

Creatinine is formed in the metabolism of muscle creatinine and phosphocreatine, and is less affected by external factors than BUN [33]. In rodents, creatinine values are affected by many drugs and compounds, including barbiturates, glucose, protein, acetone, ketones, ascorbic acid, and

Table 11.5 Normal serum chemistry values frequently associated with renal disease [20].

Species	Blood urea nitrogen (mg/dl)	Creatinine (mg/dl)	Phosphorus (mg/dl)	Total calcium (mg/dl)
Ferret	10–45	0.4–0.9	4.0–9.1	8.0–11.8
Rabbit	13–29	0.5–2.5	0.5–2.5	5.6–12.5
Guinea pig	9.0–31.5	0.6–2.2	3.0–7.6	8.2–12.0
Hedgehog	13–54	0.4–0.8	2.4–12.0	5.2–11.3
Mouse	27.5–34.7	0.74–1.01	10.4–13.8	10.7–12.4
Rat	15–21	0.2–0.8	5.3–8.3	5.3–13.0
Hamster	12–25	0.91–0.99	3.4–8.2	5–12
Gerbil	17–27	0.6–1.4	3.7–6.2	3.7–6.1

sulfo-bromophthalein [37]. Creatinine is freely filtered through the glomerulus and excreted in the urine [33]. Creatinine levels may be increased by severe renal insufficiency or severe muscle damage; however, levels are increased only in cases where greater than 50% to 70% of nephrons are lost [33].

Azotemia is an increase in serum BUN or creatinine due to decreased GFR. Azotemia can be defined as prerenal, renal, or postrenal in origin, however, urine specific gravity is essential to clinically differentiate among these three conditions [33]. Prerenal azotemia occurs when there is decreased renal perfusion, high protein diet, and gastrointestinal hemorrhage [36]. Primary or renal azotemia results from renal parenchymal and glomerular damage; the urine specific gravity is elevated [20, 33]. Isosthenuric urine or inadequately concentrated urine along with azotemia is highly suggestive of renal disease [33]. Postrenal azotemia occurs with urinary tract obstruction, most commonly due to calculi, and in these cases, the urine specific gravity may vary [20].

Renal pathology is not uncommon in the ferret and rabbit. In one retrospective study in ferrets, the most prevalent causes of renal pathology included acute nephritis (22%), renal cysts (15%), glomerulonephritis (14%), pyelonephritis (6%), glomerulosclerosis (4%), congestion (4%), and tubular atrophy (4%) [38]. Normal creatinine levels in ferrets are considerably lower than in other mammals and have a narrower range, therefore, any increase in serum creatinine above normal should be considered significant in the ferret [20]. Elevations in the concentration of BUN associated with renal failure are not always accompanied by increases in the concentration of serum creatinine above the normal range [20]. Renal disease in rabbits was reported in 32.5% of 237 rabbits found dead or euthanized because of illness and in 25% of 77 apparently healthy adults [38]. The rabbit has a limited capacity to concentrate urea; therefore, dehydration may readily result in elevated prerenal values of BUN and creatinine [20] Table 11.5.

Electrolytes

Na/Cl, K, Ca/Phos

Electrolytes are substances that exist as positive or negative charged particles in aqueous solution [25]. Sodium is the predominant cation in the body and responsible for the largest proportion of molecules and compounds determining osmolarity [14]. Hypernatremia is often seen in cases of severe water deprivation (water bottle out of reach or neurologic signs preventing access) [14]. True hyponatremia in rabbits was reported in 34% of the samples while the remaining were pseudohyponatremic [39]. Significantly higher mortality seemed to be associated with sodium levels less than 129 mEq/l. [39] Pseudohyponatremia in rabbits can be related to a high glucose value or a sodium level decrease in response to high glucose level (related to fluid shift and dilution of the sodium) [14]. Hypernatremia is less common than hyponatremia [39]. Extrarenal hypotonic water loss with resulting hypernatremia can also be associated with diarrhea, intestinal obstruction, cutaneous loss, or peritonitis [14].

Chloride is the principal anion in the extracellular fluid and is the second main contributor to plasma tonicity [40]. Chloride levels in rabbits are lower than other small mammal normal ranges, and hypochloremia is not associated with an increase in HCO_3 [14]. It was postulated that the alkalinizing effect of hypochloremia is less pronounced in rabbits [14].

Potassium is largely an intracellular ion with over 98% of the exchangeable potassium located intracellularly [25]. Potassium distribution across the cell membrane plays a critical role in the maintenance of cardiac and neuromuscular excitability [25]. Major hyperkalemia can be seen with sampling artifact (hemolysis, clotting, and improper sampling technique such as inappropriate anticoagulant) or when needles smaller than 23 gauge are used for venipuncture [14]. True hyperkalemia can be seen in cases of oliguric or anuric acute kidney injury, urinary obstruction, or severe tissue necrosis or trauma [14]. Hypokalemia is seen in cases of dysorexia, loss of digestive fluid, renal failure, and stress-induced alkalosis [14]. Persistent hypokalemia has been reported in a ferret with hyperaldosteronism [41].

In an emergency setting, electrolytes are commonly assessed using point-of-care units like the i-STAT analyzer (Abbot Point of Care Inc., Abbott Park, IL). Normal reference values for electrolytes have been reported in several species of exotic mammals [5, 39, 42–44].

Calcium is the fifth most abundant element in the body and an essential supplement in that it can only be acquired through dietary sources, while phosphorus is a structural component of nucleotide coenzymes [45]. Serum calcium, magnesium, and phosphate levels are closely regulated by the combined effects of several hormones (e.g. PTH, vitamin D, calcitonin, cortisol) on the gastrointestinal tract, bone, and kidneys [45]. Two forms of calcium are present in the body; total calcium (protein-bound) and ionized calcium. Although ionized calcium only exists in minute quantities, it is in constant and rapid exchange between extra- and intracellular pools and responsible for a wide number of vital functions that include extra- and intracellular signaling, nerve impulse transmission, and muscle contraction [45]. Hypercalcemia commonly occurs due to neoplasia, chronic renal failure, and impaired calcium excretion, or calcium-rich diets (mainly rabbits and guinea pigs). Hypocalcemia usually occurs due to increase demand associated with pregnancy. As total calcium is protein-bound, hypoalbuminemia might result in an artifactually low calcium level. Hyperphosphatemia can develop in animals fed phosphorus-rich diets, renal failure, bladder rupture, hypervitaminosis D, hypoparathyroidism, bone neoplasia, and trauma or muscle necrosis. Hypophosphatemia is usually secondary to malabsorption, hypovitaminosis D, and primary hyperparathyroidism and pseudohyperparathyroidism Tables 11.6 and 11.7.

Table 11.6 Information on origin and relevance, and potential causes for elevation of alanine aminotransferase, aspartate aminotransferase, lactate dehydrogenase, and creatine kinase.

	Origin and relevance	Elevation
Alanine aminotransferase (ALT)	• Primarily located in hepatocyte cytoplasm which leaks into the blood when hepatocyte cell membrane injury occurs • Lower concentrations in the erythrocytes and skeletal muscle • Highly liver-specific in ferrets but not in rabbits and guinea pigs	• Active hepatocellular damage (end-stage liver disease does not typically cause an increase) • Hepatic coccidiosis (rabbits) • Gastrointestinal disease with associated mild liver inflammation or bacterial infection • Occasionally elevated with adrenal gland disease, influenza (ferrets) • Fever • Myocarditis • High protein diet (rats) • Sample lipemia and hemolysis
Aspartate aminotransferase (AST)	• Found in a wide variety of tissues but has high concentrations in skeletal muscle, cardiac muscle, red blood cells, and liver • AST increase alone is not pathognomonic of damage to a particular organ or tissue • Longer-acting than CK	• Sample hemolysis • Muscle damage (seizures, trauma, exertional rhabdomyolysis, intramuscular damage) • Hepatic damage (drug-induced, endocrinopathies, hypoxia, severe lipidosis, inflammation/infection, toxicity, neoplasia) • Sample lipemia and hemolysis
Lactate dehydrogenase (LDH)	• Enzyme that catalyzes the interconversion of pyruvate and lactate • LDH is found in most cells in the body and is not organ-specific	• Myocardial disease • Hemolysis • Handling
Creatine kinase (CK)	• 3 isozymes (skeletal muscle, cardiac muscle, brain) • Specific for muscle cell damage • Relatively short half-life (<72 hr)	• Skeletal muscle damage • Myocardial disease and myositis • Hyperthermia • Hypothermia • Vitamin E/selenium deficiency • Trauma • Surgical • Ischemia • Sample hemolysis and hyperbilirubinemia

Table 11.7 Information on origin and relevance, and potential causes for elevation and decrease for alkaline phosphatase, γ-glutamyl transferase, and total bilirubin.

	Origin and relevance	Elevation	Decrease
Alkaline phosphatase (ALKP)	• Membrane-associated enzymes found in most tissues of the body that hydrolyze monophosphates at an alkaline pH • Numerous isoenzymes present in the blood; most mammals have 2 ALKP encoding genes: one intestinal, and another hepatic, renal, osseous • Limited specificity for hepatobiliary disease in most animals	• Osteogenesis in young growing animals • Hepatic necrosis or hepatocyte swelling (biliary stasis)	• No significant causes • Low levels can be seen with diarrhea and pregnancy
Gamma-glutamyl transferase (GGT)	• Catalyzes the transfer of the gammaglutamyl group from a donor peptide to an acceptor compound • Biliary system is the primary source of plasma GGT • In rabbit is found primarily in the bile duct of the epithelium and therefore is more diagnostic for hepatobiliary disease than for hepatocellular damage	• Cholestatic disorders • Biliary obstruction or damage (neoplasia, inflammation, cholelithiasis, and intra- and extra-hepatic cholestasis) • Sample lipemia and heparin	• Sample hemolysis
Total bilirubin (TBil)	• Breakdown product of heme, derived primarily from senescent erythrocytes • Carried by albumin to the liver, where it is detoxified by the glucuronic acid pathway, conjugated, and excreted into the bile • Rabbits produce biliverdin, but bilirubin occurs at measurable levels • Rabbit produces significantly more bile than a dog of equal size, but rabbits have low activity of biliverdin reductase, and only about 30% is converted	• Prehepatic is usually caused by hemolytic crisis • Hepatic is usually caused by hepatic disease and intrahepatic cholestatic disease • Post-hepatic is usually caused by bile duct obstruction • Sample hemolysis or lipemia	• Sample hemolysis • Light exposure

Liver/Muscle Enzymes

ALT, AST, LDH, CK: See Table 11.6

ALKP, GGT, TBIL: See Table 11.7

Bile Acids

Bile acids are synthesized in the liver from cholesterol and secreted via the bile. Bile acids assist with the digestion and absorption of fat and fat-soluble vitamins. Intestinal bacteria further modify bile acids. Bile acids are secreted via the bile duct into the small intestine and emulsify ingested fats to be solubilized for digestion and absorption. Fasting samples in most species should be less than 15 mmol/l. Increase bile acid concentration is usually associated with portosystemic shunts, liver failure, and cholestasis. Decreased bile acids usually are attributable to delayed gastric emptying or an ileal abnormality, acute/early liver disease, liver cirrhosis, microhepatia, and fasting [46, 47].

Cholesterol/Triglyceride

Cholesterol is either absorbed from the diet or is synthesized by the liver. The liver breaks down cholesterol and excretes it in bile. Elevated cholesterol levels are indicative of a variety of metabolic disorders such as hypothyroidism, hepatopathy, diabetes mellitus, and hyperadrenocorticism. Impaired hepatic function can lead to decreased values. Changes in serum triglyceride levels reflect a similar range of diseases. Blood levels of triglycerides increase after a meal, especially if it is a fatty meal [18].

Male rabbits have lower cholesterol levels than females and there is a diurnal variation, with higher levels occurring during the late afternoon [23]. Increase triglycerides have occurred in induced chronic renal failure in rabbits [23]. One study has shown that rabbits with hyperlipidemia is associated with markers of inflammation, severe infection/sepsis, renal failure, and hepatopathy [48]. Increased cholesterol (non-high-density lipoprotein cholesterol) and triglycerides may be indicators of disease, independent of the diet [48].

Glucose

Blood glucose concentration is important to evaluate and might provide prognostic information in several clinical conditions in small mammals. Hypoglycemia is very common in middle-aged to older ferrets with endocrine pancreatic neoplasia (insulinoma) [9, 49] with values below 60–70 mg/dl being strongly suggestive. Hypoglycemic ferrets usually present on emergency with severe lethargy or hypoglycemic seizures [16]. Other causes of hypoglycemia in ferrets include sepsis, liver disease, or prolonged food deprivation. Diabetes mellitus can occur in ferrets, mainly associated with pancreatectomy, but is commonly transient and normalizes the first few weeks after surgery [50]. Glucose metabolism in rabbits and rodents differs from carnivores [18]. Blood sugar levels can vary daily due to the circadian rhythm in rodent species, and seasonally (associated with estivation and hibernation in hamsters) [51]. Causes of hyperglycemia in rabbits and rodents include acute intestinal obstruction, early mucoid enteropathy, hepatic lipidosis, hypovolemic shock, hyperthermia, exogenous glucocorticoids, halothane, and xylazine [51, 52]. Naturally occurring diabetes mellitus has been reported in laboratory rabbits but not in pet rabbits [14, 53]. In rabbits, one study suggested that blood glucose may be a helpful indicator in differentiating GI stasis from GI obstruction (normal or decreased glucose can be seen with the former whereas hyperglycemia can be seen in the latter) [54]. Nevertheless, hyperglycemia may be caused by other conditions. Hyperglycemia in clinical practice is often associated with stress, not only in rabbits but also rodents (handling, transport, presence of other animals) [51].

Diabetes mellitus has been described in many rodent species (laboratory colony and pet guinea pigs [55, 56], Chinese hamsters [51], and gerbils [52]). In chinchillas, it has been reported in cases of anorexia and hepatic lipidosis, but is a rare finding [57]. Hypoglycemia is a common finding in most rodents after small periods of pre-surgical fasting [58].

Hypoglycemia is a common emergency finding in sugar gliders, with neurologic signs (seizures) [59]. In the rabbit, it has been reported in cases of severe starvation or sepsis, traumatic conditions, hyperthermia, chronic diseases, and liver failure [14, 18]. It is also associated with pregnancy ketosis in rabbits and guinea pigs [51, 60].

Blood glucose is important to evaluate in several clinical conditions in small mammals. For this reason, the accuracy of different devices (portable glucometers [PBGM] for human and veterinary medicine, and benchtop analyzers) have been evaluated and compared. The use of PBGM has been evaluated for ferrets, rabbits, and prairie dogs. Most of the PBGM for human use underestimate blood glucose in ferrets with a specificity of 50% (meaning half are falsely hypoglycemic, being in fact normoglycemic) [16]. PBGM intended for veterinary use provided results that are more in agreement with laboratory analyzers, presenting a negligible mean difference [16], with the PBGM coded for canine blood more accurate with better agreement [61, 62]. In one study in rabbits, the hexokinase method revealed good accuracy and was not influenced by hematocrit [63]. The use of human PBGM also underestimates blood glucose, but on the basis of the modified error grid analysis, it was acceptable for clinical use in rabbits [63]. The canine and feline settings of the veterinary PBGM did not provide clinically acceptable results in rabbits [63]. In black-tailed prairie dogs, results from human and veterinary PBGM did not provide consistently accurate blood glucose concentrations when compared with values determined with a biochemistry analyzer [64].

Amylase/Lipase

Amylase is an enzyme that catalyzes the hydrolysis of complex carbohydrates in the gastrointestinal tract [65]. Amylase is found in the pancreas and to a lesser extent in the salivary glands, liver, and small intestinal mucosa [23]. In rabbits, amylase is also produced by cecal micro-organisms and is present in cecotrophs, aiding conversion of glucose to lactic acid during digestion in the stomach and small intestine [23]. Amylase has a short half-life, is rapidly removed from the circulation, and is excreted by the kidney [23]. Elevation of amylase can be caused by pancreatic duct obstruction, pancreatic disease/neoplasia/necrosis, renal insufficiency (decreased glomerular filtration), intestinal obstruction, enteritis, zinc toxicity, hepatic disease, or diabetic ketoacidosis [65]. Low values can be related with exocrine pancreatic insufficiency and hepatoxicity [65].

Serum amylase levels are lower in rabbits than in other species [23]. Rabbits have little amylase in their salivary glands and intestines, and none is produced by the rabbit liver [35]. The salivary glands of rats and mice have amylase activity nearly as high as that seen in the pancreas [65]. It is likely that, like dogs, ferrets produce significant levels of amylase in all four tissues, with liver amylase accounting for most of the normal serum amylase levels [35]. Because ferrets tend to ingest their food quickly, it is unlikely that salivary enzymes play a significant role in digestion, as evidenced by demonstration that parotid and submandibular saliva lack amylase activity [5].

Lipase is an enzyme that breaks down triglycerides into monoglycerides and free fatty acids by hydrolyzing it [66]. Lipase is produced primarily in the pancreas, with a small amount produced by the gastric mucosa, and it is inactivated and excreted by the kidney [66]. Lipase is considered

Table 11.8 Amylase and lipase normal values.

Species	Amylase (U/l)	Lipase (U/l)	References
Ferret	34–50	131.6–338.8	[68]
Hedgehog	244–858		[69]
Rabbit	166.5–314.5		[70]
Guinea pig	0–3159	0–152	[71]
Chinchilla	478–805	N/A	[72]

a more sensitive indicator of pancreatic necrosis than amylase but can be normal with pancreatitis [66]. Elevation of lipase can be caused by acute pancreatitis, pancreatic neoplasia, pancreatic abscesses, pancreatic duct obstruction, peritonitis, and generalized gastrointestinal pathologies, while decreased lipase is usually caused by exocrine pancreatic insufficiency [66].

Increased lipase and globulin levels in ferrets might be suggestive of a chronic GI problem such as inflammatory bowel disease or enteric glial cells [66]. Epizootic catarrhal enteritis might also increase lipase in ferrets [5]. Corticosteroids may cause increased lipase levels in ferrets and rabbits [35]. Rabbits with *Microsporum canis* had significantly higher lipase activity compared to clinically unaffected rabbits [67] Table 11.8.

Urine Evaluation

Sample Collection

Manual/Voided Samples

Urine collection can be performed by manual or voided collection. By applying pressure on the bladder, urination can be induced in most small mammals. Gentle pressure should be applied and the urine is collected directly to a container. If the patient is painful on abdominal palpation, manual compression of the bladder may cause additional pain.

To collect voided samples, the animal should be placed in an empty cage without towels. Cages with mesh bottoms can also be used to facilitate urine collection. Urine can also be collected from the floor if the animal urinates while out of the cage.

This type of sample collection may provide adequate samples for simple urinalysis, however, contamination with the cage floor will impair certain procedures, particularly urine culture. The animal should be supervised to collect the urine as soon as possible [17, 23].

Cystocentesis Samples

Cystocentesis is a procedure in which a needle is inserted through the abdominal wall into the urinary bladder to withdraw urine [73]. The procedure can be performed percutaneously or if the abdomen is open (surgically), directly through the bladder wall [73]. Cystocentesis is a superior collection method as it allows the collection of "clean" urine. Therefore, this sampling method is the preferred sampling method if microbiological culture is needed.

Catheter Samples

Urinary catheters are commonly used in obstructed male ferrets to manage urolithiasis and prostatomegaly secondary to hyperadrenocorticism. Although not common in females, catheters may occasionally be necessary. Other indications for urinary catheterization include infection and post urethrotomy, among others (Figure 11.9). Although this technique is usually used for the management of urinary obstruction, it also allows the collection of clean urine if sterile technique has been used. Urine at the time of the catheter placement should be collected for urinalysis and culture. Urine can be collected using a syringe and gentle pressure should be applied.

In human medicine and small animal medicine, secondary infections associated with urinary catheters are common. The length of time the catheter is left in place increases the risk of infection. Up to 25% of hospitalized patients undergo urinary catheterization, and about 5% develop bacteriuria each day of catheterization [74]. In dogs, placement of an indwelling urinary catheter in dogs is associated with a low risk of catheter-associated UTI during the first three days after catheter placement, provided that adequate precautions are taken for aseptic catheter placement and maintenance [75]. No such information is available for exotic animals.

Volume/Appearance

Normal urine in herbivores may vary in color including red, brown, orange, and yellow (Figure 11.10). Rabbit urine

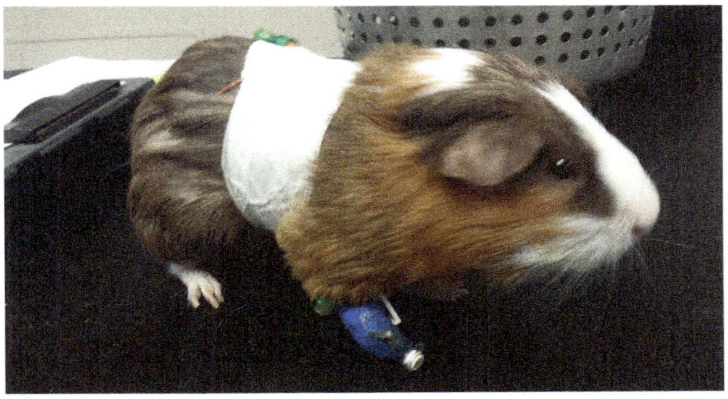

Figure 11.9 Guinea pig with urinary catheter. *Source:* Image courtesy of Mallory Keller.

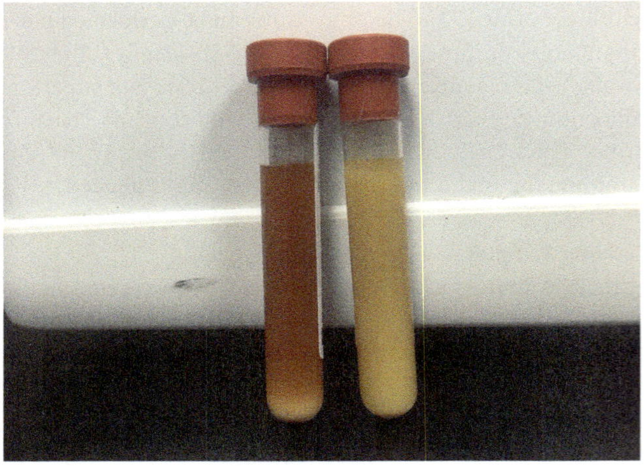

Figure 11.10 Urine from a suspected healthy rabbit.

contains mucus from mucus-secreting glands in the renal pelvis, which means there is a small amount of protein in the urine [76]. Small amounts of ammonium magnesium phosphate crystals are a normal finding [76]. Cloudy urine is common and is the result of calciuria and crystalluria [35]. Clear urine occurs in end-stage renal failure when kidneys cease to excrete calcium and can indicate a poor prognosis [74]. Ferret urine resembles dog and cat urine; therefore, it should be transparent and of varying shades of yellow [35].

Urinalysis

Dipstick

Rabbit urine can be orange-brown intermittently from porphyrin pigment. This can be distinguished from hematuria by urinalysis or dipstick [35]. Examination of the urine with a dipstick will often differentiate between blood and plant pigments; however, if the urine is concentrated and strongly colored this may affect reading the stick [23]. Test dipsticks work well to evaluate blood, glucose, ketone, and pH levels in rabbit urine but are not accurate for other parameters [18]. While glucosuria may be associated with stress hyperglycemia, ketones are always abnormal and indicate anorexia (even short duration), hepatic lipidosis, pregnancy toxemia, or diabetes [18]. In guinea pigs, urine ketones, bilirubin, and glucose should be negative [77].

Dipstick analysis of normal ferrets indicated trace protein in most of the patients (55/69), with non-statistically significant higher prevalence in males [78]. Bilirubin (+1) was detected in 11/69 ferrets [78]. Bilirubinuria in the absence of liver disease is considered normal in ferrets [78].

Dipsticks can be affected when exposed to light, and expired sticks should be discarded because results can be erroneous [35]. The urinary refractometer should be calibrated prior to use [35].

Urine Sediment Exam

Urine sediment analysis can offer information on urinary tract hemorrhage, inflammation, and bacteria [20]. Rabbits absorb more calcium from their diet than they require, and excrete surplus via urine (opposed to mammals that use bile for this purpose), therefore it is normal to contain a typical "sludge" [35, 79]. Calcium oxalates, calcium carbonate, and ammonium magnesium phosphate (triple phosphate) crystals are commonly found in normal rabbits, and the presence of these crystals does not imply urinary tract infection [35]. In guinea pigs, calcium is the major constituent of urinary calculi [80]. Ferrets appear to be more sensitive to some of the predisposing factors that increase levels of magnesium and phosphates in urine (depending on the type of diet), thus developing an alkaline urinary pH (as in urinary tract infections). Struvite (phosphate, ammonia, and magnesium hexahydrate) and cysteine are the most commonly found uroliths in ferrets [81–83]. Amorphous urates have also been reported in normal ferrets most urine samples contained mucous strands and/or protein sheaths [5].

Normal urine has few RBCs (0–3/high power field) and the presence of blood in the urine supports inflammation and/or hemorrhage [35, 77]. Grossly, rabbit and some rodent (guinea pigs, chinchillas) urine can have a red color; however, this does not imply blood in the urine. Sediment analysis can assist in distinguishing hematuria from normal pigmentation. Occasional leukocytes can be normal in the urine but increased numbers suggest inflammation [35]. Increased numbers of leucocytes in the urine sediment indicate nonspecific urinary tract inflammation, whereas WBC casts are suggestive of pyelonephritis [20]. Casts are cylindric molds of the renal tubules ("cylinduria") and are composed of aggregates of cells or proteins, and the presence of casts in the urine indicates a pathologic change in the kidneys [35]. Renal epithelial cell casts, which suggest tubular sloughing, may occur with acute tubular necrosis or pyelonephritis [20]. Casts were not reported in normal ferret urine, but a small number (0–2/high power field) was reported in healthy guinea pigs [77, 78].

If urine is collected via cystocentesis, bacteria should not be found in the urine. Bacteriuria may be an indication of upper or lower urinary tract infection but is more commonly associated with lower urinary tract disease [20]. If bacteria are found, bacterial culture and sensitivity is recommended. See Table 11.9 for normal urinalysis parameters in exotic mammals.

Table 11.9 Selected urinalysis parameters in exotic mammals.

Species	Specific gravity	Protein (mg/dl)	pH	Urine volume (ml/24 hr)	References
Ferret	Males 1.034–1.070 Females 1.026–1.060	0–33	6.5–7.5	26–140	[20, 78]
Rabbit	1.003–1.036	Trace	8.2–8.8	130/kg	[20]
Guinea pig			9.0		[20]
Mouse	1.034–1.058		7.3–8.5	0.5–2.5	[20]
Rat	1.022–1.050	<30	7.0–7.4	13–23	[20]
Hamster	1.050–1.060		Basic	5.1–8.4	[20]
Gerbil				Few drops-4 ml	[20]
Chinchilla	1.014 to >1.060	6–87	8.5		[84]
Prairie dog	1.005–1.059	6–124	8–8.5		[85]

References

1 Campbell, T.W. (2015). Exotic Animal Hematology and Cytology. Wiley.

2 Zimmerman, K., Moore, D.M., and Smith, S.A. (2015). Hematological assessment in pet Guinea pigs (*Cavia porcellus*): blood sample collection and blood cell identification. *Vet. Clin. North Am. Exot. Anim. Pract.* 18: 33–40.

3 Marshall, K.L. (2008). Rabbit hematology. *Vet. Clin. North Am. Exot. Anim. Pract.* 11: 551–567.

4 Siperstein, L.J. (2008). Ferret hematology and related disorders. *Vet. Clin. North Am. Exot. Anim. Pract.* 11: 535–550.

5 Fox, J.G. and Marini, R.P. (2014). Biology and Diseases of the Ferret. Wiley.

6 Pilny, A.A. (2008). Clinical hematology of rodent species. *Vet. Clin. North Am. Exot. Anim. Pract.* 11: 523–533.

7 Christopher, M.M., Hawkins, M.G., and Burton, A.G. (2014). Poikilocytosis in rabbits: prevalence, type, and association with disease. *PLoS One* 9: e112455.

8 Lawson, A., Lichtenberger, M., Day, T. et al. (2005). Comparison of sevoflurane and isoflurane in domestic ferrets (*Mustela putorius* furo). *Vet. Ther.* 7: 207–212.

9 Pollock, C. (2007). Emergency medicine of the ferret. *Vet. Clin. North Am. Exot. Anim. Pract.* 10: 463–500.

10 Kerr, M.G. (2008). Veterinary Laboratory Medicine. Wiley.

11 Weiss, D.J. and Wardrop, K.J. (2011). Schalm's Veterinary Hematology. Wiley.

12 Le K, Beaufrere H, Bassel L, et al. Polycythemia vera in a ferret (*Mustela putorious* furo). *Exoticscon 2016 Proceedings, Portland, August 27 to September 1 2016*: 437–438.

13 Robertson J, Musgrave K, Baumwart R, et al. Tetralogy of fallot in a 5-year-old ferret (*Mustela putorius* furo). *Exoticscon 2016 Proceedings* 2016:415.

14 Huynh, M., Boyeaux, A., and Pignon, C. (2016). Assessment and care of the critically ill rabbit. *Vet. Clin. North Am. Exot. Anim. Pract.* 19: 379–409.

15 Moore, D.M., Zimmerman, K., and Smith, S.A. (2015). Hematological assessment in pet rabbits: blood sample collection and blood cell identification. *Clin. Lab. Med.* 35: 617–627.

16 Di Girolamo, N. and Selleri, P. (2016). Medical and surgical emergencies in ferrets. *Vet. Clin. North Am. Exot. Anim. Pract.* 19: 431–464.

17 Siegel, A., Loar, A.S., and Walberg, J. (2012). Hematology and cytology of small mammals. In: Ferrets, Rabbits, and Rodents : Clinical Medicine and Surgery (eds. K. Quesenberry and J.W. Carpenter), 511–522. St. Louis, MO: Elsevier/Saunders.

18 Melillo, A. (2007). Rabbit clinical pathology. *J. Exot. Pet Med.* 16: 135–145.

19 Lindstrom, N.M., Moore, D.M., Zimmerman, K. et al. (2015). Hematologic assessment in pet rats, mice, hamsters, and gerbils: blood sample collection and blood cell identification. *Clin. Lab. Med.* 35: 629–640.

20 Fisher, P.G. (2006). Exotic mammal renal disease: diagnosis and treatment. *Vet. Clin. North Am. Exot. Anim. Pract.* 9: 69–96.

21 Melillo, A. (2013). Applications of serum protein electrophoresis in exotic pet medicine. *Vet. Clin. North Am. Exot. Anim. Pract.* 16: 211–225.

22 Harvey, J.W. (2012). Veterinary Hematology: A Diagnostic Guide and Color Atlas. Elsevier Health Sciences.

23 Varga, M. (2013). Textbook of Rabbit Medicine. Elsevier Health Sciences.

24 Cray, C., Arcia, G., Schneider, R. et al. (2009). Evaluation of the usefulness of an ELISA and protein electrophoresis in the diagnosis of *Encephalitozoon cuniculi* infection in rabbits. *Am. J. Vet. Res.* 70: 478–482.

25 Kaneko, J.J., Harvey, J.W., and Bruss, M.L. (2008). Clinical Biochemistry of Domestic Animals. Academic Press.

26 Ameri, M., Schnaars, H.A., Sibley, J.R. et al. (2011). Determination of plasma fibrinogen concentrations in

beagle dogs, cynomolgus monkeys, New Zealand white rabbits, and Sprague–Dawley rats by using clauss and prothrombin-time–derived assays. *J. Am. Assoc. Lab. Anim. Sci.* 50: 864–867.

27 Lowe, G.D., Rumley, A., and Mackie, I.J. (2004). Plasma fibrinogen. *Ann. Clin. Biochem.* 41: 430–440.

28 Georgieva, T.M., Georgiev, I.P., Tanev, S. et al. (2009). Variations of acute phase protein (haptoglobin, fibrinogen and ceruloplasmin) concentrations in weaning rabbits after experimental infection with *E. coli*. *Rev. Med. Vet.* 160: 133–139.

29 Georgieva, T., Petrov, V., Lyutsakanov, M. et al. (2016). Effect of *Staphylococcus aureus* infection on plasma creatine kinase activity in rabbits. *Trakia. J. Sci.* 14: 53.

30 Takahashi, S., Hirai, N., Shirai, M. et al. (2011). Comparison of the blood coagulation profiles of ferrets and rats. *J. Vet. Med. Sci.* 73: 953–956.

31 Benson, K.G., Paul-Murphy, J., Hart, A.P. et al. (2008). Coagulation values in normal ferrets (*Mustela putorius* furo) using selected methods and reagents. *Vet. Clin. Pathol.* 37: 286–288.

32 Matthews, M. and Eshar, D. (2016). Coagulation parameters of captive black-tailed prairie dogs (*Cynomys ludovicianus*). *Comp. Clin. Pathol.* 25: 219–223.

33 Jenkins, J.R. (2008). Rabbit diagnostic testing. *J. Exot. Pet Med.* 17: 4–15.

34 Johnson, J., Brandão, J., Perry, S. et al. (2015). Renal system of exotic species. In: Current Therapy in Exotic Pet Practice (eds. M. Mitchell and T. Tully), 494–548. Oxford: Elsevier.

35 Fudge AM. Laboratory Medicine: Avian and Exotic Pets, 2000.

36 Jenkins, J.R. (2010). Evaluation of the rabbit urinary tract. *J. Exot. Pet Med.* 19: 271–279.

37 Jenkins, J.R. (2008). Rodent diagnostic testing. *J. Exot. Pet Med.* 17: 16–25.

38 Fisher, P.G. (2006). Exotic mammal renal disease: causes and clinical presentation. *Vet. Clin. North Am. Exot. Anim. Pract.* 9: 33–67.

39 Ardiaca, M., Bonvehi, C., and Montesinos, A. (2013). Point-of-care blood gas and electrolyte analysis in rabbits. *Vet. Clin. North Am. Exot. Anim. Pract.* 16: 175–195.

40 Yunos, N.M., Bellomo, R., Story, D. et al. (2010). Bench-to-bedside review: chloride in critical illness. *Crit. Care* 14: 1.

41 Desmarchelier, M., Lair, S., Dunn, M. et al. (2008). Primary hyperaldosteronism in a domestic ferret with an adrenocortical adenoma. *J. Am. Vet. Med. Assoc.* 233: 1297–1301.

42 Eatwell, K., Mancinelli, E., Hedley, J. et al. (2013). Use of arterial blood gas analysis as a superior method for evaluating respiratory function in pet rabbits (*Oryctolagus cuniculus*). *Vet. Rec.* 173: 166.

43 Selleri, P. and Di Girolamo, N. (2014). Point-of-care blood gases, electrolytes, chemistries, hemoglobin, and hematocrit measurement in venous samples from pet rabbits. *J. Am. Anim. Hosp. Assoc.* 50: 305–314.

44 Jekl, V., Hauptman, K., Jeklova, E. et al. (2011). Selected haematological and plasma chemistry parameters in juvenile and adult degus (*Octodon degus*). *Vet. Rec.* 169: 71.

45 Brandão, J., Rick, M., and Mayer, J. (2015). Endocrine system. In: Current Therapy in Exotic Pet Practice (eds. M. Mitchell and T. Tully), 277–318. St. Louis, MO: Elsevier.

46 -Chapman, S.E. and Hostutler, R.A. (2013). A laboratory diagnostic approach to hepatobiliary disease in small animals. *Ve.t Clin. North Am. Small Anim.* 43: 1209–1225.

47 Eshar, D. (2013). Bile Acids. In: Clinical Veterinary Advisor, Birds and Exotic Pets: Clinical Veterinary Advisor (eds. J. Mayer and T.M. Donnelly), 606–607. Philadelphia, PA: Elsevier Health Sciences.

48 Sharma, D., Hill, A.E., and Christopher, M.M. (2018). Hypercholesterolemia and hypertriglyceridemia as biochemical markers of disease in companion rabbits. *Vet. Clin. Pathol.* 47: 589–602.

49 Antinoff, N. and Giovanella, C.J. (2012). Musculoskeletal and neurologic diseases. In: Ferrets, Rabbits, and Rodents : Clinical Medicine and Surgery (eds. K.E. Quesenberry and J.W. Carpenter), 132–140. St. Louis, MO: Elsevier/Saunders.

50 Rosenthal, K.L. and Wire, N.R. (2012). Endocrine diseases. In: Ferrets, Rabbits, and Rodents: Clinical Medicine and Surgery, 3e (eds. K. Quesenberry and J.W. Carpenter), 86–102. St. Louis, MO: Elsevier/Saunders.

51 McClure, D.E. (1999). Clinical pathology and sample collection in the laboratory rodent. *Vet. Clin. North Am. Exot. Anim. Pract.* 2: 565–590.

52 Harkness, J.E., Turner, P.V., VandeWoude, S. et al. (2013). Harkness and Wagner's Biology and Medicine of Rabbits and Rodents. Wiley.

53 Roth, S. and Conaway, H. (1982). Animal model of human disease. Spontaneous diabetes mellitus in the New Zealand white rabbit. *Am. J. Pathol.* 109: 359.

54 Harcourt-Brown, F. and Harcourt-Brown, S. (2012). Clinical value of blood glucose measurement in pet rabbits. *Vet. Rec.* 170: 674–674.

55 Vannevel, J. (1998). Diabetes mellitus in a 3-year-old, intact, female guinea pig. *Can. Vet. J.* 39: 503.

56 Belis, J.A., Curley, R.M., and Lang, C.M. (1996). Bladder dysfunction in the spontaneously diabetic male Abyssinian-Hartley guinea pig. *Pharmacology* 53: 66–70.

57 Mans, C. and Donnelly, T. (2012). Disease problems of chinchillas. In: Ferrets, Rabbits, and Rodents : Clinical Medicine and Surgery (eds. K. Quesenberry and J.W. Carpenter), 311–325. St. Louis, MO: Elsevier/Saunders.

58 Bennett, A. (2012). Soft tissue surgery. In: Ferrets, Rabbits, and Rodents : Clinical Medicine and Surgery (eds. K.E. Quesenberry and J.W. Carpenter), 373–291. St. Louis, MO: Elsevier/Saunders.

59 Lennox, A.M. (2007). Emergency and critical care procedures in sugar gliders (*Petaurus breviceps*), African hedgehogs (*Atelerix albiventris*), and prairie dogs (*Cynomys* spp). *Vet. Clin. North Am. Exot. Anim. Pract.* 10: 533–555.

60 Huston, S.M., Ming-Show Lee, P., Quesenberry, K.E. et al. (2012). Cardiovascular disease, lymphoproliferative disorders, and thymomas. In: Ferrets, Rabbits, and Rodents : Clinical Medicine and Surgery (eds. K.E. Quesenberry and J.W. Carpenter), 257–268. St. Louis, MO: Elsevier/Saunders.

61 Summa, N.M., Eshar, D., Lee-Chow, B. et al. (2014). Comparison of a human portable glucometer and an automated chemistry analyzer for measurement of blood glucose concentration in pet ferrets (*Mustela putorius* furo). *Can. Vet. J.* 55: 865.

62 Petritz, O.A., Antinoff, N., Chen, S. et al. (2013). Evaluation of portable blood glucose meters for measurement of blood glucose concentration in ferrets (*Mustela putorius* furo). *J. Am. Vet. Med. Assoc.* 242: 350–354.

63 Selleri, P., Di Girolamo, N., and Novari, G. (2014). Performance of two portable meters and a benchtop analyzer for blood glucose concentration measurement in rabbits. *J. Am. Vet. Med. Assoc.* 245: 87–98.

64 Higbie, C.T., Eshar, D., and Bello, N.M. (2015). Evaluation of three point-of-care meters and a portable veterinary chemistry analyzer for measurement of blood glucose concentrations in black-tailed prairie dogs (*Cynomys ludovicianus*). *Am. J. Vet. Res.* 76: 532–539.

65 Hersey-Benner, C. (2013). Amylase. In: Clinical Veterinary Advisor, Birds and Exotic Pets: Clinical Veterinary Advisor (eds. J. Mayer and T.M. Donnelly), 602. Philadelphia, PA: Elsevier Health Sciences.

66 Lipase, M.C. (2012). Clinical Veterinary Advisor, Birds and Exotic Pets: Clinical Veterinary Advisor (eds. J. Mayer and T.M. Donnelly), 624. Philadelphia, PA: Elsevier Health Sciences.

67 Cafarchia, C., Figueredo, L.A., Coccioli, C. et al. (2012). Enzymatic activity of *Microsporum canis* and Trichophyton mentagrophytes from breeding rabbits with and without skin lesions. *Mycoses* 55: 45–49.

68 Ohwada, K. and Katahira, K. (1993). Reference values for organ weight, hematology and serum chemistry in the female ferret (*Mustela putrius* furo). *Jikken. Dobutsu. Exp. Anim.* 42: 135–142.

69 Ivey, E. and Carpenter, J.W. (2012). African hedgehogs. In: Ferrets, Rabbits, and Rodents : Clinical Medicine and Surgery (eds. K. Quesenberry and J.W. Carpenter), 411–427. St. Louis, MO: Elsevier/Saunders.

70 Graham, J. and Mader, D. (2012). Basic approach to veterinary care. In: Ferrets, Rabbits, and Rodents : Clinical Medicine and Surgery (eds. K. Quesenberry and J.W. Carpenter), 174–182. St. Louis, Mo: Elsevier/Saunders.

71 Quesenberry, K., Donnelly, T., and Mans, C. (2012). Biology, husbandry, and clinical techniques of guinea pigs and chinchillas. In: Ferrets, Rabbits, and Rodents: Clinical Medicine and Surgery (eds. K. Quesenberry and J.W. Carpenter), 279–294. St. Louis, MO: Elsevier/Saunders.

72 Rivas, A.E., Mitchell, M.A., Flower, J. et al. (2014). Effects of ultraviolet radiation on serum 25-hydroxyvitamin D concentrations in captive chinchillas (*Chinchilla laniger*). *J. Exot. Pet Med.* 23: 270–276.

73 Brown, C. (2006). Diagnostic cystocentesis: technique and considerations. *Lab. Anim.* 35: 21–23.

74 Saint, S. and Lipsky, B.A. (1999). Preventing catheter-related bacteriuria: should we? Can we? How? *Arch. Intern. Med.* 159: 800–808.

75 Smarick, S.D., Haskins, S.C., Aldrich, J. et al. (2004). Incidence of catheter-associated urinary tract infection among dogs in a small animal intensive care unit. *J. Am. Vet. Med. Assoc.* 224: 1936–1940.

76 Harcourt-Brown, F.M. (2013). Diagnosis of renal disease in rabbits. *Vet. Clin. North Am. Exot. Anim. Pract.* 16: 145–174.

77 Bishop CR, Fischer J, Brossoit A, et al. Standardization of renal physiology parameters in guinea pigs via urinalysis. *Proceedings of the Association of Avian Veterinarians and Association of Exotic Mammal Veterinarians, San Diego, August 1 to august 5 2010*: 49–52.

78 Eshar, D., Wyre, N., and Brown, D. (2012). Urine specific gravity values in clinically healthy young pet ferrets (*Mustela furo*). *J. Small Anim. Pract.* 53: 115–119.

79 Clauss, M., Burger, B., Liesegang, A. et al. (2012). Influence of diet on calcium metabolism, tissue calcification and urinary sludge in rabbits (*Oryctolagus cuniculus*). *J. Anim. Physiol. Anim. Nutr.* 96: 798–807.

80 Miwa, Y. and Sladky, K.K. (2016). Small mammals: common surgical procedures of rodents, ferrets, hedgehogs, and sugar gliders. *Vet. Clin. North Am. Exot. Anim. Pract.* 19: 205–244.

81 Del Angel-Caraza, J., Chávez-Moreno, O., García-Navarro, S. et al. (2008). Mixed urolith (struvite and calcium oxalate) in a ferret (*Mustela putorius* furo). *J. Vet. Diagn. Investig.* 20: 682–683.

82 Nwaokorie, E.E., Osborne, C.A., Lulich, J.P. et al. (2011). Epidemiology of struvite uroliths in ferrets: 272 cases (1981–2007). *J. Am. Vet. Med. Assoc.* 239: 1319–1324.

83 Nwaokorie, E.E., Osborne, C.A., Lulich, J.P. et al. (2013). Epidemiological evaluation of cystine urolithiasis in domestic ferrets (*Mustela putorius* furo): 70 cases (1992–2009). *J. Am. Vet. Med. Assoc.* 242: 1099–1103.

84 Doss, G.A., Mans, C., Houseright, R.A. et al. (2016). Urinalysis in chinchillas (*Chinchilla lanigera*). *J. Am. Vet. Med. Assoc.* 248: 901–907.

85 Eshar, D., Pohlman, L.M., and Harkin, K.R. (2016). Urine properties of captive black-tailed prairie dogs (*Cynomys ludovicianus*). *J. Exot. Pet Med.* 25: 213–219.

12

Cytology

Carla Monteiro[1] and João Brandão[2]

[1] Exotic/Wild Life Consulting – Clínica Veterinária Atlântida, Porto, Portugal
[2] Department of Veterinary Clinical Sciences, College of Veterinary Medicine, Oklahoma State University, Oklahoma, USA

CONTENTS

Sample Collection

FNA/Impression Smears

Fine needle aspiration (FNA) is a simple and cost-effective procedure to obtain cytological samples that can be used for a quick presumptive or definitive diagnosis, with minimal trauma to the patient. This procedure can be performed on cutaneous, subcutaneous, or internal masses and organs [1]. There are two techniques: aspiration or non-aspiration [1]. For both techniques, hypodermic needles (usually 22-gauge, 1-in., but 25–20 gauge are also acceptable), syringe (3 ml or larger), and glass microscope slides are necessary [1]. Prior to aspiration of vascular tissues, coating the needle and syringe lumen with sterile 4% disodium EDTA reduces the possibility of clot formation [1].

Impression smear cytology is obtained by contact between the slide and the tissue, imprinting the cut surfaces of removed masses or tissues by lightly touching the glass microscope slide to the surface of the mass (and not vice-versa), to obtain monolayers of cells. If the result of the imprint is acellular, scraping the cut surface of an exposed lesion with a scalpel blade onto a glass microscope slide may improve the cellular content of the sample.

Centesis Techniques

Cystocentesis

Urine samples can be collected by cystocentesis or by free catch after natural voiding or gentle manual expression of the bladder (Figure 12.1) [2]. Cystocentesis is the preferred method to obtain urine samples, which allows the clinician to perform urinalysis as well as bacterial culture and sensitivity [2]. This technique is best performed when ultrasound-guided, although blind cystocentesis can also be done. Anesthesia or sedation in fractious animals may be necessary [2, 3]. A small-diameter needle (22- to 25-gauge) with a 3–6 ml syringe provides enough volume for a thorough urinalysis (Table 12.1) [3]. Potential complications during this procedure are accidental puncture of the intestinal tract [2]; leakage of urine into the

Exotic Animal Emergency and Critical Care Medicine, First Edition. Edited by Jennifer E. Graham, Grayson A. Doss and Hugues Beaufrère.

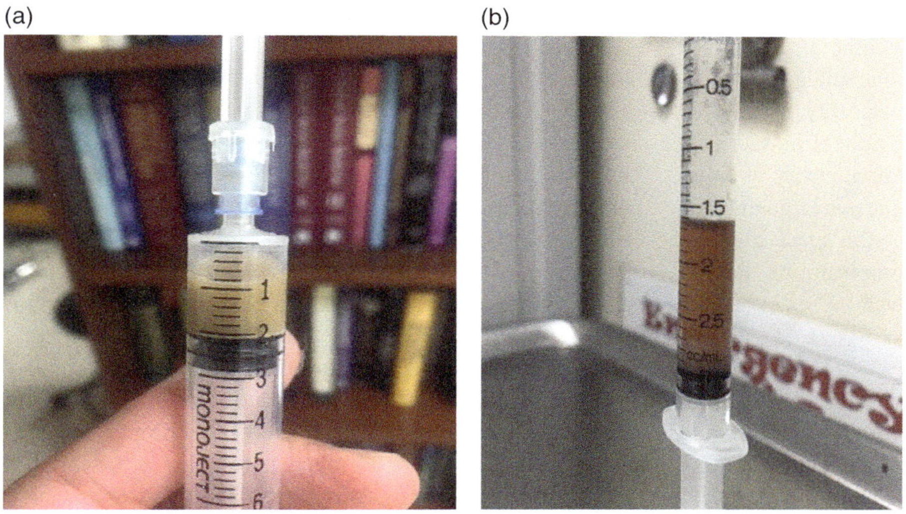

Figure 12.1 Normal color and turbidity in rabbit urine (a). Normal rabbit urine after being allowed to rest in a syringe (b).

Table 12.1 Normal urinalysis parameters in several small exotic mammal species.

Parameter	Ferrets	Rabbits	Guinea pig	Mouse	Rat	Hamster	Chinchilla
pH	6.5–7.5	8.2–8.8	9.0	7.3–8.5	7.0–7.4	Basic	8–9
Urine protein (mg/dl)	0–32 (females) 7–33 (males)	Trace	N/A	N/A	<30	10	N/A
Specific gravity	1.059 ± 0.007 (males) 1.047 ± 0.007 (females)	1.003–1.036 (fixed range 1.008–1.012)	N/A	1.034–1.058	1.022–1.050	1.050–1.060	N/A
Color/ transparency	Transparent and of varying shades of yellow	Red, orange, brown, or clear yellow, cloudy white and turbid in appearance (Figure 12.1)	Yellow/ amber Opaque		N/A	Cloudy	Yellow/ amber

Source: Refs. [3–7].

peritoneal cavity, laceration of the great vessels [8]; and calculus formation in rabbits (by repetitive puncture of the bladder) [9].

Abdominocentesis

Abdominocentesis is the collection of fluid from the abdominal cavity. It can be performed in small mammals to obtain ascitic fluid for evaluation and, as previously stated, for cystocentesis. It is preferable to collect the sample using an ultrasound guide with sedation or anesthesia in fractious patients [10]. The procedure begins by the surgical preparation of the aspiration site. A 21- to 25-gauge needle is inserted along the ventral midline of the abdomen distal to the umbilicus of mammals [1]. Other authors prefer a different approach, inserting a 20–22 G needle paramedially in the right cranial quadrant [11]. It is overall considered an uncomplicated procedure without serious hazards for the patient [11].

Diagnostic peritoneal lavage in small mammal patients is similar to that described in dogs and cats [2]. The anesthetized or sedated patient is placed in dorsal recumbency. Shave and aseptically prepare the skin caudal to the umbilicus. Local infusion with 2% lidocaine may be beneficial. Elevate the body wall with sterile forceps, and insert an 18- to 20-gauge over-the-needle catheter through the body wall, being cautious to avoid the spleen (the catheter can be sterilely fenestrated before insertion to optimize fluid recovery). Advance the catheter caudodorsally, and remove the stylet. Aspirate the catheter and if no fluid appears, instill 20–22 ml/kg of warm sterile isotonic saline. Massage the abdomen or gently rock the patient for one to two minutes. Aspirate the fluid and place into sterile containers for evaluation. If necessary, repeat fluid instillation at up to half the initial volume used. Remove the catheter, and suture or glue the incision. Treat with a systemic analgesic subsequent to the procedure. In dogs and cats, the accuracy of diagnosis is higher with diagnostic peritoneal lavage than with abdominocentesis [2]. The abdominal cavity of some mammals, such as rabbits and guinea pigs, is large and the gastrointestinal tract occupies much of the space and lies just under the body wall. Potential complications include penetration of the gastrointestinal tract or other organs of the abdominal cavity [1].

Thoracocentesis

Thoracocentesis is commonly performed to allow the aspiration of air or fluid from the pleural space through a needle inserted in the intercostal space and is performed not only as a diagnostic tool but also as a therapeutic procedure in emergency situations (Figure 12.2) [12]. The technique is similar in most species. Start by identifying the mid-thorax region for needle placement (seventh intercostal space, midway between shoulder and last rib), and prepare a hypodermic needle or a butterfly catheter attached to a three-way stopcock and syringe unit [12]. Ferrets have 14 ribs versus 13 in dogs and cats. Additionally, the ferret's heart sits much more caudally in the thorax than in other small mammals, usually extending from the sixth rib to the caudal border of the seventh or eighth rib, with the apex only 1 cm from the diaphragm. This unique anatomy makes thoracocentesis in ferrets generally more difficult than in cats and dogs. Therefore, it is essential to use thoracic radiography or thoracic ultrasonography as a guide in choosing a proper thoracocentesis site. Thoracocentesis is performed by inserting a needle at the junction of the ventral third of the thorax to remove fluid with pleural effusion [13]. In rodents, thoracocentesis should be ultrasound-guided, and it can be performed using a 25-gauge butterfly catheter with a 3 or 6 ml syringe and two-way stopcock [8, 10, 14]. Potential complications with thoracocentesis include iatrogenic hemothorax, neuritis, paralysis of the intercostal muscles, iatrogenic pneumothorax from lung laceration, and creation of a hole in the intercostal muscles and skin [13].

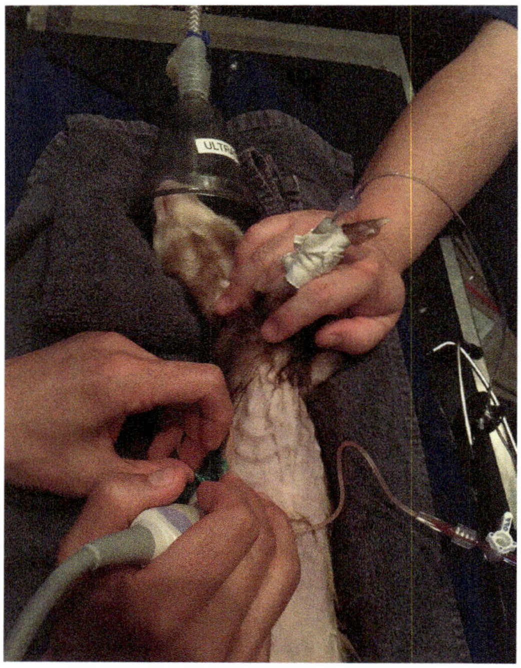

Figure 12.2 Thoracocentesis in a ferret. *Source:* Image courtesy of Miranda Sadar.

Arthrocentesis

Under normal conditions, the joints of most of the small mammals contain a fluid volume that is too small for sampling or complete evaluation. Fluid distension of a joint may occur when certain arthropathies are present, which will allow for the collection of enough synovial fluid for evaluation. A complete synovial fluid analysis should include an assessment of appearance (color and turbidity), protein content, viscosity, a mucin clot test, and a nucleated cell count, differential, and cell morphology [1]. The normal parameters are described in Table 12.2.

Gastrointestinal Sampling

Oral Cavity

Diseases of the oral cavity are common in small exotic mammals [15]. Anatomy and dentition vary significantly

Table 12.2 Normal synovial fluid analysis.

Fluid appearance	Protein content	Viscosity	Mucin clot test	Nucleated cell count	Cell differential
Clear/straw	Low (2.5 g/dl)	2 cm	Clot remains attached to the slide when the slide is inverted	<3 cells/high-power field (depending upon the thickness of the smear)	Mononuclear cells (macrophages-small and synovial lining cells-large) and granulocytes <10%(neutrophils)

Source: From Campbell [1].

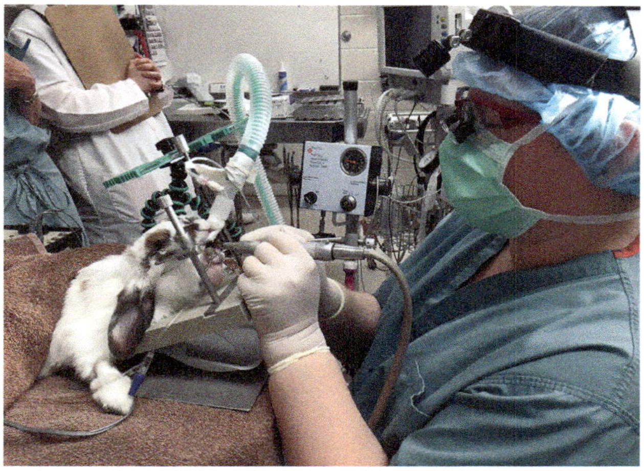

Figure 12.3 Rabbit dental occlusal surface correction using a tabletop mouth gag. *Source:* Image courtesy of Miranda Sadar.

among the species; diagnosis and treatment are often extrapolated from other species [16]. Clinical examination of the oral cavity of small herbivorous mammals needs to be species-specific, owing to differences in their oral anatomy; several methods have been described for close examination of the oral cavity, including endoscopy [15]. The intraoral examination includes a thorough evaluation of the soft tissues (lips, tongue, gingiva, and oropharynx). Common abnormalities include ulceration of the buccal mucosa, gingival hyperplasia, and gingival pockets with associated periodontal disease [17]. Complications such as infections associated with the teeth should be addressed as well [17]. Endoscopy-guided examinations are recommended for small mammals, (like guinea pigs, chinchillas, and degus) to minimize the risk of missing intraoral pathology and iatrogenic trauma during the intraoral treatment [17, 18]. Special equipment is necessary in order to perform a complete intraoral examination in non-carnivore small mammals. The tabletop mouth gag is the preferred instrument for positioning the patient (Figure 12.3). If a standard mouth gag and cheek dilators are used, an assistant is needed to position and hold the patient in place [17]. An intraoral examination in a conscious chinchilla or degu cannot rule out intraoral disease, considering that up to 50% of intraoral lesions can be missed [17], therefore anesthesia or sedation is recommended [18]. The oral cavity can be sampled in the presence of ulcerative lesions and/or masses. The techniques used include brushings, aspirates, and impressions smears. Care should be taken to ensure sampling at a depth appropriate to the lesion, as superficial sampling is often unrewarding [19]. Ferrets, like other carnivores, are capable of widely opening the oral cavity, facilitating inspection and sampling [20].

Respiratory Sampling

Nasal Swab/Flushing

Superficial and deep nasal swabs (NS) are easy to obtain, although manipulation of the nasal cavity often results in hemorrhage [19, 21]. To perform both techniques, general anesthesia (preferably with endotracheal tube in place and with packing of the oropharynx with gauze) is recommended [19]. Superficial NS can be collected by inserting a cotton-tipped swab into the nares and gently rolling it along the nasal mucosa at varying depths to obtain samples for cytological analysis. This procedure should be performed as carefully as possible to avoid trauma to the nasal cavities (particularly in obligate nasal breathers) and contamination of subsequent samples with blood [22]. The rabbit's nose is sensitive and it can be difficult to insert the swab deep into the nasal passages in the conscious animal. Superficial lesions such as fungal rhinitis can occasionally be identified [21] but mostly are limited to identifying superficial inflammation, secondary bacterial infection, hemorrhage, or necrosis, not providing much information in processes involving deeper layers of the nasal mucosa [19]. Some infectious agents including *Cryptococcus* and *Aspergillus* may be easily identified from nasal discharge, either by culture or PCR [19, 23].

The nasal flush (NF) technique is the least invasive method to obtain diagnostic samples from the nasal cavity, but only cells and debris that are easily dislodged are collected. The other disadvantage is sample contamination from outside the nasal cavity, which happens when the flushed saline is collected as it flows out of the nares [23]. To obtain a NF sample, general anesthesia and packing of the oropharynx are also recommended [22, 23]. During NF the patient should be in sternal recumbency with the nose pointing slightly downward to facilitate sample collection [22, 23]. Depending on the size of the patient, a 5, 8, or 10 French catheter is passed from the nares into the caudal nasal cavity. Prior to inserting the catheter, it is necessary to mark the distance to the medial canthus the eye (to avoid possible penetration of the cribriform plate). A syringe filled with sterile saline is attached to the catheter. The saline is then flushed into the nasal cavity and then aspirated back into the syringe.

Another sampling technique is nasolacrimal duct (NLD) flush (Figure 12.4). Flushing of the NLD is a common procedure in the rabbit and can be both diagnostic and therapeutic [2]. Topical anesthesia +/− sedation/general anesthesia is required for effective irrigation of the NLD. Good illumination is required and magnification may facilitate the performance of this technique. The *punctum lacrimale* is identified in the medial canthus by gently everything the lower lid (Figure 12.5). Forceps can be used to hold the eyelid away from the cornea. A small irrigating cannula is introduced through the *punctum lacrimale* into

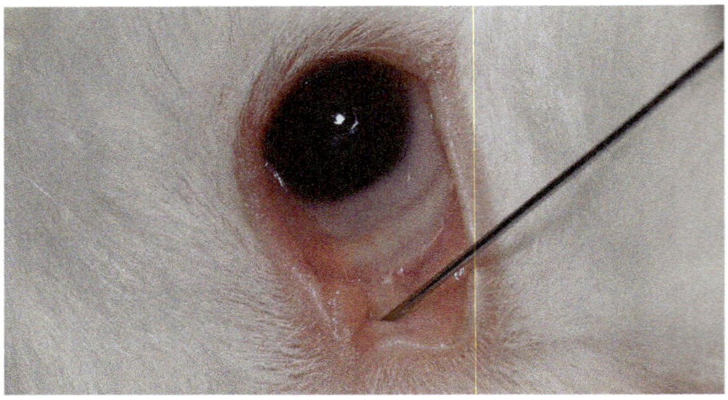

Figure 12.4 Nasolacrimal duct flush in a rabbit. *Source:* Image courtesy of Katie Lennox.

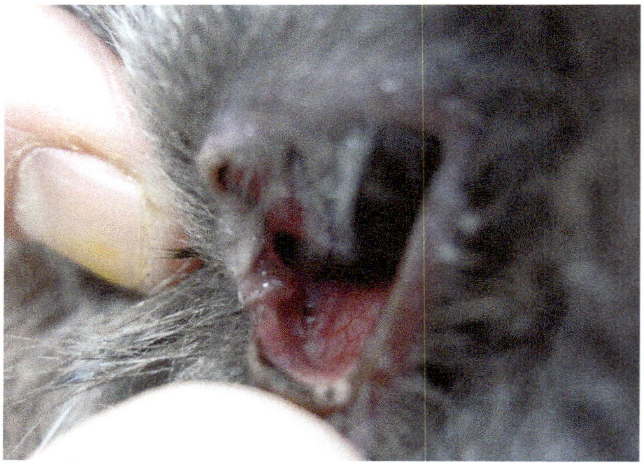

Figure 12.5 Punctum lacrimale in a rabbit. *Source:* Image courtesy of Miranda Sadar.

the lacrimal sac, and sterile water or saline can be gently flushed until it emerges in the nasal cavity at the ventromedial aspect of the alar fold, a few millimeters inside the mucocutaneous junction [9]. The irrigation should be performed gently. It is possible to cause soft tissue damage, especially with metal catheters. It is sometimes necessary to pass a cannula through the lacrimal foramen to flush purulent material from the maxillary section of the NLD. Bacterial culture of material flushed aids antibiotic selection [9]. Rupture of the duct or lacrimal sac can occur if excessive pressure is applied [9].

Tracheal Wash

Tracheal wash is a minimally invasive diagnostic test to obtain airway samples for cytology and bacterial culture [24]. This procedure involves insertion of a catheter into the airway, injection of sterile saline, and subsequent aspiration of the fluid. The catheter is inserted through a sterile endotracheal tube [23]. The procedure in the ferret is similar to that used in a cat. Anesthetize the ferret and

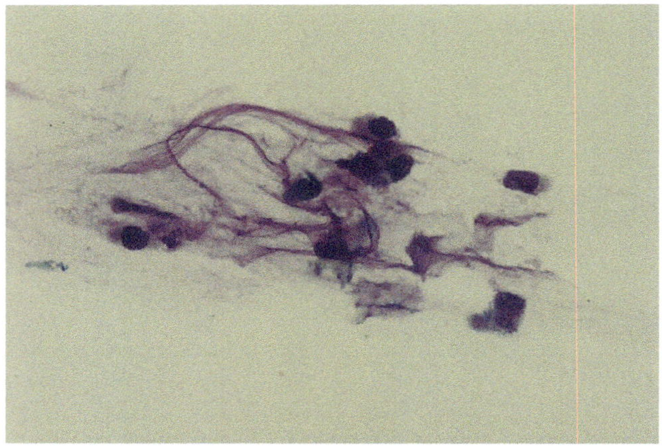

Figure 12.6 Tracheal wash from a kinkajou. The cells seen in this image are normal cells of the respiratory tract (non-ciliated) and pink staining string material is normal mucous. Some of the cells appear spindle-shaped most likely due to the process of making the smear.

intubate with a sterile endotracheal tube. An 8-French pediatric suction catheter (Safe-T-Vac Suction, Kendall Healthcare Products, Mansfield, MA) connected to a specimen container (Argyle Lukens Specimen Container, Sherwood Medical, St. Louis, MO) and attached to a wall suction outlet [2]. Pass the tip of the suction catheter through the endotracheal tube, preferably to the level of tracheal bifurcation [2]. Inject up to 2 ml of warm, sterile saline solution, then aspirate the fluid into the specimen container [2]. If the recovered tracheal fluid is cloudy or with clumps of material, direct smears or crush preparations can be made. If the obtained fluid is clear, it is probably of low cellularity and smears should be prepared from centrifugal sediment to ensure adequate material is present. Usually, tracheal washes are more rewarding and provide more information than lung aspirates (Figure 12.6) [25]. Endoscopic aided intubation may be useful when performing this technique in rabbits and rodents.

Dermatologic Sampling

The diagnostic workup in these species is very similar to that used for other small animals [26]. Diagnosis is mainly based on direct and microscopic visualization of ectoparasites, microscopy of trichograms, tape preparations, and skin scrapings [27].

Skin Scraping

Skin scraping diagnostic technique is extremely useful for ectoparasite visualization. The site of the scraping should be one that is a suspected predilection site for the ectoparasite or shows changes suspicious of ectoparasite infestation

Table 12.3 Common findings on skin scrapings, impression, and tape preparations.

	Ferrets	Rabbits	Rodents	Hedgehogs
Skin scrapings	*Sarcoptes scabiei, Lynxacarus mustelae, Otodectes cynotis* (Figure 12.7)	*Sarcoptes scabiei var. cuniculi, Notoedres cati var. cuniculi, Psoroptes cuniculi, Psorobia lagomorphae*	*Chirodiscoides caviae, Demodex caviae, Demodex criceti, Demodex aurati, Notoedres notoedres, Notoedres cati, Sarcoptes scabiei, Trixacarus caviae, Ornithonyssus bacoti, Myocoptes musculinus, Notoedres muris* (Figure 12.8), *Demodex ratticola, Liponyssus bacoti*	*Caparinia tripilis, Trombicula autumnalis*
Impression smears	Pyoderma, neoplasia	Eosinophilic granuloma	Pyoderma/abscess, sebaceous gland, and nasal dermatitis, epitheliotropic lymphoma	Neoplasia
Tape preparations		*Cheyletiella parasitovorax, Psoroptes cuniculi, Trombicula autumnalis, Leporacarus (Listrophorus) gibbus*	*Myobia musculi*	*Caparinia tripilis, Trombicula autumnalis*

Source: Refs. [26–32].

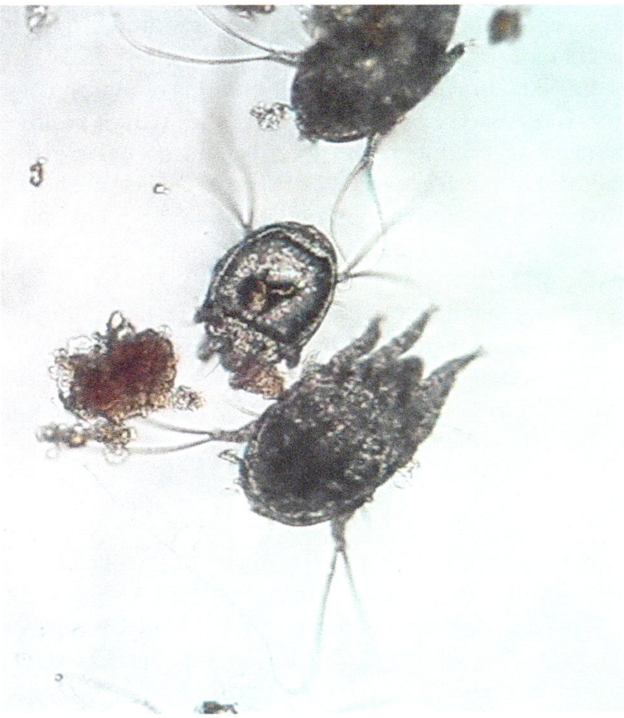

Figure 12.7 *Otodectes cynotis* in a ferret obtained from skin scraping.

and has not been traumatized by the host. In some species due to their size and temperament, anesthesia or sedation may be necessary [28]. For parasites occupying the deeper layers of the skin (e.g. burrowing mites), skin scrapes should be performed. Burrowing mites include species belonging to the family Demodectidae (*Demodex* spp.) and Sarcoptidae (*Sarcoptes* spp., *Notoedres cati*, *Trixacarus caviae*) [27].

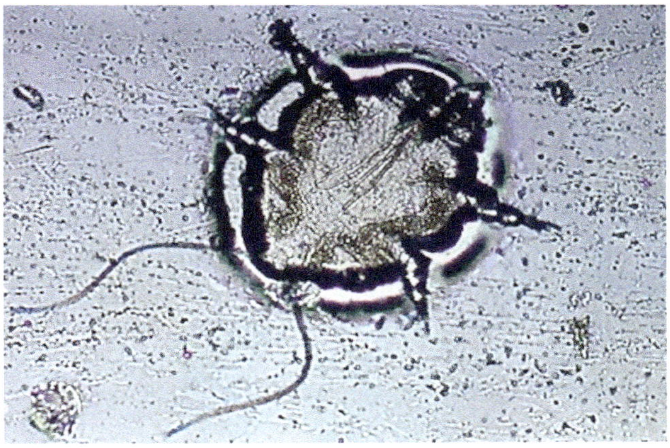

Figure 12.8 *Notoedres muris* from a pet rat on tape impression.

Impression/Tape Preps

This alternative to skin scraping has been recommended to find superficial ectoparasites such as *Cheyletiella* mites, poultry mites, and *Myobia* [26, 28]. The hair is parted and a piece of clear adhesive tape is attached to and then removed from the skin several times to collect material. It is then attached to a microscope slide and viewed under the microscope under low power [28]. It may be used to identify a lymphocytic infiltration in plaques seen with lymphoma, e.g. in the hamster. For the diagnosis of sucking parasites such as species of the families Psoroptidae (*Psoroptes* spp., *Chorioptes* spp., *Otodectes cynotis*, *Caparinia* spp.) and Listrophoridae (*Myocoptes* spp., *Myobia* spp.), skin scraping, impression smears, or tape preparations can be used [27]. For surface mites (*Cheyletiella parasitivorax*, *Leporacarus gibbus*, *Chirodiscoides caviae*) and other opportunistic parasites like poultry mites (*Ornithonyssus* spp., *Dermanyssus gallinae*), tape preparations should be used (Table 12.3) [27].

Cutaneous Neoplasia

Cutaneous tumors are frequent in exotic mammals. In ferrets, tumors of the skin are the third most common neoplasm in ferrets after endocrine and hemolymphatic neoplasms [25]. Among cutaneous tumors, 33% were mast cell tumors and 30% were sebaceous epitheliomas (more common than sebaceous adenomas) [33]. Other tumors included cutaneous hemangioma, preputial tumors, and lymphoma (cutaneous and epitheliotropic) as well as sarcomas (leiomyosarcoma and to a lower extent, fibrosarcoma) [33]. The diagnosis of spindle cell tumors based on cytology was rare. For squamous cell carcinoma (Figure 12.9), aspiration is recommended over impression smears because these lesions are commonly secondarily infected and inflamed, which will interfere with the cytologic interpretation [33]. Apocrine gland adenoma and mammary gland tumors typically result in acellular smears [25, 33]. Ferrets may have multiple cutaneous tumors of differing types at the same time [33]. In the pet rabbit, 20% of the cutaneous tumors have been reported to be trichoblastoma, followed by spindle cell sarcoma, collagenous hamartoma, squamous papilloma (rabbit papilloma virus-induced), mammary gland adenocarcinoma, and soft tissue sarcoma [33, 34]. Other tumors with less than 5% prevalence include mammary gland adenoma and carcinoma, lipoma, fibrosarcoma, carcinomas, melanoma, and lymphoma [33, 34]. Melanomas, including amelanotic melanomas, have also been reported in rabbits but appear to be rare [35, 36]. In guinea pigs, the most common cutaneous tumors were trichofolliculoma, followed by lipomas [33, 34]. Other less prevalent tumors included trichoepithelioma, mammary gland adenocarcinoma, adenoma and cystadenoma, sarcomas and carcinomas, melanoma, and epitheliotropic lymphoma [33, 34]. Overall, in ferrets, rabbits, and guinea pigs, most of the cutaneous masses were benign tumors [33]. However, malignant neoplasia was more commonly found in rabbits (46% of all cutaneous neoplasms in rabbits were malignant), followed by guinea pigs (26% malignant skin masses), and ferrets (19% malignant masses) [33]. In rats, the most common mammary tumor is the fibroadenoma [37]. Mongolian gerbils commonly develop proliferative lesions of the ventral abdominal marking gland, that can appear as hyperplasia, adenoma, adenocarcinoma, and squamous cell carcinoma [34]. Hedgehogs are well known for developing tumors, including skin tumors and associated tissues, among which mammary adenocarcinoma, cutaneous mast cell tumor, and soft tissue sarcomas are common [38].

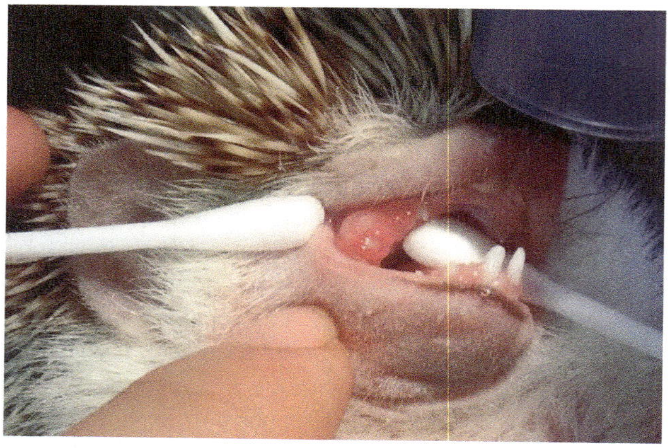

Figure 12.9 Maxillary squamous cell carcinoma in a pet hedgehog.

Ocular Sampling

Ocular cytology is a quick and simple method to characterize and, in some cases, diagnose the disease process involving the ocular surface. Although less sensitive than culture, exfoliative cytology is a very rewarding tool. It can identify organisms (e.g. bacteria, fungal hyphae, yeast bodies) and provide information in terms of morphology (e.g. rods/cocci), staining characteristics (Gram-positive or negative), number, and location (intracellular/extracellular) of the organisms [39]. Sample collection should produce minimal irritation to the animal [39]. Excessive surface debris and mucus should be removed prior to cytology [39].

With some minor variation in technique, depending on the case and patient, samples for microbiologic and cytological assessment can be collected following the application of a drop of topical anesthetic using Kimura platinum spatula, the handle-end of a scalpel blade, swab, or single-use gynecological cytobrush.

Conjunctival

For conjunctival sampling, the swab should be rolled in the lower conjunctival sac anterior to the third eyelid (using retropulsion to protrude the third eyelid) [39]. The normal cytology of a conjunctival scraping or brush specimen consists of epithelial cells and goblet cells. Scraping samples often contain cornified squamous epithelial cells derived from the margins of the eyelids (Table 12.4) [1].

Corneal

To obtain corneal material by scraping, follow the same procedure as for conjunctival samples. The blunt end of a sterile surgical blade or a Kimura spatula is used in a scraping motion, ideally in one direction to create a "pile of cells." The material is then transferred onto a sterile swab tip [39]. To obtain a corneal sample using a swab, the swab is gently rubbed or rolled over the lesion [39].

Table 12.4 Common bacterial isolates from the conjunctiva of exotic mammals.

Species	Bacteria	Notes
Rabbit	*Staphylococcus* spp., *Micrococcus* spp., *Bacillus* spp., *Stomatococcus* spp., *Neisseria* spp., *Corynebacterium* spp., and *Streptococcus* spp. [9]	Conjunctival sac, pet rabbits
Rabbit	*Bacillus subtilis* and *Staphylococcus aureus*, *Pseudomonas* spp., *Neisseria* spp., *Bordetella* spp., *Moraxella* spp., and *Pasteurella* spp. [39]	Healthy laboratory rabbits
Guinea pigs	*Corynebacterium* spp., *Streptococcus* spp., and *Staphylococcus* spp. [40]	Pet guinea pigs
Chinchillas	*Streptococcus* sp., *Staphylococcus aureus*, and coagulase-negative staphylococcus [41].	Breeding facility chinchillas
Ferrets	*Staphylococcus* sp. and *Corynebacterium* sp. [42]	Pet ferrets

Fluid Cytology

Sample Preparation

Effusions

Aspirated fluids should be evaluated for specific gravity, protein content, and cellularity, color, and character of the fluid [1]. Protein can be quantified using refractometry or by laboratorial units. For an accurate fluid evaluation, the sample should be assessed immediately and if such is not possible, the sample should be refrigerated [1]. Causes of effusions can include cardiac disease (in case of abdominal effusions), mediastinal lymphosarcoma (mediastinal effusion), and mesothelioma (this tumor can elicit an effusion in any body cavity) (Table 12.5) [25].

Fecal Cytology

Small mammals presenting with abnormal feces or GI signs should be subjected to a complete fecal evaluation, which should include wet mount, flotation, Gram's stain, and cytology.

Wet Mount/Direct

Endoparasites are uncommon in pet ferrets, but this differential diagnosis should not be ignored. Juveniles are susceptible to coccidiosis (*Isospora* and *Eimeria*) or giardiasis infestation [43]. Outbreaks of severe enteric disease associated with *Eimeria furonis* infection in ferrets has been reported [44]. Enteric coccidiosis due to infection with *E. furonis* has typically been reported to be subclinical rather than to cause severe gastrointestinal disease in ferrets [44]. *E. furonis* can also cause biliary coccidiosis, which has been associated with pure red cell aplasia [45, 46].

Coccidial infections are common when rabbits are held at high densities under inappropriate husbandry conditions (Figure 12.10). *Eimeria perforans*, *Eimeria magna*, *Eimeria media*, and *Eimeria irresidua* are among the most common [47]. *Eimeria stiedae* is the only liver coccidium [47]. Several nonpathogenic flagellates may be found in the feces of rabbits including *Monocercomonas cuniculi* and *Retortamonas cuniculi*. *Giardia duodenalis* occurs rarely in the small intestine and is not considered pathogenic [2].

Guinea pig coccidia can be found in direct fecal smear. Coccidia are usually considered nonpathogenic, however, *Eimeria caviae* infections in guinea pigs may occasionally result in diarrhea and death [48].

Protozoal parasites are a common cause of diarrhea in young rodents, particularly hamsters and chinchillas [49]. In one study, chinchillas usually harbored nonrodent-specific Giardia species, and a high positivity rate (39.4%) was found despite all animals being asymptomatic [50].

Mice commonly are affected by parasites like *Spironucleus muris* and *Giardia muris* which are commonly considered pathogenic, even though they are not associated with clinical signs in immunocompetent hosts [51]. *Aspiculuris tetraptera*, can also be found in a direct smear [51]. *Giardia muris* can also be found in rats [52].

Low levels of *Giardia* sp. appear to be common in sugar gliders but may lead to diarrhea [53, 54]. Lungworm infestation can cause pneumonia in African pygmy hedgehogs but is rarely diagnosed in the domestically raised hedgehog [51].

Flotation

Fecal flotation test is made by mixing a small amount of feces with a flotation solution. Fecal flotation relies on the differences in the specific gravity of the egg(s), fecal debris,

Table 12.5 General characteristics of effusions.

Type of effusion	Characteristics
Transudate	• Fluids that have accumulated in the serous cavities as a result of oncotic pressure changes or other circulatory disturbances (i.e. increased hydrostatic vascular pressure). • Causes of transudate formation include hypoalbuminemia (hypoproteinemia), overhydration, and lymphatic or venous congestion, cardiac insufficiency, portosystemic shunt, and hepatic cirrhosis and insufficiency.
Modified transudate	• Often associated with cardiac insufficiency, cardiomyopathy, compression of vascular structures from neoplasia, inflammation or torsion of an organ, and the presence of sterile irritants. • Grossly resemble transudative effusions and long-standing transudates become modified with the increase in the number of cells or protein content.
Hemorrhagic	• Often result from trauma or injury. • Peracute hemorrhagic effusions may resemble peripheral blood; however, the presence of platelets is suggestive of peripheral blood contamination. • Chronic and resolving hemorrhagic effusions exhibit varying degrees of erythrophagocytosis.
Exudate	• Fluids containing increased protein content and cellularity. • Vary in color and turbidity, may have a foul odor, and often clot during sample collection. • Fluid samples suggestive of an exudative effusion should be placed into a tube with anticoagulant (e.g. EDTA) to prevent clotting of the sample. • Exudates typically result from inflammatory processes or chemotactic stimulation within the peritoneal cavity that causes increased capillary permeability. • Identification of microorganisms may provide clues to the etiology of the exudative effusion. Culture and sensitivity are advisable in these cases.
Chylous	• Composed of chyle, which is a mixture of lymph and chylomicrons (triglycerides). • Typically have a "milky" white to pink-tinged appearance and contain variable cell counts and protein content. • Longstanding chylous effusions usually have a mixed population of small mature lymphocytes, vacuolated macrophages, and neutrophils. • Thoracic chylous effusions are usually caused by leakage of lymphatic vessels from trauma or obstruction due to neoplasia, cardiovascular disease, lung torsion, heartworm disease, mediastinal granulomas, and occasionally chronic coughing or vomiting. • Abdominal chylous effusion may be associated with malignant neoplasia, biliary cirrhosis, lymphatic leakage, or obstruction of the thoracic duct.
Pseudochylous	• Pseudochylous effusions are usually secondary to chronic peritonitis or pleuritis and can be distinguished from true chylous effusions by the cholesterol content.
Malignant or neoplastic	• May be caused by blood or lymphatic vessel blockage and may be similar to modified transudates, hemorrhagic effusions, or exudates. Malignant or neoplastic cells may be identified. When undifferentiated malignant cells are present in the peritoneal effusion, determination of cell origin is very difficult.

Source: From Campbell [1].

and flotation solution. For the parasite eggs to float, the specific gravity of the solution must be greater than the eggs, therefore, different flotation solutions may provide different results. Several solutions are commonly available; magnesium sulfate, zinc sulphate, sodium nitrate, saturated salt, and modified Sheather's (sugar and formaldehyde).

Although reports are rare, domestic ferrets can be infected by helminth species that occur in dogs, cats, and other animals [5]. Among these are nematodes (*Toxascaris leonina*, *Toxocara cati*, *Ancylostoma* spp., *Spiroptera nasicola*) and cestodes (*Mesocestoides* spp., *Atriotaenia procyonis*, *Dipylidium caninum*) [5].

Wild rabbits have a variety of helminth parasites but few of these afflict pet rabbits [6]. The most frequently found nematode is suggested to be *Passalurus ambiguus*, which is usually non-pathogenic [6, 55]. Other parasites that can be found in rabbits include *Taenia pisiformis*, *Multiceps serialis*, *Ascaris columnaris*, and *Cittotaenia variabilis* [55, 56]. *Capillaria hepatica* can occasionally affect rabbits [57].

In a recent study in Italy, intestinal parasites were detected in 31.7% of pet guinea pigs. *Paraspidodera uncinata* eggs were found in 13.3%, while *Nippostrongylus*-like eggs were found in 10%. None of the animals were showing signs of disease [58]. In pet rabbits, coccidia can also be

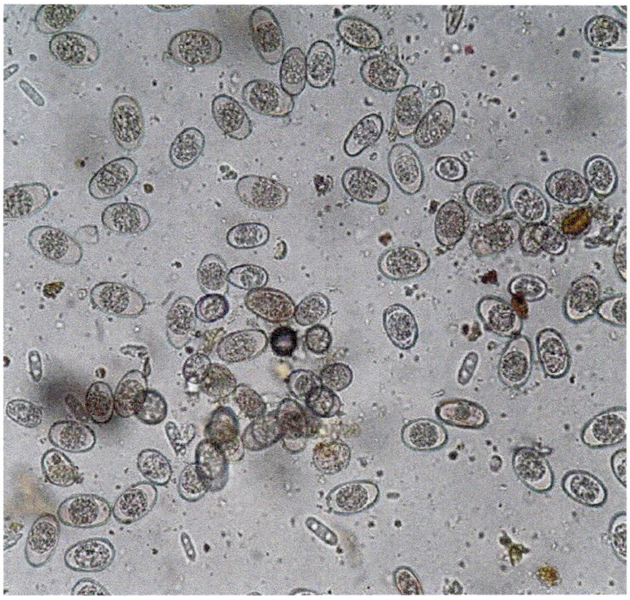

Figure 12.10 *Eimeria* sp. in a pet rabbit fecal flotation.

found in fecal flotations (Figure 12.10). Although intestinal cestodes or trematodes do not commonly cause disease in pet rabbits, these can host *Cittotaenia variabilis*, *Mosgovoyia pectinata americana*, *Mosgovoyia perplexa*, *Monoecocestus americana*, and *Ctenotaenia ctenoides*. Only *Ci. variabilis* has been found in domestic rabbits, whereas the other species are most often found in wild rabbits in North America and Europe [2, 52]. Zoonotic parasites such as *Rodentolepis (=Hymenolepis) nana* and *Rodentolepis microstoma* have been reported in rodents [59].

Gram Stain

Gram stain is used to identify microorganisms according to their staining characteristics which allow the differentiation between two large groups, Gram-positive and Gram-negative. The identification of a Gram-positive coiled and curved organisms on direct smear of the terminal ileum or cecum is suggestive of *Clostridium spiroforme*. In healthy rabbits, non-pathogenic, Gram-negative *Bacteroides* spp. predominate in a flora composed of a wide variety of Gram-positive and -negative rods, cocci, filaments, coccobacilli, and spirochetes [60]. The normal predominant bacteria in rodents' intestines are Gram-positive organisms such as Lactobacillus spp. and anaerobes such as *Bacteroides* spp.

Smear Cytology

Fecal cytology is performed by collecting a small sample of fresh fecal material. The sample should be spread on the slide making a thin layer of material. The slide is then stained with routine stains like Diff-quick. Other stains like acid-fast can also be performed. Examination of a stained smear of a fecal sample can be useful for the detection of numerous pathogens. Cryptosporidiosis commonly affects small mammals, causing chronic diarrhea, particularly in young animals. Diagnosis of cryptosporidial infection can be made from microscopic examination of concentrated fecal flotation samples or from acid-fast stains of fresh or formalin-fixed fecal smears or tissue sections [61, 62]. Intestinal candidiasis (*Candida albicans*) has been reported in a pet hedgehog [63].

Fecal cytology may also allow the identification of red blood cells which would be supportive of hemorrhage. Depending on the origin of the bleeding, the red blood cells may not be easily identified. The presence of white blood cells can also be suggestive of infection/inflammation. In ferrets, leukocytes may be seen on fecal cytology of animals with salmonellosis [64].

References

1 Campbell, T.W. (2015). Exotic Animal Hematology and Cytology. Wiley.

2 Quesenberry, K.E. and Carpenter, J.W. (2012). Ferrets, Rabbits, and Rodents : Clinical Medicine and Surgery, 3e. St. Louis, MO: Elsevier/Saunders.

3 Fisher, P.G. (2006). Exotic mammal renal disease: diagnosis and treatment. *Vet. Clin. North Am. Exot. Anim. Pract.* 9: 69–96.

4 Harcourt-Brown, F.M. (2013). Diagnosis of renal disease in rabbits. *Vet. Clin. North Am. Exot. Anim. Pract.* 16: 145–174.

5 Fox, J.G. and Marini, R.P. (2014). Biology and Diseases of the Ferret. Wiley.

6 Fudge, A.M. (2000). Laboratory Medi2cine: Avian and Exotic Pets. Philadelphia, PA: WB Saunders Company.

7 Suckow, M.A., Stevens, K.A., and Wilson, R.P. (2012). The Laboratory Rabbit, Guinea Pig, Hamster, and Other Rodents, 1e. London; Waltham, MA: Academic Press/ Elsevier.

8 Brown, C. (2006). Diagnostic cystocentesis: technique and considerations. *Lab. Anim. (NY)* 35: 21–23.

9 Harcourt-Brown, F. and Harcourt-Brown, N.H. (2002). Textbook of Rabbit Medicine. Butterworth-Heinemann.

10 Evans, E.E. and Souza, M.J. (2010). Advanced diagnostic approaches and current management of internal disorders

of select species (rodents, sugar gliders, hedgehogs). *Vet. Clin. North Am. Exot. Anim. Pract.* 13: 453–469.

11 Hauptman, K., Tichý, F., and Knotek, Z. (2001). Clinical diagnostics of hepatopathies in small mammals: evaluation of importance of individual methods. *Acta Vet. Brno* 70: 297–311.

12 Wingfield, W. and Raffe, M. (2002). The Veterinary ICU Book. Teton NewMedia.

13 Wyre, N.R. and Hess, L. (2005). Clinical technique: ferret thoracocentesis. *Semin. Avian Exot. Pet Med.*: 22–25.

14 McLaughlin, A. and Strunk, A. (2016). Common emergencies in small rodents, hedgehogs, and sugar gliders. *Vet. Clin. North Am. Exot. Anim. Pract.* 19: 465–499.

15 Jekl, V., Hauptman, K., and Knotek, Z. (2008). Quantitative and qualitative assessments of intraoral lesions in 180 small herbivorous mammals. *Vet. Rec.* 162: 442–449.

16 Lennox, A.M. and Miwa, Y. (2016). Anatomy and disorders of the oral cavity of miscellaneous exotic companion mammals. *Vet. Clin. North Am. Exot. Anim. Pract.* 19: 929–945.

17 Mans, C. and Jekl, V. (2016). Anatomy and disorders of the oral cavity of chinchillas and degus. *Vet. Clin. North Am. Exot. Anim. Pract.* 19: 843–869.

18 Legendre, L. (2016). Anatomy and disorders of the oral cavity of guinea pigs. *Vet. Clin. North Am. Exot. Anim. Pract.* 19: 825–842.

19 Barger, A.M. and MacNeill, A. (2016). Small Animal Cytologic Diagnosis. Boca Raton, FL: CRC Press.

20 Johnson-Delaney, C.A. (2016). Anatomy and disorders of the oral cavity of ferrets and other exotic companion carnivores. *Vet. Clin. North Am. Exot. Anim. Pract.* 19: 901–928.

21 Raskin, R.E. and Meyer, D. (2015). Canine and Feline Cytology: A Color Atlas and Interpretation Guide. Elsevier Health Sciences.

22 Vaden, S.L., Knoll, J.S., Smith, F.W. Jr. et al. (2009). Blackwell's Five-Minute Veterinary Consult: Laboratory Tests and Diagnostic Procedures, Canine and Feline. Wiley-Blackwell.

23 Ettinger, S.J. and Feldman, E.C. (2010). Textbook of veterinary internal medicine : diseases of the dog and the cat, 7e. St. Louis, MO: Elsevier Saunders.

24 Silverstein, D. and Hopper, K. (2008). Small Animal Critical Care Medicine. Elsevier Health Sciences.

25 Rakich, P.M. and Latimer, K.S. (2007). Cytologic diagnosis of diseases of ferrets. *Vet. Clin. North Am. Exot. Anim. Pract.* 10: 61–78.

26 Miller, W.H., Griffin, C.E., Campbell, K.L. et al. (2013). Muller and Kirk's Small Animal Dermatology 7: Muller and Kirk's Small Animal Dermatology. Elsevier Health Sciences.

27 Fehr, M. and Koestlinger, S. (2013). Ectoparasites in small exotic mammals. *Vet. Clin. North Am. Exot. Anim. Pract.* 16: 611–657.

28 Paterson, S. (2008). Skin Diseases of Exotic Pets. Wiley.

29 Gardhouse, S. and Eshar, D. (2015). Retrospective study of disease occurrence in captive African pygmy hedgehogs (*Atelerix albiventris*). *Isr. J. Vet. Med., Vet. Rec.* 143: 532–534.

30 Fredes, F. and Román, D. (2004). Fauna parasitaria en erizos de tierra africanos (*Atelerix albiventris*). *Parasitol. Latinoam.* 59: 79–81.

31 Demkowska-Kutrzepa, M., Tomczuk, K., Studzińska, M. et al. (2015). Caparinia tripilis in African hedgehog (*Atelerix albiventris*). *Vet. Dermatol.* 26: 73–75.

32 Pantchev, N. and Hofmann, T. (2006). Notoedric mange caused by *Notoedres cati* in a pet African pygmy hedgehog (*Atelerix albiventris*). *Vet. Rec.* 158: 59–60.

33 Kanfer, S. and Reavill, D.R. (2013). Cutaneous neoplasia in ferrets, rabbits, and Guinea pigs. *Vet. Clin. North Am. Exot. Anim. Pract.* 16: 579–598.

34 Garner, M.M. (2007). Cytologic diagnosis of diseases of rabbits, Guinea pigs, and rodents. *Vet. Clin. North Am. Exot. Anim. Pract.* 10: 25–49.

35 von Bomhard, W., Goldschmidt, M.H., Shofer, F.S. et al. (2007). Cutaneous neoplasms in pet rabbits: a retrospective study. *Vet. Pathol.* 44: 579–588.

36 Brandão, J., Blair, R., Kelly, A. et al. (2015). Amelanotic melanoma in the rabbit: a case report with an overview of immunohistochemical characterization. *J. Exot. Pet. Med.* 24: 193–200.

37 Vergneau-Grosset, C., Keel, M.K., Goldsmith, D. et al. (2016). Description of the prevalence, histologic characteristics, concomitant abnormalities, and outcomes of mammary gland tumors in companion rats (Rattus norvegicus): 100 cases (1990–2015). *J. Am. Vet. Med. Assoc.* 249: 1170–1179.

38 Juan-Sallés, C. and Garner, M.M. (2007). Cytologic diagnosis of diseases of hedgehogs. *Vet. Clin. North Am. Exot. Anim. Pract.* 10: 51–59.

39 Gelatt, K.N., Gilger, B.C., and Kern, T.J. (2012). Veterinary Ophthalmology. Wiley.

40 Coster, M.E., Stiles, J., Krohne, S.G., and Raskin, R.E. (2008). Results of diagnostic ophthalmic testing in healthy guinea pigs. *J. Am. Vet. Med. Assoc.* 232 (12): 1825–1833.

41 Lima, L., Montiani-Ferreira, F., Tramontin, M. et al. (2010). The chinchilla eye: morphologic observations, echobiometric findings and reference values for selected ophthalmic diagnostic tests. *Vet. Ophthalmol.* 13 (s1): 14–25.

42 Montiani-Ferreira, F., Mattos, B.C., and Russ, H.H.A. (2006). Reference values for selected ophthalmic

diagnostic tests of the ferret (*Mustela putorius* furo). *Vet. Ophthalmol.* 9 (4): 209–213.

43 Hoare, C.A. (1927). On the coccidia of the ferret. *Ann. Trop. Med. Parasitol.* 21: 313–320.

44 Sledge, D.G., Bolin, S.R., Lim, A. et al. (2011). Outbreaks of severe enteric disease associated with *Eimeria furonis* infection in ferrets (*Mustela putorius* furo) of 3 densely populated groups. *J. Am. Vet. Med. Assoc.* 239: 1584–1588.

45 Williams, B., Chimes, M., and Gardiner, C. (1996). Biliary coccidiosis in a ferret (*Mustela putorius* furo). *Vet. Pathol. Online* 33: 437–439.

46 Kaye, S.W., Ossiboff, R.J., Noonan, B. et al. (2015). Biliary coccidiosis associated with immunosuppressive treatment of pure red cell aplasia in an adult ferret (*Mustela putorius* furo). *J. Exot. Pet. Med.* 24: 215–222.

47 Pakandl, M. (2009). Coccidia of rabbit: a review. *Folia Parasitol.* 56: 153.

48 Rigby, C. (1976). Natural infections of guinea-pigs. *Lab. Anim.* 10: 119–142.

49 Hawkins, M.G. and Graham, J.E. (2007). Emergency and critical care of rodents. *Vet. Clin. North Am. Exot. Anim. Pract.* 10: 501–531.

50 Veronesi, F., Fioretti, D.P., Morganti, G. et al. (2012). Occurrence of *Giardia duodenalis* infection in chinchillas (*Chincilla lanigera*) from Italian breeding facilities. *Res. Vet. Sci.* 93: 807–810.

51 Mitchell, M. and Tully, T.N. Jr. (2008). Manual of Exotic Pet Practice. Elsevier Health Sciences.

52 Feely, D.E. and Erlandsen, S.L. (1981). Isolation and purification of giardia trophozoites from rat intestine. *J. Parasitol.*: 59–64.

53 Brust, D. and Pye, G. (2009). Sugar gliders. *Exot. DVM* 11: 32–41.

54 Brust, D.M. (2013). Gastrointestinal diseases of marsupials. *J. Exot. Pet. Med.* 22: 132–140.

55 Morrisey, J.K. (1996). Parasites of ferrets, rabbits, and rodents. *Semin. Avian Exot. Pet Med.*: 106–114.

56 Patton NM, Hagen KW, Gorham JR, et al. (2008). Domestic rabbits: Diseases and parasites: [Covallis, Or.]. Oregon State University Extension Service.

57 Mowat, V., Turton, J., Stewart, J. et al. (2009). Histopathological features of *Capillaria hepatica* infection in laboratory rabbits. *Toxicol. Pathol.*

58 d'Ovidio, D., Noviello, E., Ianniello, D. et al. (2015). Survey of endoparasites in pet guinea pigs in Italy. *Parasitol. Res.* 114: 1213–1216.

59 Macnish, M.G., Ryan, U.M., Behnke, J.M., and Thompson, R.C.A. (2003). Detection of the rodent tapeworm *Rodentolepis* (= *Hymenolepis*) microstoma in humans. A new zoonosis? *Int. J. Parasitol.* 33 (10): 1079–1085.

60 Varga, M. (2013). Textbook of Rabbit Medicine. Elsevier Health Sciences.

61 Harkness, J.E., Turner, P.V., VandeWoude, S. et al. (2013). Harkness and Wagner's Biology and Medicine of Rabbits and Rodents. Wiley.

62 Lv, C., Zhang, L., Wang, R. et al. (2009). *Cryptosporidium* spp. in wild, laboratory, and pet rodents in China: prevalence and molecular characterization. *Appl. Environ. Microbiol.* 75: 7692–7699.

63 Campbell, T. (1997). Intestinal candidiasis in an African hedgehog (*Atelerix albiventris*). *Exot. Pet. Pract.* 2: 79–79.

64 Powers, L.V. (2009). Bacterial and parasitic diseases of ferrets. *Vet. Clin. North Am. Exot. Anim. Pract.* 12: 531–561.

13

Ancillary Diagnostics

João Brandão

Department of Veterinary Clinical Sciences, College of Veterinary Medicine, Oklahoma State University, Oklahoma, USA

CONTENTS

Infectious Disease Assessments

Culture and Sensitivity Testing

Microbiological culture is a method of multiplying microbial organisms in a predetermined culture media under laboratory conditions. Antibacterial sensitivity is performed by exposing those bacteria to specific concentrations of antibiotic. Most commercially available microbiology laboratories perform bacterial culture and sensitivity in exotic species.

Although differences in the standard growth media may exist between laboratories, the most commonly used media are MacConkey agar (differential for lactose fermentation and selects Gram negative bacteria), Columbia naladixic acid agar (selects Gram positive bacteria), and blood agar (demonstrates hemolytic properties and is selective for *Streptococcus sp.*). Other specific media can be utilized depending on microbiology results or clinical indications. For examples, *Mycobacterium sp.* need specific media to provide adequate growth.

Identification of bacteria is typically performed using biochemical reactions and phenotypic characteristics which allow the differentiation of the bacteria. With the advent of molecular testing, several newer techniques can be used to identify the bacteria based on genetic sequencing. The most commonly used methods are 16S rRNA and 26S rRNA. These methods have facilitated the detection and identification of unculturable microorganisms [1]. The 16S rRNA gene sequence analysis can better identify poorly described, rarely isolated, or phenotypically aberrant strains and can lead to the recognition of novel pathogens and non-cultured bacteria [2]. These methods allow the sequence of a specific fragment which are then compared to databases. This method only allows the identification of the organism and does not provide data in terms of antibiotic sensitivity.

Most laboratories will provide standard antimicrobial sensitivities. However, this information is not necessarily applicable to exotic mammals. Many of the antibiotics that are commonly tested are not described in exotic mammals and/or may cause significant side effects. In some cases, contacting the laboratory to establish a specific antimicrobial sensitive panel may be possible. Special requests for specific antibiotics may also be beneficial.

PCR Screens

Polymerase chain reaction (PCR) methodology is a technique used in molecular biology to amplify a small number of copies of DNA pieces across several orders of magnitude, generating thousands to millions of copies of a particular DNA sequence. This may allow the identification of some specific disease related organisms, which may suggest that the patient is carrying or shedding a certain organism.

Exotic Animal Emergency and Critical Care Medicine, First Edition. Edited by Jennifer E. Graham, Grayson A. Doss and Hugues Beaufrère.

There are several tests available that can be used in exotic animal practice. Many of these tests were originally designed for laboratory animals but can be used in exotic pet mammals. Rats and mice may be the species that benefit the most. PCR can be used to test for bacteria (e.g. *Mycoplasma pulmonis*), viruses (e.g. rat coronavirus or sialodacryoadenitis virus), fungi (e.g. *Pneumocystis spp.*), or parasites (e.g. pinworms and fur mites). Other species that can benefit as well are: guinea pig (guinea pig adenovirus), hamsters (hamster parvovirus), or rabbits (*Pasteurella multocida*). Many laboratory animal specialized laboratories provide molecular testing for these diseases.

PCR has long been used to determine the health status of laboratorial animals and used to produce and maintain specific pathogen-free animals. Although the degree of health assessment and disease control in laboratory facilities cannot be expected in pet exotic animals, clinicians can also benefit from these methodologies. The most common samples submitted to be tested by PCR include blood (whole blood, serum, or plasma), feces, and/or skin swabs.

Serology

Serology is a common diagnostic test that is used to assess the presence of antibodies against specific disease. Most commercial laboratories offer enzyme-linked immunosorbent assays (ELISAs); however, immunofluorescent assays and hemagglutination inhibition assay tests are sometimes used [3]. A positive serological titer reflects only that antibody for a disease is present which may indicate exposure, but is not necessarily indicative of true active disease. The absence of antigen may not indicate the absence of disease [3, 4]. Titers correspond to the last sample dilution that resulted in a positive reaction on the ELISA plate [4]. The basis of titer analysis is that a high initial titer correlates to the severity of the infectious disease state of the patient on presentation, and a drop in titer during and after treatment is indicative of an improved health status owing to a diminished immune response because of a reduced population of organisms present in the patient's body [4]. Therefore, optimal utilization of serological tests involves paired titers to determine changes of the titer values. As for PCR, several serologic tests are commercially available. Many of these tests are available at laboratories specialized in research animals.

Toxicology Assessments

Rodenticide

Rodenticides are commonly used to reduce the number of wild rodents in the vicinity of houses or industrial areas. The same way these toxic products are efficient to kill wild rodents, and they also cause mortality among pet exotic mammals. The most common types of rodenticides are metal phosphides, hypercalcemic or cholecalciferol based, and anticoagulants. Metal phosphide rodenticides (e.g. zinc phosphide) act as a respiratory poison because once ingested are decomposed into highly toxic phosphine gas by the action of stomach hydrochloric acid [5]. Zinc phosphide is commonly used around the world due to its relative safety record, low cost, and reasonably high efficacy against a range of target rodent species [6]. Hypercalcemic rodenticides consist of cholecalciferol or other similar molecules. These products cause changes to the normal calcium metabolism, leading to a marked increase in plasma calcium levels, leading to metastatic calcification and acute renal failure[7]. In wild European rabbits, the cholecalciferol lethal dose 50 (LD_{50}) has been reported to be 9 mg/kg, while the lethal dose 95 (LD_{95}) was 18 mg/kg [8]. Wild rabbits are more sensitive to it than any other species tested [9]. For example, the rat LD_{50} is 43.6 mg/kg, while the mouse is 42.5 mg/kg [10]. This may be related to the unique calcium homeostasis of rabbits [11]. Anticoagulant rodenticides are defined as single-dose (second generation [bromadiolone, chlorophacinone, diphacinone, brodifacoum, and difethialone]) or multiple-dose (first generation [warfarin]) rodenticides. Anticoagulant rodenticides cause mortality due to effects on the coagulation cascade. These agents interfere with the liver's production of clotting factors II, VI, IX, and X and inhibit the vitamin K1 epoxide reductase, leading to internal hemorrhages approximately three to seven days after ingestion [7, 12].

Clinical signs associated with cholecalciferol rodenticide toxicity will be associated with renal disease and potential organ dysfunction due to metastatic calcification. Therefore, clinical signs will most likely be non-specific and clinical suspicion of cholecalciferol toxicity will most likely be based on history of ingestion of bait or blood chemistry. Blood chemistry will most likely show significant elevation of total and ionized calcium, elevation of phosphorus, and renal changes. On radiographs, identification of metastatic calcification (kidneys, aorta, liver) may be visible as well. Definitive diagnosis of cholecalciferol toxicity requires measurement of circulating cholecalciferol. This test is available commercially in some laboratories, mainly endocrinology specialized laboratories. Unfortunately, circulating levels of cholecalciferol are species specific and this information may not be readily available for some species. Nevertheless, after ingestion of cholecalciferol rodenticides, circulating cholecalciferol should be significantly high, which in combination with other diagnostic tests (hypercalcemia and/or metastatic calcification) should be sufficient to make a presumptive diagnosis. Reference values for calcium metabolism-related parameters (25-hydroxycholecalciferol, 1,25-dihydroxycholecalciferol,

Table 13.1 Normal prothrombin time (PT) and activated partial thromboplastin time (aPTT) for several exotic mammal species.

Species	PT (s)	PTT (s)	References	Notes
Ferret	15.7 ± 0.4 (14.4–16.5)	54.9 ± 3.7 (38.9–67.1)	[22]	Albino
	14–17	15–22	[23]	Young adult
Rat	12–18	17–27	[23]	Young adult Sprague Dawley
Mouse	7–20	7–18	[23]	Young adult CD-1
Hamster	8–15		[23]	Adult Syrian hamster
Guinea pig	20–32	20–35	[23]	Adult
Rabbit	6–9	14–22	[23]	Young adult New Zealand white rabbit

total calcium, and ionized calcium) have been reported in several species, specifically, rats [13], rabbits [14–17], chinchillas [18], and guinea pigs [19].

Anticoagulant rodenticides cause hemorrhage and blood loss. The clinical signs associated with this toxicity may be non-specific, although owners may notice spontaneous bleeding, petechia, or melena. Hematology of intoxicated animals may show hypochromic anemia, leukocytosis with neutrophilia, thrombocytopenia, enhanced erythrocyte sedimentation rate, and decreased mean corpuscular volume [20]. Chemistry may show hypoproteinemia, hypoalbuminemia, hyperglycemia, bilirubinemia, increased urea concentration, and increased alanine aminotransferase, alkaline phosphatase, and gamma glutamyltransferase [20].

Other specific methodologies can be used to investigate the coagulation profile. The most common tests include prothrombin time (PT) and activated partial thromboplastin time (aPTT). The PT measures the activity of the extrinsic and common coagulation pathways, while aPTT assesses the integrity of the intrinsic and common pathways [21]. These tests can be performed by most clinical laboratories. Although some reference values have been reported, there is limited information (Table 13.1). In the case of anticoagulant rodenticide toxicity, the PT and aPTT should be prolonged. Note that this test requires the use of sodium citrate anticoagulant.

Newer methodologies, particularly viscoelastography, are gaining popularity in small animal medicine and most likely will be commonly used in exotic mammals in the near future. While conventional hemostasis tests (PT/aPTT) evaluate individual components of coagulation without considering interaction of the blood components, viscoelastography measures the viscoelastic properties of clot formation in whole blood. Thromboelastography (TEG®), rotational thromboelastometry (ROTEM®), and dynamic viscoelastic coagulometry (Sonoclot®) provide a global assessment of coagulation, including information about clot kinetics, clot strength, and fibrinolysis [21]. To the author's knowledge, there are limited numbers of studies assessing these methodologies. Rabbits were used to investigate the influence of induced hypothermia on Sonoclot and TEG coagulation profiles [24]. Unfortunately, due to the experimental design, results are of limited clinical use. TEG reference values have been reported in rats, mice, and rabbits [25].

Heavy Metal Screening

In the strict chemical designation, heavy metals are defined as metals that do not normally occur in living organisms (e.g. mercury, lead, cadmium) and can cause illness; while in a medical context, the term heavy metal generally refers to any metal that is potentially toxic. The most common heavy metals causing disease are lead, zinc, and copper, and less commonly, mercury and iron. Heavy metal toxicity is a common problem in small animals; however, it does not seem that toxicosis in exotic animals are commonly reported to Animal Poison Control centers [26, 27].

It is said that lead toxicity is common in pet rabbits living in houses with lead paint; however, other products like golf balls, improperly glazed ceramics, linoleum glue, metallic objects containing lead, and lead soldering can also be the source of the toxin [7]. Clinical presentation includes hyporexia progressing to anorexia. Other signs include behavioral changes; neurologic abnormalities such as seizures, torticollis, and blindness; and chronic loss of body condition [7]. Protracted diarrhea has also been noted by one of the editors (JEG). Other physical examination findings may include cardiac arrhythmias and hypertension. In induced lead toxicosis in rabbits, the relative weights of the heart and liver were increased [28]. Plasma biochemistry is usually unremarkable in rabbits but hematology may reveal anemia with a reticulocytosis and nucleated erythrocytes, hypochromasia, poikilocytosis, anisocytosis, and basophilic stippling of the erythrocytes [7]. Nevertheless, none of these findings are pathognomonic for lead toxicosis. Definitive diagnosis requires determination of lead levels in the blood. As lead is present in the red blood cells, heparinized or ethylenediaminetetraacetic acid (EDTA) whole blood sample is necessary for testing (Table 13.2). It is advisable to contact the laboratory to confirm the type of samples that are needed prior to sample submission. Blood levels greater than 10 μg/dl are considered diagnostic for lead poisoning [29].

Zinc toxicity usually causes similar clinical signs to lead. Zinc toxicity has been induced in ferrets fed a variety of diets with zinc and in an outbreak of illness in ferrets fed exclusively on raw meat which was accidentally contaminated with a zinc compound [30, 31]. In groups fed 1500 and 3000 ppm of zinc, severe signs of toxicity were noted between one to two weeks, and ferrets on the 3000 ppm diet died in less than two weeks [30]. The lesions included diffuse nephrosis, hemorrhages in the intestine, and severe macrocytic hypochromic anemia [30]. This study concluded that ferrets are more susceptible to excesses of dietary zinc than other species. Interestingly, American mink (*Neovison vison*) have been shown to be significantly more resistant to dietary zinc than ferrets [32]. Although diagnostic blood levels of zinc are not reported, organ levels have been reported in sick and healthy animals. Normal ferrets had 114, 98, 90, and 85 ppm dry weight in the livers and 110, 102, 128, and 119 ppm in the kidneys, while diseased animals had 881 and 203 ppm dry weight in the livers and 943 and 785 ppm in the kidneys [31].

Rabbits are sensitive to excess copper exposure, accumulating surplus dietary copper in the liver which may lead to hepatocellular damage and acute hemolysis secondary to stress. Most common sources are diets with copper as well as food prepared in copper cookware, copper piping, and water from ornamental copper fountains [33]. Copper toxicosis was diagnosed in two sibling ferrets, based on high hepatic copper concentrations and histologic changes in hepatic tissue [34]. Clinical signs were mostly non-specific and included severe central nervous system depression with hypothermia and hyperthermia, and one was icteric [34]. Both ferrets died within a few days of presentation. A potential genetic predisposition was suggested [34]. To this date, no diagnostic copper levels have been published in ferrets but current investigations suggest that copper hepatopathy is relatively common in ferrets [35, 36]. A recent analysis of 10 ferret diets revealed a median copper concentration of 8.8 mg/1000 kcal, seven times the recommended minimum for cats (1.25 mg/1000 kcal) [37].

Table 13.2 Preferred samples for heavy metal toxicity testing.

Metal	Sample
Lead	Heparin or EDTA whole blood
Zinc	Serum or heparin plasma; do not use EDTA plasma
Copper	Liver biopsy for histology and copper quantification

Metabolic/Endocrine Assessments

Endocrine Panels

The endocrine system contains specialized tissues/cells that synthesize, store, and release their secretions directly into the bloodstream. With the exception of the pancreas, liver, and kidney, the endocrine glands lack a duct system [38]. The main function of the endocrine system is to maintain normal metabolic function through internal and external environmental variation, a balance achieved through secretion of different hormones, some antagonistic, and others synergistic [39].

Several endocrine organs are controlled by the hypothalamus–pituitary axis. The most significant of these are the hypothalamic–pituitary–thyroid (HPT), the hypothalamic–pituitary–adrenal (HPA), and the hypothalamic–pituitary–gonadal (HPG).

Thyroid

The thyroid function is controlled by a negative feedback loop that influences the HPT axis. The hypothalamus produces thyrotropin-releasing hormone (TRH), which stimulates the pituitary to produce thyrotropin or thyroid-stimulating hormone (TSH) that in turn stimulates the thyroid gland to produce thyroxine (T_4) and triiodothyronine (T_3). Commonly, thyroid function is assessed by the measurement of circulating thyroid hormones. In dogs, total thyroxine (TT_4) is only useful if the value is normal or elevated [40]. This is probably similar in exotic animals. In human medicine, TT_4 is not commonly used because it is unreliable and other non-thyroidal diseases can significantly decrease the values although the thyroid function is normal (euthyroid sick syndrome). Although in severe non-thyroidal illness, both total triiodothyronine (TT_3) and TT_4 decrease; in mild cases, only TT_3 decreases [41]. Free hormone measurement is a more sensitive test, and the decreases in free thyroxine (fT_4) and free triiodothyronine (fT_3) are usually more modest in cases of euthyroid sick syndrome [42]. In the author's opinion, complete thyroid hormone panel including TT_4, TT_3, fT_4, and fT_3 should be performed when assessing the thyroid function of exotic animals. Overall, due to the limited published information in regard to exotic animals, thyroid assessment is challenging and other diagnostic tests should also be pursued as well (e.g. scintigraphy, stimulation tests). Furthermore, single measurement of thyroid hormones may not be reliable due to physiological variations. For that reason, suspected cases should be reassessed and thyroid panels should be repeated.

Among small mammals, the guinea pig is well known to develop thyroid tumors and hyperthyroidism. Thyroid neoplasia is one of the most common neoplasms (3.6%) detected in guinea pigs by one laboratory service [43]. Two cases of idiopathic hyperthyroidism have been described in pet rabbits [44]. Concurrent diabetes mellitus and hyperthyroidism have been reported in a chinchilla [45]. Ferret hypothyroidism has been diagnosed in seven cases based on low basal TT_4 values and a limited response (<1.4-fold increase) in TT_4 after a TSH stimulation test [46]. Human recombinant TSH stimulation test has been validated in ferrets [47]. Normal reference intervals for thyroid hormones (TT_4, TT_3, fT_4, and fT_3) have been previously reported in guinea pigs [13, 47–51], rabbits [13, 52–54], rats [13, 55], and ferrets [56–58].

Glucose Metabolism

The pancreas has both exocrine and endocrine sections. The endocrine pancreas is composed of several types of cells: alpha (α) cells (glucagon), beta (β) cells (insulin and amylin), delta (δ) cells (somatostatin), pancreatic polypeptide (PP) cells, and epsilon (ε) cells (ghrelin) [59–61]. Of all the hormones produced by the endocrine pancreas, insulin is one of the most clinically relevant. A common pancreatic neoplasia in ferrets is the insulinoma. Insulinomas are endocrinologically active insulin-secreting tumor of the pancreatic β cells [62–64]. Hyperinsulinemia causes hypoglycemia by increased uptake of glucose by muscle tissue, fat, and the liver, and suppression of hepatic glycogenolysis and gluconeogenesis [65]. Neoplastic islet cells continue to produce insulin due to lack of negative feedback [65]. Among exotic species, insulinomas are one of the two most common (~25% of all neoplasms) neoplasms of middle-aged to older ferrets [66, 67]. Both spontaneous and induced insulinomas have been reported in laboratory rats. The prevalence of spontaneous islet cell adenoma in aged laboratory rats appears to be low, with pancreatic islet cell adenomas reported to represent 2–6% of all tumors [68–70]. There have been a limited number of case reports of insulinomas in guinea pigs [71, 72]. Insulinoma was incidentally detected in one rabbit during a study assessing the usefulness of blood glucose measurement in pet rabbits [73].

Hypoglycemia alone should not be considered pathognomonic of insulinoma because it can also be cause by other diseases (e.g. sepsis, hepatic disease) [63, 74, 75]. Although the definitive diagnosis of insulinoma requires histopathology, concurrent hypoglycemia with hyperinsulinemia is highly indicative of insulinoma [63, 65, 74]. Nevertheless, due to the high prevalence of insulinoma in ferrets, hypoglycemia without evidence of other diseases is highly suggestive of insulinoma, but paired measurement of insulin and glucose is recommended to determine potential paradoxical values. Fructosamine levels and fructosamine–albumin ratio do not appear useful to investigate insulinoma-associated chronic hypoglycemia in ferrets [76] (Table 13.3).

Adrenal Gland

The adrenal gland is divided into cortical and medullary regions. The adrenal medulla is composed of chromaffin cells and paraganglia, which produce epinephrine, norepinephrine, and dopamine [62, 84–86]. The adrenal cortex is comprised of three zones: zona glomerulosa, fasciculata, and reticularis [62, 87]. The different sections of the cortex produce aldosterone, cortisol, dehydroepiandrosterone, and androstenedione [62, 87]. Adrenal glands of ferrets and some other species contain unique anatomical characteristics and less prominent layers may be present: the zona intermedia, the juxtamedullaris, and the X zone [88, 89]. In mice and ferrets, the neoplastic adrenocortical cells resemble gonadal steroidogenic cells which arise from the juxtamedullary region [90].

Table 13.3 Normal values of hormones associated with glucose metabolism.

Species	Insulin (pmol/l)	Fructosamine (μmol/l)	Glucose (mg/dl)	References
Ferret	67.5–137.6		91.4–110.3	[58]
		163 (121.1–201.6)	108.1 (54–153.2)	[57]
Rabbit	~193.7		~117	[77]
	57.4 ± 14.4		131 ± 2	[78]
	19.2 ± 4.2	287 ± 25	104.3 ± 4.7	[79]
	144.2 ± 1.4	288 ± 8.6	99 ± 8	[80]
	145.7 ± 4.3	272 ± 7.8	90.1 ± 5	[80]
Guinea pig		134–271	89–287	[81]
	373.1 ± 43.1		150 ± 5	[82]
	296.3 ± 29.4		114.3 ± 3.2	[83]

Ferret adrenal gland disease is a form of hyperadrenocorticism caused by adrenal cortex tissue hypertrophy and/or neoplasm which results in the overproduction of one or more steroid hormones (e.g. glucocorticoids, mineralocorticoids, androgens) [66]. This condition differs from Cushing's syndrome because the latter is characterized by elevated cortisol levels due to adrenocorticotropic hormone (ACTH)-secreting pituitary tumor or a cortisol-secreting adrenal tumor [66]. It has been historically suggested that removal of gonadal tissue at an early age may lead to adrenal gland disease [91]. However, it has been shown that the predisposing factor related to the development of hyperadrenocorticism in ferrets is most likely the neutering procedure itself, independent of the age at which it is performed [91].

Although ultrasound is an excellent diagnostic test for adrenal gland disease, blood level measurement of estradiol, androstenedione, and 17α-hydroxyprogesterone may also be beneficial [66]. Estradiol, androstenedione, and 17α-hydroxyprogesterone, in neutered ferrets, are normally very low, but may be elevated in patients with cases of adrenocortical disease [66].

Similar diseases to ferret adrenal gland disease have been reported in rabbits. Hypertestosteronism secondary to adrenal neoplasia and hyperplasia, with increased sexual and aggressive behavior, has been reported in older neutered rabbits [92, 93]. Sex steroid panels are also available for rabbits [94].

Bone Marrow Assessments

The bone marrow is responsible for medullary hematopoiesis. Extramedullary hematopoiesis (spleen, liver, and lymph nodes) commonly occurs in a number of healthy mammals, such as rodents and ferrets [95]. Hematopoiesis begins with the pluripotent stem cell that produces the committed progenitor cells that differentiate into the different cell lines: erythrocytes, granulocytes, megakaryocytes, monocytes, and lymphocytes [95]. Pluripotent stem cells resemble lymphocytes when stained with routine Romanowsky; therefore, the bone marrow examination only differentiates cells, such as erythrocytic cell lines, granulocytic cell lines, and megakaryocytes [95].

Bone marrow aspiration may be a valuable diagnostic tool in ferrets as in other small animals [96]. The main indications for bone marrow examination include neoplasia, hematologic disorders, anemia, thrombocytopenia, gammopathies, and lymphoproliferative disorders [97]. Bone marrow examination is usually recommended when primary or secondary hematologic disorders are present but cannot be explained by peripheral blood examination alone [98]. The most common sites for bone marrow aspiration and biopsy are the proximal femur, proximal tibia, proximal humerus, and the ileum [97]. General anesthesia and local anesthetic infiltration are recommended [97]. Bone marrow aspirate and biopsy have been described for ferrets, rabbits, guinea pigs, and mice [96, 99–102]. An 18- to 20-gauge, 1.5-in. spinal needle or Jamshidi biopsy needle may be used to collect bone marrow sample into a syringe [96]. If no stylet is used, a bone core may be lodged in the hub of the needle which will prevent aspiration [96]. In this case, the original needle may be withdrawn and a new needle of equal size may be reinserted in the same site and the marrow aspirated [96]. For biopsy sample collection, penetration of both cortices and exiting the skin through the opposite side may be attempted to preserve the core [99]. A stylet can be used to push the sample out before removing the needle [99].

Examination of bone marrow should include determination of the myeloid:erythroid (M:E) ratio, which generally ranges from 0.5:1 to 3:1 (Table 13.4) [98]. The maturation index (proliferation index; the ratio of proliferating to non-proliferating cells) is useful for characterizing abnormalities of maturation and verifying subjective interpretations of ineffective hematopoiesis.

The bone marrow evaluation of exotic mammals is the same as that of small animals [95]. Bone marrow hypoplasia can result from chemical toxicity, infectious disease, estrogen toxicity, myelofibrosis, or immune-mediated disorders [98]. In ferrets, the administration of estrogen induced severe bone marrow depression independently of sex or ovariohysterectomy [103]. Pancytopenia manifested by subcutaneous petechiae, melena, hematomyelia, pale mucous membranes, pale bone marrow, centrilobular hepatic degeneration, hydrometra, and pyometra [103]. Bone marrow hypoplasia can occur secondary to pro-

Table 13.4 Normal myeloid:erythroid ratio in exotic mammals.

Species	Myeloid:erythroid ratio	References
Rat	1.16:1–1.36:1	[98]
Mice	0.75:1–2.35:1	[98]
Gerbils	0.75:1–2.35:1	[98]
Guinea pig	1.5:1–1.9:1	[81, 98]
Chinchilla	0.9:1–1.1:1	[81]
Rabbit	1 : 1	[95]
Ferret	2.3 :1–4.5:1	[95]

longed estrus [104]. The lack of cells from all cell lines is an indication of bone marrow aplasia [98]. Immune-mediated pure red cell aplasia was diagnosed in a ferret on the basis of cytological evaluation of a bone marrow biopsy [105]. Bone marrow hyperplasia is usually associated with regenerative response to peripheral blood loss [98]. Hyperplasia can also result from neoplastic disorders, such as lymphoproliferative or myeloproliferative diseases [98].

Endoscopy

Endoscopy is typically non-invasive to minimally invasive and allows the assessment of internal structures using different types of endoscopes. Flexible endoscopes are commonly used to assess the gastrointestinal tract in mammals. Animals should be anesthetized for gastroscopy and intubated. Intubation is recommended as inflation of the stomach can depress respiratory function by diaphragm compression, thus limiting the depth of inspiration, as well as reduce the risk of pulmonary aspiration (irrigation or gastric fluids) [106]. In dogs and cats, the patient is usually positioned in left lateral recumbency as this position improves the gastric examination [106]. Nevertheless, ventral recumbency can also be used [106].

In terms of emergency presentations, a common indication for endoscopy is foreign body removal. If the owners report a recent ingestion of a foreign body, endoscopy is a good minimally invasive method that may allow the retrieval of the object. Previous diagnostic tests to confirm the ingestion of the foreign body are recommended. When gastrointestinal perforation is suspected, endoscopy may be contraindicated because insufflation during the procedure can result in bacterial contamination of the peritoneum [106]. Endoscopy is also contraindicated in animals with coagulopathies [106].

Rigid endoscopes are commonly used in birds but can also be used in mammals. Oral examination is routinely performed using otoscopes or nasal specula; however, in awake animals, extensive evaluation of the oral cavity may not be possible. Alternatively, in anesthetized animals, rigid videoscopes may provide a higher quality assessment and allow data recording. Image capture can be used for future assessments and comparison. Endoscopes can also be used to assist with dental corrections. In rabbits with chronic upper respiratory disease, rhinoscopy is a diagnostic option that may help to identify granulomatous disease unlikely to respond to simple antibiotic therapy and may also identify nasal foreign bodies [107]. This procedure will most likely be limited by the size of the patient.

Although not commonly performed on emergency, transurethral cystoscopy, and endoscopic urolith removal has been reported in female guinea pigs [108, 109]. Transurethral cystoscopy is indicated in cases of lower urinary tract inflammation of unknown origin, urolithiasis, recurrent urinary tract infections, urinary incontinence, bladder and urethral masses, and anatomic abnormalities [109]. Transurethral cystoscopic urolith removal of the female guinea pig is feasible only if the calculi are smaller than the diameter of the urethra [109]. Larger calculi can be attempted to be broken with grasping forceps and potentially lithotripsy.

References

1 Baker, G., Smith, J.J., and Cowan, D.A. (2003). Review and re-analysis of domain-specific 16S primers. *J. Microbiol. Methods* 55: 541–555.

2 Clarridge, J.E. (2004). Impact of 16S rRNA gene sequence analysis for identification of bacteria on clinical microbiology and infectious diseases. *Clin. Microbiol. Rev.* 17: 840–862.

3 Jenkins, J.R. (2008). Rabbit diagnostic testing. *J. Exot. Pet. Med.* 17: 4–15.

4 Rich, G. (2010). Clinical update on testing modalities for *Encephalitozoon cuniculi* in clinically sick rabbits. *J. Exot. Pet. Med.* 19: 226–230.

5 Bumbrah, G.S., Krishan, K., Kanchan, T. et al. (2012). Phosphide poisoning: a review of literature. *Forensic Sci. Int.* 214: 1–6.

6 Staples, L., Smith, M., Pontin, K., and Hunt, W. (2003). Use of zinc phosphide to overcome rodent infestations. *Proc. Austral. Postharvest Techn. Confer. Canberra*: 110–115.

7 Johnston, M.S. (2008). Clinical toxicoses of domestic rabbits. *Vet. Clin. North Am. Exot. Anim. Pract.* 11: 315–326.

8 Eason, C. (1993). The acute toxicity of Cholecalciferol to the European rabbit, *Oryctolagus cuniculus*. *Wildl. Res.* 20: 173–176.

9 Williams, K., Parer, I., Coman, B. et al. (1995). Managing Vertebrate Pests: Rabbits. Australian Government Publishing Service.

10 Marshall, E. F. 1984. Cholecalciferol: a unique toxicant for rodent control. Proceedings of the Eleventh Vertebrate Pest Conference, March 6–8 1984, Sacramento, California. 95–98.

11 Brandão, J., Rick, M., and Mayer, J. (2015). Endocrinology of exotic species. In: Current Therapy in Exotic Pet Practice (eds. M. Mitchell and T. Tully). Elsevier.

12 Dunayer, E. (2008). Toxicology of ferrets. *Vet. Clin. North Am. Exot. Anim. Pract.* 11: 301–314.

13 Quimby, F.W. (1999). The Clinical Chemistry of Laboratory Animals. Philadelphia: Taylor & Francis.

14 Ardiaca, M., Bonvehi, C., and Montesinos, A. (2013). Point-of-care blood gas and electrolyte analysis in rabbits. *Vet. Clin. North Am. Exot. Anim. Pract.* 16: 175–195.

15 Bas, S., Aguilera-Tejero, E., Estepa, J.C. et al. (2002). The influence of acute and chronic hypercalcemia on the parathyroid hormone response to hypocalcemia in rabbits. *Eur. J. Endocrinol.* 146: 411–418.

16 Bas, S., Bas, A., Lopez, I. et al. (2005). Nutritional secondary hyperparathyroidism in rabbits. *Domest. Anim. Endocrinol.* 28: 380–390.

17 Emerson, J.A., Whittington, J.K., Allender, M.C., and Mitchell, M.A. (2014). Effects of ultraviolet radiation produced from artificial lights on serum 25-hydroxyvitamin D concentration in captive domestic rabbits (*Oryctolagus cuniculi*). *Am. J. Vet. Res.* 75: 380–384.

18 Rivas, A.E., Mitchell, M.A., Flower, J. et al. (2014). Effects of ultraviolet radiation on serum 25-hydroxyvitamin D concentrations in captive chinchillas (*Chinchilla laniger*). *J. Exot. Pet. Med.* 23: 270–276.

19 Watson, M.K., Stern, A.W., Labelle, A.L. et al. (2014). Evaluating the clinical and physiological effects of long term ultraviolet B radiation on guinea pigs (*Cavia porcellus*). *PLoS One* 9: e114413.

20 Valchev, I., Binev, R., Yordanova, V., and Nikolov, Y. (2008). Anticoagulant rodenticide intoxication in animals – a review. *Turk. J. Vet. Anim. Sci.* 32: 237–243.

21 Hyatt, C.E. and Brainard, B.M. (2016). Point-of-care assessment of coagulation. *Top. Companion Anim. Med.*

22 Thornton, P., Wright, P.A., Sacra, P., and Goodier, T. (1979). The ferret, Mustela putorius furo, as a new species in toxicology. *Lab. Anim.* 13: 119–124.

23 Gad, S.C. (2006). Animal Models in Toxicology. CRC Press.

24 Shimokawa, M., Kitaguchi, K., Kawaguchi, M. et al. (2003). The influence of induced hypothermia for hemostatic function on temperature-adjusted measurements in rabbits. *Anesth. Analg.* 96: 1209–1213.

25 Wiinberg, B. and Kristensen, A.T. (2010). Thromboelastography in veterinary medicine. In: Seminars in Thrombosis and Hemostasis, 747–756. Thieme Medical Publishers.

26 Caloni, F., Cortinovis, C., Rivolta, M., and Davanzo, F. (2012). Animal poisoning in Italy: 10 years of epidemiological data from the Poison Control Centre of Milan. *Vet. Rec.*: 170, 415–419.

27 Mclean, M.K. and Hansen, S.R. (2012). An overview of trends in animal poisoning cases in the United States: 2002–2010. *Vet. Clin. N. Am. Small Anim. Pract.* 42: 219–228.

28 Falke, H.E. and Zwennis, W.C. (1990). Toxicity of lead acetate to female rabbits after chronic subcutaneous administration. 1. Biochemical and clinical effects. *Arch. Toxicol.* 64: 522–529.

29 Fisher, P. and Carpenter, J.W. (2012). Neurologic and musculoskeletal diseases. In: Ferrets, rabbits, and rodents: clinical medicine and surgery (eds. K.E. Quesenberry and J.W. Carpenter), 245–256. St. Louis, Mo: Elsevier/Saunders.

30 Straube, E., Schuster, N., and Sinclair, A. (1980). Zinc toxicity in the ferret. *J. Comp. Pathol.* 90: 355–361.

31 Straube, E. and Walden, N. (1981). Zinc poisoning in ferrets (*Mustella putorls furo*). *Lab. Anim.* 15: 45–47.

32 Aulerich, R.J., Bursian, S.J., Poppenga, R.H. et al. (1991). Toleration of high concentrations of dietary zinc by mink. *J. Vet. Diagn. Investig.* 3: 232–237.

33 Murphy, L.A. (2015). Environmental toxicology: considerations for exotic pets. *J. Exot. Pet. Med.* 24: 390–397.

34 Fox, J., Zeman, D., and Mortimer, J. (1994). Copper toxicosis in sibling ferrets. *J. Am. Vet. Med. Assoc.* 205: 1154–1156.

35 Graham, J.E., Heinze, C., Beamer, G., and Webster, C. (2016). Management of Copper Toxicosis in a Ferret (Mustela putorius furo). Abstracts of ExoticsCon. Portland, Oregon: ExoticsCon.

36 Graham, J.E., Garner, M., Reavill, D., and Center, S.A. (2018). Preliminary Investigation into the Characterization of Hepatic Copper Concentration in Ferrets with and without Hepatobiliary Disease. Abstracts of ExoticsCon. Atlanta, GA: ExoticsCon.

37 Torkelson, M.R., Heinze, C.R., and Graham, J.E. (2019). Copper concentration in ten popular commercial ferret diets. In: Exoticscon 2019 Proceedings, 407–408.

38 Capen, C.C. (2008). Tumors of the endocrine glands. In: Tumors in Domestic Animals (ed. D.J. Meuten), 766–833. Ames, IA: Iowa State Press.

39 Marty, M.S., Carney, E.W., and Rowlands, J.C. (2011). Endocrine disruption: historical perspectives and its impact on the future of toxicology testing. *Toxicol. Sci.* 120 (Suppl 1): S93–S108.

40 Ferguson, D.C. (2007). Testing for hypothyroidism in dogs. *Vet. Clin. North Am. Small Anim. Pract.* 37: 647–669.

41 De Groot, L.J. (1999). Dangerous dogmas in medicine: the nonthyroidal illness syndrome. *J. Clin. Endocrinol. Metab.* 84: 151–164.

42 Warner, M.H. and Beckett, G.J. (2010). Mechanisms behind the non-thyroidal illness syndrome: an update. *J. Endocrinol.* 205: 1–13.

43 Gibbons, P.M., Garner, M.M., and Kiupel, M. (2012). Morphological and immunohistochemical characterization of spontaneous thyroid gland neoplasms in guinea pigs (*Cavia porcellus*). *Vet. Pathol.* 50: 334–342.

44 Brandão, J., Higbie, C., Rick, M., et al. (2015). Naturally Occurring Idiopathic Hyperthyroidism in Two Pet Rabbits. ExoticsCon 2015 Main Conference Proceedings. San Antonio, TX, USA.

45 Fritsche, R., Simova-Curd, S., Clauss, M., and Hatt, J.M. (2008). Hyperthyroidism in connection with suspected diabetes mellitus in a chinchilla (Chinchilla laniger). *Vet. Rec.* 163: 454–456.

46 Wagner, R. (2012). Hypothyroidism in Ferrets. Proceedings of the Association of Exotic Mammal Veterinary Conference, Oakland, California, October 20–October 26. 29–31.

47 Mayer, J., Wagner, R., Mitchell, M.A., and Fecteau, K. (2013). Use of recombinant human thyroid-stimulating hormone for thyrotropin stimulation testing in euthyroid ferrets. *J. Am. Vet. Med. Assoc.* 243: 1432–1435.

48 Anderson, R.R., Nixon, D.A., and Akasha, M.A. (1988). Total and free thyroxine and triiodothyronine in blood serum of mammals. *Comp. Biochem. Physiol. A Comp. Physiol.* 89: 401–404.

49 Castro, M.I., Alex, S., Young, R.A. et al. (1986). Total and free serum thyroid hormone concentrations in fetal and adult pregnant and nonpregnant Guinea pigs. *Endocrinology* 118: 533–537.

50 Fredholm, D.V., Cagle, L.A., and Johnston, M.S. (2012). Evaluation of precision and establishment of reference ranges for plasma thyroxine using a point-of-care analyzer in healthy guinea pigs (*Cavia porcellus*). *J. Exot. Pet. Med.* 21: 87–93.

51 Muller, K., Muller, E., Klein, R., and Brunnberg, L. (2009). Serum thyroxine concentrations in clinically healthy pet guinea pigs (*Cavia porcellus*). *Vet. Clin. Pathol.* 38: 507–510.

52 Brandao, J., Rick, M. and Tully, T. N. (2016). Measurement of Serum Free and Total Thyroxine and Triiodothyronine Concentrations in Rabbits. *Exoticscon 2016 Proceedings, Portland, Oregon, USA*, 485–486.

53 Mebis, L., Debaveye, Y., Ellger, B. et al. (2009). Changes in the central component of the hypothalamus-pituitary-thyroid axis in a rabbit model of prolonged critical illness. *Crit. Care* 13.

54 Mustafa, S., Al-Bader, M.D., Elgazzar, A.H. et al. (2008). Effect of hyperthermia on the function of thyroid gland. *Eur. J. Appl. Physiol.* 103: 285–288.

55 Takeuchi, A., Suzuki, M., and Tsuchiya, S. (1978). Effect of thyroidectomy on the secretory profiles of growth hormone, thyrotropin and corticosterone in the rat. *Endocrinol. Jpn.* 25: 381–390.

56 Garibaldi, B.A., Pecquet Goad, M.E., Fox, J.G., and Murray, R. (1988). Serum thyroxine and triiodothyronine radioimmunoassay values in the normal ferret. *Lab. Anim. Sci.* 38: 455–458.

57 Hein, J., Spreyer, F., Sauter-Louis, C., and Hartmann, K. (2012). Reference ranges for laboratory parameters in ferrets. *Vet. Rec.* 171: 218–223.

58 Prohaczik, A., Kulcsar, M., and Huszenicza, G. (2009). Metabolic and endocrine characteristics of pregnancy toxemia in the ferret. *Vet. Med.* 54: 75–80.

59 Andralojc, K., Mercalli, A., Nowak, K. et al. (2009). Ghrelin-producing epsilon cells in the developing and adult human pancreas. *Diabetologia* 52: 486–493.

60 Elayat, A.A., El-Naggar, M.M., and Tahir, M. (1995). An immunocytochemical and morphometric study of the rat pancreatic islets. *J. Anat.* 186: 629.

61 Wierup, N., Svensson, H., Mulder, H., and Sundler, F. (2002). The ghrelin cell: a novel developmentally regulated islet cell in the human pancreas. *Regul. Pept.* 107: 63–69.

62 Engelking, L. (2012). Metabolic and Endocrine Physiology. CRC Press.

63 Mellanby, R.J. and Herrtage, M.E. (2002). Insulinoma in a normoglycaemic dog with low serum fructosamine. *J. Small Anim. Pract.* 43: 506–508.

64 Polton, G.A., White, R.N., Brearley, M.J., and Eastwood, J.M. (2007). Improved survival in a retrospective cohort of 28 dogs with insulinoma. *J. Small Anim. Pract.* 48: 151–156.

65 Lester, N.V., Newell, S.M., Hill, R.C., and Lanz, O.I. (1999). Scintigraphic diagnosis of insulinoma in a dog. *Vet. Radiol. Ultrasound* 40: 174–178.

66 Chen, S. (2010). Advanced diagnostic approaches and current medical management of insulinomas and adrenocortical disease in ferrets (*Mustela putorius furo*). *Vet. Clin. North Am. Exot. Anim. Pract.* 13: 439–452.

67 Vinke, C.M. and Schoemaker, N.J. (2012). The welfare of ferrets (*Mustela putorius furo* T): a review on the housing and management of pet ferrets. *Appl. Anim. Behav. Sci.*

68 Bomhard, E. (1992). Frequency of spontaneous tumors in Wistar rats in 30-months studies. *Exp. Toxicol. Pathol.* 44: 381–392.

69 Bomhard, E., Karbe, E., and Loeser, E. (1986). Spontaneous tumors of 2000 Wistar TNO/W.70 rats in two-year carcinogenicity studies. *J. Environ. Pathol. Toxicol. Oncol.* 7: 35–52.

70 Walsh, K. and Poteracki, J. (1994). Spontaneous neoplasms in control Wistar rats. *Toxicol. Sci.* 22: 65–72.

71 Hess, L.R., Ravich, M.L., and Reavill, D.R. (2013). Diagnosis and treatment of an insulinoma in a guinea pig (*Cavia porcellus*). *J. Am. Vet. Med. Assoc.* 242: 522–526.

72 Künzel, F. and Mayer, J. (2015). Endocrine tumours in the guinea pig. *Vet. J.* 206: 268–274.

73 Harcourt-Brown, F. and Harcourt-Brown, S. (2012). Clinical value of blood glucose measurement in pet rabbits. *Vet. Rec.* 170: 674–674.

74 Kraje, A.C. (2003). Hypoglycemia and irreversible neurologic complications in a cat with insulinoma. *J. Am. Vet. Med. Assoc.* 223 (812–4): 810.

75 Syme, H.M. and Scott-Moncrieff, J.C. (1998). Chronic hypoglycaemia in a hunting dog due to secondary hypoadrenocorticism. *J. Small Anim. Pract.* 39: 348–351.

76 Duhamelle, A., Vlaemynck, F., Loeuillet, E., and Larrat, S. (2018). Clinical value of fructosamine measurements and fructosamine-albumin ratio in hypoglycemic ferrets (*Mustela putorius furo*). *J. Exot. Pet Med.* 27: 103–107.

77 Knudtzon, J. (1984). Plasma levels of glucagon, insulin, glucose and free fatty acids in rabbits during laboratory handling procedures. *Zeitschrift. für. Versuchstierkunde.* 26: 123.

78 Heding, L.G. and Anderson, H. (1973). Increased serum immunoreactive insulin in rabbits fed a protein- and mineral-rich diet. *Diabetologia* 9: 282–286.

79 Helfenstein, T., Fonseca, F.A., Ihara, S.S. et al. (2011). Impaired glucose tolerance plus hyperlipidaemia induced by diet promotes retina microaneurysms in New Zealand rabbits. *Int. J. Exp. Pathol.* 92: 40–49.

80 Ersan, B. and Ok, M. (2011). Importance of fasting serum glucose, haemoglobin A1c and fructosamine in the diagnosis of diabetes. *Euras. J. Vet. Sci.* 27: 13–18.

81 Quesenberry, K., Donnelly, T., and Mans, C. (2012). Biology, husbandry, and clinical techniques of guinea pigs and chinchillas. In: Ferrets, Rabbits, and Rodents: Clinical Medicine and Surgery (eds. K. Quesenberry and J.W. Carpenter), 279–294. St. Louis, Mo: Elsevier/Saunders.

82 Saudek, C.D., Finkowski, M., and Knopp, R.H. (1975). Plasma glucagon and insulin in rat pregnancy. Roles in glucose homeostasis. *J. Clin. Investig.* 55: 180.

83 Junod, A., Lambert, A.E., Stauffacher, W., and Renold, A.E. (1969). Diabetogenic action of streptozotocin: relationship of dose to metabolic response. *J. Clin. Invest.* 48: 2129–2139.

84 Fung, M., Viveros, O., and O'connor, D. (2008). Diseases of the adrenal medulla. *Acta Physiol.* 192: 325–335.

85 Hartman, F.A. and Brownell, K.A. (1930). The hormone of the adrenal cortex. *Exp. Biol. Med.* 27: 938–939.

86 Viveros, O.H., Diliberto, E.J., Hazum, E., and Chang, K.-J. (1979). Opiate-like materials in the adrenal medulla: evidence for storage and secretion with catecholamines. *Mol. Pharmacol.* 16: 1101–1108.

87 Galac, S., Reusch, C., Kooistra, H., and Rijnberk, A. (2010). Adrenals. In: Clinical Endocrinology of Dogs and Cats, 93–154. Hannover, Schlütersche.

88 Bielinska, M., Parviainen, H., Kiiveri, S. et al. (2009). Review paper: origin and molecular pathology of adrenocortical neoplasms. *Vet. Pathol. Online* 46: 194–210.

89 Deacon, C.F., Mosley, W., and Jones, I.C. (1986). The X zone of the mouse adrenal cortex of the Swiss albino strain. *Gen. Comp. Endocrinol.* 61: 87–99.

90 Bielinska, M., Kiiveri, S., Parviainen, H. et al. (2006). Gonadectomy-induced adrenocortical neoplasia in the domestic ferret (Mustela putorius furo) and laboratory mouse. *Vet. Pathol. Online* 43: 97–117.

91 Schoemaker, N.J., Schuurmans, M., Moorman, H., Lumeij, J.T., 2000. Correlation between age at neutering and age at onset of hyperadrenocorticism in ferrets. J. Am. Vet. Med. Assoc. 216, 195–197

92 Lennox, A.M. and Chitty, J. (2006). Adrenal neoplasia and hyperplasia as a cause of hypertestosteronism in two rabbits. *J. Exot. Pet. Med.* 15: 56–58.

93 Rose, J.B., Vergneau-Grosset, C., Steffey, M. et al. (2016). Adrenalectomy and nephrectomy in a rabbit (*Oryctolagus cuniculus*) with adrenocortical carcinoma and renal and ureteral transitional cell carcinoma. *J. Exot. Pet. Med.* 25: 332–341.

94 Fecteau, K.A., Deeb, B.J., Rickel, J.M. et al. (2007). Diagnostic endocrinology: blood steroid concentrations in neutered male and female rabbits. *J. Exot. Pet. Med.* 16: 256–259.

95 Campbell, T.W. (2015). Exotic Animal Hematology and Cytology. Wiley.

96 DE Matos, R.E.C. and Morrisey, J.K. (2006). Common procedures in the pet ferret. *Vet. Clin. North Am. Exot. Anim. Pract.* 9: 347–365.

97 Evans, E.E. and Souza, M.J. (2010). Advanced diagnostic approaches and current management of internal disorders of select species (rodents, sugar gliders, hedgehogs). *Vet. Clin. North Am. Exot. Anim. Pract.* 13: 453–469.

98 Pilny, A.A. (2008). Clinical hematology of rodent species. *Vet. Clin. North Am. Exot. Anim. Pract.* 11: 523–533.

99 Antinoff, N. (2001). Oncologic diagnostic sampling for the general practitioner. *Exot. DVM* 3: 37–41.

100 Palley, L., Marini, R., Rosenblad, W. et al. (1990). A technique for femoral bone marrow collection in the ferret. *Lab. Anim. Sci.* 40: 654–655.

101 Sundberg, R.D. and Hodgson, R.E. (1949). Aspiration of bone marrow in laboratory animals. *Blood* 4: 557–561.

102 Wilson, P. (1971). Bone marrow biopsy in the rabbit. *Lab. Anim.* 5: 203–206.

103 Bernard, S., Leathers, C., Brobst, D., and Gorham, J. (1983). Estrogen-induced bone marrow depression in ferrets. *Am. J. Vet. Res.* 44: 657–661.

104 Sherrill, A. and Gorham, J. (1985). Bone marrow hypoplasia associated with estrus in ferrets. *Lab. Anim. Sci.* 35: 280–286.

105 Malka, S., Hawkins, M.G., Zabolotzky, S.M. et al. (2010). Immune-mediated pure red cell aplasia in a domestic ferret. *J. Am. Vet. Med. Assoc.* 237: 695–700.

106 Pignon, C., Huynh, M., Husnik, R., and Jekl, V. (2015). Flexible gastrointestinal endoscopy in Ferrets (*Mustela putorius furo*). *Vet. Clin. North Am. Exot. Anim. Pract.* 18: 369–400.

107 Lennox, A.M. (2012). Respiratory disease and pasteurellosis. In: Ferrets, Rabbits, and Rodents: Clinical Medicine and Surgery (eds. K.E. Quesenberry and J.W. Carpenter). St. Louis, Mo: Elsevier/Saunders.

108 Pizzi, R. (2009). Cystoscopic removal of a urolith from a pet guinea pig. *Vet. Rec.* 165: 148–149.

109 Wenger, S. and Hatt, J.-M. (2015). Transurethral cystoscopy and endoscopic Urolith removal in female guinea pigs (*Cavia porcellus*). *Vet. Clin. North Am. Exot. Anim. Pract.* 18: 359–367.

Section 3

Emergency Presentations and Management by Species

14

Ferrets

Nico J. Schoemaker and Yvonne R.A. van Zeeland

Division of Zoological Medicine, Department of Clinical Sciences, Faculty of Veterinary Medicine, Utrecht University, The Netherlands

CONTENTS

Exotic Animal Emergency and Critical Care Medicine, First Edition. Edited by Jennifer E. Graham, Grayson A. Doss and Hugues Beaufrère.

Unique Species Considerations

When evaluating a ferret presented as an emergency case, several species-specific aspects should be considered. One should familiarize themselves with the natural behavior, posture, and gait of a ferret. For example, ferrets will normally sleep most of the day (~20 hours) and naturally walk with a hunched back (Figure 14.1). This gait should not be mistaken as a sign of pain or discomfort. Similarly, one should be familiar with the unique features of the ferrets' anatomy and physiology, such as the heart being positioned more caudally in the long thorax and intact jills remaining in estrus until mating occurs, thereby predisposing them to develop estrogen-related pancytopenia. In the United States, this estrogen-induced pancytopenia is not commonly seen as most ferrets are castrated prior to entering the pet trade. However, this predisposes them to develop adrenal gland tumors (see Section "Hyperadrenocorticism").

Although ferrets have been reported to live as long as 13–14 years, their typical life expectancy lies around 6–8 years. Many ferrets will develop disease well before that age, including a variety of neoplastic (e.g. lymphoma), endocrine (e.g. insulinoma, hyperadrenocorticism), cardiovascular (e.g. cardiomyopathy), gastroenteral (e.g. *Helicobacter* gastritis, foreign body ingestion), and/or urogenital diseases (e.g. renal failure, prostatic cysts). In contrast to other species, comorbidity (presence of multiple diseases) is a common finding in ferrets.

Ferrets are agile creatures that can be challenging to examine and treat. Although most ferrets have a friendly nature, they can bite fiercely without letting go, unless they are held under a running faucet. Administering tablets to ferrets is neither easy, nor accurate. Instead, drugs should be administered as a liquid or suspension which can be flavored to mask the adverse taste of medications. Some medications, e.g. metronidazole, may be difficult to mask; for such drugs, it may help to mix them with their favorite liquid food items (Figure 14.2). Forcing a ferret to swallow a liquid medication may lead to aspiration and subsequent pneumonia and should be done with caution.

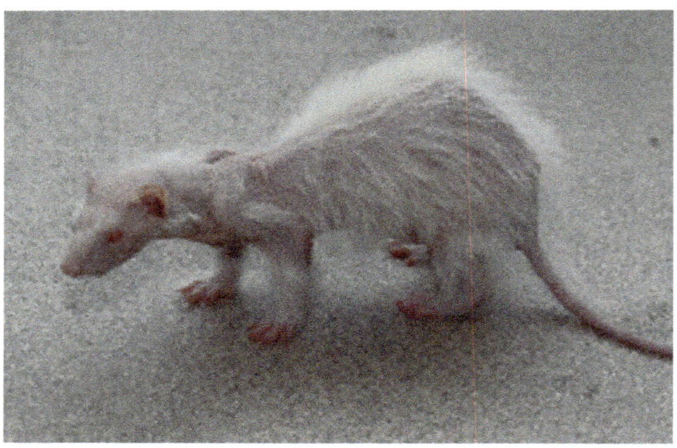

Figure 14.1 A five-year-old ferret with severe alopecia due to an adrenal tumor. Note the hunched back in this ferret, which is a normal posture for ferrets.

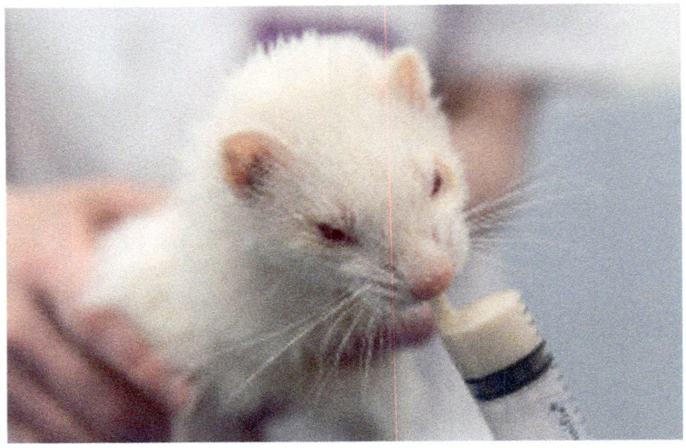

Figure 14.2 Mixing medication with a favorite liquid food item will frequently persuade ferrets to voluntarily take medications.

Common Presenting Signs

Ferrets may present with different clinical signs in the emergency clinic. Triage should always take place to determine whether immediate action is warranted. As in other animals, this includes an evaluation of the cardiovascular (mucous membrane color, capillary refill time, pulse rate, and quality), respiratory (frequency, rhythm, and depth), and central nervous (demeanor, level of consciousness) systems. If the ferret is considered unstable, further evaluation of vital physiologic parameters (i.e. blood pressure, rectal temperature, oxygen saturation, electrocardiogram, hematology, and biochemistry) is warranted to establish an adequate treatment plan. Following initial triage and stabilization of the ferret, further work-up should take place to determine the underlying cause for the presenting signs.

Anemia and Blood Loss

Introduction

Anemia is relatively common in ferrets and characterized by a reduction in the normal erythrocyte or hemoglobin value. Normal packed cell volumes (PCVs) in ferrets are higher than in most dogs and cats and vary between 45% and 65%. Aside from the bone marrow, the spleen plays an important role in the production of erythrocytes and can significantly increase in size in response to anemia.

Diagnosis

Signalment: Anemia occurs in animals of all ages and both genders. Intact females are predisposed to develop estrogen-related pancytopenia.

History: A complete and thorough history will help to identify potential underlying causes for the anemia and provide information on concurrent or underlying diseases, other animals in the household, diet, recent medication, and potential exposure to toxins or trauma.

Clinical signs:

- Lethargy
- Weakness
- Pale mucous membranes
- Anorexia
- Bounding pulse
- Tachypnea
- Tachycardia
- Systolic murmur

Differentials: Similar to dogs and cats, anemia can result from three potential etiologies (see Table 14.1 for complete list):

- Lack of production (non-regenerative anemia)
  - Neoplasia (lymphoma)
  - Endocrine disease
  - Hyperestrogenism
  - Nutritional deficiency
- Blood loss (regenerative anemia)
  - Trauma
  - Surgery
  - Gastrointestinal (GI) blood loss
    - Parasites
    - Ulcerative gastritis
    - Neoplasia
- Destruction of erythrocytes (regenerative anemia)
  - IMHA
  - Toxins
  - Infections
  - Neoplasia

Diagnostics:

- Complete blood count (CBC) (hematocrit <45%)
- Hemoglobin concentration, mean cell volume
- Reticulocyte count (normal reticulocyte count up to 10%)
- Chemistry panel
- Radiographs
- Ultrasound
- Bone marrow aspirate
- Urinalysis
- Fecal occult blood testing

Treatment

- Must identify and treat underlying cause
- Fluid therapy and nutritional support (see Chapter 8)

Table 14.1 Causes for anemia in ferrets.

Non-regenerative anemia	Regenerative anemia	
Reduced or defective erythropoiesis	**Blood loss**	**Accelerated erythrocyte destruction (hemolysis)**
• Chronic renal failure[a] • Chronic inflammation[a] • Drug toxicity (cytotoxic drugs) • Endocrine disease, e.g. hypoadrenocorticism, hypoandrogenism, hypothyroidism • Estrogen-related pancytopenia[a] • Immune-mediated disease • Myeloproliferative disorders • Neoplasia, e.g. leukemia, metastatic[a] • Nutritional deficiencies, e.g. vitamin B12, iron, copper • Radiation • Red cell aplasia	• Diffuse intravascular coagulation (DIC) • Ectoparasites (e.g. heavy flea infestation) • Endoparasitism (e.g. Coccidia) • Gastric ulcers (e.g. Helicobacter)[a] • Hematochezia, e.g. due to gastrointestinal neoplasia • Hematuria • Hemophilia • Hepatic disease (severe forms) • NSAIDS, Ibuprofen[a] • Surgery[a] • Thrombocytopenia • Trauma[a] • Toxins, e.g. rodenticide poisoning • Vascular neoplasia, e.g. hemangio(sarco)ma	• Bacterial infections, e.g. *Clostrium, Leptospira* • DIC • Fragmentation (vena caval syndrome) • Hemoparasites • Hypo-osmolality, hypotonic fluids • Hypersplenism • Immune-mediated hemolytic anemia • Metabolic, e.g. hypophosphatemia • Neoplasia, e.g. hemangiosarcoma, lymphoma • Post-parturient hemoglobinuria • Toxins, e.g. zinc, copper, onions, red maple, snake toxins, acetaminophen • Vasculitis

[a] Common in ferrets.

- Blood transfusion (if clinical signs and PCV < 20%); see Chapters 4 and 8
- Other medications as warranted: iron dextran, erythropoietin

Anorexia

Introduction

Anorexia is a common complaint mentioned by ferret owners, as almost any illness can affect the animal's appetite. In many patients, reluctance to eat may in fact be the only abnormality that is noted following the history and physical examination (see Tables 14.2 and 14.3).

Diagnosis

Signalment: Depends on the underlying cause, e.g. chronic renal disease, cardiac failure or neoplasia will generally affect middle-aged to older animals, whereas infectious diseases will be seen more commonly in (younger) animals that had contact with other animals.

History: History taking will particularly be useful to distinguish true anorexia from pseudo-anorexia (i.e. inability to prehend, chew, or swallow food). Owners should therefore be questioned about the patient's interest in food and its ability to prehend, masticate, and swallow the offered food. Moreover, a thorough history of the ferret's living environment and diet may help to reveal potential psychological causes. Questions regarding the ferret's demeanor and other disease signs can point toward specific organ systems that warrant further attention in the work-up.

Clinical Signs:

Anorexia:

- Disinterest of food, food refusal
- Weight loss

Pseudo-anorexia:

- Interested in food, unable to eat
- Halitosis
- Ptyalism
- Dysphagia
- Odynophagia (pain during eating)
- Weight loss

Differentials:

- Unpalatable diet
- Stress
- Inability to prehend/masticate/swallow
  - Gingivitis (Figure 14.3)
  - Stomatitis
  - Pharyngitis
- Gastrointestinal disease
  - Ulcerative gastritis
  - Foreign body ingestion
  - Epizootic catarrhal enteritis (coronavirus)
  - *Other:* metabolic, infectious, inflammatory, neoplasia

Table 14.2 Differential diagnosis for (pseudo)anorexia in ferrets.

List of causes resulting in anorexia	List of causes resulting in pseudo-anorexia
Any systemic disease: • Cardiomyopathy, cardiac failure • Endocrine disease, e.g. insulinoma • Gastrointestinal disease, e.g. foreign body ingestion, gastric ulceration • High environmental temperature • Infectious disease • Intoxications • Metabolic disease, especially hepatic, or renal disease • Motion sickness • Neoplasia, e.g. lymphoma • Pain • Respiratory disease, e.g. influenza • Stress • Unpalatable diet	*Diseases causing painful prehension and mastication of food:* • Dental disease • Inflammation/infection, e.g. gingivitis, glossitis, stomatitis • Musculoskeletal disorders, e.g. mandibular fractures, subluxation, myofasciitis • Neurologic disorders, e.g. rabies, tetanus, CNS lesions • Oral or glossal neoplasia, especially squamous cell carcinoma • Retrobulbar abscesses • Salivary gland disorders *Diseases resulting in dysphagia:* • Neuromuscular disorders, e.g. CNS lesions, botulism • Pharyngitis • Pharyngeal neoplasia • Retropharyngeal disorders, e.g. lymphadenopathy, abscess, sialocele, hematoma • Diseases interfering with the swallowing reflex • Esophageal diseases, e.g. esophagitis, neoplasia, neuromuscular disorders

Table 14.3 Differential diagnosis for diarrhea and vomiting in ferrets.

Differential diagnosis for diarrhea	Differential diagnosis for vomiting
• Bacterial infections, e.g. *Helicobacter*, *Campylobacter*, *Clostridium*, *Salmonella* • Viral infections, e.g. rotavirus, coronavirus (epizootic catarrhal enteritis) • Parasitic disease, e.g. coccidia, *Cryptosporidium*, *Giardia* • Inflammatory disease, e.g. proliferative bowel disease, lymphoplasmacytic or eosinophilic gastroenteritis • Metabolic disorders, e.g. hepatopathy, renal disease • Neoplasia, e.g. lymphoma, adenocarcinoma • Foreign body obstruction • Intussusception • Intoxications • Dietary, e.g. dietary intolerance, diet changes, spoiled food • Maldigestion, e.g. hepatopathy, pancreatitis	*Gastrointestinal disease*: • Bacterial gastroenteritis, e.g. *Helicobacter*, *Salmonella*, *Campylobacter*, *Clostridium* • Viral infection, e.g. ECE, rotavirus • Parasitic disease, e.g. *Giardia*, *Cryptosporidium*, Coccidia • Dietary, e.g. diet changes, spoiled food, dietary intolerance • GI obstruction (ileus), e.g. foreign body, intussusception • Inflammatory disease, e.g. lymphoplasmacytic, eosinophilic gastroenteritis • Neoplasia, e.g. lymphoma, adenocarcinoma *Metabolic disease*: • Electrolyte imbalances (e.g. hypokalemia, hyperkalemia, hypercalcemia) • Hepatic disease • Intoxications • Metabolic acidosis • Pancreatitis • Renal disease, uremia • CNS disease • Encephalomeningitis • Neoplasia, e.g. primary brain tumor • Otitis media or interna • Trauma, cerebral edema

Diagnostics:

- Varies depending on suspected underlying cause, history, and physical examination (PE) findings

Treatment

- Nutritional support (Figures 14.2 and 14.4)
  - Modify/warm diet to increase palatability (i.e. Feline a/d [Hills], Carnivore Care [Oxbow Animal Health], EmerAid Intensive Care Carnivore [Lafeber])
  - Syringe/supplemental feeding
  - Nasogastric (NG), esophagostomy, gastrotomy, or jejunostomy tube; total parenteral nutrition
- Fluid therapy
  - Correction of electrolyte imbalances

Gastroenteral Signs: Vomiting and Diarrhea

Introduction

Gastroenteral disease will commonly result in clinical signs such as vomiting and diarrhea. Similar to other animals, vomiting in ferrets occurs as a result of stimulation of the chemoreceptor trigger zone (vomiting center) in the brain (either as a result from increased intracranial pressure due to central nervous system (CNS) disease, presence of bacterial or metabolic toxins or drugs, or neurologic stimulation in case of motion sickness or vestibular disease), or from stimulation of peripheral receptors located in the gastrointestinal tract and various other organs. Diarrhea can be seen as a result of disorders affecting the digestive, absorptive, secretory, and/or motility actions of the intestinal tract.

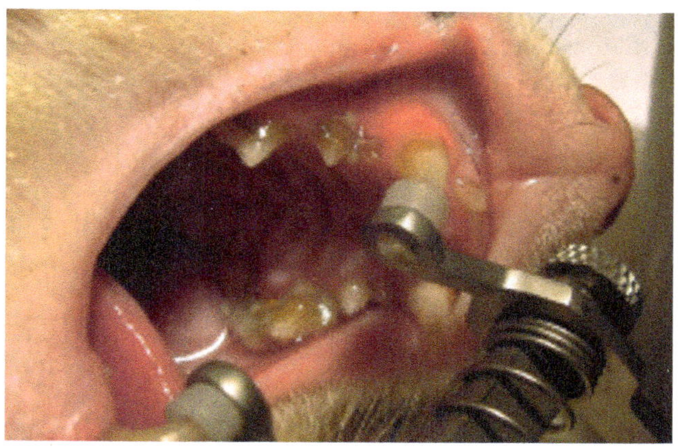

Figure 14.3 Dental disease is a common underlying cause for anorexia, as was the case in this five-year-old ferret, presented with anorexia for two days and a swelling under the right eye. Upon oral inspection, a periapical abscess was found to be the cause for the anorexia, as demonstrated by the pus seen around the first premolar on the right.

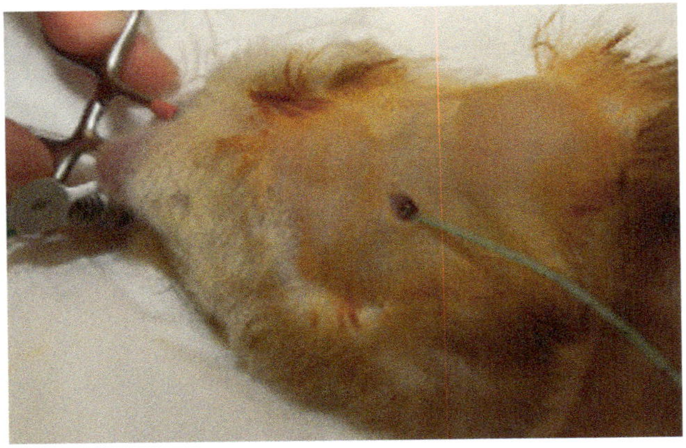

Figure 14.4 Placement of an esophagostomy tube is a relatively simple procedure in a ferret. Similar to cats, a curved mosquito forceps is placed into the esophagus, followed by a small incision over the tip of the mosquito. Next, a feeding tube is pulled back through the incision into the oral cavity and then placed retrograde into the esophagus, past the incision and into the stomach (i.e. based on the distance between the incision and last rib). Once in the correct position, the tube is sutured in place at the incision site. See Chapter 8 for more details.

Diagnosis

Signalment: No specific age or gender predilections

History: In contrast to regurgitation (which includes the passive expulsion of food from the esophagus), vomiting is usually preceded by signs indicating nausea such as ptyalism, licking the lips, pawing at the mouth, backing up, and retching. Information regarding the volume of the feces, frequency of defecation, presence of mucus or blood, and presence of weight loss, melena, tenesmus, or dyschezia may be helpful to make a distinction between small and large bowel diarrhea. Owners should also be questioned about their ferret's eating and chewing habits (e.g. chewing on food, missing toys), changes in appetite, weight loss, and changes in the diet or living environment, access to spoiled food or toxins, or exposure to other ferrets.

Clinical Signs:

- Changes in fecal volume and consistency or frequency of defecation
- Weight loss
- Hematochezia, dyschezia, tenesmus
- Colonic or rectal prolapse
- Vomiting
- Diarrhea
- Shock, dehydration
  - Dry, pale mucous membranes
  - Faint pulse
  - Hypothermia
  - Poor skin turgor

Differentials (see Table 14.3):

- Disease affecting GI tract including foreign body
- Metabolic
- Infectious
- Trauma
- Toxin
- Neurologic disease

Diagnostics:

- CBC
- Biochemistry panel
- Survey radiographs
- Abdominal ultrasound
- Fecal examination
- Gastroscopy +/− biopsy
  - Direct exam
  - Fecal flotation
  - Cytology
  - Culture/sensitivity

Treatment

- Correct fluid losses and electrolyte/acid-base disturbances (see Chapter 8)
- Symptomatic treatment as warranted
  - *Antiemetics:*
    - *Metoclopramide* (if no foreign body): 0.2–1 mg/kg PO, SC, IM q6–8h
    - *Maropitant citrate:* 1 mg/kg (dilute) SC q24h
    - *Ondansetron*: 1 mg/kg PO q12–24h
  - *Antacids:*
    - *Famotidine:* 0.25–0.5 mg/kg PO, SC, IV q12–24h
    - *Ranitidine HCl:* 3.5 mg/kg PO q12h
    - *Omeprazole:* 0.7 mg/kg PO q24h
  - Provide easily digestible, high-protein diet

Intoxications

Introduction

Because of their inquisitive nature and ability to open sealed vials and containers with their strong jaws, ferrets are likely to be exposed to toxins. Moreover, due to their relatively small size, ingestion of toxins – even in small quantities – is likely to result in intoxications (see Table 14.4). Resources may be available for recommendations on case management, for example, ASPCA Poison Control in the U.S. (1-888-426-4435).

Diagnosis

Signalment: Animals of all ages and both genders, particularly those allowed (unsupervised) time outside of their cage.

Table 14.4 Common toxins classified according to their effect.

Potentially lethal agents	• 5-Fluorouracil • Isoniazid • Metaldehyde • Strychnine • Tricyclic antidepressants (TCAs)
Seizure-inducing agents	• 5-Fluorouracil • Aminopyridine • Amphetamines • Cocaine • Metaldehyde • Nicotine • Strychnine • Tremorgenic mycotoxins
Toxins resulting in CNS depression	• Barbiturates • Benzodiazepines • Ethanol • Ethylene glycol • Ibuprofen • Ivermectin • Marijuana • Opioids • Phenothiazines • TCAs
Nephrotoxic agents	• Cadmium • Cantharidin • Cholecalciferol • Diquat herbicides • Ethylene glycol • Mercury • Nephrotoxic antibiotics (e.g. bacitracin, polymyxin-B, gentamycin, neomycin) • Non-steroidal anti-inflammatory drugs (e.g. ibuprofen) • Oxalic acid • Phenolics • Rhubarb • Zinc
Hepatotoxic agents	• Acetaminophen • Amanita mushrooms • Arsenic • Blue-green algae • Copper • Cycad species • Hepatoxic mycotoxins • Iron • Phenolics • Pyrrolizidine alkaloid plants • Tannic acid • Vitamin A
Corrosive agents	• Acids • Alkali (e.g. drain cleaners containing sodium or potassium hydroxide) • Cationic detergents • Phenolics • Petroleum distillate
Hydrocarbons, resulting in respiratory problems	• Butane • Fuel oil • Gasoline • Kerosene • Mineral spirits • Motor oil • Propane • Tar • Transmission fluid

Source: Adapted from Richardson and Balabuszko [1].

History: In any patient suspected of an intoxication, it is important to identify substances (including amounts) the animal may have had access to, and when exposure occurred, as this may help to determine when and what clinical signs are to be expected. Specific antidotes can be given based on this information.

Clinical Signs:

- Vary dependent on toxin (see Table 14.4)
- Mild GI irritation to vomiting
- Collapse
- Death

Differentials:

- Ibuprofen
- Anticoagulant rodenticide
- Many others; see Table 14.4

Diagnostics:

- Based on the history and suspected toxin; i.e. coagulation testing with rodenticide, chemistry panel with nephrotoxic or hepatotoxic compounds

Treatment

- Induce emesis if recent ingestion (i.e. <2 hours); contraindicated if caustic agent or if animal already showing symptoms
  - *Hydrogen peroxide:* 2.2 ml/kg PO
  - *Ipecac syrup* (7%)*:* 2.2–6.6 ml/animal PO
  - *Apomorphine:* 0.7–5 mg/kg SC

Table 14.6 Causes for respiratory distress (dyspnea, tachypnea) in ferrets.

Upper respiratory diseases	Lower respiratory diseases	Diseases involving the thoracic cavity	Other
Nasal obstruction • Foreign body • Granuloma • Neoplasia • Rhinitis/sinusitis (viral, bacterial, mycotic) Laryngotracheal obstruction • Foreign body • Neoplasia Trauma, e.g. airway rupture Extraluminal tracheal compression (e.g. due to lymphoma)	Neoplasia • Primary • Metastatic Pneumonia • Viral: influenza • Bacterial • Mycotic Pneumonitis • Allergic • Parasitic Pulmonary edema • Cardiogenic • Non-cardiogenic Trauma • Pulmonary contusion	• Diaphragmatic herniation • Mediastinal mass, e.g. lymphoma • Pleural effusion, e.g. due to cardiac disease, • Hemothorax, e.g. due to trauma • Chylothorax • Pyothorax • Pneumothorax • Rib fractures	Metabolic disease • Severe anemia • Acidosis • Uremia Ascites (severe forms) Organomegaly Neuromuscular disease • CNS disease (e.g. inflammation, neoplasia, trauma) • Spinal disease (e.g. intervertebral disc herniation, trauma) • Obesity • Physiologic response to, e.g. fear, pain, fever, heat stroke, physical exercise or stress

- Stress
- Pain
- Fever
- Exertion

Diagnostics:

- Thoracic or skull/neck radiographs
- Thoracic ultrasound
- CBC
- Biochemistry panel
- Thoracocentesis if effusion with cytology, C/S
- Specific testing based on differentials:
  - Heartworm testing
  - Fine needle aspirate (FNA)/biopsy of mass
  - Culture/sensitivity of nasal swab or tracheal wash

Treatment

- Based on etiology
- Supplemental oxygen
- Tracheostomy if upper airway obstruction
- Thoracocentesis

Shock and Dehydration

Introduction

Due to their small size, ferrets are particularly prone to developing dehydration and (hypovolemic) shock as a result of insufficient water intake and/or excessive fluid losses. As many diseases will be accompanied by a lack of water intake, (hypovolemic) shock and/or dehydration will be a common finding in most ferrets presented as an emergency case (see Table 14.7).

Diagnosis

Signalment: No age or gender predilections.

History: During the history taking, special attention should be paid to the water intake and presence of fluid losses which may occur as a result of vomiting, diarrhea, polyuria, hemorrhage, and/or burn wounds. In addition, history may focus on information that pertains to the underlying disease.

Clinical Signs:

- Weak pulse
- Bradycardia (<200 bpm)
- Pale, dry, or tacky mucous membranes
- Hypothermia, cold extremities
- Decreased urine output
- Decreased skin turgor
- Altered mentation: somnolence, stupor, coma
- Heart murmur or arrhythmia if cardiac disease
- Fever, muddy mucous membranes if sepsis

Table 14.7 Differential diagnosis for shock.

Hypovolemic shock	Cardiogenic shock	Obstructive shock	Distributive shock
• Blood loss • Burns • Gastrointestinal fluid loss due to vomiting or diarrhea • Hypoadrenocorticism • Heat stroke • Excess urine loss (polyuria/polydipsia), e.g. due to diabetes mellitus	• Arrhythmias • Cardiomyopathy • Congestive heart failure (CHF) • Contusio cordis • Myocardial infarction • Myocarditis • Valvular insufficiencies	• Aortic stenosis • Cardiac tamponade • Pulmonary embolism • Tension pneumothorax	• Anaphylaxis, e.g. vaccine reaction • Septic shock, e.g. due to intoxications, severe systemic infections • Neurogenic shock, e.g. due to trauma (high spinal injuries)

Differentials:

- See Table 14.7
- Hypovolemic shock
  - Blood loss (trauma, GI blood loss)
  - Fluid loss (vomiting, diarrhea, polydipsia)
- *Cardiogenic shock*: poor cardiac function
- *Obstructive shock*: blockage of circulation
- *Distributive shock*: redirection of blood to periphery

Diagnostics:

- CBC
- Biochemistry
- Radiographs
- Ultrasound
- Blood pressure measurement
- Lactate
- Fluid intake, urinary output
- Coagulation testing
- ECG

Treatment

- Identify and treat cause
- Restore circulation:
  - Control bleeding
  - Fluid therapy (crystalloids, colloids, +/− blood products; see Chapter 8)
- Oxygen supplementation
- Nutritional support
- Rewarming
- Correct glucose/electrolyte imbalance

Trauma

Introduction

Due to their inquisitive nature, ferrets are extremely prone to trauma which may vary from falling from a height, getting stuck between the door or being stepped on by the owner, getting bitten by another predator (i.e. dog or cat), or even getting stuck in a washing machine.

Diagnosis

Signalment: Animals of any age or gender.

History: During the history taking, it is important to ascertain whether trauma may have occurred, and if so, when and what type. In addition, information should be obtained on the animal's general demeanor, behavior, breathing, locomotion, micturition, and any changes therein since the accident.

Clinical Signs:

- Vary depending on type of trauma
  - Minor wound
  - Spinal/pelvic/extremity fractures
  - Internal organ damage (pulmonary contusion, splenic rupture)
  - Paresis, paralysis, coma
- Pain (tachypnea, hyperthermia)
- Pale mucous membranes

Differentials:

- Fight injury/bite wounds
- Electrocution
- Fall
- Blunt force trauma

Diagnostics:

- Assess animal's airway, breathing, and circulation
- Evaluate nervous and musculoskeletal systems, thorax, abdomen
- CBC
- Biochemistry panel
- Urinalysis
- Radiographs
- Ultrasound

Treatment

- Follow principles/guidelines as in other small animals
- Stabilize patient
  - Establish open airway
  - Restore normal breathing and circulation
  - Control bleeding
- Fluid therapy +/− blood transfusion
- Supplemental oxygen
- Analgesia

  Meloxicam: 0.1–0.3 mg/kg PO, SC, IM q24h
  Buprenorphine: 0.01–0.05 mg/kg oral transmucosal, SC, IM, IV q4–12h
  Butorphanol: 0.3 mg/kg SC, IM q2–4h
  Hydromorphone: 0.1–0.2 mg/kg SC, IM, IV
  Oxymorphone: 0.05–0.2 mg/kg SC, IM, IV q8–12h
  Tramadol: 5–10 mg/kg PO q12–24h
- Careful and continued monitoring

Urogenital Signs: Dysuria

Introduction

Dysuria (i.e. difficult and/or painful micturition) and pollakiuria (frequent voiding of small quantities or urine) are commonly seen in animals suffering from diseases affecting the urinary tract and/or prostate. When experiencing bladder fullness or pain due to presence of disease, premature micturition will follow, thereby reducing the functional capacity of the bladder. In addition, problems with micturition may result from blockage of the normal urinary outflow (e.g. due to urethral stones, plugs, strictures, or extraluminal masses compressing the urethra). Secondary complications can include uremia, hyperphosphatemia, acid-base disturbances, or electrolyte imbalances (particularly hyperkalemia).

Diagnosis

Signalment: No gender or breed predilections.

History: During the history taking, special attention should be paid to the micturition, including the frequency, volume, and macroscopic aspects of the urine. Owners should also be asked whether their ferret is still housebroken and/or showing signs of pain or discomfort when urinating or defecating (as dysuria and dyschezia can be present simultaneously in ferrets with prostatic disease). Owners should also be questioned about the ferret's water intake to rule out polyuria/polydipsia. A dietary history can be obtained in case urolithiasis is suspected, whereas specific questions can be asked about the ferret's behavior, appetite, or coat condition in case of suspected hyperandrogenism-related urogenital cystic disease.

Clinical Signs:

- Can be unremarkable
- Caudal abdominal palpable mass
  - Distended bladder
  - Prostatomegaly
- Thickened bladder wall (cystitis)
- Painful on abdominal palpation
- Lethargy
- Inappetence
- Weakness
- Cardiac arrhythmia
- Collapse
- Hematuria, dysuria, stranguria

Differentials:

- Adrenal disease with secondary prostatomegaly
- Urogenital cysts
  - Periurethral, prostatic, periprostatic
- Urolithiasis (cysteine most common)
- Urinary tract infection
- Cystitis
- Neoplasia
- Trauma (iatrogenic from catheterization, palpation, retrograde flushing)

Diagnostics:

- CBC
- Chemistry panel
- Urinalysis w/sediment evaluation
- Urine culture/sensitivity
- Radiographs
- Ultrasound
- Contrast urethrocystography
- Excretory urography

Treatment

- Based on underlying cause: see Sections "Urinary Disease" and "Endocrine Disease"
- Aggressive fluid therapy
- Correct electrolyte imbalances
- Antimicrobials if indicated

Weakness and Collapse

Introduction

Weakness is one of the most non-specific signs that can be seen in any patient. Collapse, however, represents a more severe condition of the patient which may be life-threatening.

Diagnosis

Signalment: No gender or age predilections.

History: When confronted with a collapsed ferret, it is important to find out whether the collapse had a sudden onset without prior signs or whether the animal had been sick for a longer period of time, and if so, what type of clinical signs it showed prior to the collapse. Many animals with chronic disease may eventually end up in a collapsed state following a prolonged period of anorexia or decreased water intake, resulting in shock and dehydration. During the history taking, special attention should therefore be paid to the animal's food and water intake as well as the diet provided to the animal. Other aspects to consider in the history are exposure to toxins or trauma and contact with other animals.

Clinical Signs:

- Ataxia
- Weakness
- Obtunded, minimal response
- Chronic
  - Weight loss, cachexia
  - Poor skin turgor

Differentials:

- See Table 14.8
- Anemia (severe forms)
- Cachexia, severe weight loss, e.g. due to gastrointestinal disease
- Cardiovascular disease, e.g. cardiomyopathy, arrhythmia
- Intoxications
- Metabolic disease, e.g. hypoglycemia due to insulinoma, electrolyte imbalances
- Neurologic disease, e.g. Aleutian disease virus (ADV), Canine distemper virus (CDV), trauma
- Respiratory disease, e.g. influenza, pneumonia
- Shock or dehydration
- Weakness due to systemic disease

Table 14.8 Common causes for weakness or collapse in ferrets.

Differential diagnosis for animals with signs of weakness or collapse
• Anemia (severe forms) • Cachexia, severe weight loss, e.g. due to gastrointestinal disease • Cardiovascular disease, e.g. cardiomyopathy, arrhythmia • Intoxications • Metabolic disease, e.g. hypoglycemia due to insulinoma, electrolyte imbalances • Neurologic disease, e.g. ADV, CDV, trauma • Respiratory disease, e.g. influenza, pneumonia • Shock or dehydration • Weakness due to systemic disease

Diagnostics:

- Prioritize triage and stabilization
- CBC
- Biochemistry profile
  - Especially glucose, calcium, electrolytes, liver/kidney values
- Radiographs
- Ultrasound
- ECG +/− echocardiography
- Blood pressure

Treatment

- Base on cause
- Fluid therapy and nutritional support; see Chapter 8
- Glucose administration
- Oxygen supplementation

Systemic Disease

Canine Distemper Virus (CDV)

Canine distemper is a serious infection seen in ferrets, resulting in severe respiratory, cutaneous, gastrointestinal, and neurologic signs. The disease is caused by a morbillivirus from the family paramyxoviridae. Although highly contagious (transmission may occur through inhalation or ingestion of virus particles), the disease is nowadays rarely seen in ferrets due to vaccination. Sporadically, outbreaks can be seen in unvaccinated colonies or shelters.

Diagnosis

Signalment: Ferrets of all ages and both genders that have not been vaccinated against CDV. Young animals appear more susceptible than adults.

History: History may reveal lack of adequate vaccination status as well as contact with non-vaccinated animals with CDV-infected animals (e.g. other ferrets, dogs, wild carnivores). Following an incubation period of 7–10 days, ferrets will develop characteristic respiratory and cutaneous signs as well as fever.

Clinical Signs:

- Depression
- Anorexia
- Mucopurulent ocular and nasal discharge
- Pyrexia (over 104 °F [40 °C])
- Sneezing
- Coughing
- Erythematous rash around eyes, on lips/nose/chin, inguinal region
- Hyperkeratosis of food pads ("hard pad disease")
- GI signs
  - Vomiting, diarrhea, melena

- Neurologic signs
  - Ataxia, seizures, paresis/paralysis, muscle tremors, hyperesthesia
- Death 12–35 days post-exposure

Differentials:

- Influenza
- Rabies
- Any condition causing oculonasal discharge and pyrexia

Diagnostics:

- Based on clinical signs
- Conjunctival smear (immuno fluorescence assay [IFA])
- Necropsy may be needed for definitive diagnosis

Treatment

- Isolate affected animals
- Fatal disease – no specific treatment beyond symptomatic, consider humane euthanasia
- Vaccinate to prevent
  - Purevax Ferret Distemper vaccine available (canarypox-vectored)

Heatstroke

Heatstroke can develop in any animal exposed to higher ambient temperatures. Ferrets are particularly sensitive to heat stress and heatstroke as they do not have sweat glands and have difficulty tolerating temperatures above 86 °F (30 °C), even if for a short time (~10 minutes).

Diagnosis

Signalment: No known age or gender predilection.

History: History will reveal exposure or confinement in an area with higher 86 °F (30 °C) ambient temperatures.

Clinical Signs:

- Open-mouth breathing, panting
- Red mucous membranes
- Weakness, severe depression
- Muscle cramps, diarrhea, vomiting
- If untreated can progress to seizures, shock, coma, and death
  - Death can occur in as little as 30 minutes due to multi-organ failure

Differentials:

- Sepsis (bacterial, viral)
- Myositis or other inflammatory conditions
- Other causes of hyperthermia
  - Malignant hyperthermia
  - Status epilepticus
  - Toxin inducing muscle cramps

Diagnostics:

- Based on history, ambient temperatures over 90 °F (30 °C)
- Core body temperature above 105 °F (40.6 °C)
- CBC
- Biochemistry
- Coagulation testing

Treatment

- Gradual cooling
  - Rehydration with cool intravenous fluids; see Chapter 8
  - Alcohol on foot pads
- Oxygen supplementation
- Correction of electrolyte imbalances

Sepsis

According to recently renewed definitions in human medicine, sepsis is defined as life-threatening organ dysfunction caused by a dysregulated host response to infection. Septic shock is defined as a subset of sepsis in which particularly profound circulatory, cellular, and metabolic abnormalities are associated with a greater risk of mortality than with sepsis alone.

Diagnosis

Signalment: No known age or gender predilection.

History: History will often reveal presence of a (systemic) infection.

Clinical Signs:

- Lethargy
- Anorexia
- Tachycardia
- Tachypnea
- Hyperthermia
- Vomiting, diarrhea
- Shock
- Other signs vary depending on underlying cause

Differentials:

- Any infectious or inflammatory disease process
- Intoxications or other causes of shock

Diagnostics:

- CBC
- Biochemistry profile
  - Common findings include hypoglycemia, hypoalbuminemia, hyperbilirubinemia, leukocytosis, and/or thrombocytopenia
- Coagulation testing
  - Commonly prolonged prothrombin time (PT) and aPTT (diffuse intravascular coagulation, DIC)

- Blood pressure, ECG
  - Hypotension, arrhythmias common
- Radiographs
- Ultrasound
- Sample collection for culture/sensitivity
  - Blood, urine, tracheal wash, pleural or peritoneal effusion, CSF

Treatment

- Aggressive fluid therapy
  - Colloids +/− vasopressors to correct hypotension; see Chapter 8
- Oxygen supplementation
- Antibiotics, ideally based on C/S; choose parenteral over enteral routes
  - *Amoxicillin*: 20 mg/kg PO, SC q12h
  - *Ampicillin*: 5–30 mg/kg SC, IM, IV q8–12h
  - *Enrofloxacin*: 5–10 mg/kg PO, SC, IM q12h
  - *Metronidazole*: 10 mg/kg IV; 15–20 mg/kg PO q12h
  - *Trimethoprim/Sulfa*: 15–30 mg/kg PO, SC q12h

Systemic Coronavirus Infection (Ferret Infectious Peritonitis)

Ferret systemic coronavirus (FSCV) disease is a chronic, progressive, and lethal disease that has been diagnosed worldwide in ferrets since 2002. The virus is closely related to ferret enteric coronavirus. Infection results in a systemic pyogranulomatous inflammation which shows many similarities to feline infectious peritonitis. As a result, the infection is also commonly referred to as ferret infectious peritonitis. The longest reported survival period after diagnosis is approximately seven months; however, most ferrets will die within two months.

Diagnosis

Signalment: FSCV can infect ferrets of any age or gender, but young ferrets (<1 year) appear to be more prone.

History: Animals will often have a chronic history of diarrhea (days to months) prior to developing other signs of disease. Risk factors may include post-weaning stress and immune suppression due to poor husbandry (e.g. overcrowding), transport, vaccination, and/or surgeries.

Clinical Signs:

- Usually non-specific
  - Anorexia, weight loss, diarrhea
- Fever greater than 104 °F (>40 °C)
  - Some animals normothermic

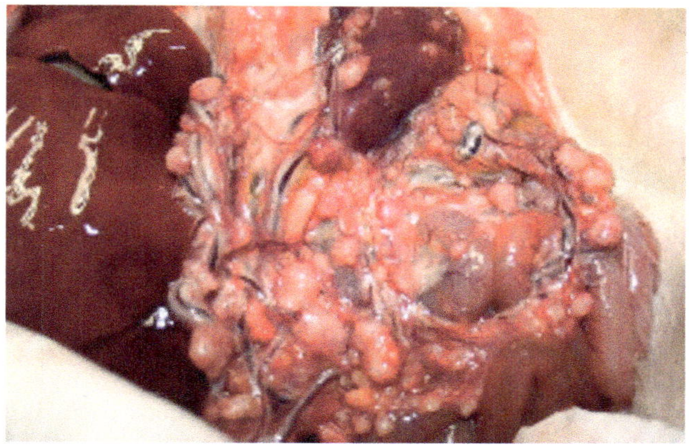

Figure 14.5 Multiple granulomas seen at post-mortem examination of a one-year-old ferret that presented with a 10-day history of anorexia, progressive weight loss, and a fever which was unresponsive to the administration of NSAIDS. These signs are consistent with a ferret systemic coronavirus infection.

- Intraabdominal masses (Figure 14.5) or splenomegaly upon abdominal palpation

Differentials:

- Any disease causing vague, non-specific symptoms, lymphadenopathy, and/or diarrhea
  - Lymphoma, proliferative bowel disease, eosinophilic gastroenteritis
- Aleutian disease if hypergammaglobulinemia and (mesenteric) lymphadenopathy

Diagnostics:

- CBC
  - May reveal mild/moderate non-regenerative anemia, thrombocytopenia, neutrophilia, lymphopenia, hyperproteinemia, and (polyclonal) hypergammaglobulinemia
- Biochemistry profile
- Abdominal ultrasonography
  - Identify spleno- or renomegaly, lymphadenopathy, and abdominal soft tissue masses
  - US-guided fine needle aspiration biopsies
- Cytology
  - Characteristic pyogranulomatous inflammation
- Post-mortem examination or surgical biopsy with immunohistochemistry (IHC) to confirm

Treatment

- Supportive care
- NSAIDs, corticosteroids, and antivirals (such as ribavirin 50 mg/kg/day combined with interferon) have been used
- Euthanasia is recommended if severe clinical disease.

Vaccine Reactions

Vaccine reactions are usually the result of a type I hypersensitivity response occurring after vaccination. Ferrets are particularly reported to be sensitive, with vaccine reactions occurring in as many as 1% of the vaccinated ferrets.

Diagnosis

Signalment: No age or gender predilections. However, incidence seems to increase with the amount of vaccinations previously received.

History: History revealed recent (<24–48 hours) vaccine administration, with most vaccine reactions occurring within 30 minutes following administering of the vaccine. Although adverse reactions can occur following any type of vaccination, they are most commonly seen following a distemper vaccination.

Clinical Signs:

- Range from mild to severe
- Pruritis, erythema
- Hypersalivation, vomiting, diarrhea
- Hyperthermia
- Ataxia
- Seizures
- Cardiovascular collapse and death

Differentials:

- All causes of shock including trauma and intoxications

Diagnostics:

- Based on history and clinical signs

Treatment

- Emergency life support
  - Open airway
  - Circulatory restoration
  - Correct physiologic abnormalities
- Diphenhydramine, epinephrine, or short-acting corticosteroid
- IV fluids
- Oxygen and aminophylline if dyspneic
- Premedicate with diphenhydramine 15 minutes prior to vaccination to decrease incidence and severity of reaction

Neurologic and Musculoskeletal Disease

Neurologic

Hypoglycemia

Hypoglycemia is the most common cause for signs resembling neurologic disease in ferrets. The most common cause for hypoglycemia in ferrets is an insulinoma, but in rare cases, liver disease, neoplasia, sepsis, starvation, and heatstroke may also be causes for hypoglycemia. In case of an insulinoma, the neurologic signs and weakness will generally disappear following the provision of a meal, while this improvement is lacking in animals with hypoglycemia due to other causes (*see further under insulinoma*).

Neurologic Toxins

Neurologic signs can result following ingestion of various toxins (see Table 14.4). The most common reported cause of neurotoxicosis in ferrets is the ingestion of ibuprofen.

Diagnosis

Signalment: No age or breed predilections are present.

History: History will reveal ibuprofen exposure due to accidental ingestion or to owners self-medicating their ferret.

Clinical Signs:

- Anorexia
- Vomiting, diarrhea, melena
- Tremors
- Ataxia
- Depression, eventual coma
- Anuria or oliguria

Differentials:

Other toxicities, including those with NSAIDs and other nephrotoxic drugs

Diagnostics:

- CBC
- Biochemistry profile
  - Usually elevated blood urea nitrogen (BUN), creatinine, and phosphorous
  - Metabolic acidosis may be seen
  - +/- elevated liver enzymes
- Ibuprofen levels
  - Serum, urine, hepatic samples

Treatment

- Induce emesis or gastric lavage and activated charcoal if ingestion within past two hours; cathartic unless dehydrated
- Prevent and/or treat gastric ulcerations, renal failure, and hepatic or CNS effects
- Intravenous fluids (see Chapter 8)
- *Sucralfate*: 25–125 mg/kg PO q8–12h

- *Misoprostol*: 1–5 µg/kg PO q8h
- *Metoclopramide*: 0.2–1 mg/kg PO, SC, IM q6–8h
  - Anti-epileptic drugs if seizures

Seizures

Although seizures are the consequence of brain abnormalities, the most commonly reported cause of seizures in ferrets is an insulinoma (see further under Section "Insulinoma"). Other causes for seizures include the ingestion of toxic substances, trauma, neoplasia, and infection or inflammation within the brain (see Table 14.5). Primary epilepsy has thus far not been described in ferrets.

Diagnosis

Signalment: Ferrets of any age, but disease appears more common in middle-aged to older ferrets.

History: History taking should focus on an accurate description of the seizure activity, including the frequency and duration of the seizures. In addition, information may be obtained regarding potential underlying causes (e.g. trauma, intoxication, dietary deficiencies, infection due to exposure to other animals).

Clinical Signs:

- Similar to dogs and cats, there are four recognizable stages of seizure activity:
  (1) the period prior to the seizure in which the animal may display signs of restlessness and/or anxiety (*prodrome*)
  (2) the start of seizure activity (*aura*) which is often marked by subtle behavioral changes and thereby difficult to recognize unless the animal starts vomiting, salivating, or urinating
  (3) the actual seizure itself (*ictus*) during which involuntary muscle activity and abnormal behavior are seen
  (4) the *post-ictal period*, which immediately follows the seizure activity in which the animal shows more atypical behavior while recovering from the seizure.

Differentials:

- Neuromuscular weakness, e.g. due to metabolic disease such as hypoglycemia
- Syncope due to cardiac disease

Diagnostics:

- Similar guidelines as those described in dogs and cats
- CBC
- Biochemistry profile
- Serologic and/or toxicologic tests
  - Toxoplasmosis
  - Lead, zinc
- MRI

Treatment

- Emergency treatment if seizuring
  - Sedative drugs (e.g. diazepam or propofol)
- Treatment for hyperthermia
- Oxygen support
- Anti-epileptic drugs (monitor plasma levels to guide optimal dosing)
  - *Levetiracetam*: 20 mg/kg PO q8h; if ineffective, increase dose in 20 mg/kg increments
  - *Phenobarbital*: 1–2 mg/kg PO q8–12h
  - *Gabapentin*: 3–5 mg/kg PO q8–24h
- Additional therapy depending on underlying cause

Spinal Cord Lesions

The most common causes for spinal cord lesions include trauma, Aleutian disease, lymphoma, chordoma, and intervertebral disk disease (see Table 14.5).

Diagnosis

- **Signalment**: No known age or gender predilection.
- **History**: Dependent on the underlying cause, history will reveal paresis/paralysis with a sudden, acute, or a more gradual onset. In many cases of focal lesions, ataxia may be the first sign that is noted by the owner, which gradually progresses into paresis or paralysis. The history may furthermore reveal the presence of trauma as the underlying cause for the lesion.

Clinical Signs:

- Ataxia
  - Paresis, paralysis
    - Usually hind leg but can be tetraparesis/paralysis
  - Other abnormal neurologic signs
    - Postural reactions, reflexes, pain perception delayed, or absent
  - Urinary or fecal incontinence

Differentials:

- Other disease resulting in weakness (see Table 14.5)
  - Insulinoma
  - Cardiac disease

Diagnostics:

- Based on clinical signs and imaging
- Radiographs +/- myelography (not without risk)
- CT/MRI

Treatment

- Supportive care
- Anti-inflammatory agents, preferentially NSAID vs. corticosteroid

- Other treatment based on underlying cause
- Regular neurologic examinations to monitor progress/deterioration

Musculoskeletal

Fractures

Ferrets are prone to orthopedic injuries due to their inquisitive nature and inability to respect heights. The sites most commonly involved include the long bones (i.e. humerus, radius ulna, femur, tibia and fibula). In addition, fractures of the mandible or maxilla can occur as a result of trauma or secondary due to bone disease.

Diagnosis

Signalment: No known age or gender predilection.

History: Trauma is usually apparent in the history, resulting in an acute onset of lameness or dysphagia, in case of mandibular or maxillary fractures.

Clinical Signs:

- Similar to those observed in dogs and cats
- Non-weight bearing lameness
- Swelling or bruising of soft tissues
- Paresis, paralysis, and urinary/fecal incontinence can be seen with spinal injury
- Difficulty eating if jaw fractures

Differentials:

- Other diseases resulting in pain and/or lameness
  - Neuromuscular disease (spinal cord lesions, peripheral neurologic or muscle diseases)
  - Joint problems (arthritis/arthrosis)
  - Metabolic disorders
  - Other bone disease (discospondylitis, neoplasia)
- Any disease resulting in dysphagia or pseudo-anorexia (see Table 14.2)

Diagnostics:

- Diagnosis based on examination
- Radiographs
- Culture/sensitivity if open fracture/wounds

Treatment

- Stabilization therapy
  - Treat respiratory compromise, shock, bleeding, thoracic/abdominal emergencies
- Fracture stabilization
  - (Sterile) bandages and/or splints
  - Internal or external coaptation may be required
- Limb amputation if severe injury/financial constraints
- Analgesia
  - *Meloxicam*: 0.1–0.3 mg/kg PO, SC, IM q24h
  - *Buprenorphine*: 0.01–0.05 mg/kg oral transmucosal, SC, IM, IV q4–12h
  - *Butorphanol*: 0.3 mg/kg SC, IM q2–4h
  - *Gabapentin*: 3–5 mg/kg PO q8–24h
  - *Hydromorphone*: 0.1–0.2 mg/kg SC, IM, IV
  - *Oxymorphone*: 0.05–0.2 mg/kg SC, IM, IV q8–12h
  - *Tramadol*: 5–10 mg/kg PO q12–24h
- Nutritional support
- Cage rest

Myofasciitis/Disseminated Idiopathic Myositis

Disseminated idiopathic myositis (DIM) or myofasciitis is a sporadically occurring, fatal condition for which no definitive cause has been identified. However, it has been hypothesized that recent vaccination may result in a delayed sensitivity reaction leading to the histological changes found at post-mortem.

Diagnosis

Signalment: Affected animals are usually younger than two years. No gender predilection has been reported.

History: Many affected animals were found to have received at least one canine distemper vaccination prior to developing clinical signs.

Clinical Signs:

- Lethargy, weakness
- Fever (temperature of up to 42 °C [108 °F] has been reported)
- Painful ambulation
- Anorexia, nausea
- Limb hyperesthesia
- Muscle wasting
- Splenomegaly
- Painful, swollen lymph nodes

Differentials:

- Non-specific signs – many differentials
- Ferret systemic coronavirus
- Distemper
- Megaesophagus

Diagnostics:

- Hx of recent vaccination and compatible clinical signs
- CBC
  - +/- profound leukocytosis (up to 100 000 ml^{-1})
  - Moderate anemia
- Chemistry profile
  - Hypoalbuminemia
  - Creatinine kinase (CK) and aspartate aminotransferase (AST) usually normal
  - Liver enzymes may be elevated
- Lymph node and skeletal muscle biopsy

Treatment

- Aggressive supportive care
- Intravenous fluids (see Chapter 8)
- Supplemental feeding
- NSAID
  - Can change to steroid after biopsy
- Moderate success using cyclophosphamide, interferon-α, chloramphenicol combination
- Treatment usually unrewarding with guarded prognosis

Cardiac Disease

AV Block

Cardiac conduction abnormalities (e.g. first-, second-, or third-degree atrioventricular blocks) will result in a decreased heart rate (bradycardia) and potentially arrhythmia, originating from the sinus, atria or ventricles. First-degree atrioventricular (AV) blocks are usually an incidental finding on an ECG and do not require any treatment. Second-degree AV blocks may also be seen in healthy ferrets. High-grade second- and third-degree AV blocks, however, may cause life-threatening bradycardia.

Diagnosis

Signalment: Disease is most commonly noted in middle-aged to older ferrets.

History: Minimal symptoms in case of a first- or second-degree AV block, or with collapse, weakness, lethargy, or dyspnea due to congestive heart failure in case of high-grade second- and third-degree AV block.

Clinical Signs:

- Asymptomatic if first- or second-degree AV block
- Irregular pulse wave or pulse deficits
- Arrhythmia or pause in heart rhythm on auscultation
- Severe bradycardia (<120 bpm) with high-grade second- or third-degree AV block
- Lethargy, weakness, exercise intolerance
- Syncope

Differentials:

- Metabolic disease
  - Hypoglycemia
  - Anemia
  - Shock
  - Neoplasia
- Congestive heart failure from structural heart disease (i.e. cardiomyopathy)
- Primary respiratory disease
- Pleural effusion
- Pneumothorax

Diagnostics:

- ECG
- Atropine response test
  - *Atropine* 0.02–0.05 mg/kg IV, IM, or SC
  - Increased heart rate within 15–30 minutes if vagal-mediated bradycardia
- Echocardiograph
- Radiographs
- CBC
- Biochemistry profile

Treatment

- Anticholinergics (e.g. propantheline)
- Beta adrenergics (e.g. terbutaline, isoproterenol) and/or phosphodiesterase inhibitors (e.g. aminophylline, theophylline)
  - May be beneficial if high-grade second- and third-degree AV block (particularly if the ferret showed an increased heart rate in response to atropine administration)
- If minimal response to above treatment, consider pacemaker if good candidate
- Attempt to eliminate underlying cause

Cardiomyopathy – Congestive Heart Failure

The most common acquired cardiac disorder in ferrets is dilated cardiomyopathy (DCM). The disease is characterized by an increased diastolic dimension and systolic dysfunction of the left and/or right ventricles and eventually valvular insufficiency. Upon progression of the disease, congestive heart failure will develop, resulting in pulmonary edema, pleural effusion, hepatosplenomegaly, and/or ascites.

Diagnosis

Signalment: Middle-aged to older ferrets of both genders.

History:

- Non-specific signs; lethargy, anorexia, weight loss
- Exercise intolerance
- Dyspnea
- Weakness/collapse

Clinical Signs:

- Respiratory distress (tachypnea, dyspnea)
- Coughing
- Pulse deficits
- Hypothermia
- Pallor, cyanosis, prolonged capillary refill time (CRT)

- Jugular vein distention
- Abdominal distention
  - Hepato(spleno)megaly
  - Ascites
- Tachycardia, systolic murmur, gallop rhythm, or arrhythmia
- Muffled heart and lung sounds if pleural effusion
- Moist rales, crackles, increased respiratory sounds if pulmonary edema

Differentials:

- Other diseases resulting in dyspnea or tachypnea
  - Primary lung disease (e.g. influenza, pneumonia, primary or metastatic neoplasia)
  - Pleural effusion (e.g. due to chylo-, hemo-, or pyothorax, heartworm disease)
  - Mediastinal masses (e.g. lymphoma)
  - Pneumothorax, diaphragmatic hernia
  - Upper respiratory disease
  - Metabolic disease (e.g. anemia, acidosis)
- Hypoproteinemia
- Hepatic cirrhosis
- Trauma (hemo or uro-abdomen)
- (Septic) peritonitis
- Neoplasia

Diagnostics:

- Radiographs
- Electrocardiography (ECG)
- Echocardiography to obtain a definitive diagnosis (see Figure 14.6).

Treatment

- Emergency treatment of ferrets with signs of congestive heart failure focuses on three aspects:

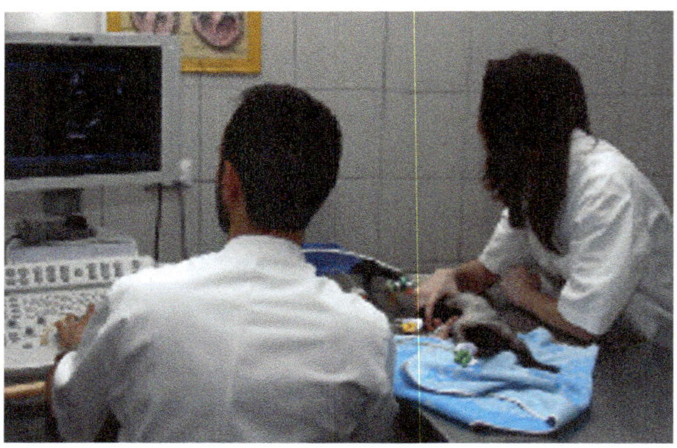

Figure 14.6 Echocardiography in ferrets is performed in lateral recumbency, like dogs and cats.

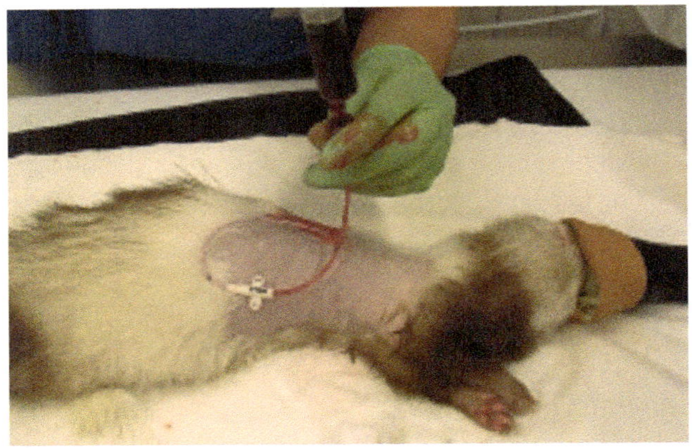

Figure 14.7 Thoracocentesis is performed by inserting a needle through the intercostal space into the thoracic cavity in a cranial direction. Care should be taken to avoid puncturing the heart. Ultrasound guidance may aid in directing the needle in a safe direction.

(1) Improving oxygenation, e.g. by placing the animal in an incubator with supplemental oxygen
(2) Reduction of the preload by provision of diuretics
Furosemide: 1–4 mg/kg PO, SC, IM, IV q8–12h
Hydrochlorothiazide: 2–4 mg/kg PO q12h
Spironolactone: 1.7–3.3 mg/kg PO q24h
(3) Reducing the afterload by providing angiotensin-converting enzyme (ACE) inhibitors (only advised in sufficiently stabilized patients due to the hypotensive effects of these drugs)
Benazepril: 0.25–0.5 mg/kg PO q24h
Enalapril: 0.25–0.5 mg/kg PO q24–48h

- Thoracocentesis if effusion (see Figure 14.7)
- *Pimobendan*: 0.25–1.25 mg/kg PO q12h
- *Digoxin*: 0.005–0.01 mg/kg PO q12–24h
  - Monitor serum concentrations (therapeutic range: 1–2 ng/ml 6–12 hours following oral administration)
  - Monitor for clinical signs of toxicity

Heartworm Disease

Heartworm disease is caused by *Dirofilaria immitis*, a filarid that is transmitted through insects. Following infection, worms will migrate to the right ventricle, cranial vena cava, or main pulmonary artery where they cause villous endarteritis. Due to the ferrets' small size, one or two worms may already result in pronounced and potentially fatal right-sided heart failure due to mechanical obstruction of the blood flow.

Diagnosis

Signalment: Ferrets that live or originate from heartworm endemic areas are considered most at risk to develop disease.

History: Animals with heartworm disease are often presented with acute onset of life-threatening respiratory distress.

Clinical Signs:

- Anorexia, lethargy, weakness, depression
- Tachycardia
- Heart murmur
- Dyspnea, tachypnea
- Coughing
- Pale mucous membranes, cyanosis
- Melena (rare)
- Crackles and moist rales (pulmonary edema)
- Decreased thoracic compliance, muffled heart, and lung sounds (pulmonary effusion)
- Abdominal distention
  - Ascites and hepatosplenomegaly (right-sided heart failure)

Differentials:

- Any cardiac, systemic or pulmonary disease resulting in dyspnea, tachypnea, and/or coughing
  - Mediastinal lymphoma
  - Dilated cardiomyopathy
  - Pyothorax

Diagnostics:

- CBC
  - Monocytosis, mild non-regenerative anemia, and (rarely) eosinophilia
- Biochemistry profile
  - Bilirubinemia
- Thoracic radiographs
  - Interstitial lung pattern secondary to pneumonitis
- Echocardiography
  - Adult worms visible in pulmonary artery, right ventricle, and/or right atrium
- Enzyme linked immunosorbent assay (ELISA)-based antigen tests
- Cytology of blood smear revealing microfilaremia

Treatment

- Stabilization care
  - Oxygen, furosemide, enalapril (see Section "Cardiomyopathy – Congestive Heart Failure")
  - *Theophylline*: 4.25 mg/kg PO q8–12h
- Thoracocentesis if pleural effusion
- Infection treatment
  - Adulticide (e.g. moxidectin) and/or microfilaricide (e.g. ivermectin, dithiazanine iodide)
  - Alternatively, transvenous heartworm extraction
  - *Prednisone* (0.5–1 mg/kg q12–24h PO) is often initiated concurrently with the adulticide treatment and continued for at least four months

Prevention

Prevention of (re)infection can best achieved through monthly administration of ivermectin, milbemycin oxime, selamectin, or moxidectin. Therapy should start one month before and continuing until one month after the heartworm season. Housing ferrets indoors, particularly during the mosquito season, may also help to minimize exposure.

Respiratory Disease

Pleural Effusion

Pleural effusion may occur due to increased production or decreased resorption of fluid from the thoracic cavity. A change in the vascular permeability or hydrostatic and oncotic pressure may also play a role. Dependent on the physical characteristics, the fluid is classified as transudate, exudates, or modified transudate. Transudate is seen in cases of heart failure, while exudate is seen in case of (bacterial) infections. Other causes for pleural effusion include overhydration, infections, hypoalbuminemia, neoplasia, and trauma (e.g. resulting in hemothorax). In rare cases, a chylothorax may be seen.

Diagnosis

Signalment: Variable, dependent on the underlying cause.

History: History will usually include acute or gradual onset of dyspnea.

Clinical Signs:

- Dyspnea and rapid, shallow respirations
- Muffled lung sounds heard ventrally
- Coughing
- Lethargy, anorexia, weakness
- Other signs may vary depending on cause
  - Febrile if infections, inflammation, and/or neoplasia
  - Heart murmur, gallops, arrhythmias, and/or jugular venous distention if heart failure

Differentials: Any other cause for respiratory disease (see Table 14.6).

Diagnostics:

- Based on clinical findings and imaging
- Radiographs
- Ultrasound
- Fluid collection for cytology and C/S

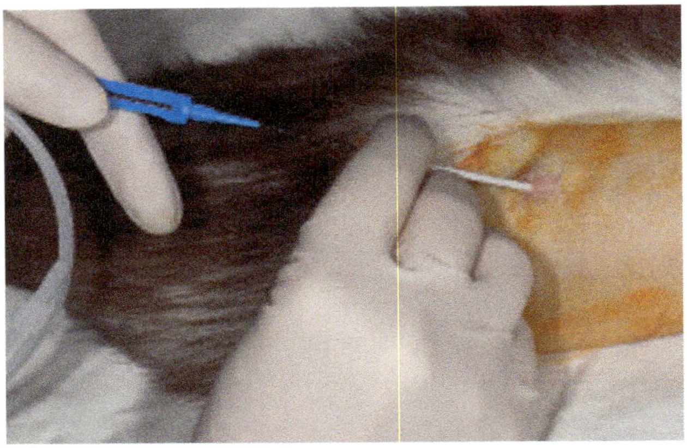

Figure 14.8 In ferrets with a pyothorax, placement of a chest drain may be considered. The technique used is like that in larger companion animals. Following placement, the drain is sutured to the skin to maintain its position.

- CBC
- Biochemistry profile
- ELISA heartworm test

Treatment

- Oxygen therapy
- Thoracocentesis or placement of chest drain to remove the excess fluid (see Figure 14.8)
- Other therapy dependent on underlying cause

Pneumonia

Aspiration pneumonia has been reported to be the most common cause of pneumonia in ferrets. Influenza is another major cause of pneumonia in ferrets. In addition, pneumonia may result from other viral (e.g. CDV), bacterial (e.g. *Streptococcus*, *Bordetella*, *Klebsiella*), and/or mycotic (e.g. *Cryptococcus*) infections.

Diagnosis

Signalment: No known age or gender predilection.

History: History will commonly reveal an acute or gradual onset of respiratory distress, lethargy, weakness, anorexia, and weight loss. In case of influenza, history will commonly reveal contact of the ferret with people showing flu-like symptoms.

Clinical Signs:

- Tachypnea
- Dyspnea
- Cyanosis
- Loud breath sounds
  - Crackles/wheezes
- +/- fever/coughing

Differentials: Any other disease resulting in dyspnea or tachypnea (see Table 14.6).

Diagnostics:

- Thoracic radiographs
  - Interstitial or alveolar pattern
- CBC
  - Leukocytosis with neutrophilia +/- left shift; normal leukocyte count does not rule out pneumonia
- Cytology or culture and sensitivity testing of samples collected via a (trans)tracheal wash and/or bronchial alveolar lavage

Treatment

- Oxygen
- Bronchodilator if respiratory distress
- Broad-spectrum antibiotics can be used, ideally based on C/S
  - *Amoxicillin/clavulanic acid*: 13–25 mg/kg PO q8–12h
  - *Doxycycline*: 10 mg/kg PO q12h
  - *Trimethoprim–sulfonamide (TMP/S)*: 30 mg/kg PO q12h
- Provision of rest and supportive care

Pulmonary Edema

Pulmonary edema may be seen in case of left-sided (congestive) heart failure. Non-cardiogenic pulmonary edema has not been reported in ferrets.

Diagnosis

Signalment: Cardiogenic pulmonary edema is most commonly seen in middle-aged to older ferrets.

History: Ferrets with cardiogenic lung edema will commonly present with a history of lethargy, anorexia, weakness, and respiratory distress.

Clinical Signs:

- (Progressive) dyspnea, tachypnea, and crackles and increased respiratory sounds on pulmonary auscultation.

Differentials: Other diseases resulting in tachypnea or dyspnea (see Table 14.6).

Diagnostics:

- Thoracic radiographs
  - Alveolar pattern
  - Cardiomegaly, pleural effusion, ascites, and/or hepatosplenomegaly if cardiogenic pulmonary edema
- Echocardiography

Treatment

Emergency treatment consists of oxygen supplementation and the administration of furosemide. In addition, the underlying cause of the pulmonary edema should be addressed.

Gastrointestinal Disease

Esophageal Disorders

Esophageal disorders are rarely seen in ferrets. Megaesophagus and foreign body ingestion have infrequently been diagnosed in ferrets. Although the underlying cause for megaesophagus in ferrets is unknown, factors attributing to the condition are likely similar to dogs and cats.

Diagnosis

Signalment: No known age or gender predilection.

History: Owners will commonly report a history of difficulty with eating, whereby the animal displays increased swallowing efforts, coughing, choking, or regurgitation.

Clinical Signs:

- Dysphagia
- Regurgitation
- Inappetence
- Weight loss
- Lethargy
- Aspiration pneumonia may occur which may lead to respiratory distress.

Differentials:

- All conditions associated with vomiting or regurgitation (see Table 14.3)
- Gastritis
- Myasthenia gravis
- Esophageal stricture
- Disease resulting in respiratory distress (e.g. influenza, [broncho]pneumonia, pleural effusion, pulmonary edema)

Diagnostics:

- Radiographs (see Figure 14.9) +/- contrast
- esophagoscopy
- Fluoroscopy
- Megaesophagus associated with myasthenia gravis has been diagnosed by radiography, combined with intravenous neostigmine methylsulfate administration and measurement of cross-reacting anti-acetylcholine receptor antibodies.

Treatment

- Correct fluid deficits and electrolyte imbalances (see Chapter 8)
- Foreign body removal via endoscopy or surgery
  - Esophageal ruptures may be sutured, but post-surgical stricture formation can occur

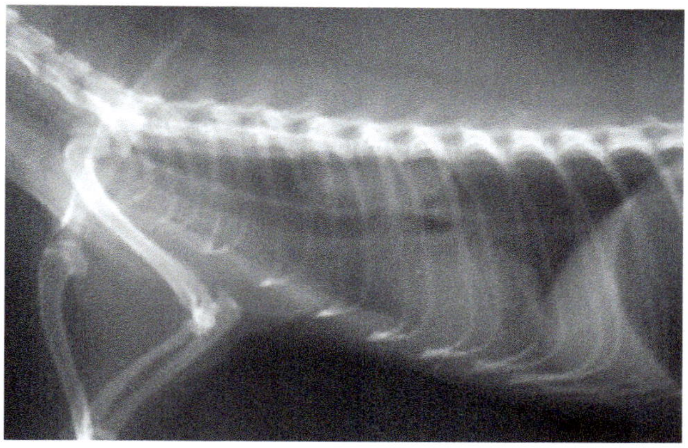

Figure 14.9 Lateral radiograph of a nine-month-old ferret presenting with anorexia, hypersalivation, and unproductive vomiting. Directly cranial to the heart a large mass is visible in the esophagus that was removed endoscopically and found to be part of a toy ball.

- Aggressive antibiotic therapy and oxygen supplementation if aspiration pneumonia
- +/- Esophagostomy tube
- Administration of pyridostigmine bromide has been found to result in a temporary remission of clinical signs of myasthenia gravis. However, managing a ferret with megaesophagus is challenging as having the animal eat from an elevation and ensuring it stays in an upright position for a sufficiently long time (10–15 minutes) after feeding is not easy. Frequent small meals and provision of soft foods is often recommended to facilitate passage of food into the stomach.

Gastritis/Gastric Ulcers/Trichobezoars

Gastritis, eventually leading to gastric ulcers is considered very common in ferrets due to either a *Helicobacter mustelae* infection or the use of NSAIDs. Irritation of the gastric wall by ingested foreign bodies or trichobezoars may also lead to gastritis.

Diagnosis

Signalment: Ferrets of any age and both genders can be affected, but disease appears to be most commonly seen in younger ferrets (<3 years).

History: Animals will commonly present with anorexia, ptyalism, pawing at the mouth, bruxism, weight loss, vomiting, diarrhea, melena, and abdominal pain. History may further reveal the presence of potential stressors resulting in gastric ulcers (e.g. overcrowding poor sanitary conditions) or intake of medications predisposing to gastric ulcers (e.g. NSAIDs, glucocorticoids).

Clinical Signs:

- May be minimal
- Signs indicating nausea (e.g. hypersalivation, pawing at the mouth, teeth-grinding), anorexia, and lethargy are commonly noted
- Vomiting and melena if GI ulcers
- Masses and/or pain on abdominal palpation

Differentials:

- Insulinoma or other causes of nausea (see Table 14.3)
- Ileus
- Liver or kidney failure
- Intracranial processes

Diagnostics:

- CBC
  - (Regenerative) anemia
  - Hemoconcentrated if dehydrated
  - +/- Leukocytosis
- Blood chemistry
  - Hypoproteinemia w/hypoalbuminemia
  - Azotemia if dehydrated
  - Hepatic enzyme elevation
- Abdominal radiographs +/- air or barium contrast
- Abdominal ultrasound
  - Can be unremarkable or reveal irregular mucosa or gastric foreign body
- Gastroscopy to confirm GI ulcers (see Figure 14.10)
- Histopathology of gastric biopsies

Treatment

- Fluid therapy (see Chapter 8)
  - Correct electrolyte or acid-base disturbances

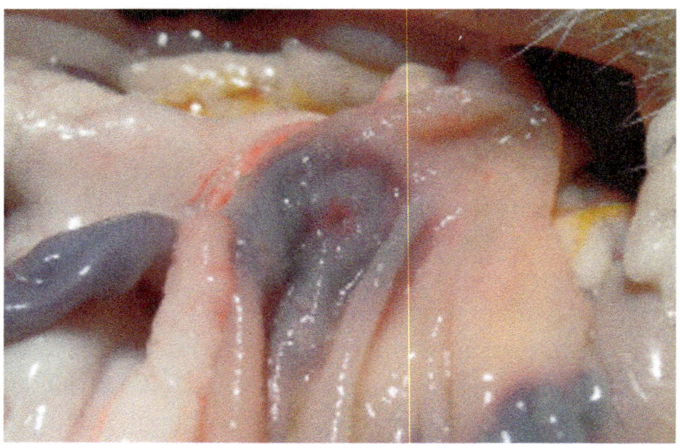

Figure 14.10 Perforating gastric ulcer diagnosed upon post-mortem examination of a four-year-old ferret that died shortly after presentation with a chronic history of persistent vomiting, melena, and regenerative anemia.

- Antacids
  - H2 receptor antagonists, i.e. ranitidine or omeprazole
    - *Ranitidine HCl*: 3.5 mg/kg PO q12h
    - *Omeprazole*: 0.7 mg/kg PO q24h
- Gastric protectants
  - *Sucralfate*: 25–125 mg/kg PO q8–12h
- Assisted feeding
- Broad-spectrum antibiotic therapy if suspected Helicobacter infection
  - *Amoxicillin/clavulanic acid:* 13–25 mg/kg PO q8–12 h × 14 days or
  - *Clarithromycin:* 50 mg/kg PO q24h or divided q12h × 14d in combination with
  - *Metronidazole*: 15–20 mg/kg PO q12h × 14 d
- Endoscopic or surgical removal of trichobezoar

Gastroenteritis

Gastroenteritis may be due to bacterial (e.g. *Salmonella*, *Campylobacter*), viral (e.g. ferret enteric coronavirus [causative agent of epizootic catarrhal enteritis or ECE], rotavirus), or parasitic (e.g. *Giardia*, *Cryptosporidium*, coccidia) infections. In addition, immune-mediated disease in the form of inflammatory bowel disease or eosinophilic gastroenteritis is frequently seen.

Diagnosis

Signalment: *Campylobacter*, proliferative bowel disease, and coccidiosis are commonly seen in younger, weanling ferrets, although these types of infections can be diagnosed in older animals as well. For many other diseases, no gender or gender predilection exists.

History: Animals suffering from *Salmonella* or *Campylobacter*-associated gastroenteritis will commonly have a history of eating raw or improperly cooked food (particularly poultry). Other risk factors include suboptimal housing conditions and exposure to other ferrets (particularly new animals). In animals with ECE, clinical signs will usually develop within 24–48 hours. Following contact with an (often asymptomatic) carrier.

Clinical Signs:

- Inappetence, weight loss
- Bruxism
- Vomiting/diarrhea
- Melena
- Thickened intestinal loops +/- enlarged abdominal lymph nodes
- +/- fever
- Severe diarrhea may result in dehydration and shock

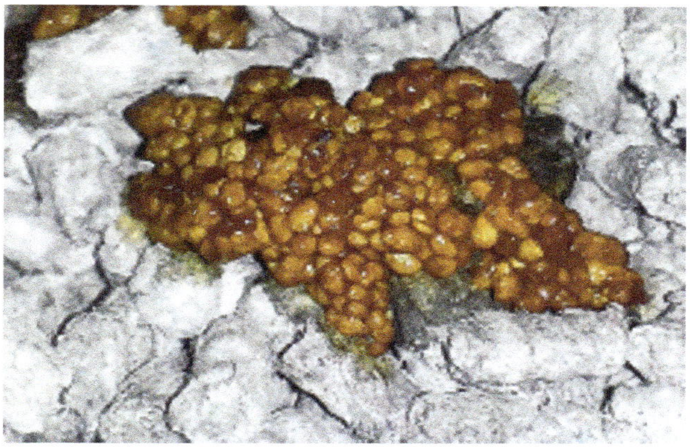

Figure 14.11 Birdseed-like feces in a ferret. This type of abnormal feces can frequently be seen in ferrets suffering from malabsorption and/or maldigestion and has been associated with inflammatory bowel disease and ferret enteric coronavirus.

- Profuse greenish to mucoid diarrhea or "birdseed-like" feces with ECE (see Figure 14.11)
- More severe signs generally seen in older vs. younger animals

Differentials: Any disease resulting in vomiting or diarrhea (see Table 14.3), especially trichobezoar and foreign body ingestion.

Diagnostics:

- CBC
  - Anemia and leukocytosis possible
- Biochemistry profile
  - r/o hypoalbuminemia and or electrolyte/acid-base disturbances
- Fecal examinations
- Fecal culture
  - Direct wet mount
  - Fecal flotation or zinc sulfate centrifugation
- Gastrointestinal biopsy to confirm immune-mediated gastritis or proliferative bowel disease (PBD)

Treatment

- Fluid therapy (see Chapter 8)
  - Parenteral if severe diarrhea
- Nutritional support
  - Diet change to primarily meat-based diet may be helpful; use reliable meat source
- Antibiotics
  - Bacterial gastroenteritis:
    - *Trimethoprim/sulfa*: 15–30 mg/kg PO q12h or
    - *Metronidazole*: 15–20 mg/kg PO q12h
  - Coccidiosis:
    - *Sulfadimethoxine*: 50 mg/kg PO, then 25 mg/kg PO q24h × 9d
    - *Amprolium*: 19 mg/kg PO q24h
  - Giardiasis:
    - *Metronidazole*: 15–20 mg/kg PO q12h or
    - *Fenbendazole*: 20 mg/kg PO q24h × 5d
  - Proliferative bowel disease (Lawsonia intracellularis):
    - *Chloramphenicol*: 25–50 mg/kg PO q12h × 14d
- Consider corticosteroids if immune-mediated disease (i.e. eosinophilic gastroenteritis)
- Proper hygiene and disinfection important; Campylobacter and cryptosporidia may be difficult to eliminate

Ileus

Foreign bodies, especially pieces of rubber toys or foam rubber, are a common cause of ileus in ferrets.

Diagnosis

Signalment: Mostly younger ferrets (<3 years).

History: Ingestion of inappropriate foods or materials is more likely to occur in animals that roam freely in the house without supervision.

Clinical Signs:

- Anorexia, lethargy
- Nausea (hypersalivation, pawing at mouth)
- Vomiting, diarrhea
- Painful on abdominal palpation +/- gas- or fluid-filled stomach
- +/- Foreign body palpation

Differentials:

- Any disease causing nausea, regurgitation, and vomiting (see Table 14.3)
  - Ulcerative gastritis, trichobezoars, and insulinoma
- Masses palpated in the abdomen can also indicate presence of a tumor, granuloma (e.g. in case of FSCV) or hyperplasia.

Diagnostics:

- Abdominal palpation
- (Contrast) radiography
- Abdominal ultrasound
  - Distended, fluid-, or gas-filled intestinal loops cranial to the obstruction. The foreign body itself may be recognized as a dense structure, filling defect, or as an intraluminal structure producing an acoustic shadow

Treatment

- Correct dehydration and fluid losses
  - Correct electrolyte and acid-base disturbances

- CBC
- Biochemistry profile
- Endoscopy, gastrotomy, or enterotomy to remove obstruction

Hepatic Disease

Although ferrets may develop hepatic disease, primary hepatic disease is not commonly seen. Hepatic tumors are seen, of which lymphoma is the most commonly found. In addition, chronic cholangiohepatitis, which has been associated with *Helicobacter* infection, can also be diagnosed in ferrets. Copper hepatopathy has also been reported.

Diagnosis

Signalment: Often involving older, neutered animals of both genders.

History: Animals will often show chronic wasting.

Clinical Signs:

- Non-specific including lethargy, anorexia, weight loss, vomiting, and diarrhea
- Icterus (see Figure 14.12) or hepatomegaly

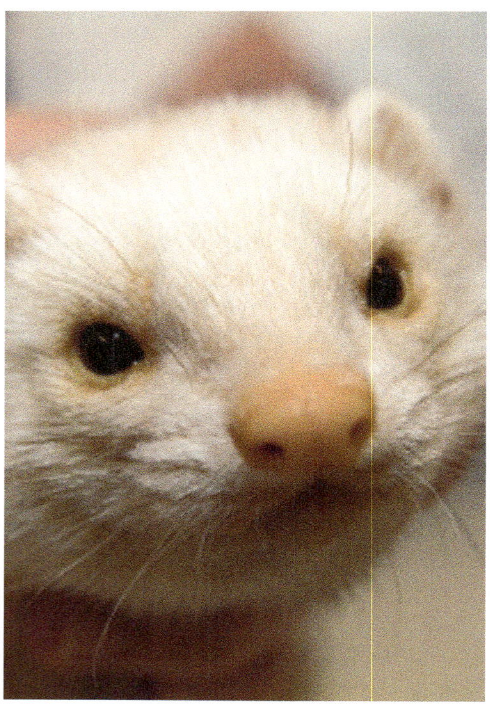

Figure 14.12 Icterus is an infrequent finding in ferrets but may be seen in advanced hepatic disease. The unpigmented nose in this two-year-old ferret with a severe hepatitis clearly shows the yellow coloration typical of icterus.

Differentials:

- Biliary obstruction
- Hepatotoxic substances
- Infectious disease: e.g. Helicobacter, Campylobacter
- Metabolic disease
- Renal disease
- Copper hepatopathy

Diagnostics:

- CBC
- Biochemistry profile
  - Elevated plasma alanine aminotransferase (ALT) concentration (> 275 IU/l)
  - Bile acid >10 μmol/l indicates loss of liver function
- Abdominal ultrasound
- Liver sampling (evaluating clotting times in advance advised)
  - Ultrasound-guided FNA
  - Tru-Cut® biopsy
  - Cytology, histopathology
  - Consider copper staining +/- quantitative copper levels if warranted

Treatment

- Fluid therapy and nutritional support (see Chapter 8)
- Additional therapy based on etiology
  - Broad-spectrum antibiotics
  - +/- Ursodeoxycholic acid if high bile acids and no biliary obstruction
  - Chelation therapy if copper hepatopathy

Pancreatitis

Pancreatitis is not well described in ferrets. It has been seen in association with insulinoma or after insulinoma surgery.

Diagnosis

Signalment: Obese ferrets appear to be predisposed, as well as those suffering from endocrine disease (e.g. diabetes mellitus, insulinoma).

History: History may reveal a recent insulinoma surgery or presence of endocrine disease.

Clinical Signs:

- Non-specific including anorexia, lethargy, nausea, vomiting, fever, and abdominal pain
- Diabetic ketoacidosis common sequelae in diabetic patients

Differentials: Any disease resulting in fever, vomiting, or abdominal pain (see Table 14.3).

Diagnostics:

- Plasma lipase or amylase elevations supportive but not sensitive/diagnostic
- Abdominal ultrasound
- Pancreatic biopsy for definitive diagnosis

Treatment

- Parenteral fluid therapy and nutritional support
- +/- broad-spectrum antibiotics and NSAID

Rectal Prolapse

A rectal prolapse is not commonly seen in ferrets, although it may be seen in ferrets with gastrointestinal (e.g. coccidiosis, proliferative bowel disease, gastrointestinal foreign body) or anal pathology (e.g. rectal or anal neoplasia), prostate enlargement or those that underwent (peri)anal or urogenital surgery (e.g. anal sacculectomy).

Diagnosis

Signalment: Usually younger animals (two to six months).

History: Animals will often present with a history of (chronic) diarrhea, tenesmus, or dyschezia.

Clinical Signs:

- Protrusion of rectal mucosa from anus
- Persistent tenesmus
- Pain while defecating

Differentials:

- Chronic diarrhea
- Inflammatory bowel disease
- Eosinophilic gastroenteritis
- Bacterial enteritis
- GI lymphoma
- Proliferative bowel disease

Diagnostics:

- Visualize prolapse
- CBC
- Biochemistry profile
- Fecal examination
  - Culture/sensitivity
  - Wet mount
  - Fecal flotation
- Abdominal radiographs
- Abdominal ultrasound
  - Ultrasound-guided FNA of affected tissue

Treatment

- Topical or systemic analgesia
- Gently replace prolapsed tissue with use of lubricants
  - 50% chilled dextrose solution can reduce swelling
  - Maintain tissue moisture to prevent desiccation
  - Purse-string suture around anus (make sure feces can still pass)
    - Non-absorbable suture material as suture may need to stay in place three weeks.
- Treat underlying cause to prevent recurrence

Urinary Disease

Acute Renal Failure: Toxins, Nephritis

The most common causes of acute renal failure are urinary obstruction (see "Urinary Obstruction") or ingestion of toxic substances such as NSAIDs (e.g. ibuprofen), and acetaminophen).

Diagnosis

Signalment: Incidence of renal disease appears to increase with age.

History: History may reveal exposure to toxins or recent medical conditions or surgery.

Clinical Signs:

- Acute onset of anorexia, lethargy, vomiting, and anuria/oliguria
- Polyuria or polydipsia possible
- Oral ulcers, diarrhea, melena, halitosis, ataxia, seizures, paresis
- Shock if acute renal failure
  - Depression, hypothermia, tachypnea, bradycardia
  - Renomegaly possible

Differentials:

- Other diseases resulting in shock (see Table 14.7)
- Disease resulting in azotemia:
  - Hypovolemia
  - Hypoadrenocorticism
  - Urinary obstruction
  - Bladder rupture
- If PU/PD: diabetes mellitus, hepatic disease, administration of diuretics, hypercalcemia, pyometra, Cushing's disease, or iatrogenic glucocorticoid administration, diabetes insipidus, and primary polydipsia
- If renomegaly: renal neoplasia, hydronephrosis, and cystic kidney disease

Diagnostics:

- Based on history and biochemistry panel
  - Uremia, hyperphosphatemia, hyperkalemia
- Urinalysis
- Abdominal radiography and ultrasound
- Blood pressure measurement

Treatment

- Intravenous fluids to restore circulation and correct electrolyte imbalances
  - Requirements range from 75 to 100 ml/kg/day based on severity of disease
  - Monitor urine production, body condition, respiratory rate, and character
- If anuria/oliguria:
  - *Dobutamine*: 0.01 ml/animal IV p.r.n. and
  - *Furosemide*: 1–4 mg/kg PO, SC, IM, IV q8–12h
- If vomiting:
  - *Metoclopramide*: 0.2–1 mg/kg PO, SC, IM q6–8h
- If NSAID ingestion:
  - *Sucralfate*: 25–125 mg/kg PO q8–12h
- Omeprazole, ranitidine, or cimetidine to reduce gastric acid production
  - *Omeprazole*: 0.7 mg/kg PO q24h
  - *Ranitidine HCl*: 3.5 mg/kg PO q12h
  - *Cimetidine*: 5–10 mg/kg PO, SC, IM q8h

Urinary Obstruction

The most common causes of urinary obstruction are urolithiasis and peri-prostatic or peri-urethral cysts and prostatic enlargement (see Section "Adrenal Masses"). If present, the most common composition of uroliths is cystine, although the more common historically was magnesium ammonium phosphate or struvite.

Diagnosis

Signalment: Mostly in male ferrets.

History: History may reveal clinical signs of adrenal disease as an underlying cause for urogenital cystic disease. In addition, dietary history may reveal feeding of dog food or plant-based protein, which can lead to development of urolithiasis.

Clinical Signs:

- Stranguria, dysuria, or anuria
- Urinary incontinence and/or urinary scalding
- In more advanced cases, may see vomiting, lethargy, anorexia, and collapse
- Distended bladder noted on abdominal palpation

Differentials:

- Territorial marking
- Urinary tract infection
- Renal disease

Diagnostics:

- Abdominal radiographs and ultrasound
  - U/S-guided FNA of cystic structures for cytology or culture
- Urinary catheterization
  - Urine or uroliths passed can be submitted for evaluation
- CBC
- Biochemistry profile

Treatment

- Urinary catheterization or cystocentesis
  - Reduce bladder volume
  - Flush intraurethral stones into bladder
- Fluid therapy
  - Correct azotemia and electrolyte imbalances
- Long-term management depends on cause
  - Urolithiasis: retrograde hydropropulsion followed by cystotomy, or urethrostomy in case of urethral stones
  - Urogenital cysts: placement of a prepubic catheter, surgical debulking of cysts combined with medical or surgical management of adrenal disease
- High-quality meat-based diet to prevent urolithiasis

Reproductive Disease

Estrogen Toxicity/Hyperestrogenism

Estrogen toxicity is a well-known condition in intact female ferrets. Unless they are bred, these females will remain in estrus when daylight lasts longer than 12 hours. The prolonged estrus and associated hyperestrogenism may result in an estrogen-induced bone marrow suppression and pancytopenia, which can result in life-threatening anemia and blood loss due to thrombocytopenia.

Diagnosis

Signalment: Sexually mature (>8–12 months), non-neutered females.

History: History will reveal a failure to breed a non-neutered female. Typically, these females will show signs of (persistent) estrus.

Clinical Signs:

- Bilateral symmetric alopecia
- Vulvar swelling

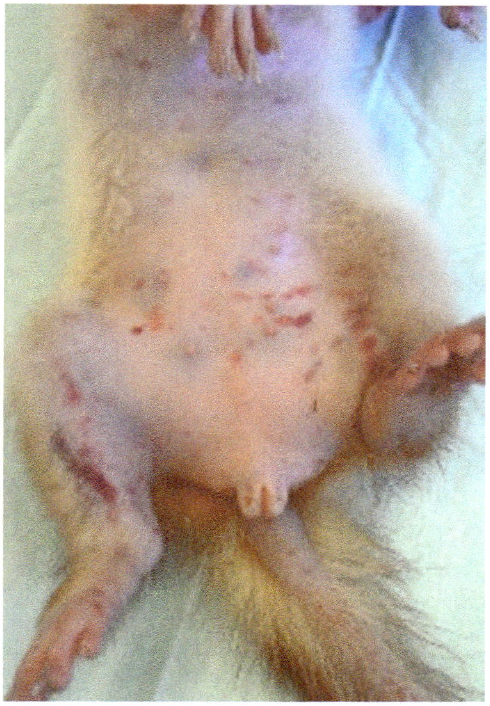

Figure 14.13 Petechial hemorrhages found on the ventral abdomen of a two-year-old, intact female ferret. These petechiae are indicative of thrombocytopenia resulting from estrogen toxicity due to prolonged estrus (as apparent from the swollen vulva).

- Pale mucous membranes
- Melena, hematuria, petechiae, ecchymosis, or other signs of hemorrhage (Figure 14.13)

Differentials:

- Adrenal gland disease
- Ovarian remnant
- Granulosa cell tumors

Diagnostics:

- Clinical signs suggestive
- CBC or bone marrow biopsy
  - Cephalic or saphenous preferred venipuncture sites to better control hemorrhage
  - Non-regenerative anemia, thrombocytopenia, leukopenia
- As swollen vulva only occurs under influence of estrogen, plasma estradiol concentrations not necessary

Treatment

- Blood transfusion if PCV drops below 15%
  - Does not address thrombocytopenia (thrombocytes aggregate w/collection)
- Cease estrogen production by inducing ovulation
  - Human chorionic gonadotropin (hCG): 100 IU/ferret IM
  - Gonadotropin releasing hormone (GnRH): 20 μg/kg IM
  - Deslorelin implant
- Prognosis better for jills with PCV >25% vs. <25%

Perinatal Complications

The most common perinatal complication seen in jills is dystocia. Duration of gestation in primiparous jills is 41 days, while jills that have delivered kits before may whelp on day 42. It is important to realize that for the initiation of parturition, a minimum of three kits is needed. If fewer than three kits are present, signs of labor and parturition may pass and the kits will likely die in the uterus after day 43. Other causes for dystocia include oversized kits, malpositioning, inadequate nutrition of the mother, abnormalities of the pelvic canal (e.g. previous pelvic fracture) or vulva (e.g. stricture), and/or prolonged labor (e.g. due to poor uterine contractions or insufficient cervical dilatation).

Diagnosis

Signalment: Intact, breeding females.

History: History will reveal mating to have occurred 41–42 days ago, with mammary gland enlargement occurring within the last week.

Clinical Signs:

- Restlessness, signs of pain and irritability, and abdominal straining for <4 hours without the delivery of the kits
- No signs in females with small litter size

Differentials: Pseudopregnancy is the most important differential diagnosis to be considered, which will occur following a failed mating.

Diagnostics:

- Clinical signs and abdominal palpation
- Abdominal radiographs to visualize number and position of kits
- Ultrasound to assess fetal viability

Treatment

- Assure kits correctly positioned in uterus prior to labor induction
- Induce labor by IM administration of prostaglandin F2α (0.5–1 mg). If this does not induce labor within three hours, oxytocin may be given IM (3 IU; dosages of up to 10 IU have been reported). Pretreatment with prostaglandin F2α has been reported to be required for oxytocin to be effective.

- Cesarean section advised if:
  - Treatment with prostaglandin F2α and oxytocin fail to result in delivery of kits within eight hours after parturition has started
  - Fetal malposition, intrauterine death, fetal stress, oversized kits

Endocrine Disease

Insulinoma

Insulinomas are one of the most commonly diagnosed tumors in ferrets. These tumors, arising from the pancreatic beta cells, are usually small (0.5–2 mm) and produce an excessive amount of insulin resulting in hypoglycemic episodes.

Diagnosis

Signalment: Middle-aged to older ferrets, with a median age of five years (range two to eight years).

History: Owners will commonly report an episodic occurrence, whereby clinical signs are most evident when the ferret has not eaten for some time and will often resolve spontaneously after providing the ferret with some food. An association with exercise or excitement may also be noticeable. Owners will often notice a glazed look in the eyes of their ferrets prior to the onset of an episode.

Clinical Signs:

- Lethargy and stargazing
- Ptyalism and pawing at the mouth (check roof of mouth for ulceration)
- Generalized seizures, collapse, and coma
- Muscle wasting in chronic cases, otherwise minimal physical examination findings may be seen

Differentials:

- Any disease resulting in weakness of the hindlimbs:
  - Spinal/orthopedic disorders
  - Cardiac disease
  - Metabolic disease including hypocalcemia and hypoglycemia
- Neoplasia
- Hepatic disease
- Sepsis
- Severe malnutrition or starvation

Diagnostics:

- Blood glucose level: Concentration below 60 mg/dl (3.3 mmol/l; reference range: 90–125 mg/dl [5.0–7.0 mmol/l]), after withholding food for four hours is highly suggestive of insulinoma
- Ultrasound may be helpful to visualize larger masses
- Plasma insulin concentration: Even values within the reference range (4.6–43.4 μU/l; 33–311 pmol/l) should be considered increased as insulin levels should normally be decreased in case of hypoglycemia.

Treatment

- 50% dextrose bolus diluted 1:1 with saline or lactated Ringer's (0.25–2.0 ml over one to three minutes, titrated to effect)
- Following initial dextrose bolus, maintenance fluids supplemented with 5% dextrose to prevent rebound hypoglycemia
- Diazepam if seizures persist despite IV dextrose
- Glucagon 15–40 ng/kg/min CRI (constant rate infusion) may be helpful in animals with an insufficient response to other types of therapy
- Once hypoglycemic crisis stabilized:
  - Surgical therapy, i.e. partial pancreatectomy or nodulectomy
  - Medical management, i.e. glucocorticoids +/- diazoxide
    - *Prednisolone*: 0.25–1 mg/kg PO divided q12h; may need to increase dose over time. Ideal to use H2 blocker concurrently
    - *Diazoxide*: 5–30 mg/kg PO q12h
  - Anecdotal reports of successful management using Palladia (toceranib phosphate)
- Dietary management important; can feed high carbohydrate liquid food in crisis but otherwise provide frequent/continuous access to high-quality protein meat-based diet

Hyperadrenocorticism

Hyperadrenocorticism is the most common endocrine disease seen in ferrets. These patients are seldom presented as emergency cases, unless suffering from severe blood loss due to hemorrhage of the adrenal tumor or from urinary blockage due to prostate enlargement in males (see Section "Adrenal Masses"). Note that clinical signs of hyperadrenocorticism in ferrets are associated with increased sex hormone production vs. cortisol elevations. As such, cortisol levels, adrenocorticotropic hormone (ACTH) stimulation tests, and dexamethasone suppression testing are not indicated.

Diagnosis

Signalment: Seen primarily in middle-aged to older neutered ferrets with a mean age of three to four years (range one to seven years).

History: Owners will commonly note progressive alopecia and pruritus as well as return of sexual behavior.

Clinical Signs:

- Symmetric alopecia (see Figure 14.1)
- Swollen vulva and occasional mammary gland enlargement in neutered females
- Return of sexual behaviors after neutering in males and females
- Pruritis
- Stranguria in males secondary to prostatic cysts or enlargement (see Section "Urinary Obstruction")
- Bone marrow suppression from estrogen toxicity in rare cases

Differentials:

- Seasonal alopecia
- Ovarian remnant
- Granulosa cell tumor
- Food intolerance (pruritis)

Diagnostics:

- Ultrasound to visualize enlarged adrenal gland in the absence of ovaries/ovarian remnant
- Radiographs rarely show adrenomegaly
- Hormone panel measuring androstenedione, estradiol, and 17-hydroxyprogesterone
- CBC
  - Rarely anemia/pancytopenia
- Biochemistry panel usually within normal limits
- In rare cases, urinalysis may show urinary tract infection concurrent with prostatic disease

Treatment

- Emergency treatment of patients with hyperadrenocorticism is rarely indicated
- Surgical resection of the affected adrenal gland(s)
  - Right adrenalectomy is high risk surgery
  - Bilateral adrenalectomy may result in hypoadrenocorticism
- Medical management with GnRH agonist (deslorelin or leuprolide acetate)
- For the treatment of hormone-induced anemia and urogenital cystic disease: see Sections "Estrogen Toxicity/Hyperestrogenism."

Neoplastic Disease

Adrenal Masses

Adrenal masses are among the most common tumors seen in ferrets. Ferrets diagnosed with these masses are frequently referred to as having adrenocortical disease, adrenal gland disease, or hyperadrenocorticism (see Section "Endocrine Disease"). Histological changes of these adrenal masses range from (nodular) hyperplasia to adenocarcinoma. Rarely, adrenal masses have been found to be associated with pheochromocytoma.

Diagnosis

Signalment: Middle aged to older, neutered ferrets of both genders.

History: Similar to hyperadrenocorticism.

Clinical Signs:

- Clinical signs resulting from adrenal masses include those described for hyperadrenocorticism (see Section "Hyperadrenocorticism")
- Dysuria due to periprostatic or periurethral cysts and/or prostatomegaly
- Abdominal distention and shock with urinary obstruction
- Large adrenal masses may be palpable in rare cases
- Shock and acute collapse with pheochromocytoma

Differentials: See Section "Hyperadrenocorticism." The most important differential of dysuria in male ferrets with an adrenal mass includes urolithiasis.

Diagnostics: See Section "Hyperadrenocorticism"

- Large adrenal masses may be palpable in some cases

Treatment

See Section "Hyperadrenocorticism"

Insulinoma

Insulinomas are tumors of the pancreatic beta cells which result in hypoglycemia due to the excessive production of insulin. Although hyperplasia, adenomas, or carcinomas may be found on histological evaluation, it is rare that these tumors will metastasize. For further information, the reader is referred to the endocrine disease section of this chapter.

Lymphoma

Lymphoma is the third most common neoplasia found in ferrets. Neoplasia may be localized in lymph nodes, spleen, liver, bone marrow, kidneys, and/or skin. These patients will not commonly present emergently, unless mediastinal involvement or paraneoplastic syndromes (e.g. hypercalcemia, anemia) are present.

Diagnosis

Signalment: Most common in ferrets of two to five years of age. Mediastinal involvement is more common in animals <1 year.

History: Clinical signs will highly vary, dependent on the anatomical location and stage of the disease.

Clinical Signs:

- Clinical signs often non-specific and may include loss of appetite, weight loss, lethargy, and peripheral lymph node enlargement or hepatosplenomegaly
- Dyspnea and coughing if pleural effusion and/or mediastinal masses present
- Vomiting, diarrhea, or melena if gastrointestinal involvement
- Solitary or multicentric pruritic masses with crusts or ulceration with epitheliotropic (cutaneous) lymphoma (see Figure 14.14)

Differentials:

- Obesity (increased fat around lymph nodes)
- Lymphadenitis
- Mediastinal lymphoma differentials include respiratory or cardiac disease (see Table 14.6)
- Gastrointestinal lymphoma differentials include gastrointestinal diseases resulting in vomiting/diarrhea
- Cutaneous lymphoma differentials include skin tumors (i.e. mast cell tumors) and infectious or inflammatory dermatologic disease

Diagnostics:

- Radiographs and ultrasound, particularly if respiratory distress
  - Visualize mediastinal masses or pleural effusion
  - Evaluate abdomen for masses or lymphadenopathy
  - Ultrasound-guided FNA to confirm diagnosis
- CBC and bone marrow aspirate
  - Anemia common, leukemic in some cases

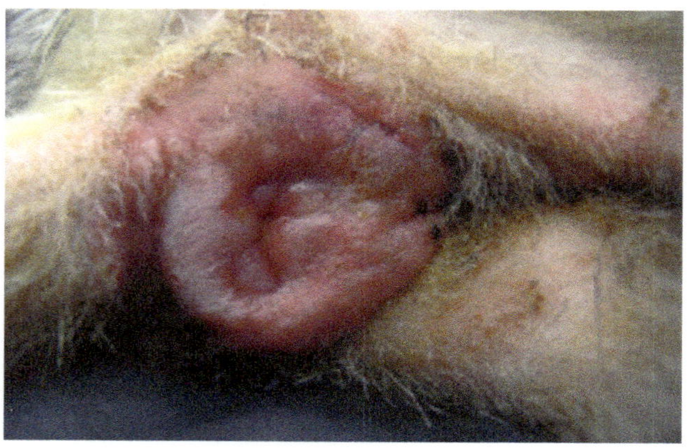

Figure 14.14 A five-year-old ferret was presented with a swelling around the anus with a duration of at least eight weeks. Aside from the swelling and frequent licking of the area, no other clinical signs such as straining were seen. Histological evaluation of the resected tissue confirmed lymphoma.

Treatment

- Oxygen therapy
- Thoracocentesis to remove/evaluate pleural effusion
- Depending on stage and owner wishes, various options including:
  - Surgery (splenectomy, lymph nodectomy) or radiation if single anatomic location
  - Multiple chemotherapy protocols have been described with variable results
  - Glucocorticoids can be considered if owners do not wish to pursue chemotherapy

Dermatologic Disease

Abscesses and Wounds

As in all animals, subcutaneous abscesses and wounds may occur in ferrets. Abscesses and wounds will generally be caused by a bite, puncture, or from eating sharp bones. Other locations where abscesses can be found include the oral cavity (i.e. dental abscesses resulting from dental disease) and perineum (i.e. abscessation of the anal glands). Although not common, mycobacteria should be considered as a differential in ferrets in association with draining wounds.

Diagnosis

Signalment: N/A

History: Owners will typically report the presence of a fast-growing swelling and/or wound as a result of previous trauma. In case of systemic infection, animals may show signs of general malaise. It is important to question the owner on how long ago the trauma has occurred in order to determine the appropriate therapeutic plan.

Clinical Signs:

- Fluctuant swelling or wound
- Pain, erythema, and/or exudate
- Fever, lethargy, and anorexia if systemic infection

Differentials:

- Neoplasia (i.e. mast cell tumor, lymphoma)
- Granuloma
- Hematoma
- Cyst
- Uncommonly, mycobacteria may be found in association with draining wounds

Diagnostics:

- Mass aspiration (purulent material may be present if open abscess)
  - Cytology
  - Culture/sensitivity

Treatment

- Use appropriate analgesia/anesthesia, surgically prepare region, and lance abscess
- Antibiotic therapy based on culture/sensitivity
- Wound management as described in other species (see Chapter 5)
  - Keep wound clean
  - Primary closure of wound can be considered if less than 6–8 hours old
  - Secondary intention healing if older wound or infection
  - Frequent monitoring on healing progress
  - Bandage may be needed to protect healing wound

Alopecia

Alopecia, which is characterized by a focal or generalized loss of hair, is a commonly seen in ferrets. Generally, it will occur secondary to other disease processes such as endocrine disease or bacterial, mycotic, or parasitic infections.

Diagnosis

Signalment: No specific gender or age predilection. Alopecia related to hyperadrenocorticism is more common in middle-aged to older, neutered ferrets.

History: Alopecia may have an acute onset or slowly progress, dependent on the underlying cause. It is important to question the owner about the initial signs and progression as well as presence of pruritus. Information should also be obtained about the animal's reproductive status, diet, exposure to contact irritants, flea control, and potential contact with other animals.

Clinical signs: Alopecia can be focal, multifocal, generalized, and occur with or without pruritus and presence of skin lesions (e.g. erythema, scaling, crusts). Dependent on the underlying cause, other clinical abnormalities may be present.

Differentials:

- Alopecia, without the presence of skin lesions, is most commonly associated with hyperadrenocorticism
- Infection (e.g. bacterial pyoderma, dermatophytosis)
- Parasitic (e.g. sarcoptic and otic mites, fleas)
- Immunologic (e.g. atopy, contact dermatitis, food allergy)
- Neoplasia (e.g. lymphoma, mast cell tumor)
- Nutritional (e.g. fat or protein deficiencies)
- Other endocrine disease (e.g. hypothyroidism, seasonal alopecia, hyperestrogenism)

Diagnostics:

- Pattern/degree of hair loss is an important feature to help distinguish causes:
  - Endocrine alopecia is generally bilaterally symmetric
  - Ear mites or fleas may be localized (e.g. ear region, tail base)
  - Dermatophyte lesions may be ring-like
- Skin sampling
  - Skin scrape
  - Bacterial or fungal culture
  - Cytology
  - Skin biopsy
- CBC
- Biochemistry profile
- Ultrasound to evaluate adrenal glands
- Elimination diet or antigen challenge

Treatment

- Varies based on cause
  - Ear mites, sarcoptic mites, fleas: Antiparasitic drugs (ivermectin, selamectin, moxidectin, fipronil)
  - Dermatophytosis: Antifungals (e.g. itraconazole, terbinafine, miconazole, lime sulfur)
  - Pyoderma: Systemic and/or topical antibiotics (amoxicillin and clavulanic acid, trimethoprim-sulfa)
- Surgical excision or chemotherapy for neoplasia
- Surgery or placement of deslorelin implant in cases of hyperestrogenism or hyperadrenocorticism
- Diet change if suspected food intolerance

Ophthalmic Disease

Corneal Ulcers

Like other animals, corneal ulcers may develop secondary to corneal trauma, e.g. scratches or puncture wounds. Due to their inquisitive nature, ferrets can easily get hurt when snooping around. Similarly, trauma can occur while playing or rough housing with ferrets or other animals.

Diagnosis

Signalment: N/A

History: History will often reveal (the nature of the) trauma resulting in corneal damage.

Clinical Signs:

- Blepharospasm (may prohibit initial view of ulcer)
- Excessive tearing or ocular discharge
- Photophobia
- Conjunctival or scleral hyperemia
- Corneal edema

Differentials:

- Bacterial, viral, or fungal infections
- Exposure to caustic substance

- Eyelid pathology (entropion, distichiasis)
- Keratoconjunctivitis sicca

Diagnostics: Diagnosis can usually be made by visualizing the ulcer during an ophthalmic examination. Fluorescein staining will enhance visualization of the ulcer.

Treatment

- Similar to those described in dogs and cats
  - Topical antibiotics
  - Systemic NSAID
  - Atropine
  - Steroids contraindicated if ulcer is present
  - Autologous serum eye drops q4–6h
- Nictitating membrane can be sutured over eyelid if deep corneal ulcer

Reference

1 Richardson, J. and Balabuszko, R. (2000). Managing ferret toxicoses. *Exotic DVM* 2 (4): 23–26.

Further Reading

Bennett, K.R., Gaunt, M.C., and Parker, D.L. (2015). Constant rate infusion of glucagon as an emergency treatment for hypoglycemia in a domestic ferret (*Mustela putorius furo*). *J. Am. Vet. Med. Assoc.* 246 (4): 451–454.

Chen, S. (2010). Advanced diagnostic approaches and current medical management of insulinomas and adrenocortical disease in ferrets (*Mustela putorius furo*). *Vet. Clin. North. Am. Exot. Anim. Pract.* 13 (3): 439–452.

Diaz-Figueroa, O. and Smith, M.O. (2007). Clinical neurology of ferrets. *Vet. Clin. North. Am. Exot. Anim. Pract.* 10 (3): 759–773.

Di Girolamo, N. and Selleri, P. (2016). Medical and surgical emergencies in ferrets. *Vet. Clin. North. Am. Exot. Anim. Pract.* 19 (2): 431–464.

Dunayer, E. (2008). Toxicology of ferrets. *Vet. Clin. North. Am. Exot. Anim. Pract.* 11 (2): 301–314.

Fox, J.G. and Marini, R.P. (eds.) (2014). *Biology and Diseases of the Ferret*. Ames, IA: Wiley.

Garner, M.M., Ramsell, K., Morera, N. et al. (2008). Clinicopathologic features of a systemic coronavirus-associated disease resembling feline infectious peritonitis in the domestic ferret (*Mustela putorius*). *Vet. Pathol.* 45 (2): 236–246.

Jekl, V. and Hauptman, K. (2017). Reproductive medicine in ferrets. *Vet. Clin. North. Am. Exot. Anim. Pract.* 20 (2): 629–663.

Johnson-Delaney, C.A. and Orosz, S.E. (2011). Ferret respiratory system: clinical anatomy, physiology, and disease. *Vet. Clin. North. Am. Exot. Anim. Pract.* 14 (2): 357–367.

Johnson-Delaney, C.A. (2016). Anatomy and disorders of the oral cavity of ferrets and other exotic companion carnivores. *Vet. Clin. North. Am. Exot. Anim. Pract.* 19 (3): 901–928.

Johnson-Delaney, C.A. (2017). *Ferret Medicine and Surgery*. Boca Raton, FL: CRC Press.

Keeble, E. and Meredith, A. (2009). *BSAVA Manual of Rodents and Ferrets*. Gloucester: British Small Animal Veterinary Association.

Langlois, I. (2005). Viral diseases of ferrets. *Vet. Clin. North. Am. Exot. Anim. Pract.* 8 (1): 139–160.

Lee, E.J., Moore, W.E., Fryer, H.C., and Minocha, H.C. (1982). Haematological and serum chemistry profiles of ferrets (*Mustela putorius furo*). *Lab. Anim.* 16 (2): 133–137.

Lennox, A.M. (2005). Gastrointestinal diseases of the ferret. *Vet. Clin. North. Am. Exot. Anim. Pract.* 8 (2): 213–225.

Moore, G.E., Glickman, N.W., Ward, M.P. et al. (2005). Incidence of and risk factors for adverse events associated with distemper and rabies vaccine administration in ferrets. *J. Am. Vet. Med. Assoc.* 226 (6): 909–912.

Oglesbee, B.L. (2006). *5-Minute Veterinary Consult: Ferret and Rabbit*. Ames, IA: Blackwell Publishing.

Orcutt, C.J. (1998). Emergency and critical care of ferrets. *Vet. Clin. North. Am. Exot. Anim. Pract.* 1 (1): 99–126.

Overman, M.C. (2015). A review of ferret toxicoses. *J. Exot. Pet Med.* 24 (4): 398–402.

Petritz, O.A., Antinoff, N., Chen, S. et al. (2013). Evaluation of portable blood glucose meters for measurement of blood glucose concentration in ferrets (*Mustela putorius furo*). *J. Am. Vet. Med. Assoc.* 242 (3): 350–354.

Pilny, A.A. and Hess, L. (2004). Ferrets: wound healing and therapy. *Vet. Clin. North. Am. Exot. Anim. Pract.* 7 (1): 105–121.

Pollock, C. (2007). Emergency medicine of the ferret. *Vet. Clin. North. Am. Exot. Anim. Pract.* 10 (2): 463–500.

Powers, L.V. (2009). Bacterial and parasitic diseases of ferrets. *Vet. Clin. North. Am. Exot. Anim. Pract.* 12 (3): 531–561.

Quesenberry, K., Orcutt, C.J., Mans, C., and Carpenter, J.W. (2020). *Ferrets, Rabbits and Rodents: Clinical Medicine and Surgery*, 4e. Philadelphia, PA: Elsevier Health Sciences.

Ritzman, T.K. and Knapp, D. (2002). Ferret orthopedics. *Vet. Clin. North. Am. Exot. Anim. Pract.* 5 (1): 129–155.

Rozengurt, N., Stewart, D., and Sanchez, S. (1995). Diagnostic exercise: ataxia and incoordination in ferrets. *Lab. Anim. Sci.* 45 (4): 432–434.

Siperstein, L.J. (2008). Ferret hematology and related disorders. *Vet. Clin. North. Am. Exot. Anim. Pract.* 11 (3): 535–550.

Schoemaker, N.J. (2017). Ferret oncology: diseases, diagnostics, and therapeutics. *Vet. Clin. North. Am. Exot. Anim. Pract.* 20 (1): 183–208.

Summa, N.M., Eshar, D., Lee-Chow, B. et al. (2014). Comparison of a human portable glucometer and an automated chemistry analyzer for measurement of blood glucose concentration in pet ferrets (*Mustela putorius furo*). *Can. Vet. J.* 55 (9): 865–869.

Van Oostrom, H., Schoemaker, N.J., and Uilenreef, J.J. (2011). Pain management in ferrets. *Vet. Clin. North. Am. Exot. Anim. Pract.* 14 (1): 105–116.

Wade, L.L. (2018). Vaccination of ferrets for rabies and distemper. *Vet. Clin. North. Am. Exot. Anim. Pract.* 21 (1): 105–114.

Wagner, R.A. (2009). Ferret cardiology. *Vet. Clin. North. Am. Exot. Anim. Pract.* 12 (1): 115–134.

Zaffarano, B. (2010). Ferrets: examination and standards of care. *J. Exot. Pet Med.* 19 (1): 73–81.

15

Rabbits

Julie DeCubellis[1] *and Jennifer E. Graham*[2]

[1] *Calgary Avian and Exotic Pet Clinic, Calgary, Alberta, Canada*
[2] *Department of Clinical Sciences, Cummings School of Veterinary Medicine, Tufts University, North Grafton, Massachusetts, USA*

CONTENTS

Unique Species Considerations

Rabbits are hindgut fermenters and engage in cecotrophy. Antibiotic-induced dysbiosis can lead to the overgrowth of pathogenic bacteria including *Escherichia coli* and *Clostridium difficile* and may result in fatal enterotoxemia. Antibiotics to be avoided in this species by any route include clindamycin, lincomycin, and erythromycin. Antibiotics unsafe to administer enterally to rabbits include penicillin, cephalosporins, streptomycin, ampicillin, and amoxicillin.

Exotic Animal Emergency and Critical Care Medicine, First Edition. Edited by Jennifer E. Graham, Grayson A. Doss and Hugues Beaufrère.

Antibiotics commonly used in rabbits include quinolones, tetracyclines, metronidazole, azithromycin, trimethoprime-sulfa, and chloramphenicol. Fipronil should not be used in rabbits.

Rabbits are prey species and can easily startle with the sounds or scents of predators, including ferrets. Caution should be used with handling to avoid iatrogenic back fractures (see Chapter 2 for information on handling rabbits). Unspayed female rabbits have a high incidence of uterine neoplasia. A complete dietary history is important as low fiber/high carbohydrate diets are a common cause of gastrointestinal pathology. Adult rabbits eating a high calcium diet (i.e. alfalfa) are prone to calcium carbonate urolithiasis.

Common Presenting Signs

As in all species, rabbits may present with a variety of different clinical signs in the emergency clinic and triage should take place to determine whether immediate action is warranted. Before taking a complete history, determine if the rabbit needs immediate care. The airway, breathing, and cardiovascular status (ABCs) should be immediately assessed with stabilization efforts made in situations of hemorrhage, respiratory distress, severe neurologic signs including seizures, open fractures, severe gastrointestinal distention, or hypothermia. Further workup can then take place once the rabbit receives initial triage and stabilization therapy.

Abnormal Droppings

Introduction

- Includes loose stool, malformed stools, and decreased stool production
- Loose stools most commonly result from inadequate dietary fiber or bacterial dysbiosis secondary to a high carbohydrate diet. They can also be caused by parasitic infection, toxins, dental disease, and systemic disease
- Malformed stools can include normal or uneaten cecotropes or indicate underlying pathologies such as megacolon or other motility disorders
- Decreased stool output can result from insufficient food intake for any reason, intestinal obstruction, and systemic disease

Diagnosis

History:

- Assess environmental changes and exposures
  - Other rabbits (infection), toxins (i.e. lead paint), ingestions
  - Unsupervised out-of-cage activity
  - Stressful events, environmental changes, or exposures
- Complete dietary history, noting any recent changes
  - Preference for soft food may indicate dental disease
  - Note time of the last intake
- Fecal output history, ensuring uneaten cecotropes are not confused with malformed stools

Signalment:

- Diarrhea in young rabbits is common with *Coccidia* infection
- Diarrhea in mature rabbits is common with husbandry-related issues, including inappropriate diet

Clinical Signs:

- Variable, from decreased appetite and behavior to normal appearing
- Teeth grinding may be a sign of pain
- Weight loss may indicate chronic disease
- Stools can be loose, malformed, or absent, cecotropes may be present
- Gastric distention, gas, borborygmus
- Doughy abdominal contents or masses

Differentials:

- Dietary imbalance
  - Insufficient dietary fiber
  - High carbohydrate diet (dysbiosis)
  - Inactivity/obesity
  - Decreased intake or ability to feed
    - A recent change in diet
    - Dental disease, upper respiratory tract disease
    - Neurologic or musculoskeletal disease
- Infections: bacterial, parasitic, viral
- Intestinal obstruction
  - Foreign body ingestion
  - Cecal impaction
  - Choke
- Gastrointestinal stasis or dysmotility
  - Ileus
  - Gastric bloat
  - Motility disorders, megacolon
- Toxin ingestion (lead, plant, other)
- Stressful events (environmental, chronic/systemic pain)
- Urinary tract disease
- Metabolic derangements and/or organ failure
- Neoplasia

STAT diagnostics:

- Radiographs
- Fecal wet mount and flotation
  - *Coccidia* (young rabbits)
  - Nematodes (rare)

Complete diagnostics:

- CBC and comprehensive blood profile
- Heavy metal (lead) testing, if indicated
- Abdominal ultrasound (obstruction, masses)

- Fecal culture and sensitivity (diarrhea)
- Continued monitoring of fecal output

Treatment

Stabilization:

- Fluids (120 ml/kg/d) SC, or IV/IO if significant dehydration
- Nutritional support (see Chapter 8)
- Surgical intervention for acute obstruction, if indicated
- Antiparasitic therapy, if indicated by fecal examination
  - *Sulfadimethoxine*: 50 mg/kg PO × 1; 25 mg/kg PO q24h × 10–20d
  - *Toltrazuril*: 20 mg/kg PO q24h × 7d
- *Chelation*: therapy for suspected heavy metal toxicosis
  - *CaEDTA*: 30 mg/kg SC q12h × 5–7d

Continued Care:

- Fluid therapy until eating/drinking
- Syringe feed until eating on own and maintaining weight
- Dietary modifications and/or weight loss, if indicated
- Chelation according to standard protocols, pending test results

Anorexia

Introduction

- Reduced or no food intake can result from stress, pain, systemic disease, and gastrointestinal and/or dental disease
- Anorexia can rapidly lead to dehydration, hypovolemia, and gastrointestinal stasis
- Anorexia >24 hours is an emergency that warrants aggressive supportive care

Diagnosis

History:

- Assess environmental changes and exposures
  - Other rabbits (infection)
  - Unsupervised out-of-cage activity (toxins, ingestions)
  - Stressful events, environmental changes, or exposures
- Complete dietary history, noting any recent changes
  - Preference for soft food may indicate dental disease
  - Note time of the last intake
- Fecal output history, presence of cecotropes

Signalment:

- Occurs at any age, more common during stressful conditions
- Rabbits with chronic painful conditions including dental disease, osteoarthritis, or spondylosis are more prone

Clinical Signs:

- Lethargic, often with signs of pain (hunched posture, teeth grinding)
- Abdominal palpation can elicit pain, but may be normal
- Note any gastric distention, gas, borborygmus, doughy abdominal contents, or masses
- Signs of dehydration, hypovolemia, and possibly hypothermia
- Weight loss may indicate chronic disease
- Stools scant and dry or absent

Differentials:

- Dental disease
- Decreased intake or ability to feed
  - Recent changes in diet
  - Upper respiratory tract disease
  - Neurologic or musculoskeletal disease
- Infections: bacterial, parasitic, viral
- Stressful events (environmental, chronic/systemic pain)
- Intestinal obstruction
- Gastrointestinal stasis or dysmotility
- Toxin ingestion (lead, plant, other)
- Urinary tract disease
- Metabolic derangements and/or organ failure
- Cardiopulmonary disease
- Neoplasia

STAT diagnostics:

- Radiographs

Complete diagnostics:

- CBC and comprehensive blood profile
- Indirect blood pressure (hypovolemic – hypotension)
- Abdominal ultrasound (obstruction, masses)
- Fecal culture and sensitivity (diarrhea)
- Continued monitoring of food intake and fecal output

Treatment

Stabilization:

- Subcutaneous fluids (120 ml/kg/d)
  - Correct for dehydration
  - IV/IO if significant dehydration
- Nutritional support (see Chapter 8)
  - Nasogastric tube feeding if oral not tolerated
- Thermal support (hypothermia)
- Analgesic drugs, if painful on exam
  - *Buprenorphine*: 0.01–0.05 mg/kg SC, IM, IV q6–12h
  - *Oxymorphone*: 0.05–0.2 mg/kg SC, IM q6–12h
  - *Hydromorphone*: 0.1 mg/kg SC, IM, IV q6–8h
- Surgical intervention for acute obstruction, if indicated
- Prokinetic drugs, if warranted (no obstruction)

- *Metoclopramide*: 0.5 mg/kg PO, SC q6–8h
- *Cisapride*: 0.5 mg/kg PO q8–12h

Continued Care:

- Fluid therapy until eating/drinking
- Syringe (or nasogastric) feed until eating on own and maintaining weight
- The treatment plan for chronic painful conditions
- Referral for dental disease or other treatments for the underlying cause

Dyspnea/Respiratory Distress

Introduction

- Can result from upper respiratory, lower respiratory, and cardiac disease
- Rabbits are obligate nasal breathers, pronounced dyspnea can result from upper airway pathology
- Open-mouth breathing is generally a poor prognostic indicator

Diagnosis

History:

- Recent exposure to other rabbits (infection)
- Ocular or nasal discharge, sneezing (acute or chronic)
- Exercise intolerance
- Complete dietary and elimination history
  - Recent changes, last food intake
  - Reduced consumption (common with respiratory distress)
  - Fecal output history, changes
- Unsupervised out-of-cage activity (possibility of electrocution)

Signalment:

- Any age; infectious disease more common in young/middle-aged rabbits
- Cardiopulmonary or neoplastic disease can be common in aged rabbits

Clinical Signs:

- Ocular or nasal discharge
  - Because of fastidious grooming, the discharge may be evident on the inside of the forefeet rather than the face
- Increased respiratory effort and rate, nostril flaring
  - Asynchronous breathing may indicate pleural disease
- Abnormal respiratory sounds
  - Coughing, while rare, can occur with tracheal disease
  - Increased airway noise or wheezing referred to the thorax with upper respiratory disease
  - Increased or decreased sounds with lower airway disease
- Chronic disease signs (lethargy, weight loss, and poor condition)

Differentials:

- Respiratory infection
  - Bacterial (most common), parasitic, viral, fungal
  - Otitis with upper respiratory extension can be seen
- Trauma, electrocution
- Dental disease
- Cardiovascular disease
- Neoplasia (upper airway, pulmonary, mediastinal)

STAT Diagnostics:

- Radiographs
  - Sedation or anesthesia and flow by oxygen ideal if severe distress

Complete Diagnostics:

- CBC/Comprehensive blood profile
- Infectious disease testing as indicated
  - Nasolacrimal duct flush (if ocular discharge) or nasal flush for C/S
  - PCR for *Bordetella bronchiseptica* and *Pasteurella multocida*
- Continued monitoring degree of respiratory distress, pulse oximetry if needed
- Thoracic ultrasound, FNA of mass/fluid for cytologic examination, C/S
- Advanced imaging (CT, endoscopy, rhinoscopy), if warranted
- Echocardiography/ECG/blood pressure if evidence of cardiovascular disease

Treatment

Stabilization:

- Intubation, LMA, or tight-fitting facemask and CPRC for rabbits in respiratory arrest
- Oxygen therapy +/− saline nebulization
- Thoracocentesis if warranted
- Subcutaneous fluids (IV or IO if necessary) (120 ml/kg/d)
- Treatment of infectious disease as warranted ideally based on C/S
  - *Enrofloxacin*: 5–10 mg/kg PO, SC, IM q12h (dilute in fluids for parenteral administration)
  - *Ciprofloxacin*: 20 mg/kg PO q24h

- *Azithromycin*: 30 mg/kg PO q24h
- *Doxycycline*: 2.5 mg/kg PO q12h
- *Trimethoprim/sulfa*: 30 mg/kg PO, SC q12h

- Analgesic drugs if painful or to obtain diagnostics
  - *Buprenorphine*: 0.01–0.05 mg/kg SC, IM, IV q6–12h
  - *Butorphanol*: 0.5–1 mg/kg SC, IM, IV q2–6h
  - *Oxymorphone*: 0.05–0.2 mg/kg SC, IM q6–12h
  - *Hydromorphone*: 0.1 mg/kg SC, IM, IV q6–8h
- Bronchodilators if the small-airway disease
  - *Terbutaline*: 0.01 mg/kg IM, SC, or via nebulization
- Management of cardiovascular disease if warranted
  - *Furosemide*: 3–4 mg/kg SC, IM
  - Nitroglycerine ointment ⅛ inch/2.5 kg on tongue or gums
  - Other cardiac medications are based on the type of disease

Continued Care:

- Continue fluid therapy until patient eating/drinking
- Continue nasogastric or syringe feeding until the patient able to eat and maintain weight on own
- Rhinotomy with surgical debridement and local therapy if warranted
- Referral for neoplasia/masses
- Manage chronic painful conditions

Neurologic Signs

Introduction

- Emergent presenting signs include seizures, head tilt, paresis, or paralysis, facial nerve paralysis, nystagmus, and behavioral changes
- Broad etiology, including trauma, infection (parasitic, bacterial, viral, *Encephalitozoon cuniculi*), degenerative/developmental problems, and toxic, metabolic, vascular, inflammatory, and nutritional causes

Diagnosis

History:

- Recent exposure to other rabbits (infection)
- Potential toxin exposure or trauma
- Complete dietary and elimination history
  - Recent changes, last food intake
  - Reduced consumption (can see with the neurologic disease)
  - Fecal output history, changes
- Behavioral changes, duration of symptoms

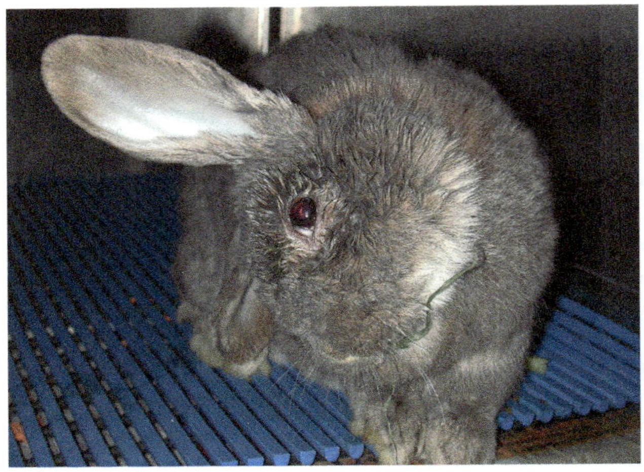

Figure 15.1 This rabbit has a right-sided head tilt. Differentials for this presentation are varied, including bacterial otitis and *Encephalitozoon cuniculi*.

Signalment:

- Any age, sex, and breed of rabbits can present with neurologic signs. Ear infection is more common in lop breeds

Clinical signs:

- Variable, including head tilt (Figure 15.1), seizures, nystagmus, paresis, paralysis, tremors, behavior changes, rolling, hyperesthesia, and ataxia
- Chronic diseases may have weight loss and lethargy

Differentials:

- Infectious disease
  - Bacterial (most common), parasitic, viral fungal
  - Otitis with upper respiratory extension can be seen
  - *E. cuniculi* infection
- Trauma
- Degenerative/developmental disease
- Toxin exposure (heavy metal, topical insecticides)
- Heatstroke
- Vascular disease, hypoxia
- Neoplasia

STAT diagnostics:

- Complete neurologic examination to localize the lesion
- Radiographs

Complete diagnostics:

- CBC/comprehensive blood profile
- Infectious/toxin screening as indicated
  - Serology (*E. cuniculi*, toxoplasmosis, pasteurellosis, etc.)
  - Lead levels
  - Bacterial cultures (deep aural, nasal, tracheal wash)

- Advanced imaging (ultrasound, CT, MRI) if warranted
- Cerebrospinal tap if warranted

Treatment

Stabilization:

- Subcutaneous fluids (IV or IO if necessary) (120 ml/kg/d)
- Anxiolytic or anti-seizure therapy:
  - *Midazolam*: 0.5 mg/kg IV, SC, IM
  - *Levetiracetam*: 20 mg/kg IV, PO q8h
- Treatment of infectious disease as warranted, ideally based on C/S
  - *Enrofloxacin*: 5–10 mg/kg PO, SC, IM q12h (dilute for parenteral route)
  - *Ciprofloxacin*: 20 mg/kg PO q24h
  - *Azithromycin*: 30 mg/kg PO q24h
  - *Doxycycline*: 2.5 mg/kg PO q12h
  - *Trimethoprim/sulfa*: 30 mg/kg PO, SC q12h
- Analgesic drugs if painful or to obtain diagnostics
  - *Buprenorphine*: 0.01–0.05 mg/kg SC, IM, IV q6–12h
  - *Butorphanol*: 0.5–1 mg/kg SC, IM, IV q2–6h
  - *Oxymorphone*: 0.05–0.2 mg/kg SC, IM q6–12h
  - *Hydromorphone*: 0.1 mg/kg SC, IM, IV q6–8h
- *E. cuniculi* treatment as warranted
  - Ideally based on positive test results after discussing risks of therapy with the owner
  - *Oxibendazole*: 15 mg/kg PO q24h × 30d
  - *Fenbendazole*: 20 mg/kg PO q24h × 30d
- Chelation therapy if heavy metal toxicosis
  - *CaEDTA*: 30 mg/kg SQ q12h × 5–7d
- Bathing and oral activated charcoal if topical insecticide

Continued Care:

- Continue fluid therapy and supplemental feeds until patient eating/drinking on own (see Chapter 8)
- Manage chronic painful conditions
- Otitis management (surgery may be necessary in some cases)
- Follow-up plan needed for seizure management, infectious therapy (*E. cuniculi*), toxin titers

Ocular Discharge

Introduction

- Normal conjunctival flora includes *Staphylococcus*, *Micrococcus*, and *Bacillus* species
- Ocular discharge can be a sign of underlying dental disease (occluding nasolacrimal duct drainage), dacryocystitis (Figure 15.2), or dacryostenosis

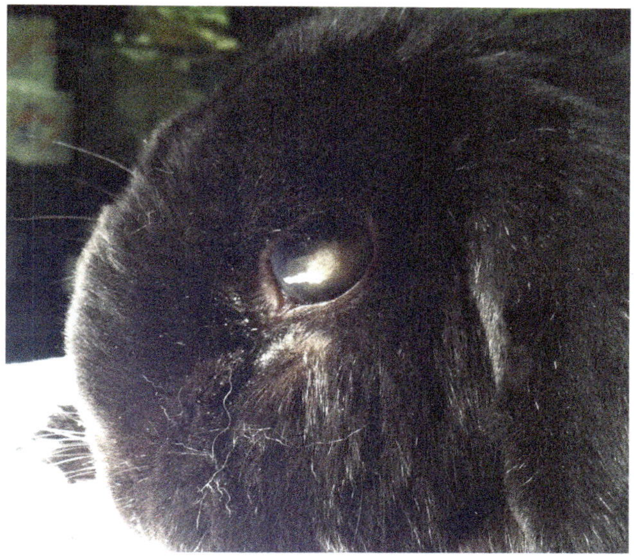

Figure 15.2 This rabbit presented for evaluation of a cataract and chronic dacryocystitis.

- Other causes include foreign body or trauma, environmental irritants (i.e. ammonia and dust), and eyelid disease

Diagnosis

History:

- Recent exposure to other rabbits (infection)
- Recent trauma or ocular foreign bodies
- Environmental assessment, noting dusty, or unsanitary conditions
- Ocular or nasal discharge and sneezing (acute or chronic)
- A complete diet and elimination history
  - Diet preference changes (dental disease), last intake
  - Characteristics of fecal output

Signalment:

- Any age; infections may be more common in young/middle-aged rabbits

Clinical Signs:

- Because of fastidious grooming, the discharge may be evident on the inside of the forefeet rather than the face
- Increased airway noise, wheezing referred to the thorax, and nasal discharge with upper respiratory disease
- Chronic ocular discharge can cause alopecia and secondary dermatitis
- Evidence of dental disease on examination

Differentials:

- Dacryocystitis: bacterial (most common), viral
  - *P. multocida*, *B. bronchiseptica*, *Staphylococcus aureus*, *Pseudomonas* sp., *Haemophilus* sp., *Treponema* sp., mycoplasma, chlamydia
  - Myxoma virus
- Eyelid infections (distichia, trichiasis, and entropion)
- Upper respiratory tract infections
- Trauma
- Dental disease
- Dacryostenosis
- Neoplasia

STAT Diagnostics:

- Ophthalmologic and oral examination
- Corneal fluorescein stain if ulceration is suspected

Complete Diagnostics:

- Complete ophthalmologic examination
  - Direct/indirect ophthalmoscopy with a slit lamp
  - Visualize punctum lacrimal and behind the third eyelid for possible foreign body (use topical local anesthetics)
- Check nasolacrimal duct patency using fluorescein dye
- Sedated examination of oral cavity if dental disease suspected
- Consider radiographic studies of skull/teeth, with multiple views and contrast dacryocystorhinography
- CBC/Comprehensive blood profile
- Infectious disease testing as indicated
  - Nasolacrimal duct flush (if ocular discharge) or nasal flush for C/S
  - PCR for *B. bronchiseptica*, *P. multocida*, chlamydia
  - Treponema serology
- Advanced imaging (CT, endoscopy, rhinoscopy) if warranted

Treatment

Stabilization:

- Saline nasolacrimal duct flush (treatment and culture)
- Local treatment as warranted, ideally based on C/S
  - Chloramphenicol ophthalmic drops q6–12h depending on the severity
  - Ofloxacin (Ocuflox, Allergan)
  - Aminoglycosides have a limited spectrum of activity
- Systemic treatment of infectious disease, ideally based on C/S
  - *Enrofloxacin*: 5–10 mg/kg PO, SC, IM q12h (dilute in fluids for parenteral administration)
  - *Ciprofloxacin*: 20 mg/kg PO q24h
  - *Azithromycin*: 30 mg/kg PO q24h
  - *Doxycycline*: 2.5 mg/kg PO q12h
  - *Trimethoprim/sulfa*: 30 mg/kg PO, SC q12h
- Local or systemic anti-inflammatories if stenosis
  - Topical flurbiprofen or diclofenac
  - *Meloxicam*: 1 mg/kg PO q24h

Continued Care:

- Environmental management (decrease ammonia, dust)
- Dental trim or other treatment based on cause of ocular discharge
- Surgery may be needed to manage eyelid abnormalities

Pigmenturia

Introduction

- Pigmenturia can be normal in rabbits due to certain plants or dietary compounds
- Normal urine color ranges from yellow to dark brown, dark orange, or even red that resembles hematuria
- True hematuria can be associated with bladder stones or masses, cystitis, uterine neoplasia, and renal disease

Diagnosis

History:

- Detailed diet history
  - Note amounts of high calcium items including alfalfa (uroliths)
  - Last food and water intake
  - Characteristics of urine and fecal output
- Potential toxin exposure or trauma
- Duration and nature of signs noted by the owner
- Determine if male or female and if spayed, neutered, or intact

Signalment:

- Any age, sex, and breed of rabbit
- Intact females are prone to uterine cancer (hematuria)

Clinical Signs:

- Discolored urine, generally asymptomatic
- Pain and weight loss may indicate chronic process (stones, uterine neoplasia)

Differentials:

- Pigmenturia
  - Dietary compounds (beta carotene), pine needle ingestion, antibiotic administration
- Hematuria
- Hemoglobinuria
- Cystitis/pyelonephritis
- Bladder polyps
- Urolithiasis
- Reproductive pathology, uterine neoplasia

STAT Diagnostics:

- For pigmenturia (fluoresce under Wood's lamp), no additional diagnostics needed
- Hematuria and hemoglobinuria (positive reaction for blood on urine dipstick) need a complete workup

Complete Diagnostics:

- Radiographs
- CBC and comprehensive blood profile
- Urinalysis and C/S
- Ultrasound of reproductive and urinary tract

Treatment

Stabilization:

- No treatment needed for pigmenturia
- Refer to urinary topics for specific treatment of causes of hematuria

Continued Care:

- No treatment is needed for pigmenturia

Rear Leg Paresis/Paralysis

Introduction

- Vertebral fracture or luxation is the most common cause of acute posterior paresis or paralysis in rabbits (Figures 15.3–15.5)

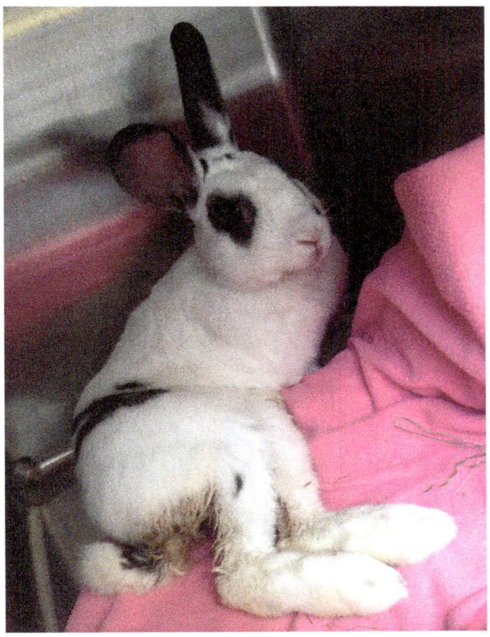

Figure 15.3 A rabbit was unable to use its hindlegs and had no deep pain present after visiting a veterinary clinic for routine castration. It is likely the rabbit fractured its back during handling or transport.

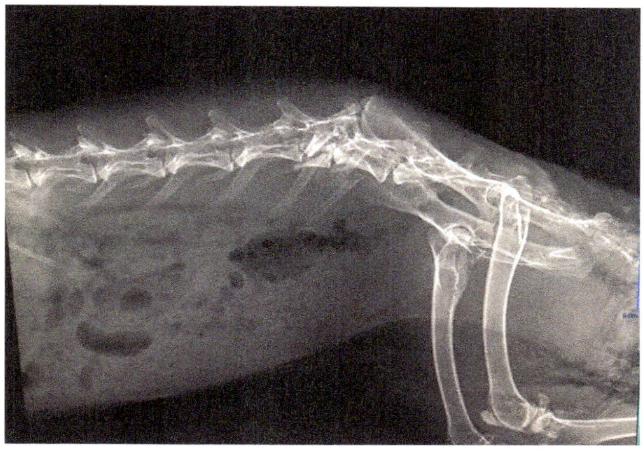

Figure 15.4 Lateral radiographic projection of the rabbit in Figure 15.3. A spinal fracture is evident at L6–L7.

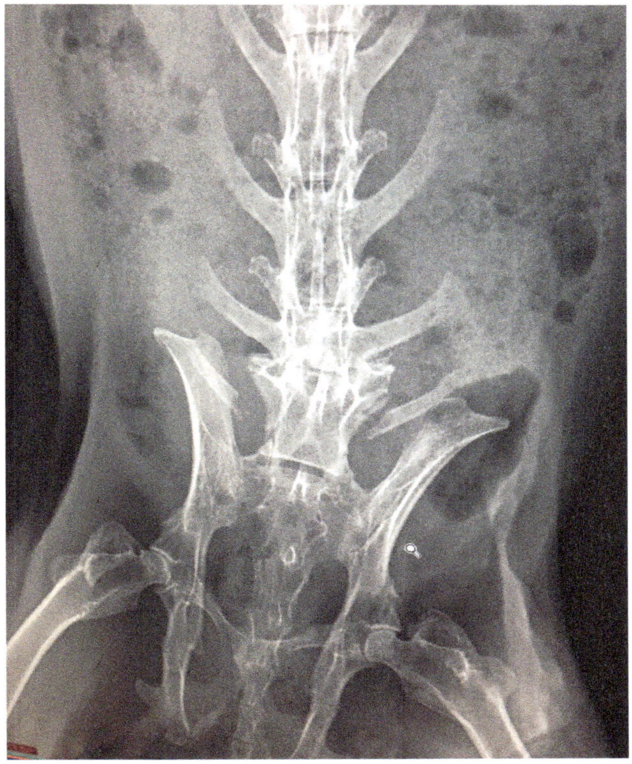

Figure 15.5 Ventrodorsal radiographic projection of the rabbit in Figure 15.3. A spinal fracture is evident at L6–L7. Note the fractured transverse processes of L7.

- Rabbits have well-developed hind limb musculature in comparison to relatively delicate bones which can predispose them to injury
- Other causes include infection (parasitic, bacterial, viral, *E. cuniculi*), degenerative/development problems, toxic, metabolic, vascular, congenital, inflammatory, and nutritional causes

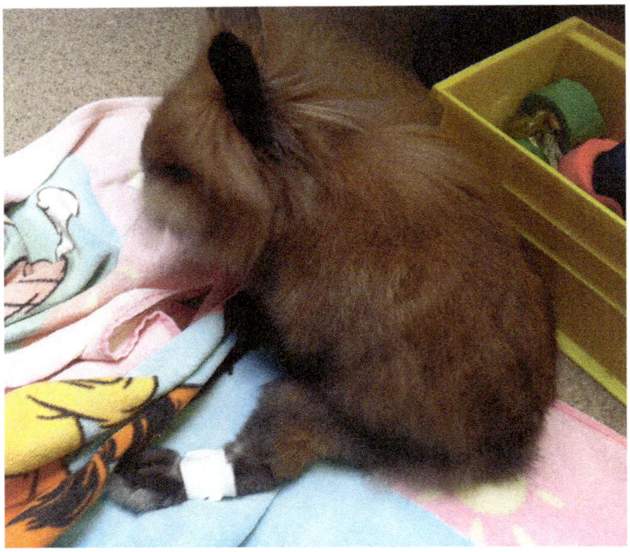

Figure 15.6 This rabbit presented for evaluation of splay leg. The left hind leg was most severely affected.

Diagnosis

History:

- Recent history of trauma or stress
- Potential toxin exposure
- Detailed diet history
  - Time of last intake
  - Painful disease etiology may cause reduced intake
  - Characteristics of fecal output
- Normal or abnormal urination and defecation
- Duration and nature of signs noted by the owner

Signalment:

- Any age, sex, and breed of rabbit
- Traumatic fractures more common in younger rabbits

Clinical Signs:

- Acute trauma often presents with paraplegia/paralysis without systemic signs
- Plegia/paralysis should be differentiated from chronic muscle wasting and/or hind limb weakness
- Cutaneous trunci response can be Lost at the level of or just caudal to the lesion
- The absence of deep pain reflexes is a poor prognostic indicator
- Urinary bladder and/or anal sphincter motor control may be lost
- Chronic painful disease may result in weight loss and lethargy
- Urine scalding and ulcerative pododermatitis may be seen

Differentials:

- Trauma
  - Vertebral fracture or luxation
- Intervertebral disk disease
- Discospondylitis
- Septic arthritis
- *E. cuniculi* infection
- Degenerative/developmental disease (Figure 15.6)
- Toxin exposure (heavy metal, topical insecticides)
- Heatstroke
- Vascular disease
- Hypoxia
- Neoplasia
- Urolithiasis

STAT Diagnostics:

- Complete neurologic examination to localize the lesion
- Radiographs (whole body, including skull, spine, affected limbs)

Complete Diagnostics:

- CBC and comprehensive blood profile
- Infectious/toxin screening as indicated
  - Serology (*E. cuniculi*, toxoplasmosis, pasteurellosis, etc.)
  - Lead levels
- Advanced imaging (ultrasound, CT, MRI, myelography) if warranted
- Aspiration of lytic/abnormal lesions or cerebrospinal tap, if indicated (cytology and/or C/S)
- Muscle and nerve biopsy for generalized lower motor neuron weakness

Treatment

Stabilization:

- Hospitalize for paralysis and determine bladder function, manual expression may be needed
- Clean/dry bedding, frequent fur cleaning, turn from side to side (if recumbent) every four hours
- Subcutaneous fluids (IV/IO if necessary) (120 ml/kg/d)
- Assisted syringe feeds for anorectic animals
- Anxiolytic therapy if distressed
  - *Midazolam*: 0.5 mg/kg IV, SC, IM
- Analgesic drugs if painful or to obtain diagnostics
  - *Buprenorphine*: 0.01–0.05 mg/kg SC, IM, IV q6–12h
  - *Butorphanol*: 0.5–1 mg/kg SC, IM, IV q2–6h
  - *Oxymorphone*: 0.05–0.2 mg/kg SC, IM q6–12h
  - *Hydromorphone*: 0.1 mg/kg SC, IM, IV q6–8h
- Anti-inflammatory therapy if indicated
  - *Meloxicam*: 1 mg/kg PO q24h

- *E. cuniculi* treatment as warranted (ideally based on positive test results after discussing risks of therapy with owner):
  - *Oxibendazole*: 15 mg/kg PO q24h × 30d
  - *Fenbendazole*: 20 mg/kg PO q24h × 30d
- Chelation therapy if heavy metal toxicosis
  - *CaEDTA*: 30 mg/kg SQ q12h × 5–7d
- Bathing and oral activated charcoal if topical insecticide
- Treatment of infectious disease as warranted ideally based on C/S
  - *Enrofloxacin*: 5–10 mg/kg PO, SC IM q12h (dilute for parenteral route)
  - *Ciprofloxacin*: 20 mg/kg PO q24h × 5–7d
  - *Azithromycin*: 30 mg/kg PO q24h
  - *Doxycycline*: 2.5 mg/kg PO q12h
  - *Trimethoprim/sulfa*: 30 mg/kg PO, SC q12h
- Surgical management could be considered in some cases but may be associated with a guarded prognosis
- Steroid therapy controversial and likely not helpful

Continued Care:

- Continue fluid therapy until patient eating/drinking
- Cage rest for four to six weeks
- Manage chronic painful conditions
- Bladder and perineal care as needed
  - Manual expression may be required
  - Wound/ulcer management if urine/fecal scalding
- Cart fitting if warranted

Trauma

Introduction

- Most commonly, the result of attacks from conspecifics or other animals in the environment or from mishandling by owners
- Self-trauma is possibly secondary to surgical procedures, behavioral abnormalities, painful conditions, neurologic damage, or entanglement in caging materials or foreign objects
- Electrocution can be a cause of edema or subcutaneous hemorrhage
- Less common causes of injury may be vehicular trauma and gunshot wounds

Diagnosis

History:

- Exposure to other rabbits or animals (probable attack)
- Unsupervised activity outside of enclosure
- Evaluate enclosure and environment for hazards
- Detailed diet and elimination history
  - Time of last food intake
  - Characteristics of fecal output
- Details of any witnessed/past trauma or aggression in environment

Signalment:

- Any age, sex, and breed of rabbit
- Conspecific aggression may be more common in intact animals

Clinical signs:

- Laceration, abrasion, or puncture wounds may be evident
- Blunt force trauma may result in neurologic signs or bleeding wounds
- Traumatic injury may result in bruising, fracture, or malpositioned limb, or paresis or paralysis
- Significant trauma can cause lethargy, recumbency, shock, coma, seizures

Differentials:

- Severe neurologic disease
- Degenerative/developmental disease
- Toxin exposure (heavy metal, topical insecticides)
- Heatstroke
- Infectious disease (bacterial, viral, fungal)
- Vascular disease
- Hypoxia
- Neoplasia

STAT Diagnostics:

- Complete physical examination and vital signs
- Wound clipping/cleaning to determine the extent of wounds
- Radiographs

Complete Diagnostics:

- CBC and comprehensive blood profile
- Infectious/toxin screening as indicated
  - Bacterial cultures if open wounds
  - Serology (*E. cuniculi*, toxoplasmosis, pasteurellosis, etc.)
  - Lead levels
- Advanced imaging (ultrasound, CT, MRI) if warranted

Treatment

Stabilization:

- Subcutaneous fluids (IV/IO if necessary) (120 ml/kg/d)
- Blood transfusion if warranted
- Oxygen therapy if respiratory distress
- Wound therapy
  - Clean and remove fur 2–3 cm from the wound

- Remove devitalized tissue and foreign material
- Lavage with 0.9% saline, LRS, dilute chlorhexidine, or povidone–iodine 1% or less
- Wound closure with primary or secondary intention
- Give broad-spectrum antibiotics
- Open wounds: apply topical ointments and occlusive dressing with 90% water (1% silver sulfadiazine cream, triple antibiotic cream – prevent ingestion)

- Prevent access with a wrap or E-collar
- Anxiolytic or anti-seizure therapy
  - *Midazolam*: 0.5 mg/kg IV, SC, IM
  - *Levetiracetam*: 20 mg/kg IV, PO q8h
- Treatment of infection as warranted ideally based on C/S
  - *Enrofloxacin*: 5–10 mg/kg PO, SC IM q12h (dilute for parenteral route)
  - *Ciprofloxacin*: 20 mg/kg PO q24h × 5–7d
  - *Azithromycin*: 30 mg/kg PO q24h
  - *Doxycycline*: 2.5 mg/kg PO q12h
  - *Trimethoprim/sulfa*: 30 mg/kg PO, SC q12h
- Analgesic drugs if painful or to obtain diagnostics
  - *Buprenorphine*: 0.01–0.05 mg/kg SC, IM, IV q6–12h
  - *Butorphanol*: 0.5–1 mg/kg SC, IM, IV q2–6h
  - *Oxymorphone*: 0.05–0.2 mg/kg SC, IM q6–12h
  - *Hydromorphone*: 0.1 mg/kg SC, IM, IV q6–8h
- Chelation therapy if heavy metal toxicosis
  - *CaEDTA*: 30 mg/kg SQ q12h × 5–7d
- Bathing and oral activated charcoal if topical insecticide

Continued Care:

- Surgical repair of wounds or fractures
- Continue fluid therapy and supplemental feeds until patient eating/drinking on own and maintaining weight
- Treatment plan for chronic painful conditions
- Continued wound management with follow-up

Systemic Disease

Heat Stroke

Diagnosis

Clinical Signs:

- Lethargy, depression
- Hyperthermia
- Ataxia, muscle tremors
- Respiratory distress
- Tachycardia, cardiac arrhythmias
- Seizures progressing to coma
- Hyperemic mucous membranes, petechiae
- Hematochezia, melena
- Oliguria/anuria
- Cardiopulmonary arrest
- Evidence of predisposing disease
  - Cardiovascular disease
  - Neuromuscular disease
  - Obesity

Differentials:

- Infection/sepsis – signs of inflammation
- Cardiopulmonary disease
- Neurologic disease
- Toxic/metabolic disease

STAT Diagnostics:

- Comprehensive physical examination
  - Vital signs elevated
  - Severity of disease
  - Evidence for predisposing disease

Complete Diagnostics:

- CBC and comprehensive blood profile
- Radiographs for suspected cardiopulmonary disease

Treatment

Stabilization:

- Correction of hyperthermia to below 103 °F
- Reduced room temperature/cooling fans, wet cold cloths/spray to body, alcohol to footpads, axilla, groin
- Supplemental oxygen (cage, mask, catheter, ventilator, as indicated)
- Aggressive fluid support for hypovolemic shock/renal insufficiency
  - LRS/crystalloid bolus 60–90 ml/kg IV/IO over 20–60 m, followed by maintenance rate
  - Or, initial crystalloid (30 ml/kg) and hetastarch (5 ml/kg) bolus
- Treatment of cardiac arrhythmia
  - Lidocaine bolus (1–2 mg/kg IV or 2–4 mg/kg IT) followed by continuous-rate intravenous infusion
- Correction of metabolic acidosis
  - Sodium bicarbonate (2 mEq/kg IV)
- Treatment of cerebral complications
  - Diazepam (1.2 mg/kg IV to effect) for seizures
  - Mannitol for cerebral edema
- Treatment of any underlying/predisposing conditions

Continued Care:

- Intensive monitoring during cooling and initial monitoring, most need several days of care

   - Monitor vital signs, blood pressure, cardiac rhythm (ECG), CBC and comprehensive profile, urine output, and urinalysis
- Education of precipitating factors (heat sources, humidity, sun exposure, ventilation, outdoor time) as these are not always obvious to the owner

Intoxications

Diagnosis

Clinical Signs:

- Temperature dysregulation (hypo/hyperthermia)
- Anorexia, hypersalivation, diarrhea
- Respiratory distress
- Seizures

Differentials:

- Diagnosis presumed from exposure, ingestion
- Ingestion of plants (outdoor/indoor), heavy metals (lead paint)
- Topical exposure to organophosphates, environmental insecticides/herbicides (lawn care products), D-limonene, permethrin, flea collars
- Antibiotics selection against Gram-positive flora can cause enteric dysbiosis and enterotoxemia

STAT Diagnostics:

- CBC and comprehensive blood profile
- Attempt to identify the specific toxin

Complete Diagnostics:

- Laboratory confirmation of toxin
- Heavy metal/lead level, if suspected
- Fecal analysis and culture for diarrhea

Treatment

Stabilization:

- Supplemental oxygen (cage, mask, catheter, ventilator, as indicated)
- Temperature regulation
- Toxin removal
   - Bathe with mild liquid detergent for topical exposures
   - Activated charcoal 1–3 g/kg slurry
   - Avoid emetics drugs in rabbits
   - Gastric lavage for lethal (non-petroleum, non-caustic) ingestions with caution
- Toxin elimination
   - LRS/crystalloid fluid therapy with two to three times maintenance rate
   - Diuresis with furosemide 1–4 mg/kg SC, IV, IM q4–6h
   - Gastric protection and prokinetics
- *Cimetidine*: 10 mg/kg PO, SC, IV, IM q8–12h
- *Sucralfate*: 25 mg/kg PO q8–12h
- *Metoclopramide*: 0.2–1.0 mg/kg PO, SC q6–8h, or *cisapride*: 0.5–1.0 mg/kg PO q8–12h
- Toxin reversal
   - *Rodenticides:* Vitamin K1 (2.5 mg/kg PO q24h for 10–30 days; oil suspension to enhance absorption), plasma or cross-matched whole-blood for significant intoxications
   - *Organophosphates:* Glycopyrrolate and 2-PAM can be tried
   - *Lead:* CaEDTA 30 mg/kg SC q12h for five to seven days
- Seizure control
   - *Diazepam*:1.2 mg/kg IV/IM to effect (1–5 mg/kg range)
- Enteritis/enterotoxemia treatment
   - Antibiotic-induced enteritis/enterotoxemia
      - *Metronidazole*: 20 mg/kg PO, IV q12h
      - *Enrofloxacin*: 5–15 mg/kg PO, IM, SC q12h; dilute for the parenteral route
      - *Trimethoprim sulfa*: 30 mg/kg PO q12h
- Analgesics for pain and prior to procedure
   - *Buprenorphine*: 0.01–0.05 mg/kg SC, IM q6–12h
   - *Meloxicam*: 1 mg/kg PO, SC q24h

Continued Care:

- Continued monitoring of vital signs and neurologic status
- Monitor hydration status and reduce fluid therapy
- Resume feeding once stabilized
   - Critical care for herbivores
   - Quality grass hay and moistened greens
- Monitor for evidence of gastrointestinal hypomotility/stasis

Sepsis

Diagnosis

Clinical Signs:

- Fever, lethargy, depression
- Anorexia, dehydration
- Diarrhea or GI stasis
- Tachycardia progressing to hypovolemic shock
- Associated infections common
- Septic mastitis
   - Firm, swollen, erythematous mammary gland(s) with purulent or hemorrhagic fluid expression
   - Postpartum or pseudopregnant does
- Septic arthritis
   - Lameness, joint pain contracture/limited mobility, effusion, thickening
   - Often associated with severe pododermatitis
- Enterotoxemia
   - Diarrhea with evidence of hypovolemia and shock
   - Associated with antibiotic administration

Differentials:

- *Generalized sepsis:* heat stroke, intoxication, metabolic disease
- *Septic mastitis:* mammary hyperplasia/tumors, subcutaneous abscessation
- *Septic arthritis:* auto-inflammatory and degenerative arthritis, trauma, neurologic disease
- *Enterotoxemia:* other infectious diarrhea/dysbiosis (bacterial, viral, parasitic)

STAT Diagnostics:

- Vitals assessment to determine stability
- Complete physical examination, assess for localized infection

Complete Diagnostics:

- CBC and comprehensive blood profile
- Aspirate and C/S of localized site (mammary, joint)
- C/S of blood, urine, and/or feces
  - Serology for *Pasteurella* of limited utility
- Radiographs (joint, uterus, intestinal tract assessment)

Treatment

Stabilization:

- Subcutaneous fluids (IV/IO, if indicated) 120 ml/kg/d
  - Correct for dehydration
  - LRS/crystalloid bolus 60–90 ml/kg IV/IO over 20–60 m, followed by maintenance rate for shock/severe hypovolemia
- Syringe feeding (see Chapter 8)
  - Nasogastric tube feeding if oral not tolerated
- Analgesia
  - *Meloxicam*: 1 mg/kg PO, SC q24h
  - *Tramadol*: 5–11 mg/kg PO q24h
  - *Buprenorphine*: 0.01–0.05 mg/kg SC, IM, IV q6–12h
  - *Oxymorphone*: 0.05–0.2 mg/kg SC, IM q6–12h
  - *Hydromorphone*: 0.1 mg/kg SC, IM, IV q6–8h
- Broad-spectrum antibiotic coverage, pending C/S
  - *Enrofloxacin*: 5–20 mg/kg PO, SC, IM q12–24h; dilute for parenteral route
  - *Trimethoprim/sulfa*: 30 mg/kg PO q12h
  - *Chloramphenicol*: 30–50 mg/kg PO q8–12h
  - *Azithromycin*: 30 mg/kg PO q24h

Continued Care:

- Continue fluid therapy and supplemental feeds until patient eating/drinking on own and maintaining weight to minimize stasis
- Treatment plan for pain management
- Continued wound management, surgical intervention if necessary
- Adjust antibiotic therapy based on C/S
  - Antibiotics may be required for a period of six to eight weeks if localized infection/abscessation present
- Environmental adjustments (isolation, disinfection) for enterotoxemia

Musculoskeletal Disease

Splay leg

Diagnosis

Clinical Signs:

- Inability to adduct one or more limbs, more common in hind limbs (Figure 15.6)
- Inability to lift body off ground or even paralysis can be seen
- Some present at an early age or during rapid early growth
  - Some autosomal recessive inheritance
  - Also diet and substrate factors in larger breeds
- Affected and unaffected limbs can have pododermatitis
- Urine scalding and perineal fecal soiling
- Anorexia and dehydration with immobility and pain

Differentials:

- Other congenital and musculoskeletal anomalies
  - Sarcocystis, spondylosis, myasthenia gravis
- Toxins
- Malnutrition, hypokalemia
- Floppy rabbit syndrome
- Traumatic injury
- Vestibular disease
- Infections (*E. cuniculi*, toxoplasmosis)

STAT Diagnostics:

- Complete neurological exam to localize the lesion
- Radiographs (anteversion/subluxation/dislocation with splay leg)

Complete Diagnostics:

- CBC and comprehensive blood profile
- Infectious and toxic workup as indicated

Treatment

Stabilization:

- Analgesia
  - *Meloxicam*: 1.0 mg/kg PO, SC q24h
- Nutritional support if anorexia and/or GI stasis is present

Continued Care:

- Address underlying cause (if present), and environmental modifications

- Monitor for complications of reduced mobility (dermatitis) and feeding (anorexia/stasis)
- Prognosis is guarded with multiple limbs affected

Spondylosis/Osteoarthritis

Diagnosis

Clinical Signs:

- Progressive degenerative abnormalities
- Spondylosis with evidence of spinal nerve root compression
  - Neurologic deficits, ataxia, rear limb weakness
- Osteoarthritis with degenerative joint disease
  - Lameness, stiff, reduced range of motion, joint swelling, and pain
- Sequelae of limited mobility: podo- and perineal dermatitis, poor grooming, mites, obesity

Differentials:

- Painful non-orthopedic conditions: pododermatitis, urolithiasis, neoplasia
- Other orthopedic conditions: spinal osteoarthritis, intervertebral disc disease, fracture non-union/complications, synovial tumors
- Septic arthritis

STAT Diagnostics:

- Complete neurological and musculoskeletal exam to localize the lesion
- Radiographs
  - Paraspinal osteophytes and fusion along the vertebral endplates, more commonly in the lumbar spine, in spondylosis
  - Degenerative articular cartilage and joint space irregularities in osteoarthritis

Complete Diagnostics:

- CBC and comprehensive blood profile
- Arthrocentesis and synovial fluid C/S and analysis if suspicion for infection
- Biopsy of proliferative synovial tissue lesions
- CT/MRI/myelogram, if warranted

Treatment

Stabilization:

- Cage rest with limited mobility
- Analgesia
  - *Meloxicam*: 1.0 mg/kg PO q24h
  - *Carprofen*: 2.2 mg/kg PO q12–24h
- Clean and treat dermatitis areas
  - *Enrofloxacin*: 5–20 mg/kg PO, SC, IM q12–24h; dilute for parenteral route
  - *Trimethoprim sulfa*: 30 mg/kg PO q12h
  - *Topical ointments*: Silver sulfadiazine cream, zinc oxide/menthol (Gold Bond)

Continued Care:

- Continue pain (NSAIDs, acupuncture) and dermatitis management
- Anecdotal use of chondroitin sulfate, polysulfate glycosaminoglycan 2.2 mg/kg SC, IM q3d × 21–28d, then q14d

Ulcerative Pododermatitis

Diagnosis

Clinical Signs:

- Plantar and palmar aspects involved, more common in hind
- Alopecia, erythema, ulceration, cellulitis, necrosis, and possible abscessation
- Secondary pain with lameness, depression, reduced intake/anorexia

Differentials:

- Traumatic fracture, abscess
- Neoplasia, granulomatous disease

STAT Diagnostics:

- Complete physical and musculoskeletal examination – other musculoskeletal, neurologic, or systemic causes of lameness
- Radiology of lesions
  - Determine bony involvement
  - Osteomyelitis has protracted/poor course

Complete Diagnostics:

- CBC and comprehensive blood profile
- Additional radiographs (spine/joints) to determine etiology if chronic limited mobility
- Ultrasonography for other painful conditions (urolithiasis, GI disease, neoplasia)
- Biopsy mass lesions, C/S of dermatitis wound

Treatment

Stabilization:

- Wound management
  - Flush and debride daily
  - Antiseptic irrigation daily (chlorhexidine, iodine)
  - Silver sulfadiazine cream
  - Wet-to-dry bandage until granulation tissue forms
- Analgesia
  - *Butorphanol*: 0.1–1.0 mg/kg SC, IM, IV q4–6h (sedating)

 - *Buprenorphine*: 0.01–0.05 mg/kg SC, IM, IV q8–12h (less sedating)
 - *Meloxicam*: 1.0 mg/kg PO q24h
- Antibiotic therapy for severe disease/osteomyelitis
 - *Enrofloxacin*: 5–20 mg/kg PO, SC, IM q12–24h; dilute for parenteral route
 - *Trimethoprim sulfa*: 30 mg/kg PO q12h
 - *Chloramphenicol*: 50 mg/kg PO q8–12h
 - *Metronidazole*: 20 mg/kg PO q12–24h
- Supplemental fluids and feeds, as needed

Continued Care:

- Continued wound care, supplemental feeding
- Surgical debridement vs. amputation for refractory osteomyelitis
- Environmental corrections: soft, dry bedding changed frequently
- Treat underlying causes to prevent recurrence

Neurologic Disease

Encephalitozoon cuniculi

Diagnosis

Clinical Signs:

- Infections marked by ocular, CNS, and renal disease
- Most asymptomatic until immunocompromised (newborn, older, chronic disease, stress)
- Ocular involvement (often unilateral) postnatal from in utero infections
 - Uveitis – aqueous flare, hypopyon, hyphema, mydriasis
 - Iriditis and iridal abscess
 - Cataracts and lens rupture
- CNS involvement with prominent vestibular signs
 - Ataxia, nystagmus, head tilt, torticollis
 - Stiff gait, paresis, paralysis
 - Tremors, seizures, incontinence
- Significant renal compromise less common
 - Dehydration, anorexia, gastrointestinal hypomotility

Differentials:

- Ocular disease
 - Bacterial uveitis, trauma/corneal ulceration with secondary inflammation/infection
- Vestibular symptoms
 - Otitis interna and/or media
   - Most common cause of vestibular signs must exclude first
 - CNS infections (toxoplasmosis, abscess), neoplasia, trauma
- Ataxia and weakness
 - Orthopedic disease – spinal (spondylosis) and developmental (splay leg) and degenerative (osteoarthritis) joint disease
 - Neurologic disease
 - Intoxications (lead)
 - Metabolic disease

STAT Diagnostics:

- Thorough physical and neurologic examination to exclude other causes
- CBC and comprehensive blood panel
 - Non-specific dehydration associated changes
- Radiographs
 - Skull to evaluate bullae
 - Spinal films to exclude degenerative disease and trauma
 - Kidneys may be small and/or misshapen

Complete Diagnostics:

- Serologic testing
 - Many North American and European rabbits will be positive, indicative of prior (in utero) exposure and not necessarily active disease
 - Definitive diagnosis based on organism (obligate intracellular microsporidian parasite) identification in affected tissues, generally postmortem
 - Positive serology and response to treatment supports presumed diagnosis, but risk/benefit discussion required prior to initiation
- Head CT/MRI is considered for excluding bulla disease, abscess, neoplasia

Treatment

Stabilization:

- Hospitalize if cannot maintain adequate intake
 - Subcutaneous (or IV) maintenance fluids (120 mg/kg/d)
 - Syringe assistance feeding (see Chapter 8) and/or offer fresh moist greens, quality grass hay, and usual diet (aspiration caution)
- Confine for severe neurologic signs (ataxia, seizures, rolling) with padded cages
- Antiparasitic therapy
 - *Oxibendazole*: 15 mg/kg PO q24h × 30d
 - *Fenbendazole*: 20 mg/kg PO q24h × 30d
 - Risk of bone marrow suppression/aplastic anemia/pancytopenia with therapy must be considered/discussed prior to therapy
- Seizures or severe vestibular signs
 - *Midazolam*: 0.5–2 mg/kg IV, IM, SC
 - *Diazepam*: 0.5–2 mg/kg IM

- Mild vestibular signs
  - *Meclizine*: 2–12 mg/kg PO q24h
- Uveitis
  - Treatment with topical corticosteroids is controversial due to significant immunosuppressive effects in rabbits that could worsen *E. cuniculi* infection

Continued Care:

- Cage modifications (padding) to avoid injury, assisted feeding at home
- Follow-up needed while on treatment
- Waxing/waning course with residual symptoms can be seen

Head Tilt/Torticollis

Diagnosis

Clinical Signs:

- Head tilt (Figure 15.1)
- Progression: rolling, eventual lateral recumbency with inability to lift head
- Other vestibular signs often present
  - Nystagmus
    - Resting-horizontal/rotational with fast phase away from tilt
    - Positional – any direction, varies with head position
  - Strabismus – often ventral deviation
  - Ipsilateral paresis and proprioceptive defects (central damage), or isolated facial nerve paralysis (peripheral damage)
  - Ataxia with falls to the side of head tilt
- Evidence of upper respiratory infection (extension into inner/middle ear)
  - Nasal, ocular, otic discharge

Differentials:

- Rule out abnormal head tilt due to pain (isolated otitis externa/media without vestibular or CNS involvement)
- Otitis media and interna
  - Central nervous system extension/encephalitis/encephalomyelitis
  - *Pasteurella* and other bacterial species more common; parasitic, fungal rare
  - *E. cuniculi* infection
- Other less common infections
  - Toxoplasmosis
  - *Baylisacaris* sp. (raccoon roundworm)
  - Rabies and herpes viruses (rare reports)
  - CNS fungal disease generally not seen in rabbits
- Trauma
  - Tympanic bulla or petrosal bone fracture
  - Fracture with brainstem injury
- Neoplasia
  - Cerebellar/brainstem tumors very rare in rabbits
  - Extension of bone or soft tissue tumor
- Metabolic
  - Hypovitaminosis A (rare)
- Toxic
  - Lead, aminoglycoside antibiotics

STAT Diagnostics:

- Otoscopic examination (see Section "Otitis Media/Interna")
- Microscopic examination and C/S of exudate, if present

Complete Diagnostics:

- Radiographs
  - Vestibular/bony destruction from infection
  - Tympanic bullae
  - Trauma
  - CT/MRI considered
- Serologic/infectious testing
  - *E. cuniculi*
  - *Pasteurella*
  - Bacterial C/S of any exudate present
  - Consider CSF analysis, C/S (cerebellomedullary cistern)
- Biopsy of mass lesions (tumors, osteomyelitis)

Treatment

Stabilization:

- Hospitalize if cannot maintain adequate intake
  - Subcutaneous (or IV) maintenance fluids (120 mg/kg/d)
  - Syringe assistance feeding (see Chapter 8) and/or offer fresh moist greens, quality grass hay, and usual diet (aspiration caution)
- Confine for severe neurologic signs (ataxia, seizures, rolling) with padded cages
- Severe vestibular signs (continuous rolling, torticollis) or seizures
  - *Diazepam*: 1–2 mg/kg IM/IV, or *midazolam*: 1–2 mg/kg IM/IV
  - *Meclizine*: 2–12 mg/kg PO q8–12h (anti-nausea, sedative effect)
- Otitis media/interna, bacterial encephalitis treatment
  - See Otitis Media/Interna

Continued Care:

- Cage modifications (padding) to avoid injury, assisted feeding at home

- Monitor for corneal ulceration if facial paralysis/vestibular episodes
- Supportive care for trauma
  - Surgical evaluation for possible ear canal ablation/bullae osteotomy
- Continue with long-term (four to six weeks minimum) antibiotic therapy

Otitis Media/Interna

Diagnosis

Clinical Signs:

- Shaking head, pawing ear, holding affected ear down
- Acute head tilt with possible progression to rolling, seizures
  - Damage to vestibular portion of acoustic nerve (otitis interna)
- Nystagmus (resting/positional), vestibular strabismus, ipsilateral leaning, ataxia (can indicate CNS extension) (see Section "Head Tilt/Torticollis")
- Ipsilateral facial nerve damage (otitis media ± interna)
  - Paresis/paralysis of ear, eyelid, nare, lip
- Anorexia, difficulty chewing
- Extension of outer ear infection (via tympanic membrane) or upper respiratory infection (via eustachian tube), with associated findings

Differentials:

- Ensure not isolated otitis externa and holding ear down from pain
- Bacterial infection (most common)
  - *P. multocida*
  - *S. aureus*
  - *Pseudomonas aeruginosa*
  - *E. coli*
  - *Listeria monocytogenes*
  - Various anaerobes
- *E. cuniculi*
- Yeast (rare as primary cause)
  - *Malassezia* sp.
  - *Candida* sp.
- Mites
  - *Psoroptes cuniculi* infestation
- Unilateral disease
  - Foreign body, trauma, tumor should be excluded
- CNS abscess
- Other – Neoplasia (rare)

STAT Diagnostics:

- Otoscopic examination
  - *Otitis externa:* thick, creamy exudate in horizontal/vertical canals, may obstruct tympanic membrane analysis
  - *Otitis interna/media without externa* (via eustachian tube)*:* dull, opaque, and bulging tympanic membrane
  - *Isolated otitis interna:* can be normal in appearance

Complete Diagnostics:

- CBC and comprehensive blood profile
- Imaging
  - Radiographs; evaluate bullae (vestibular/bony destruction from infection), trauma
  - +/− CT/MRI
- Serologic/infectious disease testing
  - *E. cuniculi*, *Pasteurella*
  - Swab exudates present (aural, nasal, ocular)
    - Microscopic examination and bacterial C/S
- Biopsy of mass lesions (tumors, osteomyelitis)

Treatment

Stabilization:

- Supportive care and vestibular therapies as in Head Tilt/Torticollis
- Antibiotic therapy for bacterial otitis ± encephalitis (four to six weeks minimum)
  - *Enrofloxacin*: 5–20 mg/kg PO, SC, IM q2–24h; dilute for parenteral route
  - *Trimethoprim sulfa*: 30 mg/kg PO q12h
  - *Chloramphenicol*: 30–50 mg/kg PO q8–12h
  - *Azithromycin*: 30 mg/kg PO q24h
  - *Metronidazole*: 20 mg/kg PO q24h
  - *Penicillin G*: 40 000–60 000 IU/kg SC, IM q24-48h
- *E. cuniculi* therapy

Continued Care:

- Cage modifications assisted feeding at home as needed for vestibular complications
- Re-evaluate for improvement of clinical symptoms in 10–14 days or sooner if not improving (re-evaluate chosen antibiotic therapy)
- Monitor for corneal ulceration if facial paralysis/vestibular episodes
- Continue with long-term (four to six weeks minimum) antibiotic therapy

Seizures/Collapse

Diagnosis

Clinical Signs:

- Sudden onset, often short duration (under two minutes)
  - More often generalized than partial
- Abrupt termination of activity with postictal period
  - Confusion, restless, or comatose, apparent blindness

- Isolated, cluster (multiple in 24 hours), or sustained (status epilepticus)
- Evidence of infection or systemic/metabolic disease in some cases
  - Head tilt and vestibular signs (*E. cuniculi*, otitis interna)

Differentials:

- Encephalitis infections
  - *E. cuniculi*
  - Toxoplasmosis
  - Baylisacaris sp. (raccoon roundworm)
  - Bacterial – *Pasteurella* sp.
- Otitis interna
- Toxin
- Metabolic
  - Hypocalcemia, lethal hypoglycemia, hepatic encephalopathy
- Hypoxic/ischemic/cardiovascular disease
- Neoplasia (rare)
- Idiopathic epilepsy (poorly documented)
- Severe vestibular disease (continuous rolling)
- Syncope/floppy rabbit syndrome

STAT Diagnostics:

- Physical exam with a comprehensive neurological exam to attempt to localize any deficits
- Otoscopic examination

Complete Diagnostics:

- CBC and comprehensive blood panel
  - Hypocalcemia, hypoglycemia, uremic encephalopathy
- Serologic testing
  - *E. cuniculi*, *Pasteurella*
- CSF analysis and C/S
- Imaging
  - Radiographs; evaluate bullae (vestibular/bony destruction from infection), trauma
  - +/− CT/MRI

Treatment

Stabilization:

- Treatment of known cause(s)
- Hospitalize for cluster seizures, rapid attention of status epilepticus
- Monitor vitals (hyperthermia), IV access, and fluids
- Treatment of severe cluster seizures and status epilepticus
  - *Diazepam*: 0.5–5 mg/kg IV bolus, start with 0.5–1.0 mg/kg
    - Repeat/increase for sustained activity after five minutes
    - Hepatic necrosis side effect in other species
  - 50% dextrose, 0.25–2.0 ml IV slow bolus in hypoglycemic animals
- Chronic recurrent seizures
  - *Phenobarbital*: 1–2.5 mg/kg PO q12h anecdotal use
    - Hepatotoxicity (not observed in rabbits)
  - *Levetiracetam*: 20 mg/kg PO q8h
- Bacterial meningoencephalitis (see Otitis Media/Interna)
- *E. cuniculi* (see Section "*Encephalitozoon cuniculi*")
- Toxoplasmosis
  - *Trimethoprim sulfa*: 30 mg/kg PO q12h
  - Sulfadiazine with pyrimethamine can also be used

Continued care:

- Varied response to drug treatment, guarded prognosis
- Overall response also depends on underlying condition (if readily identifiable)
- Require ongoing supervision at home and while boarded/hospitalized

Cardiopulmonary Disease

Congestive Heart Failure/Cardiogenic Edema

Diagnosis

Clinical Signs:

- Lethargy, weakness, exercise intolerance common findings
- Dyspnea, tachypnea (normal 30–60 breaths/min), and syncope
- Left-sided heart failure (low output, pulmonary backup)
  - Pulmonary edema
    - Tachypnea (>60 breaths/min)
    - Dyspnea, inspiratory, and expiratory
    - Pulmonary crackles increased bronchial sounds and/or wheezes on auscultation
  - Arrhythmia
    - Normal heart rate 180–330 bpm, mean 250
    - Bradycardia, tachycardia, atrial fibrillation, ventricular premature complexes possible
    - Possible murmur(s)
  - Weak peripheral pulses, prolonged capillary refill time
- Right-sided heart failure (systemic backup)
  - Ascites
  - Hepatosplenomegaly
  - Possible murmur(s)
  - Pericardial effusion with muffled heart sounds
  - Pleural effusion with rapid, shallow respiration, and muffled lung sounds

Differentials:

- Dyspnea and weakness, non-cardiac origin
  - Upper respiratory infections/obstructions
    - Sinusitis, rhinitis, laryngitis
    - Foreign body
  - Lower respiratory infections (abscess, pneumonia)
  - Pleural effusion
    - Neoplasia, infection, abscess
  - Trauma: pneumothorax, pulmonary hemorrhage, diaphragmatic hernia
  - Neoplasia: thymoma, lymphoma, cardiac tumors
- Ascites/abdominal distension
  - Nutritional deficiencies: hypoproteinemia, malnutrition
  - Renal failure: protein-losing nephropathy
  - Hepatic disease and failure
  - Peritonitis
  - Abdominal hemorrhage
  - Neoplasia
- Cardiac causes
  - Congenital heart disease (rare reports)
  - Arrhythmias (atrial fibrillation, although often secondary)
  - Cardiomyopathy/myocardial disease
    - Idiopathic, hypertrophic, and dilated (most common)
    - Vitamin E deficiency
    - Infection (*Pasteurella*, *E. cuniculi*, *Salmonella*, coronaviruses)
    - Drugs (doxorubicin, ketamine infusions)
- Valvular disease
    - Mitral and tricuspid insufficiency
    - Valvular endocarditis (*S. aureus*)
- Ischemia
    - Limited collateral myocardial circulation in rabbits
- Vascular
    - Arteriosclerosis common in older rabbits
    - Pulmonary hypertension in higher altitudes

STAT Diagnostics:

- Vital sign assessment – tachypnea, tachycardia/arrhythmia, weak pulses
- Complete physical examination with detailed thoracic auscultation
  - Mild sedation is often helpful (midazolam 0.5–1 mg/kg IM)
- Thoracic/abdominal radiographs
- Thoracic/abdominal ultrasound

Complete Diagnostics:

- Electrocardiography
- Echocardiography
- Thoracocentesis or abdominocentesis
  - Therapeutic drainage
  - Diagnostic – cytology analysis, C/S

Treatment

Stabilization:

- Minimize handling of dyspneic animals
  - Light sedation for examination and procedures is often needed (midazolam 0.5–1 mg/kg IM/IV)
- Supplemental oxygen necessary
  - Cage delivery less stressful than facemask
- Heat source for hypothermic animals
- Assisted feeding for anorexic animals
- Thoracocentesis
  - For significant pleural effusions, drain each hemithorax with 20-gauge butterfly needle under sedation
  - Anesthesia mask with isoflurane may be necessary
- Diuretic therapy (preload reduction, effusion/edema reduction)
  - *Furosemide*:
    - 1–4 mg/kg q8–12h IM/IV initially
    - 1–2 mg/kg q8–12h PO long-term therapy
    - Start at low dose unless fulminant failure
    - Potassium supplementation with long-term usage
- Venodilator therapy (preload reduction)
    - Nitroglycerin 2% ointment
    - 1/16–1/8-in. square applied to inner pinna
    - Helps to reduce the dose of diuretic needed (beneficial for dehydrated patients)
- Blood pressure reduction (ACE inhibitor – preload and afterload reduction)
  - *Enalapril maleate*:
    - Used for long-term maintenance therapy
    - 0.25–0.5 mg/kg PO q24–48h
- Other drugs to consider
  - *Digoxin*:
    - For dilated cardiomyopathy and supraventricular arrhythmias
    - 0.005–0.01 mg/kg PO q24–48h, start at the lowest dose
    - Increase gradually, monitor for toxicity (nausea)/serum levels
  - *Beta-blockers*:
    - For hypertrophic cardiomyopathy and atrial/ventricular arrhythmias in other species
    - Anecdotal use, extrapolated dosing from cats/ferrets
  - *Calcium channel blockers*:
    - For hypertrophic cardiomyopathy and atrial/ventricular arrhythmias in other species
    - Anecdotal use, extrapolated dosing from cats/ferrets

Continued Care:

- Monitor activity level, respiratory rate, and effort
- Monitor body weight and abdominal girth (ascites)
- Monitor intake/output
- Reduce stress and exercise, monitor heart rate and rhythm
- Follow-up radiographs and echocardiography to assess treatment
- Monitor electrolyte levels on therapy
- Drug toxicity concerns:
  - Anorexia can be a sign of ACE inhibitor or digoxin toxicity, lower dose if nausea suspected
  - Azotemia can develop with diuretics, requiring the lowering of dose or discontinuation if persistent
  - Monitor digoxin levels periodically
    - Extrapolated therapeutic range 1–2 ng/dl at 8–12 hours post dose

Pleural Space Disease

Diagnosis

Clinical Signs:

- Lethargy, weakness, exercise intolerance
- Dyspnea/tachypnea-rapid and shallow respirations
- Open-mouth breathing
- Nausea/anorexia
- Cardiac/congestive heart disease findings
  - See Congestive Heart Failure/Cardiogenic Edema
- Muffled/inaudible heart and breath sounds ventrally, preservation of breath sounds ventrally

Differentials:

- Congestive heart failure most common source of effusion
- Infection
  - Bacterial, viral, fungal
  - Abscess formation is common
- Neoplasia
  - Cranial mediastinal mass
    - Lymphosarcoma
    - Thymoma
  - Metastatic disease (pleural implants)
- Chylothorax
  - Congestive heart failure, cranial vena cava obstruction, neoplasia, trauma
- Hemothorax
  - Trauma, neoplasia, coagulopathy

STAT diagnostics:

- Radiographs – thoracic and abdominal
- Echocardiography
- Thoracocentesis
- CBC and comprehensive blood panel

Complete Diagnostics:

- Thoracocentesis fluid analysis and culture
  - For chyle, Sudan stain pleural fluid or send for triglyceride and cholesterol evaluations of fluid and serum (enriched in chyle vs. other effusions)
- Exploratory thoracotomy considered for thoracic masses

Treatment

Stabilization:

- Minimize handling of dyspneic animals
  - Light sedation for examination and procedures is often needed (midazolam 0.5–1 mg/kg IM/IV)
- Supplemental oxygen necessary
- Heat source for hypothermic animals
- Assisted feeding for anorexic animals
- Thoracocentesis
  - For significant pleural effusions, drain each hemithorax with 20-gauge butterfly needle under sedation
  - Anesthesia mask with isoflurane may be necessary
- Admit for stabilization and intensive monitoring
- Treatment of congestive heart failure
- Treatment of respiratory infections
- Treatment for neoplasia

Continued Care:

- Management of underlying cause of fluid accumulation
- Monitoring of activity level, respiratory rate, and effort

Pneumonia

Diagnosis

Clinical Signs:

- Lethargy, anorexia, weight loss
- Dyspnea/tachypnea in more advanced disease
- Evidence of prior oral/upper respiratory infection
  - Nasal/ocular discharge, sneezing
  - Dental disease, ptyalism, facial abscess
- Abnormal breath sounds on auscultation
  - Accentuated bronchial sounds
  - Crackles, wheezes
  - Decreased breath sounds (consolidation, abscess)
  - Concomitant upper respiratory disease referred to sounds can make thoracic auscultation difficult
- Anorectic rabbits may have dehydration, gastrointestinal hypomotility, scant dry fecal pellets

Differentials:

- Upper respiratory tract disease
  - Obligate nasal breathers; severe upper disease can mimic symptoms of pneumonia
- Pleural effusion or infection
- Congestive heart failure with pulmonary edema
- Bacterial pneumonia (most common)
  - *S. aureus*, *B. bronchiseptica*, *Moraxella catarrhalis*, *P. aeruginosa*, *Mycobacterium* sp., *P. multocida*, and various anaerobes
  - Inhalation, aspiration, or hematogenous routes of infection from environment, upper respiratory infection, oral/dental disease
  - Intraparenchymal abscess formation is common and can have initial aggressive growth pattern
- Fungal pneumonia
  - *Aspergillus* sp. and *Cryptococcus* sp. rarely reported
- Aspiration pneumonia
  - Rare as rabbits do not vomit, but can see with dysphagia
  - Following oral medications and supplemental (oral/tube) feedings

STAT Diagnostics:

- Thoracic radiographs
  - Alveolar pattern with increased pulmonary densities, air bronchograms, pulmonary consolidation
  - Intrathoracic fat in obese rabbits can mimic pneumonia/abscess

Complete Diagnostics:

- CBC and comprehensive blood panel
  - Total WBC count not always elevated, but relative neutrophilia and lymphopenia seen
- Aspirates and washings (upper and/or lower) for analysis and culture
- *Pasteurella* serology

Treatment

Stabilization:

- Minimize handling of dyspneic animals
  - Light sedation for examination and procedures is often needed (midazolam 0.5–1 mg/kg IM/IV)
- Supplemental oxygen, nebulization with bland aerosols
- Heat source for hypothermic animals
- Maintenance fluids with a balanced electrolyte solution
- Supplemental feeding for anorexic animals, monitoring intake/output
- Antimicrobial therapy with broad-spectrum antibiotics, ideally based on C/S
  - *Enrofloxacin*: 5–20 mg/kg PO, SC, IM q12–24h; dilute parenteral route
  - *Trimethoprim sulfa*: 30 mg/kg PO q12h
- If anaerobic infection suspected
  - *Chloramphenicol*: 30–50 mg/kg PO q8–12h
  - *Metronidazole*: 20 mg/kg PO q12h
  - *Azithromycin*: 30 mg/kg PO q24h (often with metronidazole)
  - *Parenteral penicillin G*: 40 000–60 000 IU/kg SC, IM q24–48h

Continued Care:

- Follow-up culture and sensitivity results
- Monitor clinical signs for improvement as radiographic improvement can be significantly delayed

Upper Respiratory Disease

Diagnosis

Clinical Signs:

- Lethargy, anorexia
- Dyspnea, stridor especially with exertion (obligate nasal breathers)
- Secretions and dried discharge on the hair around nose and eyes and on front limbs from grooming
- Sneezing and nasal discharge
  - Serous, mucoid, mucopurulent, purulent, or blood-tinged
- Ocular discharge can be mucopurulent with conjunctivitis, exophthalmos from retrobulbar abscess
- Head tilt and other vestibular signs or scratching at ears with extension into eustachian tube and ear
- Ptyalism, anorexia, and ocular/nasal discharge from concurrent dental disease

Differentials:

- Bacterial rhinitis/sinusitis (most common)
  - *Pasteurella* sp., *Bordetella* sp.
- Epiphora with ocular infection, retrobulbar abscess from nasolacrimal duct obstruction or tooth root impaction
- Epistaxis from coagulopathy, hypertension, dental abscess, neoplasia
- Dental disease
  - Tooth root impaction, malocclusion, incisor overgrowth
  - Odontogenic abscess
- Foreign body
  - Often hay/straw or bedding material
- Allergies/irritants
  - Bedding, dust, plants/soil, cat litter
- Stertor from laryngeal or pharyngeal edema/infection, neuromuscular disease
- Neoplasia
- Unilateral discharge often from non-systemic process (tumor, dental disease, foreign body)

STAT Diagnostics:

- Complete physical exam including thorough oral and otic examination

Complete Diagnostics:

- CBC and comprehensive blood panel
  - Total WBC count not always elevated, but relative neutrophilia and lymphopenia seen
- Radiographs (head and thorax) and/or CT/MRI
  - Subclinical pneumonia common with bacterial rhinitis
  - Fluid densities can obscure detail
  - Bony lysis, turbinate changes with chronic infections
  - Laryngeal soft tissue abnormalities
  - Dental disease evaluation
- *Pasteurella* serology
- Nasal discharge analysis and cultures
  - Deep cultures obtained with mini culturette tip inserted 2–4 cm into each nostril or nasal flush
  - Cytology often non-specific inflammation
  - Commonly isolated species are also commensals, rely on heavy overgrowth
  - Can be negative due to deep/inaccessible location and/or organisms difficult to culture (anaerobes, *Pasteurella*)
- Rhinoscopy with biopsy of mass lesions
- Pharyngoscopy and laryngoscopy are considered for unusual laryngeal disease/mass lesions

Treatment

Stabilization:

- For serious respiratory distress and concurrent systemic disease, hospitalized for monitoring, oxygen, and fluid administration
  - Extreme obstruction may require intubation
- Outpatient treatment for isolated infections without systemic disease or significant respiratory distress
- Offer supplemental syringe feedings and maintain hydration
- Humidification of environment and/or saline nebulization to loosen secretions
- Antimicrobial therapy (see Section "Pneumonia")
- Antihistamines
  - Allergic rhinitis and symptomatic relief with infectious rhinitis
  - Hydroxyzine or diphenhydramine at 2 mg/kg PO q8–12h
- Ciprofloxacin ophthalmic drops have been used intranasally in addition to systemic antibiotics, but require caution and restraint and are not recommended for owner administration
- For epiphora/ocular discharge without dyspnea, cannulate, and flush nasolacrimal duct
  - Topical ophthalmic anesthetic and/or midazolam
  - 23-ga lacrimal cannula or 24-ga Teflon cathether
  - Single punctum in ventral eyelid at the medial canthus
  - Flush duct out nasal meatus, instill ophthalmic antibiotic drops (ciprofloxacin, chloramphenicol, etc.) 4–6×/d for 21 days
- Topical ophthalmic antibiotic ointments for conjunctivitis

Continued Care:

- Environmental modifications to minimize allergens/irritants
- Maintain systemic antibiotics for four to six weeks
- Monitor for relapse after completion of therapy (not uncommon)
- Treat associated dental disease

Gastrointestinal Disease

Dental Disease

Diagnosis

Clinical Signs:

- Dental overgrowth and spur formation
- Malocclusion and dental asymmetry
- Tooth disfigurement/dystrophy, enamel dysplasia
- Anorexia, dysphagia, change in dietary preference (soft foods)
- Salivation, nasal, and/or ocular discharge, discharge on forearms
- Facial swelling/masses, exophthalmos, altered chewing, halitosis
- Poor grooming, uneaten cecotropes, perineal soiling
- Weight loss, change in fecal output

Differentials:

- Dental malocclusion
- Dental root impaction, infection, abscess
- Facial or jaw trauma
- Neoplasia of facial/jaw bones and soft tissue
- Metabolic bone disease (often with tooth/enamel dysplasia)
- Upper respiratory infections
- Unilateral exophthalmos
  - Retrobulbar or orbital abscess
  - Cellulitis, granuloma, cysts (i.e. cysticercosis)
  - Lacrimal or salivary obstruction/disease
  - Trauma, hemorrhage
  - Neoplasia

STAT Diagnostics:

- Thorough examination of the face, jaw, and teeth (Figure 15.7)
- CBC and comprehensive blood panel
  - +/– anemia, infection/inflammatory changes with chronic disease

Complete Diagnostics:

- Comprehensive dental evaluation under anesthesia with endoscope
  - Evaluation of incisors, cheek teeth, periapical structures, bone, tongue, and oral mucosa
- Skull radiographs are essential for evaluating dental disease
- CT to visualize extension of dental infections into nasal cavity and orbit
- Culture and sensitivity of any abscess capsule

Treatment

Stabilization:

- Supportive care
  - Subcutaneous maintenance fluid therapy (120 ml/kg/d)
  - Assisted syringe feeding (15 ml/kg PO q8h)
    - Oxbow Critical Care, Oxbow Pet Products, Murdock, N
    - Emeraid herbivore, Lafeber Vet, Cornell, IL
  - Analgesia – NSAID
    - *Meloxicam*: 1.0 mg/kg SC, PO q24h
    - *Carprofen*: 2–4 mg/kg PO, SC q24h
    - *Ketoprofen*: 1–3 mg/kg PO q12h
- Analgesia-Opioids
    - *Buprenorphine*: 0.01–0.05 mg/kg SC, IM, IV q6–12h
    - *Oxymorphone*: 0.05–0.2 mg/kg SC, IM q6–12h
    - *Hydromorphone*: 0.1 mg/kg SC, IM, IV q6–8h

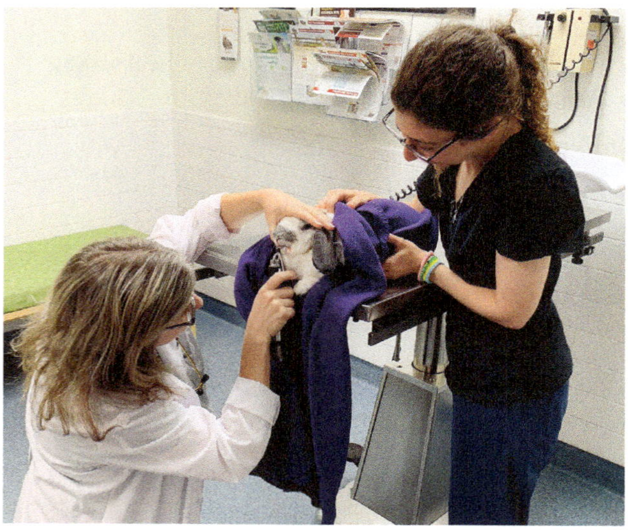

Figure 15.7 Oral examination on a non-sedated rabbit.

- Correct minor dental anomalies
  - Corrective burring of spurs and overgrown teeth
  - Diamond disc or high-speed water-cooled dental burrs
  - Avoid handheld clippers as they can induce longitudinal fractures, predisposing to periapical infection
- Dental infections
  - Antibiotics, ideally based on C/S; resolution generally requires surgery
  - *Enrofloxacin*: 5–20 mg/kg PO, SC, IM q12–24h; dilute parenteral route
  - *Trimethoprim sulfa*: 30 mg/kg PO q12h
- If anaerobic infection suspected
  - *Chloramphenicol*: 30–50 mg/kg PO q8–12h
  - *Metronidazole*: 20 mg/kg PO q12h
  - *Azithromycin*: 30 mg/kg PO q24h (often with metronidazole)
  - *Parenteral penicillin G*: 40000–60000 IU/kg SC, IM q24–48h

Continued Care:

- Referral to exotic mammal veterinarian for more extensive dental corrections, extraction of maloccluded or infected teeth, and abscess capsule removal
- Encourage a high-fiber mildly abrasive diet

Diarrhea/Dysbiosis

Diagnosis

Clinical Signs:

- Acute onset diarrhea can sometimes be without systemic illness
- More commonly evidence of infection, pain, and dietary imbalance
  - Fever
  - Hypothermia, hypotension with severe enteritis/enterotoxic shock
  - Depression, lethargy, weight loss, dehydration
  - Hunched posture, immobility, bruxism indicative of pain
  - Poor coat, fecal perineal soiling
  - Abdominal distension, gas, borborygmus
  - Fecal contents, fluid, or gas palpable in cecum
- Intermittent diarrheal illness with more mild clinical symptoms is common and evidence of intestinal dysbiosis, and can precipitate a more severe diarrheal illness

Differentials:

- Normal cecotropes
  - Nutrient and bacteria-rich soft feces formed in cecum and eliminated at night/early morning and promptly ingested
  - Chronic disease, pain, neuromuscular, and skeletal disorders may prohibit ingestion and mimic loose stool
- Improper diet
  - Most common cause of dysbiosis/intermittent diarrhea

- High simple carbohydrate diets with low coarse, indigestible fiber
  - Treats, commercial pellets, excess fruits, bread grains
  - Low in long-stemmed hay grasses
- Cause gastrointestinal hypomotility, altered acidic cecal fermentation, and selection for overgrowth of opportunistic/pathogenic bacterial species (dysbiosis)

- Dysbiosis/bacterial enteritis/enterotoxemia
  - Overgrowth of opportunistic flora or introduced pathogenic strains
  - *E. coli*, *Clostridium spiroforme*, *Clostridium piliforme* (Tyzzer's disease), *Salmonella* sp., *Pseudomonas* sp., *Campylobacter* sp.
  - Weanlings especially susceptible to *C. spiroforme* enterotoxemia
- Drug and toxins
  - Antibiotic-associated flora changes progress from dysbiosis to enterotoxemia within days of administration
  - Highest risk with agents that selectively target beneficial gram-positive bacteria (penicillins, amoxicillin-clavulanic acid, cephalosporins, ampicillin, clindamycin, and lincomycin), lowest with chloramphenicol, trimethoprim/sulfa, and fluoroquinolones
  - Ingestion of topical antibiotics (triple antibiotic ointment)
  - Some plant toxins, lead can also cause enteritis
- Other infections
  - Coronavirus ± rotavirus in neonates
  - Coccidia (*Eimeria* sp., hepatic or intestinal) in young rabbits
- Obstructions
  - Neoplasia – adenocarcinoma, leiomyosarcoma, leiomyoma
  - Foreign body – cloth, carpet, fur mat
- Chronic systemic disease and stress (via hypomotility)
  - Lack of exercise, obesity, neuromuscular, and skeletal disorders
- Metabolic disorders, hepatic, and renal disease
- Autoimmune/inflammatory bowel diseases are not described in rabbits

STAT Diagnostics:

- CBC and comprehensive blood panel
- Two view full-body survey radiographs
  - Assess gastric, cecal, and colonic contents
  - Rule-out severe gas/fluid accumulation suggestive of obstruction (surgical emergency)
- Fecal examination
  - Direct/float, Gram stain

Complete Diagnostics:

- Abdominal ultrasound for possible foreign bodies, extraluminal mass, hepatic disease
- Fecal examination
  - Cytology – Red blood cells and leukocytes suggestive of infection/invasive bacterial strains
  - Culture – Abundant growth of *E. coli* or *Clostridium* sp. significant
  - Occult blood testing for melena

Treatment

Stabilization:

- Hospitalize all juvenile rabbits, lethargic, and/or dehydrated adults with mild diarrhea, and all animals with severe diarrhea
- Maintenance fluid therapy (120 ml/kg/d), replacing losses over 24 hour period
- Assisted formula syringe feeding 15 ml/kg PO q8h
- Antibiotic therapy, ideally adjusted based on C/S
  - Broad-spectrum antibiotics for most infections
    - *Trimethoprim sulfa*: 30 mg/kg PO q12h
    - *Enrofloxacin*: 5–20 mg/kg PO, SC, IM q12–24h; dilute for parenteral route
  - *Metronidazole*: 20 mg/kg PO, IV q12h for two to three weeks (*Clostridium* sp.)
  - *Sulfadimethoxine*: 50 mg/kg PO first dose, then 25 mg/kg q24h for 10–20 days, or trimethoprim sulfa 30 mg/kg PO q12h for 10 days (*Coccidia*)
- Analgesia
  - *Buprenorphine*: 0.01–0.05 mg/kg SC, IM q6–12h
  - *Meloxicam*: 1.0 mg/kg PO q24h
  - *Carprofen*: 2.2 mg/kg PO q12–24h
- Other treatments
  - *Cholestyramine*: 2 g/20 ml water, daily gavage ×21 days has shown improved survival with acute *Clostridium* sp. enterotoxemia

Continued Care:

- Dietary modifications with enriched high insoluble fiber grains, reduction of simple carbohydrates
  - Dysbiosis, mild intermittent diarrhea should improve with dietary modifications
- Monitor appetite/intake, fecal volume and character, body weight
- Follow-up evaluation needed if diarrhea does not resolve with chosen therapy

Gastrointestinal Obstruction

Diagnosis

Clinical Signs:

- Anorexia may be acute onset
- Often history of lethargy, weakness
- Progressively reduced appetite, weight loss

- Ptyalism and repeated swallowing (esophageal obstruction)
- Reduced fecal output/small fecal pellets
- Ingestion of non-food items (cloth, carpet, fibrous objects, cat litter)
- Progressive abdominal distension
- Severe pain, hypovolemic shock, cardiovascular failure

Differentials:

- Anorexia and gastrointestinal stasis without obstruction
- Gastric bloat
  - Often combined hypomotility, stomach full of ingesta (hair and foreign material) that becomes a progressively larger, inspissated obstructing mass, and mechanical or functional pyloric obstruction (rabbits are unable to vomit)
  - Palpation reveals an enlarged doughy gas and/or fluid-filled and/or solid ingesta-filled stomach
  - Distension can occur without the mass of ingesta
  - Worsening distension causes mucosal ischemia/necrosis with systemic consequences (severe pain, shock)
- Intestinal obstruction/cecal impaction
  - With hypomotility and inspissated luminal contents ± foreign material, obstruction common in the duodenum where bowel sharply turns near the ileocecal junction
  - Chronic ingestion of scoopable cat litter ingestion can form an impacting/obstructing cecal mass
- Gastritis/gastroenteritis with *Clostridium* sp.
  - Often presents with collapse, shock
  - Palpable gas throughout the gastrointestinal tract
  - Most often the history of antibiotic use or stasis
- Heavy metal toxicity (functional ileus)
- Intussusception
- Extraluminal masses
  - Peritoneal adhesions, fibrosis, intra-abdominal masses, or abscesses
- Aerophagia
  - Respiratory disease and severe dyspnea are associated with air swallowing when nasal breathing is obstructed

STAT Diagnostics:

- CBC and comprehensive blood profile
  - Hemoconcentration/shock, electrolyte, and acid–base abnormalities
- Abdominal radiographs
  - Gastric bloat
    - Severe distension of stomach with fluid and/or gas with distal intestinal air but not significant distension
    - Expanded mass of inspissated gastric contents (trichobezoars are normally present) with surrounding fluid and gas
- Intestinal obstruction
    - Gas distension throughout the intestinal tract, including the cecum, indicating hypomotility/stasis
    - Cecal distension with ingesta and/or gas
    - Severe distension of stomach and proximal small bowel with minimal distal gas pattern with small intestinal obstruction
- Peritoneal free gas with perforation

Complete Diagnostics:

- Abdominal ultrasound
  - Gastric inspissated ingesta (foreign material vs. normal contents), duodenal or cecal obstructing mass, extraluminal obstruction, intussusception
- +/− CT if available/warranted

Treatment

Stabilization:

- Emergency management for cardiogenic shock and gastric bloat
- Fluid therapy for shock
  - LRS/crystalloid 60–90 mg/kg/h IV/IO over 20–60 minutes (or crystalloid bolus 30 ml/kg with hetastarch 5 ml/kg), followed by 120 ml/kg/d maintenance rate (±20 ml/kg/d hetastarch)
  - Maintenance plus deficit replacement for animals not in shock
- Gastric decompression
  - Orogastric intubation with light sedation
    - Midazolam 0.5–1 mg/kg IM, IV, diazepam 1–2 mg/kg IM, IV or dexmedetomidine 0.005 - 0.05 mg/kg IM
  - Securely restrain rabbit in a towel
  - An otoscope can be used as a mouth gag through which a well-lubricated, open-ended, 18-Fr flexible rubber tube is passed into the stomach . Cut additional holes at the end to allow larger volumes of fluid/gas to pass
  - Trocarization and indwelling catheters risk leakage of gastric contents into the peritoneum
- *Simethicone*: 65–130 mg q1h for two to three treatments may help alleviate painful intestinal gas
- Acute analgesia
  - *Lidocaine*: 2 mg/kg IV loading dose over 5 minutes followed by 100 ug/kg/min
  - *Buprenorphine*: 0.01–0.05 mg/kg SC, IM, IV q8–12h (pre/post decompression)
  - *Butorphanol*: 0.1–1.0 mg/kg SC, IM, IV q4–6h (sedation, short acting)
  - *Morphine*: 2–5 mg/kg SC, IM q2–4h

- +/– antibiotic treatment for shock/endotoxemia/potential surgery
  - *Trimethoprim sulfa*: 30 mg/kg PO, IM q12h
  - *Enrofloxacin*: 5–20 mg/kg PO, SC, IM, IV q12–24h; dilute for parenteral administration
  - *Metronidazole*: 20 mg/kg PO, IV q12h (*Clostridium* sp.)
  - *Cefazolin*: 20 mg/kg IV
- Thermal support as indicated
- Surgical correction
  - Most cases of gastric/small bowel obstruction require surgery to remove obstructing mass, often in duodenum where bowel sharply turns near the ileocecal junction
  - Guarded prognosis
- Emergency management for esophageal foreign bodies (as described in gastric decompression) as significant mucosal compromise can occur in short duration
- Cecal impaction in a stable rabbit can be treated urgently first with aggressive supportive care to restore motility and hydration of impacted contents

Continued Care:

- Monitor vitals and maintain blood pressure with adequate fluid support
  - Watch for recurrence of dilation and decompensation
- Monitor cardiorespiratory function for 24 hours post-surgery
- Monitor appetite (NPO until unobstructed, ideally under 12 hours) and fecal output
- Prokinetic agent once obstruction alleviated
  - *Cisapride*: 0.5 mg/kg PO q8–12h
  - *Metoclopramide*: 0.5 mg/kg PO q8–12h
- Transition to NSAIDs for pain management if renal status stable
  - *Meloxicam*: 1.0 mg/kg PO, SC, IM q24h
  - *Carprofen*: 1–4 mg/kg SC q12h
- Reduce gastric ulceration with H2-receptor antagonists
  - *Cimetidine*: 5–10 mg/kg PO, SC, IM, IV q6–12h
  - *Ranitidine*: 2 mg/kg IV q24h or 2–5 mg/kg PO q12h
- Dietary and environmental modifications to prevent recurrence
- Follow-up at several months to screen for possible post-operative adhesion/strictures

Gastrointestinal Stasis/Ileus

Diagnosis

Clinical Signs:

- Anorexia, often progressive with stopping pellets/hay and continuing to eat treats with eventual inappetence
- Often bright and alert unless acute obstruction or enterotoxemia
- Reduction in size, amount, and frequency of fecal pellets with no production in complete stasis
- Can have a history of intermittent soft, sticky stools/diarrhea
- Abdominal distension

Differentials:

- Acute gastric or intestinal obstruction/foreign body
- Anorexia
  - Dental disease, pain, stress, systemic (neurologic, musculoskeletal, cardiac, renal, respiratory) disease, metabolic disease, neoplasia, toxin (plants, lead), infections (*E. cuniculi*)
  - Progression of anorexia from these causes leads to delayed transit, hypomotility, inspissation of luminal contents to further delay motility, and can develop secondary dysbiosis/enteritis
- Gastrointestinal dysbiosis
- Mass lesions (luminal or extraluminal)
  - Adhesions, stenosis, neoplasia, abscess, hepatomegaly
- Iatrogenic
  - Prolonged opioid analgesia for painful conditions

STAT Diagnostics:

- Complete physical examination, including oral exam
  - Nearly absent abdominal sounds on auscultation
  - *Normal stomach:* Ingesta normally should be palpable and the stomach should be easily deformable, soft, and pliable
  - *GI hypomotility:* Firm, often enlarged stomach that remains pitted when compressed
  - *Complete stasis/prolonged hypomotility:* Severely distended, hard, and non-deformable stomach
  - Cecum may be filled with gas, fluid, or firm impacted contents
- CBC and comprehensive blood profile
  - Hemoconcentration, electrolyte, and acid-base abnormalities with prolonged stasis/dehydration
- Survey radiographs
  - Gastric ingesta contents are normally seen radiographically
  - Moderate to severe gastric distension with ingesta is consistent with the diagnosis of hypomotility
    - Halo of gas can be present around gastric ingesta in stasis
  - Moderate gas distension throughout intestinal tract with small or absent fecal balls is also seen
  - Exclude findings of acute obstruction/bloat

Complete Diagnostics:

- Abdominal ultrasound, if indicated

- Gastric inspissated ingesta (foreign material vs. normal contents), duodenal or cecal obstructing mass, extraluminal obstruction, intussusception

Treatment
Stabilization:

- Exclude emergent diagnoses (obstruction, enterotoxemia) and treat stasis on an urgent basis with initial hospital observation and support
- Fluid therapy key to rehydration and motility
  - Maintenance fluid therapy, LRS 120 ml/kg/d SC/IV
- Maintain oral intake to prevent worsening stasis and development of dysbiosis
  - Supplemental syringe feeds
  - Fresh, moistened greens
- Maintain physical activity (10–15 minutes hopping q6–8h) to promote motility
- Analgesia
  - *Lidocaine*: 2 mg/kg IV loading dose over 5 minutes followed by 100 ug/kg/min
  - *Meloxicam*: 1.0 mg/kg SC, PO q24h if renal status stable
  - *Buprenorphine*: 0.01–0.05 mg/kg SC, IM, IV q8–12h
- *Simethicone*: 65–130 mg q1h for two to three times to alleviate gas distension
- Prokinetic agent (after excluding the possibility of obstruction)
  - *Cisapride*: 0.5 mg/kg PO q8–12h
  - *Metoclopramide*: 0.5 mg/kg PO, SC q6–8h
- H2-receptor antagonists to ameliorate gastric ulceration
  - *Cimetidine*: 5–10 mg/kg PO, SC, IM, IV q6–12h
  - *Ranitidine*: 2 mg/kg IV q24h or 2–5 mg/kg PO q12h
- Antibiotics if presumed dysbiosis
  - *Trimethoprim sulfa*: 30 mg/kg PO q12h
  - *Enrofloxacin*: 5–20 mg/kg PO, SC, IM q12–24h; dilute for parenteral administration.

Continued Care:

- Dietary and exercise modifications to prevent a recurrence
- Address underlying causes of nausea/anorexia

Hepatic Disease

Diagnosis
Clinical Signs:

- Anorexia, lethargy, depression, weight loss
- Neurologic signs (advanced disease) – seizures, collapse
- Abdominal distension (hepatomegaly, ascites) causing dyspnea
- Jaundice is rare (heme breakdown to biliverdin, not bilirubin)
- Bleeding from coagulopathies
- Diarrhea

Differentials:

- Hepatic lipidosis
  - Anorexia, obesity, pregnancy
- Hepatic infections in young rabbits
  - Hepatic coccidiosis (*Eimeria stiedae*)
  - Tyzzer's disease (*C. piliforme*)
- Bacterial hepatitis
- Parasitic hepatic cysts
- Liver lobe torsion
- Anorexia from other causes
- GI stasis and obstruction
- Diarrhea
- Congestive heart failure
- Neurologic disease
- *E. cuniculi* infection
- Intoxication (lead)
- Pre-hepatic jaundice
  - Hemolytic anemia, bacteremia, septicemia, DIC
  - Excess brackens (kale)

STAT Diagnostics:

- CBC and comprehensive blood profile
  - Elevations in ALT, ALP, AST, GGT, and LDH
  - Elevated bilirubin, bile acids, decreased protein
  - Increased clotting times
  - PCV may be decreased with liver lobe torsion
- Survey radiographs
  - Hepatomegaly and/or abdominal effusion

Complete Diagnostics:

- Abdominal ultrasound or laparoscopy
  - Ultrasound-guided fine-needle aspiration or biopsy, if indicated
- Abdominocentesis of effusions
  - Fluid analysis (specific gravity, protein, cytology, culture)
- Fecal analysis
  - Hepatic coccidiosis, bacterial, or viral enteritis

Treatment
Stabilization:

- Supportive care
  - Maintenance fluids, assisted syringe feeding, vitamins (K)
- Analgesia
  - +/− *meloxicam*: 1.0 mg/kg PO, SC q24h if renal status stable
- Infections:
  - Hepatic coccidiosis
    - *Trimethoprim/sulfa*: 30 mg/kg PO q12h
    - *Sulfadimethoxine*: 50 mg/kg × 1, then 25 mg/kg PO q24h × 2, then repeat after five days

  - Prevent access to fresh feces
- *Taenia* sp. hepatic cysts
  - Cyst drainage
  - *Praziquantel*: 5–10 mg/kg SC, repeat in 10 days
- *Echinococcus granulosus* cyst
  - Drain cyst
  - *Albendazole*: 1.7 mg/ml injected into each cyst
- Liver fluke (*Fasciola* sp.)
  - *Triclabendazole*: 45 mg/kg/d × 2
- Bacterial hepatitis
  - *Trimethoprim sulfa*: 30 mg/kg PO q12h
  - *Enrofloxacin*: 5–20 mg/kg PO, SC, IM q12–24h; dilute for parenteral administration
  - *Metronidazole*: 20 mg/kg PO q12h for two to three weeks (*Clostridium* sp.)
  - Report zoonotic species (salmonellosis, yersiniosis, tularemia)
- Abscessation
  - Surgical removal and antibiotic treatment

- Lead toxicity
  - *CaEDTA*: 30 mg/kg SC q12h for five to seven days
- Metabolic disorders
  - Hepatic lipidosis: intravenous crystalloids with 5% dextrose
  - Pregnancy toxemia: cesarean section
- Neoplasia
  - Surgical excision is not usually performed
  - Chemotherapy for lymphoma
- Trauma (liver lobe torsion)
  - Surgical resection of torsed liver lobe. If owner declines surgery, can consider attempting general supportive care if rabbit otherwise stable

Continued Care:

- Monitor hepatic enzymes, bilirubin, clotting function
- Milk thistle (*Silybum marianum*) has been anecdotally used for hepatic regenerative properties.

Urogenital Disease

Renal Disease

Diagnosis

Clinical Signs:

- Polydipsia and polyuria with early losses of nephron reserve
- Decreased appetite, anorexia, weight loss, lethargy with development of more advanced renal insufficiency (loss of reserve capacity), and failure
- Perineal soiling, urine scalding
- Pollakiuria or hematuria with infections
- Pain, bruxism, hunched posture
- Neurologic vestibular findings (*E. cuniculi*)

Differentials:

- Infection
  - *E. cuniculi*
    - Punctate granulomatous lesions, interstitial fibrosis
    - Does not always cause renal insufficiency
  - Bacterial pyelitis, pyelonephritis, abscess
    - Ascending urinary tract infection, hematogenous
    - *E. coli* most common
- Degenerative renal disease
  - Renal calcinosis
  - Fibrosis and fatty degeneration
- Obstructive nephropathy
  - Urolithiasis, neoplasia
- Functional renal disease
  - Psychogenic PU/PD, pollakiuria
- Toxins
  - Vitamin D toxicity
    - Mineral deposition in kidneys and aorta
  - Nephrotoxicosis
    - Aminoglycosides, NASIDs, dietary mycotoxins
- Neoplasia
  - Lymphosarcoma, embryonal tumors

STAT Diagnostics:

- CBC and comprehensive blood panel
  - Renal azotemia with elevated urea and creatinine
    - Prerenal common from stress, dehydration, toxin
    - Postrenal from obstructive disease (calculi)
  - Elevated phosphorus (failure to excrete) with renal failure
  - Hemoconcentration from dehydration
  - Anemia of chronic disease
- Urinalysis
  - Analysis and culture
  - High specific gravity with prerenal causes (dehydration)
  - Elevated protein with infection or tubular damage (differ by cell composition in sediment analysis)
  - Hematuria can also be of uterine origin in females
  - Elevated pH >8 with urease-producing bacterial infections (*E. coli*)
- Abdominal radiographs
  - Kidney size, shape, calcifications, calculi
  - Bladder size, calculi

Complete Diagnostics:

- Renal ultrasound
  - Renal parenchymal assessment, definitive urolith analysis
- Contrast cystography and urethrography or intravenous pyelogram for better assessment of calculi, masses, or other obstructing lesions

- Indirect blood pressure measurement (hypertension)

Treatment

Stabilization:

- Fluid diuresis to correct azotemia and other electrolyte imbalances
  - Maintenance isotonic crystalloids at 120 ml/kg/d
  - Potassium supplementation as needed
- Discontinue any nephrotoxic drugs
- Antibiotic therapy for bacterial pyelonephritis
  - *Trimethoprim sulfa*: 30 mg/kg PO q12h
  - *Enrofloxacin*: 5–20 mg/kg PO, SC q12h; dilute for the parenteral route
- Treat associated causes of azotemia, if identified
- Assess for anorexia-induced gastrointestinal stasis

Continued Care:

- Subcutaneous fluid therapy at home to maintain diuresis
- Renal dietary changes
  - Romaine, Boston, bibb lettuce, mature (second-cut) grass hays
  - Vitamin (B, C) and omega-3 supplementation
  - Avoid high phosphorous, calcium, and protein foods
- Treat hyperphosphatemia (aluminum hydroxide)
- Antihypertensive agents, used with caution as can exacerbate renal disease
  - ACE inhibitor, *enalapril*: 0.25–0.5 mg/kg PO q24–48h

Urine Scald

Diagnosis

Clinical Signs:

- Urinary soiling, scalding, and alopecia of the perineal skin, inner thighs, rump, and tail
- Often evidence of urinary incontinence and/or obstruction

Differentials:

- Urolithiasis
  - Retention, sludging, infection, and eventual incontinence
- Mobility problems
  - Neurologic or musculoskeletal disorders
  - Ulcerative pododermatitis
  - Obesity
  - Cramped cages
- Genitourinary anatomical problems
  - Maldevelopment
  - Trauma to preputial area
  - Scarring from prior infection
- Urinary incontinence
  - Neurologic or musculoskeletal disease
  - *E. cuniculi* infection
- Increased urination
  - Renal insufficiency
  - Psychogenic polydipsia/polyuria
- Perineal dermatitis
  - Ineffective grooming, fur matted with fecal matter, neurologic disease, *Treponema paraluiscuniculi* (rabbit syphilis) infection

STAT Diagnostics:

- CBC and comprehensive blood panel
- Urinalysis
- Finings as discussed in Urolithiasis/Obstruction

Complete Diagnostics:

See Section "Urolithiasis/Obstruction"

Treatment

Stabilization:

- Address underlying condition causing inappropriate urination
- Surgical dermoplasty for deep perineal folds and corrective surgery on scarred prepuces to correct anatomical barriers to normal urination
- Carefully shave to remove all hair and clean affected areas
  - Light sedation recommended
    - Midazolam 0.5–2 mg/kg IM, diazepam 1–2 mg/kg IM, IV
  - Bathe with dilute chlorhexidine-based shampoo and thoroughly dry
  - Avoid topical antibiotics (ingestion-associated dysbiosis)
  - Topical fusidic acid, silver sulfadizine, or mupirocin ointments
  - Analgesia
    - *Meloxicam*: 1.0 mg/kg PO, SC q24h if no azotemia
    - *Carprofen*: 2–4 mg/kg PO, SC q24h if no azotemia
    - *Buprenorphine*: 0.03 mg/kg SC, IM q8h for severe pain
  - Antibiotic therapy if evidence of cystitis, urethritis (see Renal Disease)
  - Urolithiasis management

Continued Care:

- Dietary modifications (Urolithiasis)
- Urinary sphincter incompetence
  - *Diethylstilbesterol*: 0.5 mg PO 1–2×/wk
- Routine wound care of soiled areas, promptly addressing any new soiling

Urolithiasis/Obstruction

Diagnosis

Clinical Signs:

- Depression, hunched posture, bruxism
- Inappropriate urination, pollakiuria
- Stranguria, urinary sludge, hematuria
- Perineal soiling and scalding

Differentials:

- Hypercalciuria
  - Normally excessive dietary intake (alfalfa hay)
- Urinary retention
  - Obese, inactive older rabbits
  - Neurologic, musculoskeletal disorders
    - Lower motor neuron (sacral) disease with flaccid bladder
    - Upper motor neuron (suprasacral) disease with turgid bladder
  - Retention leads to the development of sabulous calcium carbonate sediment (sludge), which can lead to progression from soiling to infection to incontinence and urine scalding
- Hematuria
  - Uterine neoplasia
  - Cystitis/urethritis
  - Coagulopathy

STAT Diagnostics:

- Physical examination
  - The bladder may be distended, painful, with palpable cystoliths
  - Manual expression with thick, paste-like, brown-red urine
  - Kidneys may be enlarged or asymmetric
  - Urine soiling/scalding may be visible
- CBC and comprehensive blood panel
  - Leukocytosis with infection
  - Azotemia (elevated BUN, creatinine)
    - Prerenal (high specific gravity) with chronic disease
    - Renal (low/normal specific gravity) with renal disease
    - Postrenal/hyperkalemia with urinary obstruction
- Urinalysis
  - Hematuria ± proteinuria
  - The sediment of carbonate and phosphate crystals are normal
  - Pyuria with infection
- Radiographs
  - Ensure capture of the entire caudal half to visualize urethra, stretching hind limbs to avoid obscuring calculi
  - Uroliths are often multiple and in different locations
  - Small amount of radiodense urinary sediment is common, larger amounts suggest sludge accumulation
  - Assess spine for neuromuscular disease (spondylosis, subluxation)

Complete Diagnostics:

- Ultrasound
  - Can help visualize bladder and proximal urethra, particularly with excess sludge that can obscure calculi on radiographs
  - Assessment for ureterolithiasis and secondary hydronephrosis
- Contrast-based imaging
  - Highlight bladder wall abnormalities, reflux, obstruction

Treatment

Stabilization:

- Treatment of bladder sludge sediment
  - Sedation prior to intervention, analgesia following
    - *Midazolam*: 0.5–2 mg/kg IM, *diazepam*: 1–2 mg/kg IM, IV
    - *Buprenorphine*: 0.03 mg/kg SC, IM q8h following
  - Manual expression over several days may be successful, and/or catheterize (3–3.5 Fr) and flush with sterile 0.9% saline
  - Induce diuresis
    - Maintenance IV/SC fluids, increase oral intake (sweeten)
    - Calcium-sparing diuretic (with potassium supplement)
    - *Hydrochlorothiazide*: 0.5–2 mg/kg PO q12h
    - *Bendrofluazine*: 600 mcg/kg PO q24h
  - Inhibitor of crystal formation
    - Potassium citrate
  - Exercise as tolerated
- Surgical treatment for urolithiasis
  - Surgical removal required for cystoliths and urethroliths
  - Cystotomy with removal and flushing, send for analysis
- Antibiotic therapy for evidence of cystitis, pyelonephritis
  - See Renal Disease

Continued Care:

- Postoperative radiographs to ensure calculi removed
- Repeat radiographs and urinalysis in one to three months to screen for recurrence
- Dietary modification
  - Balanced diet without excessive calcium and phosphorous

- Too little phosphorous increases urinary calcium excretion and exacerbates hypercalciuria
  - Exclude vitamin/mineral supplements and blocks
  - Fresh low-calcium timothy hay, avoid pellets
  - *Avoid high-calcium vegetables:* kale, broccoli, turnip
  - Substitute with carrots, cabbage, celery, lettuce
- Weight loss often beneficial

- Urinary sphincter incompetence, if present
  - *Diethylstilbesterol*: 0.5 mg PO 1–2×/wk
- Routine and prompt wound care of any perineal soiling/urine scalding (see Section "Urine Scald")

Mammary Disorders

Diagnosis

Clinical Signs:

- Mastitis
  - Swollen, erythematous, ulcerated, and painful gland(s)
  - Bloody and/or purulent discharge
  - Anorexia, lethargy/depression, polydipsia
  - Death of kits can be common
- Cystic mastitis
  - Swollen glands with flocculent non-tender cysts
  - Dark/blue discoloration, clear/amber/milk colored discharge
  - Not lethargic/depressed, may show signs of pseudopregnancy
  - Hematuria (uterine pathology)
- Mammary gland dysplasia
  - One or multiple diffusely swollen gray to black teats
- Mammary gland neoplasia
  - Focal mass involving gland
  - Hematuria from uterine pathology can be seen

Differentials:

- Mastitis
  - Lactating or pseudopregnant does
  - Heavy lactation (milk retention with pseudopregnancy), nipple injury, unsanitary conditions predispose to infection.
  - *S. aureus*, *Streptococcus* sp., *Pasteurella* sp. most common organisms
- Cystic mastitis
  - Sterile mammary cysts derived from ductal epithelium
  - Can progress to benign and malignant neoplasm
  - Can have signs of pseudopregnancy
  - Associated with endometrial hyperplasia, uterine adenocarcinoma
- Mammary gland dysplasia
  - Diffuse hyperplasia, often in older, primiparous does
  - Secondary to hormonal influence (prolactin-producing pituitary adenomas in some cases)
- Neoplasia
  - Benign adenomas and papillomas, adenocarcinoma
  - Tumors may have been preceded by cystic disease
  - Regional node and lung metastases are seen

STAT Diagnostics:

- CBC and comprehensive blood panel
  - Generally normal, inflammatory changes with infection
- Mild/discharge analysis and culture/sensitivity
- Fine needle aspiration biopsy of solid or cystic masses and swollen glands for cytopathology and culture/sensitivity (for cystic disease)

Complete Diagnostics:

- Abdominal radiographs and/or ultrasound to evaluate for uterine disease
- Thoracic imaging/ultrasound to exclude metastatic disease if neoplasia expected
- Serum prolactin levels and/or brain CT for dysplasia

Treatment

Stabilization:

- Bacterial mastitis
  - General supportive care
    - Maintenance fluid therapy (120 ml/kg/d)
    - Assisted syringe feeds
  - Analgesia
    - *Meloxicam*: 1.0 mg/kg PO, SC q24h
    - *Carprofen*: 2–4 mg/kg PO, SC q24h
    - *Buprenorphine*: 0.03 mg/kg SC, IM q8h
  - Antibiotic therapy
    - *Procaine penicillin*: 40 000–60 000 IU/kg SC, IM q24–48h
    - *Trimethoprim/sulfa*: 30 mg/kg PO q12h
    - *Enrofloxacin*: 10 mg/kg + *metronidazole*: 20 mg/kg PO q12h
  - Warm compresses
  - Remove kits to prevent bacterial enteritis or starvation
- Cystic mastitis
  - Ovariohysterectomy without removal of mammary lesions usually produces regression of cystic disease
- Neoplasia
  - Complete mastectomy and ovariohysterectomy

Continued Care:

- Abscess formation in mastitis requires drainage ± removal
- Removal of mammae if cystic disease not regressed by one-month post-ovariohysterectomy to prevent development into neoplasm

Pregnancy Toxemia

Diagnosis

Clinical Signs:

- Obese does near the end of pregnancy, or recent delivery or abortion
- Depressed, weak, anorectic with rapid progression
- Dyspnea with acetone breath and urine odor
- Confusion, seizures, coma

Differentials:

- Hepatic lipidosis
  - Obesity, metabolic disease
  - Anorexia/starvation can precipitate massive mobilization of fat stores, resulting in ketoacidosis
- Ketosis
  - Metabolic disease, obesity
- Heatstroke
- Pregnancy toxemia
  - Obesity with underlying hepatic lipidosis
  - Demands of late-stage pregnancy trigger the massive mobilization of fat stores with ketosis
  - Ensuing anorexia with the development of gastrointestinal stasis

STAT Diagnostics:

- CBC and comprehensive blood panel
  - Hyperkalemia, hypocalcemia, ketonemia
- Urinalysis
  - Acidic urine with proteinuria and ketonuria

Complete Diagnostics:

- Clinical suspicion and history are primary method of diagnosis
- Findings of abundant adipose stores and hepatic lipidosis often confirmed postmortem

Treatment

Stabilization:

Supportive care
  - Environmental/supplemental heat
  - Fluid therapy with 5% dextrose IV/IO
    - Calcium supplementation as needed
  - Assisted syringe feedings
  - Prokinetic and anti-ulcer therapy with GI stasis
  - Consider Cesarean section if stable as this can improve condition

Continued Care:

- Monitor neurologic status, ketonuria, input/outputs
- Prognosis is very poor, most do not survive
- Counsel owners regarding optimal diet and fitness levels prior to future pregnancy in other does

Treponematosis

Diagnosis

Clinical Signs:

- Lesions at the mucocutaneous junctions of face (nose, lips, eyelids) and genitalia (prepuce or vulva)
  - Initially edematous, erythematous, and progress to papules that erode to form characteristic crusted lesions
  - Can have genital only lesions, occasionally face only (Figure 15.8)
- Localized lymphadenopathy
- Skin signs appear three to six weeks after infection (sexual, direct contact, birthing)

Differentials:

- *T. paraluiscuniculi*
  - Ubiquitous distribution can only infect rabbits
  - Generally, multiple animals infected in the colony
- Isolated genital lesions in individual rabbit
  - Trauma
  - Pyoderma in obese females
  - Myxomatosis

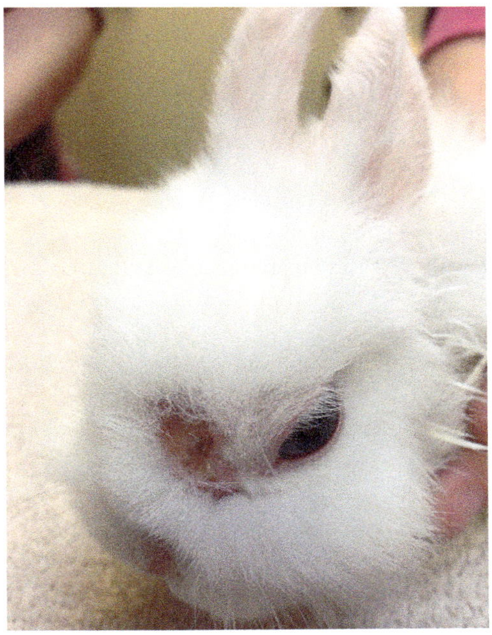

Figure 15.8 Circular lesions noted on the face of a young rabbit with treponema. Although a dermatophyte infection was initially suspected, sampling including serology confirmed treponema. The source of infection was determined to be the parents and multiple offspring were infected.

STAT Diagnostics:

- Physical examination
- Sampling/biopsy of lesion to identify organism

Complete Diagnostics:

- Histopathologic confirmation of spirochete (Warthin–Starry stain)
- Darkfield microscopy of fresh mount of lesional scrapings can also identify spiral bacterium with corkscrew motility
- Serologic testing can also be performed, but false-negatives can occur with single test

Treatment

Stabilization:

- *Parenteral benzathine penicillin G*: (42 000–84 000 IU/kg) SC, IM q7d × 3
- Treat entire colony for eradication

Continued Care:

- Lesions should resolve one to two weeks after initiation of therapy
- Monitor for signs of antibiotic-associated dysbiosis/diarrhea

Uterine/Vaginal Cranial Vena Cava Occlusion with Bilateral Pathology

Diagnosis

Clinical Signs:

- Hematuria
- Bloody vulvar discharge
- Infertility
- Swollen mammary glands
- Abdominal swelling with palpable masses cranial to the bladder
- Gastrointestinal stasis
- Dyspnea (mass effect from abdominal mass, metastatic disease)
- Acute anorexia, collapse, shock with uterine torsion, vaginal prolapse

Differentials:

- Endometrial venous aneurysm
  - Congenital vascular anomaly prone to hemorrhage
- Pyometra/endometritis
  - Infections predominately occur during periods of progesterone-induced endometrial growth and secretions, providing a favorable environment for bacterial colonization, including *Pasteurella* sp.
- Uterine torsion
- Benign/premalignant endometrial proliferations
  - Endometrial hyperplasia
  - Uterine polyps
- Uterine neoplasia
  - Adenocarcinoma, often preceded by hyperplasia and/or polyps
- Hydrometra
  - Fluid accumulation in uterus due to outflow obstruction (hyperplasia or neoplasia), most common in pseudopregnant does (elevated progesterone)
  - Fluid can be mucinous (mucometra)
- Prolapsed vagina
  - Swollen, bloody protruding mass from vulva
  - Believed complication of sexual activity
- Non-gynecologic causes of bloody vulvar discharge
  - Cystitis, nephrolithiasis/urolithiasis, coagulopathy, porphyrinuria
- Abdominal swelling
  - Pregnancy, gastric bloat, intestinal obstruction, ascites/abdominal effusions, hepatomegaly, mass lesions (abscess/neoplasia)

STAT Diagnostics:

- CBC and comprehensive chemistry panel
- Urinalysis for cytology (shed uterine carcinoma) and to exclude urinary infections
- Vulvar swab for cytology
- Abdominal and thoracic radiographs
  - Uterine masses, metastatic disease
- Abdominal ultrasound

Complete Diagnostics:

- Bacterial cultures and sensitivities of sampled fluids/discharge
  - Serologic testing for *Pasteurella* if infection suspected
- Uterine biopsy with histopathology
  - Helpful to release obstruction with hydrometra

Treatment

Stabilization:

- Aggressive fluid, supportive care, and opioid analgesia for patients with symptoms of shock (vaginal prolapse, uterine torsion)
- Fluid and nutritional support for stable patients
- Broad-spectrum antibiotic coverage pending results

 - *Enrofloxacin*: 10 mg/kg PO q12h
 - *Metronidazole*: 20 mg/kg PO q12h
 - *Trimethoprim/sulfa*: 30 mg/kg PO q12h
- Emergent evaluation and ovariohysterectomy for uterine torsion
- Surgical reduction or partial resection under anesthesia for vaginal prolapse
- Ovariohysterectomy once patient is stable for benign (hyperplasia and polyps) and malignant (adenocarcinoma) proliferative lesions (provided not planning to breed again)

Continued Care:

- Chemotherapeutic protocols for uterine adenocarcinoma not established for rabbits
- Risk of continued metastatic spread of adenocarcinoma, guarded prognosis once metastatic

Neoplasia

Lymphoma

Diagnosis

Clinical Signs:

- Anorexia, weight loss, diarrhea
- Lethargy, weakness
- Cutaneous nodules
 - Ulcerated, crusty, erythematous, alopecia, non-tender
- Peripheral adenopathy
- Dyspnea, tachypnea, possible bilateral exophthalmos with precaval syndrome (large mediastinal lymphoma)

Differentials:

- Lymphoma (multicentric forms)
 - Lymphoblastic (large cell) type
 - Lymphocytic (small cell type)
 - B- and T-cell forms
 - Skin, peripheral nodes, abdominal viscera
 - Leukemic (blood) phase possible
- Lymphoma (localized forms)
 - Cutaneous
 - Thymic (T-cell)
 - Other visceral sites
- Thymoma
 - Differentiation requires biopsy
- Cutaneous diseases
 - Infection, allergic, parasitic

STAT Diagnostics:

- CBC and comprehensive chemistry panel
 - Normal or lymphocytosis in leukemic states
 - Elevated hepatic or renal values with involvement
 - Calcium can be high in rabbits and is generally not due to paraneoplastic process
- Imaging
 - Radiographs/CT scan for visualizing thymic disease
 - Ultrasound is best for detecting abdominal visceral involvement
- Biopsy diagnosis
 - Fine needle aspirate of enlarged nodes, mediastinal mass, or cutaneous nodules useful for diagnosis of large cell lymphoblastic lymphoma
 - Core biopsy histology for the diagnosis of a small cell lymphocytic lymphoma or thymic lymphoma vs. thymoma distinction
 - Bone marrow aspirate is performed if peripheral blood suggests leukemic involvement

Complete Diagnostics:

- Complete pathology diagnosis dependent on immunohistochemistry and/or flow cytometry (aspirate) to document cellular origins
- B-cell lymphomas most common, followed by T-cell rich B-cell lymphoma

Treatment

Stabilization:

Mediastinal form (often presents with clinical compromise)
 - Radiation therapy is efficacious and well-tolerated
 - Systemic chemotherapy as an adjuvant for thymic lymphoma, as is prednisone
 - Surgical excision following staging is performed, but with a high perioperative mortality

Continued Care:

- No definitive protocols for rabbit lymphoma, most care is palliative
- Oral *prednisolone* 1–2 mg/kg PO q12–24h has been used
- Multiple-drug regimens have not been studied in rabbits, but various drugs have been used in laboratory rabbits and extrapolated for pets
- Consultation with a veterinary oncologist for further treatment options and considerations after discussion with owners (efficacy, cost, side effects, expected outcomes) as overall survival is poor

Differentials:

- Bacterial cystitis
- Urolithiasis (with or without urethral obstruction)
- Nephrolithiasis
- Neoplasia
- Renal diseases

STAT Diagnostics:

- *Whole-body radiographs*
- *Urinalysis*
- *BUN/Creatinine, PCV/TS, Electrolytes*

Complete Diagnostics:

- *Abdominal US*
- *CBC/Biochemistry*
- *Urine culture/sensitivity*

Treatment

Stabilization:

- *Fluids*: SC, IV, or IO fluids based on severity (see Chapter 8)
- *Analgesia*: See Table 16.1. Multimodal analgesia is preferred
- *Diet*: Assisted feeding as deemed appropriate (see Chapter 8)
- *Antibiotics*: Based on culture/sensitivity if underlying infectious etiology
- *Urinary catheterization*: to relieve obstruction if present (Figure 16.4)

Continued Care:

- Surgery (urolithiasis, neoplasia)
- Endoscopy-guided removal [45, 77]
- Continued supportive care including fluid therapy and antibiotics as needed
- Analgesia
- Dietary modifications
- Vitamin C 50–100 mg/kg PO, IM, SC q24h in case of lacking supplementation

Dystocia

Diagnosis

History:

- Continuous straining for 20 minutes or unproductive contractions for more than 2 hours.
- Normal parturition generally lasts less than 30 minutes with a 5-minute interval between pups.

Clinical Signs:

- Abdominal distension
- Lethargy

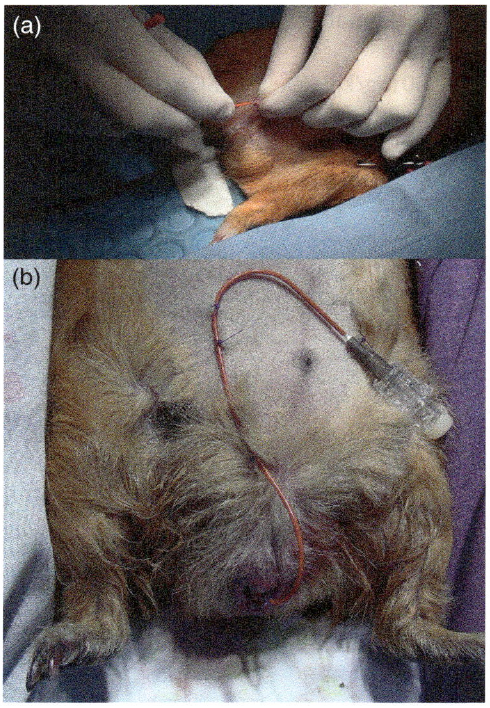

Figure 16.4 Insertion (a) and setup (b) of a urinary catheter in a guinea pig.

- Dyspnea
- Nonproductive contractions
- Hind limb paresis
- Paralysis

Differentials:

- Toxemia of pregnancy
- Ectopic pregnancy [46]
- Normal parturition
- Gastric dilatation and volvulus

STAT Diagnostics:

- *Abdominal radiographs* (Figure 16.5)
- *PCV/TS, Glu, Lactate, Blood gas including ionized calcium*

Complete Diagnostics:

- *Abdominal US*
- *CBC/Biochemistry*

Treatment [47]

Stabilization:

- *Fluids*: SC, IV, or IO fluids based on severity (see Chapter 8)

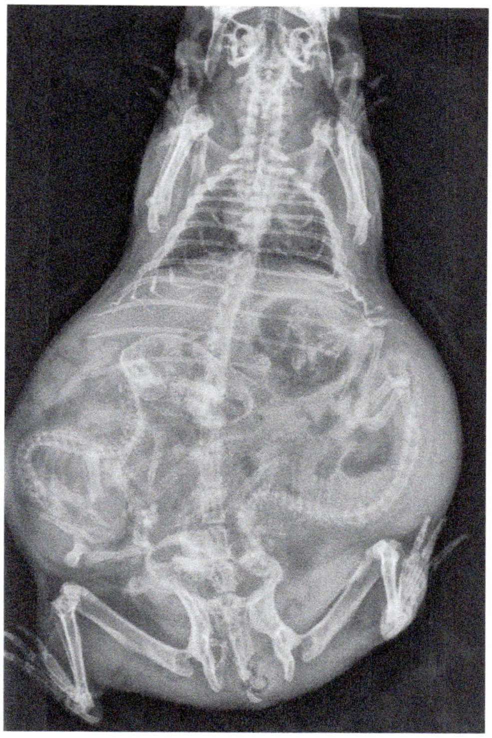

Figure 16.5 Radiographs of a female guinea pig with dystocia. One pup is engaged in the sacrum but blocked by the symphysis. Another pup is in a normal position. A third skull is visible with no associated skeleton, suggesting fetal resorption.

- *Analgesia*: See Table 16.1. Multimodal analgesia is preferred. See Chapter 7 for contraindications in pregnant and lactating females

Continued Care:

- Oxytocin (unless contraindicated)
- Cesarean-section
- Analgesia
- Assisted-feeding of the pups (Critical Care herbivore from birth has been more successful than using replacement milk in one of the authors' experience)

Toxemia of Pregnancy

Diagnosis

History:

- Pregnant females between two weeks prepartum and two weeks postpartum. Obesity has been reported anecdotally as a risk factor.

Clinical Signs:

- Abdominal distension
- Lethargy
- Dyspnea
- Ataxia
- Hind limb paresis or paralysis
- Muscle spasms
- Breath smell of ketones
- Hypertension (preeclampsia form only) [48]

Differentials:

- Dystocia
- Gastric dilation and volvulus

STAT Diagnostics:

- *Urinalysis*
- *PCV/TS, Glu, Lactate, Electrolytes, Blood gas*

Complete Diagnostics:

- *CBC/Biochemistry*
- *Abdominal US*

Treatment

Stabilization:

- *Dextrose*: 1–2 ml of 50% dextrose in 3–5 ml saline IV or IO, PO undiluted
- *Fluids*: SC, IV, or IO fluids based on severity (see Chapter 8)
- *Assisted feeding* (nasogastric, gastric, or esophagostomy tubes might be required) (see Chapter 8)
- *Emergency Cesarean-section* for ischemic forms
- Calcium gluconate 50–100 mg/kg IM (diluted 50:50), slow IV/IO, and magnesium sulfate have also been suggested

Continued Care:

- Continued supportive care
- Increase carbohydrate supplementation during the last two weeks prepartum and during the first two weeks of lactation to ensure a positive energy balance
- Dietary modifications
- Vitamin C 30 mg/kg PO, IM, SC q24h

Ovarian Cysts

Diagnosis

Clinical Signs:

- Abdominal distension
- Bilateral symmetrical flank alopecia (functional cysts only)
- Abdominal pain
- Hunched posture
- Partial/complete anorexia

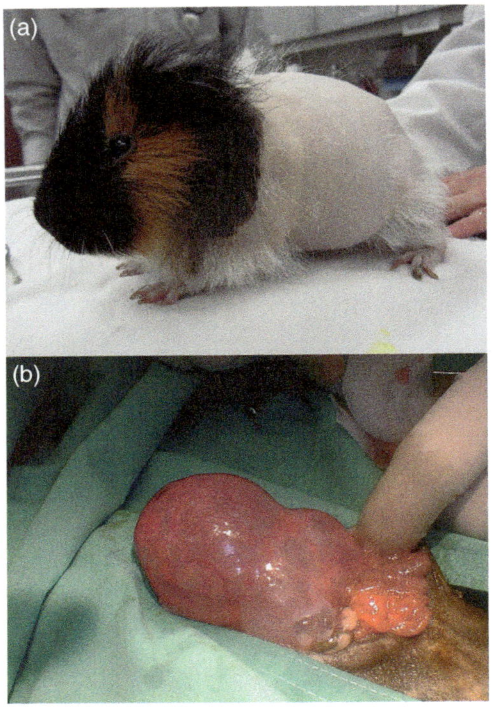

Figure 16.6 Bilaterally symmetric alopecia in a guinea pig with ovarian cysts (a). Surgical appearance of ovarian cysts during an ovariohysterectomy procedure (b).

- Lethargy
- Decline in fertility (Figure 16.6a)

Differentials:

- See Section "Abdominal Distension"
- Hyperadrenocorticism (alopecia)

STAT Diagnostics:

- *Abdominal radiographs*
- *Abdominal US*

Complete Diagnostics:

- *Preoperative CBC/Biochemistry*

Treatment

Stabilization:

- *Fluids*: SC, IV, or IO fluids based on severity (see Chapter 8)
- Percutaneous drainage of the cysts
- Hormone therapy with hCG or GnRH agonist has been cited by some authors. However, there is little evidence of their efficacy. Deslorelin implants have been shown to have no effect on the size of ovarian cysts [49].

Continued Care:

- Ovariohysterectomy (Figure 16.6b)

Endocrine Disease

Diabetes Mellitus

Diagnosis

History:

- Inquire about diet high in carbohydrates

Clinical Signs:

- Transient neurologic signs
- Obesity
- Recurring cystitis
- Polyuria/polydipsia

Differentials for Hyperglycemia:

- Diabetes mellitus (type I, type II, gestational diabetes)
- Stress
- Hypercortisolism
- *Iatrogenic*: treatment of insulinoma (diazoxide [50]), prednisolone

STAT Diagnostics:

- *Glu, Electrolytes, Blood osmolarity*
- *Urinalysis*

Complete Diagnostics:

- *CBC/chemistry*
- *Abdominal US*

Treatment

Stabilization:

- *Insulin therapy*: NPH insulin 1–2 IU SC q12h adapted based on glycemic curve and clinical response at home may be considered. Oral hypoglycemic treatments were not effective at doses used in a single case report [51].

Continued Care:

- *Dietary modifications*: hay should be the main food item
- Weight loss program
- Follow-up glycemia/urinalysis until insulin can be discontinued

Table 16.7 Investigation of hyperadrenocorticism in guinea pigs: ACTH stimulation and results obtained with various samples.

	Basal cortisol concentration	Cortisol concentration	Methodology	References
Plasma	50–80 ng/ml[a], diurnal variation, stress	After 4 h, 736 ng/ml[b]	Radioimmunoassay, n = 8	[53]
Saliva	11–25 ng/ml[a]	After 4 h, 157 ± 19 ng/ml[c]	Radioimmunoassay, n = 8	[53]
Feces	206–796 ng/g feces during diurnal phase	After 8 h, 259–2634 ng/g feces	Enzyme immunoassay, n = 12	[54]

[a] Values are provided as mean and standard range depending on available information.
[b] Values are provided as mean and standard mean depending on available information.
[c] Values are provided as mean and standard error of the mean.

Hyperadrenocorticism

Diagnosis

History:

- Bilateral hair loss without pruritus
- Muscle atrophy
- Weight gain with polyphagia
- Lethargy

Clinical Signs: Dorsolumbar bilateral apruriginous alopecia

Differentials:

- Ovarian cysts
- Dermatophytosis

STAT Diagnostics:

- *Glu* (high)
- *Urine-specific gravity*
- *Skin scrapings*

Complete Diagnostics:

- *ACTH stimulation test*: Measure saliva basal cortisol concentration (cortisol is the major corticosteroid in guinea pigs [52, 78]), administer ACTH (Synacthen depot, Novartis Pharma) 20 IU IM, saliva cortisol concentration after four hours; plasma (correlation with saliva: $R^2 = 0.88$) or feces may also be used for analysis [52] (see Table 16.7)
- *Abdominal US*: Note that guinea pig adrenals are physiologically larger compared to body weight than in domestic carnivores (length: 13–14 mm, width: 3–6 mm, $n = 2$) [55]
- *MRI* to evaluate hypophysis

Treatment

Stabilization:

- *Fluids*: SC, IV, or IO fluids based on severity (see Chapter 8)
- *Trilostane* 2–6 mg/kg PO q24h [55]

Continued Therapy:

- Adapt treatment dose based on clinical response and follow-up cortisol concentration measurements

Hyperparathyroidism

Diagnosis

History:

- Lameness without reported trauma. Satin breeds may be predisposed [56].

Clinical Signs:

- Lameness
- Muscle tremors
- Dental malocclusion

Differentials:

- Primary hyperparathyroidism (parathyroid neoplasm, breed predisposition)
- Paraneoplastic parathormone-related hormone (PTHrH) secretion
- Secondary nutritional hyperparathyroidism (phosphorous excess, vitamin D/UVB deficiency)
- Secondary renal hyperparathyroidism

STAT Diagnostics:

- *Radiographs*: Double cortical line, pathologic fractures [54]
- *Ionized calcium concentration*: Range in healthy guinea pigs: 1.29–1.74 mmol/l [57]; primary hyperparathyroidism may cause increased ionized calcium while advanced stage of secondary hyperparathyroidism may cause hypocalcemia.

Complete Diagnostics:

- *Biochemistry*, including Ca:P ratio (reference: 1.5–1 [58]); differentiate primary vs. secondary renal hyperparathyroidism

- *Cervical US/CT scan* to detect a parathyroid mass (not reported in guinea pigs): Ultrasound-guided stain injection before surgery may be useful to facilitate localization
- *Parathormone and PTHrH* concentrations measurement [56] to rule out paraneoplastic disease (lower reference intervals in Satin breeds)
- *Dual-energy X-ray absorptiometry* to confirm osteopenia [54]

Treatment

Stabilization:

- Calcium glubionate 100–150 mg/kg PO q24h (or calcium gluconate SC once in case of clinical hypocalcemia, then recheck ionized calcium)
- In case of secondary renal hyperparathyroidism, treat the renal disease (see Section "Renal Diseases")

Continued Therapy:

- Favor UVB exposure to increase vitamin D endogenous secretion [57]
- Vitamin D 1600 IU/kg food maximum (use with caution, especially with calcium supplementation) [58]
- In case of idiopathic primary hyperparathyroidism with persistent hypercalcemia, consider furosemide (1–2 mg/kg SC q12h), and bisphosphonates (risedronate 0.25 mg total PO q24h or alendronate 0.5–1 mg/kg/wk extrapolated from other species)

Hyperthyroidism

Diagnosis

History:

- Weight loss despite a good appetite
- Exercise intolerance
- Behavioral changes (hyperphagia, hyperactivity) [59]

Clinical Signs:

- Ventral cervical mass, sometimes with a palpable thyroid slip
- Polyuria/polydipsia, poor-quality haircoat [59]
- Abnormal cardiac auscultation with tachyarrhythmia

Differentials:

- Cervical lymphadenomegaly or neoplasia
- Enlarged parathyroid glands

STAT Diagnostics:

- *Radiographs*: To assess whether cardiomegaly +/− congestive heart failure are present. Note that osseous metaplasia of the thyroid gland is not a criterion for malignancy [60]

Complete Diagnostics:

- *Cervical US* with guided fine-needle aspirate (most thyroid tumors are benign) [60]
- *CT-scan or MRI* [58]
- *Serum thyroid panel* (see Table 16.8)
- *Thyroid stimulation test* with human recombinant TSH 100 μg/kg IM in case of equivocal results (reference in

Table 16.8 Reference intervals of total thyroxine (TT4), total triiodothyronine (TT3), free thyroxine (fT4), and free triiodothyronine (fT3) of guinea pigs.

Target population	Total T_4 (μg/dl)	Total T_3 (ng/dl)	Free T_4 (ng/dl)	Free T_3 (ng/dl)	Methodology
Pet	4.17 (3.01–5.33)[a]				Enzyme immunoassay [61]
Pet	0.70 (0.57–1.32)[a]				Radioimmunoassay [62]
Pet	2.1 (1.1–5.2)[a]				Chemiluminescence [53]
Laboratory	4.04 (2.26–5.82)[a]				Enzyme immunoassay [61]
Laboratory			1.17 ± 0.09[b]		Unknown [63]
Laboratory	2.5–3.2	39–44	1.26–2.03	0.221–0.260	Radioimmunoassay [64]
Unknown	4.54 ± 0.443[b]	31.7 ± 1.4[b]	0.67 ± 0.57[b]	0.224 ± 0.108[b]	Radioimmunoassay [65]
Unknown	Male 2.9 ± 0.6[b] Female 3.2 ± 0.7[b]	Males 39 ± 17[b] Females 44 ± 10[b]			Unknown [66]

Information on the different target populations (laboratory vs. pet guinea pigs) and methodology used to determine values are provided when information was available.
[a] Values are provided as mean values and reference interval.
[b] Values are provided as mean and standard error of the mean.
[c] Values are provided as reference interval. Source: Modified from Brandao et al. 2013 [58]. © 2013, Elsevier.

euthyroid cavi: increase of 2.6 times of total T_4 three to four hours post-stimulation) [62]
- *Scintigraphy* [58]
- *Cardiac ultrasound* to investigate hypertrophic cardiomyopathy
- *Biochemistry* to investigate concurrent nephropathy (systemic hypertension)

Treatment

Stabilization:

- Treat potential renal and cardiac complications
- *Diet*: Assisted feeding as deemed appropriate (see Chapter 8)

Continued Care

- Methimazole 1–3 mg/kg PO q8–24h [58, 67] or carbimazole 1–2 mg/kg PO q24h [58] with monitoring of the thyroid panel (individual dose adjustment)
- Radioactive iodine treatment administered SC or IV [58]
- Thyroidectomy
- Treatment of hypertrophic cardiomyopathy (see Section "Cardiac Diseases")

Neoplastic Disease

Lymphoma

Diagnosis

History:

- One or multiple animals may be affected in the same household as cavian retrovirus has been associated with this neoplasm [12]. This is considered the most common malignancy of guinea pigs [58].

Clinical Signs:

- Crusts, alopecia, and ulcerations with pruriginous epitheliotropic lymphoma (Figure 16.7)
- Multifocal lymphadenopathy, splenomegaly, hepatomegaly
- Non-specific signs (lethargy, weight loss, anorexia)

Differentials:

- *Other causes of pruritic alopecia*: Parasitic, fungal, bacterial dermatitis (see Section "Dermatologic Disease")
- Other causes of lymphadenopathy (see Section "Cervical Lymphadenitis")
- Other cutaneous neoplasms, including ulcerated mammary tumors, with higher prevalence of mammary tumors in male guinea pigs compared to other species [67, 68]

STAT Diagnostics:

- *Fine-needle aspirate* for cytology
- *CBC*: Leukemia may be present concomitantly or results may be within normal limits in early stages of the disease
- *Biochemistry*
- *Thoracic radiographs and abdominal US*: To assess extension: lungs, hemolymphatic organs, digestive tract, and other organs may be affected; epitheliotropic lymphoma may also metastasize systemically [69]

Complete Diagnostics:

- Cutaneous/mass biopsy for histopathology and immunohistochemistry (T-cell lymphomas are most common [69])
- Bone marrow aspirate

(a) (b)

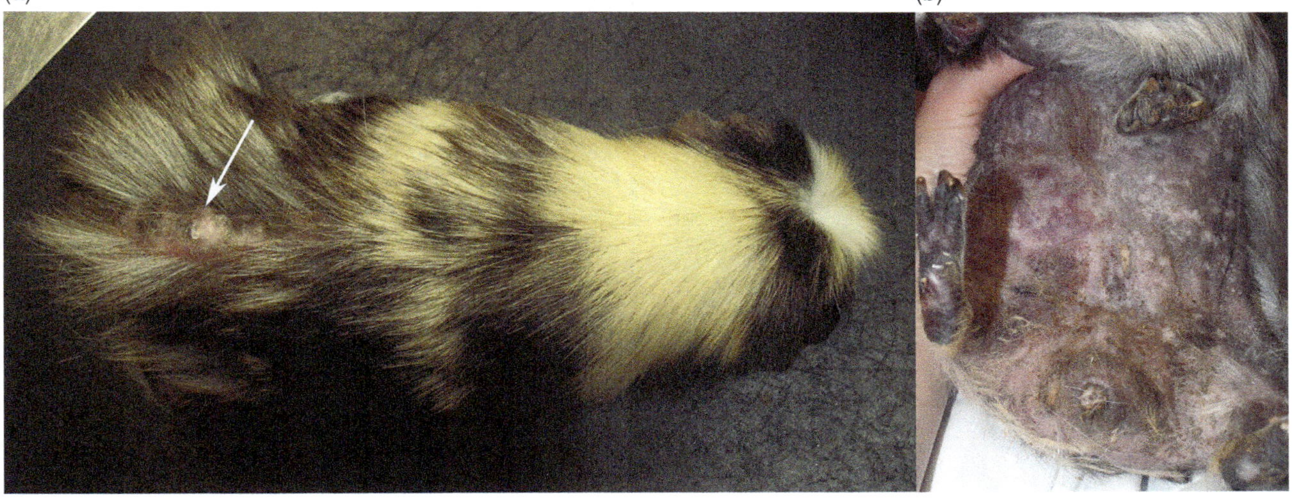

Figure 16.7 Alopecia and crusty appearance of the dorsal (a) and ventral (b) skin of a guinea pig with epitheliotropic lymphoma.

Treatment
Stabilization:

- *Antibiotics* to prevent or treat secondary infections of the skin in case of epitheliotropic lymphoma
- *Analgesia*: See Table 16.1. Multimodal analgesia is preferred
- *Diet*: Assisted feeding as deemed appropriate (see Chapter 8)
- *Chemotherapy*: By extrapolation from other species, systemic chemotherapy, and topical retinoic acid may be attempted in case of localized epitheliotropic lymphoma. The use of steroids has been reported [70]

Continued Care:

- Follow-up hematobiochemistry to assess evolution, especially if the patient is receiving steroids

Trichofolliculoma

Diagnosis
History: Slowly growing mass with/without associated ulceration. This is considered the most common cutaneous neoplasm of guinea pigs [67].

Clinical Signs:

Dorsocaudal mass central or asymmetric mass is noted. It can become very large (Figure 16.8). If ruptured trichofolliculomas may exude a creamy to gray sebaceous thick discharge (trichofolliculomas are benign hair follicle tumors).

Differentials:

- Dorsal abscess
- Other cutaneous neoplasms (lipoma, trichoepithelioma, malignant tumors)

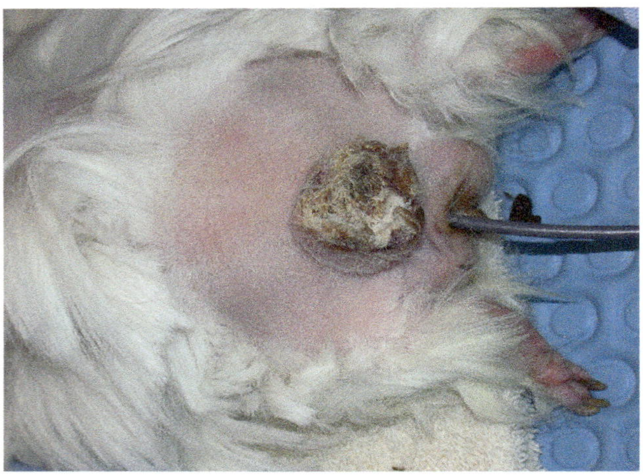

Figure 16.8 Trichofolliculoma on the ventral skin of a guinea pig.

STAT Diagnostics:

- *Cytology* of the secretions to differentiate sebaceous secretions from pus
- *CBC* if secondary infection of the mass is suspected

Complete Diagnostics:

- *Biochemistry*
- *Complete surgical excision* of the mass and histopathology

Treatment
Stabilization:

- *Analgesia*: See Table 16.1
- *Diet*: Assisted feeding as deemed appropriate (see Chapter 8)
- *SC fluids*, especially if the mass is ulcerated and fluid loss or dehydration is noted
- *Antibiotics* in case of infection of the mass, based on culture/sensitivity

Continued Care:

- Surgical excision biopsy of the mass is usually curative if margins are clean

Dermatologic Disease

Infestation with Trixacarius caviae

Diagnosis
Clinical Signs:

- Pruritus of variable intensity
- Hyperkeratosis, and crusting (Figure 16.9)
- Self-trauma
- Anorexia
- Seizures

Differentials:

- Pediculosis (*Gyropus ovalis, Gliricola porcelli*)
- Dermatophytosis (*Trichophyton mentagrophytes, Microsporum*)
- Bacterial dermatitis (*Staphylococcus* sp.)
- Hypovitaminosis C

STAT Diagnostics:

- *Multiple skin scrapings*

Complete Diagnostics:

- *Skin cytology*
- *Dermatophyte and bacterial cultures*
- *CBC, Chemistry*

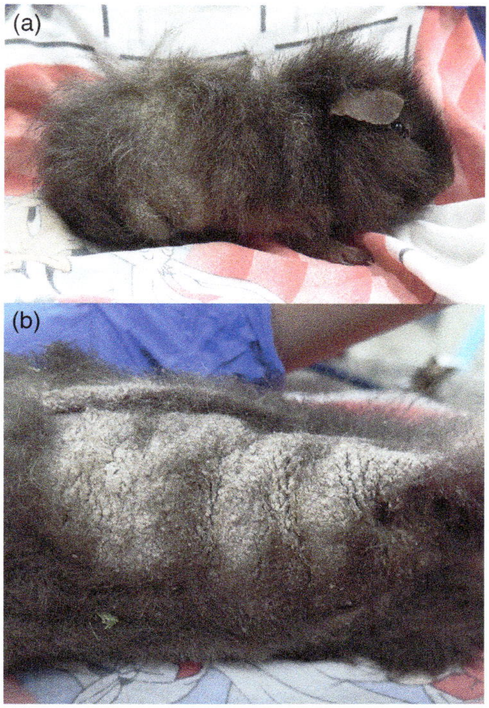

Figure 16.9 Alopecia, crusty appearance, and hyperkeratosis of the lateral (a) and dorsal (b) skin of a guinea pig with an infestation of *Trixacarus caviae*.

Treatment

- All animals in contact must be treated
- Controversial zoonotic potential [71, 72]

Stabilization:

- See Table 16.9 for various therapeutic options.
- *Analgesia*: See Table 16.1. Multimodal analgesia is preferred
- *Fluids*: SC, IV, or IO fluids based on severity (see Chapter 8)
- *Diet*: Syringe feed as deemed appropriate (see Chapter 8)

Continued care:

- Regular bedding changes/cage cleaning
- Vitamin C 50–100 mg/kg PO, IM, SC q24h in case of lacking supplementation
- Analgesia
- Fluid and nutritional support

Ophthalmic Disease

Conjunctivitis

Diagnosis

Signalment:

- *C. caviae* most common in young animals (four to eight weeks)

Clinical Signs:

- Conjunctival chemosis/hyperemia, serous/purulent discharge
- Upper/lower respiratory signs

Differentials:

- Bacterial: *C. caviae*, *B. bronchiseptica*, *Streptococcus* sp., *Salmonella* sp., *S. aureus*, *P. multocida*, *Y. pseudotuberculosis*
- Foreign body
- Dental disease
- Hypovitaminosis C
- Conjunctival lipid deposition ("Fatty eye")

STAT Diagnostics:

- *Schirmer test* (controversial) [75]
- *Fluorescein test*
- *Conjunctival swab for Chlamydia PCR*
- *Conjunctival cytology (Giemsa or Macchiavello for C. caviae)*

Complete Diagnostics:

- *CBC, Chemistry*
- *Conjunctival culture*

Treatment

Infection with *C. caviae* is most often self-limiting within 28 days after the onset of clinical signs. No treatment is required [70]

Stabilization:

- Diclofenac ophthalmic drop to improve comfort
- Ophthalmic antibiotic drops (ciprofloxacin) if condition worsens, or bacterial infection other than *Chlamydia* is confirmed

Continued Care:

- Antibiotics (doxycycline 2.5 mg/kg PO q12h) may be considered.
- Vitamin C 50–100 mg/kg PO, SC, IM q24h in case of lacking supplementation
- Analgesia
- Fluid and nutritional support

Corneal Ulceration

Diagnosis

Clinical Signs:

- Eye discharge
- White discoloration of cornea
- Blepharospasm
- Hyperemia

Table 16.9 Medical management of *Trixacarius caviae* [11].

Drug	Dosage	Comments
Ivermectin	0.2–0.5 mg/kg SC, PO q7–10d × 3–4 treatments	• Miticide
Selamectin	15–30 mg/kg topically q21–28d [73, 74]	• Miticide • Prefer ivermectin at high dosage for severe infestation
Lime sulfur dip	1:32 dilution with water q7d	• Adjunct treatment to avermectin • For immediate antiparasitic/antibacterial action/anti-inflammatory properties • Consider sedation prior to bathing
Diphenhydramine	1–5 mg/kg SC, 2–7.5 mg/kg PO	• Control pruritus and allergic response to mites
Midazolam	Midazolam 0.25–0.5 mg/kg IM, IV	• Relief anxiety associated to severe pruritus/discomfort
Trimethoprim-sulfa	15–30 mg/kg PO, SC q12h	• If concurrent bacterial dermatitis is present • Should be based on culture and sensitivity

Consider analgesia according to the patient's comfort level (see Table 16.1).

- Enophthalmia
- Exophthalmia (periapical abscess)
- Third eyelid prolapse

Differentials:

- Distichiasis and entropion (Texel guinea pigs)
- Foreign body
- Hypovitaminosis C
- Osseous choristoma
- Otitis media associated with facial paralysis

STAT Diagnostics:

- *Schirmer test (controversial)* [75]
- *Fluorescein test* (Figure 16.10)
- *Conjunctival cytology*

Complete Diagnostics:

- *CBC, Chemistry*
- *Skull radiographs/CT*
- *Endoscopic examination of the oral cavity*
- *Ocular ultrasound*

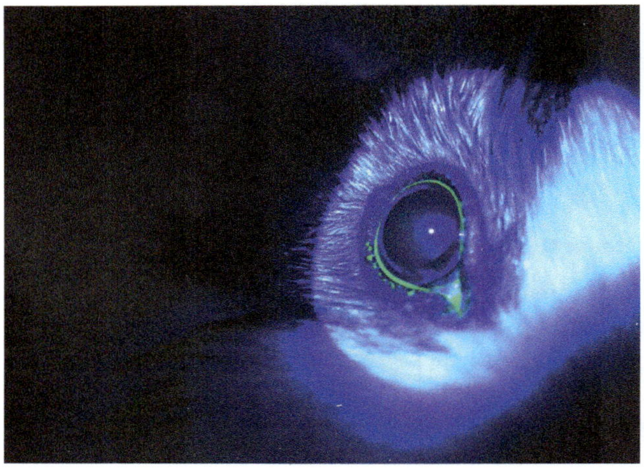

Figure 16.10 Fluorescein test in a guinea pig with right eye corneal ulceration.

Treatment

Stabilization:

- Eye lubricant
- *Topical antibiotic*: Ciprofloxacin q4–12h, tetracycline q4–6h
- *Topical analgesia*: Diclofenac q4–6h, tropicamide 0.5% q4–6h [76]
- *Anticollagenase*: *N*-Acetylcysteine q2–6h, autologous serum eye drops q4–6h
- *Systemic analgesia*: See Table 16.1. Multimodal analgesia is preferred.

Continued Care:

- Vitamin C 50–100 mg/kg PO, SC, IM q24h in case of lacking supplementation
- Analgesia
- Fluid and nutritional support
- Dental extraction

References

1 Grant, K. (2014). Rodent nutrition: digestive comparisons of 4 common rodent species. *Vet. Clin. North Am. Exot. Anim. Pract.* 17: 471–483.

2 Young, J., Hurst, W., White, W. et al. (1987). An evaluation of ampicillin pharmacokinetics and toxicity in guinea pigs. *Lab. Anim. Sci.* 37: 652–656, Erratum in: Lab. Anim. Sci. 1988; 1938(1983): 1345.

3 Morrisey, J.K. and Carpenter, J.W. (2012). Appendix. Formulary. In: *Ferrets, Rabbits and Rodents Clinical Medicine and Surgery*, 3e (eds. K.E. Quesenberry and J.W. Carpenter), 566–575. St. Louis, MO: Elsevier Saunders.

4 DeCubellis, J. and Graham, J. (2013). Gastrointestinal disease in guinea pigs and rabbits. *Vet. Clin. North Am. Exot. Anim. Pract.* 16: 421–435.

5 Dudley, E.S. and Boivin, G.P. (2011). Gastric volvulus in guinea pigs: comparison with other species. *J. Am. Assoc. Lab. Anim.* 50: 526–530.

6 Mitchell, E.B., Hawkins, M.G., Gaffney, P.M., and Macleod, A.G. (2010). Gastric dilatation-volvulus in a guinea pig (*Cavia porcellus*). *J. Am. Anim. Hosp. Assoc.* 46 (3): 174–180.

7 Nielsen, T.D., Holt, S., Ruelokke, M.L. et al. (2003). Ovarian cysts in guinea pigs: influence of age and reproductive status on prevalence and size. *J. Small Anim. Pract.* 44: 257–260.

8 Sadar, M.J., Knych, H., Drazenovich, T. et al. (2014). Pharmacokinetics of buprenorphine in the guinea pig (*Cavia porcellus*): intravenous and oral transmucosal administration. In: *Association of Exotic Mammal Veterinarians 13th Conference Proceedings, 19–24 October*, vol. 4. Orlando, Fl: AEMV.

9 Ambros, B., Knych, H.K., and Sadar, M.J. (2020). Pharmacokinetics of hydromorphone hydrochloride after intravenous and intramuscular administration in guinea pigs (*Cavia porcellus*). *Am. J. Vet. Res.* 81: 361–366.

10 Moeremans, I., Devreese, M., De Baere, S. et al. (2019). Pharmacokinetics and absolute oral bioavailability of meloxicam in guinea pigs (*Cavia porcellus*). *Vet. Anaesth. Analg.* 46: 548–555.

11 Carpenter, J.W. (2013). *Exotic Animal Formulary*, 4e. St Louis, MO: Elsevier, Saunders.

12 Percy, D. and Barthold, S. (2007). Chapter 5: Guinea pig. In: *Pathology of Laboratory Rodents and Rabbits*, 3e (eds. D.H. Percy and S.W. Barthold), 217–251. Ames, IO: Blackwell Publishing.

13 Hawkins, M. and Bishop, C.R. (2012). Chapter 23: Disease problems of guinea pigs. In: *Ferrets, Rabbits and Rodents Clinical Medicine and Surgery*, 3e (eds. K.E. Quesenberry and J.W. Carpenter), 295–310. St. Louis, MO: Elsevier Saunders.

14 Yarto-Jaramillo, E. (2011). Respiratory system anatomy, physiology, and disease: guinea pigs and chinchillas. *Vet. Clin. North Am. Exot. Anim. Pract.* 14: 339–355.

15 Greenacre, C.B. (2004). Spontaneous tumors of small mammals. *Vet. Clin. North Am. Exot. Anim. Pract.* 7: 627–651.

16 Klcalp, D. and Ms, L. (2014). ECG of a guinea pig with ventricular premature complex. *Yuzuncu Yil Univ. Vet. Fak. Derg.* 25: 51–52.

17 Illanes, O.G., Tiffani-Castiglioni, E., Edwards, J.F. et al. (1993). Spontaneous encephalitozoonosis in an experimental group of guinea pigs. *J. Vet. Diagn. Invest.* 5: 649–651.

18 Eidson, M., Matthews, S.D., Willsey, A.L. et al. (2005). Rabies virus infection in a pet guinea pig and seven pet rabbits. *J. Am. Vet. Med. Assoc.* 227 (6): 932–935.

19 Burk, R.F., Christensen, J.M., Maguire, M.J. et al. (2006). A combined deficiency of vitamins E and C causes severe central nervous system damage in guinea pigs. *J. Nutr.* 136: 1576–1581.

20 Saito, M., Muto, T., Haruzono, S. et al. (1983). An epizootic of pneumococcal infection occurred in inbred guinea pig colonies. *Exp. Anim.* 32: 29–37.

21 van der Linden, M., Al-Lahham, A., Nicklas, W. et al. (2009). Molecular characterization of pneumococcal isolates from pets and laboratory animals. *PLoS One* 4: e8286.

22 Cao, H., Wang, M.-W., Sun, L.-X. et al. (2005). Pharmacodynamic comparison of pantoprazole enantiomers: inhibition of acid-related lesions and acid secretion in rats and guinea-pigs. *J. Pharm. Pharmacol.* 57: 923–927.

23 Gruszynski, K., Young, A., Levine, S.J. et al. (2015). *Streptococcus equi* subsp. *zooepidemicus* infections associated with guinea pigs. *Emerg. Infect. Dis.* 21: 156–158.

24 Holowaychuk, M. (2006). Renal failure in a guinea pig (*Cavia porcellus*) following ingestion of oxalate containing plants. *Can. Vet. J.* 47: 787–789.

25 Kuwahara, M., Yagi, Y., Ji, B. et al. (1996). Non-invasive measurement of systemic arterial pressure in guinea pigs by an automatic oscillometric device. *Blood Press. Monit.* 1: 433–437.

26 Franklin, J.M. and Guzman, D.S. (2005). Dilated cardiomyopathy and congestive heart failure in a guinea pig. *Exotic DVM* 7: 9–12.

27 Cowan, M., Monks, D., Miles, S. et al. (2012). Thoracic diseases of guinea pigs (*Cavia porcellus*). *Assoc. Avian Vet. Australasian Committee – Unusual Exotic Pet. Vet.*: 321–325.

28 Dzyban, L., Garrod, L., and Besso, J. (2001). Pericardial effusion and pericardiocentesis in a guinea pig (*Cavia porcellus*). *J. Am. Anim. Hosp. Assoc.* 37: 21–26.

29 Quinton, J.-F. and Maguire, R. (2012). Cardiac disease in guinea pigs. *Assoc. Exot. Mamm. Vet.*: 33–35.

30 Harkness, J.E., Murray, K.A., Wagner, J.E. et al. (2002). Biology and diseases of guinea pigs. In: *Laboratory Animal Medicine (Third Edition)*, 2e (eds. J.G. Fox, L.C. Anderson, G. Otto, et al.), 247–283. Boston, MA: Academic Press.

31 Heatley, J.J. (2009). Cardiovascular anatomy, physiology, and disease of rodents and small exotic mammals. *Vet. Clin. North Am. Exot. Anim. Pract.* 12: 99–113.

32 Williams, B.H. (2012). Non-infectious diseases. In: *The Laboratory Rabbit, Guinea Pig, Hamster, and Other Rodents* (eds. M.A. Suckow, K.A. Stevens and R.P. Wilson), 685–704. San Diego, CA: Academic Press.

33 Çetin, N., Çetin, E., and Toker, M. (2005). Echocardiographic variables in healthy guineapigs anaesthetized with ketamine–xylazine. *Lab. Anim.* 39: 100–106.

34 Sisk, D.B. (1976). Physiology. In: *The Biology of the Guinea Pig* (eds. J.E. Wagner and P.J. Manning), 63–92. San Diego: Academic Press.

35 Sadar, M.J., Knych, H.K., Drazenovich, T.L., and Paul-Murphy, J.R. (2018). Pharmacokinetics of buprenorphine after intravenous and oral transmucosal administration in guinea pigs (*Cavia porcellus*). *Am. J. Vet. Res.* 79 (3): 260–266, https://doi.org/10.2460/ajvr.79.3.260.

36 Maguire, R. and Maguire, P.J. (2012). Management of dilated cardiomyopathy in a guinea pig utilizing carvedilol. *Assoc. Avian Vet.*: 31–32.

37 Brabb, T., Newsome, D., Burich, A., and Hanes, M. (2012). Part III Guinea pigs: infectious diseases. In: *The Laboratory Rabbit, Guinea Pig, Hamster and Other Rodents* (eds. M.A. Suckow, K.A. Stevens and R.P. Wilson), 638–683. SanDiego, CA: Elsevier.

38 Legendre, L.F. (2002). Malocclusions in guinea pigs, chinchillas and rabbits. *Can. Vet. J.* 43: 385–390.

39 Capello, V., Lennox, A., and Ghisleni, G. (2015). Elodontoma in two guinea pigs. *J. Vet. Dent.* 32: 111–119.

40 Schweda, M.C., Hassan, J., Böhler, A. et al. (2014). The role of computed tomography in the assessment of dental disease in 66 guinea pigs. *Vet. Rec.* 175: 538.

41 Müller, J., Clauss, M., Codron, D. et al. (2015). Tooth length and incisal wear and growth in guinea pigs (*Cavia porcellus*) fed diets of different abrasiveness. *J. Anim. Physiol. Anim. Nutr.* 99: 591–604.

42 Fisher, P.G. (2006). Exotic mammal renal disease: causes and clinical presentation. *Vet. Clin. North Am. Exot. Anim. Pract.* 9: 33–67.

43 Eshar, D., Lee-Chow, B., and Chalmers, H.J. (2013). Ultrasound-guided percutaneous antegrade hydropropulsion to relieve ureteral obstruction in a pet guinea pig (*Cavia porcellus*). *Can. Vet. J.* 54: 1142–1145.

44 Fisher, P.G. (2006). Exotic mammal renal disease: diagnosis and treatment. *Vet. Clin. North Am. Exot. Anim. Pract.* 9: 69–96.

45 Coutant, T., Dunn, M., Langlois, I., and Maccolini, E. (2019). Cystoscopic-guided lithotripsy for the removal of a urethral stone in a guinea pig. *J. Exotic Pet Med.* 28: 11–114.

46 Martinho, F. (2006). Dystocia caused by ectopic pregnancy in a guinea pig (*Cavia porcellus*). *Vet. Clin. North Am. Exot. Anim. Pract.* 9: 713–716.

47 Hawkins, M.G. and Graham, J.E. (2007). Emergency and critical care of rodents. *Vet. Clin. North Am. Exot. Anim. Pract.* 10: 501–531.

48 Seidl, D.C., Hughes, H.C., Bertolet, R. et al. (1979). True pregnancy toxemia (preeclampsia) in the guinea pig (*Cavia porcellus*). *Lab. Anim. Sci.* 29: 472–478.

49 Schuetzenhofer, G., Goericke-Pesch, S., and Wehrend, A. (2011). Effects of deslorelin implants on ovarian cysts in guinea pigs. *Schweiz. Arch. Tierheilkd.* 153: 416–417.

50 Hess, L., Ravich, M.L., and Reavill, D. (2013). Diagnosis and treatment of an insulinoma in a guinea pig (*Cavia porcellus*). *J. Am. Vet. Med. Assoc.* 242: 522–526.

51 Vannevel, J. (1998). Diabetes mellitus in a 3 year old intact, female guinea pig. *Can. Vet. J.* 39: 503–504.

52 Bauer, B., Palme, R., Machatschke, I.H. et al. (2008). Non-invasive measurement of adrenocortical and gonadal activity in male and female guinea pigs (Cavia aperea f. porcellus). *Gen. Comp. Endocrinol.* 156: 482–489.

53 Muller, K., Muller, E., Klein, R. et al. (2009). Serum thyroxine concentrations in clinically healthy pet guinea pigs (*Cavia porcellus*). *Vet. Clin. Pathol.* 38: 507–510.

54 Schwarz, T., Stork, C.K., Megahy, I.W. et al. (2001). Osteodystrophia fibrosa in two guinea pigs. *J. Am. Vet. Med. Assoc.* 219: 63–66, 49.

55 Zeugswetter, F., Fenske, M., Hassan, J. et al. (2007). Cushing's syndrome in a guinea pig. *Vet. Rec.* 160: 878–880.

56 Bishop, C.R. and Hawkins, M.G. (2015). Investigating the cause of fibrous osteodystrophy in satin cavies. *ExoticsCon*: 379.

57 Watson, M., Stern, A.W., Labelle, A.L. et al. (2014). Evaluating the clinical and physiological effects of long

term ultraviolet B radiation on guinea pigs (*Cavia porcellus*). *PLoS One* 9: e114413.

58 Brandao, J., Vergneau-Grosset, C., and Mayer, J. (2013). Hyperthyroidism and hyperparathyroidism in guinea pigs (*Cavia porcellus*). *Vet. Clin. North Am. Exot. Anim. Pract.* 16: 407–420.

59 Künzel, F., Hierlmeier, B., Christian, M. et al. (2013). Hyperthyroidism in four guinea pigs: clinical manifestations, diagnosis, and treatment. *J. Small Anim. Pract.* 54: 667–671.

60 Gibbons, P., Garner, M., and Kiupel, M. (2013). Morphological and immunohistochemical characterization of spontaneous thyroid gland neoplasms in guinea pigs (*Cavia porcellus*). *Vet. Pathol.* 50: 334–342.

61 Fredholm, D.V., Cagle, L.A., and Johnston, M.S. (2012). Evaluation of precision and establishment of reference ranges for plasma thyroxine using a point-of-care analyzer in healthy guinea pigs (*Cavia porcellus*). *J. Exot. Pet. Med.* 21: 87–93.

62 Mayer, J., Wagner, R., Mitchell, M.A. et al. (2013). Use of recombinant human thyroid-stimulating hormone for evaluation of thyroid function in guinea pigs (*Cavia porcellus*). *J. Am. Vet. Med. Assoc.* 242: 346–349.

63 Binah, O., Rubinstein, I., and Gilat, E. (1987). Effects of thyroid hormone on the action potential and membrane currents of guinea pig ventricular myocytes. *Pflugers Archiv: Eur. J. Physiol.* 409: 214–216.

64 Castro, M.I., Alex, S., Young, R.A. et al. (1986). Total and free serum thyroid hormone concentrations in fetal and adult pregnant and nonpregnant guinea pigs. *Endocrinology* 118: 533–537.

65 Anderson, R.R., Nixon, D.A., and Akasha, M.A. (1988). Total and free thyroxine and triiodothyronine in blood serum of mammals. *Comp. Biochem. Physiol. A, Comp. Physiol.* 89: 401–404.

66 Quimby, F.W. (1999). *The Clinical Chemistry of Laboratory Animals*, 2e. Philadelphia: Taylor & Francis.

67 Kanfer, S. and Reavill, D.R. (2013). Cutaneous neoplasia in ferrets, rabbits, and guinea pigs. *Vet. Clin. North Am. Exot. Anim. Pract.* 16: 579–598.

68 Suárez-Bonnet, A., Martín de Las Mulas, J., Millán, M.Y. et al. (2010). Morphological and immunohistochemical characterization of spontaneous mammary gland tumors in the guinea pig (*Cavia porcellus*). *Vet. Pathol.* 47: 298–305.

69 Martorell, J., Such, R., Fondevila, D. et al. (2011). Cutaneous epitheliotropic T-cell lymphoma with systemic spread in a guinea pig (*Cavia porcellus*). *J. Exot. Pet. Med.* 20: 313–317.

70 Williams, D. and Sullivan, A. (2010). Ocular disease in the guinea pig (*Cavia porcellus*): a survey of 1000 animals. *Vet. Ophthalmol.* 13: 54–62.

71 Beck, W. and Pantchev, N. (2008). *Trixacarus caviae* as a cause of mange in the guinea pig and pseudoscabies in a human being – a case report. *Kleintierpraxis* 53: 424–430.

72 Honda, M., Namikawa, K., Hirata, H. et al. (2011). An outbreak of *Trixacarus caviae* infestation in guinea pigs at an animal petting facility and an evaluation of the safety and suitable dose of selamectin treatment. *J. Parasitol.* 97: 731–734.

73 Eshar, D. and Bdolah-Abram, T. (2012). Comparison of efficacy, safety, and convenience of selamectin versus ivermectin for treatment of *Trixacarus caviae* mange in pet guinea pigs (*Cavia porcellus*). *J. Am. Vet. Med. Assoc.* 241: 1056–1058.

74 Fisher, M., Beck, W., and Hutchinson, M.J. (2007). Efficacy and safety of selamectin (Stronghold) used off-label in exotic pets. *Int. J. Appl. Res. Vet. Med.* 5: 87–96.

75 Coster, M.E., Stiles, J., Krohne, S.G. et al. (2008). Results of diagnostic ophthalmic testing in healthy guinea pigs. *J. Am. Vet. Med. Assoc.* 232: 1825–1833.

76 Rival F. (2007). Cochon d'Inde. In: *Atlas l'ophtalmologie des nouveaux animaux de compagnie* (ed. F. Rival), 57–66. France: Vetnac.

77 Wenger, S. and Hatt, J.M. (2015). Transurethral cystoscopy and endoscopic urolith removal in female guinea pigs (*Cavia porcellus*). *Vet. Clin. North Am. Exot. Anim. Pract.* 18: 359–367.

78 Fenske, M. (1996). Saliva cortisol and testosterone in the guinea pig: measures for the endocrine function of adrenals and testes? *Steroids* 61: 647–650.

17

Chinchillas

Jennifer E. Graham[1] *and Christoph Mans*[2]

[1] *Department of Clinical Sciences, Cummings School of Veterinary Medicine at Tufts University, North Grafton, Massachusetts, USA*
[2] *Department of Surgical Sciences, School of Veterinary Medicine University of Wisconsin–Madison, Madison, Wisconsin, USA*

CONTENTS

Unique Species Considerations

Chinchillas are becoming increasingly popular as companion animals and are frequently presented for emergency care. Chinchillas, like other rodents, are obligate nasal breathers. While closely related to guinea pigs as hystricomorph rodents from South America, the diseases occurring in chinchillas and their medical management are vastly different. Chinchillas frequently suffer from dental disorder including periodontal disease, conjunctivitis, penile disorders, and ketoacidosis associated with hepatic lipidosis secondary to anorexia. Like guinea pigs, chinchillas are hindgut fermenters that are very susceptible to changes in enteric microbial flora. Of note, giardia shedding is reported in 27–66% of healthy pet chinchillas. Antibiotics to be avoided in this species include oral penicillin, cephalosporins, erythromycin, clindamycin, and other antibiotics with a predominantly Gram-positive and anaerobic spectrum. Parenteral administration of these antibiotics can be considered. Antibiotics commonly used in chinchillas include azithromycin, chloramphenicol, quinolones, and trimethoprim-sulfa. Caution should be used with oral metronidazole in chinchillas, as food intake can be significantly reduced; total daily dose should not exceed 20 mg/kg.

Exotic Animal Emergency and Critical Care Medicine, First Edition. Edited by Jennifer E. Graham, Grayson A. Doss and Hugues Beaufrère.

Common Presenting Signs

Anorexia and Decreased Fecal Output

- This is a nonspecific finding, but often a sign of underlying pain or disease

Diagnosis

History and clinical signs:

- Partial or complete cessation of food intake and/or fecal output
- Changes in food preferences
- Other abnormalities may be seen, reflecting the primary cause of illness
- Note any recent changes in housing or offered diet

Signalment:

- Chinchillas, any age or sex

Differentials:

- Numerous, as any painful condition or illness may lead to anorexia. Dental disease is a common cause. Hepatic lipidosis and ketosis secondary to excessive fat mobilization are common

Diagnostics

STAT:

- Radiographs – dental disease and gastroenteritis common in chinchillas, will also help determine if other lesions present
- Urine dipstick testing to check for urinary ketones, decreased urine pH (normal pH: 8.5–9.5), and glucose
- PCV/TS
- Chemistry – changes will reflect primary disease

Complete:

- CT – evaluate for periodontal disease, dental disease, hepatic lipidosis or other disease
- CBC – may be normal, but may see evidence of inflammation, anemia

Treatment

Stabilization:

- Nutritional support and fluid therapy, see Chapter 8
- See "Dental Disease", "Anorexia and Decreased Fecal Output", and "Hepatic Lipidosis and Ketosis"

Continued care

- Will depend on diagnosis

Gastrointestinal Disease

- Dysbacteriosis, diarrhea, and/or tympany

Diagnosis

History and clinical signs:

- Soft feces or diarrhea, and fecal-stained perineum (Figure 17.1)
- Weight loss
- Decreased fecal output
- Inappetence or anorexia
- Distended and tense abdomen
- Dehydration and lethargy
- Constipation, intussusception, and rectal prolapse possible
- Inquire about health of past and current cage mates

Signalment:

- Chinchillas, any age or sex

Differentials:

- Infectious causes
  - *Yeast (Cyniclomyces guttulatus)* always secondary (Figure 17.2)
  - *Escherichia coli*, *Pseudomonas* sp., *Proteus* sp
  - Giardiasis (often secondary)
  - Coccidiosis (often secondary, predominately in young animals)
- Noninfectious causes
  - Sudden diet change
  - Inadequate fiber
  - Inappropriate antibiotic therapy

Diagnostics

STAT:

- Fecal cytology
- Fecal parasite examination
- Fecal culture
- Whole-body radiographs

Complete:

- CT or ultrasound to rule out torsion, intussusception

Treatment

Stabilization:

- Nutritional and fluid support, see Chapter 8
- Gastric decompression could be considered if severe tympany but may result in collapse and death in decompensated patient
- Analgesia if warranted (Table 17.1)
- Antibiotics if warranted (Table 17.2)

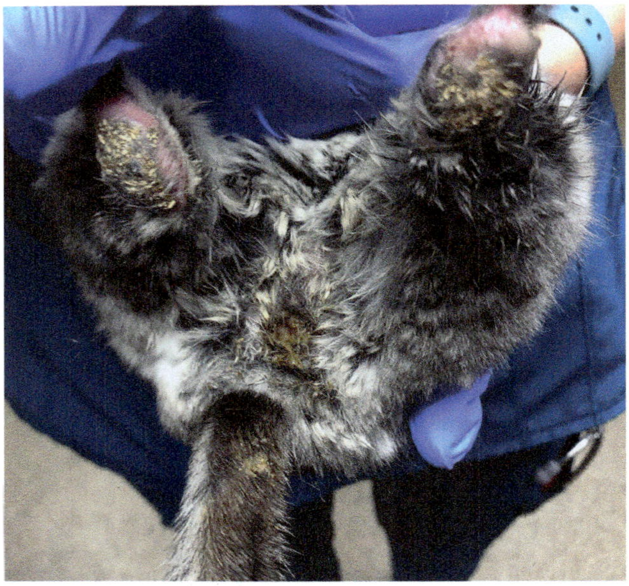

Figure 17.1 Fecal-stained perineum in a chinchilla with diarrhea. This chinchilla also has pododermatitis.

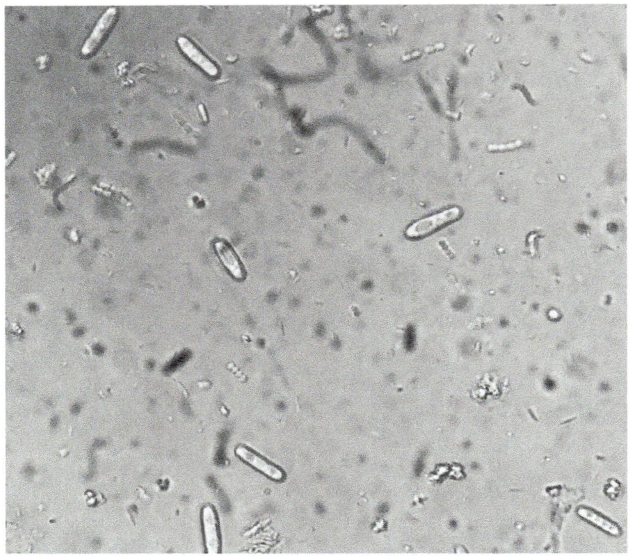

Figure 17.2 Fecal cytology from the chinchilla in Figure 17.1 showing yeast (*Cyniclomyces guttulatus)* overgrowth.

- Antiparasitic if warranted (Table 17.3)
- Avoid use of prokinetics

Continued care

- Depends on cause

Dental Disease

- Common diagnosis in chinchillas. Specialized dental instruments and general anesthesia are necessary for diagnosis and treatment of dental and periodontal disease in chinchillas. The use of a video otoscope or rigid endoscope greatly enhances the intraoral exam and aids in treatment and documentation of intraoral disease. Treatment of dental disease in chinchillas is challenging and should not be attempted without the necessary equipment (i.e. low-speed handpiece, cheek dilators, and diamond burr) and expertise

Diagnosis

History and clinical signs:

- Reduced body condition and weight loss
- Preference for softer food items
- Reduced fecal output and small/irregular feces
- Saliva-stained skin of perioral/chin region, unkempt coat, and fur chewing (Figure 17.3)
- Changes in food preferences
- Palpable irregularities of ventral borders of mandible and depigmentation of orange enamel of incisor teeth
- Periodontal disease and tooth resorption are common in chinchillas
- Sharp buccal points of the maxillary cheek teeth, often leading to ulceration of the cheek mucosa
- Widened interproximal spaces, food impaction, resorbed teeth, and gingival hyperplasia common
- Other abnormalities including ketoacidosis may be seen, reflecting the primary cause of illness

Signalment:

- Chinchillas, any age or sex

Differentials:

- Numerous, as many conditions and illness may result from dental pathology. Gastroenteritis, hepatic lipidosis, and ketosis are common secondary sequelae

Diagnostics

STAT:

- Once stable, thorough intraoral examination under general anesthesia. Isoflurane or dexmedetomidine-ketamine (0.015 mg/kg + 5 mg/kg) result in reliable and safe anesthesia
- Radiographs – skull and whole body
- Urinalysis – rule out ketoacidosis
- Chemistry – may be nonspecific

Table 17.1 Analgesic agents commonly used in chinchillas.

Agents	Dosage	Comments
Buprenorphine	0.2 mg/kg SC q4–6h	PD
Butorphanol	0.5–1.0 mg/kg SC, IM, IV q2–4h	Lower dose used in premedication combinations
Fentanyl	0.5 μg/kg/h CRI IV or IO	Anecdotal
Gabapentin	3–5 mg/kg PO q12–24h	Anecdotal
Hydromorphone	1–2 mg/kg SC, IM q6–8 h	PD
Meloxicam	≥0.5 mg/kg PO, SC q12–24h	Anecdotal, hydration status must be restored prior to administration
Tramadol	Not recommended	No analgesic effects; adverse effects at >40 mg/kg in single-dose study

Source: Refs. [1, 2].

Table 17.2 Antibiotics commonly used to treat infection in chinchillas.

Antibiotic	Dosage	Comments
Azithromycin	30 mg/kg PO q24h	Limited spectrum. Not effective against most Gram-negative aerobic bacteria. Good activity against anaerobic bacteria
Enrofloxacin	10 mg/kg PO, SC, IM q12h	Dilute 50:50 (in NaCl or LRS) for SC, IM injections. Limit SC and IM injections
Marbofloxacin	4 mg/kg PO, SC q24h	Do not give during lactation, pregnancy, or while growing; injectable can be given orally
Metronidazole	10 mg/kg PO q12h or 20 mg/kg PO q24h	Use with caution, can cause appetite suppression. Excellent anaerobic coverage
Penicillin G (benzathine and procaine)	50 000 U/kg SC q3–5d	Parenteral use only, do not give orally. Not effective against most Gram-negative aerobic bacteria. Good activity against anaerobic bacteria
Trimethoprim/sulfa	30 mg/kg PO, SC q12h	Broad-spectrum, not effective against *Pseudomonas aerguinosa*. Limited anaerobic spectrum
Tinidazole	20 mg/kg PO q12h	Treatment anerobic infections (e.g. periodontal disease). No negative effect on food intake

Source: Carpenter [1]. © 2018, Elsevier.

Table 17.3 Antiparasitic and antifungals commonly used in chinchillas.

Drug	Dosage	Comments
Fenbendazole	20 mg/kg PO q24h × 5d	Up to 50 mg/kg PO q24h × 5d used for giardiasis; treatment reduces shedding and clinical signs but does not eradicate
Sulfadimethoxine	50 mg/kg PO once, then 25 mg/kg q24h × 10–20d	Coccidiosis; may resolve clinical signs but does not eradicate
Metronidazole	10 mg/kg PO q12h or 20 mg/kg PO q24h	Use with caution, can cause appetite suppression. Treatment for giardiasis
Terbinafine	30 mg/kg PO q24h	More effective than itraconazole to treat dermatophytosis in guinea pigs
Nystatin	100 000 IU/kg PO q-8h × 5d	*Enteral C. guttulatus* (yeast) overgrowth
Tinidazole	20 mg/kg PO q12h	Treatment for giardiasis, no negative effect on food intake

Source: Carpenter [3]. © 2018, Elsevier.

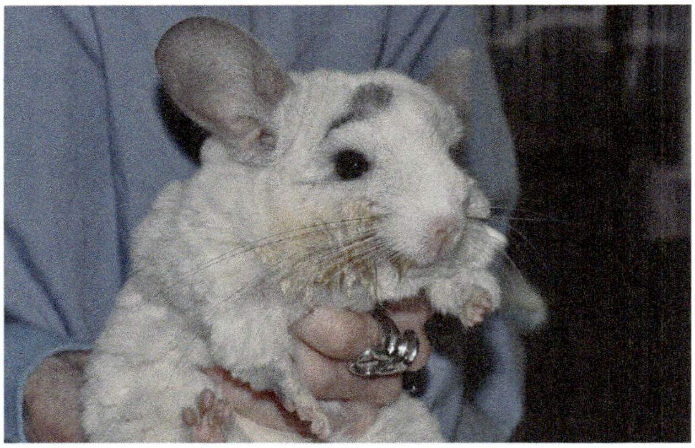

Figure 17.3 Drooling and fur staining around the mouth in a chinchilla with dental disease. Hypersalivation in chinchillas is most associated with intraoral disease and an intraoral exam should be performed under general anesthesia.

Complete:

- Head CT ideal to evaluate extent of disease
- Check urine pH and ketones to rule out ketoacidosis
- CBC – may be normal but may see evidence of inflammation or infection

Treatment

Stabilization:

- Nutritional support and fluid therapy, see Chapter 8
- Dental treatments – removal of spurs and elongated crowns and periodontal disease treatment
- Pain management (Table 17.1)

Continued care:

- Doxycycline polymer filling (Doxirobe gel) into gingival and periodontal pockets to reduce inflammation and delay reimpaction
- Systemic antibiotics as warranted; ideally based on C/S (Table 17.2)
  - Penicillin G benzathine/procaine: 50000 IU/kg SC q3–5d
  - Azithromycin 30 mg/kg PO q24h
  - Tinidazole 20 mg/kg PO q12h
- Some animals may require long-term nutritional support in form of syringe feeding, particularly if ketoacidosis and/or hepatic lipidosis is present
- Pain management

Ocular Signs

- Epiphora, conjunctivitis, and corneal disease

Diagnosis

History and clinical signs:

- Serous ocular discharge with periocular fur wetting
- Purulent ocular discharge
- Corneal opacity
- Grossly visible corneal defect
- Blepharospasm
- Chemosis
- Proptosis
- Anorexia and inactivity may be noted
- Inquire about any cage mates and interactions (possible fights)

Signalment:

- Chinchillas of any age or sex

Differentials:

- Bacterial conjunctivitis (*Pseudomonas aeruginosa* and *Staphylococcus* sp. common, others). Normal conjunctival bacterial flora consists of predominantly Gram-positive species. Most isolates in chinchillas with conjunctivitis are Gram-negative with *P. aeruginosa* frequently associated with concurrent upper respiratory signs (Figure 17.4)
- Corneal ulceration/epiphora
- Inadequate cage hygiene – excessive dust bathing, inappropriate sand for bathing, inadequate cage ventilation
- Otitis media (lack of palpebral reflex secondary to facial nerve damage)
- Dental disease
- Retrobulbar mass (rare), tooth root abscess, and neoplasia
- Nasolacrimal duct obstruction
- Herpesvirus I (rare)
- Corneal lipid keratopathy and cataracts reported in chinchillas

Diagnostics

STAT:

- Fluorescein stain to rule out corneal ulceration

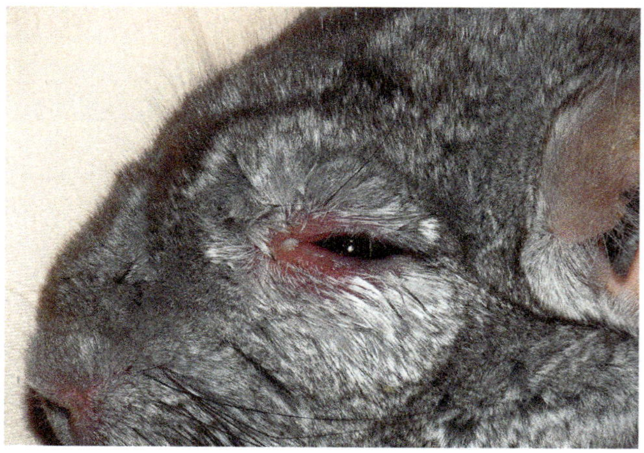

Figure 17.4 Conjunctivitis in a chinchilla with suspected *P. aeruginosa*. *Source:* Mans and Donnelly [3].

Complete:

- Conjunctival bacterial C/S if conjunctivitis
- Urinalysis, if not eating, depressed; r/o ketoacidosis
- Chemistry – generally normal
- CT/radiographs – rule out tooth root lesions, bone lysis associated with infection or neoplasia
- Ocular ultrasound
- CBC – nonspecific findings, possible inflammatory leukogram

Treatment

Stabilization:

- As described in other species. Flush excessive dust/debris from eyes; flushing nasolacrimal duct is not feasible in chinchillas
- Animals with purulent conjunctivitis, depression, and anorexia are more likely to suffer from a Pseudomonal infection and require aggressive and immediate therapy with empirically selected systemic (i.e. enrofloxacin 10 mg/kg SC, IM, q12h; ceftazidime 30 mg/kg SC, IM, q8h) and topical antibiotics (i.e. gentamicin, polymyxin B combinations), and supportive care. Animals with no signs of systemic illness should be treated with topical antibiotics only, pending culture, and susceptibility. Topical ophthalmic ointments tend to leave the surrounding fur greasy; when possible, ophthalmic solutions should be used
- Systemic analgesics if indicated (Table 17.1)

Continued care:

- Corneal ulcer and ocular trauma
  - Topical antibiotic
    - Gentamicin ophthalmic solution
    - Tobramycin ophthalmic solution
    - Neomycin–polymyxin–bacitracin ophthalmic solution. Avoid preparations with dexamethasone. Prevent ingestion
    - Ofloxacin ophthalmic solution
- Systemic antibiotic or analgesia may be indicated if significant trauma (Tables 17.1–17.2)
- Address underlying dental disease or husbandry deficiencies
- Restrict dust bathing until clinical signs resolved

Trauma

Diagnosis:

History and clinical signs:

- Traumatic incident may not be witnessed, but wounds may be noted afterward
- Owner may report the patient caught by or "playing" with a predator species (dog and cat)
- Lameness or limb paresis
- Blood may be seen on cage furnishings or substrate, but not on the patient due to grooming habits
- In some cases, a bite wound may necrose and/or abscess a few days later
- Fractures of the tibia are common

Signalment:

- Chinchillas any age or sex

Differentials:

- Limb entrapment within wire exercise wheels or cage bars may lead to secondary limb fracture, limb edema, or neurologic injury as the animal attempts to free itself
- Falls within cage, or from owner's arms or shoulder
- Crush trauma (hiding under couch or chair cushions, inside a recliner, or trapped under falling items)
- Predator trauma
- Conspecific fights
- Dermatologic disease
- IVDD, peripheral neuropathy (rare, Figure 17.5)

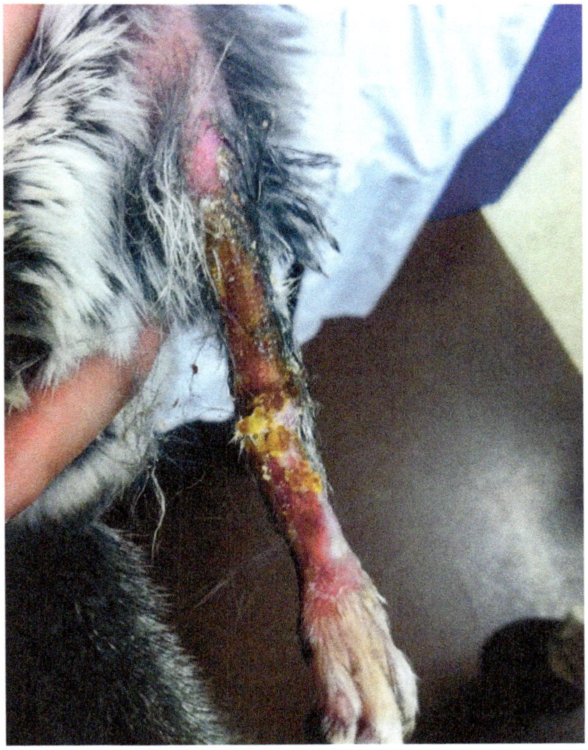

Figure 17.5 Mutilation in the left hind limb of a chinchilla following traumatic leg avulsion and subsequent neuropathy. This lesion resolved with bandaging, topical therapy, meloxicam, gabapentin, and cage rest.

Diagnostics
STAT:

- Radiographs to determine if fracture present
- Be sure to assess the entire body, as multiple injuries possible
- PCV/TS if blood loss is a concern

Complete:

- CT or thoracic and abdominal ultrasound to further identify internal injury
- Chemistry – may be normal, may see elevations in CK with muscle trauma, increased liver enzymes in crush trauma

Treatment
Stabilization:

- Analgesia (Table 17.1)
- Wound care (cleansing/lavage, shaving fur, and laceration repair) – local block and sedation may be required
- Splinting of fractured limbs (if possible) until definitive treatment can be pursued (Figure 17.6)

Continued care:

- Laceration repair
- Bandage management if secondary intention healing
- Fracture repair or limb amputation (see Musculoskeletal Disease – Fractures)
- Antibiotics as indicated (bite wounds and open wounds) (Table 17.2)

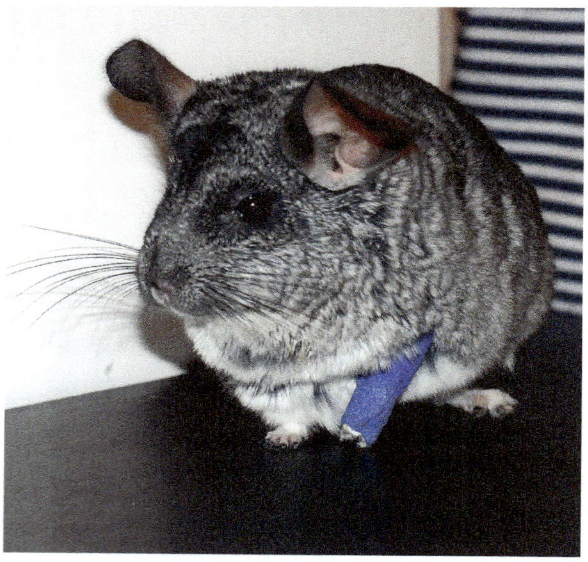

Figure 17.6 External coaptation for treatment of a left radius and ulnar fracture in a chinchilla.

Systemic Disease

Heatstroke

Diagnosis
History:

- Often seen in summer months, but possible on any warm day. The patient may have been in a warm room without air conditioning (above 77 °F; 25 °C) in a hot car (even for a short time), or in a cage located in front of a sunny window. The detrimental effects of high temperature worsen when accompanied by high humidity

Signalment:

- Chinchillas of any age or gender

Clinical signs:

- Panting, hyperthermia (rectal temperature > 101), lethargy, obtunded mentation, dyspnea, seizures, hemorrhage, ataxia, recumbency, cyanosis, and death
  - Normal rectal temperature is 94.8–100.2 °F (34.9–37.9 °C) at 2 cm insertion depth

Differentials:

- Severe fever due to inflammation or infection

Diagnostics:

STAT:

- rectal temperature and history usually suffice for diagnosis

Complete:

- CBC/chemistry ideal to assess organ function but may lead to increased morbidity if coagulopathy present

Treatment
Stabilization:

- Cooling via lukewarm water baths and cool environment via fans, removing cage linings and towels
- IV or IO fluids ideal but may not be feasible if cardiovascular instability present; otherwise SC fluids
- IV or IO mannitol if concern for increased ICP

Continued care:

- Nutritional support
- Prognosis poor, depending on degree and duration of hyperthermia – euthanasia may be warranted

Hepatic Lipidosis and Ketosis

Diagnosis

History:

- Partial or complete cessation of food intake and/or fecal output
  - Changes in food preferences
  - Note any recent changes in housing or offered diet

Signalment:

- Chinchillas, any age or sex

Clinical signs:

- Depression and dehydration, other abnormalities may be seen, reflecting the primary cause of illness

Differentials:

- Numerous, as any painful condition or illness may lead to anorexia. Dental disease and gastroenteritis are common causes. Hepatic lipidosis and ketosis occur secondary to excessive fat mobilization

Diagnostics

STAT:

- Radiographs – dental disease and gastroenteritis common in chinchillas, will also help determine if other lesions present
- Urine dipstick testing to check for urinary glucose, ketones, and decreased urine pH (normal pH: 8.5–9.5)
- Chemistry – changes will reflect primary disease. Increased ALT, ALP, AST, GGT, and totsl bilirubin may be seen. Hyperglycemia in severe cases should not be misinterpreted as diabetes mellitus
- CBC – may be normal, but may see evidence of inflammation, nonregenerative anemia

Complete:

- Abdominal ultrasound or preferably whole-body CT – evaluate for hepatic lipidosis or other disease (e.g. dental disease)

Treatment

Stabilization:

- Nutritional support and fluid therapy, see Chapter 8
  - Correct electrolyte abnormalities – hypokalemia, hypophosphatemia, and hypomagnesemia can be seen
- See "Dental Disease" and "Anorexia and Reduced Fecal Output" for more information

Continued care:

- Will depend on cause; often long-term nutritional support is necessary treat underlying primary cause
- Urinary ketone concentrations and pH monitoring to monitor response to therapy. Can be performed by owners
- Severe ketoacidosis, not responsive to initial treatment, carries a poor prognosis

Neurologic and Musculoskeletal Disease

Neurologic-Head Tilt

Diagnosis

History:

- Head tilt, rolling, circling, ataxia, and anorexia. Primary otitis externa is rare; most cases are otitis media ± perforated tympanic membrane

Signalment:

- Chinchillas of any age or sex

Clinical signs:

- Head tilt (Figure 17.7), head shaking, facial paralysis (Figure 17.8), torticollis, nystagmus, ataxia, thin body condition, purulent discharge in external ear canal, and severe neurologic deficits. Changes in vascularity or opacity or bulging of tympanic membrane are abnormal

Differentials:

- Otitis media ± perforated tympanic membrane; otitis externa rare
  - Bacterial infection; *P. aeruginosa, Proteus* spp. common
  - Neoplasia
  - Toxin, especially lead

Diagnostics

STAT:

- Radiographs, particularly skull VD – rule out otitis media
- Cytology of discharge present in the ear canal

Complete:

- CT of brain/skull (Figure 17.9)
- Cytology, culture, and sensitivity (minimally invasive transbulbar approach to sample middle ear described in chinchillas)
- Lead screening as warranted
- CBC and chemistry panel – may show nonspecific changes or concurrent disease

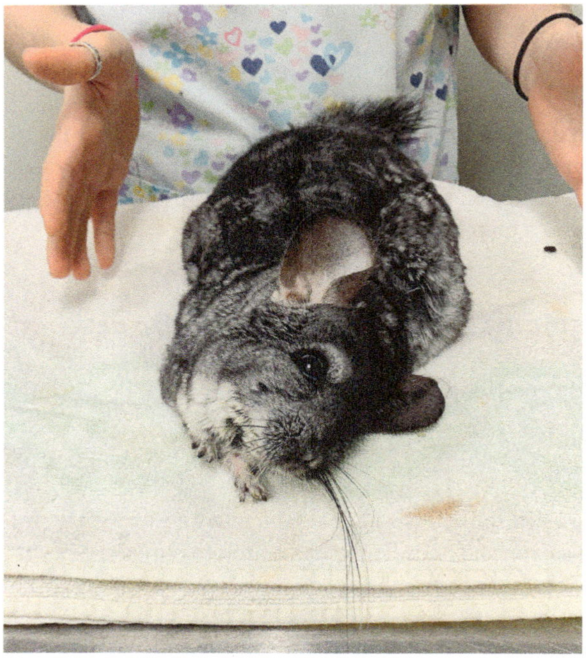

Figure 17.7 Left-sided head tilt in an eight-year-old chinchilla with otitis.

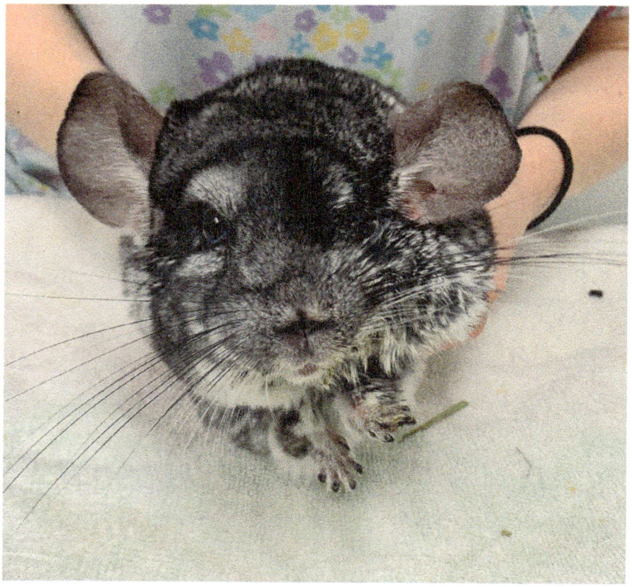

Figure 17.8 Closer view of the face of the chinchilla in Figure 17.7. Note the facial nerve paralysis; the whiskers are asymmetric and there is no palpebral reflex on the left side.

Treatment

Stabilization:

- Fluid and nutritional support if indicated, see Chapter 8
- Systemic antibiotics if otitis suspected (Table 17.2), ideally based on C/S

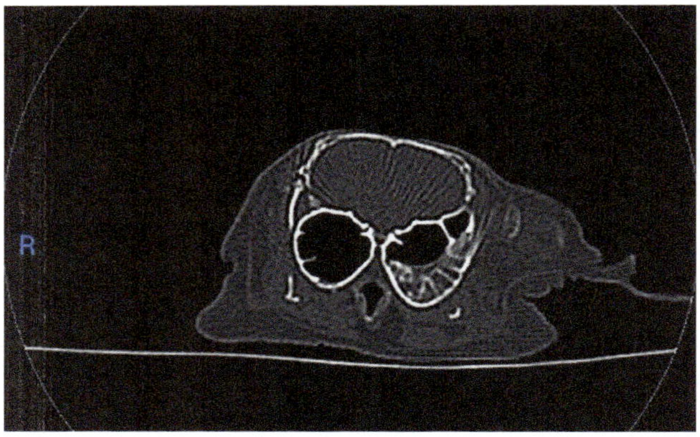

Figure 17.9 CT of the chinchilla in Figures 17.7 and 17.8. CT confirmed otitis media.

  - Azithromycin 30 mg/kg PO q24h reaches appropriate tissue levels to eliminate bacteria in middle ear if susceptible. Use enrofloxacin if *P. aeruginosa*, is suspected based on cytology, and pending C/S.

Continued care:

- Prognosis generally guarded to poor for bacterial otitis media, but some may learn to function with persistent head tilt
- Cage modification for accessibility and safety
- Surgical treatment of otitis is unrewarding in chinchillas, due to the large size and complex anatomy of the middle ear

Neurologic – Seizures

Diagnosis

History:

- Owner may witness the seizure, or may find the pet post-ictal; hot days during summer or leaving pet in car are risk factors for heat stroke

Signalment:

- Chinchillas of any age or sex

Clinical signs:

- Status epilepticus, post-ictal behavior, hyperthermia, hypersalivation, lateral recumbence, and non-responsiveness

Differentials:

- Heatstroke
- Toxicosis (lead can cause acute blindness and seizures)
- Septicemia
- Encephalitis – listeriosis, human herpes simplex virus, and cerebrospinal nematodiasis
- Dietary deficiencies
- Hypoglycemia

- Hypocalcemia may mimic seizures
- Hepatic or renal insufficiency
- Idiopathic epilepsy

Diagnostics

STAT:

- Chemistry to assess glucose, iCa, hepatic/renal enzymes
- CBC may be normal but may see evidence of inflammation or infection
- Whole-body radiographs to rule out systemic disease

Complete:

- Blood lead concentrations
- Advanced imaging (CT/MRI) can be considered

Treatment

Stabilization:

- Seizure control – sedative drugs (e.g. midazolam)
- Hyperthermia – cooling measures, IV or IO fluids if severe
- Hypoglycemia – PO dextrose, IV, IO if not responsive
- Fluid and nutritional support as warranted, see Chapter 8

Continued care

- Antibiotics if sepsis suspected (Table 17.2)
- Chelation if the blood lead level is >25 mg/dl
  - Calcium EDTA 30 mg/kg SC q12h
- Address primary causes of hypoglycemia, hypocalcemia, and other metabolic disease
- Anti-epileptic drugs (monitor plasma levels to guide optimal dosing)
  - Levetiracetam: 20 mg/kg PO q8h; if ineffective, increase dose in 20 mg/kg increment
  - Phenobarbital: 5–20 mg/kg PO q12–24 h
  - Prognosis may be guarded to poor

Musculoskeletal Disease-Fracture

- Traumatic in origin
  - Open-wire exercise wheel, entrapment in cage bars a risk factor for limb fracture, open fracture common
  - Falls from great height – dropped by human
  - Crush trauma – entrapment, under cushions on furniture

Diagnosis

History:

- Trauma may be witnessed (crush, fall)
- May or may not be found with limb trapped
- Inquire about caging and exercise wheels
- Lameness
- Dangling limb
- Hemorrhage if open fracture

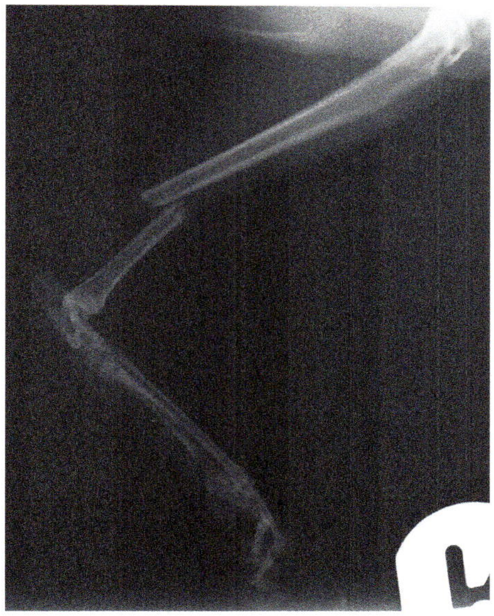

Figure 17.10 Tibial fracture in a chinchilla. These fractures are common in chinchillas and are usually transverse or short spiral.

- Tibial fractures most common; usually transverse or short spiral (Figure 17.10)
  - Tibia longer than femur, fibula virtually non-existent

Signalment:

- Chinchillas of any age or sex

Clinical signs:

- Lameness
- Palpable instability of the limb
- Crepitus
- Displacement of fragments or open fracture may be directly observed
- Dyspnea, thoracic pain if rib fracture
- Incisor fracture possible if fall involved

Differentials:

- Soft tissue trauma
- Neuropathic pain

Diagnostics

STAT:

- Radiographs to identify and characterize fractures

Complete:

- Chemistry – desirable if surgery to be performed

Treatment

Stabilization:

- Analgesia, see Table 17.1

- External coaptation if antebrachial limb fracture; not always well-tolerated by the patient (Figure 17.6)

Continued care:

- Surgical fracture repair – best for ideal alignment and preservation of limb
  - External fixation or coaptation and IM pin
  - Complications including bone-pin loosening, infection, nonunion, necrosis of distal limb, and auto-mutilation
- Limb amputation – usually well-tolerated
- External coaptation and splinting can be used for forelimb fractures distal to elbow
- Cage rest

Cardiopulmonary Disease

Respiratory Tract Disease

Diagnosis

History:

- Uncommon in chinchillas
- Inquire about cage hygiene (frequency, products used [including laundry detergents), ventilation, substrate, and location/frequency of dust bath

Signalment:

- Chinchillas of any age or sex

Clinical10 signs:

- Nasal discharge
- Tachypnea
- Dyspnea, nostril flaring
- Open mouth breathing (only in severe disease since obligate nasal breather)
- Poor body condition
- Poor haircoat
- Sneezing

Differentials – multifactorial:

- Nasal discharge – dental disease, nasal foreign body, rhinitis, megaesophagus, cleft palate, lower respiratory tract disease. If accompanying conjunctivitis, and r/o *P. aeruginosa*
- Pneumonia – usually Gram-negative organisms, *Mycobacteria genavense* reported
- Other rule outs include congestive heart failure, intrathoracic neoplasia, diaphragmatic hernia, and dyspnea secondary to severe metabolic acidosis

Diagnostics

STAT:

- Thoracic radiographs or preferably CT to rule out pneumonia, include skull to assess nasal cavity and teeth

Complete:

- Urine pH and ketones if ketoacidosis suspected
- Thoracic ultrasound to identify abscesses and aid FNA sampling
- CT
- Cytology and bacterial culture (nasal or conjunctival swabs, and aspirates of abscesses)
- CBC – may be unremarkable, may see inflammatory leukogram with monocytosis, anemia of chronic disease

Treatment

Stabilization:

- Oxygen
- Antibiotics (Table 17.2)
  - Enrofloxacin 10 mg/kg SC, IM (diluted) if pneumonia suspected

Continued care:

- Nebulization with antimicrobials (gentamicin 5 mg/ml in 0.9% saline)
- Fluid therapy and nutritional support as needed
- Prognosis may be poor if multidrug-resistant bacteria
- Treat underlying dental disease if present

Cardiac Disease

Diagnosis

History:

- Uncommon in chinchillas. Heart murmurs are a common incidental finding on physical examination in healthy and diseased chinchillas. Most heart murmurs in chinchillas are benign (physiological). Echocardiographic abnormalities are more likely to be found in chinchillas with a grade 3 or higher heart murmur compared to a chinchilla without a heart murmur. However, despite the presence of echocardiographic abnormalities, most chinchillas show no clinical signs. Therefore, the presence of a heart murmur in a chinchilla should be interpreted cautiously

Signalment:

- Chinchillas of any age or sex

Clinical signs:

- Labored breathing
- Weakness
- Lethargy
- Heart murmur

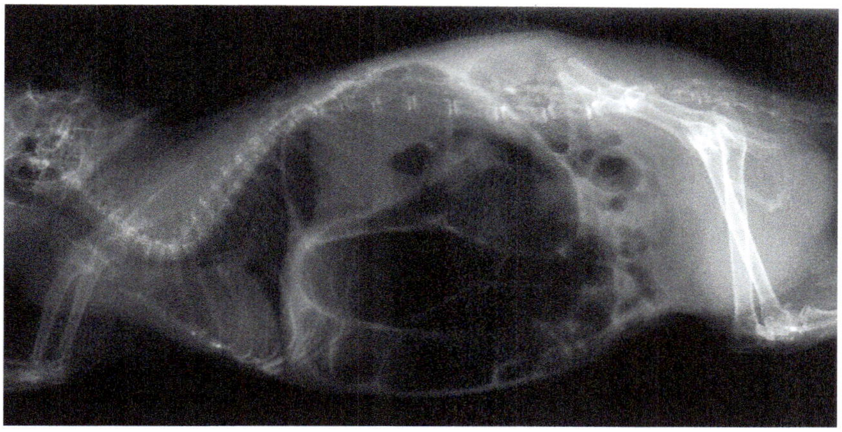

Figure 17.11 Severe tympany in a chinchilla.

Differentials:

- Mitral valve insufficiency
- Dynamic right ventricular outflow tract obstruction
- Tricuspid valve insufficiency
- Left ventricular hypertrophy
- Ventral septal defect
- Dilated cardiomyopathy

Diagnostics:
STAT:

- thoracic radiographs or CT
  - Reference intervals for vertebral heart size based on radiographs (reference interval: 7.5–10.4) or CT (reference interval: 7.1–9.4)

Complete:

- echocardiography
  - Measurements for healthy chinchillas under manual restraint and isoflurane have been published

Treatment

Stabilization:

- Oxygen
- Furosemide 2–4 mg/kg SC, IM q4–6h

Continued care:

- Clinical management not described, base treatment on other species

Gastrointestinal Disease

Dysbacteriosis and Diarrhea

Diagnosis

History:

- Diarrheic feces, feces smeared on cage floor or in the perianal fur. There may be a history of recent diet change or antibiotic use (Figure 17.1)
- Signalment – chinchillas of any age or sex
- Clinical signs – diarrhea with no other clinical signs is possible. The animal may also have reduced food intake and fecal output. Lethargy and dehydration are possible

Differentials:

- Noninfectious causes more common in pet chinchillas
  - Sudden diet change
  - Inappropriate oral antibiotic therapy (penicillins, cephalosporins, erythromycin, and clindamycin); topical therapies (e.g. bacitracin and fusidic acid)
  - Dental disease (see Common presenting signs – dental disease)
  - Constipation
  - Tympany (Figure 17.11)
  - Intussusception
  - Rectal prolapse
  - Any systemic disease processes
- Infectious (parasitic and bacterial) causes more common in farmed or research chinchillas
  - *Yeast (C. guttulatus)* always secondary (Figure 17.2)
  - Giardia
  - Eimeria
  - *Hymenolepis nana* (Mouse tape worm)
  - *Pseudomonas* sp. or Enterobacterial overgrowth (*E. coli, Proteus* sp.)

Diagnostics

STAT:

- Fecal cytology and flotation exam, direct saline smear to identify parasites and yeast
- Whole-body radiographs
- Fecal culture for enteric pathogens

Complete:

- Advanced imaging (ultrasound, CT)

Treatment

Stabilization:

- Fluid therapy and nutritional support, see Chapter 8
- Other supportive care and treatment as indicated based on primary cause

Continued care:

- Antibiotics if infectious cause suspected, ideally based on culture and sensitivity results (i.e. enrofloxacin 10 mg/kg SC diluted in fluids q12h)
- Ideal to avoid oral drug administration until animal is eating and GI function improved
- Well dried, high-quality hay when animal is eating
- If *C. guttulatus* overgrowth, consider nystatin (100000 U/kg PO q8h for 5 days)
- Treatment of endoparasites as in other species (Table 17.3)
- Use caution with metronidazole in chinchillas. Total daily dose should not exceed 20 mg/kg. Consider using tinidazole (20 mg/kg PO q12h) instead

Rectal/intestinal Prolapse

Diagnosis

History:

- Tissue prolapse from rectum noted by owner. Rectal and distal intestinal prolapse frequently occur with intestinal intussusception. The small intestine may be involved in some cases (Figures 17.12 and 17.13)

Signalment:

- Chinchillas of any age or sex; intestinal prolapse from intussusception more common in chinchillas <1 year

Clinical signs

- Straining, diarrhea, constipation, and tissue prolapse from rectum. Abdominal palpation may reveal turgid cylindrical mass reflecting intussuscepted part of intestine; this tissue is usually cyanotic, congested, and may be nonviable

Differentials:

- As under diarrhea
  - Dysbacteriosis
  - Enteritis
  - Constipation
  - Diarrhea
  - Endoparasites

Diagnostics

STAT:

- Assess prolapsed tissue for viability and trauma

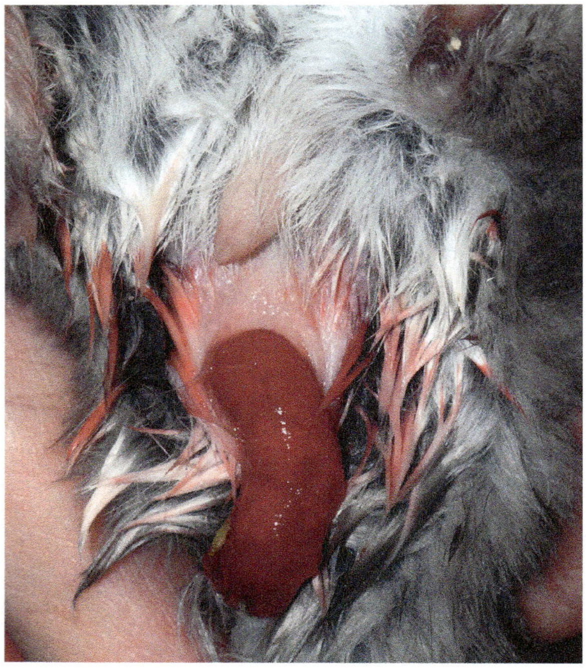

Figure 17.12 Rectal prolapse in a chinchilla with an intussusception.

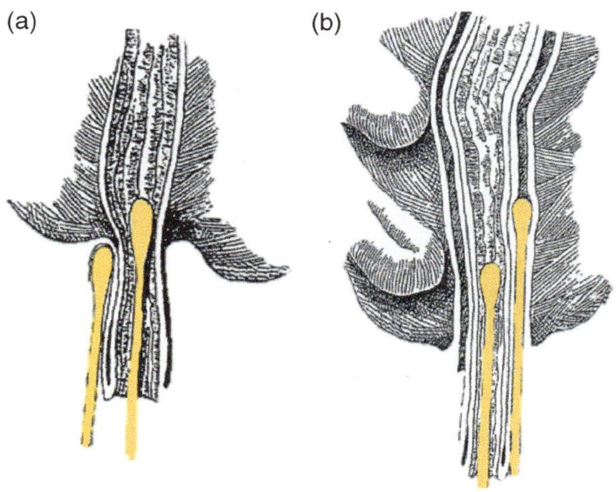

Figure 17.13 Schematic illustrating (a) rectal prolapse vs. (b) rectal prolapse with intussusception.

- If no intussusception
  - Clean and soak edematous prolapsed rectal tissue w/ 50% dextrose
  - Replace prolapsed tissue and place perianal purse-string suture
  - Ensure defecation through suture is possible
- To diagnose intussusception
  - Palpation and ultrasound or CT

- Successful outcome w/ laparotomy and manual correction of proximal intussusception has been reported but overall prognosis poor; recurrence and patient deterioration common

Complete:

- CBC and chemistry to r/o underlying disease
- As described under dysbacteriosis and diarrhea

Treatment

Stabilization:

- Fluid therapy and nutritional support, see Chapter 8
- Other supportive care and treatment as indicated based on primary cause

Continued care:

- See diagnostics for surgical options
- See diarrhea
- Prognosis is poor for intussusception

Tympany

- see also Common presenting signs – gastrointestinal disease

Diagnosis

History:

- Anorexia, lethargy, abdominal distention, recumbent, and decreased fecal output
- Signalment – chinchillas of any age and sex
- Clinical signs – distended and tense abdomen, depression, dyspnea, recumbency, (septic)shock/hypotension, and hypothermia

Differentials:

- Gastroenteritis
- Dysbacteriosis with increased intestinal gas production
- Ileus
- Luminal obstruction (rare)
- Intestinal torsion (rare)
- Others as described under dysbacteriosis and diarrhea

Diagnostics

STAT

- Whole-body radiographs (Figure 17.11)

Complete:

- CBC, chemistry panel
- Advanced imaging to rule out obstruction/torsion (ultrasound or CT)
- As described under dysbacteriosis and diarrhea

Treatment

Stabilization:

- Supportive care as warranted
  - Aggressive fluid therapy, see Chapter 8
  - Thermal support if hypothermia
  - Oxygen may be beneficial
  - Parenteral antibiotics if sepsis suspected (Table 17.2)
  - Analgesia if painful (Table 17.1)
  - Prokinetics contraindicated if infection or obstruction cannot be ruled out
- Orogastric tube placement for gastric decompression in severe cases
  - May lead to collapse and death in decompensated patient

Continued care:

- Based on underlying disease
- Prognosis depends on severity/duration but is usually poor in severe or chronic cases

Urogenital and Reproductive Disease

Urogenital Disease-Urolithiasis

Diagnosis

History:

- Owner may note straining to urinate or blood in urine, hiding behavior, decreased appetite, and fecal production possible. Risk factors for urolithiasis in chinchillas are unknown; unlikely to be high calcium diet as excess dietary calcium is excreted in the feces and not in the urine in chinchillas

Signalment:

- Predominantly male chinchillas very uncommon in female chinchillas

Clinical signs:

- Abdominal pain, stranguria, pollakiuria, enlarged urinary bladder on palpation, gross hematuria, and palpable stones
- Differentials – usually calcium carbonate stones; urinary bladder neoplasia (rare); urinary tract infection (uncommon); pyelonephritis; female – uterine disease; and male – furring, semen-matrix calculi, balanoposthitis and preputial abscesses, paraphimosis, and phimosis

Diagnostics

STAT:

- Urinalysis – hematuria, ±pyuria
- Radiographs – urolith may be identifiable

- Ultrasound – can help better differentiate if calculi are within ureters (usually not associated with lower urinary tract signs), bladder, or urethra
- CBC and chemistry panel – r/o concurrent diseases, e.g. azotemia, electrolyte imbalances, and ketoacidosis

Complete:

- Urine culture
- Stone analysis (post-treatment, usually calcium carbonate)

Treatment

Stabilization:

- Analgesia (Table 17.1)
- Antibiotics if urinary tract infection suspected – collect urine culture sample first if possible (Table 17.2)
- Urinary catheterization if possible, avoid repeated cystocentesis
  - Use caution to avoid bladder rupture during palpation or manipulation

Continued care:

- Stone removal – may only need sedation in females if distal urethra
- Urethral calculi
  - Urinary catheterization with retropulsion into bladder for cystotomy
  - Frequently urethral calculi are embedded and cannot be dislodged. Most chinchillas (75% in one retrospective) with urethral calculi are euthanized w/in 24 hours of diagnosis
- Cystotomy
  - Recommended to treat cystic calculi
  - Recurrence of stones is reported at 50% after surgery
    - Median recurrence time: 68 days
    - Median survival time: 391 days in chinchillas with calculi recurrence; six years in chinchillas without recurrence
  - Closely monitor for recurrence and re-obstruction

Male Reproductive Disease

- Furrings, paraphimosis, phimosis, balanoposthitis, and preputial abscesses

Diagnosis (Figure 17.14)

History:

- May be incidental findings on examination, particularly furrings. Excessive grooming or mutilation may be noted by the owner. Owner may note prolapsed tissue, blood, or abnormal odor. Anuria in some cases of paraphimosis

Signalment:

- Male chinchillas of any age

Clinical signs:

- No signs, hunched posture, overgrooming or mutilation, hematuria, stranguria or anuria, and blood or urine staining of perineum
- Furrings: accumulation of fur at base of glans penis within prepuce, often incidental finding. May predispose to balanoposthitis and paraphimosis with secondary bacterial infection and constriction of glans penis
- Balanoposthitis and preputial abscesses: inflammation of the prepuce and glans penis secondary to infection

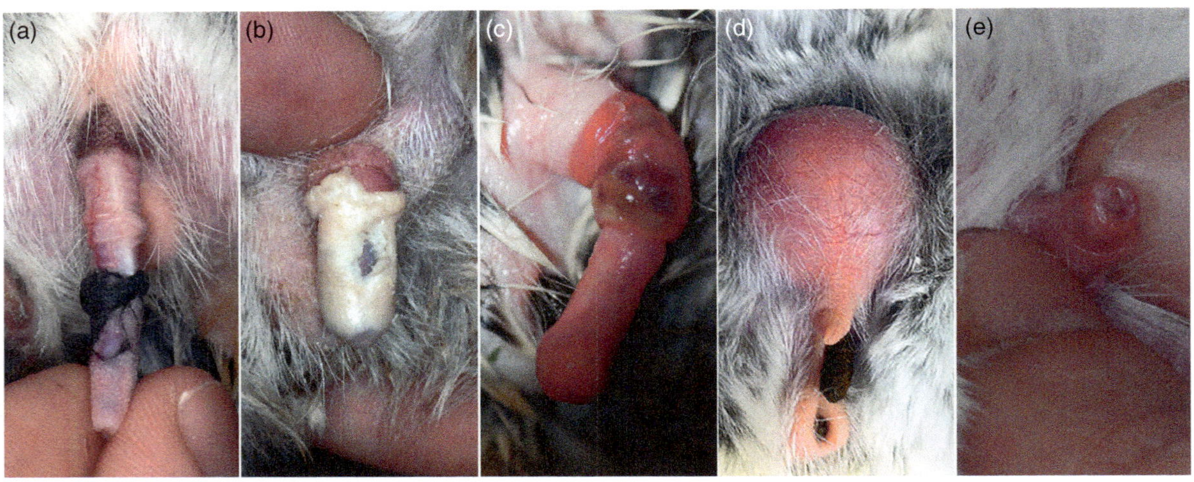

Figure 17.14 Penile disorders in chinchillas. (a) Furring. (b) Smegma accumulation. (c) Balanoposthitis and paraphimosis. (d) Preputial abscess. (e) Phimosis. Source: Mans and Donnelly [3]. Reproduced with permission of Elsevier.

- Paraphimosis: acute severe balanoposthitis or furrings leading to prolapse of the glans from the prepuce with inability to replace
- Phimosis: inability to completely protrude the glans penis from the prepuce or entrapment of the penis within the prepuce. Often subclinical unless balanoposthitis develops

Differentials:

- *Furring*: trauma, occurs most commonly in breeding males
- *Balanoposthitis and preputial abscesses*: *P. aeruginosa* or other bacterial infection, phimosis
- *Paraphimosis*: flaccid paresis of the penis secondary to excessive breeding, separation during copulation, urolithiasis, and stricture
- *Phimosis*: preputial abscesses, adhesion formation between preputial visceral layer and glans penis

Diagnostics

STAT:

- Lubrication and close examination of penis/prepuce following extrusion of glans penis from prepuce. Assess viability of tissue
- Radiographs – rule out cystic calculi, underlying disease

Complete:

- Cytology and culture/sensitivity of masses or abscesses
- Urinalysis – r/o ketoacidosis, urinary tract infection
- Chemistry – r/o concurrent diseases, e.g. azotemia and electrolyte imbalances

Treatment

Stabilization:

- Furring
  - After lubrication and extrusion of penis, remove accumulated fur or smegma and clean penis with chlorhexidine solution
- Balanoposthitis and preputial abscesses:
  - Antibiotics, ideally based on C/S (Table 17.2)
  - Surgical exploration and drainage of abscesses, clean tissue and remove debris. Aspirate preputial abscess and remove by extrusion of glans penis or surgical lancing through prepuce
- Paraphimosis:
  - If tissue viable, clean tissue with chlorhexidine and apply lubricant gel or ointment to facilitate replacement. Do not force replacement if resistance; keep lubricated with petroleum-based ointments/hydrogels three to four times daily until swelling reduced to prevent desiccation
  - Place e-collar if necessary
  - Treat with analgesic, anti-inflammatory, and antibiotic if bacterial balanoposthitis present (Tables 17.1–17.2)
  - Penile amputation and PU could be considered if prolapsed glans penis not visible, but prognosis of procedure not known in chinchillas
- Phimosis:
  - Only treat if balanoposthitis present
  - Resect adhesions between preputial visceral layer and glans penis using magnification and treat preputial abscess if present
  - After removing adhesions, evert glans from prepuce for evaluation
  - Regularly extrude penis after surgery manually and apply ointment; risk of reformation of adhesions possible

Continued care:

- Regularly examine male chinchillas with history of penile disorders and evert glans penis completely during examination

Female Reproductive Disease

- Fetal retention and abortion; endometritis and pyometra; and dystocia

Diagnosis

History:

- May be known history of breeding with fetal resorption, retention, abortion, and dystocia. Endometritis and pyometra reported in farmed chinchillas but increasingly reported in pet chinchillas

Signalment:

- Females of breeding age

Clinical signs:

- Fetal resorption, mummification, retention, and abortion: Vaginal discharge, may be hemorrhagic; soft tissue masses protruding from vaginal opening if leiomyoma. Palpable masses often noted with neoplasia
- Endometritis and pyometra: Weight loss, lethargy, reduced appetite, severe depression, dehydrated, poor body condition. Absence of the vaginal membrane and mucoid, mucopurulent, purulent, or hemorrhagic vaginal discharge that may/may not be malodorous. Note – some mucoid discharge normal during estrus and may not be pathologic

- Dystocia: Restlessness, frequent crying, constant genital attention, and widened vaginal opening. Allantoic fluid or mucohemorrhagic discharge often present

Differentials:

- Fetal resorption, mummification, retention, and abortion: Infectious and noninfectious causes; if hemorrhagic vaginal discharge, consider abortion or fetal/placental retention if housed with male. Neoplasia including leiomyosarcoma, leiomyoma, fibroma, and hemangioma
- Endometritis and pyometra: Cause often not determined. Stump pyometra secondary to incomplete ovariectomy reported
- Dystocia: Single oversized fetus or malpresentation of kit(s); uterine inertia

Diagnostics

STAT:

- Abdominal radiographs and ultrasound
- Vaginal smear to differentiate physiologic and pathologic conditions

Complete:

- Chemistry – r/o concurrent diseases, e.g. hypocalcemia, electrolyte imbalances, and ketoacidosis
- CBC – may see evidence of inflammation or infection
- Culture and sensitivity of discharge

Treatment

Stabilization:

- Treat with fluid therapy and general supportive care based on underlying pathology, administer additional therapy include calcium or dextrose as warranted
- Antibiotic therapy (Table 17.2), may resolve mild cases of endometritis and pyometra
- Dystocia: Lubrication and gentle traction
- Uterine inertia: Oxytocin (0.5–1 IU/kg SC) and calcium gluconate (25–50 mg/kg SC diluted)
- Surgical intervention imperative if labor >4 hours and kits cannot be delivered; Cesarean section survival rate of 67% reported in one study

Continued care:

- Ovariohysterectomy if the ability to breed does not need to be maintained
- Prognosis fair to good depending on concurrent disease (ketosis, sepsis, etc.)

Dermatologic Disease

Dermatophytosis

Diagnosis

History:

- Chinchillas require regular access to a dust bath in order to maintain the normal coat condition. Abnormal appearance of the fur may be caused by lack of dust bathing (greasy, unkempt appearance) or high humidity in the environment. Ectoparasites have not been reported in chinchillas, and therefore should not be included on the differential list for dermatological disorders

Signalment:

- Chinchillas of any age and breed

Clinical signs:

- Scaly patches of alopecia on nose, behind ears, on forefeet. Large, circumscribed areas of inflammation and scab formation

Differentials:

- Fur chewing
- Neoplasia
- Husbandry deficiencies, lack of dust bath

Diagnostics

STAT:

- Skin scrape or tape preparation, cytology. Ectoparasites have not been reported in captive chinchillas

Complete:

- Dermatophyte PCR or culture; ultraviolet light not useful in making diagnosis
- Diagnostic imaging – r/o painful conditions, which may lead to fur chewing, such as dental disease, otitis media
- Biochemistry – r/o underlying conditions, which could lead to fur chewing
- Bacterial culture, biopsy

Treatment

Stabilization:

- Topical therapy: Removes spores from hair shafts – antifungal wipes (i.e. chlorhexidine/2% miconazole wipes), add miconazole powder to dust bath
- Systemic therapy: Removes spores from hair follicles – terbinafine (30 mg/kg PO q24h) preferred treatment, shown to be more effective than itraconazole

Continued care:

- Continue therapy until two negative dermatophyte tests obtained
- Inform owners of zoonotic potential

Ulcerative Pododermatitis

Diagnosis

History:

- Hyperkeratosis, mild erythema, to ulceration and/or infection of the plantar aspect of the hind feet (Figure 17.1)
- Hindlimb lameness
- Risk factors
  - Age
  - Poor cage hygiene
  - Cage design (improper resting floors)
  - Obesity

Signalment:

- Chinchillas, either gender, any age but often older

Clinical signs:

- Erythema and swelling of the plantar foot
- Ulcerative lesion on the plantar metatarsus; tendon and bone involvement with progressed disease
- Lameness
- Obesity common

Differentials:

- Neoplasia
- Trauma

Diagnostics

STAT:

- Radiographs to assess possible osteomyelitis

Complete:

- Bacterial culture of tissue biopsy or aspirate, histopathology of lesion
- CBC – inflammatory leukogram
- Chemistry – usually unremarkable

Treatment

Stabilization:

- Cage modifications, application of petroleum-based ointment might be enough to resolve hyperkeratosis and mild erythema
- Surgical debridement and management of the lesions as open wounds until healing by secondary intention if severe infection
- Bandaging for wound protection and wound care

Continued care:

- Antibiotics – based on C/S, consider TMS (30 mg/kg PO q12h). Azithromycin 30 mg/kg PO q24h, enrofloxacin 10 mg/kg PO q12h (Table 17.2)
- Analgesia as warranted (Table 17.1)
- Obesity management
- Husbandry improvements

Fur Chewing and Fur Slip

Diagnosis

History:

- Fur chewing: Up to 20% of chinchillas in breeding facilities can be affected. Suspected to be maladapted displacement behavior triggered by stress and affecting predominantly stress-sensitive animals. Also common in chinchillas with dental disease or other painful conditions such as otitis media
- Fur slip: Predator avoidance mechanism in chinchillas

Signalment:

- *Fur chewing*: Chinchillas of any age and sex
- *Fur slip*: Recent history of fighting or rough handling

Clinical signs:

- *Fur chewing*: Normal fur on head and distal extremities; shortened fur on dorsum, from lumbar to tail and laterally on flanks
- *Fur slip*: Clean, smooth area of skin where large patch of fur has been released

Differentials:

- *Fur chewing*: Dental disease, otitis media, high-stress chinchilla or environment, lack of hay in diet, and dermatophytosis
- *Fur slip*: Trauma

Diagnostics

STAT:

- *Fur chewing*: See "Dental Disease" and "Head Tilt". Obtaining definitive diagnosis for fur chewing may be difficult
- *Fur slip*: None needed if no suspicion of underlying disease

Complete:

- *Fur chewing*: See "Dental Disease", "Head Tilt", and "Dermatophytosis"
- *Fur slip*: None needed if no suspicion of underlying disease

Treatment

Stabilization:

- *Fur chewing*: See "Dental Disease" and "Head Tilt". Fluoxetine reportedly ineffective in managing. Treat underlying painful conditions. Fur chewing is not a significant threat to animal's health if medical conditions ruled out
- *Fur slip*: None needed if no suspicion of underlying disease. Chinchillas should never be grasped by the fur over the back or flanks. Instead, they should be lifted from underneath. Alternatively, they can be caught by grasping them at the tail base

Continued care:

- *Fur chewing*: See "Dental Disease" and "Head Tilt". Reduce environmental stressors (reduce handling, light, noise, avoid keeping solitary, and offer enrichment items). Increase hay consumption
- *Fur slip*: Evaluate environment and handling techniques. Reduce potential for fighting between conspecifics. Hair may require several months to regrow

Ophthalmic Disease

- Epiphora, conjunctivitis, and corneal diseases: see Common Presenting Signs; Ocular signs
- Corneal trauma and keratitis

Diagnosis

History:

- Corneal surface is large and prominent, and chinchillas lack a protective nictitating membrane, factors that likely predispose chinchillas to corneal trauma. Blepharospasm, ocular discharge, ocular hemorrhage, facial pain, and rubbing at face. History of trauma or rough handling or neurologic signs

Signalment:

- Chinchillas of any age or sex

Clinical signs:

- Blepharospasm, ocular discharge, possible grossly visible corneal defect, loss of anterior chamber depth, or protruding iris if perforated, may lack palpebral reflex (Figure 17.8)

Differentials:

- Conjunctivitis (Figure 17.4), ocular foreign body, retrobulbar mass (rare), fight wound, self-trauma secondary to pruritus, otitis media, and facial nerve paralysis (Figures 17.7–17.9), excessive dust bathing, corneal lipid keratopathy, and cataracts reported in chinchillas

Diagnostics

STAT:

- Fluorescein staining, evaluate ears and examine for palpebral reflex

Complet:

- Full ophthalmologic exam, bacterial and fungal culture if nonhealing ulcer
- CBC/chemistry – unremarkable, but may help diagnosis of underlying disease
- See "Dental Disease", "Head Tilt", and "Ocular Signs"

Treatment

Stabilization:

- As reported for other species
- Topical antibiotic solutions (drops over ointment preferable, particularly if perforated)
  - Ofloxacin
  - Tobramycin
  - Gentamicin
  - Neomycin-polymyxin-bacitracin (prevent ingestion)
- E-collar to prevent self-trauma

Continued care:

- Above sufficient if simple ulceration; see "Ocular Signs"
- Chronic nonhealing ulcers may require corneal debridement or grid keratectomy after treatment of bacterial infection
- Remove access to dust bathing until resolution of signs

References

1 Carpenter, J.W. (2018). Exotic animal formulary, 5e, 460–493. St Louis, MO: Elsevier, Saunders.

2 Hawkins, M.G. and Pascoe, P.J. (2021). Anesthesia, analgesia, and sedation of small mammals. In: Ferrets, Rabbits, and Rodents, 4e (eds. K.E. Quesenberry, C.J. Orcutt, C. Mans and J.W. Carpenter), 536–558. Saint Louis: Elsevier.

3 Mans, C. and Donnelly, T.M. (2021). Chinchillas. In: Ferrets, Rabbits, and Rodents, 4e (eds. K.E. Quesenberry, C.J. Orcutt, C. Mans and J.W. Carpenter), 298–322. Saint Louis: Elsevier.

Further Reading

Doss, G.A., Mans, C., Houseright, R.A., and Webb, J.L. (2016). Urinalysis in chinchillas (*Chinchilla lanigera*). *J. Am. Vet. Med. Assoc.* 248 (8): 901–907.

Mans, C. and Jekl, V. (2016). Anatomy and Disorders of the Oral Cavity of Chinchillas and Degus. *Vet. Clin. North Am. Exot. Anim. Pract.* 19 (3): 843–869.

Fox, L., Snyder, L.B., and Mans, C. (2016). Comparison of dexmedetomidine–ketamine with isoflurane for anesthesia of chinchillas (*Chinchilla lanigera*). *J. Am. Assoc. Lab. Anim. Sci.* 55 (3): 312–316.

Ozawa, S., Mans, C., Szabo, Z., and Di Girolamo, N. (2017). Epidemiology of bacterial conjunctivitis in chinchillas (*Chinchilla lanigera*): 49 cases (2005 to 2015). *J. Small Anim. Pract.* 58 (4): 238–245.

Martel-Arquette, A. and Mans, C. (2016). Urolithiasis in chinchillas: 15 cases (2007 to 2011). *J. Small Anim. Pract.* 57 (5): 260–264.

Mans, C. and Donnelly, T.M. (2013). Update on diseases of chinchillas. *Vet. Clin. North Am. Exot. Anim. Pract.* 16 (2): 383–406.

Kraft, H. (1987). Diseases of Chinchillas, 141. T.F.H. Publications Inc.

Doerning, B.J., Brammer, D.W., and Rush, H.G. (1993). *Pseudomonas aeruginosa* infection in a *Chinchilla lanigera*. *Lab. Anim.* 27 (2): 131–133.

Fehr, M. (2015). Chinchilla [German]. In: Krankheiten der Heimtiere, 8e (eds. M. Fehr, L. Sassenburg and P. Zwart), 207–237. Hannover: Schluetersche.

Pignon, C., Sanchez-Migallon Guzman, D., Sinclair, K. et al. (2012). Evaluation of heart murmurs in chinchillas (*Chinchilla lanigera*): 59 cases (1996–2009). *J. Am. Vet. Med. Assoc.* 241 (10): 1344–1347.

18

Rats and Mice

Kristin M. Sinclair

Kensington Bird and Animal Hospital Kensington, Connecticut, USA

CONTENTS

Unique Species Considerations

Rats and mice can be a challenge to diagnose and treat, given their small size and agility. Diagnostics such as radiographs and venipuncture often require sedation, and only a limited volume of blood may be spared even in a healthy rodent. Oral medications should ideally be very palatable or concealed within a delicious vehicle (applesauce, peanut butter, etc.). They may have a limited patience for handling and restraint, making advance preparation and consolidation of treatments key to success.

Common Presenting Signs

Anorexia

- This is a nonspecific finding, but often a sign of significant pain or disease

Diagnosis

History:

- Partial or complete cessation of food intake
- Changes in food preferences
- Other abnormalities may be seen, reflecting the primary cause of illness

Exotic Animal Emergency and Critical Care Medicine, First Edition. Edited by Jennifer E. Graham, Grayson A. Doss and Hugues Beaufrère.

- Note any recent changes in housing or offered diet

Signalment:

- Rats and mice, any age or sex

Differentials:

- Numerous, as any painful condition or illness may lead to anorexia

Diagnostics

STAT:

- *CBC*: May be normal, but may see evidence of inflammation, anemia
- *Chemistry*: Changes will reflect primary disease
- *Radiographs*: Pneumonia common in rats, will also help determine whether other lesions present

Complete:

- *Thoracic and abdominal ultrasound*: Follow-up on STAT diagnostic findings
- *Urinalysis*: UTI not common, but may find evidence of urolithiasis or to support renal disease

Treatment

Stabilization:

- *Nutritional support*: Offer favorite food items, syringe feed as needed. Some owners report success using a small amount of peanut butter, applesauce, or strawberry or banana-flavored nutritional beverages to entice a rat to eat
- Fluid therapy, see Chapter 8
- Analgesics as indicated
  - Meloxicam 1–2 mg/kg PO or SC q24h
  - Buprenorphine 0.02–0.5 mg/kg SC, IV, or IM q6–12h
  - Hydromorphone 0.1–0.5 mg/kg SC or IM q6–8h
  - Tramadol 5–20 mg/kg PO q12–24h
  - Gabapentin: 10–30 mg/kg PO q8h

Continued care:

- Will depend on diagnosis.

Dyspnea

- Most common emergency presentation for rats, often pneumonia

Diagnosis

History:

- Labored breathing
- Grossly audible respiratory noise (wheezing, stertor, and sneezing)
- Fluffed haircoat
- Weight loss
- Inappetence or anorexia
- Inquire about cage hygiene (frequency of cleaning, products used), substrate, use of scented items in the vicinity of the cage, and number of animals in the cage
- Inquire about health of past and current cage mates

Signalment:

- Rats and mice, often older but any age possible, any sex

Differentials:

- Pneumonia
- Congestive heart failure
- Pulmonary or intranasal neoplasia
- URI
- Inadequate cage hygiene

Diagnostics

STAT:

- *Thoracic radiographs*: May see evidence of pneumonia (though pulmonary parenchyma may appear normal), pulmonary nodules or other soft tissue masses, and cardiomegaly

Complete:

- Thoracic ultrasound if pulmonary masses identified
- Fine-needle aspirate of masses or abscesses for cytology +/or culture
- Echocardiogram
- Infectious disease serology

Treatment

Stabilization:

- Oxygen
- Nebulization – 0.9% saline a reasonable initial choice
- Nutritional and fluid support, see Chapter 8
- Sedation may be helpful if the patient is significantly dyspneic and agitated

Continued care:

- Antibiotics if pneumonia or URI suspected
  - Enrofloxacin 5–20 mg/kg PO or SC q12h (limit SC use and/or dilute with SC fluids to avoid tissue inflammation)
  - Doxycycline 5 mg/kg PO q12h
  - Azithromycin 15–30 mg/kg PO q24h (once-daily dosing may be ideal for patients that are difficult to medicate)
- Bronchodilator helpful in pneumonia cases
  - Aminophylline 50 mg/kg PO or SC
  - Theophylline 10 mg/kg PO q8–12h
  - Albuterol inhaler can help if tolerated
- Nebulization if tolerated

- Sildenafil citrate (5 mg/kg PO q24h) has been reported to protect pulmonary vasculature in *Mycoplasma* pneumonia
- Treatment of congestive heart failure if present
  - Furosemide 0.3–4 mg/kg PO, SC, IM, IV q12–24h
  - Enalapril 0.5–1 mg/kg PO q24h
  - Pimobendan 0.2–0.4 mg/kg PO q12h

Neurologic Signs

- Uncommon, prognosis often poor

Diagnosis

History:

- Ataxia
- Pelvic limb paresis or paralysis more common than pectoral limb
- Facial paralysis
- Seizures
- Head tilt, torticollis, and circling

Signalment:

- Rats and mice, any sex, any age possible but generally older

Differentials:

- Pituitary adenoma
- Otitis media, otitis interna
- Spinal cord degeneration of elder rats
- Hypoglycemia
- Hepatic encephalopathy
- Trauma
- Heat stroke
- Lymphocytic choriomeningitis virus (mice)

Diagnostics

STAT:

- *CBC*: May be normal, may see inflammatory leukogram with otitis or trauma
- *Chemistry*: Blood glucose and hepatic parameters of biggest concern
  - i-STAT or glucometer will suffice for blood glucose (BG) measurement if blood sample is small
- *Radiographs*: Rule out spinal fracture, hepatomegaly

Complete:

- CT of skull

Treatment

Stabilization:

- *Seizure control*: Midazolam 0.5 mg/kg IM
- Fluid support, see Chapter 8
- Dextrose (IV, PO) as indicated for hypoglycemia

Continued care:

- Padded and safe caging to prevent self-injury
  - Owner may need to renovate home cage to remove ramps, high hammocks, and wheels; cover wire floors, eliminate, or limit opportunity to climb
- Nutritional support if anorectic
- Trauma or otitis
  - Meloxicam 1–2 mg/kg PO or SC q24h
  - Enrofloxacin 5–20 mg/kg PO or SC q12h
- Cabergoline (pituitary adenoma) 0.6 mg/kg PO or SC q72h

Ocular Signs

- Chromodacryorrhea, ocular trauma, and conjunctivitis

Diagnosis

History:

- Unilateral or bilateral red non-hemorrhagic oculonasal discharge (Figure 18.1)
- Epiphora
- Mucoid ocular discharge (Figure 18.2)
- Corneal opacity
- Grossly visible corneal defect
- Blepharospasm
- Chemosis
- Proptosis
- May note predisposing lesion such as exophthalmia or facial paralysis (Figure 18.1)
- Inquire about any cage mates and interactions (possible fights)

Signalment:

- Rats and mice, any age or sex

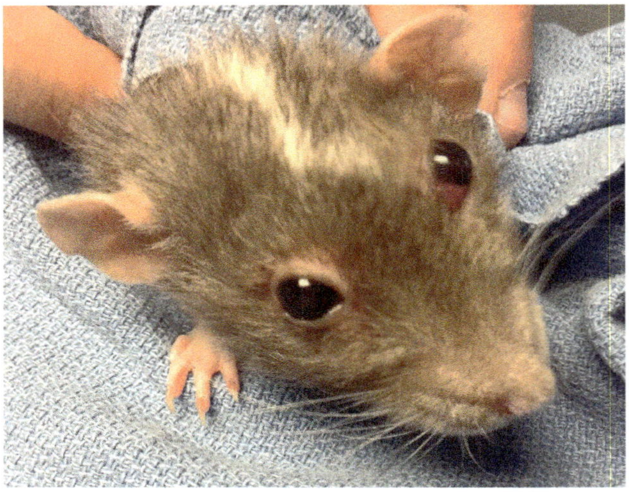

Figure 18.1 Chromodacryorrhea in a rat, right eye. Note the exophthalmia on the left side (suspected retrobulbar abscess).

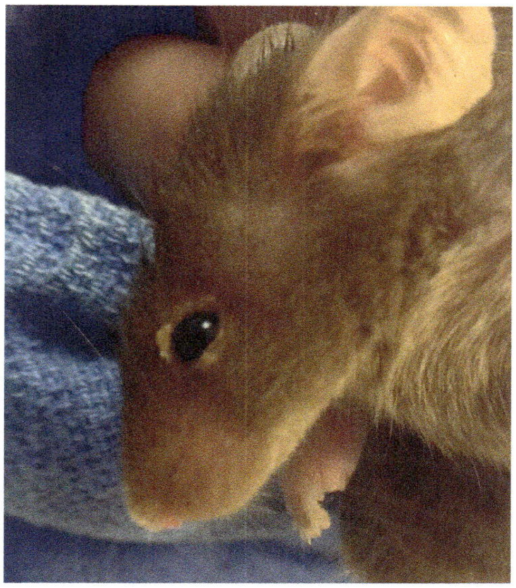

Figure 18.2 Mucoid ocular discharge in a mouse.

Differentials:

- Conspecific trauma to eyelids
- Corneal ulceration
- Inadequate cage hygiene
- Retrobulbar mass
  - Neoplasia
  - Tooth root abscess
- Sialodacryoadenitis virus (SDAV)
- Bacterial conjunctivitis (*Streptococcus* spp., *Mycoplasma pulmonis*, and others)
- Chromodacryorrhea is generally secondary to other stressors

Diagnostics

STAT:

- Fluorescein stain to rule out corneal ulceration

Complete:

- *CBC*: Nonspecific findings, possible inflammatory leukogram
- *Chemistry*: Generally normal, ideal if surgery required
- *Radiographs*: Rule out tooth root lesions, bone lysis associated with infection or neoplasia
- *Thoracic and abdominal ultrasound*: While not specific to the eye, useful in detecting disease processes leading to chromodacryorrhea

Treatment:

- Topical ophthalmic ointments tend to leave the surrounding fur greasy and encourage the rat to groom the area; when possible, ophthalmic solutions may be ideal to avoid inadvertent corneal self-trauma

Stabilization:

- Topical ±systemic analgesics if ulceration identified
  - Meloxicam 1–2 mg/kg PO or SC q24h
  - Tramadol 5–20 mg/kg PO q12–24h
  - Gabapentin 10–30 mg/kg PO q8h
  - Atropine ophthalmic solution
- Flurbiprofen ophthalmic solution may be used if no ulceration identified

Continued care:

- Corneal ulcer, ocular trauma
  - Topical antibiotic
    - Neomycin–polymyxin–bacitracin ophthalmic solution
      - Avoid the preparation with dexamethasone due to risk of localized immunosuppression
    - Tobramycin ophthalmic solution
    - Gentamicin ophthalmic solution
    - Ofloxacin ophthalmic solution
  - Systemic antibiotic may be indicated if significant trauma to globe or conjunctiva
    - Enrofloxacin 5–20 mg/kg PO q12h
    - Trimethoprim-sulfa 15–30 mg/kg PO q12h
- Chromodacryorrhea – focus on treating primary lesion, reducing stress

Trauma

Diagnosis

History:

- Traumatic incident may not be witnessed, but wounds may be noted afterwards
- Owner may report the patient caught by or "playing" with a predator species (dog, cat)
- Lameness or limb paresis
- Blood may be seen on cage furnishings or substrate, but not on the patient due to grooming habits
- In some cases, a bite wound may necrose and/or abscess a few days later

Signalment:

- Rats and mice, any age or sex

Differentials:

- Conspecific fights
- Falls within cage, or from owner's arms or shoulder
- Crush trauma (hiding under couch or chair cushions, inside a recliner, or trapped under falling items)
- Predator trauma

- Limb entrapment within wire exercise wheels or cage bars may lead to secondary limb fracture, limb edema, or neurologic injury as the animal attempts to free itself
- Ulcerative dermatitis
- Acariasis and self-excoriation
- Intervertebral disk disease (IVDD), peripheral neuropathy

Diagnostics

STAT:

- Radiographs to determine if fracture present
  - Be sure to assess the entire body, as multiple injuries possible
- PCV if blood loss is a concern

Complete:

- Thoracic and abdominal ultrasound to further identify internal injury
- *Chemistry*: May be normal, may see elevations in CK with muscle trauma, increased liver enzymes in crush trauma

Treatment

Stabilization:

- *Analgesia*
  - Meloxicam 1–2 mg/kg PO or SC q24h
  - Buprenorphine 0.02–0.5 mg/kg SC or IM q6–12h
  - Hydromorphone 0.1 mg/kg SC or IM q8–12h
  - Gabapentin 10–30 mg/kg PO q8h
  - Tramadol 5–20 mg/kg PO q12–24h
- Wound care (cleansing/lavage, shaving fur, and laceration repair) – local block and sedation may be required
- Splinting of fractured limbs (if possible) until definitive treatment can be pursued

Continued care:

- Laceration repair
- Bandage management if secondary intention healing
- Fracture repair, limb amputation
- Antibiotics as indicated (bite wounds and open wounds)
  - Trimethoprim-sulfa 15–30 mg/kg PO q12h
  - Enrofloxacin 5–20 mg/kg PO q12h
  - Amoxicillin-clavulanic acid 20 mg/kg PO q12h

Systemic Disease

Heat Stroke

Diagnosis

History:

- Often seen in summer months, but possible on any warm day. The patient may have been in a warm room without air conditioning (above 75–77 °F) in a hot car (even for a short time), or in a cage located in front of a sunny window

Signalment:

- Any age, gender, or species

Clinical signs:

- Hyperthermia (rectal temperature > 100), lethargy, obtunded mentation, tachypnea, dyspnea, seizures, hemorrhage, and death
- Normal rectal temperature is approximately 98–100 °F

Differentials:

- Severe fever due to inflammation or infection

Diagnostics

STAT:

- Rectal temperature and history usually suffice for diagnosis

Complete:

- CBC/chemistry ideal to assess organ function, but may lead to increased morbidity if coagulopathy present

Treatment

Stabilization:

- Cooling via lukewarm water baths, fans, and removing cage linings and towels
- IV or IO fluids ideal but may not be feasible if cardiovascular instability present
- SC fluids
- IV or IO mannitol if concern for increased intracranial pressure (ICP)

Continued care:

- Prognosis poor, depending on degree and duration of hyperthermia – euthanasia may be warranted
- Gastrointestinal protectants
  - Sucralfate 25–100 mg/kg PO q8–12h
- Nutritional support

Neurologic and Musculoskeletal Disease

Neurologic-Head Tilt

Diagnosis

History:

- Head tilt, rolling, circling, ataxia, and anorexia

Signalment:

- Rats, less commonly mice; older rats more common with neoplasia

Clinical signs:

- Head tilt, torticollis, nystagmus, ataxia, and thin body condition

Differentials:

- *M. pulmonis* – rats, less likely mice; extension of respiratory infection into otitis media/interna
- *Streptococcus pneumonia* – otitis media in rats
- Zymbal's gland neoplasia – can lead to secondary otitis if it is large enough to impede drainage from ear or allow debris retention
- Pituitary neoplasia – older rats, especially females

Diagnostics

STAT:

- Radiographs – rule out otitis media, pulmonary disease (*M. pulmonis*)

Complete:

- CT of brain/skull
- Serology (*M. pulmonis*)
- Culture and sensitivity (myringotomy)

Treatment

Stabilization:

- Meloxicam 1–2 mg/kg PO or SC q24h
- Enrofloxacin (5–20 mg/kg PO q12h) +/or doxycycline (5 mg/kg PO q12h) if *M. pulmonis* suspected
- Fluid and nutritional support if anorectic

Continued care:

- Prognosis generally guarded to poor, but some may learn to function with persistent head tilt
- Cage modification for accessibility and safety
- Enrofloxacin (5–20 mg/kg PO q12h) may be useful with otitis
- Cabergoline for pituitary neoplasia (0.6 mg/kg PO q72h)
- Dietary restriction and low-protein diet might influence development of pituitary neoplasia

Neurologic-Hindlimb Paresis

Diagnosis

History:

- May be traumatic or degenerative in origin, but latter may have a seemingly rapid onset, progressive hindlimb paresis, and paralysis in older rats; traumatic injury may or may not be seen but onset acute

Signalment:

- Trauma may entail any age, sex, and both rats and mice; degenerative tends to be seen in older (>2 years) rats, males more commonly than females

Clinical signs:

- Loss of proprioception, hindlimb ataxia, hindlimb motor deficits, hindlimb muscle atrophy

Differentials:

- Degenerative disease, radiculoneuropathy of elder rats – spinal nerve root degeneration and demyelination, generally progressive
- Spinal trauma
- IVDD
- Spinal neoplasia
- Osteoarthritis or ulcerative pododermatitis may mimic clinical signs

Diagnostics:

STAT:

- Radiographs to rule out spinal trauma

Complete:

- CBC, chemistry – unremarkable

Treatment

Stabilization:

- Analgesia if known or suspected trauma
  - Meloxicam 1–2 mg/kg PO or SC q24h
  - Buprenorphine 0.02–0.5 mg/kg SC or IM q6–12h
  - Hydromorphone 0.1 mg/kg SC or IM q8–12h
  - Tramadol 5–20 mg/kg PO q12–24h

Continued care:

- Physical therapy
- Cage ameliorations to accommodate limited mobility
- Hygienic care

Neurologic-Seizures

Diagnosis

History:

- Owner may witness the seizure, or may find the pet postictal; hot days during summer or leaving pet in car are risk factors for heat stroke

Signalment:

- No age, gender, and species predilection

Clinical signs:

- Status epilepticus; postictal behavior; hyperthermia

Differentials:

- Heat stroke
- Lead toxicosis
- Lymphocytic choriomeningitis virus (LCMV) – zoonotic, often asymptomatic in rodents, uncommon in rats but mice can be carriers
- Hypoglycemia
- Hypocalcemia may mimic seizures
- Hepatic encephalopathy

Diagnostics

STAT:

- Chemistry or i-STAT to assess glucose, iCa, liver enzymes

Complete:

- Serology or PCR testing (rodent infectious disease panels available)
- Blood lead concentrations
- Radiology to rule out other systemic disease
- Abdominal ultrasound

Treatment

Stabilization:

- *Seizure control*: Midazolam 0.5 mg/kg IM
- *Hyperthermia*: IV or IO fluids, cooling measures
- *Hypoglycemia*: IV or PO dextrose

Continued care:

- *LCMV*: Euthanasia indicated
- *Chelation*:
  - Calcium EDTA 30 mg/kg SC q12h
- Address primary causes of hypoglycemia, hypocalcemia, and hepatic encephalopathy

Musculoskeletal Disease-Fracture

- Traumatic in origin
  - Open-wire exercise wheel, entrapment in cage bars a risk factor for limb fracture, open fracture common
  - Falls from great height – dropped by human
  - Crush trauma – entrapment, under cushions on furniture

Diagnosis

History:

- Trauma may be witnessed (crush, fall)
- May or may not be found with limb trapped
  - Inquire about caging, exercise wheels
- Lameness
- Dangling limb
- Hemorrhage if open fracture

Signalment:

- Any age or sex, rats or mice

Clinical signs:

- Lameness
- Palpable instability of the limb
- Crepitus
- Displacement of fragments or open fracture may be directly observed
- Dyspnea, thoracic pain if rib fracture
- Tooth crown fracture if fall involved

Differentials:

- Soft tissue trauma
- Neuropathic pain

Diagnostics

STAT:

- Radiographs to identify and characterize fractures (Figure 18.3)

Complete:

- *CBC*: Inflammatory leukogram, anemia if significant blood loss

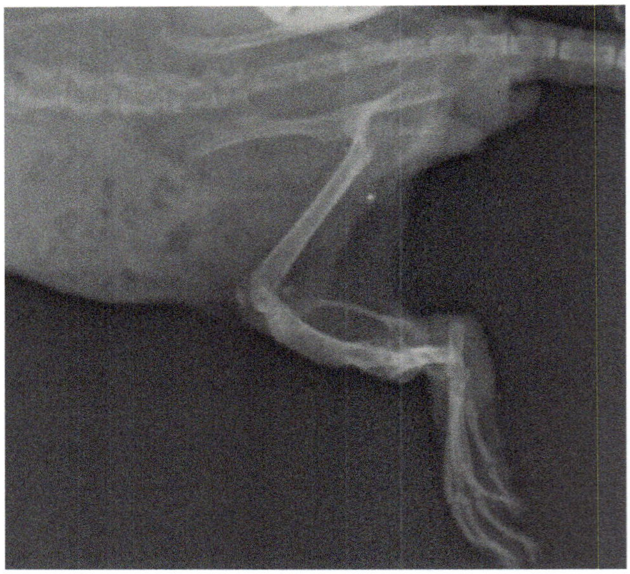

Figure 18.3 Malunion healing of a tibial and fibular fracture in a mouse. This mouse was presented for other reasons, but the fracture was noted on examination.

- *Chemistry*: Unremarkable, but desirable if surgery to be performed.

Treatment

Stabilization:

- *Analgesia*:
  - Meloxicam 1–2 mg/kg PO or SC q24h
  - Hydromorphone 0.1 mg/kg SC or IM q8–12h
  - Tramadol 5–20 mg/kg PO q12–24h
  - Gabapentin 10–30 mg/kg PO q8h
- External coaptation of limb fracture – not always well-tolerated by the patient

Continued care:

- Surgical fracture repair – best for ideal alignment and preservation of limb
- Limb amputation – usually well-tolerated
- External coaptation – not generally feasible but may be tolerated by some patients.
- Cage rest

Cardiopulmonary Disease

Respiratory Disease-Pneumonia

Diagnosis

History:

- Sneezing, cough, grossly audible wheezing and rhonchi (owners often describe "snuffling" or "rattling" noises), dyspnea, weight loss, and chromodacryorrhea
- Inquire about cage hygiene (frequency, products used [including laundry detergents]), substrate

Signalment:

- Any age, gender, or breed, but severity tends to increase with age in rats

Clinical signs:

- Dyspnea, cough, sneezing, nasal discharge, tachypnea, rales, rhonchi, audible respiratory stertor, chromodacryorrhea, and nasal discharge (*Corynebacterium kutscheri*); some rats asymptomatic in the face of severe pulmonary lesions

Differentials:

- Multifactorial
  - *Mice*: *M. pulmonis*, Sendai virus in neonates and weanlings, pneumonia virus of mice
  - *Rats*: *M. pulmonis*, *S. pneumonia*, and *C. kutscheri* are the more important pathogens; Sendai virus, CAR bacillus, others are minor copathogens
  - *Husbandry*: Bedding, cage hygiene, and ventilation
  - Immune response to infection may lead to airway destruction with loss of villi, bronchiectasis, abscess formation
  - *Rule outs*: Upper respiratory infection, congestive heart failure, and intrathoracic neoplasia

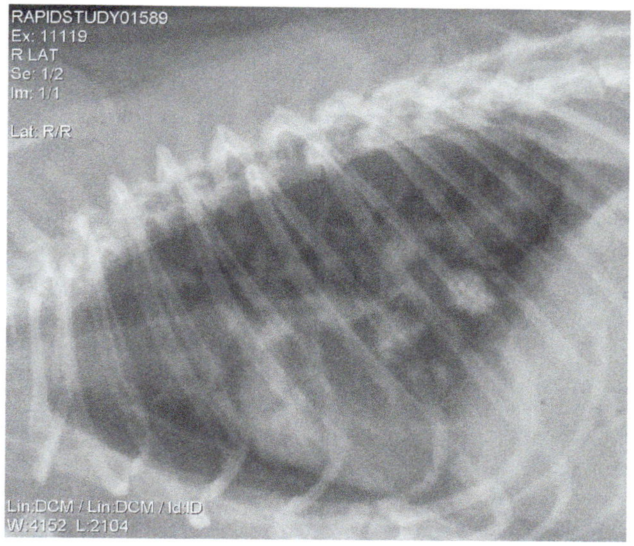

Figure 18.4 Thoracic radiograph of a rat with severe *Mycoplasma pneumonia* and abscess formation. On necropsy, the nodules noted on this radiograph were found to be pulmonary abscesses.

Diagnostics

STAT:

- Radiographs – may be unremarkable, may see nodules corresponding to abscessation, pulmonary infiltrates (Figure 18.4)

Complete:

- CBC – may be unremarkable, may see inflammatory leukogram with monocytosis, anemia of chronic disease
- Thoracic ultrasound to identify abscesses and aid fine needle aspirate (FNA) sampling
- CT to identify pulmonary lesions
- Serology/PCR (*M. pulmonis*, viral etiologies)
- Culture (aspirates)
- Gram stain of nasal discharge (*C. kutscheri*)

Table 18.1 Drugs commonly used in the management of respiratory disease in rats and mice.

Drug	Dosage	Notes
Antibiotics		
Doxycycline	5 mg/kg PO q12h	Often used concurrently with enrofloxacin
Doxycycline, long-acting formulation	70–100 mg/kg SC or IM q7d	Can be advantageous with dyspneic rodent that cannot tolerate oral dosing; dose volume is often large and may need to be split into several injection sites if administered IM
Enrofloxacin	5–20 mg/kg PO q12h	Often used concurrently with doxycycline
Azithromycin	15–30 mg/kg PO q24h	Once-daily dosing advantageous with dyspneic or fractious rodent
Chloramphenicol	30–50 mg/kg PO q8–12h	Warn owner of human risk
Amoxicillin-clavulanic acid	20 mg/kg PO q12h	Ineffective against *M. pulmonis*, but may control secondary bacterial infection
Bronchodilators		
Aminophylline	50 mg/kg PO or SC	
Theophylline	10 mg/kg PO q8–12h	Commercially available pediatric suspension; dosing volume tends to be large and may be unacceptable to dyspneic rats
Albuterol	0.05 mg/kg PO q12h	
Nebulizing agents		
Isotonic saline 0.9%	15 min q8–12h	
Hypertonic saline 7%	15 min q12h	
Albuterol	One puff into nebulizing chamber	
Aminophylline	3 mg/ml in sterile water or saline[a] or 25 mg/ml in 9 ml sterile water	
Acetylcysteine	22 mg/ml in sterile water[a]	
Terbutaline	0.02 mg/kg in 9 ml sterile saline[a]	
		General notes on nebulization: This is often best accomplished by placing the rodent in a chamber apparatus rather than holding a mask or mouthpiece to their face
Miscellaneous		
Meloxicam	1–2 mg/kg PO or SC q24h	Commercially available oral suspension and injectable formulations very amenable to use in rats and mice
Carprofen	2–5 mg/kg PO or SC q12h	
Sildenafil citrate	5 mg/kg PO q24h	Protects pulmonary vasculature from structural changes and fibrosis

[a] Extrapolated from avian nebulization doses.

Treatment

Stabilization:

- Oxygen
- Nebulization (see Table 18.1)
- Bronchodilator (see Table 18.1)

Continued care:

- Antibiotics (doxycycline and enrofloxacin usually the first choice – see Table 18.1)
- Bronchodilators
- Nebulization
- Fluid therapy and nutritional support as needed

Respiratory Disease-Upper Respiratory Infection

Diagnosis

History:

- Sneezing, dyspnea, weight loss, chromodacryorrhea, and anorexia

Signalment:

- Any age, gender, or species

Clinical signs:

- Dyspnea, sneezing, respiratory stertor, and stridor
- Obligate nasal breathers – eating and drinking difficult if severe congestion

Differentials:

- Similar spectrum of pathogens as seen with pneumonia
  - *Mice*: Sendai virus in adults, *M. pulmonis* can cause suppurative rhinitis
  - *Rats*: Sialodacryoadenitis virus
  - *Rule outs*: Neoplasia, tooth root abscess

Diagnostics

STAT:

- Thoracic radiographs to rule out pneumonia, include skull to assess nasal cavity and tooth roots

Complete:

- CBC (inflammatory leukogram)
- Chemistry (nonspecific)

Treatment

Stabilization:

- Oxygen, nebulization if in respiratory distress.

Continued care:

- Antibiotics (doxycycline, enrofloxacin, and others – see Table 18.1)
- NSAID may help if significant congestion
  - Meloxicam 1–2 mg/kg PO q24h
- Nebulization – see Table 18.1
- Fluid therapy, nutritional support as needed

Gastrointestinal Disease

Diarrhea

Diagnosis

History:

- Diarrheic feces, appetite, and attitude generally remain normal if dietary; those with infectious causes may be anorectic

Signalment:

- Young rodents more common with infectious disease, whereas dietary factors can affect any age, no gender predilection

Clinical signs:

- Diarrhea, dehydration, and weight loss

Differentials:

- Tyzzer's disease (*Clostridium piliforme*)
- Other bacterial pathogens (many)
- Viral (rats) – infectious diarrhea of infant rats, coronavirus; rare in mice outside lab setting
- Cestodiasis – potential zoonosis
- Spironucleus, Giardia
- Cryptosporidiosis (mice)

Diagnostics

STAT:

- Fecal flotation examination, direct saline smear to identify protozoa or cestodes

Complete:

- Fecal culture
- Serology (*C. piliforme*)
- Intestinal histopathology, culture

Treatment

Stabilization:

- Fluid therapy
- Nutritional support
- Other supportive care as indicated

Continued care:

- Antibiotics based on culture and sensitivity results
- Cestodiasis – Praziquantel 6–10 mg/kg PO or SC, repeated in 10 days
- Protozoa
  - Metronidazole 20 mg/kg PO q12h
  - Tetracycline 10–20 mg/kg PO q12h
  - Fenbendazole 20 mg/kg PO q24h for five days.
- Analgesia may be beneficial if abdominal pain present
  - Meloxicam 1–2 mg/kg PO q24h (avoid if GI ulceration suspected)
  - Buprenorphine 0.02–0.5 mg/kg SC or IM q6–12h
  - Tramadol 5–20 mg/kg PO q12–24h

Urogenital and Reproductive Disease

Urogenital Disease-Urolithiasis

Diagnosis

History:

- Dysuria, hematuria, and bloody discharge may be mistaken for vaginal discharge in females

Signalment:

- Any age or gender

Clinical signs:

- Abdominal pain, stranguria, enlarged urinary bladder on palpation, and gross hematuria. May be able to grossly distinguish hemorrhage from urethra vs. vulva (external orifices are separate in rats and mice)

Differentials:

- Urinary bladder neoplasia, UTI, uterine disease (females), and pyelonephritis

Diagnostics

STAT:

- *Urinalysis*: Hematuria, ±pyuria
- *Radiographs*: Urolith may be identifiable (Figures 18.5 and 18.6)

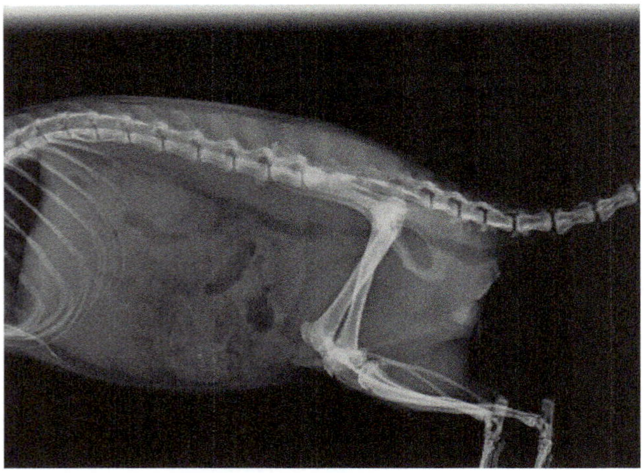

Figure 18.5 Abdominal radiograph of a female rat with an urethrolith.

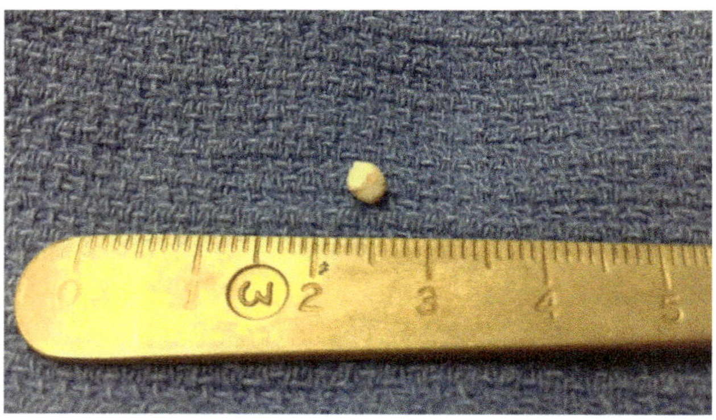

Figure 18.6 This is the urethrolith identified radiographically in Figure 18.5.

- ±Ultrasound

Complete:

- CBC, chemistry – azotemia if obstructed, inflammatory leukogram
- Urine culture
- Stone analysis

Treatment

Stabilization:

- *Analgesia*:
  - Meloxicam 1–2 mg/kg PO or SC q24h
  - Buprenorphine 0.02–0.5 mg/kg SC, IV, or IM q6–12h
  - Hydromorphone 0.1 mg/kg SC or IM q6–8h
  - Tramadol 5–20 mg/kg PO q12–24h
  - Gabapentin 10–30 mg/kg PO q8h
- Antibiotics (collect urine culture sample first if possible)
  - Enrofloxacin 5–20 mg/kg PO q12h
  - Amoxicillin-clavulanic acid 20 mg/kg PO q12h
  - Choice ideally determined by urine culture and sensitivity results
- Urinary catheterization if possible, avoid repeated cystocentesis unless necessary

Continued care:

- Stone removal – may only need sedation in females if distal urethra
- Cystotomy
- Urethrotomy

Renal Failure

Diagnosis

History:

- Many causes are more chronic in nature; presentation may be acute-on-chronic, polyuria, polydipsia, weight loss, anorexia, hematuria, and abnormal posture

Signalment:

- Older rats and mice; males prone to obstruction secondary to preputial and bulbourethral gland abscessation; female rats more prone to nephrocalcinosis

Clinical signs:

- Hunched posture, abdominal pain, hematuria, stranguria, polyuria, and thin body condition

Differentials:

- Hydronephrosis
- Pyelonephritis – *Pseudomonas aeruginosa*, *Proteus mirabilis*, *Staphylococcus aureus*, LCMV, *Leptospira* spp.
- Amyloidosis

- Chronic progressive glomerulopathy/nephropathy (CPN) – older rats, often male
- Obstruction
- Nephocalcinosis – female rats more common

Diagnostics

STAT:

- *Chemistry*: Elevations in BUN, creatinine, phosphorus; hypokalemia
- *CBC*: anemia of chronic disease, inflammatory leukogram if acute
- *Urinalysis*: proteinuria normal but can see severe proteinuria, isosthenuria in chronic disease; pyuria, hematuria if more acute
- *Radiographs*: rule out cystic calculi, renomegaly

Complete:

- Urine culture
- Abdominal ultrasound
- Serology, PCR (leptospirosis)

Treatment

Stabilization:

- Fluid therapy
- Nutritional support
- Broad-spectrum antibiotics if pyelonephritis suspected
  - Amoxicillin-clavulanic acid 20 mg/kg PO q12h
  - Enrofloxacin 5–20 mg/kg PO or SC q12h

Continued care:

- Antibiotics based on culture and sensitivity results
- Phosphate binders
  - Aluminum hydroxide 20–40 mg/animal PO
- Potassium supplementation
- Nutritional support – calorie restriction and low-protein diets can reduce severity of CPN

Uterine Disease

- Dystocia, neoplasia, endometrial disease, and pyometra

Diagnosis

History:

- May note bleeding or discharge from the vulva, owner may assume bleeding is hematuria. May be accompanied by mammary neoplasia. Weight loss or abdominal distension may be noted

Signalment:

- Intact female, often older. May or may not have a known history of breeding.

Clinical signs:

- Frank hemorrhage from the vulva, mucoid vulvar discharge or crusting, possible palpable caudal abdominal mass
  - Hormonal influence may also cause mammary neoplasia development
  - Dystocia may already have given birth to some of the litter

Differentials:

- Dystocia, pyometra, uterine neoplasia, endometritis, and endometrial hyperplasia
  - Must differentiate from urolithiasis or other source of urinary hemorrhage – the urethral and vulvar orifices are separate in rats and mice
  - *M. pulmonis* has been associated with endometritis

Diagnostics

STAT:

- *Radiographs*: Rule out dystocia and determine how may feti remain, evaluate pulmonary tissues for metastasis
- *Ultrasound*: Determine if feti are viable, rule out uterine mass

Complete:

- PCV if nothing else available
- CBC to determine if anemia present, may see inflammatory leukogram
- Chemistry ideal if surgery indicated

Treatment

Stabilization:

- Fluid therapy (see Chapter 8)
- Analgesics
  - Select with caution in cases of dystocia with viable feti, as transplacental drug distribution may occur – avoid NSAIDs, consider sedative and respiratory depressant effect on neonates
  - Buprenorphine 0.02–0.05 mg/kg SC, IV, or IM q6–12h
  - Hydromorphone 0.1 mg/kg SC or IM q6–8h
  - Gabapentin 10–30 mg/kg PO q8h
  - Meloxicam (after surgery if dystocia) 1–2 mg/kg PO or SC q24h

Continued care:

- *Surgery*:
  - Caesarian section indicated if dystocia present and breeding future to be preserved
  - Ovariohysterectomy generally preferred, concurrent with Caesarian section in cases of dystocia
- *Antibiotics*: Indicated if endometritis or pyometra suspected
  - Enrofloxacin 5–20 mg/kg PO q12h

- Amoxicillin-clavulanic acid 20 mg/kg PO q12h
- Consider doxycycline (5 mg/kg PO q12h) if *M. pulmonis* a concern

Endocrine Disease

- Rare in the emergency setting – diabetes is reported in rats and mice but generally only in certain lab strains.

Neoplastic Disease

Mammary Fibroadenoma

Diagnosis

History:

- While not a true emergency by itself, a mammary mass will often grow to such large sizes that mechanical abrasion becomes a problem, leading to acute presentations for bleeding, ulceration, or infection. Large, often rapidly growing mass on the ventrum or flanks; bleeding, discharge, odor, or eschar may be noted

Signalment:

- Female, usually 1+ years of age. Intact females are most common, as mass growth is under hormonal influence (estrogens), but spayed females are also possible (prolactin-secreting pituitary mass).

Clinical signs:

- Large soft subcutaneous mass(es); may be ulcerated, hemorrhaging, ulceration may become infected or matted with bedding material. (Figures 18.7 and 18.8)

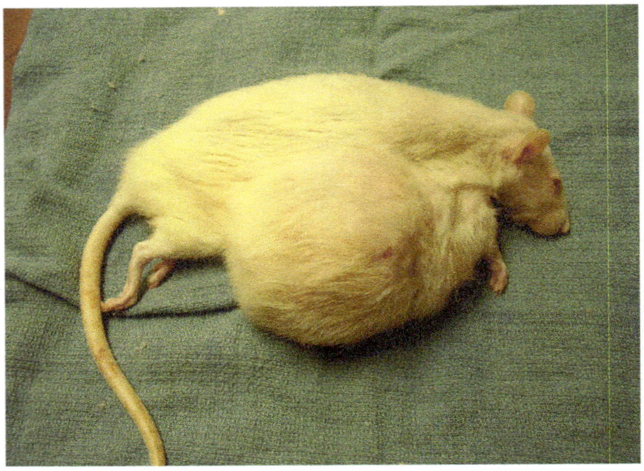

Figure 18.7 Female rat with a large mammary mass.

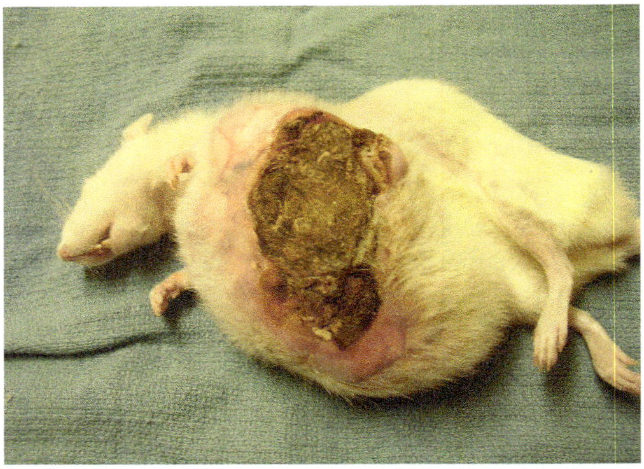

Figure 18.8 This is the same rat as Figure 18.7. Note how the dependent portion of the mass has ulcerated from chronic abrasion, with a thick eschar and embedded bedding covering the surface.

Differentials:

- Any other soft tissue neoplasia (many)

Diagnostics

STAT:

- Usually not needed

Complete:

- Radiographs to assess for concurrent disease
- CBC, chemistry – unremarkable unless concurrent disease

Treatment

Stabilization:

- *Analgesics*: Usually not painful unless ulcerated
  - Meloxicam 1–2 mg/kg PO or SC q24h
  - Buprenorphine 0.02–0.5 mg/kg SC, IV, or IM q6–12h
  - Tramadol 5–20 mg/kg PO q12–24h
  - Gabapentin 10–30 mg/kg PO q8h
- Wound care if ulcerated
- Hemostasis

Continued care:

- Antibiotics if indicated
  - Amoxicillin-clavulanic acid 20 mg/kg PO q12h
  - Enrofloxacin 5–20 mg/kg PO q12h
  - Trimethoprim-sulfa 15–30 mg/kg PO q12h
- Surgical excision of mass (Figure 18.9)

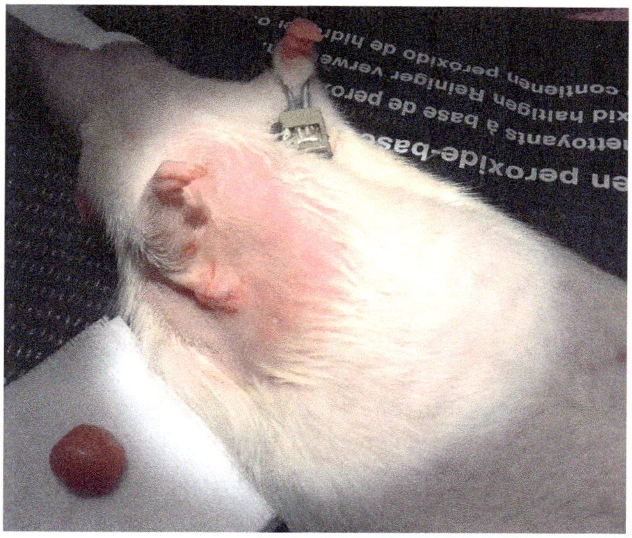

Figure 18.9 Female rat, post-operative mammary mass removal.

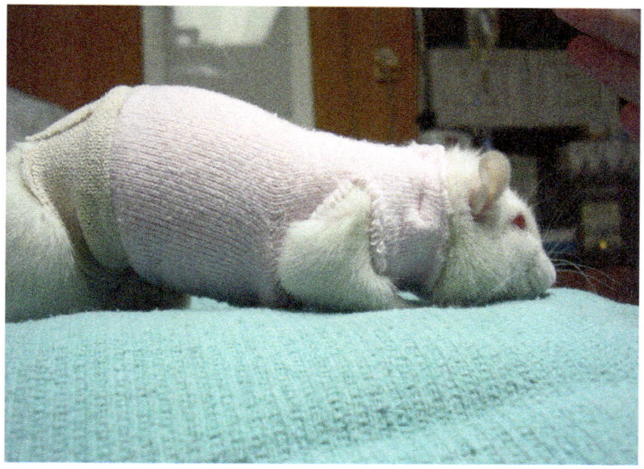

Figure 18.10 This rat is wearing a "preemie" baby sock, modified into a tunic to protect dermal lesions from further self-trauma.

- Client education: New masses may develop; early spay significantly reduces risk of mammary tumor development

Dermatologic Disease

Pruritus

Diagnosis

History:

- Not always emergent, but pruritus may lead to excoriation and self-mutilation if severe, or secondary bacterial infection. Pruritus may be severe, or may not be witnessed by the owner (may see only the dermal lesions). Multiple animals may be affected if mites are present

Signalment:

- Mites – any age, gender, and species
- Idiopathic ulcerative dermatitis reported in black mice (C57BL strain in particular)

Clinical signs:

- Pruritus, excoriation, superficial or deep ulceration of the dermis, and alopecia

Differentials:

- Acariasis (*Myobia musculi*, *Myocoptes musculinus*, *Radfordia affinis* most important in mice, *R. ensifera*, and *Ornithonyssus bacoti* in rats)
- Idiopathic ulcerative dermatitis (mice) – vasculitis
- Ulcerative dermatitis – *Staphylococcus aureus* (rats and mice), Group G Streptococcus (mice)
- Pinnal necrosis (mice)

Diagnostics:
STAT:

- Microscopic examination of hair pluck or skin scraping to identify mites/eggs, and skin cytology

Complete:

- Fungal culture, bacterial culture, and dermatohistopathology

Treatment

Stabilization:

- May need sedation if pruritus severe, or a protective body bandage or collar (Figure 18.10)

Continued care:

- *Antibiotics*:
  - Amoxicillin-clavulanic acid 20 mg/kg PO q12h
  - Enrofloxacin 5–20 mg/kg PO q12h
  - Trimethoprim-sulfa 15–30 mg/kg PO q12h
- Analgesics if significant ulcerative lesions present
  - Meloxicam 1–2 mg/kg PO or SC q24h
  - Buprenorphine 0.02–0.5 mg/kg SC, IV, or IM q6–12h
  - Tramadol 5–20 mg/kg PO q12–24h
  - Gabapentin 10–30 mg/kg PO q8h
- Antiparasitics

- Selamectin 15–30 mg/kg topically
- Ivermectin 0.2–0.4 mg/kg SC q7–14d

- Idiopathic dermatitis may respond to supplementation with omega-3 fatty acids and vitamin E
- Pinna necrosis may respond to topical cyclosporine/lidocaine/gentamicin

Abscessation

Diagnosis

History:

- May be result of fight wounds or other penetrating wound
- Preputial gland abscess in males
- Focal swelling anywhere on the body, may be history of fighting or other trauma

Signalment:

- Any age or gender; males for preputial gland abscess

Clinical signs:

- Discrete focal dermal swelling, may have draining tract, crusting, and dermal necrosis (Figure 18.11)

Differentials:

- Neoplasia

Diagnostics

STAT:

- Fine-needle aspirate may yield thick purulent material

Complete:

- CBC – may be normal, possible inflammatory leukogram

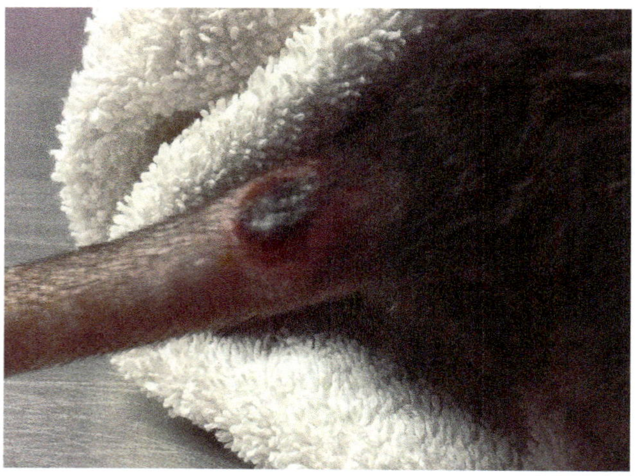

Figure 18.11 Abscessed and necrosed fight wound on the tail of a rat. The owner noted a small bite wound a few days before.

- Chemistry – unremarkable, may see azotemia if preputial gland abscess with secondary urinary obstruction (see urogenital diseases)
- Radiographs if concern for deeper involvement
- Aerobic and anaerobic bacterial culture

Treatment

Stabilization:

- Wound care if ruptured
- Analgesics
  - Meloxicam 1–2 mg/kg PO or SC q24h
  - Tramadol 5–20 mg/kg PO q12–24h
- ± Antibiotics if ruptured
  - Amoxicillin-clavulanic acid 20 mg/kg PO q12h
  - Enrofloxacin 5–20 mg/kg PO q12h
  - Trimethoprim-sulfa 15–30 mg/kg PO q12h
  - Ideally guided by culture and sensitivity results

Continued care

- Surgical excision preferred; debridement if not in a location amenable to complete excision

Fight wounds

Diagnosis

History:

- May be conspecific trauma
- Rodents that "play" with cats or dogs also at risk
- Incident may be witnessed, or the owner may see blood or the wound afterward

Signalment:

- Any age or gender

Clinical signs:

- Laceration, deep abrasion, hemorrhage, puncture wounds, may develop an abscess or necrose after a few days (Figures 18.11 and 18.12)

Differentials:

- Self-excoriation due to pruritus
- Ulcerative dermatitis (rats)
- Pinna necrosis (mice)

Diagnostics

STAT:

- Not necessary for diagnosis

Complete:

- CBC – normal if acute, later may see inflammatory leukogram, anemia if significant blood loss
- Chemistry – unremarkable but desirable if surgery indicated

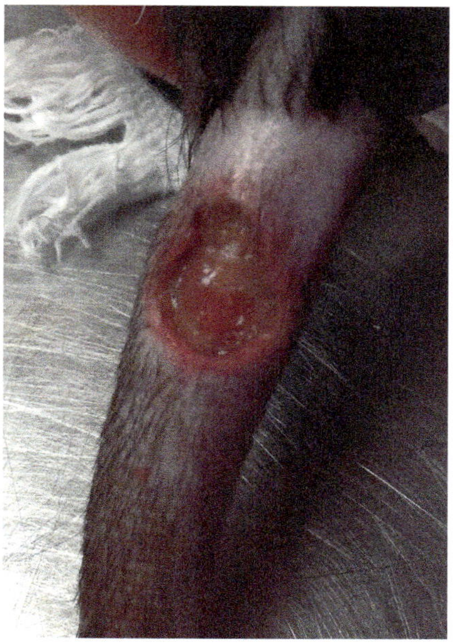

Figure 18.12 This is the same rat as in Figure 18.11, with the necrotic crust and purulent material debrided.

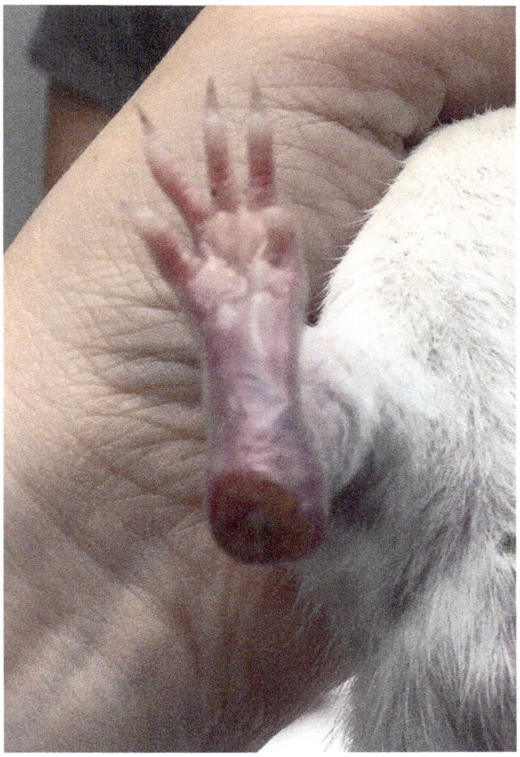

Figure 18.13 Rat with ulcerative pododermatitis.

- Radiographs if concern for underlying structures

Treatment
Stabilization:

- Antibiotics – any wounds involving a predator species need to start broad-spectrum antibiotics ASAP
  - Amoxicillin-clavulanic acid 20 mg/kg PO q12h
  - Enrofloxacin 5–20 mg/kg PO q12h
  - Trimethoprim-sulfa 15–30 mg/kg PO q12h
- Fluid therapy, see Chapter 8
- Analgesia
  - Meloxicam 1–2 mg/kg PO or SC q24h
  - Buprenorphine 0.02–0.5 mg/kg SC or IM q6–12h
  - Tramadol 5–20 mg/kg PO q12–24h
- Wound care – shave fur, gentle scrub ±debridement

Continued care:

- Laceration repair if needed

Ulcerative Pododermatitis

Diagnosis
History:

- Swellings or ulcerations on the plantar foot, may be erythematous or hemorrhaging
  - Owner may mistake them for tumors
- Lameness – usually hindlimb, but forelimb possible
- Risk factors
  - Poor cage hygiene
  - Cage design (wire floors)
  - Obesity

Signalment:

- Rats, either gender, any age but may be older

Clinical signs:

- Erythema and swelling of the plantar foot in early cases
- Ulcerative lesion on the plantar metatarsus (Figure 18.13)
- May be a proliferative granulating lesion
- Lameness
- Obesity common

Differentials

- Neoplasia
- Trauma

Diagnostics
STAT:

- Radiographs to assess possible osteomyelitis

Complete:

- CBC – inflammatory leukogram
- Chemistry – usually unremarkable
- Bacterial culture of tissue biopsy or aspirate
- Histopathology of lesion

Treatment

Stabilization:

- *Analgesics*:
  - Meloxicam 1–2 mg/kg PO q24h
  - Tramadol 5–20 mg/kg PO q12–24h
- Hemostasis
- Bandaging for wound protection and wound care

Continued care:

- *Antibiotics*: – Ability to penetrate bone is ideal
  - Amoxicillin-clavulanic acid 20 mg/kg PO q12h
  - Enrofloxacin 5–20 mg/kg PO q12h
  - Chloramphenicol 30–50 mg/kg PO q8–12h (warn owner of human risk)
- Obesity management
- Husbandry improvements
- Surgical debridement may help if severe

Ophthalmic Disease

Chromodacryorrhea

- Not primary disease, but sign of other disease, stress, and environmental issues
- May be reported by owner as "bleeding from the eyes" (Figure 18.1)
- Increased secretions from Harderian gland in response to stress, systemic illness, SDAV infection

Corneal Ulceration/Perforation

Diagnosis

History

- Globe tends to be protuberant in small rodents and is easily traumatized
  - Blepharospasm, ocular discharge, ocular hemorrhage, facial pain, and rubbing at face (Figure 18.1)

Signalment:

- Any age or gender; hairless rats predisposed due to lack of protective facial hairs

Clinical signs:

- Blepharospasm, ocular discharge, possible grossly visible corneal defect, loss of anterior chamber depth, or protruding iris if perforated

Differentials:

- Conjunctivitis, ocular foreign body, retrobulbar mass, fight wound, and self-trauma secondary to pruritus

Diagnostics

STAT:

- Fluorescein staining

Complete:

- Full ophthalmologic exam
- CBC/chemistry – unremarkable, but desirable if surgery indicated

Treatment

Stabilization:

- *Analgesics*:
  - Meloxicam 1–2 mg/kg PO q24h
  - Tramadol 5–20 mg/kg PO q12–24h
  - Gabapentin 10–30 mg/kg PO q8h
  - Topical ophthalmic analgesic solutions such as atropine or proparacaine
- Topical antibiotic solutions (avoid ointment if perforated)
  - Ofloxacin
  - Tobramycin
  - Gentamicin
  - Neomycin–polymyxin–gramicidin
- E-collar to prevent self-trauma

Continued care:

- Above sufficient if simple ulceration
- Deep ulcerations may require conjunctival pedicle graft, corneal repair, or enucleation

Proptosis

Diagnosis

History:

- Globe easily proptoses in these species, ocular hemorrhage, ocular discharge, rubbing at the face, and displaced globe

Signalment:

- Any age or sex

Clinical signs:

- Proptosed globe readily evident, distinguish from exophthalmos

Differentials:

- Trauma, retrobulbar abscess, and retrobulbar neoplasia

Diagnostics

STAT:

- Usually not required for initial diagnosis

Complete:

- Skull/whole-body radiographs – tooth root abscess
- CT – retrobulbar mass, tooth root abscess
- CBC – may be normal, may see inflammatory leukogram, anemia of chronic disease, or acute blood loss
- Chemistry – unremarkable, desirable if surgery indicated

Treatment

Stabilization:

- *Analgesia*:
  - Meloxicam 1–2 mg/kg PO or SC q24h
  - Buprenorphine 0.02–0.5 mg/kg SC or IM q6–12h
  - Tramadol 5–20 mg/kg PO q12–24h
  - Gabapentin 10–30 mg/kg PO q8h
- Lubrication of globe
- Topical antibiotics
  - Ofloxacin
  - Tobramycin
  - Gentamicin
  - Neomycin–polymyxin–gramicidin
- Systemic antibiotics
  - Amoxicillin-clavulanic acid 20 mg/kg PO q12h
  - Enrofloxacin 5-20 mg/kg PO q12h

Continued care:

- Surgical reduction
- Enucleation if the globe is ruptured, dessicated, or otherwise severely traumatized

Further Reading

Beaumont, S. (2002). Ocular disorders of pet mice and rats. *Vet. Clin. North Am. Exot. Anim. Pract.* 5: 311–324.

Brown, C. and Donnelly, T.M. (2013). Disease problems of small rodents. In: Ferrets, Rabbits, and Rodents: Clinical Medicine and Surgery, 3e (eds. K.E. Quesenberry and J.W. Carpenter), 354–372. St. Louis, MO: Elsevier.

Eguchi, K., Kawamoto, K., Uozumi, T. et al. (1995). in vivo; effect of cabergoline, a dopamine agonist, on estrogen-induced rat pituitary tumors. *Endocr. J.* 42 (2): 153–161.

Fisher, P. (2006). Exotic mammal renal disease: causes and clinical presentation. *Vet. Clin. North Am. Exot. Anim. Pract.* 9: 33–67.

Fisher, P. (2006). Exotic mammal renal disease: diagnosis and treatment. *Vet. Clin. North Am. Exot. Anim. Pract.* 9: 69–96.

Hawkins, M.G. and Graham, J.E. (2007). Emergency care and critical care of rodents. *Vet. Clin. North Am. Exot. Anim. Pract.* 10: 501–531.

Herbert, S. (2012). The challenges of rodent medicine can leave you and your pet gasping. An overview of respiratory disease and its sequelae in pet rats. *Proceedings of Association of Avian Veterinarians (AC) & Unusual and Exotic Pets Conference 2012*, Melbourne, Australia.

Hoefer, H. and Latney, L. (2009). Rodents: urogenital and reproductive system disorders. In: BSAVA Manual of Rodents and Ferrets (eds. E. Keeble and A. Meredith), 150–153. Gloucester, UK: British Small Animal Veterinary Association.

Hollamby, S. (2009). Rodents: neurological and musculoskeletal disorders. In: BSAVA Manual of Rodents and Ferrets (eds. E. Keeble and A. Meredith), 161–168. Gloucester, UK: British Small Animal Veterinary Association.

Goodman, G. (2009). Rodents: respiratory and cardiovascular system disorders. In: BSAVA Manual of Rodents and Ferrets (eds. E. Keeble and A. Meredith), 142–149. Gloucester, UK: British Small Animal Veterinary Association.

Knafo, S.E. (2014) Sildenafil citrate as a pulmonary protectant in chronic murine *Mycoplasma pulmonis* infection. *Proceedings of Association Exotic Mammal Veterinarians Conference 2014*, New Orleans, LA.

Longley, L. (2009). Rodents: dermatoses. In: BSAVA Manual of Rodents and Ferrets (eds. E. Keeble and A. Meredith), 107–122. Gloucester, UK: British Small Animal Veterinary Association.

Mayer, J. and Mans, C. (2018). Rodents. In: Exotic Animal Formulary, 5e (eds. J.W. Carpenter and C.J. Marion), 459–493. St. Louis, MO: Elsevier.

McLaughlin, A. and Strunk, A. (2016). Common emergencies in small rodents, hedgehogs, and sugar gliders. *Vet. Clin. North Am. Exot. Anim. Pract.* 19: 465–499.

Monks, D. and Cowan, M. (2009). Chronic respiratory disease in rats. *Proceedings of Association of Avian Veterinarians (AC) & Unusual and Exotic Pets Conference 2009*, North Sydney, Australia.

Montiani-Ferrera, F. (2009). Rodents: ophthalmology. In: BSAVA Manual of Rodents and Ferrets (eds. E. Keeble and A. Meredith), 169–180. Gloucester, UK: British Small Animal Veterinary Association.

Orr, H. Rodents: neoplastic and endocrine disease. In: BSAVA Manual of Rodents and Ferrets (eds. E. Keeble and A. Meredith), 181–184. Gloucester, UK: British Small Animal Veterinary Association.

Otto, G.M., Franklin, C.L., and Clifford, C.B. (2014). Biology and diseases of rats. In: Laboratory Animal Medicine, 3e (eds. J.G. Fox, L.C. Anderson, G.M. Otto, et al.), 151–208. Oxford, UK: Elsevier.

Sayers, I. and Smith, S. (2010). Mice, rats, hamsters, and gerbils. In: BSAVA Manual of Exotic Pets, 5e (eds. A. Meredith and C. Johnson-Delaney), 1–27. Gloucester, UK: British Small Animal Veterinary Association.

Tully, T. (2009). Mice and rats. In: Manual of Exotic Pet Practice (eds. M. Mitchell and T. Tully), 326–344. St Louis, MO: Saunders Elsevier.

Ward, M.L. (2009). Rodents: digestive system disorders. In: BSAVA Manual of Rodents and Ferrets (eds. E. Keeble and A. Meredith), 123–141. Gloucester, UK: British Small Animal Veterinary Association.

Whary, M.T., Baumgarth, M., Fox, J.G., and Barthold, S.W. (2014). Biology and diseases of mice. In: Laboratory Animal Medicine, 3e (eds. J.G. Fox, L.C. Anderson, G.M. Otto, et al.), 34–150. Oxford, UK: Elsevier.

19

Hamsters and Gerbils

Andrew D. Bean

Avian & Exotic Medicine Service, Animal Emergency and Referral Center of Minnesota, Oakdale, Minnesota, USA

CONTENTS

Unique Species Considerations

- Hamsters and gerbils are prey animals. Veterinary visits cause a substantial stress response, exacerbating already compromised pets. Consider sedation to facilitate extensive restraint/handling. Midazolam +/− opioids useful [1]
- Glucocorticoids typically avoided – risk of profound immunosuppression. Limit use to confirmed steroid-responsive diseases when alternatives do not exist

Common Presenting Signs

Diarrhea

Introduction

- True emergency – rapid fluid loss, metabolic derangements, intussusception, bowel prolapse, and GI dysbiosis with circulatory translocation of the GI flora

Exotic Animal Emergency and Critical Care Medicine, First Edition. Edited by Jennifer E. Graham, Grayson A. Doss and Hugues Beaufrère.

Diagnosis

History:

- Husbandry and environmental factors (Table 19.4)
- Inappropriate antibiotic use (Table 19.2)

Signalment: [7–9]

- Juveniles (4–8 weeks) or young adults

Clinical Signs: [7–10]

- Weight loss
- Liquid, unformed stool
- Perineal fecal staining (Figure 19.1)
- Hunched posture/abdominal pain
- Rectal/intestinal prolapse
- Abdominal distention

Differentials: [8, 10–15]

- Enteritis: Bacterial, parasitic (see Gastrointestinal Disease)
- Nutritional: Inappropriate diet, sudden diet change
- Stress
- Neoplasia (see Neoplastic Disease)

STAT Diagnostics: [7, 9, 15]

- PCV/TS/glucose (GLU)

Complete Diagnostics: [7, 11, 13–15]

- Fecal analysis (see Gastrointestinal Disease)
- Tape cytology (perineal – evaluate for pinworms)
- CBC/Chem
- POCUS
- FNA/cytology (masses)

Treatment

Stabilization: [7, 8, 15]

- Supportive care (fluids, nutrition, analgesia; see Chapters 7–8)
- Antibiotics: Metronidazole, doxycycline, chloramphenicol, enrofloxacin, TMS (Table 19.2)
- Antiparasitics PRN (Table 19.3)
- Discontinue inappropriate antibiotics

Continued Care: [7, 10, 14]

- As above until patient is eating and drinking normally (usually 1–2 weeks)

Neurologic Signs

Introduction

- Complete neurologic examination difficult due to size, restraint. Observe movement, note mentation, placing reactions, muscle strength, pain responses [18]
- Primary neurologic origin generalized seizures have been reported in gerbils (see Neurologic and Musculoskeletal Disease)
- Torpor/hibernation may be confused with neurologic disease (see Torpor/Hibernation)
- Rabies highly unlikely in hamsters/gerbils

Diagnosis

History:

- Husbandry and environment (Table 19.4)
- Toxin exposure (see Toxins)

Signalment:

- No predilections

Clinical Signs: [18, 19]

- Mentation changes
- Ataxia
- Tremors
- Head tilt
- Nystagmus
- Circling
- Paresis/paralysis
- Seizures

Differentials: [11, 13, 19, 20]

- Vestibular disease, seizures, paresis/paralysis (see Neurologic and Musculoskeletal Disease)
- Mentation changes: General malaise, pain, behavioral, neoplasia (CNS, endocrine), hepatic/renal dysfunction, infection
- Blindness, anisocoria: Trauma, neoplasia, nutritional deficiency, infection

STAT Diagnostics:

- PCV/TS/GLU

Complete Diagnostics: [18]

- Electrolytes + iCa
- CBC/Chem
- Radiographs – skull and spine
- Anesthetized otoendoscopic examination +/– culture
- Serial neurologic exams
- Blood lead

Treatment

Stabilization:

- Supportive care (fluids, nutrition, analgesia; see Chapters 7–8)
- Anticonvulsant therapy (Table 19.1)
  - Consider hyperosmolar therapy if head trauma suspected and neurologic status deteriorates

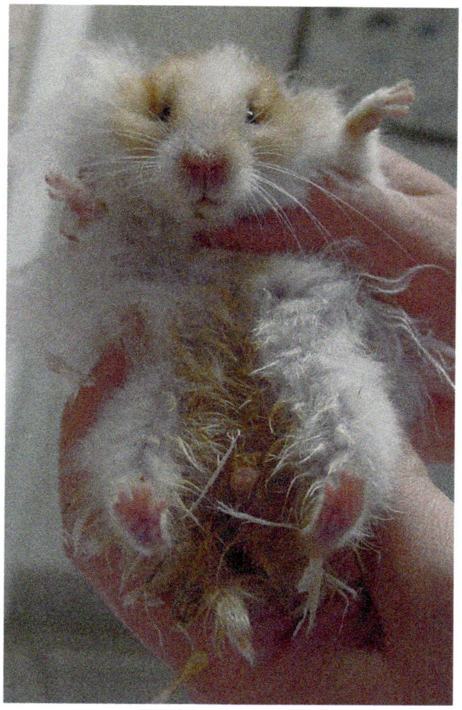

Figure 19.1 Severe perineal fecal staining secondary to diarrhea in a Syrian hamster. *Source:* Courtesy of Peter G. Fisher.

Continued care:

- Seizures (see Neurologic and Musculoskeletal Disease)
- Antimicrobials as warranted (Table 19.2)
- Nutritional correction
- Lead chelation – see Toxins
- Surgical treatment as indicated
- Referral to neurologist and/or exotics specialist

Ocular Signs

Introduction

- Environmental issues and trauma often lead to ocular problems

Diagnosis

History:

- Husbandry and environment (Table 19.4)

Signalment:

- Chinese hamsters (*Cricetulus griseus*) predisposed to diabetic cataracts [26, 27]
- Djungarian hamsters (*Phodopus songurus cambelli)* may develop idiopathic glaucoma [28]
- Syrian hamsters (*Mesocrecitus auratus*) not housed solitarily at risk for trauma

Clinical signs: [8, 27, 29–31]

- Blepharospasm, conjunctivitis, oculonasal discharge (may be red in hamsters)
- Corneal opacity/vascularization
- Dysphagia
- Hypersalivation
- Incisor malocclusion
- Facial swelling
- Buphthalmos/exophthalmos
- Proptosis
- Hypopyon and hyphema (Figure 19.2)
- Phthisis bulbi (Figure 19.3)

Differentials: [8, 27, 32]

- Exophthalmos, proptosis (see Ophthalmic Disease)
- Buphthalmos: Glaucoma

Table 19.1 Anticonvulsant drugs in hamsters and gerbils (H = hamster, G = gerbil).

Drug	Dosages	Comments
Alfaxalone	5 mg/kg IP (H) [21]	Acute seizure control only
Diazepam	0.2–1 mg/kg IM, IP (G) [22, 23]	Acute seizure control only
Gabapentin	15–33 mg/kg PO (G) [24]	Single dosage evaluated. Pharmacokinetic, pharmacodynamic, safety profiles not established. May cause sedation
Levetiracetam	30–100 mg/kg IP (H) [25]	Variable efficacy. Sedation, ataxia observed at higher doses
Phenobarbital	7–15 mg/kg IP, PO (G) [23, 24]	Anticonvulsant activity wanes dramatically after first few days; not recommended for long-term management
	10–20 mg/kg IP (H) [25]	For acute seizure control only, serum levels undetectable after 30 minutes
Zonisamide	112–144 mg/kg PO (G) [24]	Single dosage evaluated. Pharmacokinetic, pharmacodynamic, safety profiles not established. Side effects not reported

Table 19.2 Antibiotic and antifungal drugs in hamsters and gerbils (H = hamster, G = gerbil).

Drug	Dosages	Comments
Amikacin	16 mg/kg SC, IM divided q8–24h (H, G) [2]	Once daily dosing may offer greater efficacy, safety [2]
Azithromycin	15–35 mg/kg PO q24h (H, G) [3]	
Chloramphenicol palmitate	30–50 mg/kg PO q8–12h (H, G) [3]	Wear gloves when handling – may cause bone marrow suppression in humans [4]
Chloramphenicol succinate	30–50 mg/kg PO q8–12h (H, G) [3] 0.83 mg/ml drinking water (G) [3]	Wear gloves when handling – may cause bone marrow suppression in humans [4]
Doxycycline	2.5–5 mg/kg PO q12h (H, G) [3]	Contraindicated in young or pregnant animals [3]
Enrofloxacin	5–20 mg/kg PO, SC, IM q12h (H, G) [3] 0.05–0.2 mg/ml drinking water × 14d (H, G) [3]	Avoid high doses in young animals. SC/IM injections may cause tissue irritation/necrosis – recommend dilution in normal saline or LRS Pasteurellosis
Griseofulvin	25 mg/kg PO q24h (H, G) [2]	Teratogenic – do not use in pregnant animals. Should not be handled by pregnant women. Bone marrow suppression not documented in rodents [2, 5]
Ketoconazole	10–40 mg/kg PO q24h (H, G) [2]	Potentially teratogenic/embryotoxic. Caution in patients with hepatic disease, thrombocytopenia [6]
Lime sulfur dip	Dip q7d × 4–6 treatments (H, G) [3]	Dermatophytosis; dilute 1 : 40 w/ water [3]
Marbofloxacin	4 mg/kg PO, SC q24h (H, G) [3]	Contraindicated in pregnant, lactating, growing animals [3]
Metronidazole	20 mg/kg PO q12h(H, G) [2]	
Neomycin	100 mg/kg PO SC q24h (H, G) [3] 0.4 mg/ml drinking water (H) [3]	Proliferative ileitis
Terbinafine	10–30 mg/kg PO q24h × 4–6 wks (H, G) [3]	Dermatophytosis
Trimethoprim/sulfamethoxazole	15–30 mg/kg PO, SC q12h (H, G) [3]	Tissue necrosis possible w/ SC administration [3]
Penicillins, cephalosporins, macrolides, lincosamides, (dihydro)streptomycin, gentamicin (oral)	Do not use	Toxic – result in GI dysbiosis, septicemia, death

- Blepharospasm, ocular discharge, conjunctivitis, corneal opacity/vascularization: Infection (*Pasteurella* spp., *Streptococcus* spp.), entropion, foreign body, other trauma, keratoconjunctivitis sicca, intraocular neoplasia, environmental irritants
- Ocular signs + dysphagia, hypersalivation, incisor malocclusion, facial swelling: Dental disease, oral trauma, neoplasia

STAT Diagnostics: [27, 33–35]

- Assess vision
- Fluorescein stain

Complete Diagnostics: [31, 33]

- Intraocular pressure
  - Rebound tonometry normal = 2–8 mmHg
- Tear production evaluation
  - Phenol red thread test normal = 3–11.5 mm/15 s
  - Schirmer tear test not recommended – poor sensitivity
- Fundic examination
  - Induce mydriasis with 1.0% tropicamide (nonpigmented animals) or 2.5% phenylephrine (pigmented animals). May require 10% phenylephrine. Mydriasis achieved within 20 minutes
- Corneal/conjunctival scraping cytology +/− culture

Table 19.3 Antiparasitic drugs in hamsters and gerbils (H = hamster, G = gerbil).

Drug	Dosages	Comments
Amitraz	0.013% topical bath (H) [16]	Demodicosis. Apply with cotton ball or brush [3]
Fenbendazole	20–50 mg/kg PO q24h × 5d (H, G) [2]	Giardia, nematodes
Fipronil	7.5 mg/kg topically q30–60d (H, G) [3]	Flea adulticide
	Soaked swab wiped over whole body 2 times 10d apart (H) [16]	Tropical rat mite
Imidacloprid	20 mg/kg topically q30d [3]	Flea adulticide/larvicide
Ivermectin	0.2–0.4 mg/kg SC q5–7d (H) [3]	Demodicosis
	0.3 mg/kg PO q24h (H) [17]	
	0.2 mg/kg SC q7d (G) [16]	
	0.2–0.4 mg/kg SC q7–14d (H, G) [2]	Sarcoptiform mites, tropical rat mite
Metronidazole	70 mg/kg PO q8h (H) [3]	
	20–50 mg/kg PO q8h (H, G) [2]	
Nitenpyram	1 mg PO once (H, G) [3]	Flystrike
Praziquantel	6–10 mg/kg PO, SC once, repeat in 10 days (H, G) [3]	Cestodes
	30 mg/kg PO q14d × 3 Tx (G) [3]	
Pyrantel pamoate	50 mg/kg PO once [3]	Nematodes
Selamectin	15–30 mg/kg topically q21–28d (H, G) [3]	Sarcoptiform mites (use 30 mg/kg), tropical rat mite, flea adulticide
Sulfadimethoxine	25–50 mg/kg PO q24h × 10–14d (H, G) [2]	Coccidia
Toltrazuril	25 mg/kg PO q24h × 3d, off 3d, on 3d [3]	Coccidia

- Anesthetized oral examination
- Radiographs – skull
- GLU

Treatment [28, 29, 33]

Stabilization:

- Cleaning, lubrication of eye
- Foreign body removal
- See Exophthalmos/Proptosis (see Ophthalmic Disease)

Continued care:

- Conjunctivitis/keratitis: Antibiotics, supportive care (fluids, nutrition, analgesia; see Chapters 7–8)
- See Dental Disease
- Retrobulbar neoplasia/abscess: Enucleation
- Glaucoma: As for other species

Respiratory Distress

Introduction

- Rodents are obligate nasal breathers [36]
- Pneumonia (bacterial, viral) common in hamsters, especially juveniles [12, 37]
- Congestive heart failure has been reported in hamsters/gerbils [38–40]

Diagnosis

History:

- Husbandry and environment (Table 19.4)
- Exposure to other animals, especially potential carriers of *Bordetella bronchiseptica* and *Pasteurella* spp. (e.g., dogs, rabbits, guinea pigs) [13]

Signalment:

- Infections more common in juveniles, geriatrics [12]

Clinical Signs: [8, 11, 13, 41, 42]

- Oculonasal discharge (may be noted on forepaws) (Figure 19.4)
- Tachypnea, dyspnea
- Coughing, sneezing
- Collapse/syncope

Table 19.4 Environmental/nutritional factors and their health impacts on hamsters and gerbils.

Environmental/nutritional factor	Health impact
Infrequent cage cleaning	Irritation of ocular and upper airway mucus membranes, palmar/plantar paws Predisposes to secondary infection
Inadequate depth of bedding	Stress Stereotypic behavior
Inappropriate temperature	Stress Low: torpor High: heat stroke (esp. gerbils)
Inappropriate diet (high sugar, fat; excessively sticky; pieces too large/small)	Nutritional inadequacies Dental caries or abscesses Cheek pouch impaction (hamsters) Obesity Diabetes
Exercise wheels without solid flooring	Traumatic injuries
Airborne particulate matter (smoke, dust)	Irritation of ocular and upper airway mucus membranes Predisposes to secondary infection
Bedding with aromatic oils (cedar, lavender) Nearby aromatherapeutic diffusers	Irritation of ocular and upper airway mucus membranes Predisposes to secondary infection
High-density housing	Variable stressor High exposure to infectious disease
Transport High noise levels	Stress
Excessive humidity	Stress Oculonasal discharge with secondary dermatitis (gerbils)
Exposure to predator species	Stress Traumatic injuries
Outdoor exposures	Infectious disease Traumatic injuries Toxin exposure
Chewing excessively hard objects	Incisor fracture, malocclusion

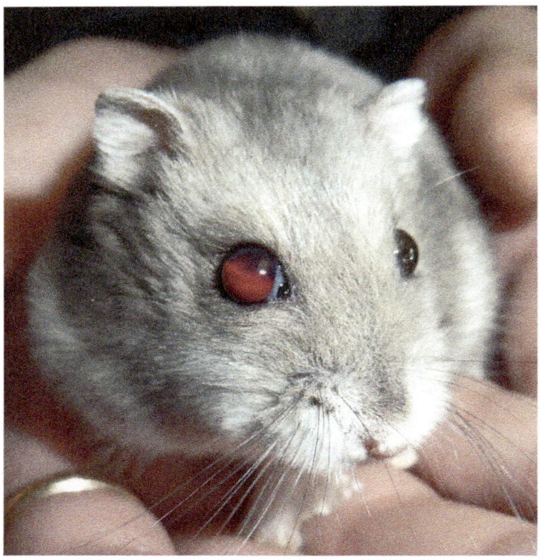

Figure 19.2 Hyphema in a Russian dwarf hamster. *Source:* Courtesy of Peter G. Fisher.

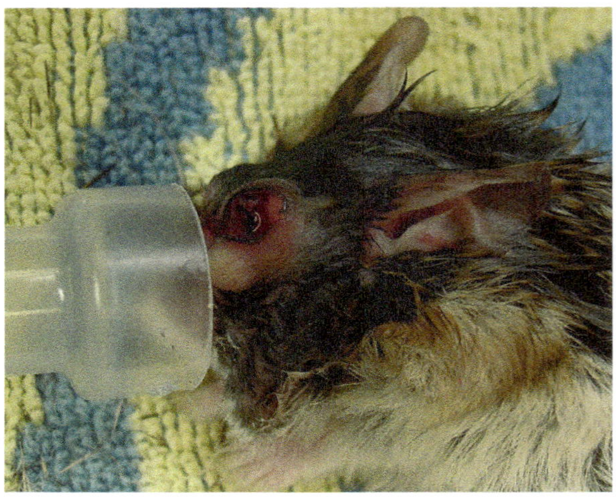

Figure 19.3 Phthisis bulbi in a hamster. *Source:* Courtesy of Peter G. Fisher.

- Abdominal distention
- Oral ulcers

Differentials: [8, 11, 13, 36, 38, 40, 41, 43–45]

- Infection (bacterial, viral)
- Neoplasia
- Cardiac disease (see Cardiopulmonary Disease)
- Dental disease
- Trauma
- Pain
- Foreign body
- Electrocution
- Anticoagulant rodenticide

STAT Diagnostics:

- SpO_2

Complete Diagnostics:

- Radiographs
- Cytology, culture (nasal discharge, aspirate)
- CBC/Chem
- Thoracic ultrasound

Treatment

Stabilization:

- Supportive care, esp. O_2 supplementation
- Terbutaline 0.01 mg/kg IM (diluted 1:10 in sterile water) [46]
- Nebulization 30–45 minutes q4–12h PRN (doses extrapolated from birds) [47]
  - Amikacin, gentamicin: 50 mg in 10 ml saline; may add 1 ml 20% acetylcysteine
  - Enrofloxacin: 100 mg in 10 ml saline
  - Terbutaline: 0.01 mg/kg in 9 ml saline

Continued Care:

- Antimicrobials PRN
- Terbutaline 0.3–0.4 mg/kg PO q12h [3]
- Theophylline 10 mg/kg PO q12h [48]

Trauma (Predator, Self, Fall, Conspecific, Crushing, Cage)

Introduction

- Patients may self-traumatize in response to pain or stress
- Common sources of trauma: Children, predators, exercise wheels without solid floors

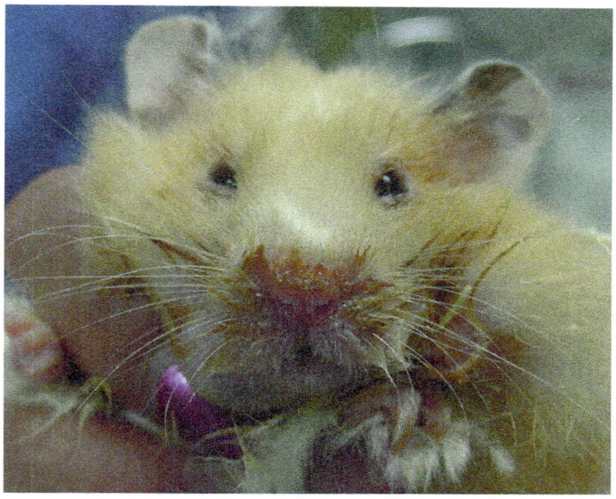

Figure 19.4 Purulent nasal discharge in a Syrian hamster. *Source:* Courtesy of Peter G. Fisher.

Diagnosis

History:

- Husbandry and environment (Table 19.4)
- Potential predator exposures

Signalment:

- Syrian hamsters are solitary animals and may fight if multiple animals are housed in a single cage.

Clinical Signs: [31]

- Alopecia
- Hunched posture
- Perineal soiling
- Wounds
- Lameness/paresis
- Exophthalmos/proptosis
- Tachypnea, dyspnea
- Muffled heart sounds
- Head tilt
- Abdominal distention
- Asynchronous breathing patterns

Differentials:

- Respiratory signs: Hemo/pneumothorax, pain, diaphragmatic hernia, costal fractures, congestive heart failure, neoplasia, infection, acid–base derangement
- Lameness/paresis: Fracture/dislocation, soft tissue injury, neoplasia, metabolic disease

- Abdominal distention: Hemoabdomen, gastrointestinal gas accumulation, cystic viscera (hamsters), congestive heart failure, hyperadrenocorticism (hamsters)
- Exophthalmos/proptosis: See Ophthalmic Disease
- Depressed mentation, anisocoria: Head trauma, neoplasia, postictal phase of seizure, torpor
- Head tilt: See Neurologic and Musculoskeletal Disease
- Perineal soiling: Fear, diarrhea, pain/malaise, spinal trauma/neoplasia
- Tail degloving, wounds, fractures: Inappropriate handling, predator/conspecific attack, fall, entrapment
- Seizures: Idiopathic (gerbils), intoxication, head trauma, infection, neoplasia, hepatic/renal dysfunction

STAT Diagnostics:

- Point-of-care ultrasound (POCUS)
- SpO_2

Complete Diagnostics:

- CBC/Chem
- Radiographs
- Thoraco/abdominocentesis, fluid analysis
- Culture/sensitivity
- Serial neurologic examinations

Treatment

Stabilization: [1, 49]

- External coaptation (short term)
- Wound care
- Head trauma: Minimize movement, keep head and neck at ~30° angle to avoid jugular vein occlusion

Continued Care: [1, 31, 49]

- Fractures
  - Limb: Rodents generally intolerant of bandages; long-term external coaptation often fails. Modified Robert–Jones bandage or tape splint may be attempted.
    Surgical fracture repair.
    Last resort (closed Fx only): Strict cage rest on soft bedding, removal of all climbable structures in the cage x 6wks. Prognosis for return to full function poor, substantial risk of malunion/nonunion, progression to open fracture
  - Skull: Nondisplaced fractures treated supportively. Displaced fractures may require referral
  - Spinal: Surgical stabilization (unlikely to be feasible); alternatively cage rest, supportive care. Prognosis guarded to poor
  - Dental: Fractured incisors will regrow. Fractured cheek teeth require extraction
- Wounds:
  - Open wounds: Lavage +/− surgical debridement. Drains not used – often removed prematurely by patients, rodent pus very thick. Antibiotics (e.g., potentiated sulfas) pending culture
  - Abscesses: See Dermatologic Disease
- Head trauma: Continued supportive care with frequent monitoring. Consider mannitol if neurologic status declines

Neurologic and Musculoskeletal Disease

Seizures: Gerbil Epilepsy/Seizures

Diagnosis

History:

- Inciting causes/scenarios. Seizures in gerbils may be induced by sudden auditory/physical stimuli, changes in environment
- Toxin exposures

Signalment:

- Epileptic seizures manifest in young animals, often by two months of age. Seizures in adults raise concern for non-epileptic causes. [7]
- Prevalence in laboratory gerbils 10–80% [50, 51]. Prevalence in pet gerbils unknown, anecdotally uncommon. Cause of epileptic seizures in gerbils believed to be reduced glutamate synthetase activity in the CNS. [52]

Clinical Signs: [51]

- Seizures (focal to *grand mal*). Manifestations like those reported in other species

Differentials:

- Gerbil epilepsy
- Other primary neurologic disease
- Toxin (e.g., lead, rodenticides, insecticides)
- Nutritional deficiency (e.g., hypocalcemia)
- Heat stroke
- Systemic disease

STAT Diagnostics:

- PCV/TS/GLU
- Rectal temp

Complete Diagnostics:

- CBC/Chem +/− iCa
- Blood lead
- Radiographs

Treatment

Stabilization:

- Anticonvulsant therapy (Table 19.1)

Continued care:

- Continued anticonvulsant therapy for epilepsy generally not recommended – anecdotal evidence that seizures do not have lasting effects, severity may diminish with time [8]
- Frequent handling during first three weeks of life believed to reduce seizure frequency, severity [42]

Torpor/Hibernation

Diagnosis

History:

- Husbandry and environment (Table 19.4)
- Torpor: State of physical and mental dormancy lasting <24 hours. Hibernation: Prolonged state of torpor [53]
- Hamsters readily enter torpor under proper conditions, including: [54]
  - Photoperiod – shorter periods of light, longer dark periods
  - Low ambient temperature – varies by species, temperatures below 8 °C (46 °F) likely to induce torpor
  - Inadequate food availability
  - Gonadectomy

Signalment:

- Hamsters enter torpor much more readily than gerbils.

Clinical Signs:

- Minimal responsiveness
- Bradycardia
- Hypopnea
- Hypothermia

Differentials:

- Hypoglycemia
- Shock
- Death

STAT Diagnostics:

- Temp
- ECG
- GLU
- Response to warming and physical stimulation – patient should arouse in 5–10 minutes

Complete Diagnostics:

- Per underlying disease

Treatment

Stabilization:

- Supportive care +/− oral dextrose
- Per underlying disease

Continued Care:

- Husbandry correction
- Per underlying disease

Toxins

Diagnosis

History: [55]

- Toxin exposures:
  - Rodenticides
  - Lead: Paint, solder, fishing sinkers, ammunition, toys, linoleum, batteries, foil from champagne bottles, drapery weights, improperly glazed bowls
  - Insecticides (organophosphates and carbamates)
  - Herbicides
  - Toxic plants – assume any plant that is toxic to other species to be a potential toxin

Signalment:

- No predilections.

Clinical Signs:

- Lead [56, 57]
  - Emaciation
  - Rough coat
  - Lethargy
  - Diarrhea
  - Neurologic signs
- Anticoagulant rodenticides: Similar to other mammals [55]
- Organophosphates and carbamates [57]
  - Hypersalivation
  - Bradycardia
  - Muscle tremors
  - Seizures
  - Death

Differentials:

- Variable

STAT Diagnostics:

  - Variable
  - Organophosphate/carbamate: Response to atropine administration (see Treatment)

Complete Diagnostics:

- CBC/Chem
  - RBC basophilic stippling normal in gerbils [58]
- Blood lead
- Urinalysis
- Radiographs

Treatment

Stabilization:

- Dermal exposures:
  - Bathe with mild detergent and warm water. Use of spray bottle may be less stressful than running water [55]
  - Glue traps: Use oily substances (e.g., mineral oil, cooking oil), then bathe as above. Caution with commercial adhesive removers – may be toxic [57]
- Ocular exposures: Flush with warm saline [55]
- Oral exposures [55]
  - Emetics contraindicated – rodents cannot vomit
  - Hamsters: Remove all material from cheek pouches using cotton swabs (anesthesia recommended)
  - Corrosive substances: Dilute toxicant with milk; nonacidic, juicy fruits (e.g., cantaloupe, pears, watermelon); saline
  - Activated charcoal: 1 g/kg (1–3 mg/g)
  - Cathartics may cause severe dehydration
  - Bulking agents for removal of ingested toxins (anecdotal)
  - Psyllium powder: 1/2 tsp in 60 ml baby food
  - Peanut butter: Small amount PO
- Chelation (lead toxicity):
  - Ca EDTA: 25–30 mg/kg SC q6–12h × 5 days (extrapolated from chinchillas) [59]
    - May enhance heavy metal absorption from GI tract if source still present
  - Succimer (DMSA): 30 mg/kg PO q12h × 21 days (extrapolated from rats) [60]
- Anticoagulant rodenticides: [61]
  - Vitamin K1 2.5–5 mg/kg IM q24h × 4–6 days (warfarin), × 21–28 days (brodifacoum)
- Organophosphates/carbamates
  - Atropine 10 mg/kg SC q20 minutes [3]

Continued Care:

- As indicated

Vestibular Signs

Diagnosis

History:

- See Neurologic Signs

Signalment:

- No predilections.

Clinical Signs: [18, 19]

- Head tilt
- Circling
- Ataxia
- Nystagmus

Differentials: [18–20]

- Otitis media/Internet
- Aural neoplasia (gerbils)
- Head trauma
- Clostridium piliforme infection
- CNS neoplasia
- Aminoglycoside ototoxicity

STAT Diagnostics:

- Otoscopic examination

Complete Diagnostics:

- Cytology
- Skull radiographs
- Bacterial culture

Treatment

Stabilization:

- None

Continued Care:

- Meclizine 2–12 mg/kg PO q8–24h (extrapolated from guinea pigs, chinchillas) [62]
- Per underlying disorder

Cardiopulmonary Disease

Congestive Heart Failure

Diagnosis

History:

- Lethargy common. Owners may not notice respiratory signs until advanced

Signalment:

- >1 year
- Intact male hamsters overrepresented [38]

Clinical Signs: [38, 39]

- Tachycardia
- Tachypnea

- Cyanosis
- Cold extremities
- Generalized edema

Differentials: [13, 38, 40]

- Thrombosis
- Degenerative conditions (calcifying vasculopathy, myocardial fibrosis, etc.)
- Infection (myocarditis, endocarditis)
- Congenital anomalies
- Hyperadrenocorticism
- Cardiovascular disease complex of breeding gerbils

STAT Diagnostics:

- SpO_2

Complete Diagnostics:

- Radiographs
- CBC/Chem
- ECG
- Echocardiography

Treatment

Stabilization:

- Furosemide: 1–10 mg/kg SC, IM, PO q4–12h [38, 63]
- Nitroglycerin ointment 2%: 1/16 in. per kg, apply to hairless region q12–24h [38]
- Thoracocentesis/abdominocentesis – ultrasound, sedation advised

Continued Care:

- In addition to furosemide (doses for hamsters; no published dosages for gerbils):
  - Diltiazem: 25 mg/kg PO q24h [64]
  - Pimobendan
    - 0.2–0.4 mg/kg PO q12h [65]
    - ~2.8 mg/kg daily in food [66]
  - Enalapril
    - 0.5–1 mg/kg PO q24h [3]
    - 20 mg/kg/day in food [67]
  - Amlodipine: 10 mg/kg/day in food [67]
  - Digoxin: 0.05–0.1 mg/kg PO q12–24h. Reserve for nonresponsive cardiomyopathy, right-sided CHF, DCM, atrial fibrillation [38]

Pneumonia

Diagnosis

History:

- Husbandry and environment (Table 19.4)

Signalment:

- No predilections

Clinical Signs: [41]

- Oculonasal discharge
- Coughing
- Sneezing
- Tachypnea
- Dyspnea

Differentials:

- See Respiratory Distress; Congestive Heart Failure

STAT Diagnostics:

- SpO_2

Complete Diagnostics:

- Radiographs
- CBC/Chem
- Thoracic ultrasound
- Cytology, culture (nasal discharge swab, thoracic aspirate)

Treatment

Stabilization:

- Supportive care (fluids, nutrition, analgesia; see Chapters 7–8)
- Terbutaline: 0.01 mg/kg IM (dilute 1:10 w/ sterile water) [46]
- Nebulization
- Antimicrobials PRN

Continued Care:

- Antibiotic therapy, ideally guided at least by cytology if not culture
- Terbutaline: 0.3–0.4 mg/kg PO q12h [46]
- Theophylline: 10 mg/kg PO q12h (extrapolated from prairie dogs) [3]

Upper Respiratory Infection/Inflammation V. Nasal Dermatitis

Diagnosis

History:

- Husbandry and environment (Table 19.4)
- Gerbils housed without sand baths, on wood shavings, or in excessively humid environments (>50% humidity) predisposed to increased nasolacrimal secretions, causing secondary pyoderma (nasal dermatitis)

Signalment:

- Nasal dermatitis common in gerbils

Clinical Signs: [8, 11, 13, 44]

- Oculonasal discharge (Figure 19.4)
- Sneezing
- Nasal/facial ulcerations
- Facial swelling/asymmetry

Differentials: [11, 13, 32, 43, 44, 68]

- Infectious: *Pasteurella* spp., *Streptococcus* spp
- Environmental irritants
- Dental abscess
- Nasal foreign body
- Neoplasia/polyps

STAT Diagnostics:

- Wood's lamp – porphyrin from Harderian gland secretions will fluoresce

Complete Diagnostics:

- Cytology
- Anesthetized oral examination
- Bacterial culture
- Skull radiographs

Treatment

Stabilization:

- Supportive care (fluids, nutrition, analgesia; see Chapters 7–8)
- Antimicrobials PRN

Continued Care:

- As indicated

Gastrointestinal Disease

Cheek Pouch Eversion

Diagnosis

History:

- Husbandry and environment (Table 19.4)
  - Predisposing factors: Trauma (falls), overfeeding, sticky foods, very large/small foods [69, 70]

Signalment:

- Hamsters only – gerbils do not have cheek pouches
- Russian dwarf hamsters (*Phodopus* spp.) may be predisposed [71]
- Compromised forelimb function may predispose [70]

Clinical Signs: [72]

- Everted cheek pouch: Pedunculated soft tissue originating from distolateral oral cavity. Ulceration, masses, or adhered food possible findings
- Underweight
- Firm swelling on lateral head/neck
- Dental abnormalities

Differentials: [72, 73]

- Inappropriate nutrition
- Neoplasia (Figure 19.5)
- Abscess
- Dental disease
- Foreign body

STAT Diagnostics:

- Anesthetized oral exam

Complete Diagnostics: [72]

- FNA/cytology
- Skull radiographs
- Histopathology
- Bacterial culture

Treatment

Stabilization:

- Supportive care (fluids, nutrition, analgesia; see Chapters 7–8)

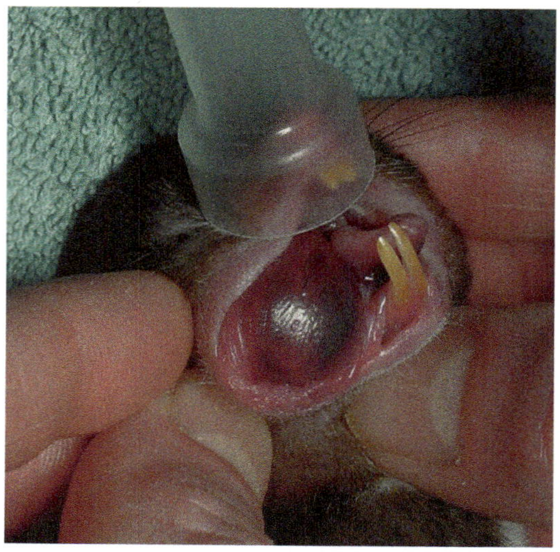

Figure 19.5 Cheek pouch prolapse secondary to neoplasia in a hamster. *Source:* Courtesy of Peter G. Fisher.

Continued Care:

- Replacement: Anesthetize, lavage with warm saline, debride as necessary, apply lubricant, replace. Manipulate with cotton swabs. Percutaneous stay suture using 4–0 or 5–0 suture (absorbable or nonabsorbable). Suture removal 10–14 days [69, 70]
- Resection: Place hemostat across pouch proximal to lesion, transect distal to clamp, close with 5–0 or 6–0 absorbable suture. Remove all cage bedding, hand feed 24–36 hours. Post-op [69, 70]

Dental Disease

Diagnosis

History: [32, 74]

- Husbandry and nutrition (Table 19.4)

Signalment:

- Prior trauma
- Cage chewing
- Gerbils fed non-gerbil diets [15]

Clinical Signs: [32, 49, 74, 75]

- Underweight
- Dental abnormalities (Figure 19.6)
- Ptyalism
- Dysphagia
- Halitosis
- Oculonasal discharge
- Facial swelling, draining tract
- Exophthalmos

Differentials: [32, 49, 74, 75]

- Full cheek pouch
- Abscess
- Trauma
- Neoplasia
- Congenital malocclusion
- Cheek pouch disorders (see above)

STAT Diagnostics:

- Anesthetized oral exam

Complete Diagnostics: [75–77]

- Skull radiographs
- FNA/cytology
- Bacterial culture
- Histopathology

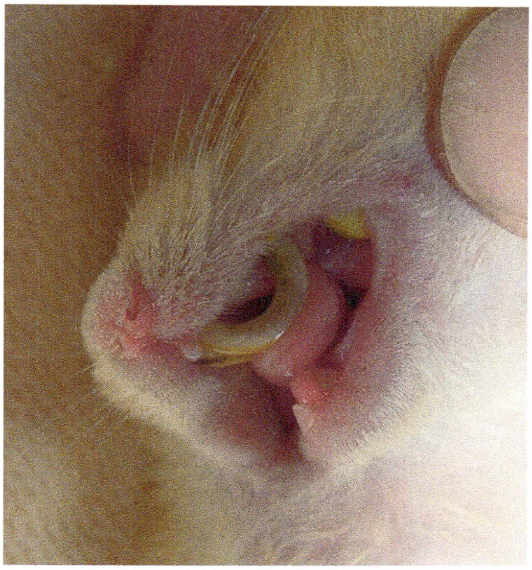

Figure 19.6 Fractured mandibular incisors with secondary maxillary incisor overgrowth in a Syrian hamster. *Source:* Courtesy of Peter G. Fisher.

Treatment

Stabilization:

- Supportive care (fluids, nutrition, analgesia; see Chapters 7–8)
- Reduction of incisor length: Sedate/anesthetize, cut incisors with cross-cut high-speed dental burr, use spatula to protect lips/tongue. Do not use nail trimmers, other manual cutting instruments – potential for vertical fractures, damage to germinal epithelium
- Antimicrobials PRN

Continued Care:

- Periapical abscesses: Extraction of affected teeth
- Surgical treatment of masses
- Mandibular symphyseal fractures: Suture rostral hemimandibles together with 4–0 or 5–0 absorbable suture [76]
- Supportive care until eating on own
- Chronic incisor malocclusions may require trimming ≥ every two weeks

Enteritis: Bacterial, Parasitic

Diagnosis

History:

- See Diarrhea

Signalment:

- See Diarrhea

Clinical Signs:

- See Diarrhea

Differentials [7–15]

- Hamsters:
  - Bacterial: *Lawsonia intracellularis, Clostridium difficile, C. piliforme, Campylobacter jejuni, Salmonella* spp., *Escherichia coli, Helicobacter* spp.
  - Parasitic
    - Helminths
      - Tapeworms (*Rodentolepis* spp., *Hymenolepis diminutia*), pinworms (*Syphacia* spp.)
    - Protozoa
      - *Giardia* spp., *Spironucleus muris* (flagellate), *Cryptosporidium* spp.
- Gerbils
  - Bacterial: *Clostridium piliforme, C. difficile, Citrobacter rodentium, Salmonella* spp., *Helicobacter* spp.
  - Parasitic: *Giardia* spp., pinworms, tapeworms (*Rodentolepis nana, Hymenolepis diminutia*), coccidia (*Eimeria* spp.), *Trichomonas* spp., *Entamoeba muris*

STAT Diagnostics:

- See Diarrhea

Complete Diagnostics: [7, 11, 13–15]

- Fecal cytology (note that *Hymenolepis* is zoonotic and inform owners if found)
- *Giardia* ELISA
- *C. difficile* toxins ELISA
- Fecal PCR
- Fecal culture
- Necropsy

Treatment

Stabilization:

- See Diarrhea
- Antibiotics: Metronidazole, doxycycline, chloramphenicol, enrofloxacin, TMS (see Table 19.2)
- Antiparasitics: Metronidazole, fenbendazole, praziquantel (see Table 19.3)

Continued Care:

- See Diarrhea

Prolapsed Bowel

Diagnosis

History:

- See Diarrhea

Signalment:

- Hamsters with intestinal disease

Clinical Signs:

- See Diarrhea
- Prolapsed bowel (Figure 19.7)

Differentials:

- See Diarrhea (Enteritis – Bacterial, Parasitic)

STAT Diagnostics:

- Verify the identity of prolapsed tissue (bowel v. polyp/mass). If bowel, pass small blunt probe (tom cat catheter, cotton swab) adjacent to/alongside prolapsed tissue
  - If probe passes into pelvic canal, prolapse is intestinal; if not, prolapse is rectal [69]

Complete Diagnostics:

- See Diarrhea (Enteritis – Bacterial, Parasitic)

Treatment

Stabilization:

- Supportive care (fluids, nutrition, analgesia; see Chapters 7–8)
- Prolapse is a surgical emergency; prognosis is poor to grave [49, 69, 70]
- Rectal prolapses
  - Replacement: [69]
    - Lubricate and reduce tissue into pelvic canal using small cotton swabs, soft urinary catheters
    - Pass 5-Fr red rubber catheter into anus, place, anal purse string suture (5–0 or 6–0 nonabsorbable material; snug, not tight)
    - Remove catheter
    - Suture removal 3–5 days

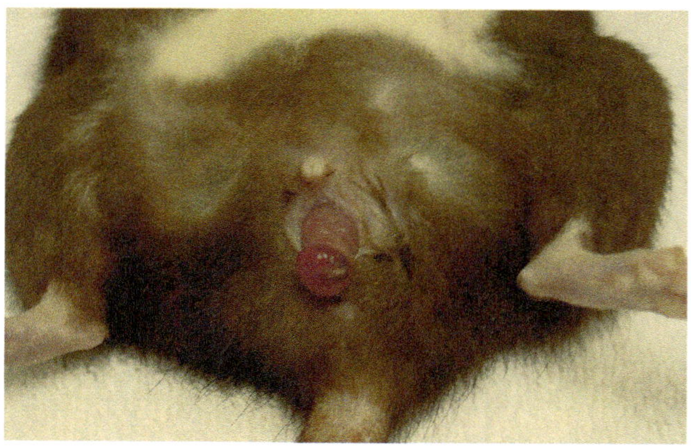

Figure 19.7 Bowel prolapse in a Syrian hamster. *Source:* Courtesy of Peter G. Fisher.

- Necrotic tissue resection: [69]
  - Find segment with healthy tissue around >50% of circumference and make full-thickness incision
  - Suture healthy rectum to healthy anus using 6–0 synthetic absorbable monofilament suture
  - Resect necrotic tissue, suture remaining tissue to anus. No purse string suture needed
- Intestinal prolapses require celiotomy for reduction of intussusceptions, resection of compromised bowel [69]

Continued Care:

- Supportive care (fluids, nutrition, analgesia; see Chapters 7–8)
- Per underlying cause(s)

Urogenital and Reproductive Disease

Ovarian Cysts

Diagnosis

History:

- Recent reduction in litter size [13]

Signalment:

- Gerbils predisposed – prevalence 47% of females >400 days of age [78]
- Prevalence in hamsters unknown [69]

Clinical Signs: [69, 79]

- Abdominal distention, pain
- Dyspnea

Differentials:

- Ovarian cysts
- Ascites
- Neoplasia: Ovarian, adrenal, other [80]
- Polycystic disease (hamsters)

STAT Diagnostics:

- POCUS

Complete Diagnostics:

- Abdominal radiographs, ultrasound
- FNA/cytology
- CBC/chem
- Histopathology

Treatment

Stabilization:

- Supportive care (fluids, nutrition, analgesia; see Chapters 7–8)

Percutaneous drainage of cysts – will refill (days to weeks) [69]

Continued Care:

- Ovariectomy, ovariohysterectomy [69]

Endocrine Disease

Diabetes Mellitus

Diagnosis

History:

- Environment and husbandry (Table 19.4)

Signalment:

- High-fat diet [81]
- Chinese hamsters (*Cricetulus griseus*) may be predisposed
- Rare in gerbils [14]

Clinical Signs:

- Obesity
- Recent weight loss
- Polyuria/polydipsia

Differentials:

- Diabetes mellitus
- Renal disease
- Hyperadrenocorticism
- Neoplasia

STAT Diagnostics:

- GLU

Complete Diagnostics:

- CBC/Chem
- Urinalysis
- Urine culture
- Abdominal radiographs/ultrasound

Treatment

Stabilization:

- Supportive care (fluids, nutrition, analgesia; see Chapters 7–8)
- Insulin: 2 U/animal SC [3]

Continued Care:

- Dietary change – high fiber, high protein, low fat
- Guidelines for treatment of diabetes mellitus in rodents are sparse to nonexistent. Follow general principles for management

Hyperadrenocorticism (Hamster)

Diagnosis [82–84]
History:

- PU/PD

Signalment: [83, 84]

- Hamsters >1.5 years of age

Clinical Signs: [83, 84]

- Alopecia (nonpruritic)
- Skin hyperpigmentation
- Comedones
- Thin skin
- Pyoderma
- Abdominal distention

Differentials: [8, 82]

- Hyperadrenocorticism
- Demodicosis
- Dermatophytosis
- Satin gene carrier (thin/sparse coat)
- Neoplastic/Cystic: Adrenal, lymphoma, hepatic cysts

STAT Diagnostics:

- Skin scraping, cytology

Complete Diagnostics:

- CBC/chem – elevated ALP may be present
- Urinalysis
- DTM
- Abdominal radiographs, ultrasound
- Bacterial culture
- Serum cortisol levels – hamsters secrete both cortisol and corticosterone, limiting utility of cortisol assays alone [85]
- FNA/cytology
- Histopathology

Treatment
Stabilization:

- Supportive care

Continued Care:

- Reports on treatment of hyperadrenocorticism are sparse. Metyrapone 8 mg PO q24h resolved clinical signs in one of two animals [84]

Neoplastic Disease

Cutaneous/Multicentric: Lymphoma

Diagnosis
History:

- Lymphoma in patient's littermates suggests underlying hamster polyomavirus infection

Signalment: [86]

- Young hamsters – secondary to hamster polyomavirus infection
- Older hamsters – primary lymphoma

Clinical Signs: [8, 87–89]

- Lymphadenomegaly
- Cutaneous masses
- Patchy alopecia
- Organomegaly
- Exfoliative erythroderma
- Tachypnea
- Dyspnea

Differentials: [87–89]

- Lymphoma
- Trichoepithelioma (secondary to hamster polyomavirus infection)
- Dermatophytosis
- Ectoparasitism
- Congestive heart failure
- Polycystic disease (hamsters)
- Hyperadrenocorticism
- Nephrotic syndrome

STAT Diagnostics:

- FNA/cytology – microscopic appearance of lymphoma similar to other species [90]

Complete Diagnostics [8, 88]

- CBC/Chem
- Urinalysis
- Whole-body radiographs, ultrasound
- Histopathology +/– IHC, PCR for hamster polyomavirus

Treatment
Stabilization:

- Supportive care (fluids, nutrition, analgesia; see Chapters 7–8)

Continued Care:

– No published treatment regimens for hamster lymphoma. Consider extrapolation of protocols from other species (with caution)

Ascites/Hemoabdomen

Diagnosis
History:

- Exposure to other animals, small children, rodenticide

Signalment:

- No predilections

Clinical Signs: [8, 91]

- Pallor
- Abdominal distention (Figure 19.8)
- Cachexia
- Tachypnea
- Dyspnea

Differentials: [11, 91–93]

- Trauma
- Anticoagulant rodenticide
- Ruptured neoplasm
- Polycystic disease (hamsters)
- Congestive heart failure
- Nephrotic syndrome
- Hepatic failure

STAT Diagnostics:

- Abdominal radiographs, ultrasound
- Fluid analysis

Complete Diagnostics:

- CBC/Chem
- Urinalysis
- Histopathology

Treatment

Stabilization: [8]

- Supportive care (fluids, nutrition, analgesia; see Chapters 7–8)
- Therapeutic abdominocentesis/cyst drainage
  - Anecdotally reported to cause hypovolemia [94]

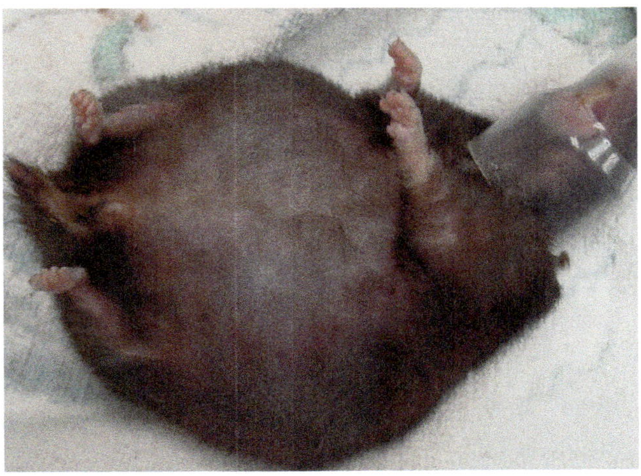

Figure 19.8 Severe ascites secondary to nephrotic syndrome in a Syrian hamster. *Source:* Courtesy of Peter G. Fisher.

Continued care: [8, 69]

- Rodenticide: See Toxins
- Trauma: Surgical emergency – locate, stop hemorrhage
- Neoplasia: Surgery, referral for chemotherapy, radiation
- Polycystic disease: Surgical resection of smaller cysts
- Congestive Heart Failure: See Cardiopulmonary Disease

Dermatologic Disease

Abscesses

Diagnosis

History:

- See Trauma; Dental Disease

Signalment:

- See Trauma; Dental Disease

Clinical Signs: [69, 82]

- Swelling(s), draining tract(s)
- Hunched posture, squinting eyes (pain)
- Alopecia
- Ptyalism
- Exophthalmos

Differentials:

- Trauma
- Periapical infection
- Neoplasia
- Hematogenous spread

STAT Diagnostics:

- FNA/cytology

Complete Diagnostics:

- Bacterial culture
- Radiography
- CBC/Chem
- Histopathology

Treatment

Stabilization:

- Supportive care (fluids, nutrition, analgesia; see Chapters 7–8)

Continued Care: [69]

- Antimicrobials PRN
- Surgical resection of abscess with capsule intact. Lance/flush therapy often fails
- If complete resection impossible, may use Doxirobe or antimicrobial-impregnated poly(methyl methacrylate) (PMMA) beads

Alopecia

Diagnosis

History:

- Husbandry and environment (Table 19.4)
- Pruritus

Signalment:

- Demodicosis common in hamsters, rare in gerbils [16]

Clinical Signs: [16, 82]

- Hair loss (Figure 19.9)
- Pruritus
- Erythema
- Crusts (Figure 19.9)
- Scaling
- Hyperpigmentation
- Excoriations
- Visible ectoparasites

Differentials: [16, 82, 84, 87, 93, 95]

- Demodex mites (Figure 19.9)
  - Adults develop clinical disease secondary to immunosuppression
- Sarcoptiform mites (*Notoedres cati*)
- Tropical rat mite (*Ornithonyssus bacoti*)
  - Grossly visible (0.7–1.1 mm long), easily squashed, may have red appearance due to recent blood meal
- Fleas
- Dermatophytosis (*Trichophyton* spp., *Microsporum* spp.)
- Trauma
- Hyperadrenocorticism
- Cutaneous lymphoma
- Nutritional deficiency
- Satin gene carrier (Syrian hamsters)

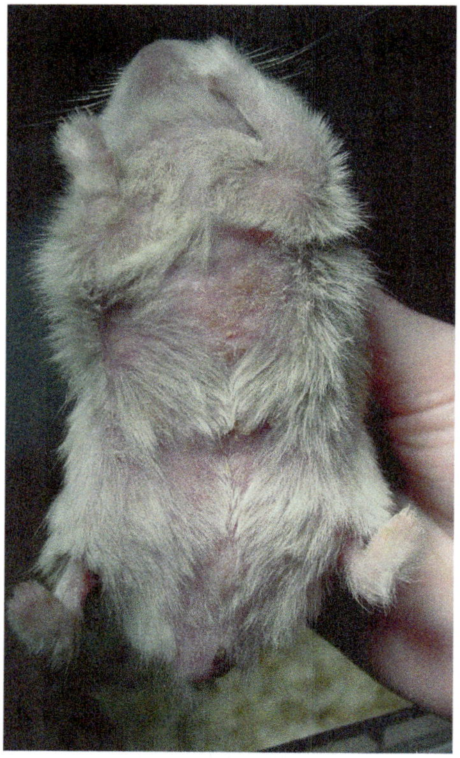

Figure 19.9 Demodicosis with secondary pyoderma in a dwarf hamster. *Source:* Courtesy of Peter G. Fisher.

STAT Diagnostics:

- Skin scraping, cytology
- Wood's lamp examination

Complete Diagnostics:

- Bacterial culture
- DTM
- CBC/Chem
- Radiography
- Ultrasonography

Treatment

Stabilization:

- Supportive care (fluids, nutrition, analgesia; see Chapters 7–8)

Continued care: [16]

- Anti-infectives PRN (Tables 19.2 and 19.3)
  - Avoid pyrethrin powders – may cause neurologic signs
- Environmental treatment
  - Dispose of bedding or wash at >60 °C (140 °F)
  - Disinfect cage
  - Tropical rat mite: Premises treatment by professional exterminator

Tail-Slip/Degloving Injuries

Diagnosis

History:

- See Trauma

Signalment:

- Gerbils restrained by tails
- See Trauma

Clinical Signs:

- Degloving injury
- Self-mutilation
- See Trauma

Differentials:

- See Trauma

STAT Diagnostics:

- Radiography of affected areas – evaluate for fractures

Complete Diagnostics:

- See Trauma

Treatment

Stabilization:

- Supportive care (fluids, nutrition, analgesia; see Chapters 7–8)

Continued Care:

- Tail slip: Partial/complete caudectomy. Technique same as larger animals. Close SC tissues with 5–0 or 6–0 absorbable suture, close skin with tissue adhesive or intradermal suture [69]
- Other sites: Bandaging if wounds are fresh, blood supply adequate, but bandages may not be well-tolerated. Amputation may be required

Ventral Gland Lesions

Diagnosis

History:

- Husbandry and environment (Table 19.4)

Signalment:

- Ventral gland neoplasia – gerbils [42]

Clinical Signs:

- Mass associated with gland
- Ulceration (Figure 19.10)
- Purulent discharge (Figure 19.10)

Differentials:

- Neoplasia [96, 97]
- Infection

STAT Diagnostics:

- FNA/impression, cytology

Complete Diagnostics:

- Histopathology
- Bacterial culture
- Thoracic radiographs

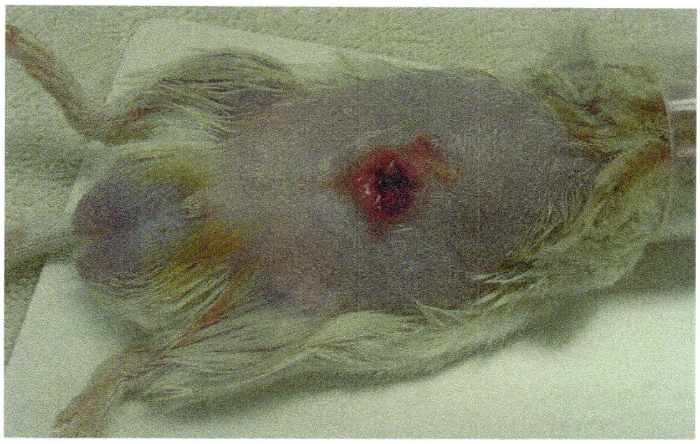

Figure 19.10 Infected ventral gland in a gerbil. *Source:* Courtesy of Peter G. Fisher.

Treatment

Stabilization:

- Supportive care (fluids, nutrition, analgesia; see Chapters 7–8)

Continued Care:

- Neoplasia: Surgical removal, referral for chemotherapy, radiation
- Antimicrobials PRN

Ophthalmic Disease

Exophthalmos/Proptosis

Diagnosis

History:

- Husbandry and environment (Table 19.4)
- Recent restraint by holding the skin of the dorsal neck

Signalment:

- Hamsters presented more often than gerbils [69]

Clinical Signs:

- Exophthalmos
- Proptosis

Differentials:

- See Ocular Signs; Trauma; Dental Disease

STAT Diagnostics:

- Assess vision

Complete Diagnostics:

- See Ocular Signs; Trauma; Dental Disease

Treatment

Stabilization:

- Supportive care (fluids, nutrition, analgesia; see Chapters 7–8)
- Traumatic exophthalmos: Cleanse globe with ophthalmic rinse and apply sterile lubricant. Retract palpebrae around globe until it falls back into position. Temporary tarsorrhaphy with 6–0 suture if needed [8]
- Retrobulbar abscess/neoplasia: Exenteration using similar technique to larger mammals. See Abscesses [69]
- Proptosis:
  - If patient presented immediately post-proptosis and eye remains visual, replacement with temporary tarsorrhaphy may be attempted
  - If salvage not possible, enucleation indicated. Transpalpebral or transconjunctival approaches have been described. Major hemorrhage often occurs with removal of the Harderian gland; advise starting palpebral closure prior to removal of the gland [69, 98]
- Avoid damaging the large retroorbital venous sinus. Control of hemorrhage achieved by placement of cellulose sponge within the orbit and applying pressure for five minutes [69]

Continued Care:

- After reduction of exophthalmos: Ophthalmic antibiotics (without glucocorticoids) for at least 7–10 days [8]

References

1 Johnson DH. Critical care in rodents and how to get them to survive [Internet]. American board of veterinary practitioners symposium; 2013 Oct 31 – Nov 3; Phoenix, AZ. [place unknown]: American Board of Veterinary Practitioners. 2013 [cited 2016 May 13]. Available from: http://www.vin.com/doc/?id=5959784.

2 Morrisey, J.K. and Carpenter, J.W. (2012). Formulary. In: Ferrets, Rabbits, and Rodents: Clinical Medicine and Surgery, 3ee (eds. K.E. Quesenberry and J.W. Carpenter), 566–575. St. Louis: Saunders.

3 Mayer, J. (2013). Rodents. In: Exotic Animal Formulary, 4ee (eds. J.W. Carpenter and C.J. Marion), 476–516. St. Louis: Saunders.

4 Plumb DC. Plumb's veterinary drug handbook [Internet]. 8th ed. Stockholm: PharmaVet Inc; 2015. Chloramphenicol; [cited 2016 June 8]. Available from: http://www.vin.com/doc/?id=4692110&pid=451.

5 Plumb DC. Plumb's veterinary drug handbook [Internet]. 8th ed. Stockholm: PharmaVet Inc; 2015. Griseofulvin; [cited 2016 June 8]. Available from: http://www.vin.com/doc/?id=5070108&pid=648.

6 Plumb DC. Plumb's veterinary drug handbook [Internet]. 8th ed. Stockholm: PharmaVet Inc; 2015. Ketoconazole; [cited 2016 June 8]. Available from: http://www.vin.com/doc/?id=4692306&pid=451.

7 Keller, D.L. (2013). Small mammals: hamsters – intestinal disorders. In: Clinical Veterinary Advisor: Birds and Exotic Pets (eds. J. Mayer and T.M. Donnelly), 291–293. St. Louis: Saunders.

8 Brown, C. and Donnelly, T.M. (2012). Disease problems of small rodents. In: Ferrets, Rabbits, and Rodents: Clinical Medicine and Surgery, 3e (eds. K.E. Quesenberry and J.W. Carpenter), 354–372. St. Louis: Saunders.

9 Reavill, D. (2005). Diagnosing the unexpected in exotic patients. *Exot. DVM* 7 (3): 16–23.

10 Fiskett, R.A.M. (2011). *Lawsonia intracellularis* infection in hamsters (*Mesocrecitus auratus*). *J. Exot. Pet Med.* 20 (4): 277–283.

11 Percy, D.H. and Barthold, S.W. (2007). Hamster. In: Pathology of Laboratory Rodents and Rabbits, 3e, 179–205. Ames: Blackwell Publishing Professional.

12 Reavill D. Disease conditions of young rodents with diagnostic and therapy options [Internet]. Association of exotic mammal veterinarians scientific program; 2011 Aug 7; Seattle, WA. [place unknown]: Assoc of Exotic Mammal Veterinarians. 2011 [cited 2016 May 31] Available from: http://tinyurl.com/hqzlulu.

13 Percy, D.H. and Barthold, S.W. (2007). Gerbil. In: Pathology of Laboratory Rodents and Rabbits, 3e, 207–216. Ames: Blackwell Publishing Professional.

14 Johnson DH. The gastrointestinal tract of the mouse, gerbil, and hamster: health and disease. American board of veterinary practitioners symposium [Internet]; 2012 April 12–15; San Antonio, TX. [place unknown]: American Board of Veterinary Practitioners. 2012 [cited 2016 May 31]. Available from: http://www.vin.com/doc/?id=5349776.

15 Huynh, M. and Pignon, C. (2013). Gastrointestinal disease in exotic small mammals. *J. Exot. Pet Med.* 22: 118–131.

16 Fehr, M. and Koestlinger, S. (2013). Ectoparasites in small exotic mammals. *Vet. Clin. North Am. Exot. Anim. Pract.* 16: 611–657.

17 Tani, K., Iwanaga, T., Sonoda, K. et al. (2001). Ivermectin treatment of demodicosis in 56 hamsters. *J. Vet. Med. Sci.* 63 (11): 1245–1247.

18 Mancinelli, E. (2015). Neurologic examination and diagnostic testing in ferrets, rabbits, and rodents. *J. Exot. Pet Med.* 24: 52–64.

19 Meredith, A.L. and Richardson, A. (2015). Neurological diseases of rabbits and rodents. *J. Exot. Pet Med.* 24: 21–33.

20 Chole, R.A., Henry, K.R., and McGinn, M.D. (1981). Cholesteatoma: spontaneous occurrence in the Mongolian gerbil *Merones unguiculatis*. *Am. J. Otol.* 2 (3): 204–210.

21 Guinjoan, S.M., Golombek, D.A., and Cardinali, D.P. (1992). Time-dependent anesthetic and anticonvulsant activities of alphaxalone in Syrian hamsters. *Life Sci.* 51: 2089–2095.

22 Frey, H.H., Löscher, W., Reiche, R. et al. (1983). Anticonvulsant potency of common antiepileptic drugs in the gerbil. *Pharmacol. Ther. Part A* 27: 330–335.

23 Löscher W, Nolting B, Hönack D. Evaluation of CPP, a selective NMDA antagonist, in various rodent models of epilepsy. Comparison with other NMDA antagonists, and with diazepam and phenobarbital.

24 Bartoszyk, G.D. and Hamer, M. (1987). The genetic animal model of reflex epilepsy in the Mongolian gerbil: differential efficacy of new anticonvulsive drugs and prototype antiepileptics. *Pharmacol. Res. Commun.* 19 (6): 429–440.

25 Barrera-Bailón, B., Oliveira, J.A.C., López, D.E. et al. (2013). Pharmacological and neuroethological studies of three antiepileptic drugs in the genetic Audiogenic seizure hamster (GASH:Sal). *Epilepsy Behav.* 28: 413–425.

26 Percy, D.H. and Barthold, S.W. (2007). Hamster: nutritional and metabolic disorders. In: Pathology of Laboratory Rodents and Rabbits, 3e, 198–199. Ames: Blackwell Publishing Professional.

27 Keller, D.L. (2013). Small mammals: hamsters – ocular disorders. In: Clinical Veterinary Advisor: Birds and Exotic Pets (eds. J. Mayer and T.M. Donnelly), 293–295. St. Louis: Saunders.

28 Ekesten, B. and Dubielzig, R.R. (1999). Spontaneous buphthalmos in the Djungarian hamster (*Phodopus sungorus cambelli*). *Vet. Ophthalmol.* 2: 251–254.

29 Millichamp, N.J. (2002). Ophthalmic disease in exotic species. *Vet. Clin. North Am. Exot. Anim. Pract.* 5: 223–241.

30 Verstraete, F.J.M. (2003). Advances in the diagnosis and treatment of small exotic mammal dental disease. *Semin. Avian Exot. Pet* 12 (1): 37–48.

31 Johnson, D.H. (2012). Emergency presentations of the exotic small mammalian herbivore trauma patient. *J. Exot. Pet Med.* 21: 300–315.

32 Legendre, L.F.J. (2003). Oral disorders of exotic rodents. *Vet. Clin. North Am. Exot. Anim. Pract.* 6: 601–628.

33 Donnelly TM. Exotic animal ophthalmology [Internet]. Association of exotic mammal veterinarians conference; 2011 Aug 6–12; Seattle, WA. [place unknown]: Assoc of Exotic Mammal Veterinarians. 2011 Aug 6 [cited 2016 June 1]. Available from: http://tinyurl.com/h5lxfho.

34 Rajaei, S.M., Mood, M.A., Sadjadi, R. et al. (2016). Results of selected ophthalmic diagnostic tests for clinically normal Syrian hamsters (*Mesocrecitus auratus*). *Am. J. Vet. Res.* 77 (1): 72–76.

35 Rajaei, S.M., Sadjadi, R., Sabzevari, A. et al. (2013). Results of phenol red thread test in clinically normal Syrian hamsters (*Mesocrecitus auratus*). *Vet. Ophthal.* 16 (6): 436–439.

36 Kling, M.A. (2011). A review of respiratory system anatomy, physiology, and disease in the mouse, rat, hamster, and gerbil. *Vet. Clin. North Am. Exot. Anim. Pract.* 14: 287–337.

37 Renshaw, H.W., Van Hoosier, G.L., and Amend, N.K. (1975). A survey of naturally occurring diseases in the Syrian hamster. *Lab. Anim.* 9: 175–191.

38 Heatley, J.J. (2009). Cardiovascular anatomy, physiology, and disease of rodents and small exotic mammals. *Vet. Clin. North Am. Exot. Anim. Pract.* 12: 99–113.

39 Liu, S.K. and Tilley, L.P. (1980). Animal models of primary myocardial diseases. *Yale J. Biol. Med.* 53: 191–211.

40 Reavill, D.R. and Schmidt, R.E. (2007). Cardiovascular disease in hamsters: review and retrospective study. *J. Exot. Pet Med.* 16 (1): 49–51.

41 Johnson DH. Pneumonia in small mammals. Association of exotic mammal veterinarians conference; 2011 Aug 6–12; Seattle, WA. [place unknown]: Assoc of Exotic Mammal Veterinarians; 2011 Aug 6. 413–418.

42 Heatley, J.J. and Harris, M.C. (2009). Hamsters and gerbils. In: Manual of Exotic Pet Practice (eds. M.A. Mitchell and T.N. Tully), 406–432. St. Louis: Saunders.

43 Pour, P., Mohr, U., Cardesa, A. et al. (1976). Spontaneous tumors and common diseases in two colonies of Syrian hamsters II. Respiratory tract and digestive system. *J. Natl. Cancer Inst.* 56 (5): 937–948.

44 Mohr, U. (1982). Tumours of the respiratory tract. In: Pathology of Tumors in Laboratory Animals. Vol. III – Tumors of the Hamster (eds. V.S. Turusov, G. Della Porta, C.F. Hollander, et al.), 115–145. Lyon: International Agency for Research on Cancer.

45 Frisk, C.S. (1987). Bacterial and mycotic diseases. In: Laboratory Hamsters (eds. G.L. Van Hoosier and C.W. McPherson), 112–133. Orlando: Academic Press.

46 Gentz N, Gwaltney-Brant S. VIN Formulary for Exotic Animals [Internet]. Davis: Veterinary Information Network; 2014. Terbutaline; [cited 2016 June 1]. Available from: http://www.vin.com/doc/?id=6461581&pid=648.

47 Hawkins, M.G., Barron, H.W., Speer, B.L. et al. (2013). Birds. In: Exotic animal formulary, 4e (eds. J.W. Carpenter and C.J. Marion), 184–437. St. Louis: Saunders.

48 Gentz N, Gwaltney-Brant S. VIN Formulary for Exotic Animals [Internet]. Davis: Veterinary Information Network; 2012. Theophylline; 2012 [cited 2016 June 1]. Available from: http://www.vin.com/doc/?id=5070265&pid=648.
49 Hawkins, M.G. and Graham, J.E. (2007). Emergency and critical care of rodents. *Vet. Clin. North Am. Exot. Anim. Pract.* 10: 501–531.
50 Bertorelli, R., Adami, M., and Ongini, E. (1995). The Mongolian gerbil in experimental epilepsy. *Ital. J. Neurol. Sci.* 16: 101–106.
51 Loskota, W.J., Lomax, P.J., and Rich, S.T. (1974). The Mongolian gerbil as a model for the study of epilepsies. *Epilepsia* 15: 109–119.
52 Laming, P.R., Cosby, S.L., and O'Neil, J.K. (1989). Seizures in the Mongolian gerbil are related to a deficiency in cerebral glutamate synthetase. *Comp. Biochem. Physiol.* 94C (2): 399–404.
53 Wilz, M. and Heldmaier, G. (2000). Comparison of hibernation, estivation, and daily torpor in the edible dormouse, *Glis glis*. *J. Comp. Physiol. B* 170: 511–521.
54 Newcomer, C.E., Fitts, D.A., Goldman, B.D. et al. (1987). Experimental biology: other research uses of Syrian hamsters. In: Laboratory Hamsters (eds. G.L. Van Hoosier and C.W. McPherson), 264–299. Orlando: Academic Press.
55 Lichtenberger, M. and Richardson, J.A. (2008). Emergency care and managing toxicoses in the exotic animal patient. *Vet. Clin. North Am. Exot. Anim. Pract.* 11: 211–228.
56 Port, C.D., Baxter, D.W., and Richter, W.R. (1974). The Mongolian gerbil as a model for lead toxicity, I. studies of acute poisoning. *Am. J. Pathol.* 76: 79–94.
57 Wismer T. Managing toxicoses in exotic animals [Internet]. Wild west veterinary conference; 2009 Oct 14–18; Reno, NV. [place unknown]: Wild West Veterinary Conference. 2009 [cited 2016 June 1]. Available from: http://www.vin.com/doc/?id=5672258.
58 Lindstrom, N.M., Moore, D.M., Zimmerman, K. et al. (2015). Hematologic assessment in pet rats, mice, hamsters, and gerbils: blood sample collection and blood cell identification. *Vet. Clin. North Am. Exot. Anim. Pract.* 18 (1): 21–32.
59 Gentz N, Gwaltney-Brant S. VIN Formulary for Exotic Animals [Internet]. Davis: Veterinary Information Network; 2012. Calcium versenate (CaEDTA); 2012 [cited 2016 June 1]. Available from: http://www.vin.com/doc/?id=5069996&pid=648.
60 Smith, D., Bayer, L., and Strupp, B.J. (1998). Efficacy of succimer chelation for reducing brain Pb levels in a rodent model. *Environ. Res. A* 78: 168–176.
61 Gentz N, Gwaltney-Brant S. VIN Formulary for Exotic Animals [Internet]. Davis: Veterinary Information Network; 2012. Viamin K1; 2012 [cited 2016 June 1]. Available from: http://www.vin.com/doc/?id=5070292&pid=648.
62 Gentz N, Gwaltney-Brant S. VIN Formulary for Exotic Animals [Internet]. Davis: Veterinary Information Network; 2012. Meclizine; 2012 [cited 2016 Sept 14]. Available from: http://www.vin.com/doc/?id=5070156&pid=648
63 Keller, D.L. (2013). Small mammals: hamsters – cardiac disease. In: Clinical Veterinary Advisor: Birds and Exotic Pets (eds. J. Mayer and T.M. Donnelly), 287–288. St. Louis: Saunders.
64 Bhattacharya, S.K., Palmieri, G.M.A., Bertorini, T.E. et al. (1982). The effects of diltiazem in dystrophic hamsters. *Muscle Nerve* 5: 73–78.
65 Mitchell EB, Zehnder AM, Hsu A, et al. Pimobendan: treatment of heart failure in small mammals. Association of exotic mammal veterinarians conference; 2008 Aug 10; Savannah, GA. [place unknown]: Assoc of Exotic Mammal Veterinarians; 2008. 71–79.
66 Van Meel, J.C.A., Mauz, A.B.M., Wienen, W. et al. (1989). Pimobendan increases survival of cardiomyopathic hamsters. *J. Cardiovasc. Pharmacol.* 13: 508–509.
67 Watanabe M, Kawaguchi H, Onozuki H, et al. Chronic effects of enalapril and amlodipine on cardiac remodeling in cardiomyopathic hamster hearts.
68 Bornstein, S. and Iwarsson, K. (1980). Nasal mites in a colony of laboratory hamsters (*Mesocrecitus auratus*). *Lab. anim.* 14: 31–33.
69 Bennett, R.A. (2012). Small rodents: soft tissue surgery. In: Ferrets, Rabbits, and Rodents: Clinical Medicine and Surgery, 3e (eds. K.E. Quesenberry and J.W. Carpenter), 373–391. St. Louis: Saunders.
70 Capello, V. (2003). Surgical techniques in pet hamsters. *Exot. DVM* 5 (3): 32–37.
71 Capello, V. (2001). Pet hamster medicine and surgery – part II: clinical evaluation and therapeutics. *Exot. DVM* 3 (4): 33–39.
72 Evans, B.A. and Keller, D.L. (2013). Small mammals: hamsters – cheek pouch disorder. In: Clinical Veterinary Advisor: Birds and Exotic Pets (eds. J. Mayer and T.M. Donnelly), 288–290. St. Louis: Saunders.
73 Emminger, A. and Mohr, U. (1982). Tumours of the oral cavity, cheek pouch, salivary glands, oesophagus, stomach and intestines. In: Pathology of Tumors in Laboratory Animals. Vol. III – Tumors of the Hamster (eds. V.S. Turusov, G. Della Porta, C.F. Hollander, et al.), 45–68. Lyon: International Agency for Research on Cancer.
74 Capello, V. and Lennox, A.M. (2012). Small mammal dentistry. In: Ferrets, Rabbits, and Rodents: Clinical Medicine and Surgery, 3e (eds. K.E. Quesenberry and J.W. Carpenter), 452–471. St. Louis: Saunders.

75 Keller, D.L. (2013). Small mammals: hamsters – dental disease. In: Clinical Veterinary Advisor: Birds and Exotic Pets (eds. J. Mayer and T.M. Donnelly), 290–291. St. Louis: Saunders.

76 Capello, V. (2008). Diagnosis and treatment of dental disease in pet rodents. *J. Exot. Pet Med.* 17 (2): 114–123.

77 Capello, V. (2008). Clinical technique: application of computed tomography for diagnosis of dental disease in the rabbit, Guinea pig, and chinchilla. *J. Exot. Pet Med.* 17 (2): 93–101.

78 Norris, M.L. and Adams, C.E. (1972). Incidence of cystic ovaries and reproductive performance in the Mongolian gerbil, *Merones unguiculatus*. *Lab. Anim.* 6: 337–342.

79 Lewis, W. (2003). Cystic ovaries in gerbils. *Exot. DVM* 5 (1): 12–13.

80 Rowe, S.E., Simmons, J.L., Ringler, D.H. et al. (1974). Spontaenous neoplasms in aging gerbillinae: a summary of forty-four neoplasms. *Vet. Path.* 11: 38–51.

81 Li, G., Liu, X., Zhu, H. et al. (2009). Insulin resistance in insulin-resistant and diabetic hamsters (*Mesocrecitus auratus*) is associated with abnormal hepatic expression of genes involved in lipid and glucose metabolism. *Comp. Med.* 59 (5): 449–458.

82 Keller, D.L. (2013). Small mammals: hamsters – skin diseases. In: Clinical Veterinary Advisor: Birds and Exotic Pets (eds. J. Mayer and T.M. Donnelly), 297–299. St. Louis: Saunders.

83 Martinho, F. (2006). Suspected case of hyperadrenocorticism in a golden hamster (*Mesocrecitus auratus*). *Vet. Clin. North Am. Exot. Anim. Pract.* 9: 717–721.

84 Bauck, L., Orr, J.P., and Lawrence, K.H. (1984). Hyperadrenocorticism in three teddy bear hamsters. *Can. Vet. J.* 25: 247–250.

85 Ottenweller, J.E., Tapp, W.N., Burke, J.M. et al. (1985). Plasma cortisol and corticosterone concentrations in the golden hamster, (*Mesocrecitus auratus*). *Life Sci.* 16: 1551–1558.

86 Kashuba, C., Hsu, C., Krogstad, A. et al. (2006). Small mammal virology. *Vet. Clin. North Am. Exot. Anim. Pract.* 9: 717–721.

87 Fisher, P.G. (2006). Exotic mammal renal disease: causes and clinical presentation. *Vet. Clin. North Am. Exot. Anim. Pract.* 9: 33–67.

88 Beck, A.P., Compton, S.R., and Zeiss, C.J. (2014). Pathology in practice: HaPyV infection in a pet Syrian hamster. *J. Am. Vet. Med. Assoc.* 244 (9): 1037–1039.

89 Simmons, J.H., Riley, L.K., Franklin, C.L. et al. (2001). Hamster polyomavirus infection in a pet Syrian hamster (*Mesocrecitus auratus*). *Vet. Pathol.* 38: 441–446.

90 Garner, M.M. (2007). Cytologic diagnosis of diseases in rabbits, Guinea pigs, and rodents. *Vet. Clin. North Am. Exot. Anim. Pract.* 10: 25–49.

91 Keller, D.L. (2013). Small mammals: hamsters – abdominal distention. In: Clinical Veterinary Advisor: Birds and Exotic Pets (eds. J. Mayer and T.M. Donnelly), 285–287. St. Louis: Saunders.

92 Fisher, P.G. (2013). Small mammals: hamsters – renal disease. In: Clinical Veterinary Advisor: Birds and Exotic Pets (eds. J. Mayer and T.M. Donnelly), 295–297. St. Louis: Saunders.

93 Somvanshi, R., Iyer, P.K.R., Biswas, J.C. et al. (1987). Polycystic disease in golden hamsters. *J. Comp. Pathol.* 97: 615–618.

94 Lewis W. Rodents [Internet]. British small animal veterinary congress; 2011 March 31 – April 3; [place unknown]. [place unknown]: British Small Animal Veterinary Association. 2011 [cited 2016 June 7]. Available from: http://www.vin.com/doc/?id=4823274.

95 Fehr, M. (2015). Zoonotic potential of dermatophytosis in small mammals. *J. Exot. Pet Med.* 24: 308–316.

96 Pogosianz, H.E. (1975). Djungarian hamster – a suitable tool for cancer research and cytogenic studies. *J. Natl. Cancer Inst.* 54 (3): 659–664.

97 Meckley, P.E. and Zwicker, G.M. (1979). Naturally-occurring neoplasms in the Mongolian gerbil, *Meriones unguiculatus*. *Lab. Anim.* 13: 203–206.

98 Holmberg, B.J. (2007). Enucleation of exotic pets. *J. Exot. Pet Med.* 16 (2): 88–94.

20

Hedgehogs

Rina Maguire[1], Ali Anwar bin Ahmad[2], and Trent Charles van Zanten[3]

[1] Owner and Veterinarian, Beecroft Bird & Exotics Veterinary Clinic, Singapore
[2] Department of Veterinary Services Singapore Zoological Gardens, Singapore
[3] Conservation, Research and Veterinary Services, Jurong Bird Park, Wildlife Reserves Singapore, Singapore

CONTENTS

Unique Species Considerations

- Shy nocturnal species that will curl into a defensive position exposing quills when scared
- Full physical examination and diagnostics usually performed on anesthetized patients
- Intubation is technically difficult and injectable sedation or anesthesia box induction followed by mask maintenance is more feasible
- Peripheral veins are small, limiting intravenous catheter placement and curling will dislodge most catheters
- When curled into a defensive position, oral medications and assisted feeding is challenging
- Placement of an esophagostomy tube can be well-tolerated [1]
- Radiodense spines should be retracted with a bulldog or plastic bag clip when imaging
- Neoplasia is very common in this species and should be considered a potential differential in all sick hedgehogs

Exotic Animal Emergency and Critical Care Medicine, First Edition. Edited by Jennifer E. Graham, Grayson A. Doss and Hugues Beaufrère.

Common Presenting Signs

Anorexia

Introduction

- This species commonly presents for anorexia and other non-specific clinical signs

Diagnosis

History:

- Environmental factors (see Box 20.3)
- Concurrent clinical signs

Signalment:

- No sex or age predilection
- Recently acquired

Clinical signs:

- Decreased or complete cessation of food intake, fecal, and/or urine output
- Decreased activity levels

Differentials:

- Medical causes
  - Systemic disease
  - Dehydration
  - Infection
  - Organ dysfunction
  - See Trauma
  - See Neoplasia
  - See Parasites
- Non-medical causes

STAT Diagnostics:

- Fecal direct and floatation
- PCV/TS/Glucose (Glu)/Lactate (if blood limited)
- Blood smear

Full Diagnostics:

- CBC/biochemistry panel
- Thoracic and abdominal radiographs
- Abdominal ultrasound

Treatment

Stabilization:

- Fluid therapy as indicated (Box 20.1)
- Nutritional support (Box 20.2)
- Hospital cages should include hide boxes, appropriate heat support, and replication of the home fed diet if appropriate

Continued Care:

- Correction of the underlying medical cause if present
- Address environmental stressors (Box 20.3)

Diarrhea

Introduction

- Commonly seen in hedgehogs
- Transit time averages 12–16 hours [4]
- Normal stool appearance varies from pellet-like to soft formed consistency
- Green coloration of stools may be the result of over-excretion of bile into the stool secondary to decreased food intake, not pathognomonic for any disease

Box 20.1 Fluid Therapy

- Subcutaneous isotonic fluids can be administered at up to 100 ml/kg/day [2] divided over 2 areas given 2–3 times daily
- The junction between spined and furred skin is the ideal area to administer fluids as it is most quickly absorbed [3]. However, in practice, this may not be possible
- Fluids are most easily administered by inserting a butterfly catheter into the subdermal space between the quills while the animal is curled
- In debilitated and collapsed animals, IV or IO fluid administration is preferred
  - The placement and maintenance of IV catheters are difficult and seldom utilized [3]
  - The preferred technique would be IO catheterization through the proximal tibia or proxim0al femur. The 0procedure is usually performed under anesthesia
- Fluid therapy using a slow bolus or syringe pump of balanced isotonic or colloidal fluids can be administered until hydration is achieved
- Maintenance fluid rate is estimated at 50-100 ml/kg/day and adjustments can be made accordingly for dehydration deficits

Box 20.2 Nutritional Support

List of soft foods that can be offered by hand or syringe feeding

- Hills A/D can food or critical care diet for carnivores
- Ground up kibble – use coffee grinder to produce a fine grind. Re-constitute to a slurry with warm water. A few drops of omega oil can be added to the mixture
- Frozen insects such as mealworm or crickets can also be mashed up
- Cooked shredded chicken meat
- Baby food – chicken, sweet potato flavor, apple favors
- Eggs – cook in microwave or soft scrambled

Box 20.3 Environmental Stressors

- Poor nutritional content of diet
- Abrupt diet change
- Inappropriate ambient temperature (ideally 72–80 F)
- Overcrowded housing (ideally housed individually otherwise compatible females or neutered male/female pairs if tolerated, males should not be housed together)
- Housing near other predator species pets
- Poor cross-flow ventilation
- Inappropriate dusty substrate such as sand, wood shaving, sawdust
- Poor cage hygiene

Diagnosis

History:

- Recent changes in diet, environment, or stressors
- Determine duration, severity, and frequency of the diarrhea
- In some instances, green diarrhea may present only at the veterinarian's office, may be stress-induced
- Mild acute diarrhea may be self-limiting due to a passing hypermotility

Signalment:

- All ages and sexes but young animals are more commonly affected by stress, diet intolerances, or infectious agents

Clinical signs:

- Unformed stools with possible mucus or blood varying in color from tan, brown to green
- Decreased appetite
- Decreased activity
- Pyrexia
- Hunched posture due to abdominal pain

Differentials:

Infectious:

- Bacterial (common), parasites (less common), and fungi (rare)

Non-infectious:

- Gastrointestinal neoplasia
- Lymphosarcoma, adenocarcinoma, acinic cell carcinoma [5]
- Dietary intolerance
- Environmental factors (Box 20.3)
- Malnutrition
- Pyloric or intestinal obstruction
- Hepatic lipidosis

STAT Diagnostics:

- Fecal floatation/direct
- Fecal culture – aerobic/anaerobic/salmonella testing

Full Diagnostics:

- CBC/biochemistry panel
- Abdominal radiographs
- Abdominal ultrasound
- Cryptosporidium PCR
- Intestinal biopsy
- Fungal culture

Treatment

- **Stabilization:**
  - Treat clinical hypoglycemia with 12.5% dextrose slow IV to effect. 2.5–7% dextrose infusion as required
  - H2 blocker for secondary gastritis
    Famotidine: 1 mg/kg PO/SC q24h
  - Analgesia
    Buprenorphine: 0.01–0.5 mg/kg IM q12h
  - Antibiotics – generally not required unless the patient is systemically unwell
  - Antifungals for systemic candidiasis; see Enteritis
  - Anti-parasitic drugs; see Enteritis
- **Continued Care**
  - Fluid therapy (see Box 20.1)
  - Nutritional support (see Box 20.2)
  - Serial blood glucose levels if anorexic
  - Repeat fecal salmonella culture after one month of antibiotic therapy

Respiratory Distress

Introduction

- Pre-oxygenate prior to exam, diagnostics, or procedures
- Stress-induced physiologic tachypnea is difficult to differentiate from distress

- Most commonly dyspnea is due to CHF (Dilated cardiomyopathy [DCM]) or pneumonia
- Hedgehogs routinely make snuffling, chuffing, grunting like noises, especially when fearful or agitated, that should not be confused with respiratory signs
- Hedgehogs exhibit a unique behavior known as "self-anointing" or "anting" where frothy saliva is produced and spread on the spines near the face. This is triggered by novel objects/smells and should not be interpreted as airway secretions or fulminant pulmonary edema

Diagnosis

History:

- Environmental factors (see Box 20.3)
- Confirm respiratory signs noted at home, usually with lethargy
- Reports of vomiting noted with aspiration pneumonia

Signalment:

- CHF common in geriatric males but can occur adults >1 year old
- General incidence of cardiac disease 40%

Clinical signs:

- Dyspnea, tachypnea
- Pulmonary crackles, rales
- Cyanosis (MM, lips, feet)
- Coughing
- Stertor
- Upper respiratory signs (nasal discharge, sneezing)
- Sudden death

Differentials:

- Pneumonia
  - Hematogenous (bacterial most common)
  - Aspiration
- Pulmonary edema/CHF
  - Dilated cardiomyopathy (DCM most common)
  - Valvular endocardiosis
- Pulmonary neoplasia
  - Primary: Bronchoalveolar carcinoma
  - Secondary: LSA, metastatic SCC, adrenocortical carcinoma
- Thoracic trauma
  - Pulmonary contusions, pneumothorax, hemothorax
- Intra-thoracic disease
  - Pleural effusion; see DCM or Neoplasia
  - Pneumothorax; see Trauma
  - Mediastinal mass(es); see Neoplasia
- Upper respiratory tract disease
  - Can mimic and/or progress to respiratory distress
  - Usually infectious or environmental

STAT Diagnostics:

- POCUS (TFAST/AFAST)
- Pulse oximetry
- ECG
- PCV/TS/Glu/Lactate (if limited blood sample)
- Blood smear

Complete Diagnostics:

- Thoracic and abdominal radiographs
- Thoracocentesis with fluid analysis
- CBC/biochemistry panel
- Echocardiogram
- Complete thoracic ultrasound
  - Ultrasound-guided transthoracic lung/mass aspirates
    - Cytology
    - Aerobic/anaerobic bacterial cultures
- *Trans*-oral tracheal wash (infrequently performed)

Treatment

Stabilization:

- Oxygen supplementation (see Chapter 3)
- Furosemide: 3–5 mg/kg SC, IM, IV, IO (See CHF management)
- Empiric antibiotics:
  - Trimethoprim-Sulfa: 30 mg/kg PO, SC, IM q12h
  - Enrofloxacin: 5–10 mg/kg PO, SC, IM q12h
- Therapeutic thoracocentesis
- Pneumothorax or large volume pleural effusion

Continued care:

- See pneumonia/URI for further management
- See DCM–CHF for further management
- General in-hospital supportive care
- Nutritional support (Box 20.2)
- Fluid therapy-high rates contraindicated in CHF (Box 20.1)
- Environmental management (Box 20.3)
- Referral to exotics specialist +/− cardiologist ideal for long-term care

Neurologic Signs

Introduction

- Neurologic disease is challenging in this species, it is not possible to conduct a full neurological exam and there is limited species-specific information on neurological diagnostic workup

- Prognosis is poor as many animals will not recover from neurologic disease [3]
- Wobbly hedgehog syndrome is a relatively common cause of ataxia and paralysis [6]
- Another disease reported to cause similar signs is intervertebral disk disease [3]

Diagnosis

History:

- Paralysis in genetically related animals
- No trauma
- Recent exposure to wildlife

Signalment:

- WHS is more likely in a young animal (average of 18 months old) compared to intervertebral disc disease (average of four years old) [7]

Clinical signs:

- Tremors
- Inability to curl into a ball
- Weight loss
- Dysphagia
- Hypothermia
- Lameness
- Ataxia
- Proprioceptive deficits
- Dysphagia
- Seizures
- Muscle atrophy
- Paresis
- Urinary stasis

Differentials:

- Genetic
  - Intervertebral disc disease
  - Wobbly hedgehog syndrome
- Neoplasia
  - Brain or spinal cord astrocytoma [8, 9]
- Bacterial
  - Otitis media or interna
  - Meningoencephalitis
- Parasitic
  - *Baylisascaris procyonis*
- Virus
  - Rabies virus
  - Polioencephalomyelitis virus
- Metabolic
  - Hepatic encephalopathy
  - Hypoglycemia
  - Torpor

STAT Diagnostics:

- PCV/TS/Glu/Lactate
- Check core temperature
- Otic examination

Full Diagnostics:

- CBC/biochemistry panel
- Aerobic bacterial culture of ear swab
- Radiographs
- CT/MRI (rare)

Treatment

Stabilization:

- NSAID or steroid can be considered for IVVD patients (not concurrently)
  - Meloxicam: 0.2 mg/kg SC, PO q24h OR
  - Prednisolone: 1 mg/kg q12h
- Antibiotic therapy: For otitis media/interna or bacterial meningoencephalitis ideally using culture and sensitivity
- Hepatic encephalopathy: See hepatic lipidosis management

Continued Care:

- See WHS for further management
- See intervertebral disc disease for further management
- See hepatic lipidosis for further management
- Fluid therapy: (Box 20.1)
- Nutritional support: (Box 20.2)

Quill Loss

Introduction

- Quill loss can be a part of normal biologic process termed quilling. Animals are typically young and new quill growth is noted
- Examination of shed quills will indicate healthy quills are smaller, more delicate with a normal root at the end as compared to diseased quills which have a flaky or soft root and may appear distorted
- Mites are the most common cause of abnormal quill loss

Diagnosis

History:

- Seasonal loss-likely quilling
- Other clinical signs and pruritus are common when dealing with medical causes of quill loss
- Environmental stressors (Box 20.3)

Signalment:

- Quilling common in animals <1 year of age

Clinical signs:

- Quill loss
- Dry flaky skin
- Hyperkeratosis
- Lichenification
- Nodules or masses
- Ulcerations
- Cellulitis
- Myositis

Differentials:

- Mites (common)
- Skin neoplasia
  - Squamous cell carcinoma, lymphosarcoma, sebaceous gland carcinoma
- Bacterial dermatitis
  - *Staphylococcus simulans* [10]
- Immune-mediated skin disease
- Pemphigus foliaceus
- Fungal dermatitis
  - Dermatophytosis
- Abscesses
- Mycobacteriosis
- Papillomas
- Cuterebrae larvae
- Fleas and ticks

STAT Diagnostics:

- Skin scraping
- Microscopic examination of skin crusts, quills, and ears
- Wood's lamp
- Fine needle aspirate and cytology

Full Diagnostics:

- CBC/biochemistry
- Dermatophyte culture
- Aerobic bacteria culture
- Radiographs
- Surgical excision and biopsy

Treatment

Stabilization:

- Anti-parasitic agent: See ectoparasite section for management
- Anti-fungal: See dermatophytosis section for management
- Steroid: For auto-immune disease (rare); prednisolone 1 mg/kg PO q24h

Continued Care:

- Enclosure disinfection and frequent bedding changes
- No treatment for mycobacteriosis – euthanasia recommended

Torpor

Introduction

- Hypothermic animals may enter a natural state of torpor, a form of hibernation and may suffer potentially fatal health complications
- Ambient temperatures should be maintained between 72 and 90F [3]
- External heat using a heating pad or ceramic heater on one side of the enclosure allows generation of heat gradient

Diagnosis

History:

- Inadequate external heat
- Clinical signs seen in cold climate

Signalment:

- Younger animals may be more susceptible

Clinical signs:

- Lethargy
- Ataxia
- Decreased appetite and water consumption
- Hypothermia (<95F)
- Cold extremities

Differentials:

- Shock
  - Hypovolemic
  - Hypoglycemic
  - Cardiogenic
  - Neurogenic

STAT Diagnostics:

- PCV/TP/Glu/lactate (if limited blood sample)
- Check body temperature

Full Diagnostics:

- CBC/biochemistry panel
- Radiographs

Treatment

Stabilization:

- Provide external heat to 85F using a heating pad; recovery within a few hours

Continued Care:

- Fluid therapy (Box 20.1)
- Syringe feed once normothermic (Box 20.2)

Trauma

Introduction

- Inappropriate bedding or cage furniture frequently leads to trauma in hedgehogs
- Entanglement in loose towel or hair strands have caused strangulation of digits and limbs
- Cornea or facial injuries can occur when animals rub against sharp corners in cages or due to irritation from sawdust or wood shavings

Diagnosis

History:

- Recent introduction of new type of bedding or cage furniture
- Usage of towels or blankets in cage

Signalment:

- No age or sex predilection

Clinical signs:

- Open wounds
- Abscesses
- Lameness
- Weakness
- Self-mutilation
- Anorexia
- Corneal ulcer
- Keratitis
- Proptosis

Differentials:

- Mite infestation
- Dermatophytosis
- Dermal neoplasia
- Mycobacteriosis
- Neurologic disease

STAT Diagnostics:

- PCV/TP/Glu/lactate (if limited blood sample)
- Ophthalmic examination
- Fluorescein eye stain
- Impression smear and cytology of open wounds

Full Diagnostics:

- Aerobic bacterial culture if wounds appear infected
- CBC/biochemistry panel
- Radiographs

Treatment

Stabilization:

- Surgical debridement and removal of foreign material if embedded or strangulating the limb/digit
- Wound dressing, topical antibiotics, and bandage placement:
  - Pododermatitis
  - Prevention of self-mutilation
- Antibiotic therapy: based on results of culture and sensitivity testing if available
  - Amoxicillin-clavulanate: 12.5 mg/kg PO q12hr
  - Enrofloxacin: 5–10 mg/kg IV/IM/PO q12hr
  - Chloramphenicol: 50 mg/kg PO q12hr
- Analgesia
- Opioids: for moderate-to-severe pain
  - Buprenorphine: 0.01–0.5 mg/kg IM/SC q6–12hr
  - Butorphanol: 0.1–0.4 mg/kg IM/SC q6–12hr [11]
- NSAIDs: can be used if patient is hydrated, eating, and kidney function is normal
  - Meloxicam: 0.2 mg/kg PO/SC q24hr
  - Carprofen: 1.0 mg/kg PO/SC q12–24 hr

Continued Care:

- Fluid therapy Box 20.1
- Nutritional support Box 20.2
- Animals that are lame or ataxic should not be allowed to climb or use exercise wheels

Systemic/Neurologic

Intervertebral Disk Disease

Diagnosis

Clinical Signs:

- Lameness
- Progressive ataxia
- Proprioceptive deficits
- Bladder atony, urinary stasis

Differentials:

- Wobbly hedgehog disease
- Spinal/brain neoplasia

- Otitis media or interna
- Infectious encephalitis – rabies, *Baylisascaris*
- Polioencephalomyelitis
- Hepatic encephalopathy
- Hypoglycemia
- Torpor
- Cardiac disease

STAT diagnostics:

- PCV/TP/Glu/lactate (if limited blood sample)
- Blood smear
- Check core body temperature
  - < 95F hypothermia
- Otic examination and cytology

Full diagnostics:

- CBC/biochemistry
  - Stress leukogram may be seen
- Radiographs
  - Multiple disks typically affected, spondylosis, narrowing of intervertebral space and disk mineralization seen
  - Cervical vertebrae were affected in 3 animals and lumbar vertebra was affected in one in a single report [7]
- Myelogram (not been attempted in this species)
- CT/MRI (not been attempted in this species)

Treatment

Stabilization:

- Fluid therapy: (Box 20.1)
- Nutritional support: (Box 20.2)
- NSAID or steroid:
  - Meloxicam 0.2 mg/kg PO, SC q24h OR
  - Prednisolone 1 mg/kg q12h but high rate of recurrence [12]
- Removal of exercise wheels and climbing structures in cage for several weeks to reduce excessive movement
- Spinal decompression: not described in this species

Continued Care:

- Daily bathing to prevent excessive soiling and moist dermatitis
- Physiotherapy to prevent pressure sores and muscle atrophy
- Manage secondary complications such as urinary tract infections
- Euthanasia if severely compromised quality of life

Wobbly Hedgehog Syndrome

Diagnosis

Clinical signs:

- Ataxia/wobbling
- Tremors
- Exophthalmos
- Scoliosis
- Seizures
- Proprioceptive deficits
- Muscle atrophy
- Dysphagia
- Emaciation
- Ascending tetraplegia
- Self-mutilation

Differentials:

- Intervertebral disc disease
- Spinal/brain neoplasia
- Otitis media or interna
- Infectious encephalitis – rabies, *Baylisascaris*
- Polioencephalomyelitis
- Hepatic encephalopathy
- Hypoglycemia
- Torpor
- Cardiac disease

STAT diagnostics:

- PCV/TP/Glu/lactate (if limited blood sample)
- Blood smear
- Otoscopic exam and cytology

Complete diagnostics:

- CBC/biochemistry
  - Stress leukogram may be seen
- Radiography to rule out IVDD
- CT/MRI: (not been attempted in this species) to rule out IVDD
- Histopathology:
  - Only means to achieve a definitive diagnosis
  - Vacuolization of white matter tracts of cerebellum and brainstem, spinal cord and neurogenic muscle atrophy [7]

Treatment

Stabilization:

- No effective treatment. Animals will progress to tetraplegia and death

- Medical trials with interferon beta-1a and steroids have shown no efficacy
- Fluid therapy: (Box 20.1)
- Nutritional support: (Box 20.2)
- Vitamin and mineral supplements: may slow progression [13, 14]
  - Vitamin E/Selenium: 0.1 ml/100–250 g SC once
  - Vitamin B: 1 mg/kg SC or IM SID for three days
  - Calcium glubionate: 50 mg/kg PO SID for three days

Continued care

- Daily bathing to prevent excessive soiling and moist dermatitis
- Physiotherapy to prevent pressure sores and muscle atrophy
- Multi-vitamin supplement for remainder of life
- Euthanasia if severely compromised quality of life

Cardiopulmonary Disease

Dilated Cardiomyopathy (CHF)

Diagnosis

Clinical Signs:

- Dyspnea, tachypnea
- Pulmonary crackles, rales
- Cyanosis (MM, lips, feet)
- Coughing
- Cardiac murmur
- Pleural effusion
- Ascites
- Progressive lethargy, anorexia, weight loss
- Sudden death

Differentials:

- Valvular endocardiosis (less common cause of CHF)
- Endocarditis
- See dyspnea/respiratory distress for other common causes

STAT Diagnostics:

- POCUS
  - TFAST-Pleural effusion and ULRs in lung fields with pulmonary edema, subjective left atrial enlargement, and poor contractility may be appreciated
  - AFAST-Hepatic congestion and abdominal effusion likely
- Pulse oximetry
  - Serial assessments may be useful in monitoring progress with therapy
- ECG
  - Monitor for significant arrhythmias – such as atrial fibrillation, ventricular premature complexes (VPCs), and ventricular tachycardia
  - Abnormal amplitude or duration of P-QRS complex indicating chamber enlargement common [15]
- PCV/TS/Glu/Lactate (if limited blood sample)
  - Assessment of hydration/hemoconcentration status
  - Monitoring for hypoglycemia
  - Evaluation of hypoperfusion due to cardiogenic shock
- Blood smear
  - Stress may increase WBC counts, non-specific findings

Complete Diagnostics:

- Thoracic radiographs
  - Cardiomegaly: increase in the vertebrae heart score (normal 7.25–8.75) [16], dorsal tracheal displacement
  - Left atrial enlargement
  - CHF Signs: pulmonary edema, pleural effusion (Figure 20.1)
- Abdominal radiographs
  - Loss of abdominal detail (ascites), hepatomegaly (due to hepatic congestion)
- Thoracocentesis with fluid analysis
  - Typically, transudate or modified transudate consistent with CHF
- CBC/biochemistry
  - Assess for pre-existing dehydration/hemoconcentration, azotemia, electrolyte derangements, liver enzyme elevations, and hyperbilirubinemia frequently noted

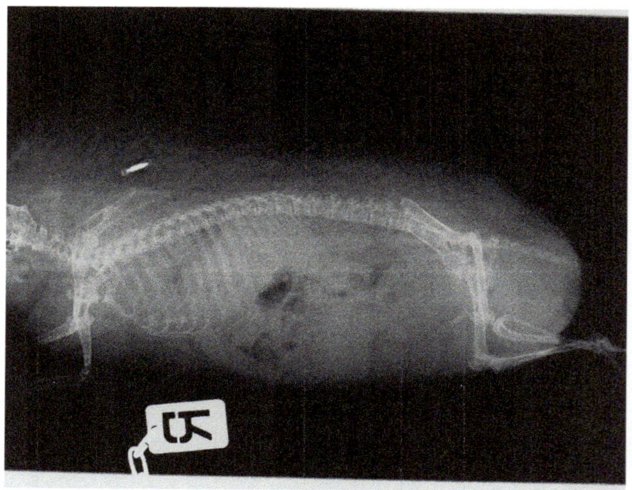

Figure 20.1 Right lateral radiograph of an African pygmy hedgehog (*Atelerix albiventris*) with congestive heart failure secondary to dilated cardiomyopathy. The radiographs reveal generalized cardiomegaly, pulmonary edema, and hepatomegaly. *Source:* Photo courtesy of Wildlife Reserve Singapore.

- Echocardiogram
  - DCM criteria: left ventricular dilation, decreased systolic function, and rounding of the left ventricle [17–19]
  - Left or bi-atrial enlargement may also be present [19]
- Complete thoracic ultrasound
  - Usually not indicated if overt signs of DCM on echocardiogram

Treatment

Stabilization:

- Oxygen supplementation (See Chapter 3)
- Furosemide: 3–5 mg/kg SC, IM, IV, IO q4–8h until CHF signs improve
- Therapeutic thoracocentesis
  - Consider for large volume pleural effusion

Continued care:

- DCM-CHF management
  - Furosemide: 3–5 mg/kg q4–8h initially, and reduce to 2 mg/kg PO, SC q8–12h once CHF signs stabilized [3]
  - Pimobendan: 0.3 mg/kg PO q12h [3]
  - Enalapril: 1 mg/kg PO q24h
- General in-hospital supportive care (Boxes 20.1 and 20.2)
- Nutritional support
  - Ensure taurine and L-carnitine supplement in animals on natural diets [20] or include formulated cat or hedgehog kibble [21]
  - Reduce sodium intake by avoiding treats, processed meats, and high sodium content cat kibble
  - Switch animal to a low sodium cat food if tolerated (e.g. Science Diet Senior, Hills K/D or Purina Proplan Kidney function)
- Aggressive fluid therapy-contraindicated in CHF
- Long-term prognosis for DCM–CHF is poor
- Referral to exotics specialist +/− cardiologist ideal for long-term care

Valvular Endocardiosis (CHF)

Diagnosis

Clinical Signs:

- See DCM-CHF
- Hind limb weakness

Differentials:

- Dilated cardiomyopathy (most common cause of CHF)
- Endocarditis
- See dyspnea/respiratory distress for other common causes
- See neurologic signs for other causes of hind limb weakness

STAT Diagnostics:

- POCUS
  - TFAST-pleural effusion and ULRs in lung fields with pulmonary edema, subjective left atrial enlargement
  - AFAST-hepatic congestion and abdominal effusion possible
- Pulse oximetry
  - Serial assessments may be useful in monitoring progress with therapy
- ECG
  - Sinus arrhythmia, atrial fibrillation, or atrial flutter [15]
- PCV/TS/Glu/Lactate (if limited blood sample)
  - See DCM-CHF
- Blood smear
  - See DCM-CHF

Complete Diagnostics:

- Thoracic radiographs
  - Cardiomegaly: increase in the vertebrae heart score (normal 7.25–8.75) [17], dorsal tracheal displacement
  - Left atrial enlargement-left atrial and/or left ventricular border may appear enlarged due to mitral regurgitation
  - Dilation of the right atrium +/− ventricle may occur secondary to tricuspid regurgitation
  - Concurrent pulmonary arterial hypertension can cause pulmonary artery enlargement
  - CHF Signs: pulmonary edema, pleural effusion
- Abdominal radiographs
  - Loss of abdominal detail (ascites), hepatomegaly (due to hepatic congestion) may occur
- Thoracocentesis with fluid analysis
  - See DCM-CHF
- CBC/biochemistry
  - See DCM-CHF
- Echocardiogram
  - Mitral or tricuspid regurgitation seen on Doppler color flow
  - Thickening or prolapse of the valve leaflets, left atrial, or right atrial enlargement, ventricles may also be enlarged

Treatment

Stabilization:

- See DCM-CHF

Continued care:

- See DCM-CHF

Respiratory Disease

Pneumonia

Diagnosis

Clinical Signs:

- Dyspnea, tachypnea
- Pulmonary crackles, rales
- Cyanosis (lips, feet)
- Coughing
- Progressive lethargy, anorexia, weight loss
- Stertor
- Upper respiratory signs (nasal discharge, sneezing)
- Hindlimb weakness
- Sudden death

Differentials:

- Hematogenous pneumonia
  - Most commonly bacterial pathogens
    - *Bordetella bronchiseptica*, *Pasteurella multocida*, *Corynebacterium* sp. routinely isolated
    - *Haemophilus*, *Staphylococcus,* and *Salmonella* strains less frequently isolated [22, 23]
  - Fungal (disseminated histoplasmosis), viral, parasitic: rare [24]
- Aspiration pneumonia
  - Concurrent vomiting and/or megaesophagus may be risk factor
  - Food material lodged in hard palate can cause choking, tachypnea, vomiting and may be a risk factor
- Dilated cardiomyopathy (most common cause of CHF)
- See dyspnea/respiratory distress for other common causes

STAT Diagnostics:

- POCUS
  - TFAST-ULRs in lung fields with pneumonia, with severe consolidation, may see tissue sign, cardiac assessment-unremarkable
  - AFAST-Usually unremarkable
- Pulse oximetry
  - Serial assessments may be useful in monitoring progress with therapy
- PCV/TS/Glu/Lactate (if limited blood sample)
  - Assessment of hydration/hemoconcentration status
  - Monitoring for hypoglycemia
  - Evaluation of hypoperfusion due to sepsis
- Blood smear
  - Consistent with inflammatory leukogram

Complete Diagnostics:

- Thoracic radiographs
  - Alveolar to interstitial pattern, focal to diffuse
  - Cranio-ventral distribution may suggest aspiration pneumonia
  - Assess for concurrent megaesophagus
- Abdominal radiographs
  - Gastric distention +/− signs of GI obstruction more commonly seen with concurrent aspiration pneumonia
  - Assess for evidence of concurrent neoplasia
- CBC and chemistry panel
  - Inflammatory leukogram due to infectious pneumonia
  - Liver enzyme changes if concurrent hepatic lipidosis
- Complete thoracic ultrasound
  - Evidence of consolidated lung tissue +/− ULRs from infiltrates
  - Ultrasound-guided transthoracic lung/mass aspirates with cytology
  - Rule out neoplasia vs. pneumonia with consolidation
  - Aerobic/anaerobic bacterial culture and sensitivities
- *Trans*-oral tracheal wash (*infrequently performed)

Treatment

Stabilization:

- Oxygen supplementation (see Chapter 3)
- Empiric antibiotics: Broad-spectrum combination initially
  - Trimethoprim-Sulfa: 30 mg/kg PO, SC, IM q12h
  - Enrofloxacin: 5–10 mg/kg PO, SC, IM q12h

Continued care:

- Pneumonia on-going management
  - *Antimicrobial therapy*: broad-spectrum initially (see above), then based on results of culture and sensitivity testing if available
  - *Bronchodilators*: theophylline 10 mg/kg PO, IM q12h
  - *Nebulization:* saline +/− the following:
    - Mucolytics: acetylcysteine 1 ml in 50 ml saline [11, 25]
    - Antibiotics: gentamicin 5 mg/ml in 50 ml saline or enrofloxacin 10 mg/ml in 50 ml saline [11, 25]
  - Environmental stress management (Box 20.3)
- Fluid therapy (Box 20.1)
- Nutritional support (Box 20.2)
- Serial thoracic radiographs for monitoring/follow-up q two weeks
- Referral to exotic specialist ideal for long term care

Upper Respiratory Tract Disease

Diagnosis

Clinical Signs:

- Dyspnea, tachypnea
- Coughing
- Sneezing
- Stertor associated with rhinitis

- Stridor associated with laryngitis, tracheitis
- Oculo-nasal discharge: clear to mucoid
- Presence of discharge on medial aspect of forelimbs
- Lethargy, anorexia

Differentials:

- Upper respiratory infection
  - Most commonly bacterial pathogens:
    - *Bordetella bronchiseptica*, *Pasteurella multocida*, *Corynebacterium* sp. [22, 23]
- Upper airway inflammation
  - Environmental factors (Box 20.3)
- Upper airway aspiration and associated rhinitis
  - Concurrent vomiting and/or megaesophagus may be risk factor
  - Food material lodged in hard palate can cause choking, tachypnea, vomiting and may be a risk factor
- Upper airway or oral neoplasia
- See dyspnea/respiratory distress for other common causes

STAT Diagnostics:

- POCUS
  - TFAST-if URI only – usually unremarkable
  - AFAST – usually unremarkable
- Pulse oximetry
  - Likely WNL – if concurrent pneumonia then serial assessments ideal
- PCV/TS/Glu/Lactate (if limited blood sample)
  - Assessment of hydration/hemoconcentration status
  - Glu and lactate – likely WNL
- Blood smear
  - Consistent with inflammatory leukogram

Complete Diagnostics:

- Thoracic radiographs
  - If URI only – likely unremarkable
  - Rule out concurrent aspiration pneumonia
  - Assess for concurrent megaesophagus
- Abdominal radiographs
  - Gastric distention +/− signs of GI obstruction more commonly seen with concurrent aspiration pneumonia
  - Assess for evidence of concurrent neoplasia
- CBC and chemistry panel
  - Inflammatory leukogram with infectious etiologies
  - Assess kidney function prior to administering NSAIDS
- Sedated oral exam
  - Assessment of oral cavity for neoplasia, food material, or FB
- Nasal flush exudate/deep nasal swab
  - Cytology
  - Aerobic/anaerobic bacterial culture and sensitivities
- CT Scan: nasal cavity, sinuses, skull recommended in refractive cases

Treatment

Stabilization:

- Oxygen supplementation (see Chapter 3)
- Empiric antibiotics: if purulent nasal discharge
  - Trimethoprim-Sulfa: 30 mg/kg PO, SC, IM q12h
  - Enrofloxacin: 5–10 mg/kg PO, SC, IM q12h
- *NSAIDS*: If patient is hydrated, eating, and kidney function is normal
  - Meloxicam: 0.2 mg/kg PO, SC q24hr
  - Carprofen: 1.0 mg/kg PO, SC q12–24 hr [11]

Continued care:

- If concurrent pneumonia (see Pneumonia)
- Environmental management (Box 20.3)
- Nutritional support (Box 20.2)
- Fluid therapy-SC usually adequate (Box 20.1)
- Prevent re-exposure: Limit contact with dogs, cats, and rabbits that may carry *Bordetella bronchiseptica*
- Referral to exotic specialist ideal for refractory cases

Gastrointestinal Disease

Dental Disease

Diagnosis

Clinical Signs:

- Loose or missing teeth (Figure 20.2)
- Deep periodontal pockets
- Dental caries
- Gingival hyperplasia
- Worn down teeth surfaces, loss of molar cusps
- Tooth fractures of canines
- Favoring one side of the jaw
- Reluctance to consume hard foods
- Progressive weight loss, anorexia
- Ptyalism
- Halitosis
- Pawing at the mouth

Differentials:

- Oral neoplasia
- Stomatitis/oral trauma
- Oral foreign body (FB)

STAT diagnostics:

- PCV/TS/Glu/Lactate (if limited sample)

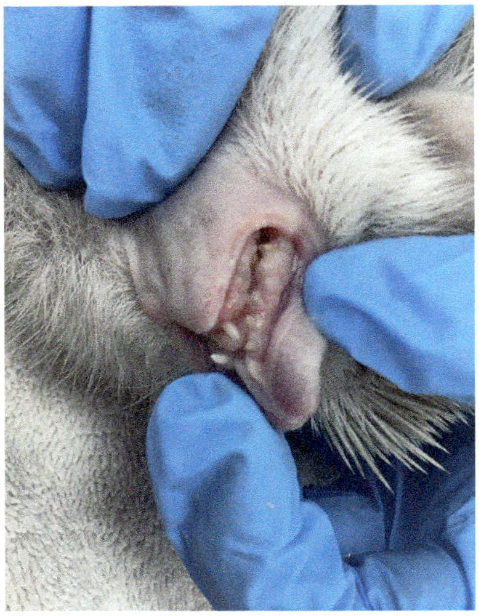

Figure 20.2 Oral examination of an African pygmy hedgehog (*Atelerix albiventris*) with severe dental disease. There were missing teeth, plaque, and gingival hyperplasia. *Source:* Photo courtesy of Wildlife Reserve Singapore.

  - Assessment of hydration/hemoconcentration
  - Monitoring for hypoglycemia
- Blood smear
  - Inflammatory leukogram possible

Full diagnostics:

- CBC/Biochemistry
  - Inflammatory leukogram with infectious etiologies
  - Assess kidney function prior to administration of NSAIDS
- Dental radiographs
  - Lucent halo surrounding tooth root
- Skull radiographs
  - Osteomyelitis of mandible or maxilla may be seen in severe periodontitis
  - Extent of abscess capsule and disruption of normal dentition and bone can be assessed
  - Lysis of bone may be seen in neoplastic processes
- Sedated Oral Exam
  - Assessment of oral cavity for dental disease, neoplasia, food material, or FB
- Aerobic and anaerobic cultures
  - Perform deep cultures of periodontal pockets and abscess walls
  - *Actinomyces* sp. has been associated with dental abscess causing osteomyelitis and cellulitis [26]

Treatment

Stabilization:

- Dental extraction and scaling
- Debride and flush abscesses
- Opioids:
  - Buprenorphine 0.01–0.5 mg/kg IM/SC q6–12h
  - Butorphanol 0.1–0.4 mg/kg IM/SC q6–12h [11]
- NSAIDs: If patient is hydrated, eating, and kidney function is normal
  - Meloxicam 0.2 mg/kg PO/SC q24h
  - Carprofen 1.0 mg/kg PO/SC q12–24 h [11]
- Empiric antibiotics
  - Indicated for abscesses and periodontal infection
  - Start therapy perioperative and postoperative for dental extractions [27]
  - Amoxicillin clavulanic acid: 14 mg/kg PO q12h
  - Chloramphenicol: 50 mg/kg PO q12h
  - Enrofloxacin: 5–10 mg/kg PO q12h [11]

Continued Care:

- Fluid therapy (Box 20.1)
- Nutritional support (Box 20.2)
- Offer permanent soft moist food diet if many teeth are missing or have worn down teeth surfaces
- Prevent further caries: provide proper diet and reduce sweet treats

Enteritis

Diagnosis

Clinical Signs:

- Diarrhea
- Anorexia
- Vomiting
- Hematemesis
- Hunched posture
- Rapid weight loss
- Emaciation
- Dehydration
- Collapse
- Neurological signs
- Frank blood from mouth and anus (due to *Clostridium perfringens*) [28]

Differentials:

- Diet indiscretion
- Recent diet change
- Malnutrition
- Pyloric or intestinal obstruction
- Gastrointestinal neoplasia
- Endoparasites
- Cryptosporidium
- Hepatic disease

STAT diagnostics:

- PCV/TS/Glu/Lactate (if limited blood sample)
  - Assessment of hydration/hemoconcentration status

- Blood smear
  - Possible inflammatory leukogram
- Direct fecal smear
  - *Giardia* sp
- Fecal floatation
  - *Capillaria* sp, *Crenosoma* sp, Isospora
- Fecal acid fast
  - *Mycobacterium bovis, Mycobacterium avium*
- Fecal cytology
  - *Clostridium perfringens*, *Candida albicans, RBCs*

Complete diagnostics:

- CBC/biochemistry
  - Leukocytosis, heterophilia, left shift, with infectious etiologies
  - Elevation in HCT, TP, BUN, and creatinine due to dehydration
- **Abdominal radiographs:**
  - Gaseous *dilation* of stomach and the intestinal tract commonly seen due to ileus [3]
- Ultrasound
  - Assess thickness of gastrointestinal tract and presence of free fluid. Aspirate and perform cytology and fluid analysis of free fluid
- Salmonella culture
  - Can be salmonella carriers and testing advocated due to zoonotic risks
- Aerobic/ anaerobic culture of feces
  - Necessary if diarrhea is protracted or if bloody stools are seen – *Clostridia*
- Cryptosporidium PCR

Treatment

Stabilization:

- Antibiotics
  - Not necessary unless systemically depressed, septic, or salmonella positive
  - Choice based on culture and sensitivity results if available
- Analgesia
  - Avoid NSAIDs if gastritis and gastric ulcer suspected
  - Buprenorphine: 0.01–0.5 mg/kg IM/SC q6–12h
  - Butorphanol: 0.1–0.4 mg/kg IM/SC q6–12h [11]
- H2 blocker for gastritis
  - Famotidine: 0.5 mg/kg IM/PO q12h [11]
- GI protectant for gastritis
  - Sucralfate:100 mg/kg PO q6–8h [11]
- Antiemetic
  - Metoclopramide: 0.5 mg/kg IV/IM q12h [11]
- Anti-parasitic
  - Ivermectin: 0.4 mg/kg SC q10 days for three to five treatments
  - Praziquantel: 7 mg/kg PO/SC q14 days for two treatments [11]
- Anti-fungal for systemic candidiasis (poor prognosis supplement with probiotics)
  - Amphotericin B: 1 mg/kg IV q24h
  - Fluconazole: 25–43 mg/kg IV q12h
  - Itraconazole: 5–10 mg/kg PO q12–24 h [11]

Continued Care:

- Fluid therapy (Box 20.1)
- Nutritional support (Box 20.2)
- Extend antibiotic coverage to minimum of one month for clinical salmonella infections

Gastrointestinal Neoplasia

Diagnosis

Clinical Signs:

- Dysphagia
- Anorexia
- Anemia
- Constipation or tenesmus
- Diarrhea
- Abdominal pain
- Ascites
- Progressive weight loss, lethargy
- Exophthalmos

Differentials:

- Gastrointestinal neoplasia [29, 30]
  - Lymphosarcoma (most common)
  - Adenocarcinoma
  - Plasmacytoma
  - Acinic cell carcinoma – seen as a retrobulbar mass [31]
- Bacterial gastroenteritis (see Enteritis)
- Gastrointestinal parasites (see Enteritis)
- Gastritis and gastric ulcer
- Esophageal disease:
  - Esophagitis, stricture, megaesophagus, neoplasia [32]
- Foreign body obstruction

STAT diagnostics:

- PCV/TS/Glu/lactate (if limited blood sample)
  - Assessment of hydration/hemoconcentration status
- Blood smear – likely normal
- POCUS
  - AFAST – hepatic metastasis and abdominal effusion possible

- TFAST – pulmonary metastasis and pleural effusion possible

Complete diagnostics:

- CBC/biochemistry
  - Possible hypercalcemia (paraneoplastic syndrome), elevated BUN and creatinine, elevated liver values
- Abdominal radiographs
  - Assess for abdominal masses, metastasis in lungs or liver
- Contrast radiographs
  - Contrast may reveal masses, filling defects, or ulcers
- Abdominal ultrasound
  - Focal or diffuse thickening of intestines
  - Loss of normal layers in the gastric or intestinal walls
  - Splenomegaly or hepatomegaly
  - Lymphadenomegaly
  - Gastric or intestinal masses
- Ultrasound-guided fine needle aspirates or biopsy
- Endoscopic gastroscopy
  - Limited by size of patient but can be attempted
  - Evaluation of gastric and intestinal lining
  - Obtain partial-thickness biopsies of suspicious lesions
- Abdominal exploratory
  - Full-thickness gastric and intestinal biopsies, biopsy of regional lymph nodes, assess liver for metastasis

Treatment

Stabilization:

- Opioids: for moderate-to-severe pain
  - Buprenorphine: 0.01–0.5 mg/kg IM/SC q6–12 h
  - Butorphanol: 0.1–0.4 mg/kg IM/SC q6–12 h [11]
- NSAID: can be used if patient is hydrated, eating, and kidney function is normal
  - Meloxicam: 0.2 mg/kg PO/SC q24h
  - Carprofen: 1.0 mg/kg PO/SC q12–24 h [11]
- H2 blocker for gastritis:
  - Famotidine: 0.5 mg/kg IM/PO q12h [11]
- GI protectant for gastric ulceration
  - Sucralfate: 100 mg/kg PO q6-8h [11]

Continued Care:

- Fluid therapy: (Box 20.1)
- Nutritional support: (Box 20.2)
- Chemotherapy for lymphoma and lymphosarcoma:
  - Currently no recognized protocols exist for chemotherapy in hedgehogs
  - L-Asparaginase: 400 U/kg SC once followed by prednisolone 1 mg/kg PO BID can be attempted
- Surgery
  - If detected early, plasmacytoma can be treated by surgical resection and anastomosis. Additional radiation therapy or chemotherapy can be considered, but there are no reports of successful treatments [29]
  - Surgical resection of retrobulbar acini cell tumor proved unsuccessful and recurrence and death occurred three months later [31]
- Bi- or tri-annual health checks: poor prognosis

Hepatic Lipidosis

Diagnosis

Clinical signs:

- Anorexia
- Progressive weight loss and lethargy
- Icterus
- Hepatomegaly (Figure 20.3)
- Diarrhea
- Neurological signs due to hepatic encephalopathy

Differentials:

- Hepatic neoplasia (see Neoplasia)
- Infectious hepatitis – bacterial, viral
- Hepatic necrosis – human herpes simplex virus [33]

STAT diagnostics:

- PCV/TS/Glu/Lactate (if limited blood sample)
  - Assessment of hydration/hemoconcentration status
  - Lactate may be elevated due to tissue hypoperfusion and hepatic dysfunction
  - Glucose may be low due to hepatic failure

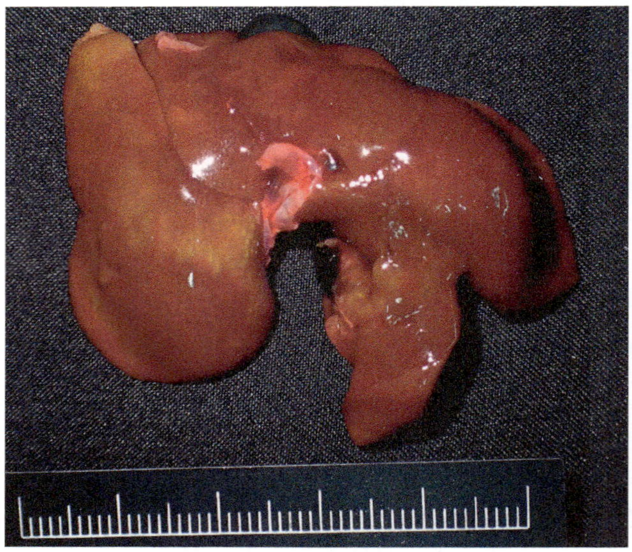

Figure 20.3 Postmortem finding of an African pygmy (*Atelerix albiventris*) hedgehog with chronic inappetence. The liver was enlarged, pale, and greasy in appearance diagnostic of hepatic lipidosis. *Source:* Photo courtesy of Wildlife Reserve Singapore.

- Blood smear: stress leukogram
- Urinalysis
  - Bilirubinuria and urobilinogen uria
- POCUS
  - AFAST – hepatic vacuolation and ascites may be present

Complete diagnostics:

- CBC/biochemistry panel
  - Elevated bilirubin, ALP, ALT, AST, and bile acids
  - Non-regenerative normochromic, normocytic anemia
  - Stress leukogram
  - Less commonly; low BUN, cholesterol, and albumin
- Abdominal radiographs
  - Hepatomegaly
- Abdominal ultrasound
  - Homogeneous hyperechoic hepatic parenchyma, hyperechoic kidneys
- Ultrasound-guided fine needle aspiration and cytology
  - Numerous hepatocytes with vacuolar degeneration
  - Homogeneous hyperechoic hepatic parenchyma compared to falciform fat and spleen is suggestive of hepatic lipidosis
- Liver biopsy and histopathology:
  - Not necessary unless animal is undergoing exploratory for other causes, as FNA is diagnostic

Treatment

Stabilization:

- Analgesia if necessary
  - Buprenorphine: 0.01–0.5 mg/kg IM/SC q6–12h [11]
- Multi-vitamin therapy
  - Carnitine, taurine, vitamin C, vitamin E, Zinc
  - < 1 drop/kg q 24 h
- H2 blocker for gastritis
  - Famotidine 0.5 mg/kg IM/PO q12hr [11]
- GI protectant for gastritis
  - Sucralfate100 mg/kg PO q6–8hr [11]
- Hepatic encephalopathy
  - Aggressive fluid therapy
  - Warm water enema
  - Lactulose: 0.3 ml/kg q12h [11]
  - Lactobacillus: ½ tsp/kg q24h [11]
  - Metronidazole: 20 mg/kg PO BID [11]

Continued Care:

- Fluid therapy: supplement fluids with 1 ml/kg SC vitamin B complex (Box 20.1)
- Nutritional support (Box 20.2)
- Address underlying medical disease that cause anorexia
- After a full recovery, gradual weight loss recommended
- Avoid environmental stressors (Box 20.3)

Megaesophagus

Diagnosis

Clinical Signs:

- Thin
- Dyspnea
- Vocalization
- Nasal discharge
- Coughing
- Dysphagia
- Hypersalivation
- Regurgitation

Differentials:

- Dysphagia due to oral foreign body
- Gastric dilatation
- Pneumonia
  - Aspiration
  - Bacterial
- Lead toxicity
- Dilated cardiomyopathy
- Lung neoplasia

STAT diagnostics:

- PCV/TS/Glu/Lactate (if limited blood sample)
  - Anemia observed with chronic disease and lead toxicity
  - Elevated lactate levels indicate poor tissue perfusion and hypoxia
- Pulse oximetry
  - Serial assessments may be useful in monitoring progress with therapy
- POCUS
  - TFAST-ULRs in lung fields/lung consolidation with concurrent aspiration pneumonia
  - AFAST – unremarkable
- Blood smear
  - Basophilic stippling of red blood cells in lead toxicity
  - Leukocytosis may be present

Complete diagnostics:

- Thoracic radiographs
  - Diffuse dilated esophagus along large portion and soft tissue opacity striations of esophagus cranial to the diaphragm [32]
- CBC/biochemistry
  - Leukocytosis with neutrophilia if aspiration pneumonia occurred
- Blood lead levels
  - Rule out lead toxicity as cause of megaesophagus

Mammals

- Contrast Radiography
  - High risk of aspiration pneumonia
  - Contraindicated unless confirmation of diagnosis is necessary [34]
- Esophagoscopy
  - Adjunct test to evaluate any esophagitis, stricture of the esophagus, gastric esophageal intussusception [35]
- Fluoroscopy
  - Definitive test, evaluates esophageal dysmotility [35]

Treatment
Stabilization:

- Oxygen supplementation (see Chapter 3)
- Empiric antibiotics for aspiration pneumonia
  - Start prior to any surgical intervention
  - Enrofloxacin: 5–10 mg/kg PO, SC IM q12h
  - Trimethoprim sulfa: 30 mg/kg PO, SC, IM q12h [11]
- Antiemetic
  - Metoclopramide: 0.5 mg/kg PO BID if vomiting
- Gastroprotectants
  - Ranitidine: 2 mg/kg PO SID
  - Famotidine: 1 mg/kg PO SID
  - Omeprazole: 0.7 mg/kg PO SID
  - Sucralfate: 10 mg/kg PO BID-TID [11]

Continued Care:

- Determine the cause of the megaesophagus and address accordingly
  - One report of gastric-esophageal intussusception-induced megaesophagus [32]
  - Esophageal reduction for gastric-esophageal intussusception was attempted. Technique is contraindicated if gastric mucosa is compromised [35]
  - Recommended treatment involves repositioning stomach and gastropexy [34]
- Fluid therapy (Box 20.1)
- Nutritional support (Box 20.2)
  - Elevated feedings may not be practical in this species. Offer multiple high caloric small feedings to prevent regurgitation

Obesity

Diagnosis
Clinical signs:

- Inability to curl completely into a ball (Figure 20.4)
- Large axillary deposits of fat
- Pendulous abdomen

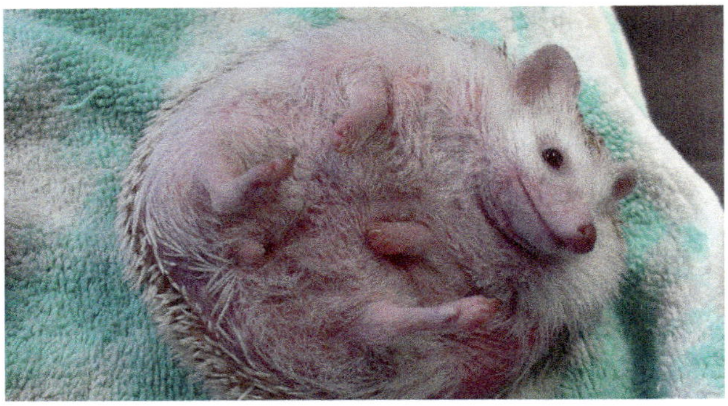

Figure 20.4 Obesity in an African pygmy hedgehog (*Atelerix albiventris*). The hedgehog was not able to roll up completely. *Source:* Photo courtesy of Angela Lennox.

Differentials:

- Free abdominal fluid
- Abdominal neoplasia
- Hepatomegaly
- Pregnant females

STAT diagnostics:

- PCV/TP/Glu/Lactate (if limited blood sample)
- Urinalysis
  - Bilirubin and urobilinogen may be positive if animal has concurrent hepatic lipidosis

Complete diagnostics:

- CBC/biochemistry: elevation of liver values due to hepatic lipidosis-common sequelae in obese patients [6]
- Radiograph
  - Large abdominal fat deposits seen with obesity
- Ultrasound
  - Large abdominal fat deposits, assess liver echotexture (see Hepatic lipidosis)

Treatment
Continued Care:

- Offer restricted high-quality insectivore/hedgehog or senior cat kibble and gradual weight reduction
- Limit high-fat food items such as mealworms and waxworms
- Replace freeze-dried insects with live ones to promote hunting and burrowing
- Encourage foraging of hidden kibble

Oral Foreign Body

Diagnosis
Clinical signs:

- Hypersalivation
- Tachypnea

- Halitosis
- Vomiting
- Choking
- Anorexia
- Dysphagia
- Glossitis

Differentials:

- Mass/foreign body embedded in tongue, or lodged in hard palate
- Oral neoplasia
- Stomatitis
- Dental disease

STAT diagnostics:

- Sedated oral examination:
  - Assess buccal cavities, sub-lingual area, and hard and soft palates
  - Assess dentition
  - Utilize endoscope if foreign body is suspected but not clearly visible
- POCUS
  - TFAST – assess for concurrent aspiration pneumonia (see Pneumonia)
- Pulse oximetry
  - Monitor oxygenation if animal is tachypneic
- PCV/TP/Glu/Lactate (if limited blood sample)
  - Assessment of hydration
  - Monitoring for hypoglycemia

Complete diagnostics:

- CBC and Chemistry panel
  - Stress leukogram possible
- Thoracic radiographs
  - Assess for concurrent aspiration pneumonia (see Pneumonia)
  - Complete thoracic ultrasound (see Pneumonia)

Treatment

Stabilization:

- Oxygen supplementation (see Chapter 3)
- Analgesia
  - Opioids: for moderate-to-severe pain
    - Buprenorphine: 0.01–0.05 mg/kg IM/SC q6–12 h
    - Butorphanol: 0.1–0.4 mg/kg IM/SC q6–12 h [11]
  - NSAIDS: if patient is hydrated, eating, and kidney function is normal
    - Meloxicam: 0.2 mg/kg PO/SC q24h
    - Carprofen: 1.0 mg/kg PO/SC q12–24 h [11]
- Foreign body removal
  - Use grabbing forceps or if embedded in the tongue or cheek, curettage, and surgical repair may be required
  - Disinfect the area with chlorhexidine
- Empiric antibiotic therapy
  - Enrofloxacin: 5–10 mg/kg PO, SC IM q12h
  - Trimethoprim sulfa: 30 mg/kg PO, SC, IM q12h
  - Amoxicillin clavulanic acid: 14 mg/kg PO q12h [11]

Continued Care:

- Fluid therapy (Box 20.1)
- Nutritional support (Box 20.2)
- Advise owners to cut food into smaller pieces and avoid items such as seeds and nuts
- Dispose of human hair and loose fibers regularly, if animal wanders on the ground
- Provide soft foods for animals with periodontal disease or oral tumors due to tendency to swallow foods whole
- Check mouths of breeding males regularly as quills may become lodged when they bite the female during mating

Pyloric and Intestinal Obstruction

Diagnosis

Clinical Signs:

- Dyspnea
- Vomiting
- Decreased stool production
- Melena
- Anorexia
- Collapse

Differentials:

- Gastrointestinal neoplasia
- Gastritis or gastric ulcer
- Esophageal disease
- Gastroesophageal intussusception
- Pneumonia
- Oral foreign body
- Cardiac disease

STAT diagnostics:

- PCV/TP/Gluc/Lactate (if limited blood sample)
  - Assessment of hydration/hemoconcentration
  - Monitoring for hypoglycemia
- Blood smear
- POCUS
- Pulse oximetry

Complete diagnostics:

- CBC/Chemistry
  - Leukocytosis and neutrophilia

 - Hemoconcentration
 - Electrolyte disturbances such as hypokalemia, hypochloremia, hyponatremia, or hypernatremia
- Abdominal radiographs
 - Gaseous dilation of stomach and the intestinal tract due to ileus is common and may hinder a diagnosis of obstruction [3]
 - Survey films may show free air due to perforation and free fluid may be present secondary to peritonitis
- Thoracic radiographs
- Abdominal US
 - Assess if free fluid or gas is present
 - Dilated loops of bowel may indicate obstruction
 - Peritoneal fluid analysis, gram stain, glucose, bacterial culture, and sensitivity
- Contrast Radiography
 - Poor diagnostic yield, ileus difficult to distinguish from an obstruction
- Gastroscopy
 - Visualize and retrieve any gastric foreign body, diagnose outflow obstruction due to pyloric neoplasia, assess appearance of gastric and intestinal wall
- Endoscopy guided biopsies
 - Partial wall thickness biopsies of gastric and intestinal tissue
- Exploratory laparotomy
 - Most effective way of diagnosing gastrointestinal obstruction [3]
 - Perform full-thickness biopsies from several sites

Treatment

Stabilization:

- Aggressive fluid therapy: pre-operative IO fluid therapy with both hetastarch 5 ml/kg and 10–15 ml/kg isotonic crystalloids
- Analgesia
 - Opioids: Pre- and post-operatively
  - Buprenorphine: 0.01–0.5 mg/kg IM/SC q6–12 h
  - Butorphanol: 0.1–0.4 mg/kg IM/SC q6–12 h [11]
 - NSAIDS: if patient is hydrated, eating, and kidney function is normal post-operatively
  - Meloxicam: 0.2 mg/kg PO/SC q24h
  - Carprofen: 1.0 mg/kg PO/SC q12–24 h [11]
- Antibiotic therapy
- Surgical intervention
 - Enterotomy or gastrostomy to remove the foreign body
 - Perform resection and anastomosis of necrotic bowel
 - Excise and biopsy any suspicious gastrointestinal masses in gastric wall, pylorus, and intestines
- H2 blocker for gastritis
 - Famotidine: 1.0 mg/kg SID PO
 - Ranitidine: 2.0 mg/kg IM/PO q12hr [11]
- GI protectant for gastritis
 - Sucralfate:100 mg/kg PO q6–8hr [11]

Continued Care

- Continue fluid therapy (Box 20.1)
- Nutritional support (Box 20.2)
 - Offer small meals of soft foods for a few days post-operatively
- Prevent future accidental ingestion of foreign material
 - Dispose of human hair, rubber, and carpet fibers regularly
 - Avoid providing towels with loose fibers and large food items such as cockroaches or meat items with tendons or ligaments

Urogenital and Reproductive Disease

Chronic Kidney Disease

Diagnosis

Clinical Signs:

- Polyuria and polydipsia
- Anorexia
- Weight loss
- Weakness
- Dehydration
- Anemia
- Small firm kidneys
- Vomiting
- General malaise and head pressing – due to uremic encephalopathy [36]

Differentials:

- Acute kidney failure
- Congenital: polycystic kidney disease; rare
- Glomerular disease: glomerulonephritis, amyloidosis
- Infectious: pyelonephritis, ascending lower urinary tract infections, interstitial nephritis, nephrolithiasis [37]
- Immune-mediated: glomerulosclerosis, chronic vasculitis
- Metabolic: hyperphosphatemia, hypertension
- Renal neoplasia
- Vascular: chronic renal infarcts
- Renal toxins and ischemia

STAT Diagnostics:

- PCV/TP/lactate
 - Chronic anemia, TP can be reduced in cases of protein-losing nephropathies mild metabolic acidosis
- BUN and Creatinine
 - Elevated levels
- USG
 - Dilute urine to isosthenuria

Complete Diagnostics:

- CBC/biochemistry
  - Stress leukogram or leukocytosis associated with infectious causes
  - Hypokalemia, hyperphosphatemia, azotemia; low albumin/TP, variable calcium
- Reticulocyte count
  - Expect non-regenerative anemia
- Complete urinalysis
  - Urine ideally collected via cystocentesis
  - Inflammatory urine sediment seen in infectious causes
  - Proteinuria may be present
- Abdominal radiographs
  - Renomegaly, shrunken or abnormally shaped kidneys; radiopaque renal calculi occasionally detectable
- Intravenous pyelograms and excretory urethrography
- Urine aerobic bacterial culture/sensitivity
- Abdominal ultrasound
- Renal biopsy

Treatment

Stabilization:

- Discontinue nephrotoxic drugs
- Antibiotics for pyelonephritis
  - Based on results of urine culture and sensitivity testing
  - If unavailable, enrofloxacin: 5–10 mg/kg PO, SC, IM q12h [11]

For gastritis:

- Famotidine: 1.0 mg/kg SID PO
- Ranitidine: 2.0 mg/kg IM/PO q12hr [11]
- For hyperphosphatemia
  - Calcium gluconate: 50 mg/kg IM q24 hr [11, 36]

For anemic patients:

- Vitamin B complex:1 ml/kg SC/IM and vitamin C 50–200 mg/kg SC/PO [11]
- Iron dextran: 25 mg/kg IM q 7 days
- Human recombinant erythropoietin: 100 U/kg SC q48–72 hrs in refractory severe anemia [11]
- In weak anemic patients (PCV below 12%) that do not respond, a blood transfusion may be necessary [38]

Continued care:

- Fluid therapy (Box 20.1)
  - Aggressive fluid therapy initially
  - Long-term SC fluid therapy: up to 25 ml divided twice daily [36]
- Assist syringe feeding (Box 20.2)
- Provide multiple water bowls and increasing proportion of wet food
- Offer feline prescription urinary diets, reduce or remove insects, and increase the proportion of egg, fruit, and vegetable matter [36]
- Addition of omega-3 fatty acid supplements
- Monitor disease progression-every three months, guarded prognosis

Cystitis

Diagnosis

Clinical Signs:

- Stranguria
- Dysuria
- Pollakiuria
- Genital discomfort – increased licking of prepuce or vulva
- Anorexia
- Lethargy
- Weakness
- Weight loss
- Pyrexia
- Dehydration
- Painful abdomen
- Distended, easily palpated bladder
- Small bladder and gentle palpation elicits voiding
- Changes in urine color, often associated with hematuria

Differentials:

- Urolithiasis/crystalluria
- Urethral blockage
- Urinary tract infections
- Trauma to the urinary tract
- Idiopathic cystitis
- Neoplasia of the genitourinary tract
- Neurologic disorders

STAT Diagnostics:

- PCV/TP/Lactate
  - Assessment of hydration/hemoconcentration status
- USG
  - Will be normal unless renal insufficiency has occurred

Complete Diagnostics:

- CBC/biochemistry
  - Assess if azotemic
- Complete urinalysis
  - Generally acidic urine
  - Crystalluria, white blood cells, red blood cells, and bacteria may be observed in sediment
  - May be present with urinary tract infections
- Urine aerobic bacterial culture/sensitivity
- Abdominal radiographs
  - Assess for evidence of neoplasia or uroliths

- Abdominal ultrasound
  - Uroliths, masses, echogenic sediment, and bladder wall changes
- Urolith analysis
- Contrast cystourethrography
  - Localize bladder wall lesions, urethral, and ureteral disease (rarely performed)
- Surgical biopsy and histopathology of the bladder
  - Indicated if cause of cystitis is unable to be determined (rarely performed)

Treatment

Stabilization:

- Analgesia
  - Opioids: for moderate-to-severe pain
    - Buprenorphine 0.01–0.5 mg/kg IM/SC q6–12 hr
    - Butorphanol 0.1–0.4 mg/kg IM/SC q6–12 hr [11]
  - NSAIDs: can be used if patient is hydrated, eating, and kidney function is normal
    - Meloxicam 0.2 mg/kg PO/SC q24hr
    - Carprofen 1.0 mg/kg PO/SC q12–24 hrs [11]
- Urethral catheterization
- Antibiotic therapy
  - Based on results of culture and sensitivity testing
  - Amoxicillin-clavulanate: 12.5 mg/kg PO q12hr
  - Enrofloxacin: 5–10 mg/kg IM/PO q12hr [11]
- Urethral smooth and skeletal muscle relaxants
  - Diazepam: 0.5–1 mg/kg IM/PO q 8 hr
  - Phenoxybenzamine: 3.75–7.5 mg PO q24–72 hr [3]

Continued care:

- Fluid therapy (Box 20.1)
- Nutritional support (Box 20.2)
- Environmental stress reduction
- Supplements
  - Omega-3 fatty acids reduce bladder wall inflammation
  - Glycosaminoglycan improve barrier function of bladder wall, reduces bacterial and crystal adherence [39]

Hematuria

Diagnosis

Clinical Signs:

- Red colored urine or gross hemorrhage
- Stranguria
- Dysuria
- Pollakiuria
- Genital discomfort – licking the prepuce or vulva
- Anorexia
- Lethargy
- Weight loss
- Pyrexia

Differentials:

- Urolithiasis/crystalluria
- Cystitis
- Uterine infections or prostatic infections or abscesses [40]
- Trauma within the urinary or reproductive tracts
- Neoplasia of the genitourinary tract
- Congenital or acquired abnormalities: endometrial polyps and cystic ovaries, polycystic kidneys, glomerulonephritis, and granulomatous urethritis, prostatic cysts [37, 41]
- Vascular disorders: renal infarcts, renal pelvic hematomas, and bleeding disorders [42]
- Myoglobinuria or hemoglobinuria

STAT Diagnostics:

- PCV/TP/Glu/Lactate (if limited blood sample)
  - Assessment of hydration/hemoconcentration status
  - Anemia may be present due to chronic bleeding
- USG
  - Urine generally well-concentrated but may decline in chronic disease
- Assess nature of hematuria
  - Start of voiding suggests hemorrhage of lower urinary tract
  - Hemorrhage at the end of voiding often from upper urinary tract [41]
  - Dripping blood from prepuce/vulva suggests bleeding distal to the urethral sphincter [43]

Complete Diagnostics:

- Complete urinalysis
  - Gross hematuria >150 RBCs/HPF, occult hematuria >5 RBCs/HPF
  - Differentiate from hemoglobinuria and myoglobinuria
    - Hemoglobinuria will not sediment with concurrent high serum hemoglobin concentration
    - Myoglobinuria will not sediment with concurrent elevated blood creatine kinase
  - Low urine pH is common
  - Crystalluria in sediment may indicate urolithiasis
  - Active sediment consistent with infectious process
- Abdominal radiographs
  - Genitourinary neoplasia, uroliths, prostatic, or kidney enlargement
- Coagulation testing
  - Indicated if animal is also bleeding from non-urinary sites
- CBC/biochemistry

  - Inflammatory leukogram indicates infectious processes
  - Anemia may indicate chronicity of bleeding
  - High BUN and creatinine may differentiate renal vs extra-renal disorders
- Abdominal ultrasound
  - Uroliths, mass lesions, echogenic sediment, and bladder wall changes
- Ultrasound-guided renal biopsy
- Urine aerobic bacteria culture/sensitivity
  - Performed via cystocentesis
- Urolith analysis
- Contrast cystourethrography
  - Localize bladder wall lesions, urethral, and ureteral disease, rarely performed
- Surgical biopsy and histopathology of urinary tract and reproductive tract
  - Indicated if the cause of the hematuria is not detected

Treatment

Stabilization:

- Analgesia
  - Opioids: for moderate-to-severe pain
    - Buprenorphine: 0.01–0.5 mg/kg IM/SC q6–12 hr
    - Butorphanol: 0.1–0.4 mg/kg IM/SC q6–12 hrs [11]
  - Non-steroidal anti-inflammatories: can be used if patient is hydrated, eating, and kidney function is normal
    - Meloxicam: 0.2 mg/kg PO/SC q24hr
    - Carprofen: 1.0 mg/kg PO/SC q12–24 hrs
- Antibiotic therapy
  - Only when indicated; drug choice based on the results of culture and sensitivity testing if possible
  - Amoxicillin-clavulanate: 12.5 mg/kg PO q12hr
  - Enrofloxacin: 5–10 mg/kg IM/PO q12hr [11]
  - Trimethoprim-Sulfa: 30 mg/kg PO q12hr
- Surgery
  - Surgical repair of trauma to urinary tract
  - Ovariohysterectomy – treat ovarian tumors and endometrial polyps [44]
  - Cystotomy – remove uroliths and allow retrograde flushing of the urethra of all sediment involved in urethral traumatization/blockage [45]
  - Partial cystectomy for bladder wall tumors – if surgical margins can be identified however tumors involving the ureters and urethra not amenable to surgery [45]

Continued care:

- (See Cystitis management)

Posthitis

Diagnosis

Clinical Signs:

- Dysuria
- Excessive grooming of preputial area
- Abdominal pain
- Occasionally a distended bladder
- Generalized swelling and inflammation of prepuce and penis

Differentials:

- Paraphimosis – stricture, swelling, neurologic disease, or hair ring
- Balanitis
- Neoplasia of penis or prepuce
- Cystitis

STAT Diagnostics:

- PCV/TP/Glu/Lactate (if limited blood sample)
  - Assessment of hydration/hemoconcentration status
- Blood smear
  - Likely normal until animal is septic and has ascending infection
- USG
  - Urine generally well-concentrated unless animal is obstructed and develops azotemia
- Examine prepuce (under anesthesia)
  - Posthitis often a result of substrate entrapment within prepuce [46]

Complete Diagnostics:

- Cytology
  - Preputial area mostly neutrophils, some macrophages, and intracellular bacteria if infection present
- Bacterial aerobic culture and sensitivity of urine if animal has trouble urinating

Treatment

Stabilization:

- Maintain a urinary catheter for a few days if animal has trouble urinating [47, 48]
- Analgesia
  - Opioids: for moderate-to-severe pain
    - Buprenorphine: 0.01–0.5 mg/kg IM/SC q6–12 hr
    - Butorphanol: 0.1–0.4 mg/kg IM/SC q6–12 hr [11]
  - NSAIDs: can be used if patient is hydrated, eating, and kidney function is normal
    - Meloxicam: 0.2 mg/kg PO/SC q24hr
    - Carprofen: 1.0 mg/kg PO/SC q12–24 hrs [11]

- Disinfect preputial area under anesthesia
  - Remove debris, disinfection of the skin surface with 0.01–0.05% dilute chlorhexidine or povidone-iodine solution
- Topical antibiotics
  - Thin layer of Intrasite gel (Smith & Nephew) to assist in rehydration and debridement of any necrotic tissue
  - Avoid repeated applications as animal may lick area excessively [41]
- Systemic empiric antibiotics
  - Enrofloxacin: 5–10 mg/kg IV/IM/PO q12hr
  - Trimethoprim-Sulfa: 30 mg/kg PO q12 hr
  - Amoxicillin-clavulanate: 12.5 mg/kg PO Q12hr [11]

Continued care:

- Fluid therapy (Box 20.1)
- Nutritional support (Box 20.2)
- Avoid fine sawdust or wood shavings and sand bedding

Urolithiasis

Diagnosis

Clinical Signs:

- Stranguria
- Dysuria
- Pollakiuria
- Anorexia
- Lethargy
- Weakness
- Weight loss
- Pyrexia
- Painful abdomen on palpation
- Palpable bladder with granular sensation when moved between fingers
- Changes in urine color, often associated with hematuria

Differentials:

- Urinary tract infections
- Uterine infections
- Prostatic infections or abscesses
- Iatrogenic trauma within the urinary or reproductive tract
- Neoplasia of the genitourinary tract
- Congenital or acquired conditions: bleeding disorders, urethral scarring, or strictures [40]

STAT Diagnostics:

- PCV/TP/Glu/Lactate (if limited blood sample)
  - Assessment of hydration/hemoconcentration status
- Anemia may be present due to chronic bleeding from hematuria
- USG
  - Usually well-concentrated unless kidney function is affected

Complete Diagnostics:

- Complete urinalysis
  - pH is generally alkaline for struvite and calcium oxalate, but acidic for cystine and urate urolith formation
  - Crystalluria in sediment can indicate urolithiasis/crystalline matrix plug formation
  - White blood cells and bacteria indicate infectious process
- Abdominal radiographs
  - Radio-opaque uroliths within the bladder or in the urethra
- Abdominal ultrasound
  - May identify uroliths, mass lesions, echogenic sediment, and bladder wall changes
- Urine culture/sensitivity
  - Performed via cystocentesis
- Urolith analysis
- Contrast cystourethrography
  - Localize bladder wall lesions and differentiate from urolithiasis (rarely performed)

Treatment

Stabilization:

- Analgesia
  - Opioids: for moderate-to-severe pain
    - Buprenorphine: 0.01–0.5 mg/kg IM/SC q6–12hr
    - Butorphanol: 0.1–0.4 mg/kg IM/SC q6–12hr [11]
  - NSAIDs: can be used if patient is hydrated, eating, and kidney function is normal
    - Meloxicam: 0.2 mg/kg PO/SC q24hr
    - Carprofen: 1.0 mg/kg PO/SC q12–24 hrs [11]
- Antibiotic therapy: drug choice based on the results of culture and sensitivity testing if possible
  - Enrofloxacin: 5–10 mg/kg IV/IM/PO SID q12hr
  - Trimethoprim-Sulfa: 30 mg/kg PO q12hr
  - Amoxicillin-clavulanate: 12.5 mg/kg PO Q12hr [11]

Continued care:

- Fluid therapy: (Box 20.1)
- Nutritional support: (Box 20.2)
- Struvite uroliths
  - Manage medically if cystotomy not possible
  - Reduce dietary intake of magnesium, protein, and phosphorus. Also treat cystitis which may be inciting cause [36]
- Calcium oxalate uroliths
  - Manage with cystotomy
  - Post urolith removal; reduce protein, calcium, oxalate, vitamin D, and sodium in diet
  - Supplement adequate phosphorus, magnesium, and vitamin B6, alkalinizing diet [36]
- Cystine uroliths
  - Manage medically

- Reduce protein and sodium, urine alkalinizing diet. 2-mercaptopropionylglycine can be given [49]
- Prevent recurrence
  - Dietary management with high moisture content food. Supplement with omega-3 fatty acids (See Cystitis)

Uterine Disease

Diagnosis

Clinical Signs:

- Vaginal bleeding – may be confused for hematuria or hematochezia
- Hematuria: typically present at the initial phase of voiding
- Single or multiple solid, mobile masses maybe palpated
- Painful abdomen
- Stranguria
- Dysuria
- Pollakiuria
- Progressive anorexia, weight loss, and lethargy

Differentials:

Neoplastic causes:

- Adenosarcoma, leiomyosarcoma, adenoma, granulosa cell tumor, adenocarcinoma, adenoleiomyoma/adenoleiomyosarcoma, endometrial/fibroadenomatous polyps, and spindle cell tumor have all been described in hedgehogs

Non-neoplastic causes:

- Urolithiasis
- Lower urinary tract infections
- Pyometra/metritis (less common): animals are systemically unwell, purulent vaginal discharge and pyrexia [50]
- Iatrogenic trauma to the reproductive and urinary tract
- Cystic ovaries [41]
- Polycystic kidneys, glomerulonephritis, and granulomatous urethritis [37]
- Vascular disorders: renal infarcts, renal pelvic hematomas, and bleeding disorders [4]

STAT Diagnostics:

- PCV/TP/Glu/Lactate (if limited blood sample)
  - Assessment of hydration/hemoconcentration status
  - Anemia may be present
- USG
  - Usually well-concentrated unless kidney function is affected

Complete Diagnostics:

- Urinalysis
  - Well-concentrated urine, acidic pH, bacteria, and neutrophils in sediment if secondary lower UTI is present
  - Neoplastic cells may rarely exfoliate into the urine
- CBC/biochemistry
  - Inflammatory leukogram can indicate infectious processes
  - Anemia may result due to hematuria or chronic disease
- Radiographs
  - Uterine masses – soft tissue density structure in the caudal abdomen displacing the gastrointestinal structures cranially [51]
  - Evidence of metastases may be present
- Abdominal ultrasound
  - Assess if the primary mass derives from the uterus/ovaries, if there is generalized thickening to uterine wall, or focal growths are filled with fluid, or soft tissue [51]
  - US-guided aspirates can provide a definitive diagnosis in some cases, however, often are insufficient for tumor classification
- Biopsy and histopathology
  - Exploratory laparotomy generally required

Treatment

Stabilization:

- Analgesia
  - Opioids: for moderate-to-severe pain
    - Buprenorphine: 0.01–0.5 mg/kg IM/SC q6–12hr
    - Butorphanol: 0.1–0.4 mg/kg IM/SC q6–12hr [11]
  - Non-steroidal anti-inflammatories: can be used if patient is hydrated, eating, and kidney function is normal
    - Meloxicam: 0.2 mg/kg PO/SC q24hr
    - Carprofen: 1.0 mg/kg PO/SC q12–24 hr [11]
- Ovariohysterectomy
  - If no metastases present, generally curative [52] with average median survival times post-surgery of approximately one year [44]

Continued care:

- Fluid therapy (Box 20.1)
- Nutritional support (Box 20.2)
- Prophylactic antibiotic coverage applied post-operatively
  - Trimethoprim-Sulfa: 30 mg/kg PO q12hr
  - Amoxicillin-clavulanate: 12.5 mg/kg PO q12hr [11]
- Chemotherapy and radiation therapy not required for uterine neoplasia

Neoplasia

Intra-Abdominal and Systemic Neoplasia

Diagnosis

Clinical Signs:

- Diarrhea
- Hematochezia and melena – common with gastrointestinal lymphosarcoma
- Vomiting – can be associated with hepatocellular carcinoma [40]

- PU/PD (rare)
- Hypocalcemic seizure (rare) [42]
- Abdominal mass [53]
- Free abdominal fluid – hemorrhagic or clear
- Submandibular lymphadenopathy – may present with lymphosarcoma [54]
- Non-specific signs – progressive weight loss, anorexia, lethargy, and pyrexia [30]

Differentials:

Neoplastic

- Hepatocellular carcinoma
  - Several cases reported, present with anorexia and diarrhea and can be associated with hepatic lipidosis. Highly metastatic and malignant; metastases to lung, spleen, kidneys, and mesentery [42]
- Lymphosarcoma
  - Alimentary and multicentric forms both reported frequently, malignant, and commonly metastatic
  - Possible association with retroviral infection [30]
- Other less common neoplasia
  - Islet cell tumor, adenocarcinoma, plasmacytoma, myelogenous leukemia, C-cell carcinoma, follicular/pancreatic/adrenal adenoma [42]

Non-neoplastic

- Enteritis
- Gastrointestinal foreign body
- Hepatitis
- Hepatic lipidosis
- Peritonitis
- Septicemia

STAT Diagnostics:

- PCV/TP/Glu/Lactate (if limited blood sample)
  - Assessment of hydration/hemoconcentration status
  - Anemia may be present
- Blood smear
- POCUS (AFAST)

Complete Diagnostics:

- CBC/ Biochemistry
  - Lymphosarcoma patients may observe leukocytosis, neutrophilia with a regenerative left shift, lymphocytosis, and atypical lymphocytes on blood smear evaluation [5]
  - With hepatocellular carcinoma – may see elevated liver enzymes, and reduced production of glucose, cholesterol, bilirubin, and albumin. May also see signs of hepatic lipidosis (poikilocytosis, hypertriglyceridemia, hyperbilirubinemia, elevated GGT, and ALP)
- Radiography
  - Allows evaluation of primary neoplastic masses and metastases
- Ultrasound
  - Assess liver for nodules or discrepancies in normal architecture and can provide information on the location of alimentary masses, metastases [3]
- Ultrasound-guided fine needle aspirate
  - Sample size and quality of cells is often poor [47]
- Biopsy and histopathology
  - Will provide definitive diagnosis and allow staging and grading
  - Obtained percutaneously (submandibular lymph nodes), via ultrasound guidance (liver), laparoscopically, or through exploratory laparotomy [52]
  - Caution when sampling from liver of animals suspected of hepatic disease due to possible prolonged clotting times

Treatment

Stabilization:

- Analgesia
  - Opioids: for moderate-to-severe pain
    - Buprenorphine: 0.01–0.5 mg/kg IM/SC q6–12hr
    - Butorphanol 0.1–0.4 mg/kg IM/SC q6–12hr [11]
  - NSAIDs: can be used if patient is hydrated, eating, and kidney function is normal
    - Meloxicam: 0.2 mg/kg PO/SC q24hr
    - Carprofen: 1.0 mg/kg PO/SC q12–24 hrs [11]
- Treat secondary hepatic lipidosis (see Hepatic lipidosis)
- Drain free abdominal fluid
- Perform free fluid analysis and cytology
- Surgical debulking of abdominal mass, if possible, will increase the median survival time

Continued care:

- Fluid therapy: IV/IO fluids generally required (Box 20.1)
- Nutritional support (Box 20.2)
- Post-operative prophylactic antibiotics
  - Generally, only required after gastrointestinal surgery
    - Chloramphenicol: 50 mg/kg PO q12hr
    - Enrofloxacin: 5–10 mg/kg IV/IM/PO q12hr [11]
- Chemotherapy
  - Currently no recognized protocols exist, some practitioners do trial chemotherapeutic options extrapolated from ferrets, cats, and dogs [55]
    - Anecdotally, L-Asparaginase 400 U/kg SC once followed by prednisolone 1 mg/kg PO q 12 hr can be attempted for lymphosarcoma
- Cancer recurrence is very likely long term and prognosis is often poor
- Euthanasia of animals with obvious metastases or that are clinically unwell is recommended

Oral Neoplasia

Diagnosis

Clinical Signs:

- Deviation of the mandible or maxilla
- Dyspnea [56]
- Gingivitis/gingival hyperplasia [42]
- Ptyalism
- Swelling along the jaws – usually unilateral, maybe ulcerated. Squamous cell carcinomas are frequently reported around incisor teeth, and on the maxilla [57]
- Teeth loss [42]
- Non-specific signs – progressive weight loss, anorexia, and lethargy

Differentials:

Neoplastic

- Oral squamous cell carcinoma (Figure 20.5)
  - Very common in oral cavity however occasionally cutaneous or intranasal [31, 58, 59]
  - Malignant, locally invasive, not highly metastatic but occasionally metastasize to lymph nodes and lungs [60]
- Fibrosarcoma
  - Less frequent, malignant, locally invasive, generally not metastatic [53]

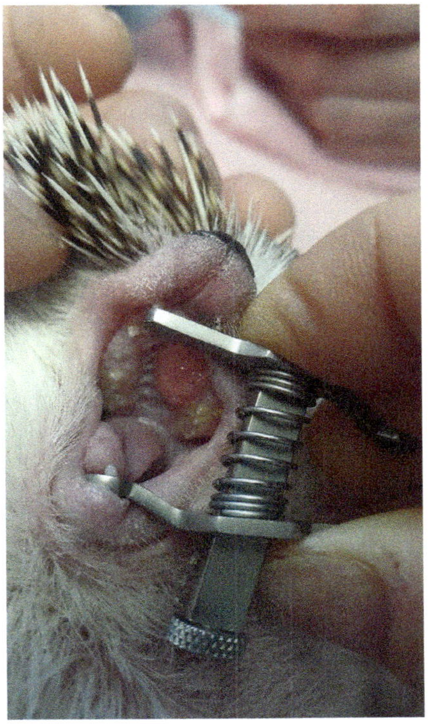

Figure 20.5 Oral squamous cell carcinoma on the hard palate of an African pygmy hedgehog (*Atelerix albiventris*). *Source:* Photo courtesy of Heidi Hoefer.

- Other oral tumors
  - Cutaneous mast cell tumor (malignant and metastatic), osteosarcoma (frequently, malignant, and metastatic), and peripheral odontogenic fibroma/fibromatous epulis (benign, proliferative mass) [37, 61]

Non-neoplastic

- Oral abscess
- Bony cysts
- Dental disease
- Rhinitis/sinusitis
- Trauma

STAT Diagnostics:

- PCV/TP/Glu/Lactate (if limited blood sample)
  - Assessment of hydration/hemoconcentration status
  - Anemia may be present
- Blood smear

Complete diagnostics:

- CBC/biochemistry: mild inflammatory leukogram, anemia
- Radiography: extent of osteolysis and to determine metastases to chest/submandibular lymph nodes [47]
- Fine needle aspirate: neoplastic squamous cells with varying levels of anisocytosis, anisokaryosis, pleomorphism, and mitosis [60]. Can be difficult to differentiate from squamous cell hyperplasia/dysplasia seen in chronic hyperplastic gingivitis, very poor cell yield [62]. FNA of the ipsilateral submandibular lymph node recommended to assess for metastases
- Biopsy and histopathology: definitive technique. Sample can be taken percutaneously, preferably via incisional or excision biopsy [42]
- CT allows assessment of bone loss and neoplastic infiltration, not widely available and expensive [47]

Treatment

Stabilization:

- Analgesia
  - Opioids: for moderate-to-severe pain
    - Buprenorphine 0.01–0.5 mg/kg IM/SC q6–12hr
    - Butorphanol 0.1–0.4 mg/kg IM/SC q6–12 hrs [11]
  - NSAIDs: can be used if patient is hydrated, eating, and kidney function is normal
    - Meloxicam: 0.2 mg/kg PO/SC q24hr
    - Carprofen: 1.0 mg/kg PO/SC q12–24 hr [11]
- Prophylactic pre-operative antibiotic therapy
  - Amoxicillin-clavulanate: 12.5 mg/kg PO q12hr
  - Enrofloxacin: 5–10 mg/kg IV/IM/PO q12hr [11]
- Surgical resection
  - Where complete resection is achievable, surgery alone is often curative [52], but complete excision is rarely possible [63]

- Incomplete resection is of questionable benefit

Continued care:

- Fluid therapy: IV/IO fluids generally required (Box 20.1)
- Nutritional support (Box 20.2)
- Chemotherapy
  - Currently no recognized protocols exist, some practitioners do trial chemotherapeutic options extrapolated from ferrets, cats, and dogs [55]
- Radiation therapy
  - Efficacy unknown, provided remission for amelanotic melanoma in a different hedgehog species [64]
- Cancer recurrence very likely, prognosis is often poor. Euthanasia of animals with extensive destruction of bone, metastases or are clinically unwell is recommended

Skeletal Neoplasia

Diagnosis

Clinical Signs:

- Hyperesthesia – osteoclastic lesions are painful [17]
- Non-mobile mass – either on the appendicular skeleton, along the ribs, fixed to the mandible or dorsal aspect of the vertebrae [65]
- Gait abnormalities – paretic, limping, dragging the legs or completely non-ambulatory
- Neurological abnormalities – proprioceptive deficits, ataxia, and reduced reflexes [66]
- Referred pain/paresthesia – one report documents a hedgehog with spinal osteosarcoma exhibiting self-mutilation of feet [66]
- Respiratory distress – one case of skeletal osteosarcoma extending from the ribs resulted in dyspnea due to compression against lungs, causing atelectasis [17]
- Non-specific signs – progressive weight loss, anorexia, lethargy, and pyrexia [30]

Differentials:

Neoplastic:

- Osteosarcoma (Figure 20.6)
  - Frequently reported, malignant, invasive, and highly metastatic
  - Several forms exist – skeletal, multicentric, subcutaneous
  - Reported locations – ribs, caudal vertebral column, distal limbs, and the mandible
  - Possible retroviral infection association [65]
- Other tumors
  - Less commonly reported, mesenchymal and epithelial cell tumors of the musculoskeletal and neuroendocrine system (such as fibrosarcoma, neurofibroma, neurofibrosarcoma, schwannoma, malignant peripheral nerve sheath tumor, fibrous histiocytoma, astrocytoma, cortical carcinoma) [42, 51]

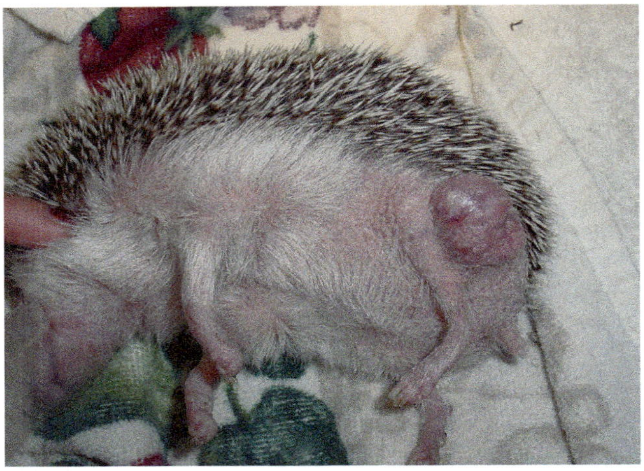

Figure 20.6 Dermal osteosarcoma on the left thigh of an African pygmy hedgehog (*Atelerix albiventris*). *Source:* Courtesy of Peter Fisher.

Non-neoplastic:

- Abscesses
- Arthritis
- Bony cysts
- Fractures
- Nutritional secondary hyperparathyroidism
- Hypocalcemia induced neuropathy
- Trauma
- Annular fiber constriction
- Wobbly hedgehog syndrome
- Intervertebral disc disease

STAT Diagnostics:

- PCV/TP/Glu/Lactate (if limited blood sample)
  - Assessment of hydration/hemoconcentration status
  - Anemia may be present
- Blood smear

Complete Diagnostics:

- CBC/Biochemistry
  - Moderate increase in ALP, hypoalbuminemia, hypercalcemia with osteosarcoma [17, 66]
- Radiography
  - Osteolysis, disorganized proliferation associated with skeletal neoplasia
- Assess metastases to the chest, liver, and vertebral column [47]
- Needle aspirate
- Tend not to exfoliate well, and can be difficult to differentiate tumor types [17]
- Biopsy and histopathology
  - Definitive diagnosis and allow staging and grading of the tumor
  - Utilize incisional/excisional biopsy, core biopsy, or Jamshidi bone needle [52]

- CT
  - Complete evaluation of bone destruction, locating metastases and for differentiating skeletal neoplasia from other causes of neurologic dysfunction; infrequently performed

Treatment

Stabilization:

- Analgesia
  - Opioids: for moderate-to-severe pain
    - Buprenorphine: 0.01–0.5 mg/kg IM/SC q6–12hr
    - Butorphanol: 0.1–0.4 mg/kg IM/SC q6–12hr [11]
  - NSAIDs: can be used if patient is hydrated, eating, and kidney function is normal
    - Meloxicam 0.2 mg/kg PO/SC q24hr
    - Carprofen 1.0 mg/kg PO/SC q12–24 hr [11]
- Treat hypercalcemia if present
  - Diuresis with fluids and furosemide: 1–5 mg/kg q8h PO, IM, or SC [11]
- Amputation of a limb containing a primary osteosarcoma may prolong the animal's life but is not typically curative [52]
- Complete resection is not possible in regions of the body such as vertebrae, the ribcage, or the mandible

Continued care:

- See continued care for oral neoplasia

Integumentary Neoplasia

Diagnosis

Clinical Signs:

- Cutaneous or subcutaneous mass
- Skin discoloration
- Foci of hemorrhage and necrotic exudates if infected
- Focal quill loss
- Peripheral lymphadenopathy
- Non-specific signs – progressive weight loss, anorexia, lethargy, and pyrexia are common findings [30]

Differentials:

Neoplastic:

- Mammary adenocarcinoma – most frequently reported neoplasm in hedgehogs [57]. Malignant, locally invasive and frequently metastasize to lymph nodes [67]; concurrently found with uterine tumors [42, 68]
- Mastocytoma – mast cell tumors, most commonly reported cutaneous mass, malignant frequently metastasizes [67]
- Fibrous histiocytoma – few reported cases; malignant non-metastatic [69]
- Neurofibroma – several reported cases, malignant, metastatic, highly invasive [42]

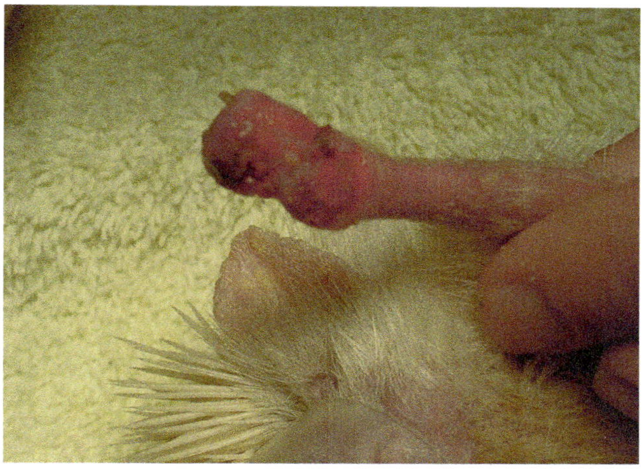

Figure 20.7 Squamous cell carcinoma on the pedal region of the left foreleg of an African pygmy hedgehog (*Atelerix albiventris*). Note the ulcerative appearance on plantar surface that may resemble severe pododermatitis. *Source:* Courtesy of Peter Fisher.

- Cutaneous squamous cell carcinoma – not frequently reported, less common than oral form, malignant, highly invasive, non-metastatic (Figure 20.7) [58]
- Many others reported infrequently [42, 70–72]

Non-neoplastic:

- Abscess
- Bacterial pyoderma
- Cuterebra larvae
- Contact dermatitis
- Dermatophytosis
- Papillomas
- Mycobacteriosis
- Trauma

STAT diagnostics:

- PCV/TP/Glu/Lactate (if limited blood sample)
  - Assessment of hydration/hemoconcentration status
  - Anemia may be present
- Blood smear

Complete diagnostics:

- CBC/biochemistry
  - Paraneoplastic hypercalcemia is suspected in mammary adenocarcinoma [71]
- Radiography
  - Evaluate metastases to lymph nodes, lungs, or other abdominal organs [47]
- Fine needle aspirate
  - Good cellular yield, no grading or staging possible, and in some cases, insufficient to provide definitive diagnosis [42]

- Biopsy and histopathology
  - Definitive diagnosis, allow staging and grading of the tumor
  - Obtain biopsy from both from the mass and nearby lymph nodes if metastases suspected

Treatment

Stabilization:

- Analgesia
  - Opioids: for moderate-to-severe pain
    - Buprenorphine: 0.01–0.5 mg/kg IM/SC q6–12hr
    - Butorphanol: 0.1–0.4 mg/kg IM/SC q6–12hr [11]
  - NSAIDs: can be used if patient is hydrated, eating, and kidney function is normal
    - Meloxicam: 0.2 mg/kg PO/SC q24hr
    - Carprofen: 1.0 mg/kg PO/SC q12–24 hr [11]
- Treat hypercalcemia if present: diuresis via fluids and furosemide: 1–5 mg/kg q8h PO, IM, or SC [11]
- Antihistamine therapy in mast cell tumors
  - Pre-operative diphenhydramine: 1.25 mg/kg q24h PO [73]
  - Reduce risk of mast cell degranulation during surgical excision [42]
- Surgical mass resection:
  - Widest surgical margins possible are recommended due to invasive nature of most cutaneous masses [52]
  - Intact females with mammary cancer should undergo ovariohysterectomy to reduce the risk of recurrence of mammary cancer and remove potential uterine/ovarian tumors

Continued Care:

- See continued care for Oral neoplasia

Dermatology

Dermatophytes

Diagnosis

Clinical signs:

- Non-pruritic
- Dry scaly skin
- Quills drop easily
- Bald patches and spine loss

Differentials:

- Mites – *Caparinia* spp., *Notoedres* spp., *Ornithonyssus bacoti*
- Bacterial dermatitis
- Normal quilling

STAT diagnostics:

- Skin scrape to rule out ectoparasites
- Microscopy of quills
  - Spores/hyphae may be seen
- Wood's Lamp
  - Positive fluorescence with some fungal infections
  - False negatives may be observed [74]

Complete diagnostics:

- Dermatophyte culture of quills or scabs
- Dermatophyte test medium (DTM) of quills or scabs
- Bacterial aerobic culture of moist exudative areas
- CBC/serum biochemistry
  - Normal liver values should be evident prior to starting animal on systemic anti-fungals

Treatment

Stabilization:

- Oral anti-fungals
  - Itraconazole: 5–10 mg/kg PO q24hr for six weeks [13]
  - Terbinafine: 100 mg/kg PO q12h
- Topical anti-fungal
  - Miconazole or clotrimazole spray applied once daily on skin
  - Topicals should be used sparingly as they may encourage excessive licking
  - Creams can be greasy and should be avoided
- Antifungal wash (Enilconazole 10%, Bayer)
  - Dilute in 50 parts water and spray entire animal for first application followed by subsequent localized application
  - Remove hard crusts on skin once softened
  - Repeat for four treatments four days apart [75]
- Lyme sulfur dip
  - Once weekly for four weeks
- Antibiotic therapy
  - Indicated only if secondary bacterial infection is present
  - Trimethoprim-sulfa: 30 mg/kg PO q12hr
  - Amoxicillin-clavulanate: 12.5 mg/kg PO q12hr

Continued Care:

- Repeat dermatophyte cultures after six weeks or after clinical signs have resolved. Two negative cultures, two weeks apart is ideal due to zoonotic potential
- Prevent re-exposure: Disinfection of environment and examine and treat all in contact animals

Ectoparasites

Diagnosis

Clinical Signs:

- Brown crusts and hyperkeratosis on dorsal back, ear pinnae, footpad, periocular areas
- Crusty exudate or brown debris in ears
- Live mites, ticks, and fleas may be seen crawling on skin
- Flaky and dry skin

- Pruritus
- Failure to roll up effectively

Differentials:

- Mites – *Caparinia* spp., *Notoedres* spp., *Ornithonyssus bacoti, Notoedres cati*
- Fleas and ticks – if housed outdoors (rare) [6]
- Cuterebrae larvae – if animal is housed outdoors (rare)
- Normal quilling
- Bacterial dermatitis – unsanitary bedding, *Staphylococcus simulans* caused quill loss and alopecia [10]
- Immune mediated skin disease – pemphigus foliaceus
- Dermatophytosis
- Mycobacteriosis [76]
- Skin neoplasia
- Abscesses

STAT diagnostics:

- Skin scraping
  - Microscopic visualization of eggs, larva, and adult mites [77]
- Skin cytology
  - Impression smears of exudative areas, to rule out secondary bacterial or yeast overgrowth
- Observation for other ectoparasites
  - Fleas and flea dirt, ticks, and cuterebra (rare)
- Otoscopic examination
  - Microscopic visualization of ear mites (*Notoedres cati*)

Complete diagnostics:

- Complete mite check (rarely performed)
  - Examine skin scraping with 0.5% KOH that has been heated gently [78]
  - Boil skin scraping in 10% KOH [79] and examine the sediment after 30 minutes [75]
- Dermatophyte culture
- CBC and Chemistry panel
  - Eosinophilia may be present
  - Assess dehydration/hemoconcentration

Treatment

Stabilization:

- Dressing and disinfection of any secondary wounds
  - Clean with chlorhexidine and apply topical antibiotics/astringents
- Antibiotic therapy: required only if wounds are extensive
  - Trimethoprim-sulfa: 30 mg/kg PO q12hr
  - Amoxicillin-clavulanate: 12.5 mg/kg PO Q12hr
  - Enrofloxacin: 5–10 mg/kg IV/IM/PO q12hr [11]
- Acaricides for mite treatment
  - Ivermectin: 0.5 mg/kg SC q 10 days × 3 treatments (effectiveness may not be 100%) [3]
  - Amitraz: (0.3% topically q 7 d) × 2–3 treatments in addition to ivermectin 0.4 mg/kg PO, SC q 10 days × 3–5 treatments may produce better results [3]
  - Selamectin: 6 mg/kg topically repeat in 14 days
  - Combination 10% Imidacloprid and 1% moxidectin: 0.1 ml/kg and repeat in 10 days [80]
  - Moxidectin: 0.3 mg/kg q 10 days × 2 treatments [75]

Continued Care:

- Prevent re-exposure: disinfect and clean the enclosure to get remove mite eggs and treat all other hedgehogs in the household
- Frequent changing of bedding recommended during mite treatment (Figures 20.8 and 20.9)

Trauma

Diagnosis

Clinical signs:

- Open injuries or wounds
- Lameness
- Blood loss
- Anorexia
- Depression

Differentials:

- Constriction injuries
- Ocular injuries
- Fractures (rare)
- Soft tissue injuries

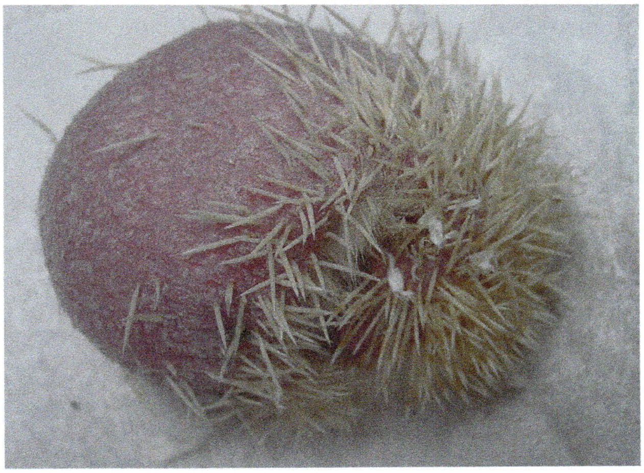

Figure 20.8 An African pygmy hedgehog (*Atelerix albiventris*) with severe mite infestation. There is extensive loss of quills on the dorsum and the skin appearance is very dry and flaky. *Source:* Courtesy of Peter Fisher.

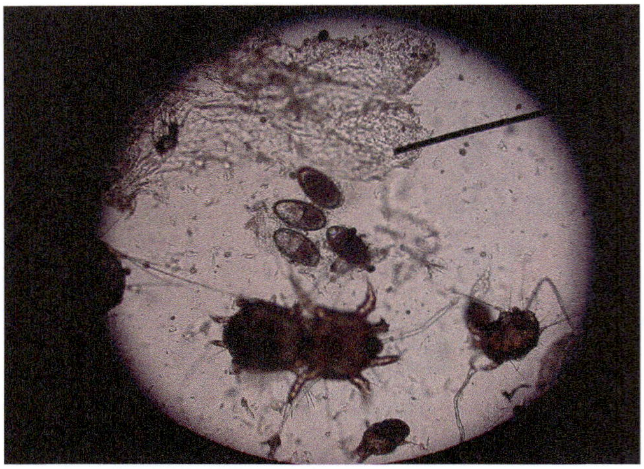

Figure 20.9 Light microscopy shows several life stages of *Caparinia* sp. in an African pygmy hedgehog (*Atelerix albiventris*). Note the presence of embryonated eggs, larva, and an attachment pair of adult male (right) and pubescent female (left). *Source:* Courtesy of Peter Fisher.

- Pododermatitis
- Contact dermatitis
- Ingrown nails
- Self-mutilation
- Osteoarthritis
- Wobbly hedgehog syndrome
- Intervertebral disc disease

STAT diagnostics:

- PCV/TP/Glu/Lactate (if limited blood sample)
  - Assessment of hydration/hemoconcentration status
  - Anemia may be present
- Blood smear
- Impression smear and cytology of the any ulcerated extensive wounds

Complete diagnostics:

- CBC/biochemistry
  - Inflammatory leukogram may be present
- Radiographs
  - Assess for fractures, osteomyelitis, and underlying osteoarthritis or neoplasia
- Aerobic and anaerobic culture
  - Open wounds that appear to be exudative

Treatment

Stabilization:

- Analgesia
  - Opioids: for moderate-to-severe pain
    - Buprenorphine 0.01–0.5 mg/kg IM/SC q6–12hr
    - Butorphanol 0.1–0.4 mg/kg IM/SC q6–12hrs [11]
  - NSAIDs: can be used if patient is hydrated, eating, and kidney function is normal
    - Meloxicam: 0.2 mg/kg PO/SC q24hr
    - Carprofen: 1.0 mg/kg PO/SC q12–24 hr
- Empiric antibiotics therapy
  - Pending culture results if available
    - Amoxicillin-clavulanate: 12.5 mg/kg PO q12hr
    - Enrofloxacin: 5–10 mg/kg IV/IM/PO q12hr
    - Chloramphenicol: 50 mg/kg PO q12hr
- Wound treatment:
  - Surgical closure is reserved for clean lacerations with large defects in normal tissue
  - Healing by secondary intention is best option for infected wounds
  - Address any ingrown nails, lance abscesses, remove any constricting foreign material and debride necrotic material
  - Thorough disinfection of the area with chlorhexidine or dilute iodine
  - Topical medication with astringents or antibiotic cream/powder
  - Avoid repeated application of topicals as animal may lick excessively
- Bandage placement on limbs
  - For moderate-to-severe pododermatitis
  - For animals that self-mutilate

Continued Care:

- Fluid therapy: as required (Box 20.1)
- Nutritional support (Box 20.2)
- Prevent recurrence
  - Remove inappropriate bedding that could cause pododermatitis
  - Improve bedding hygiene

Ophthalmic

Corneal Ulceration

Diagnosis

Clinical Signs:

- Blepharospasm
- Buphthalmos
- Corneal edema
- Epiphora
- Hyphema
- Hypopyon
- Mucopurulent discharge
- Mydriasis – unilateral, noted in ulcers resulting from retrobulbar masses
- Hunched appearance, inactivity, and anorexia sequelae to the pain

Differentials:

- Corneal perforation

- Incipient anterior cortical cataracts
- Ocular proptosis
- Orbital cellulitis
- Panophthalmitis
- Acute uveitis
- Glaucoma

STAT Diagnostics:

- Focal light examination and under magnification
- PCV/TP/Glu/Lactate
  - Assessment of hydration/hemoconcentration status
- Blood smear
  - Inflammatory leukogram may be present

Complete Diagnostics:

- Fluorescein stain
  - Stain uptake and fluorescence over the corneal defect
- Bacterial aerobic culture and sensitivity of cornea defect (for indolent ulcers)
- Skull radiographs
  - If exophthalmia is present
  - Assess for evidence of retrobulbar mass
- Ultrasound of globe if retrobulbar mass is suspected
- Fine needle aspirate and cytology of mass
- CBC and chemistry panel

Treatment

Stabilization:

- Analgesia
  - NSAIDs: can be used if patient is hydrated, eating, and kidney function is normal
    - Meloxicam: 0.2 mg/kg PO/SC q24hr
    - Carprofen: 1.0 mg/kg PO/SC q12–24 hr
- Topical antibiotics
  - Neomycin, polymyxin B and bacitracin ophthalmic ointment, ofloxacin, or ciprofloxacin drops applied to the surface of the cornea or conjunctiva q2-3hr for 24–48 hours then decrease to q8-12hr [11]
  - May require hospitalization for successful daily application
- Grid keratotomy
  - Utilized for superficial non-healing ulcers
- Third eyelid flap procedure and conjunctival graft
  - Indolent, deep, or perforating ulcers (rarely performed)
- Eye enucleation
  - Salvage procedure of end-stage corneal ulceration or globe rupture
  - Ocular neoplasia or retrobulbar mass excision

Continued care:

- For prevention of recurrence
  - Dusty substrates to be removed
  - Abrasive or sharp enclosure furnishings should be swapped for safer items

Ocular Proptosis

Diagnosis

Clinical Signs:

- Hyphema
- Pain on palpation near head/eyes
- Panophthalmitis
- Aqueous flare
- Inability to retropulse globe
- Corneal perforation
- Conjunctival trauma/hemorrhage
- Exophthalmos – all hedgehogs predisposed to the condition due to the shallow orbits surrounding the eye [3]
- Incipient anterior subcapsular cataracts
- Orbital cellulitis
- Orbital fat – increase risk of exophthalmos
- Ocular abduction – secondary to retrobulbar masses [31]
- Concurrent neurological disease – likely to result in eye trauma [81]

Differentials:

- Blepharitis/blepharoconjunctivitis
- Corneal ulceration
- Ocular lens luxation
- Orbital cellulitis
- Retrobulbar neoplasia
  - Acinic cell carcinoma and hemangioma has been reported [31, 42]
- Trauma

STAT Diagnostics:

- PCV/TP/Glu/Lactate
  - Assessment of hydration/hemoconcentration status
- Focal light examination
  - Lack of pupillary light reflexes, aqueous flare, hyphema, trauma to corneal surface, injected sclera
- Tonometry
  - Increased IOP

Complete Diagnostics:

- Skull radiographs (or CT if available)
  - If exophthalmia is present
  - Assess for evidence of retrobulbar mass
- Ultrasound of globe if retrobulbar mass is suspected
- Fine needle aspirate and cytology of mass
- CBC/biochemistry

- Fundic examination (rarely done)
  - Retinal detachment
- Histopathology
  - Determine the origin of a retrobulbar mass

Treatment

Stabilization:

- Analgesia
  - Opioids: for moderate-to-severe pain
    - Buprenorphine: 0.01–0.5 mg/kg IM/SC q6–12hr
    - Butorphanol: 0.1–0.4 mg/kg IM/SC q6–12 hr [11].
  - NSAIDs: can be used if patient is hydrated, eating, and kidney function is normal
    - Meloxicam: 0.2 mg/kg PO/SC q24hr
    - Carprofen: 1.0 mg/kg PO/SC q12–24 hr
- Eye enucleation
  - Primary method of treatment as proposed eye is typically not salvageable [82]
  - Gelfoam or similar hemostatic agents should be available during surgery to minimize hemorrhage [41]
- Excision of retrobulbar mass
  - Typically, in combination with enucleation
  - Wide margins generally necessary as neoplasia associated with proptosis is generally very invasive [31]
- Empiric antibiotic therapy
  - Amoxicillin-clavulanate: 12.5 mg/kg PO q12hr
  - Enrofloxacin: 5–10 mg/kg IV/IM/PO q12hr
  - Chloramphenicol: 50 mg/kg PO q12hr

Continued care:

- Fluids (Box 20.1)
- Nutritional support (Box 20.2)
- Lateral tarsorrhaphy
  - Performed prophylactically if the contralateral eye is also exophthalmic [81]
  - Butterfly catheter tubing can be used as stents on the palpebrae for the tarsorrhaphy sutures for 2 weeks [41]
- Prevention of recurrence (see Corneal ulceration)

References

1 Adamovicz, L., Bullen, L., Korinn, S., and Grunkemeyer, V. (2016). Use of an esophagostomy tube for management of traumatic subtotal glossectomy in an African pygmy hedgehog. *J. Exot. Pet Med.* 25: 231–236.

2 Johnson-Delaney, C.A. (2006). Common procedures in hedgehogs, prairie dogs, exotic rodents, and companion marsupials. *Vet. Clin. North Am. Exot. Anim. Pract.*; Exotic Animal Practice 9(2): 415–435.

3 Ivey, E. and Carpenter, J.W. (2012). African hedgehogs. In: Ferrets, Rabbits and Rodents Clinical Medicine and Surgery, 3e (eds. K.E. Quesenberry and J.W. Carpenter), 411–425. St. Louis, MI: Elsevier.

4 Heatley, J.J. (2009). Hedgehogs. In: Manual of Exotic Pet Practice (eds. M.A. Tully and T.N. Mitchell), 433–455. St Louis: WB Saunder.

5 Helmer, P.J. (2000). Abnormal hematologic findings in an african hedgehog (*Atelerix albiventris*) with gastrointestinal lymphosarcoma. *J. Can. Vet.* 41: 489–490.

6 Johnson, D. (2009). African pygmy hedgehogs. In: BSAVA Manual of Exotic Pets, 5e (eds. A. Meredith and C. Johnson-Delaney), 139–147. Gloucester: British Small Animal Veterinary Association.

7 Raymond, J.T., Aguilar, R., Dunker, F. et al. (2009). Intervertebral disc disease in african hedgehog (*Atelerix albiventris*): four cases. *J. Exot. Pet Med.* 18 (3): 220–223.

8 Gibson, C.J., Parry, N.M.A., Jakowski, R.M., and Eshar, D. (2008). Anaplastic astrocytoma in the spinal cord of an african pygmy hedgehog (*Atelerix albiventris*). *Vet. Pathol.* 45: 934–938.

9 Nakata, M., Miwa, Y., Itou, T. et al. (2011). Astrocytoma in an african hedgehog (*Atelerix albiventris*) suspected wobbly hedgehog syndrome. *J. Vet. Med. Sci.* 73 (10): 1333–1335.

10 Han, J.K., Lee, S.J., Jang, H.J. et al. (2011). Isolation of *Staphylococcus simulans* from dermatitis in a captive african pygmy hedgehog. *J. Zoo Wildl. Med.* 42 (2): 277–280.

11 Carpenter, J.W. and Marion, C.J. (2013). Hedgehogs. In: Exotic Animal Formulary, 4e (ed. J.W. Carpenter), 444–455. St. Louis: Elsevier Saunders.

12 Srugo, I., Chai, O., Yaakov, D. et al. (2010). Successful medical management of lumbar intervertebral disc prolapse in a ferret. *J. Small Anim. Pract.* 51 (8): 447–450.

13 Carpenter, J.W. (2005). Hedgehogs. In: Exotic Animal Formulary, 3e, 361–369. St. Louis: Elsevier Saunders.

14 Graesser, D., Spraker, T.R., Dressen, P. et al. (2006). Wobbly hedgehog syndrome in african pygmy hedgehog (*Atelerix* spp). *J. Exot. Pet Med.* 15 (1): 59–65.

15 Haggstrom, J., Kvart, C., and Pedersen, H.D. (2005). Acquired valvular heart disease. In: Textbook of Veterinary Internal Medicine Disease of the Dog and Cat, 6e (eds. S.J. Ettinger and E.C. Feldman), 1022–1039. St. Louis: Elsevier Saunders.

16 Black, P.A., Marshall, C., Seyfried, A.W., and Bartin, A.M. (2011). Cardiac assessment of african hedgehogs (*Atelerix albiventris*). *J. Zoo Wildl. Med.* 49 (1): 49–53.

17 Benoit-Biancamano, M.O., d'Anjou, M.A., Girard, C., and Langlois, I. (2006). Rib osteoblastic osteosarcoma in an african hedgehog (*Atelerix albiventris*). *J. Vet. Diagn. Invest.* 18 (4): 415–418.

18 Burgdorf-Moisuk A, Whittington JK, Mitchell MA, et al. Echocardiographic measurements in clinically healthy African hedgehogs (*Atelerix albiventris*) anesthetized with isoflurane, in Proceedings of the AAZV/AAWV Joint Conference. Tulsa, OK. 2009, p 188.

19 Dukes-McEwan, J., Borgarelli, M., Tidholm, A. et al. (2003). Proposed guidelines for the diagnosis of canine idiopathic dilated cardiomyopathy. *J. Vet. Cardiol.* 5 (2): 7–19.

20 Hedberg, G.E., Dierenfeld, E.S., and Rogers, Q.R. (2007). Taurine and zoo felids: considerations of dietary and biological tissue concentrations. *Zoo Biol.* 26: 517–531.

21 Freeman, J.M., Rush, J.E., and Markwell, P.J. (2006). Effects of dietary modification in dosg with early chronic valvular disease. *J. Vet. Intern. Med.* 20 (5): 1116–1126.

22 Johnson, D.H. (2011). Hedgehogs and sugar gliders: respiratory anatomy, physiology, and disease. *Vet. Clin. North Am. Exot. Anim. Pract.* 14 (2): 267–285.

23 Mori, M. and O'Brien, S.E. (1997). Husbandry and medical management of African hedgehogs. *Iowa State Univ. Vet.* 59 (2): 64–71.

24 Snider, T.A., Joyner, P.H., and Clinkenbeard, K.D. (2008). Disseminated histoplasmosis in an african pygmy hedgehog. *J. Am. Vet. Med. Assoc.* 232 (1): 74–76.

25 Robinson, I. and Routh, A. (1999). Veterinary care of the hedgehog. *In Practice* 21 (3): 128–137.

26 Martínez, L.S., Juan Sallés, C., and Cucchi-Stefanoni, K. (2005). Actinomyces naeslundii infection in an african hedgehog (*Atelerix albiventris*) with mandibular osteomyelitis and cellulits. *Vet. Rec.* 157: 450–451.

27 Vestraete, F.J.M. (2003). Advances in diagnosis and treatment of small exotic mammal dental disease. *Semin. Avian Exot. Pet Med.* 12 (1): 37–48.

28 Bunnell, T. (2001). The importance of faecal indices in assessing gastrointestinal parasite infestation and bacterial infection in the hedgehog (*Erinaceus europaeus*). *J. Wildl. Rehab.* 24 (2): 13–17.

29 Ramos-Vara, J.A., Miller, M.A., and Craft, D. (1998). Intestinal plasmacytoma in african hedgehog. *J. Zoo Wildl. Med.* 34 (2): 377–380.

30 Raymond, J.T., Clarke, K.A., and Schafer, K. (1998). Intestinal lymphosarcoma in captive african hedgehogs. *J. Wildl. Dis.* 34 (4): 801–806.

31 Fukuzawa, R., Fukuzawa, K., Abe, H. et al. (2004). Acinic cell carcinoma in an african pygmy hedgehog (*Atelerix albiventris*). *Vet. Clin. Path.* 33 (1): 39–42.

32 Lee, S.Y. and Park, H.M. (2012). Gastroesophageal intussusception with megaesophagus in a hedgehog (*Atelerix albiventris*). *J. Exot. Pet Med.* 21: 168–171.

33 Allison, N., Chang, T.C., Steele, K.E., and Hilliard, J.K. (2002). Fatal herpes simplex infection in a pygmy african hedgehog (*Atelerix albiventris*). *J. Comp. Pathol.* 126: 76–78.

34 Callan, M.B., Washabau, R.J., Saunders, H.M. et al. (1993). Congenital esophageal hiatal hernia in the chinese shar-pei dog. *J. Vet. Intern. Med.* 7 (4): 210–215.

35 Mc Gill, S.E., Lenard, Z.M., See, A.M., and Irwin, P.J. (2009). Non-surgical treatment of gastroesophageal intussusception in a puppy. *J. Am. Anim. Hosp. Assoc.* 45: 185–190.

36 Fisher, P.G. (2006). Exotic mammal renal disease: causes and clinical presentation. *Vet. Clin. North Am. Exot. Anim. Pract.* 9 (1): 33–67.

37 Raymond, J.T., White, M.R., and Janovitz, E.B. (1997). Malignant mast cell tumor in an african hedgehog (*Atelerix albiventris*). *J. Wildl. Dis.* 33 (1): 140–142.

38 Antinoff, N. (1998). Small mammal critical care. *Vet. Clin. North Am. Exot. Anim. Pract.* 1 (1): 153–175.

39 Panchaphanpong, J., Asawakarn, T., and Pusoonthornthum, R. (2011). Effects of oral administration of N-acetyl-d-glucosamine on plasma and urine concentrations of glycosaminoglycans in cats with idiopathic cystitis. *Am. J. Vet. Res.* 72 (6): 843–850.

40 Heatley, J.J. (2009). Cardiovascular anatomy, physiology, and disease of rodents and small exotic mammals. *Vet. Clin. North Am. Exot. Anim. Pract.* 12 (1): 99–113.

41 McLaughlin, A. and Strunk, A. (2016). Common emergencies in small rodents, hedgehogs, and sugar gliders. *Vet. Clin. North Am. Exot. Anim. Pract.* 19 (2): 465–499.

42 Heatley, J.J., Mauldin, G.E., and Cho, D.Y. (2005). A review of neoplasia in the captive African hedgehog (*Atelerix albiventris*). *Semin. Avian Exot. Pet Med.* 14 (3): 182–192.

43 Plunkett, S.J. (2000). Emergencies in exotic species. In: Emergency Procedures for the Small Animal Veterinarian, 2e (ed. S.J. Plunkett), 220. Oxford: WB Saunders.

44 Done, L., Deem, S.L., and Fiorello, C.V. (2007). Surgical and medical management of a uterine spindle cell tumor in an african hedgehog (*Atelerix albiventris*). *J. Wildl. Dis.* 38 (4): 601–603.

45 Miwa, Y. and Sladky, K.K. (2016). Small mammals: common surgical procedures of rodents, ferrets, hedgehogs, and sugar gliders. *Vet. Clin. North Am. Exot. Anim. Pract.* 19 (1): 205–244.

46 Lennox, A.M. (2007). Emergency and critical care procedures in sugar gliders (*Petaurus breviceps*), african hedgehogs

(*Atelerix albiventris*) and prairie dogs (*Cynomys* spp). *Vet. Clin. North Am. Exot. Anim. Pract.* 10 (2): 533–555.

47 Evans, E.E. and Souza, M.J. (2010). Advanced diagnostic approaches and current management of internal disorders of select species (rodents, sugar gliders, hedgehogs). *Vet. Clin. North Am. Exot. Anim. Pract.* 13 (3): 453–469.

48 Simone-Freilicher, E.A. and Hoefer, H.L. (2004). Hedgehog care and husbandry. *Vet. Clin. North Am. Exot. Anim. Pract.* 7 (2): 257–267.

49 Kupersmith, D.S. (1998). A practical overview of small mammal nutrition. *Semin. Avian Exot. Pet Med.* 7 (3): 141–147.

50 Done L. What you don't know about hedgehog diseases. Proc. N. Am. Vet. Conf. East. States Vet. Assoc., (1999) Gainesville, Florida

51 Greenacre, C.B. (2004). Spontaneous tumors of small mammals. *Vet. Clin. North Am. Exot. Anim. Pract.* 7 (3): 627–651.

52 Mehler, S.J. and Bennett, R.A. (2004). Surgical oncology of exotic animals. *Vet. Clin. North Am. Exot. Anim. Pract.* 7 (3): 783–805.

53 Raymond, J.T. and Garner, M.M. (2001). Spontaneous tumour in captive african hedgehogs (*Atelerix albiventris*): a retrospective study. *J. Comp. Pathol.* 124: 128–133.

54 Garner, M.M. (2011). Diseases of pet hedgehogs, chinchillas, and sugar gliders. In: Proceedings of the Association of Avian Veterinarians, 351–359. Seattle, WA: Association of Avian Veterinarians.

55 Kent, M.S. (2004). The use of chemotherapy in exotic animals. *Vet. Clin. North Am. Exot. Anim. Pract.* 7 (3): 807–820.

56 Reams Rivera, R.Y. and Janovitz, E.B. (1992). Oronasal squamous cell carcinoma in an african hedgehog (*Erinaceus-albiventris*). *J. Wildl. Dis.* 28 (1): 148–150.

57 Reavill D. The pathology of common diseases in small exotic mammals. Proceedings of the Western Veterinary Conference. 2009, Las Vegas, NV.

58 Couture, E.L., Langlois, I., Santamaria-Bouvier, A., and Benoit-Biancamano, M.O. (2015). Cutaneous squamous cell carcinoma in an african pygmy hedgehog (*Atelerix albiventris*). *Can. Vet. J.* 56 (12): 1275–1278.

59 Gal, J., Landauer, K., Palade, E.A. et al. (2009). Squamous cell carcinoma and consequent otitis in a long-eared hedgehog (hemiechinus auritus) - case report. *Acta Vet. Hung.* 57 (1): 69–73.

60 Cho, H., Choi, U., and Lee, H. (2013). Cytologic aspects of oral squamous cell carcinoma in a captive african hedgehog (*Altelerix albiventris*). *J. Vet. Clin.* 30 (3): 214–217.

61 Wozniak-Biel, A., Janeczek, M., Janus, I., and Nowak, M. (2015). Surgical resection of peripheral odontogenic fibromas in african pygmy hedgehog (*Atelerix albiventris*): a case study. *BMC Vet. Res.* 11 (145).

62 Juan-Salles, C. and Garner, M.M. (2007). Cytologic diagnosis of diseases of hedgehogs. *Vet. Clin. Exot. Anim.* 10: 51–59.

63 Graham, J.E., Kent, M.S., and Théon, A. (2004). Current therapies in exotic animal oncology. *Vet. Clin. North Am. Exot. Anim. Pract.* 7 (3): 757–781.

64 Harrison, T.M., Dominguez, P., Hanzlik et al. (2010). Treatment of an amelanotic melanoma using radiation therapy in a lesser Madagascar hedgehog tenrec (*Echinops telrairi*). *J. Zoo Wildl. Med.* 41 (1): 152–157.

65 Peauroi, J.R., Lowenstine, L.J., Munn, R.J., and Wilson, D.W. (1994). Multicentric skeletal sarcomas associated with probable retrovirus particles in 2 african hedgehogs (*Atelerix albiventris*). *Vet. Pathol.* 31 (4): 481–484.

66 Rhody, J.L. and Schiller, C.A. (2006). Spinal osteosarcoma in a hedgehog with pedal self-mutilation. *Vet. Clin. North Am. Exot. Anim. Pract.* 9 (3): 625–631.

67 Raymond, J.T. and Garner, M.M. (2000). Cardiomyopathy in captive african hedgehogs (*Atelerix albiventris*). *J. Vet. Diagn. Invest.* 12: 468–472.

68 Wellehan, J.F.X., Southorn, E., Smith, D.A., and Taylor, W.M. (2003). Surgical removal of a mammary adenocarcinoma and a granulosa cell tumor in an african pygmy hedgehog. *Can. Vet. J.* 44 (3): 235–237.

69 Hruban, Z., Vardiman, J., Meehan, T. et al. (1992). Haematopoietic malignancies in zoo animals. *J. Comp. Pathol.* 106 (1): 15–24.

70 Finkelstein, A., Hoover, J.P., Caudell, D., and Confer, A.W. (2008). Cutaneous epithelioid variant hemangiosarcoma in a captive african hedgehog (*Atelerix albiventris*). *J. Exot. Pet Med.* 17 (1): 49–53.

71 Matute, A.R., Bernal, A.M., Lezama, J.R. et al. (2014). Sebaceous gland carcinoma and mammary gland carcinoma in an african hedgehog (*Ateletrix albiventris*). *J. Zoo Wildl. Med.* 45 (3): 682–685.

72 Ramos-Vara, J.A. (2001). Soft tissue sarcomas in the african hedgehog (*Atelerix albiventris*): microscopic and immunohistologic study of three cases. *J. Vet. Diagn. Invest.* 13 (5): 442–445.

73 Huang, J., Eshar, D., Andrews, G., and Delk, K.W. (2014). Diagnostic challenge. *J. Exot. Pet Med.* 23 (4): 418–420.

74 English, M.P., Evans, C.D., Hewitt, M., and Warin, R.P. (1962). Hedgehog ringworm. *BMJ*: 149–150.

75 Pantchev, N. and Hofmann, T. (2006). Notoedric mange caused by Notoedres cati in a pet african pygmy hedgehog (*Atelerix albiventris*). *Vet. Rec.* 158: 59–60.

76 Riley, P.Y. and Chomel, B.B. (2005). Hedgehog zoonoses. *Emerg. Infect. Dis.* 11 (1): 1–5.

77 Gerson, L. and Boever, W.J. (1983). Acariasis (*Caparinia* sp.) in hedgehogs (*Erinaceus* spp.): diagnosis and treatment. *J. Zoo Wildl. Med.* 14 (1): 17–19.

78 Brockie, R.E. (1974). The hedgehog mange mite (*Caparinia tripilis*) in New Zealand. *N. Z. Vet. J.* 22 (12): 243–247.

79 Demkowska-Kutrzepa, M., Tomczuk, K., Studzińska, M., and Szczepaniak, K. (2015). Caparinia tripilis in african hedgehog (*Atelerix albiventris*). *Vet. Dermatol.* 26 (1): 73–75.

80 Kim, K.R., Ahn, K.S., Oh, D.S., and Shin, S.S. (2012). Efficacy of a combination of 10% imidacloprid and 1% moxidectin against *Caparinia tripili* in african pygmy hedgehog (*Atelerix albiventris*). *Parasit. Vectors* 5: 1–8.

81 Wheler, C.L., Grahn, B.H., and Pocknell, A.M. (2001). Unilateral proptosis and orbital cellulitis in eight african hedgehogs (*Atelerix albiventris*). *J. Zoo Wildl. Med.* 32 (2): 236–241.

82 Diehl, K.A. and McKinnon, J.A. (2016). Eye removal surgeries in exotic pets. *Vet. Clin. North Am. Exot. Anim. Pract.* 19 (1): 245–267.

21

Sugar Gliders

Dan H. Johnson

Avian and Exotic Animal Care, Raleigh, North Carolina, USA

CONTENTS

Unique Species Considerations

- Basal metabolic rate is about 30% lower than for placental mammals of similar size [1]
- May present in torporous state when ill, appearing moribund, yet exhibit a dramatic response to fluids and thermal support
- Are nocturnal, exhibiting more activity, normal behavior, and food intake at night
- In the wild, feed on plant exudates, mainly sap and gum, as well as insects. Considered a gumivore rather than an insectivore by some [2]

Common Presenting Signs

Anorexia

Introduction

- Captive diet should include nectar replacement, insects, and other protein sources, plant gums, and limited amounts of fruits and vegetables [2]
- Food consumption is normally 15–20% of body weight per day [1, 3]

Exotic Animal Emergency and Critical Care Medicine, First Edition. Edited by Jennifer E. Graham, Grayson A. Doss and Hugues Beaufrère.

Diagnosis

History:

- New or inexperienced owner

Signalment:

- Young, newly purchased gliders; however, all ages and both sexes susceptible

Clinical Signs:

- Weakness
- Inactivity
- Weight loss
- Reduced or abnormal feces

Differentials:

- Almost any illness can lead to anorexia

STAT Diagnostics:

- Fecal examination
- Complete blood count (CBC) and chemistry
- Radiography

Complete Diagnostics:

- Ultrasound

Treatment

Stabilization:

- Syringe-feed with commercial omnivore/carnivore formulas (e.g. Emeraid, Critical Care Omnivore, and Ensure Plus) and fruit/vegetable puree (Figure 21.1)
- Address concurrent dehydration with oral and subcutaneous (SC) fluids (Figure 21.2) (see Chapter 8)

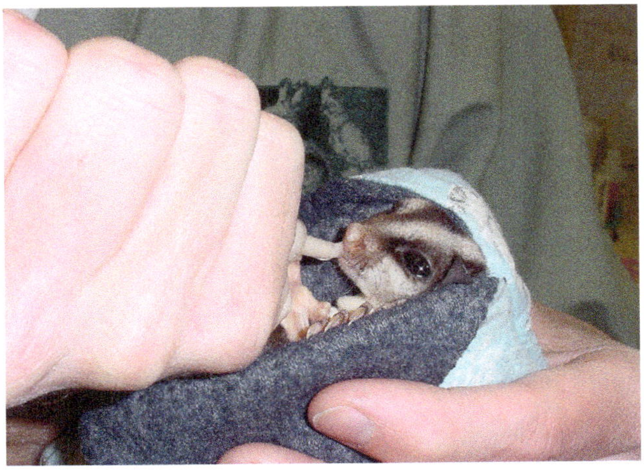

Figure 21.1 Restraint of a sugar glider for syringe-feeding a mixture of Emeraid Omnivore and Ensure Plus.

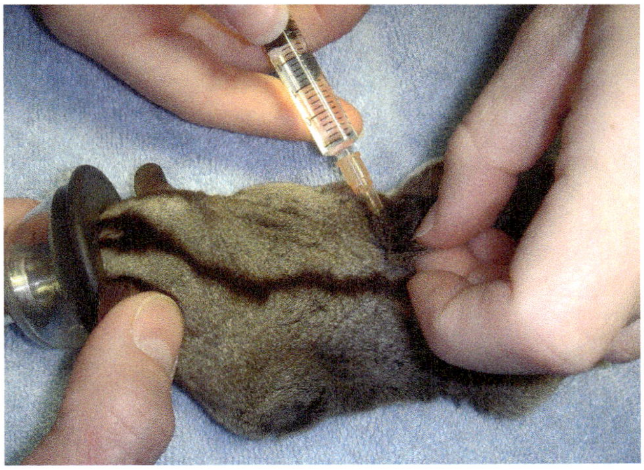

Figure 21.2 Technique for injection of subcutaneous fluids into the loose skin of the flank region in a sugar glider.

Continued Care:

- Correction of diet and husbandry

Dyspnea/Respiratory Distress

Introduction

Primary respiratory disease is considered rare in marsupials. Instead, respiratory conditions are usually associated with another disease process or an opportunistic pathogen [4]

Diagnosis

History:

- Newly purchased, recently weaned joeys
- Inappropriate/husbandry
- Environmental stress

Signalment:

- All ages and both sexes susceptible

Clinical Signs:

- Bilateral nasal discharge
- Sneezing
- Anorexia
- Coughing
- Labored breathing, often with head extended (Figure 21.3)

Differentials:

- Trauma
- Bacterial pneumonia
- Cardiac disease
- Heat stress
- Abdominal distension

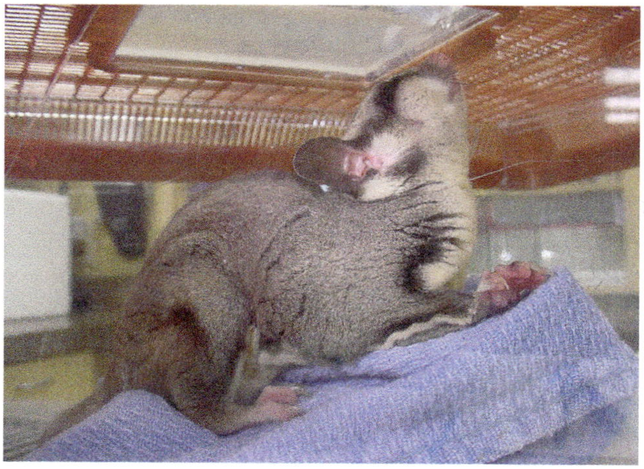

Figure 21.3 Posture of a sugar glider exhibiting severe respiratory distress.

STAT Diagnostics:

- Radiographs
- CBC and chemistry

Complete Diagnostics:

- Bacterial culture and sensitivity

Treatment

Stabilization:

- Supplemental oxygen (see Chapter 3)
- Thermal support
- Nutritional support (see Chapter 8)
- Nebulization with saline and antibiotics (see Table 21.2)
- +/− bronchodilators and +/− mucolytics
- Injectable antibiotics (see Table 21.1)

Continued Care:

- Oral antibiotics (see Table 21.1)

Generalized Muscle Tremors/Seizures

Introduction

- Tremors and seizures are most commonly caused by inappropriate nutrition, e.g. diets rich in lean meat, insects, fruit, and deficient in calcium
- May be accompanied by hind limb paresis/paralysis (see Section "Hind Limb Weakness") [5]

Diagnosis

History:

- Inappropriate diet and nutritional deficiencies

Signalment:

- Young, growing individuals, or reproducing females
- All ages and both sexes susceptible

Clinical Signs:

- Weakness
- Lethargy
- Debilitation
- Ataxia
- Muscle tremors
- Tetany
- Seizures
- Acute collapse

Differentials:

- Hypoglycemia
- Hypocalcemia
- Cranial trauma
- Parasitic central nervous system (CNS) disease
- Disseminated fungal disease
- Bacterial meningitis
- Toxin exposure
- Neoplasia

STAT Diagnostics:

- CBC and chemistry (esp. glucose, calcium [total/ionized], and phosphorus)

Complete Diagnostics:

- Radiographs

Treatment

Stabilization:

- Treat seizures with benzodiazepines (i.e. diazepam or midazolam) [10] (see Table 21.1)
- Warm fluids (SC, intravenous [IV], or intraosseous [IO]), thermal, and nutritional support (see Chapter 8)
- Correct hypoglycemia and/or hypocalcemia, if present (see Table 21.1)

Continued Care:

- Correction of inappropriate husbandry and nutrition

Hind Limb Weakness

Introduction

- Hind limb paresis/paralysis is usually a symptom of nutritional secondary hyperthyroidism associated with a calcium deficient, fruit- and protein-dominated diet, leading to osteoporosis of the vertebral column [3]

Table 21.1 Medications commonly used in sugar gliders [6–8].

Antibiotics		
Amikacin sulfate	3–10 mg/kg SC, IM q12h	Severe Gram-negative infections
Amoxicillin	30 mg/kg PO, SC, IM q12–24h	
Amoxicillin–clavulanate	12.5 mg/kg PO, SC q12–24h	
Chloramphenicol	50 mg/kg PO, SC, IM q12h	
Ciprofloxacin	10 mg/kg PO q12h	
Clindamycin	5.5–10 mg/kg PO q12h	
Enrofloxacin	2.5–5 mg/kg PO, SC, IM q12–24h	Tissue necrosis possible with parenteral injection; dilute for SC injection
Metronidazole	25 mg/kg PO q12–24h	CNS toxicity possible at high doses or if underlying hepatic disorder
Trimethoprim–sulfamethoxazole	10–20 mg/kg PO q12–24h	Monitor hydration
Penicillin	22 000–25 000 IU/kg SC, IM q12–24h	
Diazepam	0.5–2.0 mg/kg SC, IM, IV, intrarectally	
Midazolam	0.25–0.5 mg/kg IM, SC, intranasally, or intrarectally	
Calcium gluconate	100 mg/kg SC q12h	Dilute in saline to a concentration of 10 mg/ml
Calcium glubionate	100 mg/kg PO q12–24h	
Ivermectin	0.2–0.4 mg/kg PO, SC q7–14d	
Praziquantel	5–10 mg/kg PO, SC q10–14d	
Fenbendazole	20–50 mg/kg PO q24h × 3d, repeat in 14 d	
Selamectin	6–18 mg/kg topically, repeat in 30 d	
Metoclopramide	0.05–0.1 mg/kg PO, SC, IM q6–12h	
Furosemide	1–5 mg/kg PO, SC q12h	
Enalapril	0.5 mg/kg PO q24h	
Pimobendan	0.3–0.5 mg/kg PO q12h	
Cisapride	0.25 mg/kg PO, SC, IM q8–24h	

Sources: Brust and Mans [6], Raftery [7], Morrisey and Carpenter [8].

Table 21.2 Agents used in nebulization [9].

Agent	Concentration
Acetylcysteine	22 mg/ml saline
Aminophylline	3 mg/ml saline
Amikacin	5–6 mg/ml saline
Gentamicin	3–6 mg/ml saline
Enrofloxacin	10/mg/ml saline

Source: Hawkins et al. [5]. © 2017, Elsevier.

- May be accompanied by ataxia, tremors, tetany, and seizures (see Section "Generalized Muscle Tremors/Seizures") [11]
- Spinal fractures secondary to nutritional secondary hyperthyroidism are considered rare [12]

Diagnosis

History:

- Diet of mostly fruit and vegetables, muscle meat, and insects, without a dietary source of calcium [11]

Signalment:

- Young and pregnant/lactating individuals are particularly at risk
- All ages and both genders susceptible

Clinical Signs:

- Acute onset of hind limb paresis or paralysis (Figure 21.4)
- Tremors, tetany, and seizures

Differentials:

- Spinal trauma, infection, or neoplasia

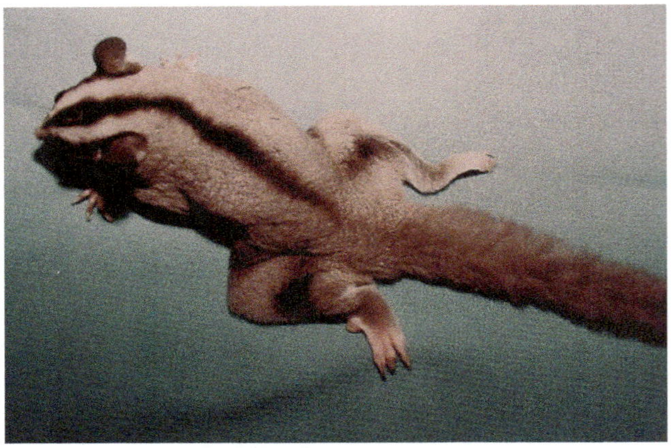

Figure 21.4 Hind limb paresis/paralysis in a sugar glider.

STAT Diagnostics:

- Serum calcium (total/ionized)
- Radiography

Complete Diagnostics:

- CBC and chemistry

Treatment

Stabilization:

- Calcium gluconate 100 mg/kg SC (diluted in saline to a concentration of 10 mg/ml) q12h for three to five days

Continued Care:

- Oral calcium supplementation (calcium glubionate 100 mg/kg PO q12–24h for 30–90 days)
- Dietary correction
- Cage rest

Neurologic Signs

Introduction

Common conditions include hind limb weakness/paralysis, ataxia, tremors, and seizures

Diagnosis

History:

- Imbalanced, inappropriate diet
- Young, breeding, or recently acquired individuals
- New/inexperienced owners
- Recent trauma
- Exposure to toxins (lead, insecticide) or potential pathogens (*Toxoplasma, Baylisascaris*)

Signalment:

- Any age and both genders susceptible
- Young and reproducing/lactating individuals are at greater risk of hypoglycemia, hypocalcemia, and nutritional secondary hyperparathyroidism

Clinical Signs:

- Weakness
- Proprioceptive deficit
- Tremors
- Ataxia
- Blindness
- Seizures

Differentials:

- Trauma
- Otitis
- Bacterial meningitis
- Toxoplasmosis
- *Baylisascaris*
- Vitamin E deficiency encephalomalacia
- Cryptococcosis

STAT Diagnostics:

- Neurological examination
- CBC and chemistry
- Radiography

Complete Diagnostics:

- Serology and cerebrospinal fluid analysis in specific cases [13]

Treatment

Stabilization:

- Supportive care
- Control seizures
- Provide fluid and nutritional support (see Chapter 8)
- Nonsteroidal anti-inflammatory drugs (NSAIDs) (e.g. meloxicam 0.1–0.2 mg/kg PO, SC q12–24h) [6] in cases of inflammation

Continued Care:

- Correction of diet and husbandry
- Specific treatments depending on etiology

Ocular Signs

Introduction

- Sugar gliders have prominent eyes that are prone to trauma from cage mates and accessories [10, 11, 14] (Figure 21.5)
- Complicated dietary requirements increase the risk of ocular disease due to nutritional cause [10]

Diagnosis

History:

- May include trauma, swelling (abscess or tumor) next to or behind the eye, nutritional deficiency, or bottle-raised joey
- Fighting between cage mates may be reported

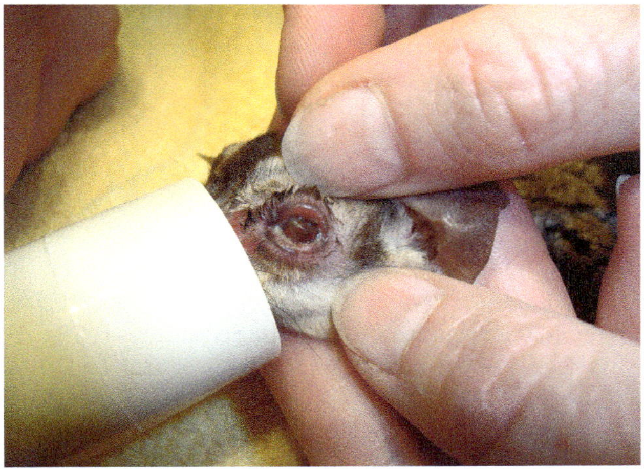

Figure 21.5 Panophthalmitis secondary to trauma in a sugar glider.

Signalment:

- No age or gender predilection

Clinical Signs:

- Periocular swelling
- Exophthalmos
- Proptosis
- Blepharospasm
- Corneal opacity
- Corneal ulceration
- Conjunctivitis
- Epiphora
- Cataracts
- Hyphema
- Hypopyon
- Uveitis

Differentials:

- Trauma
- Foreign body
- Neoplasia
- Infection
- Retrobulbar abscess
- Nutritional (hypovitaminosis A)
- Hyperglycemia
- Congenital
- Hereditary

STAT Diagnostics:

- Eye examination
- Oral examination
- Radiography

Complete Diagnostics:

- Ophthalmic examination
- Fluorescein stain
- Tonometry
- Skull radiography
- CBC and chemistry
- Bacterial culture and sensitivity
- Ultrasonography

Treatment

Stabilization:

- Topical and systemic antibiotics and analgesics are routine
- Temporary tarsorrhaphy [3]

Continued Care:

- Enucleation by subconjunctival approach (preferred to reduce risk of severe hemorrhage) [15]
- Treatment for retrobulbar abscess in certain cases [10]
- Correction of underlying nutritional imbalance [10]

Trauma

Introduction

- Are susceptible to bite wounds from dogs, cats, and other predators; secondary infections are potentially deadly
- Falls may occur secondary to generalized weakness
- Household hazards include drowning in toilets/tubs, chewing on electrical cords, being stepped or sat upon, being shut in a window or door, and landing on light bulbs or other hot surfaces
- Because of their prominent eyes, corneal trauma occurs easily (see Section "Ocular Signs")
- Constricting injuries from tattered, frayed, stringy fabrics, and natural fibers are common [11, 14] (Figure 21.6)
- Become hyperthermic and begin to pant when the ambient temperature rises above 87.8 °F (31 °C). They sprawl with their limbs extended and their patagium exposed, and they spread saliva on their forelimbs, but they do not sweat [4]
- Self-injury is regarded as a sign of stress and is sometimes seen where one sugar glider is kept on its own [7, 12]. However, *Baylisascaris*, toxoplasmosis, and listeriosis have produced CNS disease with self-mutilation in glider colonies [12]

Diagnosis

History:

- Time spent out of the cage, exposure to household hazards, or known traumatic event
- Recent injury or fighting among cage mates
- Car ride or time spent outdoors (hyperthermia)
- Solitary pet, sexual frustration in males, overcrowded or unsanitary conditions (self-mutilation)

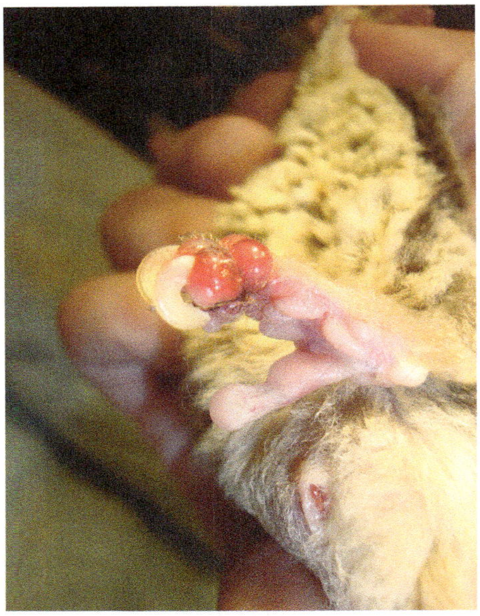

Figure 21.6 Strangulating injury to several toes of the left rear foot of a sugar glider by human hairs.

Signalment:

- No gender or age predilection

Clinical Signs:

- Pain
- Swelling
- Open wounds
- Bleeding
- Self-mutilation

Differentials:

- Infection
- Neoplasia
- Internal parasites

STAT Diagnostics:

- Radiography

Complete Diagnostics:

- Ultrasound

Treatment

Stabilization:

- Supplemental heat
- Fluid support (see Chapter 8)
- Opioid analgesics
  - Buprenorphine 0.01–0.03 mg/kg SC, IM q12h
  - Butorphanol 0.1–0.5 mg/kg SC, IM q6–8h [7, 12]
- Antibiotics; injuries by a cat or other pet should be treated with
  - Amoxicillin–clavulanate 12.5 mg/kg PO, SC q12–24h or
  - Penicillin procaine–benzathine combination 22 000–25 000 IU/kg SC, IM q12–24h to prevent/treat *Pasteurella* infection [4]

Continued Care:

- NSAIDs (e.g. meloxicam 0.1–0.2 mg/kg PO, SC q12–24h)
- General anesthesia with isoflurane or sevoflurane via mask is appropriate for most wound care procedures [3, 12]
- Allow wounds to heal by second intention; however, if suturing is necessary, use 4–0 or smaller absorbable monofilament suture and place buried sutures [7]
- Bandages and external fixation are poorly tolerated

Systemic Disease

Malnutrition

Diagnosis

History:

- Recent purchase
- Novice owner
- Inappropriate diet of fruit, insects, meat, or even commercial pellets

Signalment:

- Young, growing, and reproducing animals are most at risk
- All ages and both sexes susceptible

Clinical Signs:

- Lethargy
- Weakness
- Debilitation
- Collapse
- Hypothermia
- Weight loss
- Dehydration
- Muscle wasting
- Anemia
- Hypocalcemia
- Hypoproteinemia
- Blindness
- Cataracts
- Ataxia
- Tremor
- Tetany
- Rear-limb paresis/paralysis
- Neurological signs
- Lameness
- Reluctance to move
- Inability to support own weight
- Osteoporosis
- Pathologic fracture
- Dental disease

Differentials:

- Infection
- Neoplasia
- Toxin exposure
- Trauma
- Degenerative disease
- Metabolic disorder

STAT Diagnostics:

- Clinical presentation
- Review of diet and husbandry
- CBC and chemistry
- Urinalysis

Complete Diagnostics:

- Radiography
- Ultrasound

Treatment

Stabilization:

- Fluid and nutritional support (see Chapter 8)
- Thermal support
- Symptomatic treatment

Continued Care:

- Correction of underlying dietary problems [11]

Stress-Related Disease

Diagnosis

History:

- Isolation
- Overcrowding
- Unnatural social structure
- Sexual frustration
- Unsanitary conditions
- Perceived threat

Signalment:

- Any age and either gender
- Sexual frustration/genital self-mutilation frequently in adult males [16, 17] (Figure 21.7)

Clinical Signs:

- Self-mutilation of the tail, limbs, or genitalia
- Aggressive behavior
- Eating disorders (e.g. coprophagy, hyperphagy, and polydipsia)
- Cannibalism of young
- Excessive grooming
- Fur-pulling/alopecia (Figure 21.8)

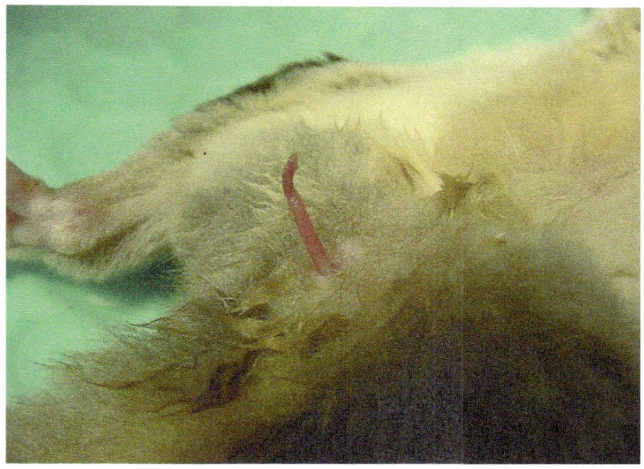

Figure 21.7 Genital self-mutilation in a male sugar glider resulting in trauma to one fork of its bifid penis and loss of the other.

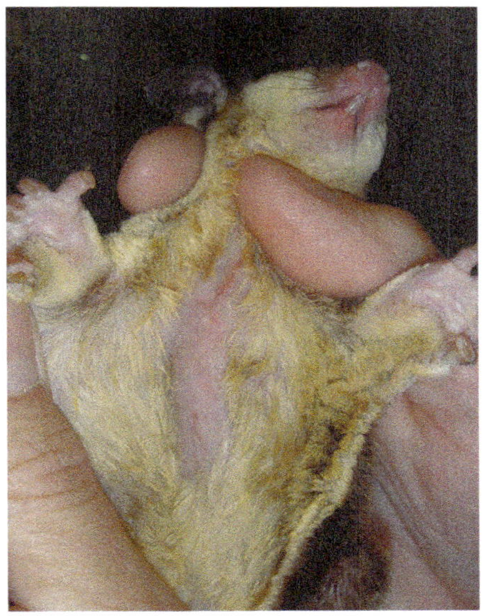

Figure 21.8 Alopecia secondary to excessive grooming attributed to stress in a solitary sugar glider.

- Stereotypic behavior/pacing

Differentials:

- Infection
- Parasitism

STAT Diagnostics:

- CBC and chemistry

Complete Diagnostics:

- Fecal flotation and direct
- Skin scrape
- Dermatophyte culture

Treatment

Stabilization:

- Provide appropriate wound care where indicated (see Section "Trauma")
- NSAIDs (e.g. meloxicam 0.1–0.2 mg/kg PO, SC q12–24h)
- Antibiotics (see Table 21.1)

Continued Care:

- Proper nutrition and good hygiene
- Normal social grouping
- Adequate cage space
- Appropriate nesting areas and cage accessories [7, 11]
- Castration of males with genital self-mutilation [16, 17]
- Amputation of bifid portion of penis may be indicated (solo males) and usually does not affect the ability to urinate since males urinate from the base of the penis; monitor urethral opening for swelling and obstruction postoperatively

Neurologic and Musculoskeletal Disease

Neurologic

Hypocalcemia

Diagnosis

History:

- Diet consisting mostly of fruit and vegetables, muscle meat and insects without a source of supplemental calcium

Signalment:

- Young, growing, and reproducing animals are at greatest risk

Clinical Signs:

- Generalized weakness
- Ataxia
- Cachexia
- Tremors
- Tetany
- Paresis
- Paralysis
- Seizures
- Pathologic fractures

Differentials:

- Nutritional secondary hyperparathyroidism
- Renal secondary hyperparathyroidism
- Primary hyperparathyroid disease

STAT Diagnostics:

- Clinical history
- Nutritional analysis
- Blood calcium level (ionized and complete)
- Blood glucose

Complete Diagnostics:

- CBC and chemistry
- Radiographs

Treatment

Stabilization:

- Emergency treatment includes calcium gluconate 100 mg/kg SC (diluted in saline to a concentration of 10 mg/ml) q12h for three to five days [11]

Continued Care:

- Calcium glubionate 100 mg/kg PO q12–24h for 30–90 days
- Adjustment Ca/P ratio to 1 : 1 to 2 : 1 [1]

Hypoglycemia

Diagnosis

History:

- Recent purchase
- New owner
- Inappropriate diet
- Failure to thrive (joeys)
- Chronic disease (adults)

Signalment:

- Recently weaned joeys at greatest risk

Clinical Signs:

- Lethargy
- Depression
- Hypothermia
- Inappetence
- Anorexia
- Weight loss
- Seizures

Differentials:

- Malnutrition
- Concurrent illness
- Hypothermia
- Liver disease
- Sepsis

STAT Diagnostics:

- Clinical history
- Nutritional analysis
- Calcium level (ionized and complete)

- Glucose

Complete Diagnostics:

- CBC and chemistry

Treatment

Stabilization:

- Dextrose in IV fluids (ideally) and by mouth
- Fluid and nutritional support (see Chapter 8)
- Thermal support
- Anticonvulsants for seizuring animals

Continued Care:

- Husbandry and diet correction
- Elimination of concurrent disease

Seizures

Diagnosis

History:

- Inadequate nutrition
- Trauma
- Toxin exposure
- Preexisting illness

Signalment:

- All ages and both genders affected

Clinical Signs:

- Tetany
- Tremors
- Convulsions
- Opisthotonus

Differentials:

- Trauma
- Hypoglycemia
- Hypocalcemia
- Liver disease
- Kidney disease
- Malnutrition
- Infection

STAT Diagnostics:

- Calcium level (ionized and complete)
- Glucose
- Packed cell volume (PCV)/total solids (TS)

Complete Diagnostics:

- CBC and chemistry
- Radiography
- Pathogen-specific testing

Treatment

Stabilization:

- Address primary disease
- Midazolam

Continued Care:

- Long-term anticonvulsant medication if indicated

Self-Mutilation Syndrome: Parasitic and Infectious

Diagnosis

History:

- Potential exposure to feces and/or fecal residue of raccoons and cats
- Potential exposure to contaminated soil, water or meats, vegetables, or dairy products

Signalment:

- All ages and both genders potentially susceptible
- Wild-caught gliders and those consuming wild-caught prey

Clinical Signs:

- Self-trauma
- Lethargy
- Depression
- Ataxia
- Seizures

Differentials:

- Stress (see Section "Stress-Related Disease")
- Sexual frustration/genital self-mutilation frequently in adult males [17]
- *Baylisascaris*
- *Toxoplasma*
- *Listeria*
- Aberrant migration of duodenal nematode [11]

STAT Diagnostics:

- CBC and chemistry

Complete Diagnostics:

- Fecal exam
- Fecal culture
- Skin scrape
- Dermatophyte culture
- Necropsy

Treatment

Stabilization:

- Appropriate wound care where indicated (see Section "Trauma")
- NSAIDs (e.g. meloxicam 0.1–0.2 mg/kg PO, SC q12–24h)
- Antibiotics (see Table 21.1)

Continued Care:

- Deworming (see Table 21.1)
- Clindamycin (5.5–10 mg/kg PO q12h) if toxoplasmosis suspected

Torpor

Diagnosis

History:

- Induced in wild gliders by reduction in food availability rather than low environmental temperatures [4]
- In captive individuals, will likely include concurrent illness, inappetence, reduced caloric intake, and weight loss

Signalment:

- Both genders and all ages

Clinical Signs:

- Moribundity
- Somnolence
- Hypothermia

Differentials:

- Malnutrition
- Infection
- Systemic disease
- Environmental problems
- Toxin exposure

STAT Diagnostics:

- Glucose
- Calcium (ionized and complete)
- PCV/TS

Complete Diagnostics:

- CBC and chemistry
- Radiography

Treatment

Stabilization:

- Thermal, fluid, and nutritional support (see Chapter 8)
- Treat primary conditions once affected glider becomes responsive

Continued Care:

- Correction of improper husbandry and diet
- Supplemental heat source recommended for healthy gliders

Musculoskeletal

Fractures

Diagnosis

History:

- Trauma
- Injury
- Malnutrition

Signalment:

- No age or gender predilection

Clinical Signs:

- Acute lameness
- Swelling
- Reluctance to move

Differentials:

- Infection
- Neoplasia
- Nutritional secondary hyperthyroidism

STAT Diagnostics:

- Radiography

Complete Diagnostics:

- CBC and chemistry

Treatment

Stabilization:

- Treat open wounds
- Antibiotics if indicated (see Table 21.1)
- Opioid analgesics
  - Buprenorphine 0.01–0.03 mg/kg SC, IM q12h
  - Butorphanol 0.1–0.5 mg/kg SC, IM q6–8h) [7, 12]
- NSAIDs (e.g. meloxicam 0.1–0.2 mg/kg PO, SC q12–24h)

Continued Care:

- Cage rest
- Internal fixation
- Amputation
- External fixation and bandages are poorly tolerated [3]

Generalized Tremors

Diagnosis

History:

- Inappropriate diet
- Trauma
- Toxin exposure

Signalment:

- Young, growing individuals
- Reproducing females
- All ages and both sexes susceptible

Clinical Signs:

- Weakness
- Lethargy
- Debilitation
- Ataxia
- Muscle tremors
- Tetany
- Seizures
- Acute collapse

Differentials:

- Hypoglycemia
- Hypocalcemia
- Cranial trauma
- Parasitic CNS disease
- Disseminated fungal disease
- Bacterial meningitis
- Toxin
- Neoplasia

STAT Diagnostics:

- Glucose
- Calcium (ionized and complete)
- Phosphorus
- CBC and chemistry

Complete Diagnostics:

- Radiography

Treatment

Stabilization:

- Warm fluids (see Chapter 8)
- Thermal and nutritional support
- Supplemental glucose or calcium as indicated (see Table 21.1)

Continued Care:

- Correct underlying nutritional and metabolic problems

Hind Limb Weakness

Diagnosis

History:

- Diet mostly of fruit, vegetables, meat, and insects without adequate supplemental calcium [11]

Signalment:

- All ages and both genders are susceptible; however, young and pregnant/lactating gliders particularly at risk

Clinical Signs:

- Sudden onset hind limb paresis or paralysis
- Tremors or tetany

Differentials:

- Spinal trauma
- Infection
- Neoplasia

STAT Diagnostics:

- Calcium
- Glucose

Complete Diagnostics:

- Radiography

Treatment

Stabilization:

- Calcium supplementation (e.g. calcium glubionate 100 mg/kg PO q12–24h for 30–90 days)
- NSAIDs (e.g. meloxicam 0.1–0.2 mg/kg PO, SC q12–24h)

Continued Care:

- Cage rest

Cardiopulmonary Disease

Cardiac

Diagnosis

History:

- Cardiac disease and myonecrosis have been reported in sugar gliders in association with malnutrition [18]
- Obesity in sugar gliders may also lead to cardiac disease [14]

Signalment:

- Adults of both genders are more likely to be affected than young

Clinical Signs:

- Weakness
- Lethargy
- Respiratory distress

Differentials:

- Pulmonary disease
- Pleural effusion
- Intrathoracic mass

STAT Diagnostics:

- Auscultation
- Radiography

Complete Diagnostics:

- Ultrasound
- Electrocardiogram (ECG)
- Normal parameters for imaging and ECG in this species have not been established [14]

Treatment

Stabilization:

- Oxygen
- Furosemide (1–5 mg/kg PO, SC q12h)

Continued Care:

- Enalapril (0.5 mg/kg PO q24h)
- Pimobendan (0.3–0.5 mg/kg PO q12h)

Respiratory

Bacterial Infection

Diagnosis

History:

- Recent stress such as weaning, shipping, overcrowding, chilling, malnutrition, change of ownership, or diet/husbandry changes
- Pneumonia is generally more common than upper respiratory infection [4]

Signalment:

- All ages and both genders may be affected
- Hand-reared infant gliders are particularly susceptible [11]

Clinical Signs:

- Sneezing
- Bilateral, clear, or mucopurulent nasal discharge
- Coughing
- Audible respiratory noises
- Anorexia

Differentials:

- Environmental irritants
- Dust
- Foreign body
- Allergy
- Neoplasia
- Cardiac disease

STAT Diagnostics:

- Radiography
- CBC and chemistry

Complete Diagnostics:

- Culture/sensitivity

Treatment

Stabilization:

- Oxygen
- Thermal support
- Fluid support (see Chapter 8)

Continued Care:

- Bactericidal antibiotics with good Gram-negative coverage (e.g. amoxicillin 30 mg/kg PO, SC, IM q12–24h or enrofloxacin 2.5–5 mg/kg PO, SC, IM q12–24h) (see Table 21.1)
- Nebulization +/−bronchodilators and/or mucolytics. (see Table 21.2)
- Corticosteroids or NSAIDs may be indicated in the early stages of aspiration pneumonia in joeys [4] (see Table 21.1)
- Husbandry problems should be corrected

Gastrointestinal Disease

Dental Disease

Diagnosis

History:

- Affected gliders have often been maintained on a soft, high-sugar diet

Signalment:

- All ages and both genders affected

Clinical Signs:

- Inappetence
- Dysphagia
- Ptyalism
- Weight loss
- Tartar accumulation
- Periodontal disease
- Tooth fractures
- Abscesses

- Osteomyelitis

Differentials:

- Trauma
- Neoplasia
- Bacterial infection
- Nutritional secondary hyperparathyroidism

STAT Diagnostics:

- Radiography of affected teeth/jaw bones
- Fine needle aspirate biopsy (FNAB) and cytology of swelling

Complete Diagnostics:

- Bacterial culture/sensitivity of abscesses

Treatment

Stabilization:

- NSAIDs (e.g. meloxicam 0.1–0.2 mg/kg PO, SC q12–24h)
- Antibiotics effective against anaerobic bacteria (see Table 21.1)
- Fluid and nutritional support (see Chapter 8)

Continued Care:

- Dental extraction(s) (Figure 21.9a–c)
  - Great care is needed in removing the mandibular incisors, as fracture of the symphysis during extraction has frequently been reported [3, 7]
  - Note that incisor teeth should never be trimmed on sugar gliders
- Dental scaling and improved diet

Constipation

Diagnosis

History:

- Dietary history may indicate insufficient roughage in the diet (e.g. excessive dry cat food) [11]

Signalment:

- Most often observed in adult gliders of either gender

Clinical Signs:

- Straining to defecate
- Reduced fecal output

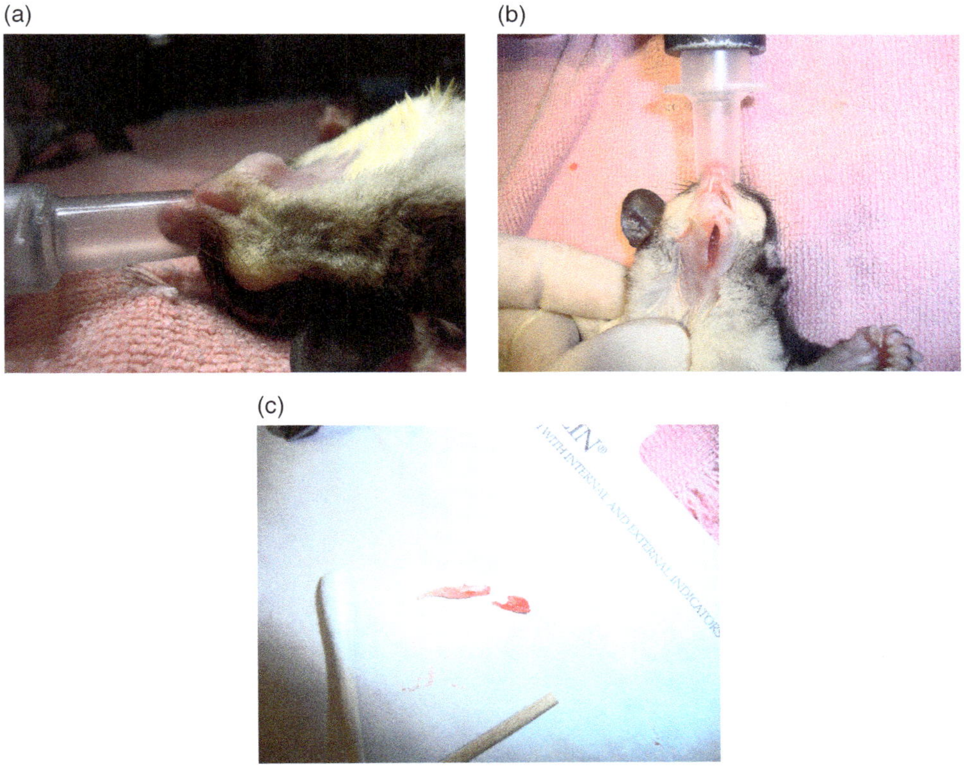

Figure 21.9 Abscess of left lower incisor and subsequent extraction in a sugar glider: (a) odontogenic abscess swelling on lower law, (b) surgical approach to the affected tooth root, and (c) extracted incisor.

- Pasty or hard feces
- Rectal prolapse (see Section "Rectal Prolapse")
- Palpable fecal impaction

Differentials:

- Gastrointestinal (GI) foreign body
- Bowel obstruction
- Impaction/megacolon (see Section "Impaction/Megacolon")
- Intussusception
- Neoplasia
- Improper nutrition

STAT Diagnostics:

- Fecal examination
- Plain and contrast radiography

Complete Diagnostics:

- Ultrasound examination

Treatment

Stabilization:

- Fluid and nutritional support (see Chapter 8)
- Thermal support
- Enemas
- Stool softeners
- Prokinetics (i.e. metoclopramide, cisapride) (see Table 21.1)
- Surgical removal of impacted feces in extreme cases (see Section "Impaction/Megacolon")

Continued Care:

- Addition of fiber (e.g. canned pumpkin, prunes) to the diet
- Diet correction

Impaction/Megacolon

Diagnosis

History:

- Affected gliders may have had a history of constipation (see Section "Constipation") and insufficient roughage in the diet [11]

Signalment:

- Adults of either gender are most often affected

Clinical Signs:

- Distended abdomen
- Depression
- Anorexia
- Hypothermia
- Pasty or hard feces
- Palpable fecal impaction
- Straining
- Rectal prolapse (see Section "Rectal Prolapse")

Differentials:

- Bowel obstruction
- Gastric dilatation and volvulus (GDV) [19, 20]
- Intestinal intussusception [19]
- Neoplasia

STAT Diagnostics:

- Fecal examination
- Plain and contrast radiography [21]

Complete Diagnostics:

- Ultrasound examination
- Necropsy
- Colon and the cecum are often filled with a thick, pasty fecal material

Treatment

Stabilization:

- Fluid and nutritional support (see Chapter 8)
- Thermal support
- Enemas
- Stool softeners
- Prokinetics (as for Section "Constipation")

Continued Care:

- Addition of fiber (e.g. canned pumpkin, prunes) to the diet
- Surgical removal of impacted feces in extreme cases
- Diet correction
- Megacolon generally carries a poor prognosis [11]

Diarrhea

Diagnosis

History:

- Dietary indiscretion
- Sudden change in diet
- New environment
- Poor husbandry
- Stressful event

Signalment:

- Any age and either gender

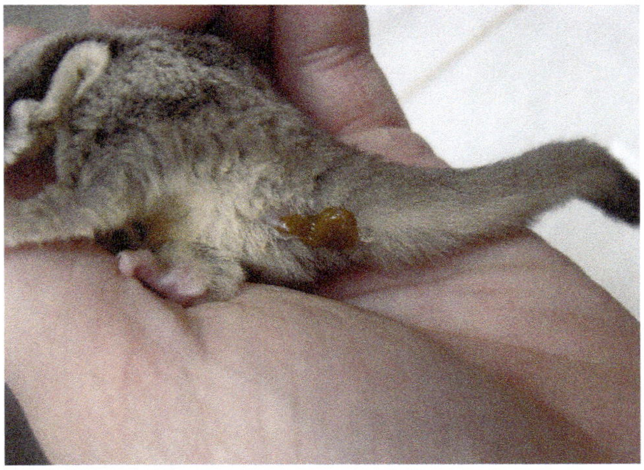

Figure 21.10 Diarrhea in a sugar glider.

- Joeys transitioning to a new diet or new home are particularly susceptible [19]

Clinical Signs:

- Lethargy
- Weight loss
- Runny stool (Figure 21.10)
- Dehydration
- Tenesmus
- Rectal prolapse (see Section "Rectal Prolapse")
- Death

Differentials:

- Dysbiosis [7]
- Bacterial infection (*Salmonella* [19, 22], *Clostridium piliforme* [11, 19, 20])
- Internal parasites (*Giardia*, coccidiosis, cryptosporidiosis, trematodes [11, 19, 20], *Simplicomonas* [16])
- Concurrent systemic disease [20]
- Toxin exposure

STAT Diagnostics:

- Fecal flotation
- Direct smear
- Gram staining

Complete Diagnostics:

- Culture/sensitivity
- Fecal polymerase chain reaction (PCR) for *Simplicomonas* [16]
- CBC and chemistry
- Radiography

Treatment

Stabilization:

- Warm fluids and nutritional support (see Chapter 8)
- Antibiotics (see Table 21.1)
- Antiparasitics (see Table 21.1)

Continued Care:

- Rectal prolapse reduction (see Section "Rectal Prolapse")
- Prevention by adhering to strict hygiene protocols and reducing stress [19]

GI Parasites

Diagnosis

History:

- Improper diet or husbandry
- Unsanitary conditions
- Wild-caught
- Housed outdoors
- Consuming wild-caught prey

Signalment:

- All ages and both genders susceptible

Clinical Signs:

- Lethargy
- Weight loss
- Decreased appetite
- Diarrhea or other changes in feces
- Joeys in the pouch may present ungroomed, covered in tacky mucus
- "Sticky joeys" affected by "ick" [16] (Figure 21.11)

Differentials:

- *Giardia* [22]
- *Simplicomonas* [16]
- Trematodes [20]
- Nematodes
- Cestodes
- Coccidia
- Cryptosporidiosis [11]

STAT Diagnostics:

- Fecal flotation
- Direct smear
- Fecal acid fast

Complete Diagnostics:

- Fecal PCR for *Simplicomonas* [16]

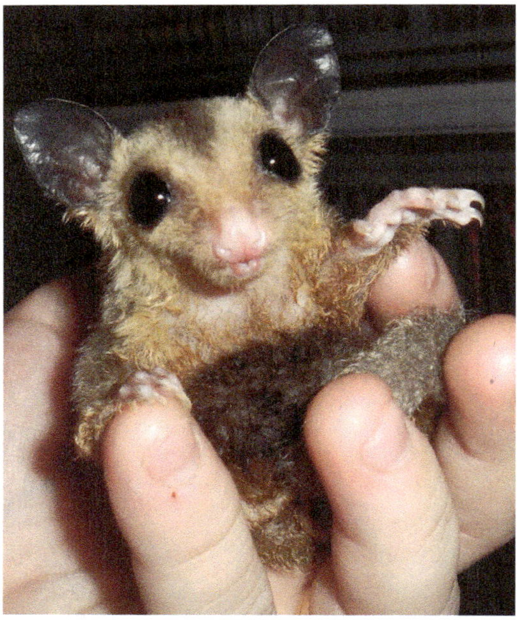

Figure 21.11 Appearance of "sticky joey" affected by "ick" (*Simplicomonas*) infection. Source: Image courtesy of Cathy Johnson-Delaney.

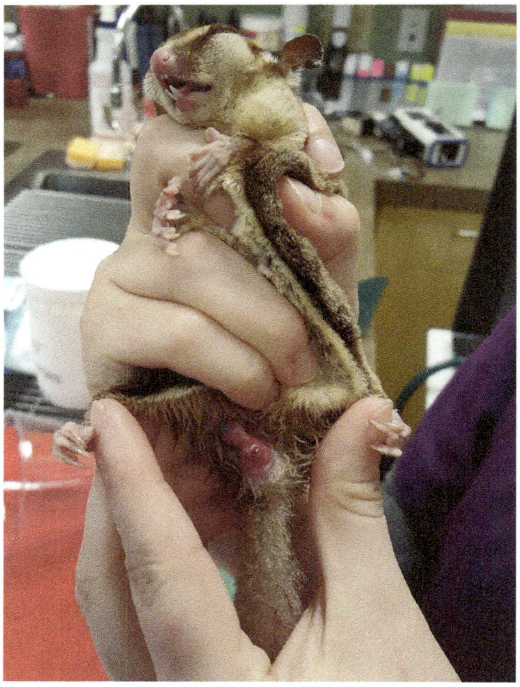

Figure 21.12 Rectal prolapse with secondary self-trauma in a sugar glider.

Treatment

Stabilization:

- Warm fluids and nutritional support (see Chapter 8)
- Antibiotics (see Table 21.1)
- Antiparasitics (see Table 21.1)

Continued Care:

- Prevention by adhering to strict hygiene protocols
- Feed captive-raised prey from a reputable source

Rectal Prolapse

Diagnosis

History:

- Inappropriate diet
- Straining
- Constipation
- Impaction
- Diarrhea

Signalment:

- All ages and both genders affected

Clinical Signs:

- Prolapse of rectal tissue (Figure 21.12)
- Tenesmus

Differentials:

- Improper diet and husbandry
- Parasites
- Protozoa
- Bacterial infection
- Reduced anal sphincter muscle tone

STAT Diagnostics:

- Fecal floatation
- Direct smear
- Fecal Gram stain
- Fecal culture

Complete Diagnostics:

- Radiography
- Ultrasound

Treatment

Stabilization:

- Address underlying etiology of tenesmus [11]
- Prolapsed rectal tissue should be gently cleaned, debrided, and replaced. Recurrence is prevented by placing two vertical sutures on the lateral aspects of the anus without reducing the patency of the cloaca or urogenital slit

- Antibiotic cream may be instilled into cloaca following reduction

Continued Care:

- NSAIDs and systemic antibiotics are indicated in most cases [10, 19] (see Table 21.1)
- A custom E-collar is advocated by some [19]

Paracloacal Gland Infection/Impaction/Neoplasia

Diagnosis

History:

- Straining to defecate
- Decreased appetite
- Perineal swelling, self-mutilation

Signalment:

- Abscessation and impaction may occur in adults of either gender
- Two case reports of neoplasia involved adult males [23, 24]

Clinical Signs:

- Perineal swelling/mass
- Straining to defecate
- Decreased appetite
- Self-mutilation of the perineal skin [17]
- Abdominal distention

Differentials:

- Paracloacal gland infection/impaction/neoplasia
- Constipation
- Large bowel impaction
- Perineal hernia
- Sexual frustration/genital self-mutilation frequently in adult males [17]

STAT Diagnostics:

- FNAB/cytology
- Culture and sensitivity

Complete Diagnostics:

- Surgical biopsy/histopathology
- Radiography

Treatment

Stabilization:

- Enemas
- Stool softeners
- Expressing infected and impacted glands
- NSAIDs and appropriate antibiotic therapy (see Table 21.1)

Continued Care:

- Surgical removal of glands is recommended in cases of paracloacal gland neoplasia and chronic infection or impaction [10, 19]

Urogenital and Reproductive Disease

Urinary System

Cystitis/Crystalluria/Urolithiasis

Diagnosis

History:

- Poor nutrition
- Inadequate hydration
- Inactivity
- Improper husbandry conditions, especially those that disrupt normal urine marking behavior

Signalment:

- Any age and either gender may be affected

Clinical Signs:

- Hematuria
- Stranguria
- Dysuria

Differentials:

- Cystitis
- Crystalluria
- Urolithiasis

STAT Diagnostics:

- Urinalysis
- Radiography

Complete Diagnostics:

- Culture and sensitivity
- CBC and chemistry

Treatment

Stabilization:

- Fluid and nutritional support (see Chapter 8)
- NSAIDs (e.g. meloxicam 0.1–0.2 mg/kg PO, SC q12–24h)
- Antibiotics (See Table 21.1)

Continued Care:

- Surgery
- Correction of causative husbandry factors [10]

Reproductive

Mastitis and Pouch Infection

Diagnosis

History:

- Pouch exudate
- Foul odor
- Mammary swelling
- Sick joeys

Signalment:

- Lactating females with joeys are most often affected

Clinical Signs:

- Exudative, malodorous material coming from the pouch
- Firm painful mammary glands
- Teats without milk
- Joeys of affected females may be dehydrated or septicemic

Differentials:

- Bacterial and yeast infection
- *Simplicomonas* infection (i.e. "ick" or "sticky joey") [16]
- Mammary neoplasia [25, 26]

STAT Diagnostics:

- Pouch cytology
- Fecal wet mount from affected joeys

Complete Diagnostics:

- CBC and chemistry
- Pouch culture and sensitivity

Treatment

Stabilization:

- Antibiotics (see Table 21.1)
- Antifungals (see Table 21.1)
- NSAIDs (e.g. meloxicam 0.1–0.2 mg/kg PO, SC q12–24h)
- Disinfection of the pouch with dilute chlorhexidine solution

Continued Care:

- Joeys of affected dams may need to be bottle-fed and may also require antimicrobial therapy [10, 16] (see Table 21.1)

Pouch Prolapse

Diagnosis

History:

- Excessive grooming
- Pouch infection
- Mastitis

Signalment:

- Adult females

Clinical Signs:

- Eversion and prolapse of pouch tissue (Figure 21.13a,b)

Differentials:

- Mastitis
- Bacterial or yeast infection
- Mammary neoplasia [25, 26]
- Excessive grooming

STAT Diagnostics:

- Cytology of pouch

Complete Diagnostics:

- Culture and sensitivity

(a) (b)

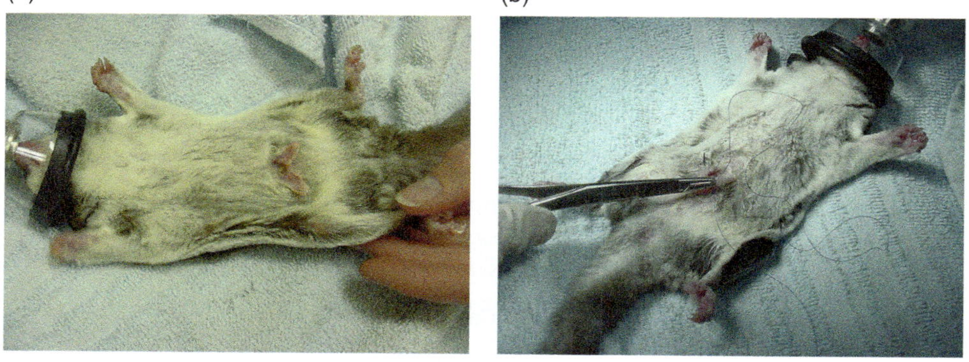

Figure 21.13 Prolapse of pouch tissue (a) and (b) subsequent replacement of pouch tissue with temporary sutures.

Treatment

Stabilization:

- Gently clean the pouch with warm, dilute chlorhexidine solution
- NSAIDs (e.g. meloxicam 0.1–0.2 mg/kg PO, SC q12–24h)
- Antibiotic/antifungals as indicated (see Table 21.1)

Continued Care:

- Replace pouch tissue with temporary sutures until inflammation resolves [11]

Neoplastic Disease

Lymphoma/Lymphosarcoma

Diagnosis

History:

- Is the most common neoplasia, representing approximately 50% of all neoplasia cases in gliders [3, 19]
- Swollen lymph nodes, abdominal mass, or cutaneous ulceration [19, 27]

Signalment:

- Adults of either gender affected

Clinical Signs:

- Lymphadenopathy
- Abdominal mass (commonly in liver or spleen)
- Limb swelling
- Ulcerative skin lesion

Differentials:

- Other neoplasia such as duodenal or hepatic adenocarcinoma [19, 26]; hemangiosarcoma [28]; mammary carcinoma [26]; mammary adenocarcinoma [25]; vascular hamartoma; cutaneous leiomyoma [26]; adrenocortical carcinoma and hepatocellular carcinoma [29]
- Infection
- Impaction/megacolon (see Section "Impaction/Megacolon")
- Self-mutilation (see Sections "Trauma", "Stress-Related Disease", and "Self-mutilation Syndrome: Parasitic and Infectious")

STAT Diagnostics:

- FNAB (with ultrasound guidance where appropriate)
- Cytology

Complete Diagnostics:

- Radiography
- Ultrasound
- Surgical biopsy
- Histopathology

Treatment

Stabilization:

- Fluid, nutritional, and thermal support (see Chapter 8)
- NSAIDs (e.g. meloxicam 0.1–0.2 mg/kg PO, SC q12–24h)

Continued Care:

- Management following standard protocols used for domestic species [19]

Dermatologic Disease

Ectoparasites

Diagnosis

History:

- Unsanitary conditions
- Exposure/proximity to various other small mammals
- Wild-caught animals

Signalment:

- Both genders and any age

Clinical Signs:

- Pruritis
- Alopecia
- Erythema
- Dandruff
- Excessive grooming
- Self-trauma

Differentials:

- Bacterial
- Fungal
- Neoplastic
- Endocrine alopecia [10]
- Stress and other causes of self-trauma (see Sections "Trauma", "Stress-Related Disease", and "Self-mutilation Syndrome: Parasitic and Infectious")

STAT Diagnostics:

- Skin scrape
- Cellophane tape preparation

Complete Diagnostics:

- Bacterial and fungal culture
- Skin biopsy

Treatment

Stabilization:

- Ivermectin injection (0.2–0.4 mg/kg PO, SC q7–14d)
- Selamectin topically (6–18 mg/kg topically, repeat in 30 days)

Continued Care:

- Improved sanitation
- Cleaning nest box

Wounds

Diagnosis

History:

- Injury
- Fighting
- Self-trauma

Signalment:

- Both genders and all ages

Clinical Signs:

- Lameness
- Swelling
- Lacerations, punctures (Figure 21.14)
- Hemorrhage
- Excessive grooming and/or self-trauma at sites of injury

Differentials:

- Bite wounds
- Self-mutilation (see Sections "Trauma", "Stress-Related Disease", and "Self-mutilation Syndrome: Parasitic and Infectious")

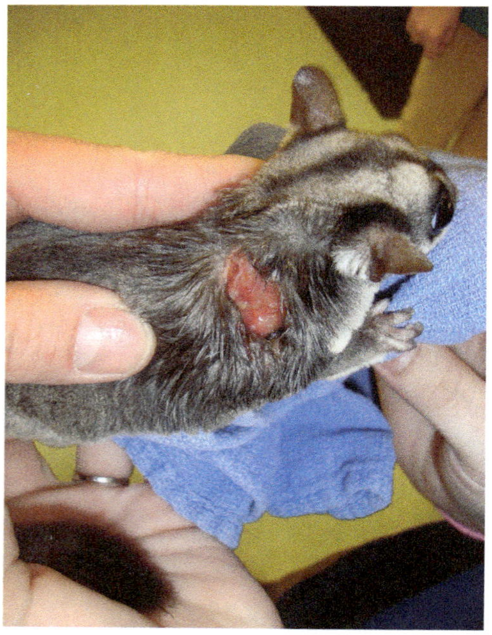

Figure 21.14 Laceration caused by fighting among cage mates.

- Burns
- Neoplastic processes

STAT Diagnostics:

- Skin scrape
- Bacterial/fungal culture

Complete Diagnostics:

- Radiography (see Section "Trauma")
- Ultrasound

Treatment

Stabilization:

- Antibiotics (see Table 21.1)
- NSAIDs (e.g. meloxicam 0.1–0.2 mg/kg PO, SC q12–24h)
- Allow most mild-to-moderate self-mutilation wounds to heal by second intention
- Modified E-collar or "straight jacket" fabricated from bandage material [7, 13, 17]
- Treat self-trauma with fluoxetine 1–5 mg/kg PO q8–12h [13, 30–32]

Continued Care:

- Treat wounds as in other species [17, 32] (see Sections "Trauma" and "Wounds")

Ophthalmic Disease

Cataracts/Blindness

Diagnosis

History:

- Trauma
- Improper diet/husbandry

Signalment:

- Cataracts in hand-reared joeys and young of obese dams (Figure 21.15)
- Blindness in any age and either gender

Clinical Signs:

- Visual impairment
- Change in activity, behavior, or eating habits
- Ocular lesions
  - Cataracts
  - Corneal opacity/lipid deposits, uveitis, ocular trauma

Differentials:

- Hypovitaminosis-A
- Bacterial infection
- Toxoplasmosis

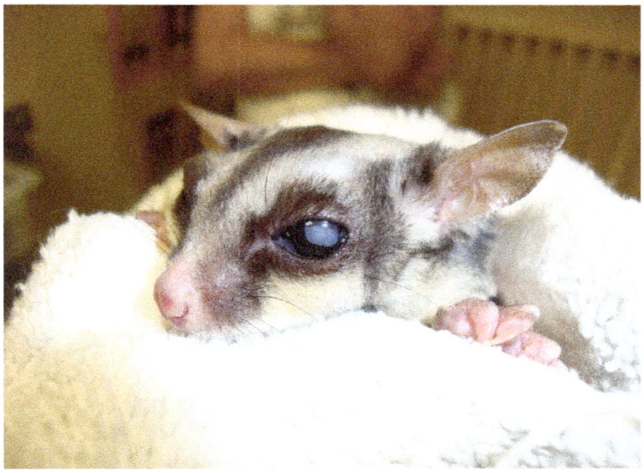

Figure 21.15 Cataracts in a young sugar glider.

- Ocular injury
- Idiopathic uveitis
- Idiopathic or senescent cataracts [31]
- Nutritional problems (milk replacers containing high levels of lactose, sucrose, or other oligosaccharides [1])
- Hyperglycemia
- Congenital and hereditary factors [33]

STAT Diagnostics:

- Ophthalmic examination
- Fluorescein stain
- Tonometry

Complete Diagnostics:

- Bacterial culture and sensitivity
- Skull radiography
- *Toxoplasma* serology
- CBC and chemistry
- Ultrasonography

Treatment

Stabilization:

- If corneal damage or uveitis, treat as for other small animals

Continued Care:

- Correction of diet and husbandry [11]
- Vitamin A supplementation for cataracts [31]

References

1 Johnson-Delaney, C.A. (2014). Captive marsupial nutrition. *Vet. Clin. Exot. Anim.* 17: 415–447.

2 Dierenfeld, E.S. (2009). Feeding behavior and nutrition of the sugar glider (*Petaurus breviceps*). *Vet. Clin. Exot. Anim.* 12: 209–215.

3 Booth, R. (2003). Sugar gliders. *Semin. Avian Exot. Pet. Med.* 12 (4): 228–231.

4 Johnson, D.H. (2011). Hedgehogs and sugar gliders: respiratory anatomy, physiology, and disease. *Vet. Clin. Exot. Anim.* 14: 267–285.

5 Wojick, K.B. (2013). Small mammals: sugar gliders – nutritional disorders. In: *Clinical Veterinary Advisor: Birds and Exotic Pets* (eds. J. Mayer and T.M. Donnelly), 320–330. St. Louis: Elsevier. 6 Brust, D.M. and Mans, C. (2018). Sugar gliders. In: *Exotic Animal Formulary*, 5e (ed. J.W. Carpenter), 432–442. St. Louis: Elsevier.

7 Raftery, A. (2015). Sugar gliders (*Petaurus breviceps*). *Companion Anim.* 20 (7): 422–426.

8 Morrisey, J.K. and Carpenter, J.W. (2020). Appendix: formulary. In: *Ferrets, Rabbits, and Rodents: Clinical Medicine and Surgery*, 4e (eds. K.E. Quesenberry, C.J. Orcutt, C. Mans and J.W. Carpenter), 620–630. St. Louis, MO: Elsevier.

9 Hawkins, M.G., Guzman, D.S., Beaufrere, H. et al. (2017). Birds. In: *Exotic Animal Formulary*, 5e (eds. J. Carpenter and C. Marion), 247–248. St Louis, MO: Elsevier.

10 Johnson-Delaney, C.A. (2020). Sugar gliders. In: *Ferrets, Rabbits, and Rodents: Clinical Medicine and Surgery*, 4e (eds. K.E. Quesenberry, C.J. Orcutt, C. Mans and J.W. Carpenter), 385–400. St. Louis, MO: Elsevier.

11 Raftery, A. (2010). Sugar gliders. *British Veterinary Zoological Society Proceedings*, Birmingham (7 April 2010), pp. 13–18

12 Lennox, A.M. (2007). Emergency and critical care procedures in sugar gliders (*Petaurus breviceps*), African hedgehogs (*Atelerix albiventris*), and prairie dogs (*Cynomys* spp.). *Vet. Clin. Exot. Anim.* 10 (2007): 533–555.

13 Ness, R.D. and Johnson-Delaney, C.A. (2012). Sugar gliders. In: *Ferrets, Rabbits, and Rodents: Clinical Medicine and Surgery*, 3e (eds. K.E. Quesenberry and J.W. Carpenter), 393–410. St. Louis: Saunders.

14 Johnson, D. (2012). Emergency presentations of the exotic small mammalian herbivore trauma patient. *J. Exot. Pet. Med.* 21 (4): 300–315.

15 Diehl, K.A. and McKinnon, J. (2016). Eye removal surgeries in exotic pets. *Vet. Clin. Exot. Anim.* 19: 245–267.

16 Johnson-Delaney, C. (2014). Common diseases of sugar gliders. *BSAVA Companion* (November), pp. 20–21.

17 Miwa, Y. and Sladky, K.K. (2016). Small mammals: common surgical procedures of rodents, ferrets, hedgehogs, and sugar gliders. *Vet. Clin. Exot. Anim.* 19: 205–244.

18 Heatley, J.J. (2009). Cardiovascular anatomy, physiology, and disease of rodents and small exotic mammals. *Vet. Clin. Exot. Anim.* 12: 99–113.

19 Brust, D.M. (2013). Gastrointestinal diseases of marsupials. *J. Exot. Pet. Med.* 22: 132–140.

20 Reavill, D. (2014). Pathology of the exotic companion mammal gastrointestinal system. *Vet. Clin. Exot. Anim.* 17: 145–164.

21 Evans, E.E. and Souza, M.J. (2010). Advanced diagnostic approaches and current management of internal disorders of select species (rodents, sugar gliders, hedgehogs). *Vet. Clin. Exot. Anim.* 13: 453–469.

22 Pignon, C. and Mayer, J. (2011). Zoonoses of ferrets, hedgehogs, and sugar gliders. *Vet. Clin. Exot. Anim.* 14: 533–549.

23 Marrow, J.C., Carpenter, J.W., Lloyd, A., and Bawa, B. (2010). A transitional cell carcinoma with squamous differentiation in a pericloacal mass in a sugar glider (*Petaurus breviceps*). *J. Exot. Pet. Med.* 19 (1): 92–95.

24 Chen, J.C., Yu, P.H., Liu, C.H. et al. (2018). Paracloacal gland carcinoma in a sugar glider (*Petaurus breviceps*). *J. Exot. Pet. Med.* 27: 36–40.

25 Keller, K.A., Nevarez, J.G., Rodriguez, D. et al. (2014). Diagnosis and treatment of anaplastic mammary carcinoma in a sugar glider (*Petaurus breviceps*). *J. Exot. Pet. Med.* 23: 277–282.

26 Churgin, S.M., Deering, K.M., Wallace, R., and Clyde, V.L. (2015). Metastatic mammary adenocarcinoma in a sugar glider (*Petaurus breviceps*). *J. Exot. Pet. Med.* 24: 441–445.

27 Hough, I., Reuter, R.E., Rahaley, R.S. et al. (1992). Cutaneous lymphosarcoma in a sugar glider. *Aust. Vet. J.* 69 (4): 93–94.

28 Rivas, A.E., Pye, G.W., and Papendick, R. (2014). Dermal hemangiosarcoma in a sugar glider (*Petaurus breviceps*). *J. Exot. Pet. Med.* 23: 384–388.

29 Lindemann, D.M., Carpenter, J.W., DeBey, B.M., and Ryseff, J.K. (2016). Concurrent adrenocortical carcinoma and hepatocellular carcinoma with hemosiderosis in a sugar glider (*Petaurus breviceps*). *J. Exot. Pet. Med.* 25: 144–149.

30 Tully, T.N. and Mitchell, M.A. (2012). Sugar gliders. In: *A Veterinary Technician's Guide to Exotic Animal Care*, 2e (eds. T.N. Tully and M.A. Mitchell), 187. Lakewood: American Animal Hospital Association.

31 Jepsen, L. (2016). *Exotic Animal Medicine: A Quick Reference Guide*, 2e, 231–257. St. Louis: Elsevier.

32 Hernandez-Divers, S.M. (2004). Principles of wound management of small mammals: hedgehogs, prairie dogs, and sugar gliders. *Vet. Clin. Exot. Anim.* 7: 1–18.

33 Johnson-Delaney, C. (2010). Marsupials. In: *BSAVA Manual of Exotic Pets*, 5e (eds. A. Meredeth and C. Johnson-Delaney), 103–126. Quedegley: British Small Animal Veterinary Association.

Part 2

Avian

Section 1

Triage and Stabilization

22

History and Clinical Exam

Grayson A. Doss and Christoph Mans

Department of Surgical Sciences, School of Veterinary Medicine, University of Wisconsin-Madison, Madison, Wisconsin, USA

CONTENTS

Initial Phone Consultation

Is it an Emergency?

Oftentimes, what owners perceive as an acute illness is actually a chronic disease process, and the patient is decompensating. Depending on owner knowledge and experience level, they may not realize that the acute onset of a "tail bob" in their pet bird is a true emergency or that sitting fluffed on the bottom of the cage doesn't simply constitute an animal that is feeling a little tired. Fractures or luxations, hemorrhage, dyspnea, egg binding, anorexia, predator attacks, non-behavioral regurgitation or vomiting, and overt lethargy constitute emergencies.

Having contact with the client in the early stages of the emergency before the patient arrives at the hospital also affords the clinician the chance to have the owner bring all relevant husbandry items, including diets or toxic items the pet bird may have been exposed to. Obtaining information on signalment can help the clinician discern possible differentials before patient presentation.

Stress should be minimized, if at all possible, in the clinically ill pet bird, as rapid decompensation or death can occur with minimal disturbance. Making the trip to the hospital can be stressful to a bird not used to car rides, and minimizing audiovisual stimuli may be helpful. For birds with active, life-threatening hemorrhage, application of digital pressure using a clean object like a small towel, cotton ball, or gauze until arrival at the hospital may be lifesaving. For bleeding pinfeathers or nails, application of clean cornstarch, flour, or styptic powder can slow bleeding until the bird reaches the hospital.

History

The anamnesis provides invaluable information regarding the patient and assists the clinician in making critical decisions regarding treatment. During immediate triage of an unstable patient, having a second person available to obtain a history allows for simultaneous focused attention on the patient and gathering of potentially useful information about the presentation (see Avian History Form at end of this chapter and a downloadable form is available at www.wiley.com.). If trauma is the presenting complaint, it is crucial to ask questions pertaining to the incident early on in order to guide specific therapy. For instance, initial therapy for a bird that has collided with a stationary object may differ than those utilized in a patient who has been bitten by the family cat. Determining the duration, severity, and progression of clinical signs can also assist diagnostic and treatment decisions.

Exotic Animal Emergency and Critical Care Medicine, First Edition. Edited by Jennifer E. Graham, Grayson A. Doss and Hugues Beaufrère.

Husbandry

Many avian emergencies are directly related to improper husbandry, and a clinician must focus on obtaining a detailed account of the owner's husbandry while also discerning their level of expertise regarding the proper care of their pet. Discussing husbandry with the owner can be a lengthy yet rewarding process. For routine bird appointments, premade questionnaires with detailed avian husbandry questions that the owner can fill-out ahead of time can be beneficial for maximizing appointment time [1, 2].

Enclosure

Enclosures that are too small for the animal can lead to sanitation issues, damaged tail feathers, or environmental stress, predisposing an animal to disease. Often, pet owners have photographs on their mobile phones, allowing for quick inspection of the cage size, type, and furnishings. The location of the enclosure is also important. Cages should not be located in drafty areas or near the kitchen to limit the potential for exposure to toxic fumes. Use of aerosols in the environment should be limited or avoided, in order to prevent airway irritation or intoxication. Owners should also be aware of potentially toxic plant species to prevent exposure. While access to a window is often stimulating, visualization of outdoor birds or animals might be a source of constant stress. If the bird is flighted, making sure ceiling fans are not located nearby or at least turned off is of utmost importance.

Cage Materials Galvanized wire is used in the construction of some caging, leaving behind a white powder coating that can contain high levels of zinc [3, 4]. Inquiry into the type, size, and location of perches can reveal an underlying source of foot issues, including pododermatitis. Ideally, perches should have varying diameters appropriate for the size of the bird and consist of different materials to provide different perching textures, limiting the potential for development of integumental disorders of the plantar surface.

Toys Toys are a potential source for intoxication, depending on the materials used. Bird shows and fairs often sell custom-made or homemade designs, which may include toxic metals or natural items unfit for consumption. Additionally, toys ordered online may contain questionable elements and owners should be instructed to explore purchasing toys from reputable dealers and companies. Toys with chains or string can result in entanglement and trauma in birds. Nests made of fine fibers can result in toe constriction in small bird species, like finches. In the authors' experience, owners are frequently unaware of sources of heavy metals in the home, despite a diagnosis of acute or chronic intoxication in their pet. While central neurologic signs are commonly reported, pet psittacine birds with lead intoxication may present with peripheral neuropathy alone [5]. See Box 22.1 for a list of common sources of heavy metal intoxication in pet birds.

Box 22.1 Sources of Heavy Metal Intoxication In Pet Birds

Zinc

- New or improperly cleaned galvanized wire
- Pennies (U.S.) minted after the year 1982
- Metal hardware
- Inappropriate toys containing metal

Lead

- Toys containing metal or lead-based paints
- Metal hardware
- Lead-based paints, Venetian blinds, or linoleum in older homes or buildings
- Stained-glass hobby materials
- Solder
- Fishing or curtain weights

Source: Adapted from Lightfoot and Yeager [6]

Table 22.1 Substrates for avian enclosures.

Appropriate	Inappropriate
• Newsprint or other available paper • Recycled paper or paper fiber products	• Corn cob or walnut shell-based bedding • Shavings made of woods containing aromatic oils • Materials producing excessive amounts of dust or strong scents

Substrate The enclosure substrate or ground covering should be easy to clean and not promote growth of mold or bacteria when soiled. See Table 22.1 for a list of appropriate and inappropriate substrates for bird enclosures.

Diet

Proper nutrition is a major component of avian health, and the conveyance of its importance to owners is a constant struggle. Vitamin and mineral deficiencies or excessive fat intake can lead to a variety of medical problems, which often manifest as emergent problems. For most pet bird species, a balanced pelleted diet should make up the majority of their diet, and supplemental foodstuffs appropriate for the species should also be provided. Commonly encountered toxic foods in birds include avocado, chocolate, and *Allium* plant species like garlic and onion [6]. While beyond the scope of this chapter, there are many excellent resources for proper pet bird nutrition available to the clinician [2, 7].

Owner Interaction

Discussing how the owner interacts with their pet bird can often reveal information about a clinical problem. For example, male birds (cockatoos may be overrepresented) can present with acute-onset or chronic cloacal prolapse, which may ultimately be attributed to excessive sexual stimulation secondary to an owner's inappropriate interaction with their pet [8]. While sometimes awkward, questioning the owner on how they interact with their bird may reveal an underlying etiology to a clinical problem.

Clinical Exam

The clinical examination offers immediate information about the health status of the avian patient and consists of the visual and physical examinations.

Visual Examination

First, visually inspect the patient, preferably at a distance if the animal appears stable. A healthy bird should be perched or climbing the walls of its enclosure all-the-while keeping a watchful eye on you or its new surroundings. Birds that are lethargic, weak, or dyspneic on presentation should be quickly placed into a quiet, warmed incubator with oxygen supplementation as necessary. Handling should be minimized in these patients. By the time a bird has become outwardly ill, there are often substantial physiologic changes present and even short-term handling may result in death. See Table 22.2 for information regarding approach to the clinical examination based on patient stability. Inspection of the cage/carrier may also provide useful information such as fecal abnormalities (polyuria, hematochezia), bleeding (feces, hemoptysis), or regurgitation. Active hemorrhage and seizures should be addressed immediately. If handling or manipulation of an unstable patient is needed for treatment (e.g. significant hemorrhage, open fractures), determine whether the benefit of immediate care outweighs the risk of handling. If required, consider handling after administering sedation.

Table 22.2 Approach to avian clinical examinations based on patient presentation.

Unstable (lethargic, weak, dyspneic)	Stable (fluffed but active, alert, responsive)
• Provide immediate supportive care • Minimize handling • Discuss prognosis with owner • Pursue physical exam once bird is more stable • Consider staging physical exam to limit induced stress • Sedation is recommended for dyspneic patients	• Perform visual ("hands-off") exam • Perform physical examination if bird remains visibly stable • Consider sedation or postponing exam if you are suspicious the bird has occult significant illness based on anamnesis

Physical Examination

The physical examination should be performed in a systematic fashion and in a consistent order to prevent inadvertent omission. Overt abnormalities are ideally examined last in order to prevent overlooking other significant findings. All necessary equipment should be assembled prior to restraint in order to minimize handling time and patient stress level. See Box 22.2 for a checklist of materials needed for a detailed avian physical examination. While under manual restraint, examine the bird's attitude. Healthy parrots will often vocalize during capture and handling and actively try to bite the handler or towel surrounding them.

Box 22.3 contains a list of focus areas for the avian physical examination.

Box 22.2 Equipment List for the Detailed Avian Physical Examination

- Infant or pediatric-sized stethoscope
- Ophthalmoscope, penlight, transilluminator, or headlamp
- Tape strips, paperclip, or oral speculum
- Cotton-tipped applicator for visualizing the ear canals
- Sterile lubricant and sterile cotton-tipped applicators for examining the cloacal mucosa in South American parrot species

Box 22.3 Focus Areas for an Avian Physical Examination

- Hydration status
- Body condition or keel score
- Respiratory effort
- Auscultation of the heart, lungs, and air sacs
  - Respiratory rate and sounds
  - Heart rate and sounds
- Symmetry of head and beak
- Nares
- Oral cavity
- Eyes
- Ears
- Crop palpation and visualization
- Palpation of long bones
- Feather condition
- Wings
- Legs
- Skin of legs and feet
- Coelomic palpation
- Uropygial gland
- Vent
- Eversion of the cloacal mucosa in select species

Dorsally deviating the skin overlying a superior palpebra and watching for the speed of return can give an indication of hydration status (Figure 22.1a); this is similar to a skin tent evaluation in mammals. A sluggish return to normal position or an eyelid that remains in the abnormal position suggests a clinically dehydrated animal (Figure 22.1b). The skin over the edge of the keel can also be utilized to judge hydration. In a well-hydrated animal, the skin should easily slide from side-to-side over the bony protuberance of the keel. In dehydrated birds, the skin often requires more force to move it from one side to the other and often feels less elastic. In the authors' experience, these techniques are best suited for serial evaluations in a single animal, as variation can exist between individuals making interpretation subjective. The position of the eyes within the bony orbits can also give an indication of hydration status.

The basilic vein (synonym: ulnar or wing vein) can provide information regarding patient perfusion. First, wet the feathers over the elbow in order to visualize the basilic vein where it courses over the proximal ulna (Figure 22.2); place slight pressure over this point, compressing the vessel between a finger and the bone. After release, assess the speed in which the vessel refills. In a healthy animal, the vein will refill so fast that it is often difficult to see. In a bird with perfusion deficits, there may be a visible lag before the occluded portion of the vessel refills. Blanching of the cloacal mucosa may also be used to assess perfusion, as well as the comb in poultry.

Nares, Sinuses, Eyes, Ears, Beak, Oral Cavity, and Crop

Examine the head and face from a craniocaudal direction to evaluate symmetry. All structures should be symmetrical with deviations indicating an underlying abnormality. Sinusitis can result in facial deformation or periorbital swellings. The nares should be clear and free of debris. Active hemorrhage or dried blood may be present in or around the nares after a traumatic incident.

Evaluation of the lens and anterior chamber is possible using direct ophthalmoscopy or biomicroscopy. If trauma is suspected, a detailed ophthalmologic examination including evaluation of the fundi should be performed.

The ear canals are easily examined by lifting the feathers located caudoventral to the eyes up with a cotton-tipped applicator. The canals should be clear and the surrounding skin normal in color (Figure 22.3). Canals that are stenotic, filled with debris, or surrounded by hyperemic skin indicate an underlying disorder or inflammation.

The beak is a common site of injury in birds attacked by dogs or larger bird species. Active hemorrhage from beak fractures can be controlled using digital pressure, styptic powder, or cyanoacrylate glue (i.e. tissue glue).

The oral cavity can be opened using avian oral metallic speculums, tape strips, or simply by hand in docile patients. Use of metal avian oral speculums can result in beak fractures if not used properly, particularly in larger unsedated parrots (e.g. macaws). For this reason, tape strips may be

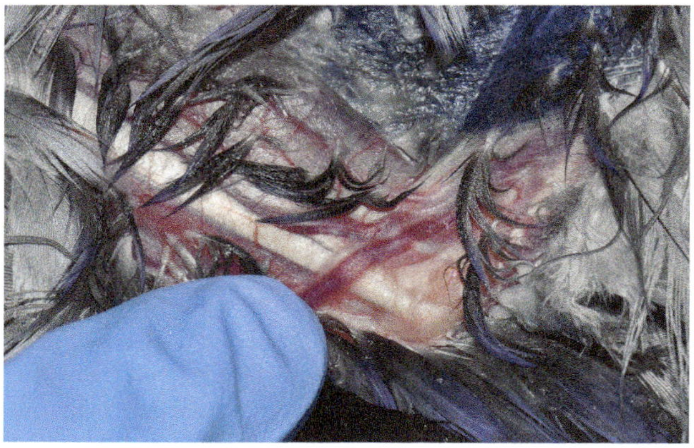

Figure 22.2 Basilic vein coursing over the ulna just distal to the elbow joint.

(a)

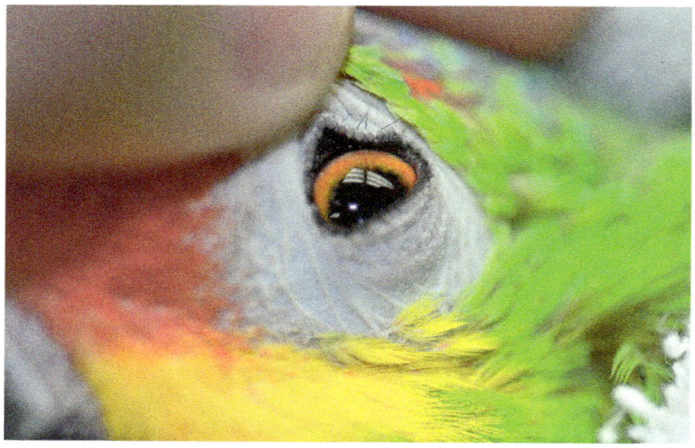

(b)

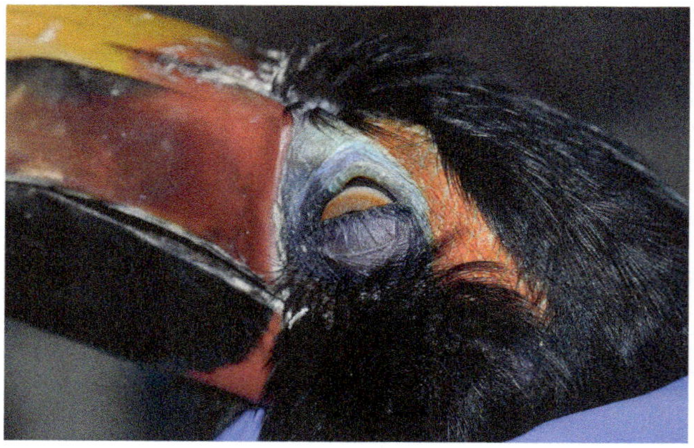

Figure 22.1 Using the elasticity of the superior palpebra to assess hydration status in an Amazon parrot (a); poor elasticity of the superior palpebra in a dehydrated green aracari (*Pteroglossus viridis*) (b).

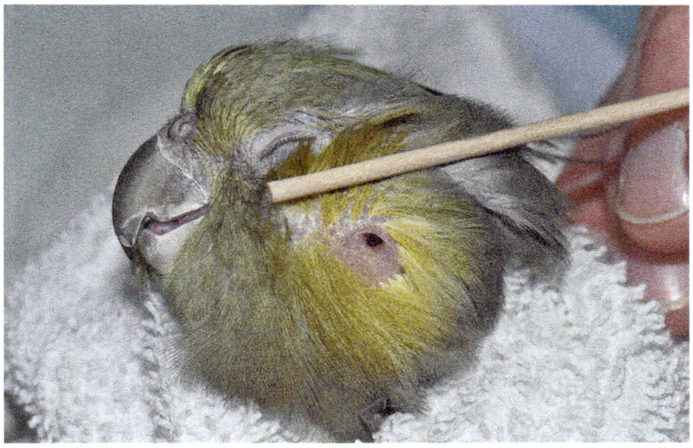

Figure 22.3 External ear canal in a cockatiel (*Nymphicus hollandicus*); note position caudoventral to the eye.

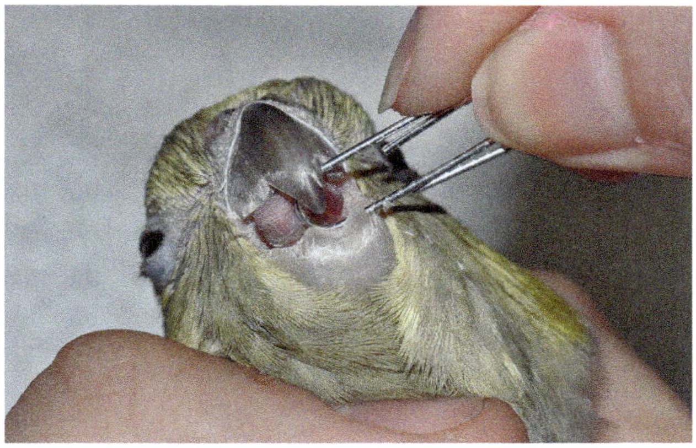

Figure 22.5 Small paperclips can be utilized for oral examination in small parrot species, like this cockatiel (*Nymphicus hollandicus*).

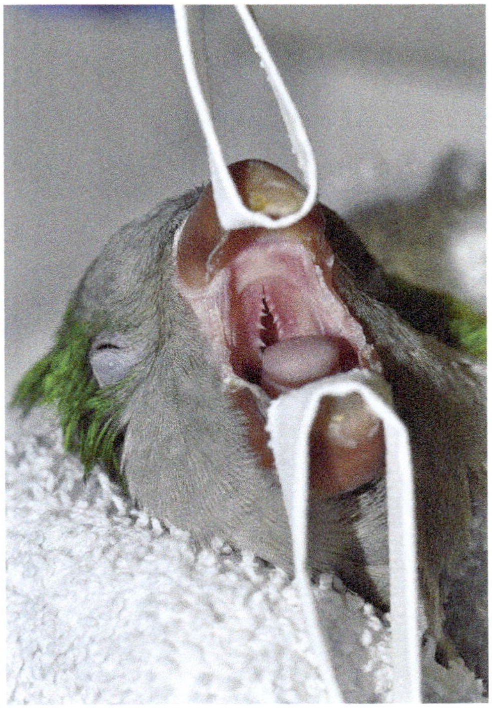

Figure 22.4 Use of tape strips to perform an oral exam in a quaker parrot (*Myiopsitta monachus*); note the sharp choanal papillae, a normal finding.

considered instead for these patients (Figure 22.4), but requires the presence of an assistant. Separate tape loops (medical-grade white tape) are used to pull apart the rhinotheca and gnathotheca simultaneously. Once purchase has been obtained, gentle but firm traction is applied until the beak is opened and the bird no longer resists the procedure. Using focused lighting allows for inspection of the choana, infundibular cleft, and oropharyngeal cavity, while the mouth is held open. A small, clean paperclip can be useful for examining the oral cavity in smaller parrots like budgerigars and cockatiels (Figure 22.5). Breaking a cotton-tipped applicator in half creates a small point that helps open the bill of small passerine species.

The choanal papillae should be sharp (Figure 22.4) and the structures within the oropharyngeal cavity symmetrical. Blunted choanal papillae, loss of choanal papillae, exudate within the choanal slit, or hyperemic choanal mucosa can indicate stomatitis, rhinitis, sinusitis, or hypovitaminosis A [1].

The ingluvies or "crop" is a diverticulum of the esophagus used for food storage in many bird species. Palpation of the caudal cervical area cranial to the sternum may reveal the thin-walled crop filled with fluctuant food material. The wall of the crop and its contents can be examined by using alcohol to part the feathers. Transillumination of the ingluvies can allow assessment of its vasculature and wall thickness [1, 9]. Marked distension of the crop with fluid or food material most likely signals an abnormality with crop emptying, commonly seen with crop infections, lead intoxication and other disorders [1]. Foreign bodies and masses may also be palpated in the crop.

Musculoskeletal

Palpation of the pectoral musculature surrounding the keel (Figure 22.6) is used to estimate the bird's body condition. The edge of the keel should be palpable, but you should not be able to grab and hold it in between two fingers (poor body condition score) or barely feel it (excessive body condition score).

The clinician should palpate all long bones. In small species, fractures or luxations may not be easily appreciated on the physical exam and diagnostic imaging is often required for a diagnosis. The humerus should be supported while extending the wing for examination to prevent trauma upon sudden wing flapping. The coracoid can be palpated in large birds by inserting a finger between the clavicle.

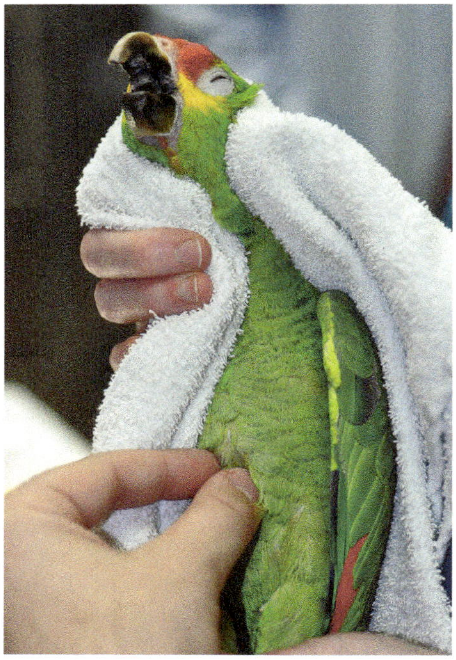

Figure 22.6 Palpation of the edge of the keel and adjacent pectoral musculature provides an estimate of body condition, although species-specific differences exist.

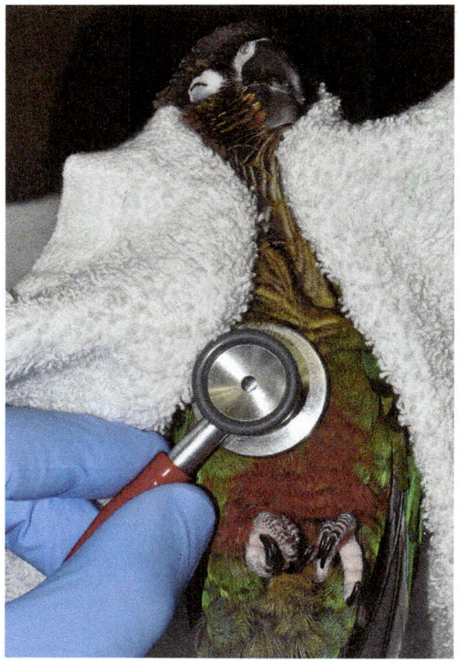

Figure 22.7 Use of an infant-sized stethoscope for auscultation of a restrained conure; the small size helps improve localization of sounds.

Birds may be presented for keel wounds after a recent wing trim. In overweight birds or in species that are relatively heavy for their body size (e.g., *Amazona* spp.), an overly aggressive wing trim can result in a hard fall if the bird is not used to being flight restricted.

Cardiorespiratory

Auscultation of the heart and airways is most easily accomplished using a stethoscope with a small diaphragm (Figure 22.7). The stethoscope is placed over the pectoral muscles to either side of the edge of the keel; the heartbeat is usually the loudest in the area of the cranial portion of the keel. The heart may also be ausculted over the dorsum in the area of the lungs, which is a helpful approach for bird species with thick, downy, breast feathers. Murmurs may be difficult to appreciate in most species, simply due to the rapid heart rate.

By tilting the bird into a normal standing position, one can easily auscult the lungs in the interscapular area (Figure 22.8). Listen to the trachea in the area of the clavicle and along the sides of the bird to evaluate the air sacs. Wheezing, popping, or harsh lung sounds are indicative of an abnormality. End-expiratory crackles are often auscultated in the caudal air sacs of birds with a coelomic mass effect or effusion.

Any dyspnea should be characterized (inspiratory, expiratory, mixed).

Coelomic Cavity

The coelomic cavity can be accessed in the small region caudal to the sternum and cranial to the vent. This area should normally be a smooth, concave slope. The edge of the sternum should be readily palpable, and coelomic distension may result in disappearance of this normal protuberance. Hepatomegaly, space-occupying masses, or ascites may result in abnormalities on coelomic palpation. The right liver lobe lies the most caudally and is often palpated first in cases of hepatomegaly [9]. Palpate the pubic bones in the caudal coelomic area; birds in dystocia or preparing for oviposition may have an enlarged interpubic width. Using isopropyl alcohol to wet the feathers over the coelom in passerines facilitates examination of organs through their nearly translucent coelomic wall [1, 9].

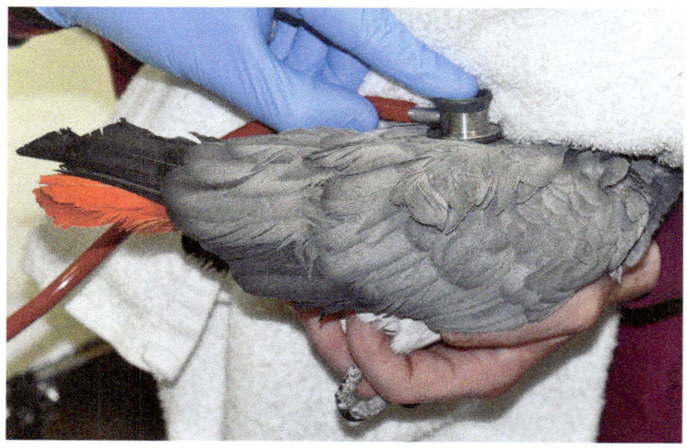

Figure 22.8 Positioning a restrained parrot with its keel parallel to the floor facilitates lung auscultation.

Cloaca and Vent

If not readily apparent on the bird's ventral surface due to heavy feathering, the vent lies just caudal to the pubic bones, which can be easily palpated. The feathers surrounding the vent should be free from fecal material and there should be tone present when the vent is manipulated.

Eversion of the proctodeal mucosa (Figure 22.9) should be performed in species susceptible to developing cloacal papillomas, such as Amazon parrots and macaws. This can be performed by gently inserting a cotton-tipped applicator coated with a sterile lubricant into the cloaca and rolling the mucosa outward, examining around the entire orifice.

Cloacal prolapse is a frequent presenting sign and should be characterized for viability, the presence of ulceration, and origin of the prolapse (coprodeum, oviduct, rectum).

Integument

Feathers from all parts of the body should be examined for abnormalities. The feather quality may reflect the overall chronic health status of the bird as well as the quality of its diet. While examining the flight feathers, look for the presence of pinfeathers (Figure 22.10).

While rarely a true emergency, feather-destructive behavior can rapidly progress to self-mutilation of the soft tissues in some birds and may be related to an acute increase in the affected bird's environmental stress level.

Smoothing of the plantar skin of the foot (Figure 22.11) can be an indication of an underlying nutritional deficiency or improper perch surfaces [2]. If unilateral, this can indicate uneven weight bearing, and examination of the bird perching or ambulating may be useful in ruling out unilateral leg lameness.

Examine the uropygial or "preen" gland located cranial to the tail base for asymmetry, discomfort, or an abnormal appearance. Its location can be easily estimated by manipulating the tail feathers up and down; the preen gland lies just cranial to this area of mobility (pygostyle) on the dorsal surface of the bird. Disorders include impaction or obstruction, infection, and neoplasia. The uropygial gland is absent in Amazon parrots, pionus parrots, and blue macaws.

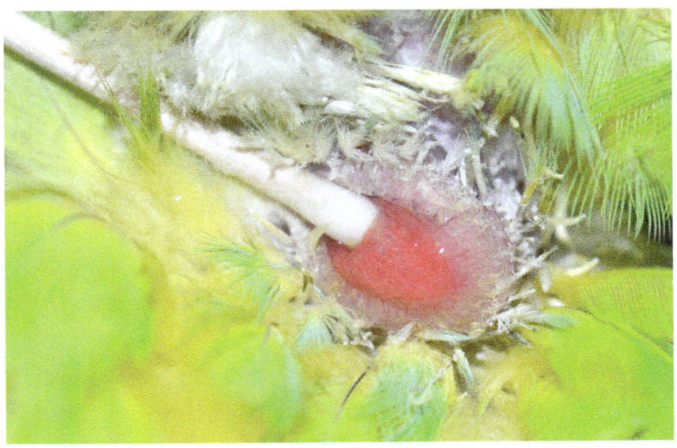

Figure 22.9 Eversion of the cloacal mucosa in an Amazon parrot using a sterile, lubricated cotton-tipped applicator.

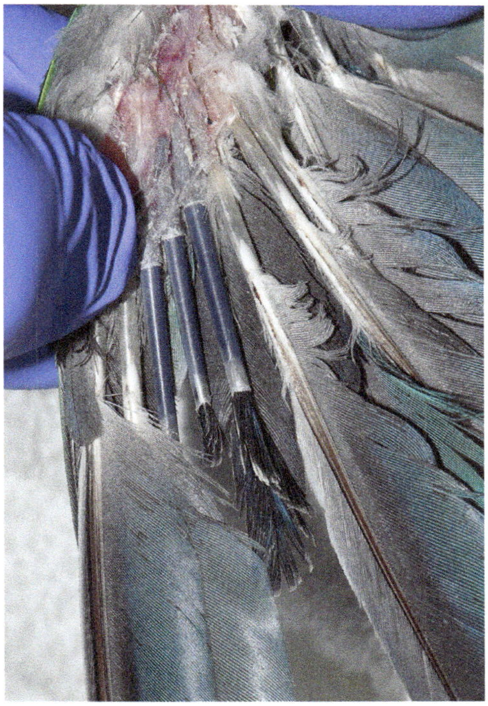

Figure 22.10 Three pinfeathers noted during examination of the primary flight feathers.

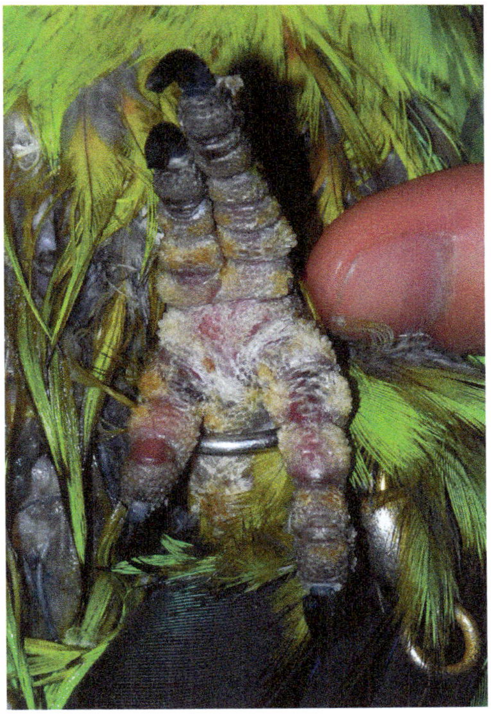

Figure 22.11 Excessive smoothing of the plantar surface in an overweight Amazon parrot on a poor diet.

Birds

Stool Appearance

Birds are often presented for changes in their droppings. When a bird with a history of changes in the droppings arrives at the clinic for examination, remove the substrate of the caging and replace it with clean paper to observe a fresh sample for abnormalities. Make sure to examine the excrement left on the used substrate. In the exam room, the stools may contain a larger liquid component; polyuria is a common finding in birds secondary to the stress of transport or from being in a new environment.

The excrement normally consists of fecal, urine, and urate components. Bright green to yellow feces or urates may indicate a liver abnormality or hemolysis (Figure 22.12). Undigested seed or other food material in the droppings indicates an abnormality within the gastrointestinal system. Hemoglobinuria or porphyrinuria may occur secondary to heavy metal toxicosis [6]; this may manifest as chocolate colored or blood tinged stools in some parrot species. Dark-colored feces may be indicative of melena or a diet containing highly pigmented berries or fruits. Although uncommon, the presence of gas bubbles with the excrement is highly suggestive of diarrhea [9].

The cloaca accepts material from several different sources, including the urinary, reproductive, and gastrointestinal tracts, which can make determination of the origin of fresh blood in the droppings a challenge.

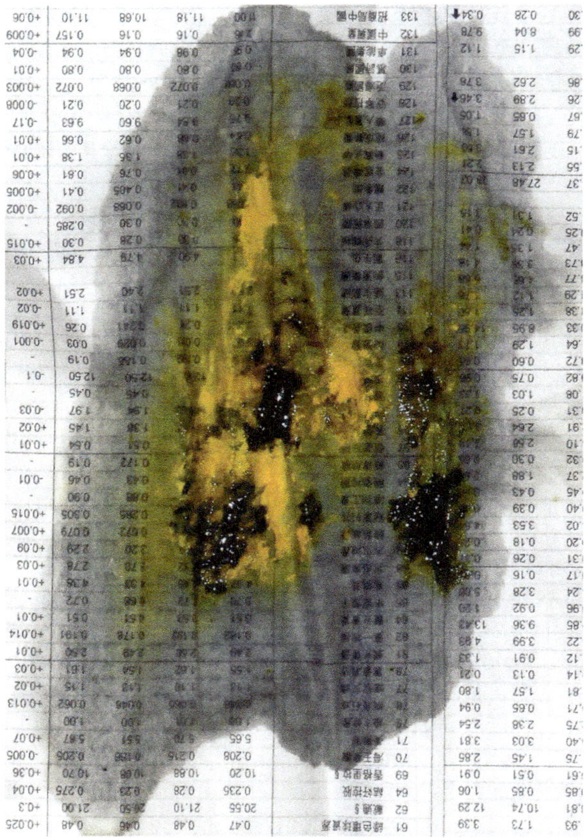

Figure 22.12 Abnormal droppings in an Amazon parrot with a hepatopathy; note the bright yellow urates.

Conclusion

Obtaining an excellent patient history is important for a tailored physical exam, proper diagnostic work-up, and overall patient care. It assists clinicians in identifying potential life-threatening problems in emergent cases and helps guide conversations regarding preventable problems. A thorough clinical examination provides a large amount of information within a relatively short period of time. The clinician should approach the examination systematically and quickly in order not to overlook subtle abnormalities or cause undue stress from handling. Together, the clinical history and examination comprise the foundation of avian medicine.

References

1 Hillyer, E. (1997). Physical examination. In: Avian Medicine and Surgery (eds. R. Altman, S. Clubb,G. Dorrestein and K. Quesenberry), 125–141. Philadelphia: WB Saunders.

2 Tully, T. Jr. (2009). Birds. In: Manual of Exotic Pet Practice (eds. M. Mitchell and T. Tully Jr.), 250–298. St. Louis: Saunders Elsevier.

3 Bauck, L. and LaBonde, J. (1997). Toxic diseases. In: Avian Medicine and Surgery (eds. R. Altman, S. Clubb, G. Dorrestein and K. Quesenberry), 604–613. Philadelphia: WB Saunders.

4 Holz, P., Phelan, J., Slocombe, R. et al. (2000). Suspected zinc toxicosis as a cause of sudden death in orange-bellied parrots (*Neophema chrysogaster*). *J. Avian Med. Surg.* 14 (1): 37–41.

5 Martel, A.K., Doss, G.A. and Mans, C. (2020). Suspected peripheral neuropathy secondary to lead intoxication in three psittacine birds. *J. Exot. Pet. Med.* 32: 13–17.

6 Lightfoot, T.L. and Yeager, J.M. (2008). Pet bird toxicity and related environmental concerns. *Vet. Clin. North Am. Exot. Anim. Pract.* 11 (2): 229–259.

7 Orosz, S.E. (2014). Clinical avian nutrition. *Vet. Clin. North Am. Exot. Anim. Pract.* 17 (3): 397–413.

8 Bowles, H., Lichtenberger, M., and Lennox, A. (2007). Emergency and critical care of pet birds. *Vet. Clin. North Am. Exot. Anim. Pract.* 10 (2): 345–394.

9 Harrison, G. and Ritchie, B. (1994). Making distinctions in the physical examination. In: Avian Medicine: Principles and Application (eds. B. Ritchie, G. Harrison and L. Harrison), 144–175. Lake Worth: Wingers Publishing.

Avian History Form

A detailed history is essential to provide the most appropriate veterinary care for your animal. Please complete this form as accurately as possible. If there is anything you are unsure about you can discuss it in more depth with the veterinary staff during your appointment.

Animal Details

Avian name or identification: ____________________

Common or scientific species name: ____________________

Date of birth: ____________________

Sex: M F neutered/spayed unknown Determined by: DNA endoscopy visual other: ____________________

Origin: captive bred wild caught import unknown

How long have you had this bird? ____________________

From where did you obtain this bird? ____________________

Does this bird have a reproductive history? N / Y please give details ____________________

When did your bird last molt? ____________________

How often has your bird been molting? ____________________

Is your bird vaccinated? N / Y please give details ____________________

Does your bird get wing trimmed? N / Y if yes, please give details ____________________

Do you have other birds or pets? N / Y please give details: ____________________

Have you or your bird had any contact with other birds in the last 30 days? N / Y please give details ____________________

____

When was the last bird added to your collection? ____________________

Reason for Presentation Today

What is the primary complaint or what signs have you noticed? ____________________

How long have these problems been present? ____________________

What health problems has your bird had previously? ____________________

Has your bird received any treatment in the last 30 days? N / Y If yes, please give details (what was used, dosage, how often, duration): ____________________

Have you noticed any change in your bird's behavior? N / Y please give details ____________________

Have any other animals or persons in the household had any illness in the last 30 days? N / Y

Diet

How often do you feed your animal? ____________________

Indicate which foods are eaten and in what amounts (by number, weight, or approx. volume):

Seed mixtures: __________ Brand? __________ Amount? ____________________

Pellets: __________ Brand? __________ Amount? ____________________

Fruits and/or vegetables: __________ Type? __________ Amount? ____________________

Meat (type and amount) Freshly killed Frozen/thawed Live prey Amount? ____________________

____

Treats: __________ Brand? ____________________

Other: ____________________

What water supply do you provide? tap water bottled water rain/river water

How is water provided? Bowl dripper system spray How often? _______ How often is the water changed? __________

Do you use any water supplements? N / Y please give details: ________ Have you noticed any changes in feeding or drinking behavior? N / Y

Please give details: ____________________

Have you noticed any changes in droppings (fecal material, urine and urates)? N / Y

Please give details: ____________________

Do you use any nutritional supplements? N / Y , if yes what, how much, and how often? ____________________

____

(Continued)

Avian History Form (Continued)

Cage Environment

Cage size: ______________________________

Where is the cage located? inside outside Please give details______________________________

What is the cage made of? ______________________________

What kind of bedding is used? ______________________________

What décor and furnishings are present? nest box perches swings toys other

Please give details: ______________________________

Are bathing/spraying facilities provided? ______________________________

How often is the cage cleaned? ______________________________

What cleaning/disinfectant agents are used? Please give details: ______________________________

What percentage of time does your bird spend inside and outside of its cage? ______________________________

Is the animal supervised when out of the cage? N Y Please give details: ______________________________

Does your bird have regular exposure to sunlight? N Y Frequency and length of time ______________________________

Is your bird exposed to full spectrum (UVA and UVB) lighting? N Y Brand? ______________________________

What is your bird's light/dark cycle? ______________________________

Does anyone in the household smoke? N Y Do you use any aerosolized products? N Y

Do you use Teflon pans? N Y Do you use a self cleaning oven? N Y Last self-clean cycle? ______________________________

Have there been changes in the bird's environment in the last 3 months? N Y Please give details: ______________________________

____

23

Restraint and Handling

Grayson A. Doss and Christoph Mans

Department of Surgical Sciences, School of Veterinary Medicine, University of Wisconsin-Madison, Madison, Wisconsin, USA

CONTENTS

Overview and Indications

Restraint refers to control of the patient, either by physical or chemical means, or a combination of both, and is commonly utilized in veterinary medicine as a means to facilitate safe interaction with a patient, either during transport, examination, or various medical procedures. Proper restraint accomplishes enough immobility to complete the intended task in the shortest time possible, while remaining safe for both the handler and the patient. Physical restraint includes manual restraint, where a handler manually controls a patient, and other types of restraint (e.g. mechanical) in which the animal remains conscious yet safely controlled.

Strongly consider postponing restraint or using sedation to facilitate handling in birds that are critically ill, as the stress of restraint alone could result in patient death.

Transport

Minimizing or removing cage furniture prior to the car ride is important to prevent trauma from falling perches or swinging toys. In weak or ataxic birds, removal of high perches can prevent serious falls. Birds that are flighted should be properly enclosed to prevent escape. A travel-sized birdcage, ventilated plastic container, or cardboard box lined with a soft cloth can be used to transport most species.

Manual Restraint

Manual restraint is used for a variety of procedures including physical examination, cosmetic procedures like nail, beak, and wing trims, sample collection such as venipuncture and swabs, non-invasive diagnostic tests such as ultrasound examination and even radiographs in critically ill animals, and basic treatments such as gavage feeding and drug administration. In most companion birds, manual restraint is possible using simple equipment like towels. Care must be taken to prevent a struggling patient from overheating in a thick towel, however. A list of items required of restraint is summarized in Box 23.1. Important tips for avian restraint are listed in Box 23.2.

With most companion bird species, control of ambient light can have a dramatic effect on restraining a patient. Passerine species tend to freeze when room lights are turned out suddenly, facilitating a quick capture. Most parrots will also freeze for a moment when confused by a rapid decrease in ambient light, allowing for a brief moment to quickly restrain an animal.

Passerines, Columbids, and Poultry

Passerine species, like finches and canaries, are usually caught from a small enclosure with a bare hand or using a towel. Small, soft nets can also be used. Passerine birds, especially small species, are less likely to bite a handler than parrots. Passerines may be held with the neck held

Exotic Animal Emergency and Critical Care Medicine, First Edition. Edited by Jennifer E. Graham, Grayson A. Doss and Hugues Beaufrère.

Box 23.1 Checklist for Avian Restraint By Group

Passerines
- Small towel
- Net

Psittacines, Columbids
- Towel

Poultry
- Usually no specific equipment required

Box 23.2 Important tips during avian restraint

- Have all necessary items for a procedure ready prior to initiating restraint
- Immobilize the head of parrots first to prevent injury
- Avoid touching the featherless facial skin in macaws and African gray parrots during restraint
- Allow the patient's keel to move normally
- Remove towel if patient begins to overheat
- If a bird becomes dyspneic during an exam, abort restraint
- Communicate constantly with restrainer during examination to prevent injury

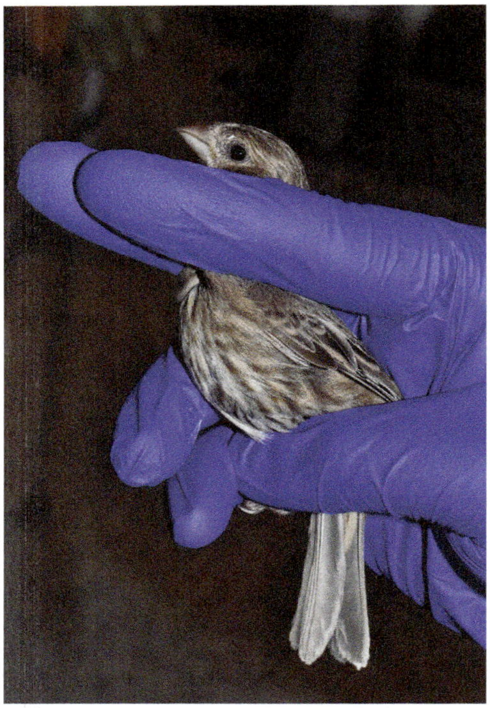

Figure 23.1 Manual restraint of a passerine bird; note how the keel remains free to move normally.

between the pointer and middle fingers, and the legs held still with the thumb and ring finger; this allows for easy access to a large portion of the body for the physical examination and ensures the keel is able to move freely (Figure 23.1). Due to the small size and fragile skeleton of most passerine species, care must be taken when manipulating limbs as fractures can occur with rough handling. Passerines can be very difficult to catch if they escape from restraint, and can fly into unseen spaces high in a room. Escaped birds may also fly into windows or other solid objects, resulting in serious injury. Use of long-handled nets or low ambient light is helpful for re-capture.

Columbids (e.g. pigeons and doves), while larger than passerines, do not inflict painful bites and are easily restrained. However, it is common for pigeons and doves to shed feathers during attempted restraints. A small towel may be used to keep the wings close to the body, or the handler may hold the bird one-handed; this is accomplished by placing the palm over the bird's dorsum and the base of its neck between the pointer and middle fingers, using the remaining digits to wrap underneath the patient and keep the wings in place next to the body.

Poultry, including domestic chickens, turkeys, and waterfowl like ducks and geese, are typically restrained without the use of special equipment, and the majority of the physical examination and blood collection can be performed with minimal restraint. Often, forceful manual restraint or placing the bird in dorsal body position will make restraint more challenging, because of the increased struggling caused. Long-necked species are often restrained against the side of the handler, with an arm wrapped around the bird at mid-body, supporting the weight of the animal. The head may be covered or restrained with the other hand depending on the individual patient. Large species like turkeys may be restrained with their dorsum pressed against the front of the handler and the handler holding a leg in each arm; alternatively, both legs may be controlled with a single hand, leaving an arm free to wrap around the bird to keep the wings from flapping. Chickens are often most calm when minimally restrained and held in place while standing on a stable surface (Figure 23.2). Because of a propensity for biting, control of or covering the head is recommended for geese and swans when performing procedures or administering treatments. It is important to control the legs in male chickens and turkeys to prevent injury from large, tarsometatarsal spurs. Turkeys and swans are powerful animals and may require a second handler for safe restraint.

Psittacines

A parrot's main mechanism of defense is biting, owing to its sharp beak and incredible jaw pressure that can lead to serious bite wounds to the handler. Even small psittacine species can inflict painful bites.

The least intrusive methods should be attempted first. Some parrots will step onto a stranger's hand or a held perch, which can facilitate obtaining a body weight or closer visual exam. Some birds will accept having the towel lightly placed over their head if approached carefully. However, many birds will be leery of the new environment, and restraint is often required for moving them. *Never let owners restrain their own bird, regardless of experience level.*

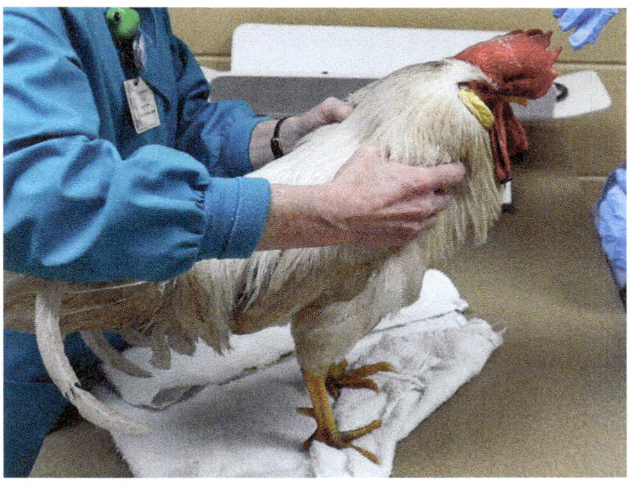

Figure 23.2 Manual restraint of a rooster using a firm surface for the animal to stand on.

Most parrot species can be safely restrained using towels. Depending on the bird's anxiety level and behavior prior to being restrained, several toweling methods may be used. In all cases, the handler should focus on the head. Birds naïve to towel restraint may show more anxiety to being wrapped up. For calm birds, they can be toweled while perched on the handler's hand or arm or while seated with the bird. Many non-flighted birds are easily toweled after being placed on the ground. If inside an enclosed space, many birds will back into a corner. In this situation, the handler can either force the bird to move into an easier-to-catch position when approaching with the towel or have the bird bite the side of a large towel while catching the head with the other side. Some birds (e.g. macaws and Amazon parrots) have a tendency to back into a corner and lie on their back, making any sort of restraint attempt difficult. In these situations, waiting until the bird stands up and moves out of a corner or begins climbing the side of a cage allows for safer restraint attempts. The handler should be swift and decisive when going for the head as hesitancy and a slow grab may result in being bitten. A thick blanket, fleece, or multiple layers of towels are often easier to use for large macaw restraint.

The head should be restrained using a collar-like grip around the neck at the base of the head (Figure 23.3a) or by using a three-fingered technique to immobilize the skull (Figure 23.3b). A towel between the restraining hand and the bird helps with grip and provides a barrier should the patient bite. Birds possess closed tracheal rings making it unlikely for a gentle yet firm grip to result in tracheal

(a) (b)

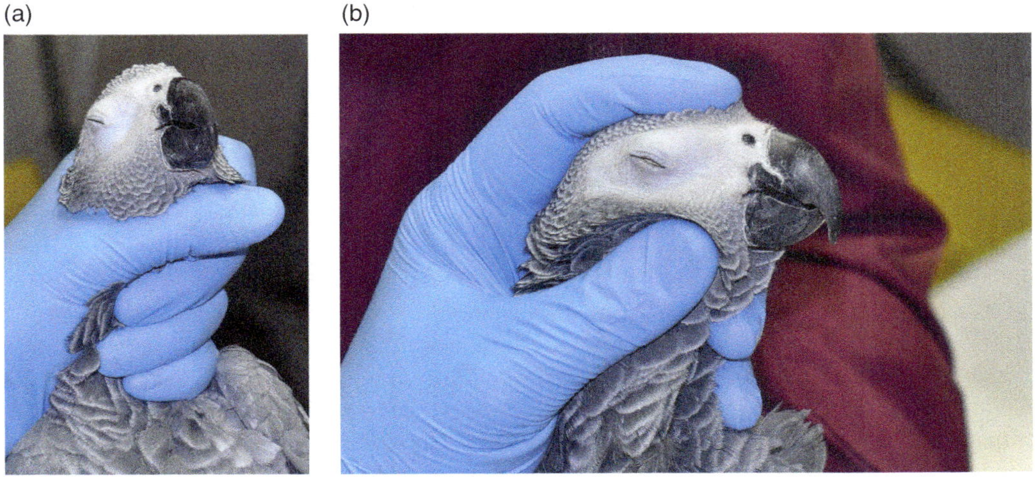

Figure 23.3 Proper restraint of the psittacine head to prevent biting of the handler during manual restraint. Shown are the Elizabethan collar-like grip (a) and the three-fingered grip (b) of a grey parrot (*Psittacus erithacus*).

Birds

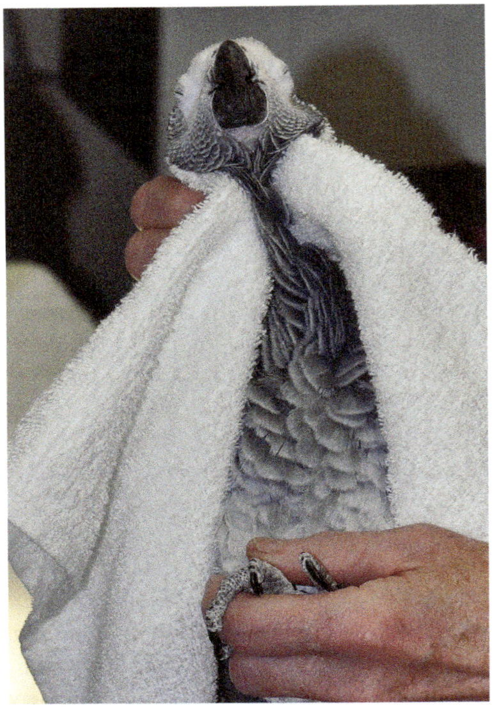

Figure 23.4 Towel restraint of a grey parrot (*Psittacus erithacus*) demonstrating open access to the front of the bird for examination.

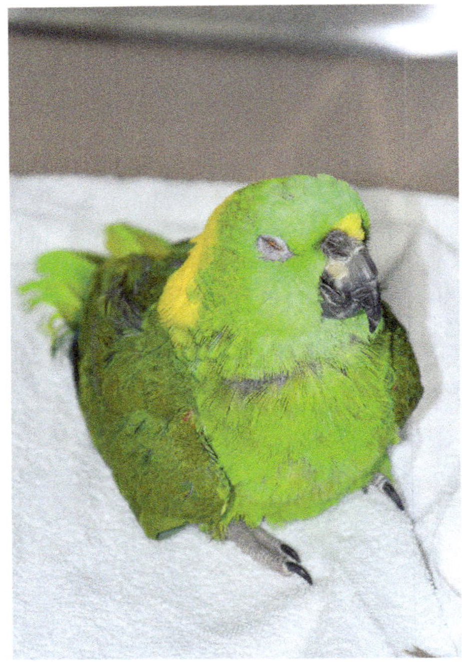

Figure 23.5 Amazon parrot administered intranasal midazolam and butorphanol showing the closed eyes and relaxed body typical of sedation.

injuries during handling. Care should be taken in parrots with featherless facial skin (e.g. macaws, grey parrots), to avoid excessive pressure on these areas, as they will readily bruise. Pressure should not be exerted on the keel to allow for unrestricted breathing. The opening of the towel should face the keel to allow for the physical examination and prevent overheating (Figure 23.4). The wings and caudal half of the bird are held together with the restrainer's other hand. When releasing a parrot from restraint the feet are first placed on a steady, solid surface and the head is released last.

Sedation

Procedural sedation is commonly used in pet birds [1–7] and can facilitate safe handling of aggressive animals and result in life-saving modulation of the stress response in some critical patients. Sedation also facilitates a variety of procedures such as taking radiographs with improved radiosafety compared with manual restraint, safer, and more efficient venipuncture techniques, and many others.

Injectable drugs can be quickly administered intramuscularly in the pectoral muscles to severely ill animals, while they remain in an oxygen cage or incubator. Within 5–10 minutes after administration, gentle restraint can be attempted while monitoring the patient closely for signs of distress.

The authors routinely use midazolam (2–4 mg/kg) with or without butorphanol (1–3 mg/kg) for procedural sedation in healthy and ill companion birds. Smaller birds, such as passerines, budgerigars, or cockatiels, often require higher doses of midazolam (passerines >4–6 mg/kg). Reversal of midazolam with flumazenil (0.05 mg/kg IM, IN, IV) results in rapid recovery, if needed. Butorphanol is not routinely reversed. Sedation often results in a relaxed patient that struggles and vocalizes less (Figure 23.5), making the restraint process, diagnostic sample collection and therapeutic interventions (e.g. subcutaneous fluids, gavage feeding) less stressful, reducing the risk of injury to the patient and handler, and shortening the time the bird requires restraint.

Some injectable agents, including diazepam, midazolam, and butorphanol, can be administered intranasally, if needed. Intramuscular administration, however, may be preferred in dyspneic patients or birds with small, non-spherical, or obstructed nares. Intranasal sedation is preferred when blood samples are collected to avoid biochemical artifacts associated with IM injections.

Reversal of sedation is recommended in most instances, except if an e-collar, bandage, or splint was placed or if the patient was sedated for seizure management. Never discharge a bird, which has not received reversal of its sedation. Some birds may mildly to moderately re-sedate later as the half-life of flumazenil is shorter than that of midazolam.

Hospitalization

Hospital caging should be simple yet provide avian patients with necessary comfort. All species should be supplied with appropriate perches for their size. A variation in texture and size of perches is recommended to prevent fatigue. High perches or tall caging should be avoided with ataxic or neurologic birds. Covering or providing a visual barrier for at least a portion of the enclosure is recommended to minimize patient stress, especially in non-pet birds. Cage bar spacing should be appropriate for the size of the animal to prevent escape. Ill birds benefit from increased environmental temperature and humidity, which is provided with most veterinary critical care incubators. Substrate should be easy to clean and afford inspection of patient droppings. Ideally, caging should allow for full extension of the wings for comfort and provide several different perching areas. Avian patients should be housed in quiet, non-drafty areas, away from excessive audiovisual stimuli. Fresh standing water should be provided for all birds, in addition to diet offerings appropriate for the species and feeding history of the patient. Provision of a variety of feedstuffs throughout the enclosure may help promote foraging activity and encourage eating.

Daily Monitoring

Serial physical examinations are recommended to ensure proper therapeutic response. Food and water intake and body weight should also be monitored to ensure appropriate supportive care is administered. Droppings within the enclosure can provide an idea of patient mobility during unobserved periods. Cage humidity and temperature should be monitored hourly to observe for malfunction of equipment and subsequent patient injury.

Birds

References

1. Sadegh, A.B. (2013). Comparison of intranasal administration of xylazine, diazepam, and midazolam in budgerigars (Melopsittacus undulatus): clinical evaluation. *J. Zoo Wildl. Med.* 44 (2): 241–244.
2. Hornak, S., Liptak, T., Ledecky, V. et al. (2015). A preliminary trial of the sedation induced by intranasal administration of midazolam alone or in combination with dexmedetomidine and reversal by atipamezole for a short-term immobilization in pigeons. *Vet. Anaesth. Analg.* 42 (2): 192–196.
3. Schäffer, D.P., Raposo, A.C.S., Libório, F.A. et al. (2016). Intranasal administration of midazolam in blue-and-yellow macaws (Ara araruana): evaluation of sedative effects. *Vet. Anaesth. Analg.* 43 (4): 459–460.
4. Vesal, N. and Eskandari, M.H. (2006). Sedative effects of midazolam and xylazine with or without ketamine and detomidine alone following intranasal administration in ring-necked parakeets. *J. Am. Vet. Med. Assoc.* 228 (3): 383–388.
5. Vesal, N. and Zare, P. (2006). Clinical evaluation of intranasal benzodiazepines, alpha-agonists and their antagonists in canaries. *Vet. Anaesth. Analg.* 33 (3): 143–148.
6. Mans, C. (2014). Sedation of pet birds. *J. Exot. Pet. Med.* 23 (2): 152–157.
7. Mans, C., Guzman, D.S.-M., Lahner, L.L. et al. (2012). Sedation and physiologic response to manual restraint after intranasal administration of midazolam in Hispaniolan Amazon parrots (Amazona ventralis). *J. Avian Med. Surg.* 26 (3): 130–139.

24

Oxygen Therapy

Hugues Beaufrère

Department of Medicine and Epidemiology, School of Veterinary Medicine, University of California-Davis, Davis, California, USA

CONTENTS

Indications for Oxygen Therapy

The goal of oxygen supplementation is to increase the oxygen concentration of inspired air (fraction of inspired O_2: FiO_2) to improve blood oxygenation and increase tissue delivery of O_2. General hypoxia may be due to anoxic hypoxia (low FiO_2, hypoventilation, diffusion impairment, ventilation/perfusion mismatching), anemic hypoxia (anemia, methemoglobinemia, CO poisoning), stagnant hypoxia (low blood flow due to cardiac failure or hemorrhage), and histiocytic hypoxia (cyanide poisoning) [1]. Common indications of oxygen therapy include severe anemia, hemodynamic compromise, and hypoxemia (decreased blood oxygen concentration) due to pulmonary and obstructive airway diseases [2].

The respiratory anatomy and physiology of birds is very different from mammals. Birds have the highest metabolism among vertebrates, hence the highest oxygen consumption. A fundamental understanding of avian respiratory anatomy and physiology is vital in diagnosing respiratory diseases, interpreting diagnostic tests pertaining to the respiratory system or hypoxemia, and devising a plan for emergency stabilization and treatment of underlying conditions. In contrast to mammals, the avian lungs do not participate in ventilation, which is performed by the air sac system, which in turn does not play any direct role in gas exchange. Air sacs act as bellows to ventilate the lungs. Avian lungs are also unique in that ventilation is both tidal as in mammals (bidirectional in neopulmo part of the lungs) and through-flow (unidirectional in paleopulmo part of the lungs). The lungs are formed of a complex network of parabronchi and air capillaries, where gas exchange takes place. The avian lungs generate much greater exchange surface for a comparable volume than mammalian lungs (about 15% more), have a thinner blood–air barrier (about 2.5 times thinner), and harvest oxygen through diffusion in a cross-current exchange system maximizing oxygen uptake [3]. The air sacs are functionally divided into two groups: the cranial group of air sacs composed of the cervical, interclavicular, and cranial thoracic air sacs receiving expiratory air and the caudal group of air sacs that include the caudal thoracic and abdominal air sacs, which receive inspiratory air [4, 5]. Two respiratory cycles are necessary for a given volume of inspired air to move across the avian respiratory system. In birds, both inspiration and expiration are active and the relaxed sternal position is at midpoint between end-inspiration and end-expiration. In addition, the thoracic cavity is not at subatmospheric pressure as in mammals and a large number of muscles participate in ventilation. Ventilation is regulated by various mechanisms in birds, which are important to understand in order to treat hypoxemia and perform diagnostic tests in dyspneic birds. Central chemoreceptors are present in birds and initiate an increase in ventilation when $PaCO_2$ increases. Arterial chemoreceptors located at the carotid bodies, near the parathyroid glands, and innervated by the vagus nerve modulate ventilation in response to changes in PaO_2, $PaCO_2$, and pH. Another group of

Exotic Animal Emergency and Critical Care Medicine, First Edition. Edited by Jennifer E. Graham, Grayson A. Doss and Hugues Beaufrère.

chemoreceptors, unique to birds and reptiles, known as the intrapulmonary chemoreceptors, are found in the lungs and are innervated by the vagus nerve. In contrast to arterial chemoreceptors, intrapulmonary chemoreceptors are stimulated by hypocapnia (overall decreases in lung PCO_2), leading to decreases in ventilatory drive. Finally, air sac mechanoreceptors are also present. In summary, changes in ventilation occur in response to changes in $PaCO_2$, intrapulmonary PCO_2, PaO_2, and pH. The unique anatomy of the lung–air sac system allows for the provision of anesthetic and respiratory gases through a cannula in the caudal or abdominal air sacs, effectively bypassing the trachea.

As a consequence of these differences, oxygen therapy seems extremely beneficial to birds, which have higher metabolic demand for oxygen and may take extra advantage of an increased FiO_2 due to their more efficient gas exchange mechanisms. On the down side, birds are more susceptible to air borne toxins and respiratory lesions may be more likely to cause clinical respiratory signs in birds than in other terrestrial vertebrate species. Indeed, the high efficiency of the avian pulmonary cross current gas exchange makes birds more susceptible to ventilation/perfusion mismatching and hypoxemia may consequently develop more readily with respiratory diseases than in mammals [3]. In addition, extra-respiratory diseases may decrease ventilation capabilities by decreasing air sac volume, blocking air sac ostia, and impairing ventilation as both inspiration and expiration are active processes and ventilatory muscles are numerous. Thus, any bird presenting with a disease that results in a decrease in air sac volume (e.g. ascites, coelomic organomegaly) may benefit from oxygen supplementation. Finally, due to the increased metabolic state induced by diseases and the high oxygen consumption and extensive respiratory system of birds, birds may still benefit from oxygen supplementation even when not appearing clinical dyspneic. For these reasons, initial stabilization, pending further diagnostics and assessment, may include oxygen therapy in most avian emergency presentations.

Assessing the hypoxemic status of birds may not be clinically feasible so oxygen therapy may be started pre-emptively. Specific history of respiratory diseases that may prompt pre-emptive oxygen therapy may include nasal or ocular discharge, sneezing, coughing, dyspnea, collapse, exercise intolerance, voice changes, voice loss, respiratory noises, tail-bobbing, open-mouth breathing, subcutaneous emphysema, ataxia, lethargy, anorexia, and weight loss. Increased respiratory frequencies and efforts may be noted on examination. Increases in ventilatory efforts and volume are achieved in birds in part by using additional muscle groups, which include the tail depressor and suprapubic muscles [6]. The increased activity of these muscles under certain conditions leads to the clinical manifestations of tail-bobbing in dyspneic birds.

Pulmonary auscultation is not very sensitive in birds but wheezes, crackles, and other pulmonary noises may be detected. The stethoscope is placed over the dorsum right over the lungs or on different areas of the abdomen to auscultate the air sacs. As with the type of dyspnea, increased inspiratory noises may correlate with upper respiratory diseases and increased expiratory noises with lower respiratory diseases. Cardiac auscultation should also be performed. Assessment of cyanosis may also be difficult. However, in chickens, the comb and wattles or unfeathered skin of the face or periorbital areas in some parrots may clinically appear cyanotic. Weight loss may indicate a chronic respiratory disease. In a normal bird, normal respiration should return within minutes after restraint or a short period of wing flapping [7].

Arterial blood gases are impractical to take in most awake birds, typically requiring deep sedation or anesthesia. As in mammals, the normal PaO_2 of birds is around 95–100 mmHg and the SaO_2 is around 97–100%. Under anesthesia, PaO_2 may be as high as 300–500 mmHg due to the concurrent supplementation of 100% oxygen associated with inhalant anesthesia. On the other hand, venous blood gases are easily performed in most medium to large size birds and may give a clue on the hypoxemic status of a bird when the PvO_2 is less than 30 mmHg and the $ScvO_2$ is lower than 50% [8]. In addition, pulse oximetry may be difficult to place in the awake birds and is likely not reliable owing to calibration having been performed based on a mammalian hemoglobin dissociation curve [9]. As a result, avian SpO_2 values tend to be underestimated by current pulse oximeters [9].

Response to therapy should also be used for monitoring and to titrate the oxygen flow. It is ideal to monitor the SpO_2 or PaO_2 during oxygen supplementation but this is rarely practical in most birds. The response to oxygen therapy may be poor depending on the disease. For instance, a poor to fair response may be seen in diseases producing a low ventilation/perfusion mismatch (perfusion predominates with decreased supply in O_2 to the exchange surface) such as pulmonary edema, pneumonia, asthma, pulmonary neoplasia, and atelectasis. In extreme cases of these diseases (severe pneumonia), oxygen therapy may not be efficacious because blood makes no contact with ventilated lungs. Response is good in diseases with a high ventilation/perfusion mismatch (low perfusion in normally ventilated lungs) such as pulmonary thromboembolism [1]. Improving cardiac function and fluid resuscitation are best to correct stagnant hypoxemia. While the degree of response to oxygen therapy may be variable, regardless of the underlying conditions, any patient with acute respiratory distress and signs of hypoxia (cyanosis, dyspnea, tachypnea, open-mouth breathing) may benefit from supplemental oxygen. In addition, birds may show a more consistent or noticeable response to oxygen supplementation than mammals with comparable diseases.

Due to the extensive nature of the air sac system in birds in the abdomen and thorax, any extra-respiratory disease resulting in reduction of air sac volume or occlusion of major airways may result in respiratory clinical signs. A significant reduction in air space may occur with fluid accumulation in the coelomic cavities of birds such as ascites resulting from cardiac, hepatic, or neoplastic diseases, and egg yolk coelomitis. Severe respiratory complications may arise if the fluid/yolk gains access to the inside of the respiratory system. Space-occupying masses are also associated with impairment of abdominal ventilation and are encountered with large tumors (e.g. budgerigars), granuloma, eggs, and organomegaly.

If ascites is suspected and associated with significant dyspnea, a coelomocentesis should be performed (see Figure 33.13). A small needle or a small butterfly catheter mounted on a syringe is inserted in the abdomen around the midline and directed to either side, and fluid is aspirated. A preliminary ultrasound may be performed to select the area over the ventro-caudal coelom where most fluid is present (see Chapter 30 for further details on point of care ultrasound). Sometimes, the area with the most fluid can be directly visualized through the skin.

Oxygen Toxicity

The most common complication associated with oxygen therapy is oxygen toxicity because oxygen is a potent oxidizing agent. The degree of toxicity is related to the level of oxygen and duration, and the lung is the most vulnerable organ to oxygen radicals. General guidelines recommend not to supplement oxygen at 60–100% for more than 24–48 hours in mammals [1, 2]. Depletion of endogenous antioxidant levels may also promote oxygen toxicity at lower oxygen percentages. Oxygen toxicity has been reported in birds. A study demonstrated oxygen toxicity in canaries and budgerigars on 68–100% oxygen after three to eight days [10]. In another experiment, budgerigars were found to have mild pulmonary lesions in as little as three hours after exposure to 100% oxygen but more severe lesions after 24 hours [11]. In the same study, birds exposed to 100% oxygen for three hours or three hours per day for three days did not show any clinical signs. On the other hand, birds exposed to oxygen supplementation for 72 hours developed respiratory distress after 24 hours and some birds died. Acute repeated exposure to three hours resulted in mild lesions consisting of mild thickening of gas exchange barriers and increased numbers of endothelial cells and heterophils. Chronic exposure resulted in more severe changes, most prominent within parabronchi, with severe edema, increased inflammation and decreasing number of endothelial cells. In different studies, chronic exposure also resulted in depletion in antioxidant mechanisms in budgerigars, which indicated the progression from oxygen stress to oxygen toxicity [12, 13]. In addition, oxygen exposure leads to significant respiratory alkalosis and reduced respiratory function in chronic exposure and repeated acute expose to oxygen supplementation [12].

Methods of Oxygen Supplementation

Non-Invasive Methods

Oxygen Chamber/Cage

Oxygen may be delivered to an oxygen chamber or an anesthetic machine through high pressure oxygen cylinders, a central oxygen supply system in universities and large veterinary hospitals, or stationary or portable oxygen concentrators. Oxygen concentrators are especially useful when anesthetizing birds in the field or when supplying oxygen to an oxygen chamber for several days without access to a central oxygen line. Oxygen therapy is typically implemented using an oxygen cage in avian patients because it is low-stress and non-invasive. For small to medium birds, the travel cage or carrier may be placed in the oxygen chamber prior to restraint for pre-oxygenation. It is best if the oxygen chamber is also an incubator where temperature and humidity can be controlled to provide additional support to the patient.

The authors strongly encourage veterinarians to measure the FiO_2 that can be achieved in their oxygen cages using an oxygen sensor to verify their performance before administering supplemental oxygen to patients. The FiO_2 is typically between 30 and 60% in most incubators depending on oxygen flow and seal.

Flow-By and Facemask Oxygen

An FiO_2 of 25–45% may be reached using flow-by of oxygen and 35–60% using facemasks [1, 2]. While these methods are frequently employed in sedated or anesthetized unintubated patients, they are rarely practical in awake birds, except when moribund. Most pet birds will not tolerate having their head in an oxygen mask or even have a flow by oxygen tube without significant restraint. However, in birds that are significantly depressed, oxygen supplementation provided either via facemask or flow by should be given while performing other procedures (e.g. IV or IO catheter placement). The oxygen flow rate should be high enough when using a facemask to prevent CO_2 rebreathing. Corneas should be lubricated to avoid corneal dryness.

Invasive Methods

Oral Endotracheal Intubation

Endotracheal intubation is relatively easy in most birds. The glottis is located at the base of the tongue and the avian larynx lacks the epiglottic and thyroid cartilages as well as the vocal cords. The trachea is longer in birds than in mammals. The increased tracheal length in birds is compensated by an increased tracheal diameter resulting in a resistance to tracheal airflow similar to mammals. However, the tracheal dead space is about four times that of mammals, which is compensated by a larger tidal volume.

It can be more challenging to visualize the glottis in small psittacine birds as the tongue can be bulky and the oral cavity small. Pulling the tongue gently with atraumatic plastic forceps will facilitate the visualization of the glottis in most instances. In several species (e.g. pelicans, hornbills, kiwis, penguins, some ducks), a median crest, the *Crista ventralis*, arises ventrally from the cricoid cartilage inside the glottis and should be avoided during endotracheal intubation (Figure 24.1) [14, 15].

Birds have complete tracheal rings and, in order to reduce tracheal trauma, uncuffed endotracheal tubes should be used (Figure 24.2). Since the tubes are uncuffed, significant air leakage or problems with capnography during spontaneous or manual ventilation may be encountered. Standard plastic Magill tubes are typically used for avian endotracheal intubation. Endotracheal Cole tubes are wider several centimeters distally in such a way that they seal the glottis upon intubation. Lightly wrapping vetrap or other materials around standard Magill tubes a few centimeters distally may provide the same results. In smaller birds, IV catheters or similar diameter tubes may be used for intubation. Airway resistance increases dramatically when intubating small birds as it increases with the fourth power of the tracheal radius [16]. These small diameter tubes may also obstruct more easily with tracheal secretions. As a consequence, routine intubation of small birds may lead to more severe ventilation problems if frequent manual or artificial ventilations are not provided. It may be best not to intubate small birds such as budgerigars or passerines for routine procedures.

Laryngospasm is infrequent in birds but may be encountered in larger birds. A drop of lidocaine may be applied on the glottis prior to intubation if necessary. As birds are small, lidocaine may have to be diluted to provide a safe dose (around 1–2 mg/kg). Lidocaine sprays are not recommended as the total dose of lidocaine may be far greater than required and may lead to toxic doses. As the trachea significantly narrows down in most species after a few centimeters, the endotracheal tube should not be introduced too far. Intubation-induced tracheal stenosis is not uncommon in birds and has been reported in multiple species [17–22]. It typically presents with coughing or acute inspiratory dyspnea about one to two weeks after an intubation event. Endotracheal treatments or tracheal resection and anastomosis are required to remove the lesions. Tracheal stenosis secondary to trauma may recur after surgical correction. A retrospective study in a zoo including birds that underwent surgical treatments reported a mortality rate of 70% overall [17]. Specific risk factors that are associated with secondary tracheal stenosis are unknown but suspected to include physical trauma, chemical insult (from sterilizing agents), and focal tracheal desiccation from the oxygen flow. In order to minimize tracheal trauma, care should be taken to intubate gently and not too deeply and to be extremely cautious

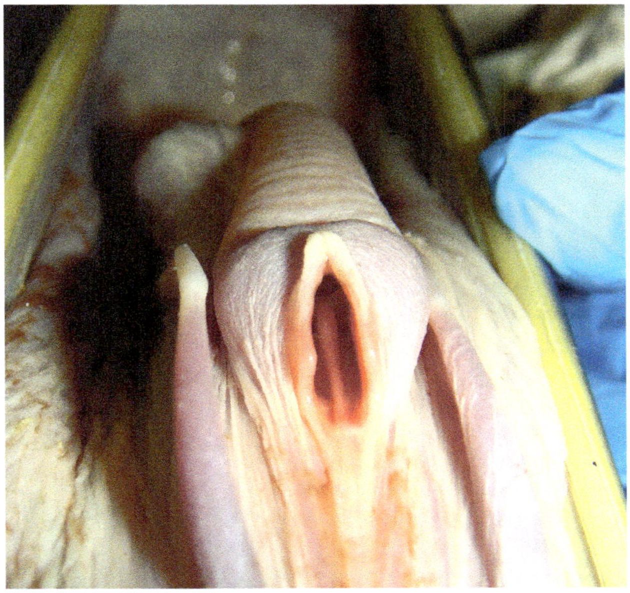

Figure 24.1 Glottis with *Crista ventralis* in its center in a brown pelican (*Pelecanus occidentalis*). This structure is only present in select species such as some ducks and it should not be damaged during endotracheal intubation.

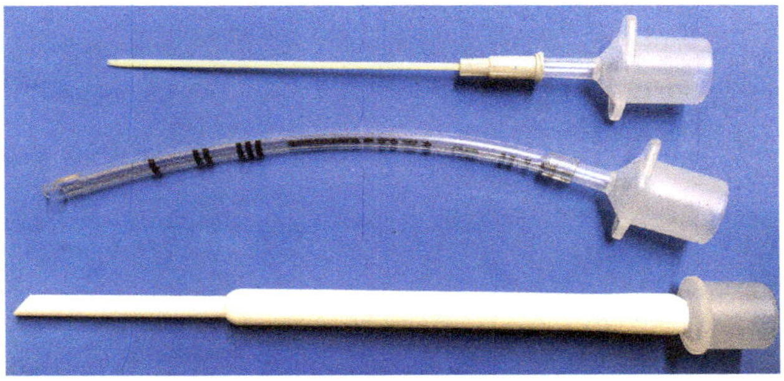

Figure 24.2 Different types of endotracheal tubes that can be used in birds. From top to bottom: intravenous catheter, Magill endotracheal tube, Cole endotracheal tube.

Birds

when moving the head and neck of intubated birds. The tip of the endotracheal tubes should be lubricated, as for other species. Sterile tubes may also be used to intubate birds. Some birds, such as waterfowl (Anseriformes), may produce relatively thick tracheal mucus that may obstruct the tubes [23]. In these species, it is best to replace the tube every hour. An obstructed endotracheal tube typically presents as birds with difficulties exhaling or capnography not recording any CO_2 (see Chapter 28). Birds in which the crop is not fully emptied should have their head elevated to prevent regurgitation.

Air Sac Tube Placement

When tracheal obstruction is suspected, an air sac tube may be placed either in the caudal thoracic or abdominal air sac. Placement in the cranial air sacs is not recommended as they contain expiratory air. Most common causes of tracheal obstruction in birds include post-intubation tracheal stenosis, tracheal foreign body, tracheal or syringeal aspergilloma, tracheal trauma, and a mass occluding the trachea at the thoracic inlet. The tube is placed between the last two ribs with the leg positioned caudally or behind the last rib with the leg positioned cranially usually on the left side such as during a conventional endoscopic approach (Figure 24.3). A left sided approach prevents iatrogenic trauma to the larger right liver lobe. A small skin incision is made, and the muscular wall is exposed (Figure 24.4). The abdominal wall is then punctured with a small hemostat, while the respiratory system is distended by the anesthetist to prevent the puncture of the abdominal organs. The principal organ that can be punctured during this procedure is the proventriculus, which can be distended due to aerophagia caused by open-mouth breathing. The proventriculus can also be large in some diseases (e.g. proventricular dilation disease) or in certain species (e.g. Eclectus parrots). It is best to obtain radiographs prior, but this is not always practical in emergency presentations. The hemostat is then open and held in place to guide the insertion of a tube between its jaws. The tube used may be a cut sterile endotracheal tube (Figure 24.5) (see Table 27.1 for sizes). The tubes frequently get obstructed so it is advisable to fenestrate its extremity. During the placement of the air sac tube, if

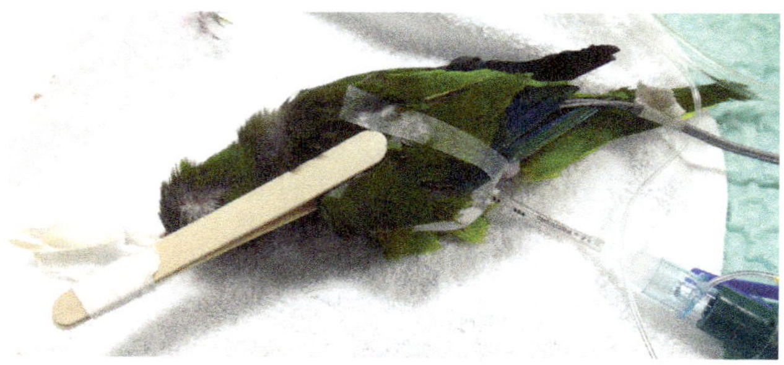

Figure 24.3 A Quaker parrot being anesthetized through an air sac cannula. This parrot had papillomatous lesions inside the oral cavity and around the larynx that obstructed the glottis. As the bird was open mouth breathing and could not initially be intubated, an air sac tube was placed to secure an emergency airway pending the treatment of the oral lesions.

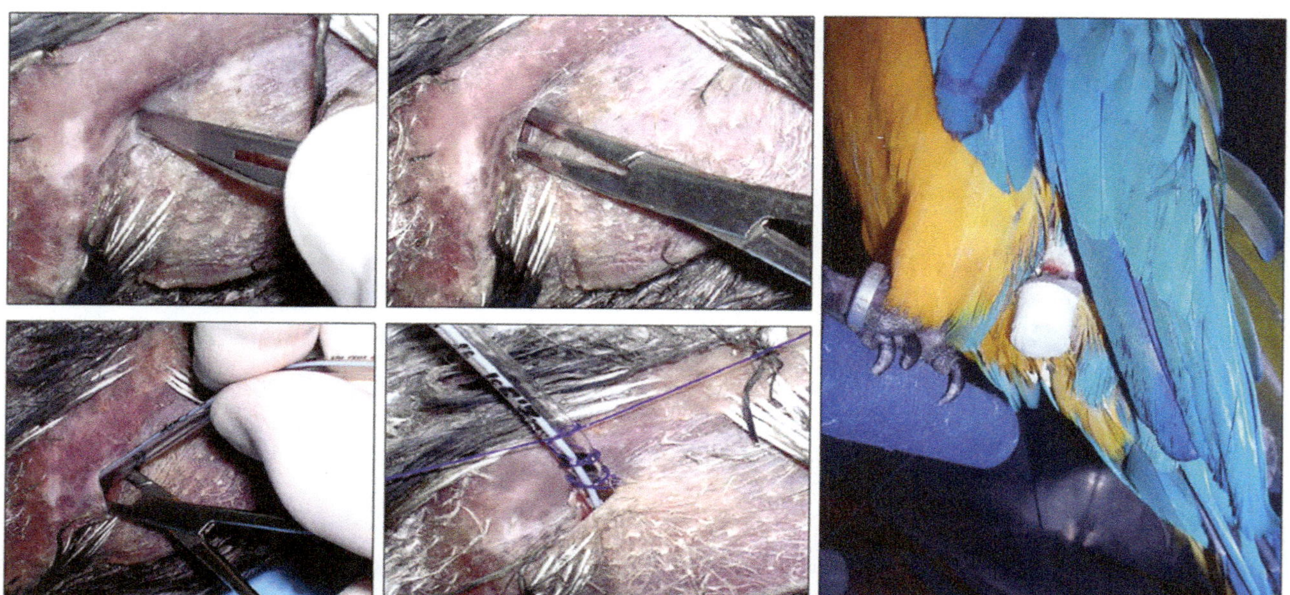

Figure 24.4 Step-by-step placement of an air sac tube in a bird. The skin is first incised and then slightly enlarged with a hemostat. The hemostat is then pushed into the caudal thoracic or abdominal air sac and then secured in place with a Chinese-finger trap suture. A filtering system may also be added.

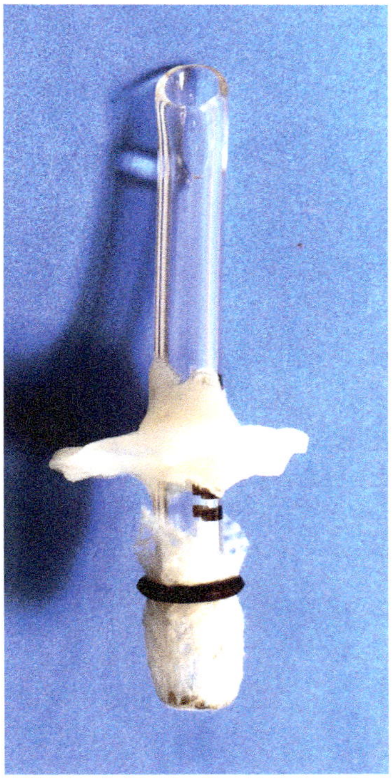

Figure 24.5 Air sac tube made from a cut endotracheal tube with a custom-fitted retention disc made from moldable thermoplastic and a filter made from surgical mask and a plastic o-ring.

endoscopy equipment is available, it is best to perform a brief endoscopic examination through the tube to both ensure correct placement in regard to the caudal ostia and perform an examination of the air sac, lung, and coelomic organs. Correct placement can also be ascertained by the presence of air flow (a small down feather can be plucked and placed in front of the tube to visualize airflow). The tube is sutured to the skin using a retention disc, tape, or directly onto the tube using a Chinese finger-trap suture. A cruciate suture is placed over the musculocutaneous incision around the tube. A filtering system should be placed on the tip of the tube to avoid inhalation of dust and feather debris. Several materials may be used for this purpose such as found in surgical or facial masks or using filter paper (see also Chapter 27).

Upon insertion of an air sac tube, the capnograph may stop measuring end tidal CO_2 as air escapes through the tube or the body wall incision. In addition, birds may stop breathing due to a CO_2 wash-out induced by the flow of oxygen.

Air sac tubes are far from being innocuous, and every effort should be made to re-establish a normal tracheal airway as soon as possible to reduce the time an air sac tube is present. The tube is kept for a maximum of five days, and another tube should be placed in the contralateral air sac if needed. Air sac tubes should be cleaned once a day using sterile cotton tip applicators until their removal to prevent obstructions by exudates and secretions. When the air sac tube is removed, it is recommended to culture its tip and to perform a brief endoscopic examination of the area. Air sac tubes induce a lot of inflammatory reaction, and it is not uncommon to diagnose focal aspergillosis upon their removal. If such lesions are observed, a topical instillation of amphotericin B is recommended. The stoma should be left patent until it heals by secondary intention. Topical ointment may be used to prevent or treat local infections of the site. Subcutaneous emphysema is a potential complication and is usually self-limiting.

References

1 Manning, A.M. (2002). Oxygen therapy and toxicity. *Vet. Clin.* 32 (5): 1005–1020.

2 Hopper, K. (2010). Oxygen therapy. In: *Textbook of Veterinary Internal Medicine*, 7e (eds. S. Ettinger and E. Feldman), 516–519. St Louis, MO: Saunders Elsevier.

3 Powell, F. (2015). Respiration. In: *Sturkie's Avian Physiology*, 6e (ed. C. Scanes), 301–336. San Diego, CA: Academic Press.

4 Maina, J. (2005). Qualitative morphology. In: *The Lung-Air Sac System of Birds* (ed. J. Maina), 65–124. Berlin, Heidelberg: Springer.

5 Powell, F. (2000). Respiration. In: *Sturkie's Avian Physiology*, 5e (ed. G. Whittow), 233–264. San Diego, CA: Academic Press.

6 Baumel, J., Wilson, J., and Bergren, D. (1990). The ventilatory movements of the avian pelvis and tail: function of the muscles of the tail region of the pigeon (Columba livia). *J. Exp. Biol.* 151 (1): 263–277.

7 Tully, T. and Harrison, G. (1994). Pneumonology. In: *Avian Medicine: Principles and Applications* (eds. B. Ritchie, G. Harrison and L. Harrison), 559–581. Palm Beach, FL: Wingers Publishing.

8 Beaufrere, H. (2016). Blood gases and critical care hematology and chemistry analyses. In: *Avian Medicine*, 3e (ed. J. Samour), 112–117. St Louis, MO: Elsevier.

9 Schmitt, P., Gobel, T., and Trautvetter, E. (1998). Evaluation of pulse oximetry as a monitoring method in avian anesthesia. *J. Avian Med. Surg.* 12 (2): 91–99.

10 Stauber, E. (1991). Effects of increased concentration of inspired oxygen. *Proc. Eur. Assoc. Avian Vet.*: 105–114.
11 Jaensch, S.M., Cullen, L., and Raidal, S.R. (2001). The pathology of normobaric oxygen toxicity in budgerigars (Melopsittacus undulatus). *Avian Pathol.* 30 (2): 135–142.
12 Jaensch, S., Cullen, L., Morton, L., and Raidal, S.R.R. (2001). Normobaric hyperoxic stress in budgerigars: non-enzymic antioxidants. *Comp. Biochem. Physiol. Part C Toxicol. Pharmacol.* 128 (2): 181–187.
13 Jaensch, S., Cullen, L., and Raidal, S.R. (2001). Normobaric hyperoxic stress in budgerigars: enzymic antioxidants and lipid peroxidation. *Comp. Biochem. Physiol. C Toxicol. Pharmacol.* 128 (2): 173–180.
14 King, A. (1993). Apparatus respiratorius. In: *Handbook of Avian Anatomy: Nomina Anatomica Avium*, 2e (eds. J. Baumel, A. King, J. Breazile, et al.), 257–300. Cambridge, MA: The Nuttal Ornithological Club, N 23.
15 McLelland, J. (1985). Larynx and trachea. In: *Form and Function in Birds Volume 3* (eds. A. King and J. McLelland), 69–104. London, UK: Academic Press.
16 Hawkins, M., Zehnder, A., and Pascoe, P. (2014). Cagebirds. In: *Zoo Animal and Wildlife Immobilization and Anesthesia*, 2e (eds. G. West, D. Heard and N. Caulkett), 399–433. Ames, IA: Wiley-Blackwell.
17 Sykes, J.M., Neiffer, D., Terrell, S. et al. (2013). Review of 23 cases of postintubation tracheal obstructions in birds. *J. Zoo Wildl. Med.* 44 (3): 700–713.
18 Jankowski, G., Nevarez, J.G., Beaufrere, H. et al. (2010). Multiple tracheal resections and anastomoses in a blue and gold macaw (Ara ararauna). *J. Avian Med. Surg.* 24 (4): 322–329.
19 de Matos, R.E.C., Morrisey, J.K., and Steffey, M. (2006). Postintubation tracheal stenosis in a blue and gold macaw (Ara ararauna) resolved with tracheal resection and anastomosis. *J. Avian Med. Surg.* 20 (3): 167–174.
20 Evans, A., Atkins, A., and Citino, S.B. (2009). Tracheal stenosis in a blue-billed currasow (Crax alberti). *J. Zoo Wildl. Med.* 40 (2): 373–377.
21 Monks, D.J., Zsivanovits, H.P., Cooper, J.E., and Forbes, N.A. (2006). Successful treatment of tracheal xanthogranulomatosis in a red-tailed hawk (Buteo jamaicensis) by tracheal resection and anastomosis. *J. Avian Med. Surg.*. Association of Avian Veterinarians; 20 (4): 247–252.
22 Clippinger, T. and Bennett, R. (1998). Successful treatment of a traumatic tracheal stenosis in a goose by surgical resection and anastomosis. *J. Avian Med. Surg.* 12 (4): 243–247.
23 Backues, K. (2015). Anseriformes. In: *Fowler's Zoo and Wild Animal Medicine*, 8e (eds. R. Miller and M. Fowler), 116–126. St Louis, MO: Elsevier.

25

Catheterization and Venipuncture

Rodney Schnellbacher[1] *and Hugues Beaufrère*[2]

[1]*Associate Veterinarian, Zoo Miami, One Zoo Boulevard, Florida, USA*
[2]*Department of Medicine and Epidemiology, School of Veterinary Medicine, University of California-Davis, Davis, California, USA*

CONTENTS

Venipuncture

Phlebotomy for drug administration, or to investigate hematological and biochemical profiles, or serological testing is a useful tool in avian medicine. Collection site selection depends upon the size of the bird, its health status, volume of sample needed, and the experience of the phlebotomist. Circulating blood volumes in birds, depending on species, are about 10% of the body weight. Approximately 10% of the blood volume, or 1% of the body weight (1 ml/100 g), may be removed during phlebotomy in healthy patients without risk of hypovolemic compromise. Studies in chickens and quail have shown that avian species are better able to compensate for blood loss than mammals (see CPR section) [1]. Although only a minimal amount of blood may be collected in smaller avian species, generally 0.2–0.3 ml of blood is sufficient to perform a full CBC and a reduced biochemical panel. A sample volume of 1 ml is ideal to perform a CBC and a full-panel biochemical profile, depending on PCV and whether some tests require dilution or re-analysis.

Avian veins tend to be fragile and moveable. Hematomas can occur more readily in avian versus mammalian species. Although phlebotomy is common and relatively safe in awake patients, some risk accompanies the procedure [1]. Typically, manual restraint may cause stress for patients, which can lead to higher blood pressure and prolongation of the time necessary to apply hemostatic pressure. Thus, stress increases the risk of hematoma formation. Movement of the animal during the procedure can lead to more vascular trauma or lacerations and can make blood collection more technically challenging. Anesthesia or sedation can make blood collection easier and less stressful to the animal. The risks of anesthesia, therefore, should be weighed against the benefits of venous access. If animals are compromised, and there is concern about the stress of manual restraint or anesthesia, sedation with intranasal or intramuscular midazolam at 0.5–3 mg/kg may be beneficial. Midazolam has a limited effect on the cardiovascular and respiratory systems and it can be easily reversed with flumazenil [2].

In general, it is recommended that blood collection be done as early as possible, even before a complete physical examination is performed. This limits stress-induced changes on the hemogram and biochemical profiles. General anesthesia has been shown to induce various hematological changes [3]. Restraint of most birds is performed using an appropriately sized towel. Place the towel over the dorsum and then gently wrap it around the wings to restrict flapping (Figure 25.1). This procedure should be quick, quiet, and gentle, so as to reduce unnecessary stress. For raptors, the animal's talons must be considered. The authors recommend use of a raptor glove to restrain the raptor's feet. Vet wrap around the talons may also be used to secure the feet. For long-legged birds such as Ciconiiformes, Gruiformes, and Phoenicopteriformes, the legs should be restrained by an assistant with a finger between the animal's hocks to prevent dermal abrasions [4].

Usually, 22–27-gauge needles are used for avian phlebotomy. Although smaller needles reduce the chances of vascular damage, they can increase the likelihood of hemolysis, which can interfere with a variety of laboratory tests. The size of the syringe can also affect blood collection. Larger syringes can

Exotic Animal Emergency and Critical Care Medicine, First Edition. Edited by Jennifer E. Graham, Grayson A. Doss and Hugues Beaufrère.

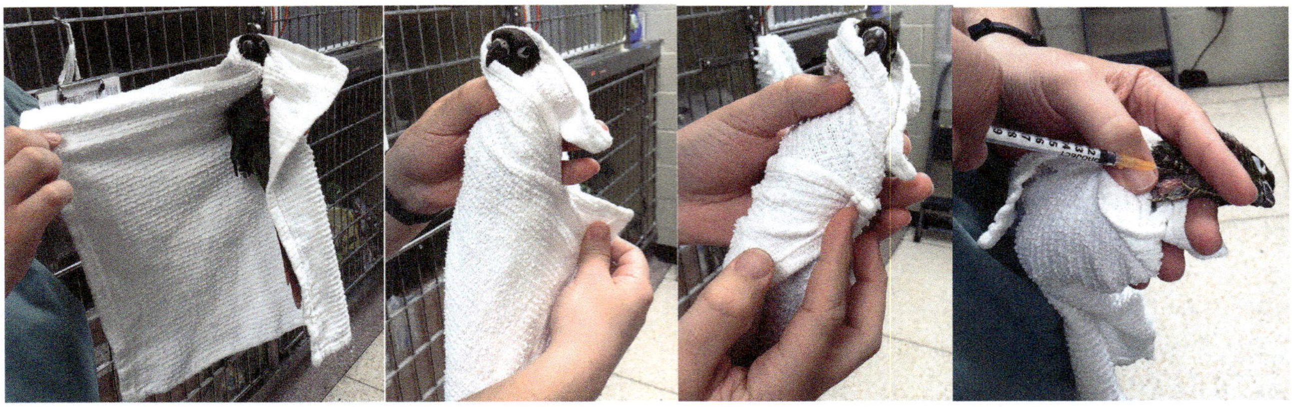

Figure 25.1 Restraint with a towel on a green-cheeked conure (*Pyrrhura molinae*) for venipuncture shown as step-by-step pictures.

cause excess negative pressure, which can lead to the collapse of the vein during phlebotomy. This author has not found differences with the rotation of the bevel during the procedure. However, some clinicians believe that if the needle bevel faces down, it can reduce the frequency of vessel collapse due to negative pressure when aspirating the syringe [1]. When inserting the needle into the vein, it is important to keep it parallel to the vein to limit the likelihood of going through the vessel, especially when the bird struggles. The needle may be slightly bent to facilitate this, while keeping the syringe at a comfortable angle for the phlebotomist. Preheparinization of syringes is not recommended as it will result in over heparinization and dilution of the samples and potentially interfere with hematologic and biochemical values.

In most birds, the right jugular vein is the largest and most easily accessible vein and is commonly used for phlebotomy or for emergency drug administration [5]. The feathers of the neck can be parted with alcohol to expose the jugular apterium where the jugular vein is located. Water or long neck birds such as Anseriformes, Sphenisciformes, Pelecaniformes, Ciconiiformes, Phoenicopteriformes, and Gruiformes may or may not have this featherless tract. Given the size of the animal, the jugular may still be palpated and identified [4]. In some birds, such as penguins, jugular venipuncture is blind. Although the right jugular vein is preferred over the left jugular vein, the left jugular vein is also an acceptable collection site [6]. In smaller species, the jugular vein may be the only site large enough to collect a significant amount of blood for diagnostic testing [7]. For phlebotomy, the animal should be manually restrained in lateral recumbency with the neck extended (Figure 25.2). A single person can perform jugular venipuncture under manual restraint for most birds under 500–700 g and most sedated birds under 1–1.5 kg. An additional person may be needed to perform the restraint for fractious birds and un-sedated larger birds such as macaws. The vein should be occluded with a thumb or forefinger at the level of the thoracic inlet with the skin stretched prior to venipuncture. Supporting the animal's neck on the opposing side will usually help to stabilize the vein. With gentle pressure at the base of the neck, the vein can be raised. Then, a needle should be inserted at a shallow angle for phlebotomy. The phlebotomist should restrain small birds such as passerines and small psittacines with the head between the thumb and forefinger, and the body within the palm. Alternatively, some clinicians prefer a three-point technique with thumb and middle finger supporting the mandible, and the index finger on top of the head [8]. When performing jugular venipuncture in long-necked and water birds, care must be taken to palpate and move the trachea away from venipuncture site [4]. Bruising of the face is possible in large macaws, so only the minimum force necessary to restrict movement should be applied [6]. In some cases, if the cervicocephalic diverticulum of the infraorbital sinus or the esophagus is also punctured, free blood may enter the upper respiratory tract or esophagus and can be visualized as blood in the mouth. An

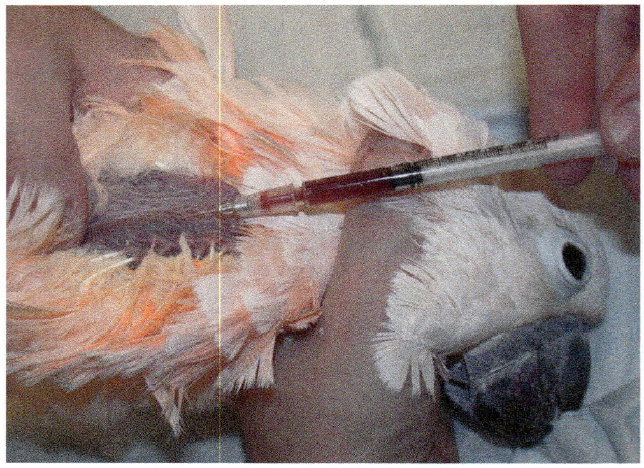

Figure 25.2 Manual restraint and blood collection from a Moluccan cockatoo (*Cacatua moluccensis*). *Source*: Courtesy of Kristina Palmer.

easily distensible subcutaneous space surrounding the jugular vein seems to precipitate hematoma formation. Because of the thin nature of avian skin and the relatively small size of the jugular vein, it is easy to puncture through both walls of the vein and potentially create such a hematoma. To minimize this potential, the authors recommend introducing the needle at a shallow 30° angle. Following phlebotomy, digital pressure should be maintained on the site to reduce the risk of hemorrhage or hematoma formation [1]. Some Columbiformes, such as pigeons, possess a venous plexus (*plexus venosus intracutaneous collaris*) that extends as a web of fine vessels from the cranium to the crop. This vascular network makes jugular venipuncture challenging and the vein difficult to identify [1].

The basilic vein, also called the ulnar vein or wing vein, lies over the medial aspect of the elbow joint (Figure 25.3). Contour feathers often need to be wetted with alcohol or plucked for visualization. Because of the vessel size, basilic venipuncture is usually reserved for medium to large birds when jugular venipuncture is not feasible. It can be a preferred site of blood collection in some species such as birds that lack a jugular apterium, patients who are anesthetized in dorsal recumbency, animals who have recently undergone jugular venipuncture, or for younger birds that resist handling in lateral recumbency for jugular venipuncture [6]. Conscious basilic blood collection usually takes at least two people to restrain the animal. Birds should be wrapped in a towel to secure the legs and the opposite wing that is not being used for venipuncture. They are usually placed on their backs with a wing extended. Great care must be implemented to firmly stabilize the extended wing (at the elbow) and prevent any attempts at wing movement. Digital pressure with the thumb at the proximal humerus will usually help dilate the vein. Using the free hand, a needle should be introduced parallel to where the vein crosses the elbow. Postvenipuncture hematoma formation is common and a longer period of digital pressure is needed for hemostasis (at least 30–120 seconds) [1]. The site should be closely monitored to ensure that all bleeding has stopped. Excessively flapping or poorly restrained patients increase the risk of soft tissue injuries, fractures, and venous lacerations. In most cases, this technique should be reserved for patients under anesthesia, while the patient is not moving. On the other hand, field biologists studying passerine birds commonly perform ulnar venipuncture using the prick technique. However, it is not recommended on pet birds.

The medial metatarsal, or caudal tibial vein, is located along the medial aspect of the tibiotarsus, crosses over the medial aspect of the tarsal joint, and progresses down to the dorsomedial aspect of the foot (Figure 25.4). This location is commonly preferred for Galliformes, Anseriformes, Columbiformes, and Accipitriformes. The vein is raised by

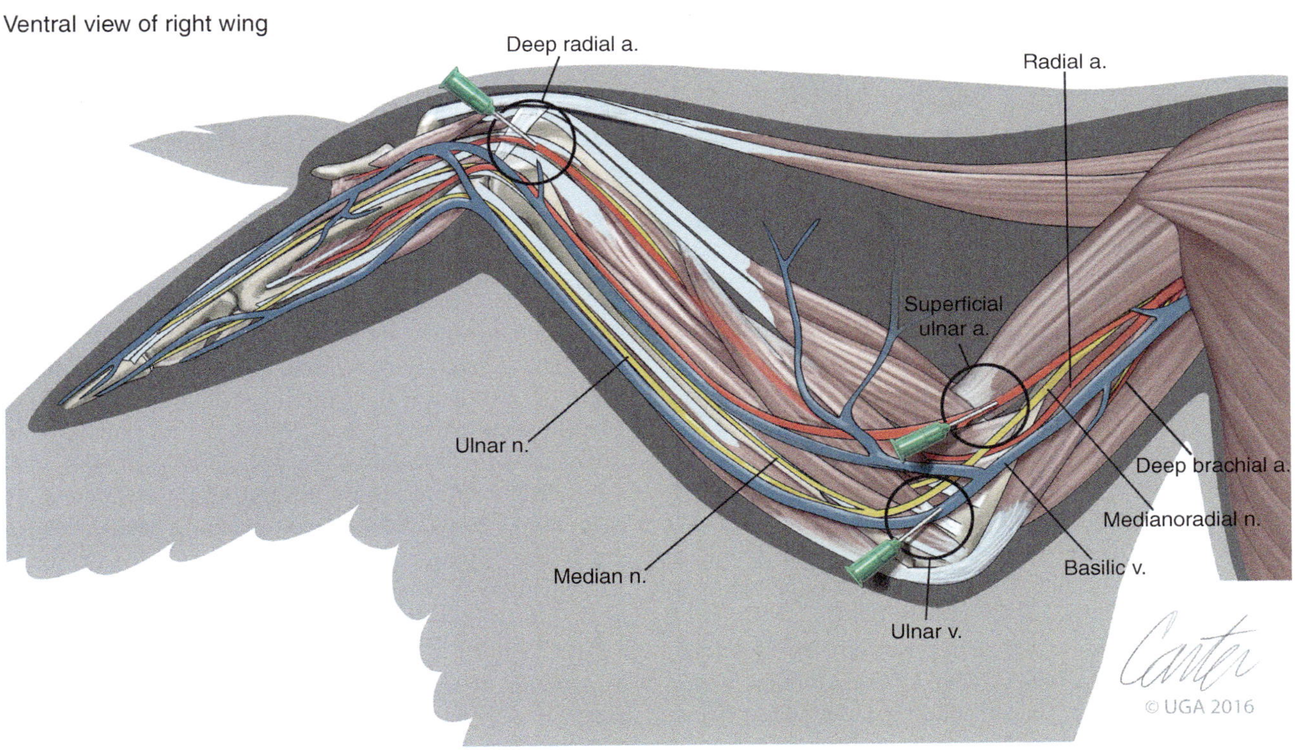

Figure 25.3 Anatomic of location of the ulnar vein and superficial ulnar and deep radial artery of the wing for venous and arterial catheterization and blood collection. *Source*: Illustration by Kip Carter. Reproduced with permission of the University of Georgia.

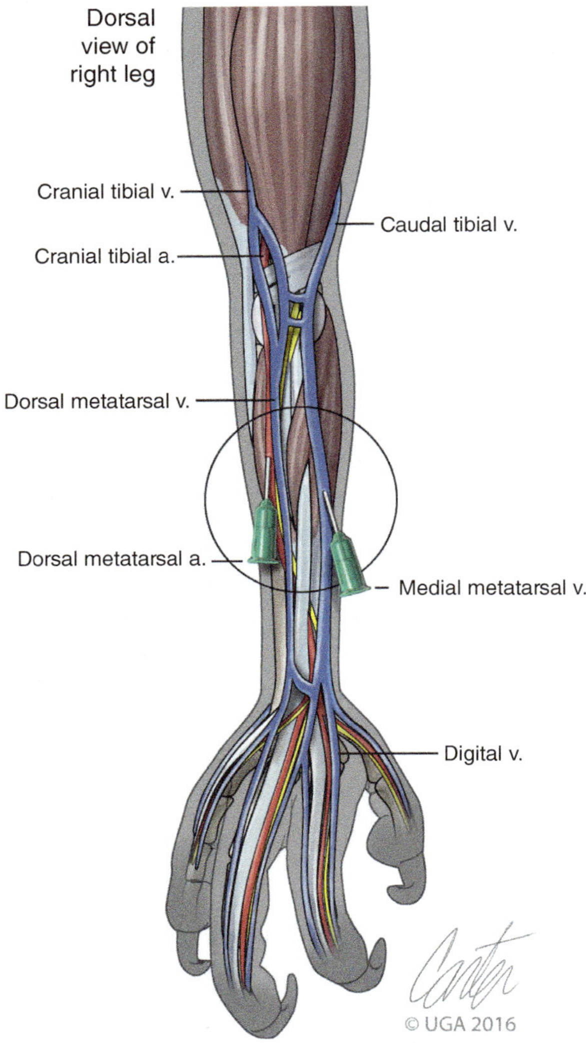

Figure 25.4 Anatomic location of the cranial tibial and metatarsal arteries and metatarsal vein for venous and arterial catheterization and blood collection. *Source*: Illustration by Kip Carter. Reproduced with permission of the University of Georgia.

applying pressure over the medial distal tibiotarsus. The area of venipuncture should be cleaned thoroughly with chlorhexidine and alcohol due to fecal and urate contamination. The medial metatarsal vein is very superficial. Thus, during venipuncture the needle should be introduced at a very shallow angle. Proper manual restraint is necessary to prevent excessive flailing and vascular injuries. Hematomas are less likely to form at this site due to the presence of scaly skin, but hemorrhage often occurs, so prolonged digital pressure or a constrictive dressing is needed temporarily [1].

Although in the past toenail clipping has been used for blood collection, it has been shown to be an unreliable and more painful method of blood collection. Cellular artifacts from microclotting and urofeces or debris have been shown to lead to erroneous results and bacterial contamination of the sample [3].

The occipital sinus has also been historically used for blood collection. However, in the author's opinion, it should only be used as the last resort in birds 40 g or less where vascular access is limited, or in cases of euthanasia. All animals must be anesthetized. Complications and risks of the procedure must be discussed with the owners. [1]

Catheterization

Although avian species present unique challenges due to their anatomic and physiologic differences, similar principles of stabilization used in mammalian species should be applied in emergency situations. Initial evaluation should always be performed to determine mental status, hydration, and cardiovascular and respiratory stability. Administration of fluids at an appropriate rate to rehydrate a patient represents one of most important procedures in emergency medicine (see Nutrition and Fluid Therapy). When patients present for dehydration and/or shock, fluid therapy can be administered by oral, subcutaneous, intravenous, or intraosseous routes. Although multiple methods can be used, selection should be based on level of dehydration, health status of the animal, size, and temperament. Oral and subcutaneous fluid administration is usually reserved for stable patients, with dehydration less than 5%. With severe and critical animals, vascular access should be established to assure intravascular fluid support. Catheter placement can sometimes be difficult in different species, and practice is required to gain the technical skills and finesse that is required to perform this procedure [9]. Magnifying glasses can be used to facilitate catheter placement in small birds.

Intravenous Catheter Placement

The most common catheter sites include the proximal basilic and medial or dorsal metatarsal veins (Figures 25.5–25.7) The jugular vein, although large, is less frequently used due its difficulty to maintain in active patients and the need to immobilize the neck. However, the jugular vein can be used to place vascular access ports. Although avian skin is thin and transparent, it is also strong and pliable. In order to reduce the risk of hematomas and placement failure, a small dermal cut down with the edge of a beveled 22–25-gauge needle should be performed to prevent burring and bending of the catheter. Owing to vessel fragility and the technical difficulty of catheterization, birds should be sedated or anesthetized before catheter placement, except in very lethargic and moribund patients [10]. Like phlebotomy sites, the vein should be visualized by wetting down or plucking the feathers. The area should be aseptically prepared and the catheter should be inserted parallel

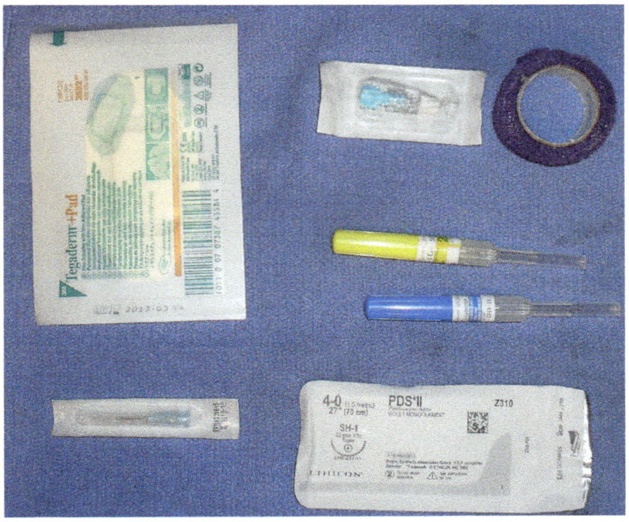

Figure 25.5 Materials needed for arterial and venous catheter placement: a 22, 24-gauge catheter, 25-gauge needle, injection cap, a piece of tegaderm, and suture material.

to the vessel. Before placement, the authors prefer to flush the catheter with heparinized saline to prevent clot formation. The catheter should be inserted into the vein at a steep angle and then flattened against the skin surface parallel with the longitudinal axis of the vein, so that the tip of the needle penetrates the most superficial wall of the vein. Once the catheter has entered the vein, a flash of blood in the hub should be visualized or a change in resistance should be felt. It should then be introduced a few millimeters more, so that the tip of the catheter itself enters the vessel. A T-port or stop cock should be attached to the catheter and the catheter should again be flushed to ensure its patency. Basilic vein catheters should be secured with skin sutures around the hub of the catheter and stop cock [10]. Authors also use a piece of tegaderm to help secure the catheter to the skin and surrounding feathers. If the catheter is intended to remain while the animal is conscious, the catheter should be incorporated into a figure-of-eight bandage and tape guards should be used to distract the animal from chewing on the bandage. The superficial plantar metatarsal (medial metatarsal) vein is useful for catheterization, particularly in birds with longer legs. This vein can also be used in most birds over 300 g and can be seen as it courses along the dorsomedial aspect of the tarsometatarsus. As with all catheterizations, the area should be aseptically prepared and an 18- to 26-gauge over-the-needle catheter should be inserted parallel to the vessel. Compared to other veins, the metatarsal vein is more stable. The tough scaly skin of the feet helps to hold the catheter firmly in place. Catheters should be secured using adhesive tape and a light dressing. For long-term placement, a catheter guard consisting of a plastic syringe cap may be used to protect the catheter [6]. In large palmate birds, interdigital veins may also be used for intravenous (IV) catheterization.

Intraosseous Catheter Placement

Although intravenous access is a standard technique in small animal medicine, it becomes increasingly more demanding with avian patients due to their relatively smaller size. Intraosseous catheterization provides an effective and better alternative when intravenous catheterization becomes difficult, impractical, or the risk of hemorrhage upon removal by the bird is too great. Intraosseous catheterization is a method to gain access to the vascular system by catheterizing the medullary canals of long bones. It is typically well tolerated in most avian patients. It tends to be

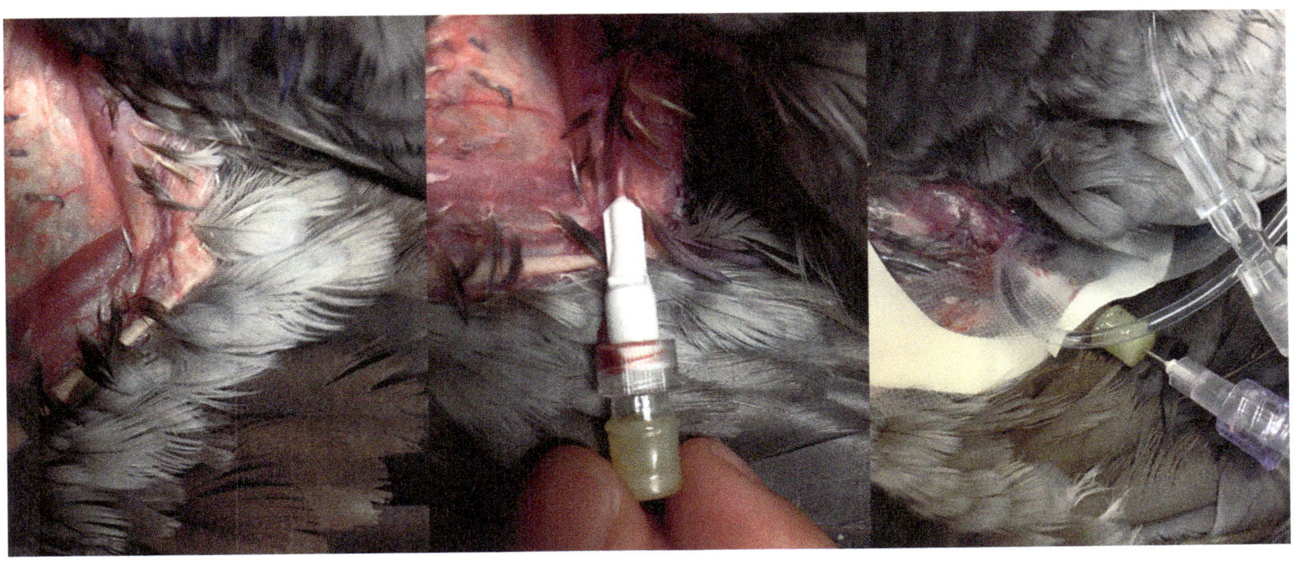

Figure 25.6 Venous catheter placement of the ulnar vein in a grey parrot (*Psittacus erithacus*).

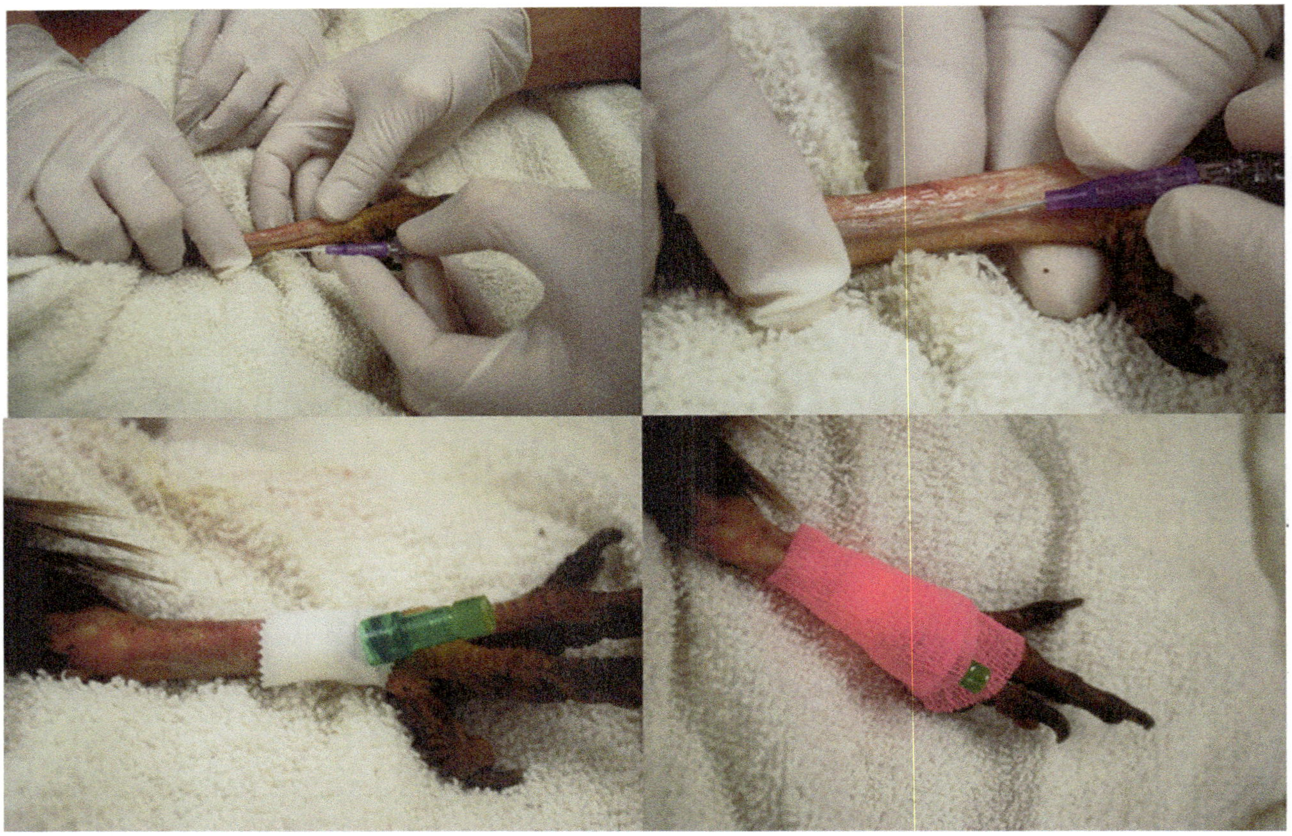

Figure 25.7 Venous catheter placement of the medial metatarsal vein in a domestic chicken (*Gallus gallus domesticus*). *Source*: Courtesy of Joao Brandao.

more advantageous in that it is less challenging to place, maintenance is less problematic, and less dangerous if it accidently removed by the avian patient. It is particularly useful when vascular access is a challenge due to size or when peripheral vasoconstriction or cardiovascular compromise occurs. It is considered the standard of care in small birds weighing less than 60g. Fluids administered into the bone marrow cavity are rapidly absorbed into the systemic circulation. Administration of crystalloid and/or colloidal fluids through the intramedullary cavity has the same efficacy and an equivalent absorption rate as the intravenous route. One study showed that over 50% of the administered intraosseous fluid passes into the central circulation within 30 seconds of it being introduced into the patient. Mild resistance may occur when injecting a large volume which may be minimized by using small-volume syringes or by giving fluids via constant rate infusion with a fluid pump. With regular maintenance and appropriate sterility, intraosseous catheters can be used for up to three days. Complications such as iatrogenic fractures may occur and placement is not advisable in osteoporotic birds.

The distal ulna or proximal tibiotarsal bone is commonly used for intraosseous catheter placement (Figures 25.8 and 25.9). Pneumatic bones, such as the humerus, and in some birds, the femur, should not be used with intraosseous fluids as their use can lead to air sacculitis, pneumonia, or asphyxiation. In some birds such as members of the order Cathartiformes and potentially some Pelecaniformes, the ulna is a pneumatized bone and should not be catheterized. Similar techniques used for introducing intraosseous catheters in small mammal medicine are applicable to avian species. Depending on the size of the animal, 20-, 22-, and 25-gauge, 1 to 1-, and 1/2-in. spinal needles should be used with a stylet to prevent bone from obstructing the needle (Figure 25.10). However, if these needles are not available or the animal size is too small for a spinal needle, hypodermic needles may be used. If the needle becomes occluded, appropriately sized sterilized cerclage wire can be inserted into the needle to remove the obstruction. Insertion of intraosseous catheters tends to be painful and stressful and often necessitates anesthesia for placement, except in moribund birds [5].

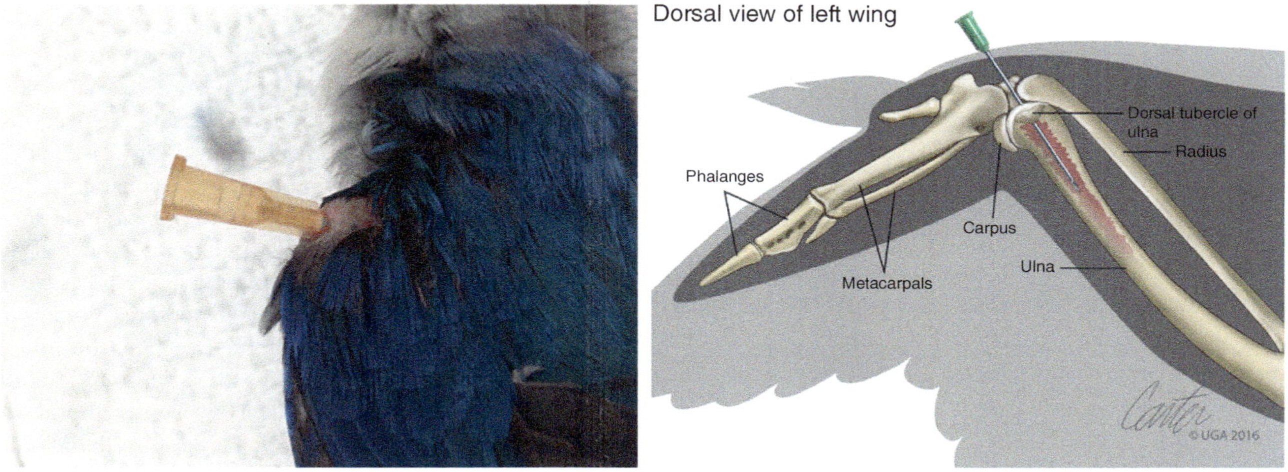

Figure 25.8 Intraosseous catheter in the distal ulna of a lovebird (*Agapornis roseicollis*). *Source*: Illustration by Kip Carter. Reproduced with permission of the University of Georgia.

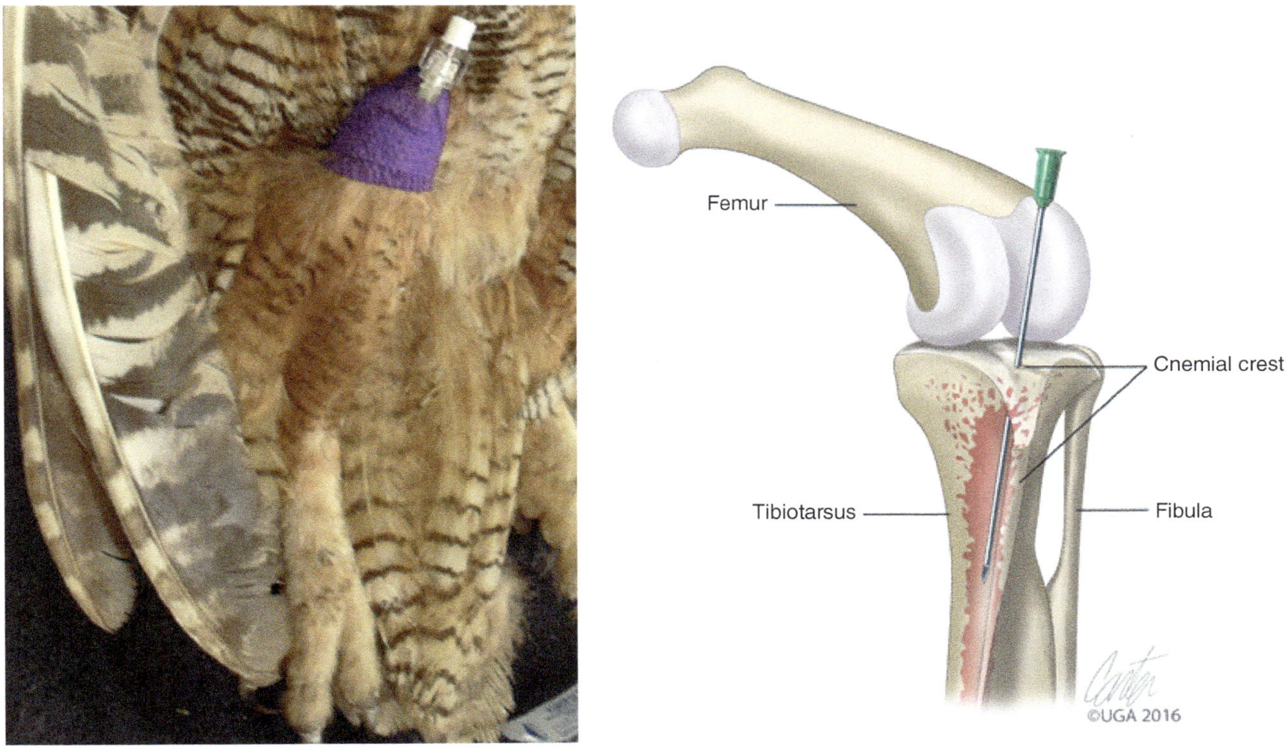

Figure 25.9 Intraosseous catheterization of the proximal tibiotarsus in a great horned owl (*Bubo virginianus*). *Source*: Illustration by Kip Carter. Reproduced with permission of the University of Georgia.

For placement of ulnar intraosseous catheters, the dorsal tubercle of the distal ulna should be located and palpated and the manus slightly pronated. The feathers should be plucked over this area and the area aseptically prepared for better visualization of the landmark. Lidocaine may be used to block the skin and periosteum over the site. Grasping the ulna between the fingers of one hand, the spinal needle is situated over the distal ulna and directed between the fingers holding the ulna. With a small amount of pressure, the needle is rotated through the cortex of the bone, slowly working the needle along the medullary canal until it is seated. Patency then should be tested with a small amount of saline [9]. Upon injection, the ulnar vein should blanch as the fluid passes through the vasculature. Catheter confirmation can be determined by radiographs

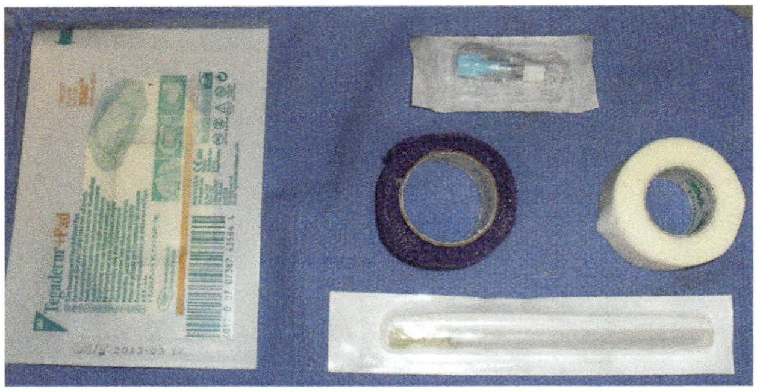

Figure 25.10 Materials needed for intraosseus catheter placement: a spinal needle, injection cap, a piece of tegaderm, vet wrap, and tape.

(lateral and anterior/posterior views) or by palpation with similar movement of the needle with the bone. It can be secured by butterfly taping or by suturing it to the skin. The movement of the wing can cause the perforation of the catheter in the bone to widen which can lead to fluid leakage. For long-term intraosseous placement, a figure-of-eight wing bandage should be used to minimize wing movement.

Another common site for intraosseous catheterization is the proximal tibiotarsus. With catheterization, the leg should be extended and flexed at the knee. The cnemial crest should be palpated at the cranial and proximal portion of the tibiotarsus, and the area should be plucked and aseptically prepared. The needle should then be slowly introduced in a cranio-medial direction into the cnemial crest at the insertion of the patellar tendon taking care to avoid this tendon. Once through the cortical bone, the catheter should slide in easily into the medullary cavity. Patency can be confirmed through radiographs with two different views, injecting of a small amount of fluid, or by palpation. A padded bandage or lateral splint can be placed to stabilize the catheter [10].

Arterial Catheter Placement

In veterinary medicine, there are typically two techniques available for measuring blood pressure: invasive and noninvasive methods. Invasive techniques require an arterial catheter. Noninvasive techniques include Doppler, photoplethysmographic/photoacoustic probes with a sphygmomanometer, and oscillometric monitors. In previous studies, noninvasive techniques have been reported to be inaccurate in measuring blood pressure in birds when compared with invasive blood pressure monitoring [11]. The technique using a Doppler unit and a sphygmomanometer has shown to vary in reliability, being more reliable in large birds. However, oscillometric units have consistently shown to be unreliable and should not be used in birds.

Unlike domestic mammals, there are only a few placement sites available for arterial catheterization in birds. For medium to large birds, the deep radial artery is the preferred site. However, for smaller birds the authors favor catheterization of the superficial ulnar artery. For water birds or long-legged birds, the cranial tibial or dorsal metatarsal arteries are acceptable choices for catheterization. Catheterization of the external carotid artery has also been described in birds, but it is usually more invasive and requires a cut down procedure for proper visualization [12].

The authors prefer the deep radial artery to the other sites for arterial catheterization because of its minimal mobility. The deep radial artery lies just between the tendons of the *extensor digitorum longus* and the *flexor digitorum profundus* in the distal wing of most birds. Catheter placement should occur where the artery is most superficial at the radial carpal bone or at the distal head of the ulna (Figure 25.11). At this location, the deep radial artery can be readily found and palpated on the medial side of the wing. At a more proximal location, the artery dips deeper and

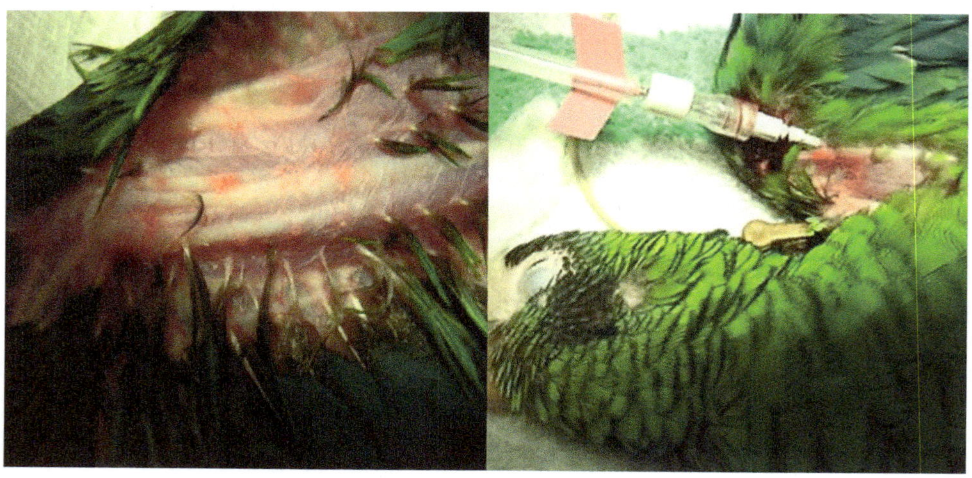

Figure 25.11 Catheter placement of deep radial artery in a Hispaniolan Amazon parrot (*Amazona ventralis*).

runs along the radius. Proximal placement of the catheter becomes more reliant on palpation skills of the veterinarian as the artery becomes less visible. Moreover, with a more proximal placement, additional care is required during catheter insertion because of the close association of the deep radial artery with the median nerve. The superficial ulnar artery, along with the recurrent ulnar artery, branches off from the ulnar artery at the elbow. The superficial ulnar artery then runs medially over the *extensor metacarpi radialis*, *pronator superficialis*, and *pronator profundus* muscles before dipping along the ulna and crossing the carpus and terminating at the base of the distal phalanx of the major digit. Although more prominent in size, the superficial ulnar artery is very mobile and crosses the elbow, thus increasing the technical difficulty of placement without inducing hematoma. Furthermore, owing to the wing's unique anatomy, securing the catheter at this location can also be problematic [12].

The cranial tibial artery is the major vascular supply to the lower leg and its digits. As the artery dorsolaterally crosses the hock, it becomes the metatarsal artery, which then travels medially across the tarsometatarsus. The artery is more prominent and easier to visualize and palpate in long-legged birds. As the artery moves distally, catheterization becomes more problematic because of the keratinized scales on the bird's legs. As most bird scales do not significantly overlap, catheterization may be attempted between scutes. The cranial tibial and metatarsal artery offer advantages over other locations recommended for arterial catheterization in that the leg arteries are much easier to secure and maintain once placed. Care must be taken when inserting the catheter into either the cranial tibial artery or the metatarsal artery; it should not be placed too close to the tarsal joint, as movement of the leg may cause positional occlusion leading to inconsistent readings. Owing to vessel fragility and the technical difficulty of catheterization, all birds should be anesthetized before catheter placement [12].

For the superficial ulnar and deep radial artery, patients should be positioned in dorsal recumbency with their wings extended. The insertion site should be aseptically prepared and the catheter should be flushed with heparinized saline (1 U/ml). Without entering the artery, a relief hole or cut down should be made completely through the dermis with a beveled edge of a hypodermic needle just distal to where the arteries are readily palpated. Arterial location can be confirmed by applying a Doppler transducer over the site and listening for the pulse. Once the artery is palpated and mentally traced, the catheter should be subcutaneously positioned, superficial to the artery. The catheter needs to be inserted into the artery at a steep angle and then flattened against the skin surface parallel with the longitudinal axis of the artery, so that the tip of the needle penetrates the most superficial wall of the artery. As both arteries are very superficial, the catheter should be very slowly inserted, watching carefully for blood within the catheter. The catheter then can be gently advanced off the stylet to its full length, and the stylet removed. Advancement should be smooth with little or no resistance. Unless the patient is extremely hypotensive, pulsatile blood flow should be noted from the catheter once the needle stylet has been removed. Owing to the size of these animals, care must be taken to avoid blood loss and a heparin overdose. The authors have had limited success using adhesive tape to securing both the deep radial or superficial catheters. For temporary anesthetic placement, tissue glue and/or clear adherent adhesive dressing may be used; for conscious animals, the catheter should be sutured in place and incorporated into a figure-of-eight bandage. Bandaging material should be carefully selected to readily reveal if bleeding occurs due to catheter dislodgement. However, consideration must be made if the catheter is placed in the avian wing. If the transducer is too close to the patient, its weight may act as a fulcrum and dislodge the catheter [12].

For the cranial tibial or metatarsal artery, catheterization can be performed with the animal in ventral or lateral recumbency while caudally extending its leg. After the insertion site is properly prepared, the thumb and middle finger of one hand locate the artery and the leading edge of the same hand can be used to stabilize catheter placement. Once placed, however, the catheter is best secured with white adhesive tape. After the arterial catheter has been successfully placed and secured, it can be connected and operated as in other species.

Arterial catheterization is generally considered a safe and useful technique that is associated with few serious complications. Around-the-clock supervision is imperative for the management to ensure that an animal does not endanger itself by pulling out its catheter. Circumstances permitting, the authors rarely keep avian arterial lines in place for more than 12 hours. In addition to iatrogenic hemorrhage, there is an increased risk of infection, thromboembolism, and hematoma formation associated with long-term arterial catheter usage. Moreover, frequent administration of heparin can lead to iatrogenic coagulation abnormalities, especially in smaller patients. Sepsis is also more prevalent when local inflammation is present. Although rare, other complications such as cellulitis, abscess formation, temporary occlusion of the artery, nerve paralysis, suppurative thromboarteritis, arteriovenous fistulas, and pseudoaneurysm have been reported in domestic animals. Fluids and medications should never be administered via the arterial catheter because of the potential risk of vascular damage and subsequent tissue necrosis [13]. After removing the catheter, pressure should be applied over the insertion site with dry cotton swabs or gauze. It usually takes three to five minutes for complete hemostasis after catheter removal. Patients should be monitored until no bleeding is observed.

Protective Devices

Catheter maintenance may be difficult, especially if the bird is prone to chew at the site and may require the placement of a mechanical barrier to prevent self-trauma. Sectioned syringe cases or dental acrylics may be used to protect the area. Anti-siphon valve (NP medical) may be connected to the catheter to prevent blood loss from sectioning the IV line. However, anti-siphon valves will not reduce blood loss if the bird removes its catheter. Bandages around the catheter area can be modified to include tape tabs to serve as a distraction. A restraint collar may also be necessary, but may add to the stress of an already critical patient.

Normal Arterial Blood Pressure in Birds

Multiple studies on avian arterial blood pressure measurements have demonstrated that arterial blood pressure in most avian species is significantly higher than mammals [11, 14–19]. However, there have only been a few studies in birds that have determined the correlation between measured blood pressure values and the inhibition and autoregulation of the vascular system. A study performed on anesthetized Galliformes comparing glomerular filtration rate and blood pressure found that Galliformes were able to maintain their glomerular filtration rate when mean arterial pressure (MAP) ranged between 60 and 110 mmHg [20]. When MAP decreased to less than 50 mmHg, chickens were unable to sustain glomerular filtration and urine output ceased. Unlike chickens that have normal systolic, mean, and diastolic arterial blood pressures of 99 ± 13, 84 ± 13, and 69 ± 5 mmHg, respectively, values for normotension are higher in Psittaciformes, Gruiformes, Falconiformes, Accipitriformes, Strigiformes, and other Galliformes (e.g. turkeys) [18, 21] (Table 25.1). In Hispaniolan Amazon parrots anesthetized with 2.5% isoflurane, the systolic, mean, and diastolic arterial blood pressures were 132.9 ± 22.1, 116.9 ± 20.5, and 101.9 ± 22.0 mmHg, respectively [22]. Additionally, most baseline avian blood pressure values are obtained from birds under anesthesia, where materials such as inhalant gases can cause significant depressant effects and can alter arterial blood pressure, either through reduction in systemic vascular resistance or a reduction in cardiac output. Therefore, avian blood pressure measurement and monitoring have to be interpreted in this context and with the reference values corresponding to measurement conditions.

Table 25.1 Previous published direct blood pressure (DBP) values in avian species.

Species	SAP ± SD	MAP ± SD	DAP ± SD	Experimental methods	References
Chicken	99 ± 13	84 ± 13	69 ± 15	Sevoflurane	Naganobu et al. [20]
Pigeon	93 ± 10	82 ± 14	72 ± 13	Isoflurane	Touzot-Jourde et al. (2005)
	88 ± 11	75 ± 10	60 ± 11	Isoflurane	Touzot-Jourde et al. (2005)
Sandhill crane		205 ± 29		1× MAC isoflurane	Ludders et al. [19]
Cockatoo		143 ± 4		Isoflurane	Curro et al. (1994)
Amazon parrots	163 ± 18	155 ± 18	148 ± 18	2% Isoflurane	Acierno et al. [11]
	132.9 ± 22	116.9 ± 20.5	101.9 ± 22.0	2.5% Isoflurane	Schnellbacher et al. [22]
Great horned owl	232 ± 37	203 ± 28	178 ± 25	Baseline awake values	Hawkins et al. [14]
Red-tailed hawk	220 ± 51	187 ± 42	160 ± 45	Baseline awake values	Hawkins et al. [14]
Bald eagle	194 ± 13		158 ± 13*	Isoflurane	Joyner et al. [16]
	146 ± 13		135 ± 13*	Sevoflurane	Joyner et al. [16]

Mean ± SD values for systolic arterial pressure (SAP), mean arterial pressure (MAP), and diastolic arterial pressure (DAP) are presented.

Birds

References

1 Kramer, M.H. and Harris, D.J. (2010). Avian blood collection. *J. Exot. Pet Med.* 19 (1): 82–86.

2 Mans, C., Guzman, D.S., Lahner, L.L. et al. (2012). Sedation and physiologic response to manual restraint after intranasal administration of midazolam in Hispaniolan Amazon parrots (Amazona ventralis). *J. Avian Med. Surg.* 26 (3): 130–139.

3 Beaufrere, H. and Ammersbach, M. (2016). Variability and limitations in clinical avian hematology. In: *Current Therapy in Avian Medicine and Surgery* (ed. B. Speer), 467–485. Elsevier.

4 MacLean, R.A. and Beaufrère, H. (2015). Gruiformes (cranes, limpkins, rails, gallinules, coots, bustards). In: *Fowler's Zoo and Wild Animal Medicine*, vol. 8 (eds. R.E. Miller and M.E. Fowler), 155–165.

5 de Matos, R. and Morrisey, J.K. (2005). Emergency and critical care of small psittacines and passerines. *Semi. Avian. Exot. Pet Med.* 14 (2): 90–105.

6 Quesenberry, K.E. and Hillyer, E.V. (1994). Supportive care and emergency therapy. In: *Avian Medicine: Principles and Application* (eds. B.W. Ritchie, G.J. Harrison and L.R. Harrison), 382–416. Wingers Publishing.

7 Kerlin, R.E. (1964). Venipuncture of small birds. *J. Am. Vet. Med. Assoc.* 144: 870.

8 Low, A. (2012). Practical avian venipuncture: how to take blood from birds. *Vet. Nurs. J.* 3 (7): 446–448.

9 Briscoe, J.A. and Syring, R. (2004). Techniques for emergency airway and vascular access in special species. *Semi. Avian. Exot. Pet Med.* 13 (3): 118–131.

10 Dubé, C., Dubois, I., and Struthers, J. (2011). Intravenous and intraosseous fluid therapy in critically ill birds of prey. *J. Exot. Pet. Med.* 20 (1): 21–26.

11 Acierno, M.J., Da Cunha, A., Smith, J. et al. (2008). Agreement between direct and indirect blood pressure measurements obtained from anesthetized Hispaniolan Amazon parrots. *J. Am. Vet. Med. Assoc.* 233 (10): 1587–1590.

12 Schnellbacher, R., da Cunha, A., Olson, E.E., and Mayer, J. (2014). Arterial catheterization, interpretation, and treatment of arterial blood pressures and blood gases in birds. *J. Exot. Pet Med.* 23 (2): 129–141.

13 Hall, L.W., Clarke, K.W., and Trim, C.M. (2001). Patient monitoring and clinical measurement. In: *Veterinary Anaesthesia* (ed. J.G. Adams), 29–57.

14 Hawkins, M.G., Wright, B.D., Pascoe, P.J. et al. (2003). Pharmacokinetics and anesthetic and cardiopulmonary effects of propofol in red-tailed hawks (Buteo jamaicensis) and great horned owls (Bubo virginianus). *Am. J. Vet. Res.* 64 (6): 677–683.

15 Goelz, M.F., Hahn, A.W., and Kelley, S.T. (1990). Effects of halothane and isoflurane on mean arterial blood pressure, heart rate, and respiratory rate in adult Pekin ducks. *Am. J. Vet. Res.* 51 (3): 458–460.

16 Joyner, P.H., Jones, M.P., Ward, D. et al. (2008). Induction and recovery characteristics and cardiopulmonary effects of sevoflurane and isoflurane in bald eagles. *Am. J. Vet. Res.* 69 (1): 13–22.

17 Lichtenberger, M. (2007). Emergency and critical care. *Vet. Clin. North Am. Exot. Anim. Pract.* 10 (2): 275–712.

18 Lichtenberger, M. (2005). Determination of indirect blood pressure in the companion bird. *Semi. Avian. Exot. Pet Med.* 14 (2): 149–152. WB Saunders.

19 Ludders, J.W., Rode, J., and Mitchell, G.S. (1989). Isoflurane anesthesia in sandhill cranes (Grus canadensis): minimal anesthetic concentration and cardiopulmonary dose-response during spontaneous and controlled breathing. *Anesth. Analg.* 68 (4): 511–516.

20 Naganobu, K., Fujisawa, Y., Ohde, H. et al. (2000). Determination of the minimum anesthetic concentration and cardiovascular dose response for sevoflurane in chickens during controlled ventilation. *Vet. Surg.* 29 (1): 102–105.

21 Fricke, C., Schmidt, V., Cramer, K. et al. (2009). Characterization of atherosclerosis by histochemical and immunohistochemical methods in African grey parrots (*Psittacus erithacus*) and Amazon parrots (*Amazona* spp.). *Avian Dis.* 53 (3): 466–472.

22 Schnellbacher, R.W., Da Cunha, A.F., Beaufrère, H. et al. (2012). Effects of dopamine and dobutamine on isoflurane-induced hypotension in Hispaniolan Amazon parrots (Amazona ventralis). *Am. J. Vet. Res.* 73 (7): 952–958.

26

Wound Care and Bandaging Techniques

Anna Martel and Christoph Mans

Department of Surgical Sciences, School of Veterinary Medicine, University of Wisconsin–Madison, Madison, Wisconsin, USA

CONTENTS

Introduction

Injuries or trauma are common reasons for avian patients to present as emergencies. Whether due to an attack by animal (dog, cat, or bird), owner-induced trauma (e.g. stepped on), cage-related trauma (stuck between bars, hooked to toy, etc.), or self-mutilation, soft tissue injuries, and bone and joint trauma should be appropriately diagnosed and treated.

Initial Wound Assessment and Management

Pet birds are prey species and therefore of a more delicate nature than dogs and cats. Care must be taken to minimize stress and evaluate the whole patient prior to initiation of treatment. Staged examination, sedation, and/or supplemental oxygenation may be required to safely examine and treat the avian patient. Blood loss should also be considered during the evaluation (due to the small size of some avian patients), and patients may need to be supplemented with fluid therapy as needed to restore volume. Blood transfusion should be considered if blood loss is severe. Because avian skin is very thin and fragile, it is common for fractures to be open, in particular fractures of the humerus, antebrachium, and distal to the stifle. Antibiotic therapy is indicated for all contaminated or infected wounds or may be considered as a prophylactic measure if the risk of wound infection exists. Self-mutilation is also common after injury, and some species are more likely to self-mutilate (e.g. Quaker parrots and cockatoos). Due to the small size of pet birds, care must be taken that the applied bandages, wound dressings, or splints are of appropriate size and weight, and do not interfere negatively with food intake, ambulation, and other normal behaviors. Further, bandages, sutures, and splints may be manipulated by birds, using their beaks, and therefore, placement of an e-collar is often necessary. Ensuring proper adjustment to the e-collar prior to discharge from the hospital is critical. Sufficient food and water intake should be witnessed while the e-collar is in place. Birds wearing e-collars should be prevented from climbing, due to the risk of falling and inflicting further injury. Therefore, maintaining birds with e-collars in smooth-walled enclosures (e.g. plastic tubs and boxes) is recommended.

Because of the presence of air sacs in the coelom and direct communication of the pneumatized humerus and femurs with the air sacs, great care should be taken when lavaging coelomic wounds and open humeral and femoral fractures. Air sacs are present throughout the entire coelom, and lavage with fluids is contraindicated with coelomic wounds that have penetrated an air sac. If it cannot

Exotic Animal Emergency and Critical Care Medicine, First Edition. Edited by Jennifer E. Graham, Grayson A. Doss and Hugues Beaufrère.

be established if an air sac has been entered, lavage should not be performed and instead gentle cleansing with moistened gauze (either with sterile saline and/or an antiseptic agent) is recommended. Antibiotics are indicated for all wounds entering the coelom or open fractures. Systemic antifungal treatment is also recommended as prophylaxis, in particular in species prone to development of respiratory fungal infections (e.g. African gray parrots, pionus parrots, and waterfowl). When applying a body wrap or bandage, the ability to breathe can be easily compromised if the bandage is too tight and constricts the keel. Because birds do not possess a diaphragm, any body wrap which restricts free movement of the keel can restrict respirations and lead to significant respiratory distress in the avian patient.

Initial Wound Assessment

Most wounds are preferably assessed with the patient under sedation, in order to minimize manual restraint-induced stress and to provide analgesia. Combination of midazolam (2–4 mg/kg) and butorphanol (2–3 mg/kg) administered intramuscular or intranasal provide sedation, anxiolysis, and analgesia. Meloxicam (1–1.5 mg/kg IM, SC, PO q12–24h) can be administered to provide longer-lasting pain relief and anti-inflammatory action, since butorphanol requires very frequent administration (q2–4h). Ensure proper hydration prior to administration of meloxicam. Once sedation and analgesia have been induced, assessment and cleaning of the wound should be performed. The feathers may be cut away from the wound or carefully plucked. Feathers that are cut will take longer to regrow (until the next molt cycle). Gross debris should be removed manually. Lavage is the most effective way to reduce bacterial counts. However, as stated previously, this is contraindicated with air sac penetration or open fractures of the humerus or femur. Debridement of non-vital tissue should be performed as indicated, similar to mammalian patients.

Wound Management

Similar considerations as in mammals guide wound management decisions in avian patients. If the wound is fresh, has not been caused by a predator (e.g. dog/cat) bite, and there is limited contamination, the wound may be closed, following thorough cleaning, with sutures or surgical glue as appropriate. An extensive wound may also be partially closed if skin tension is an issue. Delayed closure should be considered with cases of extensive tissue damage and necrosis. Management of a contaminated wound with an open technique is commonly recommended for avian patients. Birds form granulation tissue quickly and can heal well by second intention.

Superficial Wounds

Most superficial wounds can be managed with cleaning, a layer of topical antimicrobial (such as silver sulfadiazine cream, triple antibiotic ointment), a non-adherent pad, and a transparent adhesive film (e.g. Tegaderm, 3M, St. Paul, MN). Follow-up should be scheduled in two to three days for re-assessment and bandage change.

Full Thickness Wounds

Larger or deeper tissue wounds require additional, more extensive bandaging with more frequent re-assessment and bandage changes. Drains are generally not used in birds, since wound exudates are typically not a concern. Options for dressing for deeper or more extensive wounds include placing suture as tie-over loops on the periphery of the wound (Figure 26.1). Umbilical tape is commonly used to hold bandages in place using the tie-over loops, especially in larger birds including chickens, waterfowl, and large parrots.

Wet-to-dry bandaging may be considered with extensive necrotic tissue, but are rarely used in birds due to the high frequency of changes required and bulkiness. Honey and sugar bandages can also be used for infected wounds, but patient size and wound location are often limiting factors. Deeper wounds should be filled with a material hydrogel or hydrocolloid. Several sustained-release ionic silver hydrogel products are available as gels and sheets and are used

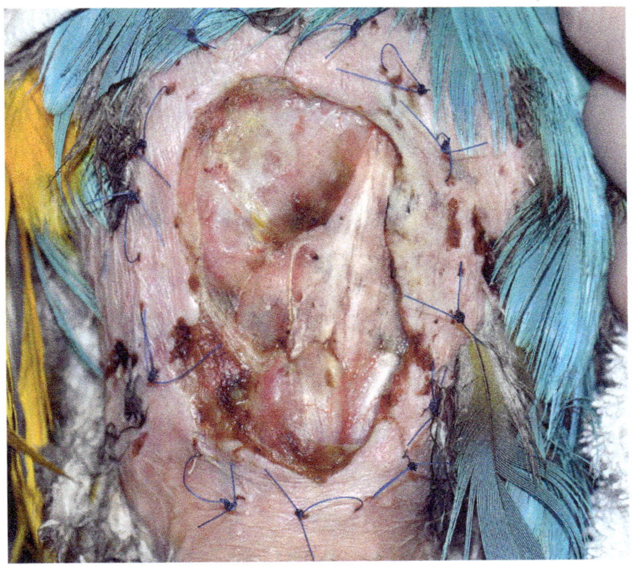

Figure 26.1 Full-thickness wound in a macaw over the back. Note the loops of suture placed along the periphery of the wound, which allow the use of umbilical tape to tie down wound dressing material.

frequently for soft tissue wounds by the authors (Figure 26.2). The prolonged antimicrobial action of these products allows for less frequent bandage changes, which minimize stress and discomfort for the avian patient, and allows for many patients to be managed on an outpatient basis.

Bite Wounds

All bite wounds inflicted by dogs or cats are considered infected wounds, regardless or the age of the wound, and should be treated aggressively, since the risk for sepsis is high in birds. Systemic administration of broad-spectrum antibiotics is critical and the antibiotics should have a broad coverage against gram-negative bacteria (e.g. *Pasteurella* sp. and *Pseudomonas* sp.) as well as anaerobic bacteria (Table 26.1). Enrofloxacin, while often prescribed in avian patients, is an inappropriate choice if given alone, since it does not have any activity against anaerobic bacteria. Injectable antibiotics are recommended for initial therapy and the patient should remain hospitalized for observation and treatment. Bites inflicted by other pet birds (usually parrots) are less of a concern, since the risk of contamination of the wound with pathogenic bacteria is much lower.

External Coaptation of Fractures

External coaptation of fractures of the wings and legs can be used as a temporary measure to stabilize fractures until further assessment and potentially surgical stabilization is performed or it can be used as the definitive treatment for many types of fractures, particularly in small birds. Specific recommendations for fracture stabilization in avian patients can be found in Table 26.2. Most uncomplicated

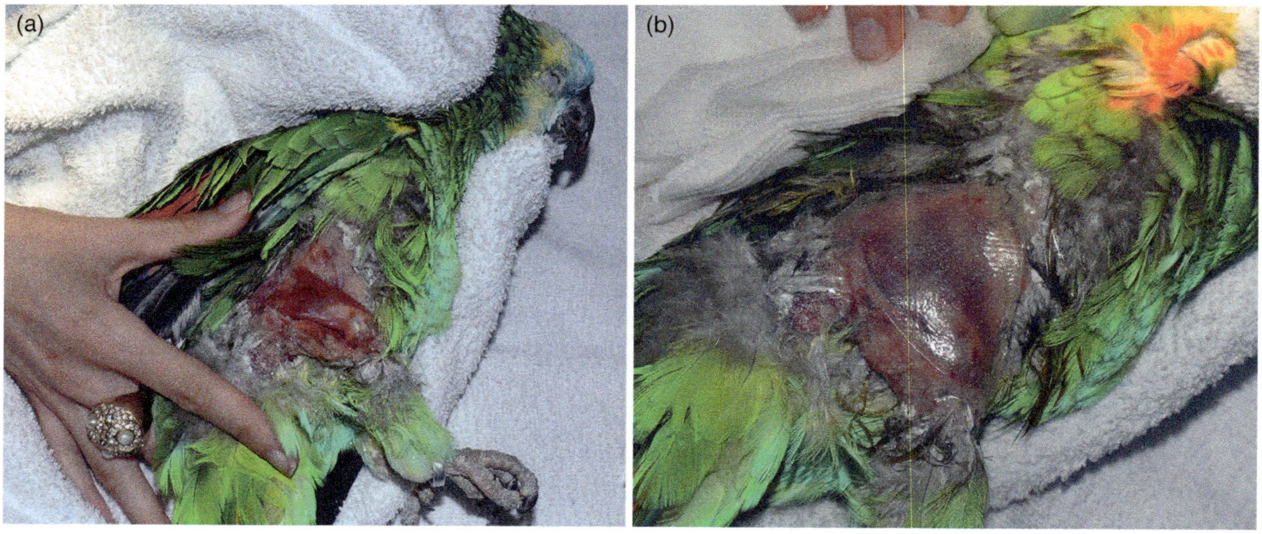

Figure 26.2 (a) Full-thickness traumatic wound of the right lateral thigh area in a parrot. (b) A sustained-release silver hydrogel sheet was applied to the wound following lavage. An adherent clear film bandage has been placed over the hydrogel sheet.

Table 26.1 Recommended antibiotics for birds with bite wounds inflicted by predators (i.e. dogs, cats, ferrets, wild carnivores).

Drug	Dosage	Frequency	Comment
Piperacillin/Tazobactam	100–200 mg/kg IM, IV	q6–12h	
Ticarcillin/Clavulanic acid	100–200 mg/kg IM, IV	q4–12h	PD Amazon parrot, 100 mg/kg IM q2–4 h
Enrofloxacin	25 mg/kg SC (diluted), IV, PO	q24 h	Not in waterfowl or poultry, always combine with antibiotic which provides coverage against anaerobic bacteria (e.g. penicillins and metronidazole)
Metronidazole	30–50 mg/kg IM, PO	q12 h	Not in waterfowl or poultry, always combine with antibiotic which provides coverage against aerobic bacteria (enrofloxacin)
Trimethoprim/ Sulfonamide	30 mg/kg PO	q12 h	Poor coverage against Pseudomonas and anaerobic bacteria

Table 26.2 Recommended treatment for common fractures in birds.

Type of fracture	External coaptation	Surgical treatment
Coracoid, clavicle, scapula	Body wrap[a], or cage rest only	Not recommended
Humerus	Body wrap[a]	IM pinning +/− external fixation
Radius, ulna, metacarpus	Figure of 8[a]	IM pinning +/− external fixator
Femur	Ehmer sling (foot sling) or no coaptation	IM pinning +/− external fixator
Tibiotarsus	<200 g: tape splint >200 g: tape splint enforced with syringe case, etc., or Robert-Jones bandage	IM pinning +/− external fixator
Phalanges	Shoe bandage or ball bandage	

[a] Physical therapy of the wing under sedation or anesthesia is recommended every five to seven days.

fractures in birds are stable within three weeks, if properly immobilized. Therefore, most splints and bandages can be removed after three weeks.

Bandages and splints in birds should be lightweight and avoid bulk as much as possible. Materials frequently used for bandages and splints in mammals, such as cast padding and stretch gauze wrap, should be avoided when possible in avian patients, in order to minimize the bulkiness of the bandage. Elastic bandages (e.g. Vetwrap), non-adherent pads (Telfa, Medline Industries, Inc., Mundelein, Illinois), adhesive films (Tegaderm, 3M, St. Paul, MN), and different tapes are most frequently used. Materials can be cut to size in order to more appropriate for smaller avian patients

Immediately after applying any bandage, the bird should be observed for a period of time to determine whether an e-collar is necessary. It may take some time for the bird to become accustomed to the bandage. The bird should not be discharged until after becoming accustomed to the bandage and before the need for an e-collar is determined. Maintaining mild sedation often helps birds to adjust to the placed bandages or splints.

External Coaptation: Wing

Body Wrap

Body wrap (Figure 26.3e,f) is indicated for treatment of fractures of the shoulder girdle and humeral fractures. The equivalent of this bandaging technique is an arm sling in humans, and it should be kept in mind when applying this bandage. The primary purpose is to stabilize the shoulder joint and humeral fractures. If open wounds are present, then they should be managed as described above and covered prior to applying further bandaging material. While the placement of a figure-of-eight bandage was previously recommended in addition to the body wrap, a body wrap alone is now the preferred option. The figure-of-eight bandage tends to further distract humeral fracture fragments and leads to patagial tendon contraction toward the fracture site (Julia Ponder, 2020, personal communication). Likewise, for fractures of the bones of the shoulder girdle, it does not provide additional stability when compared to a body wrap alone. For the body wrap, either elastic bandage or silk tape can be used. As stated previously, with any body wrap in a bird, the bandage must allow free movement of the keel in order to prevent any respiratory difficulty.

Figure of 8 Bandage

Figure of 8 bandage (Figure 26.3a–d) is indicated for fractures of the bones distal to the elbow. Cast padding is not usually applied, in order to limit the bulkiness of the bandage. Instead, an elastic bandage material (e.g. Vetwrap) is applied to the wing in the figure 8 pattern (Figure 26.3); however, the bird should be monitored closely to ensure it does not tighten the bandage and create a tourniquet affect if cast padding is omitted under this layer. This process may take a few trials in order to support the wing in a neutral, stable position without creating too much weight or bulk to the wing. The bandage should be placed initially on the distal antebrachium (Figure 26.3a), then applied in a circumferential fashion around the distal antebrachium. The second, or bottom of the "figure of 8" should be placed as high up into the axilla as possible to prevent slipping and to ensure effective immobilization. This loop should be around the elbow joint, or the proximal antebrachium and the distal humerus. The most frequent mistakes made applying figure of 8 bandages are placing the bandage below the elbow joint and applying the bandage too tightly, which results in perfusion issues and discomfort. The flight feathers of the wing should be positioned parallel to each other, if the bandage is applied correctly. If the bandage is too tight, the flight feathers will be crossed and the bandage should be replaced.

Physical therapy (PT) should be performed carefully with the bird under sedation or anesthesia, if a figure of 8 bandage has been applied. The initial PT should be performed five to seven days after bandage application, in order to minimize interruption of the forming callus. The wing web and tendons will contract if PT is not performed, which may lead to the inability to fly once the fracture is healed.

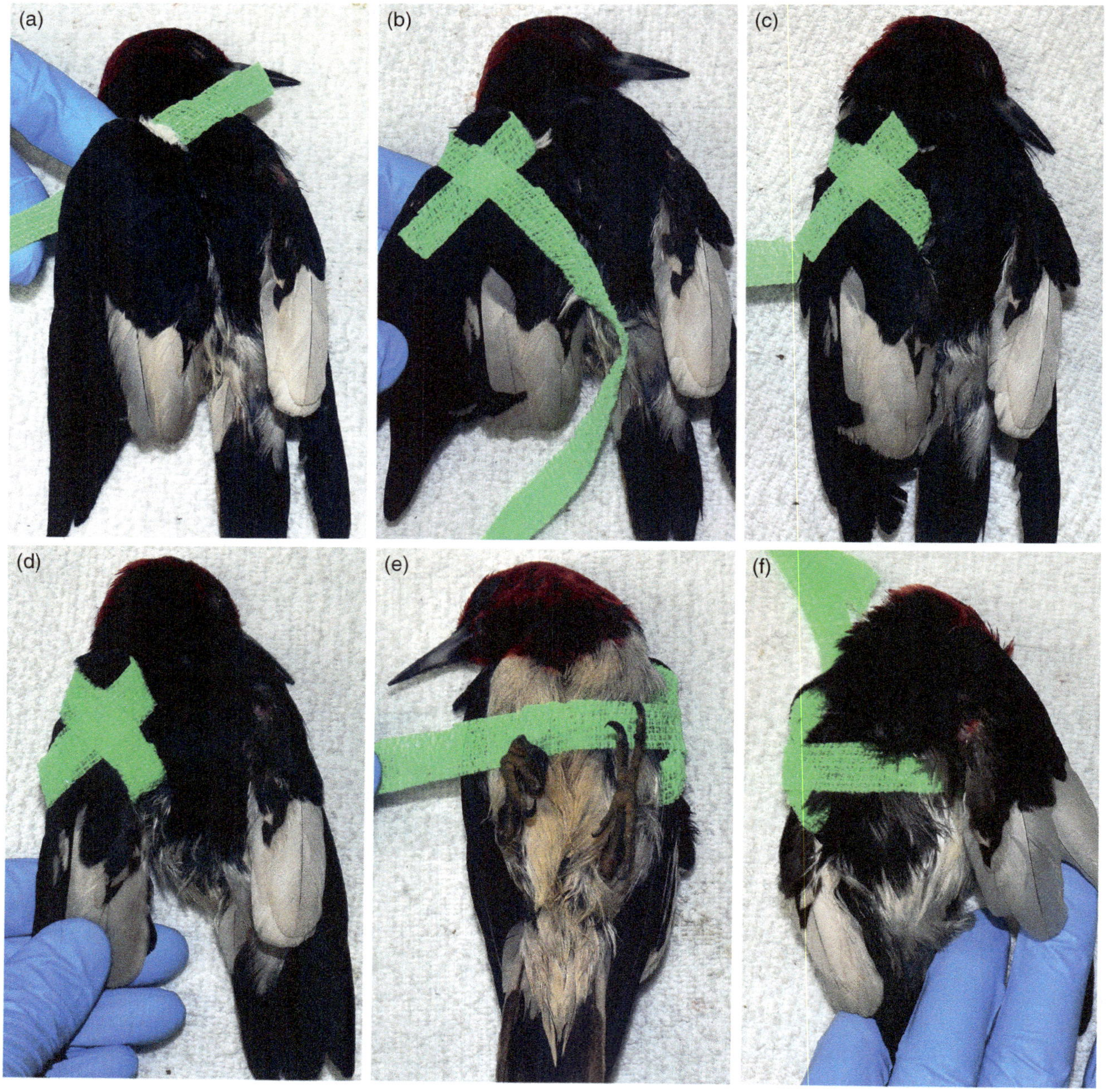

Figure 26.3 Figure of 8 bandage (a–d) for stabilization of fractures distal to the elbow joint, which can be combined with a body wrap (e, f) in order to immobilize the shoulder joint as well as stabilize fractures of the humerus and shoulder girdle.

External Coaptation: Leg

Foot Sling (Ehmer Sling) (Figure 26.4)

This technique is used for fractures of the femur or proximal tibiotarsal factures which cannot be effectively treated with a tape splint. The fracture can be immobilized by applying tape in a fashion which immobilizes the affected leg against the body. All the joints will be immobilized in a flexed position and birds are able to cope well with this type of bandage.

Tape Splint (Altman Splint) (Figure 26.5)

This splint can be utilized with tibiotarsal or tarsometatarsal fractures in birds with a body weight of less than 200 g. The feathers on the affected leg are carefully plucked or carefully cut off. A layer of elastic bandage (e.g. Vetwrap) should be applied as the primary layer around the leg, in order to protect the skin from the adhesive tape applied on top. Pieces of white medical tape are used to create the splint. Care should be taken to immobilize the joints above and below the fracture. Typically, two to three

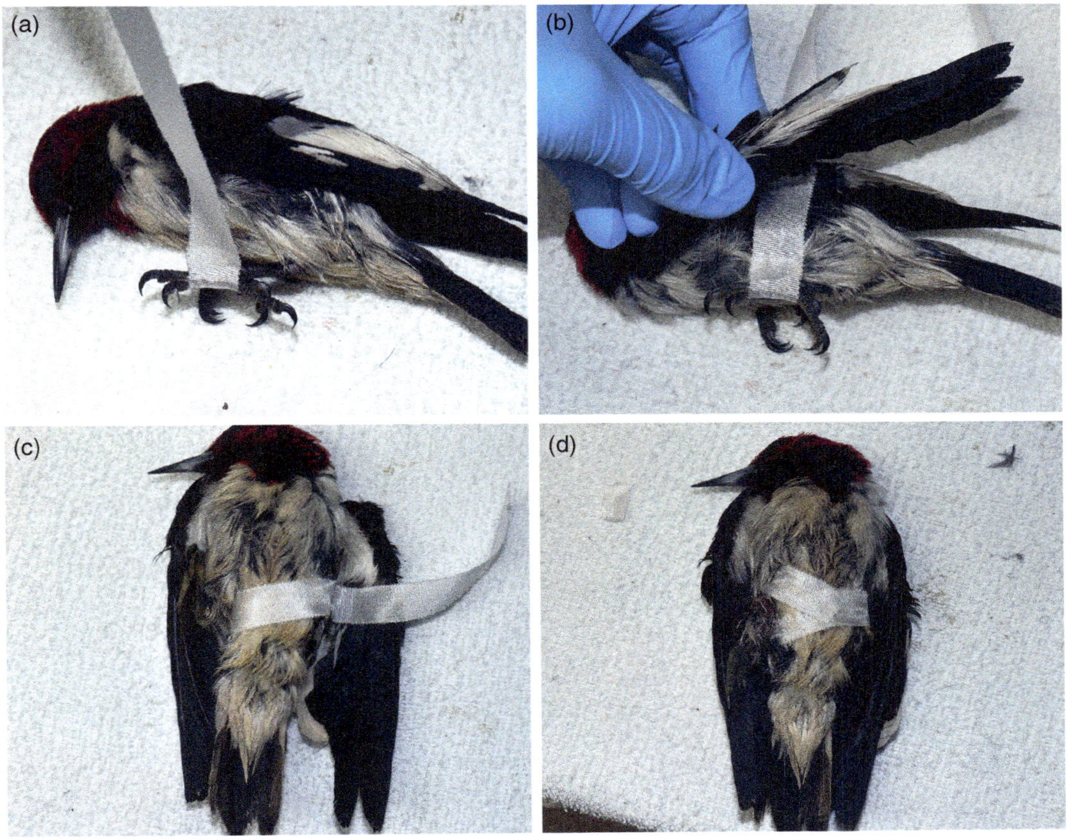

Figure 26.4 Foot sling (Ehmer sling) for stabilization of femoral fractures in birds. Care should be taken to place the tape in a fashion that does not compromise the movement of the opposite leg and does not compress the caudal coelom and cloaca. (a) A loop of tape is first applied circumferentially to the foot with the digits in a natural position, (b–d) The limb is flexed fully to the ventrum and a body wrap performed, which immobilizes the limb.

pieces of white medical tape are layered on top of each other and placed medially and laterally on the tibiotarsus, making sure that the fracture has been reduced and the ends opposed. This is repeated with several of these pieces to increase the strength of the bandage. The medial and lateral pieces are pressed together carefully using hemostats (Figure 26.5c). Excess tape can be trimmed. Superglue or tissue glue should be applied to the trimmed edges of the splint and the glue can also be applied parallel to the leg, in order to increase the stiffness of the splint (Figure 26.5d). The tape splint should be removed three weeks after initial placement. More frequent replacement of the splint is only recommended if complications occur, since manipulation of the leg and replacement of the splint can lead to disruption of the fracture healing. For birds that weigh more than 200 g, tape splints alone are often insufficient and therefore a modified and reinforced Robert-Jones bandage should be considered for temporary stabilization of the fracture, until surgical treatment can be performed.

Shoe Splints (Figure 26.6)

Shoe splints are indicated for fractures of the toes. The phalanges can be splinted by fashioning a “shoe” or “sandal.” Cardboard or thick paper is used to form the “sole.” Shorter, multilayered pieces are used for the dorsal surface, front, and back.

Ball Bandages

Ball bandages can be used to immobilize toe fractures. Cotton balls or gauze applied to the bottom of the foot and the foot including all the toes are wrapped with an elastic bandage material.

Interdigitating Bandage (Figure 26.7)

For pododermatitis wound (i.e. bumble foot), the interdigitating bandages provide protection of the plantar foot pad and allows application of wound dressings as well as

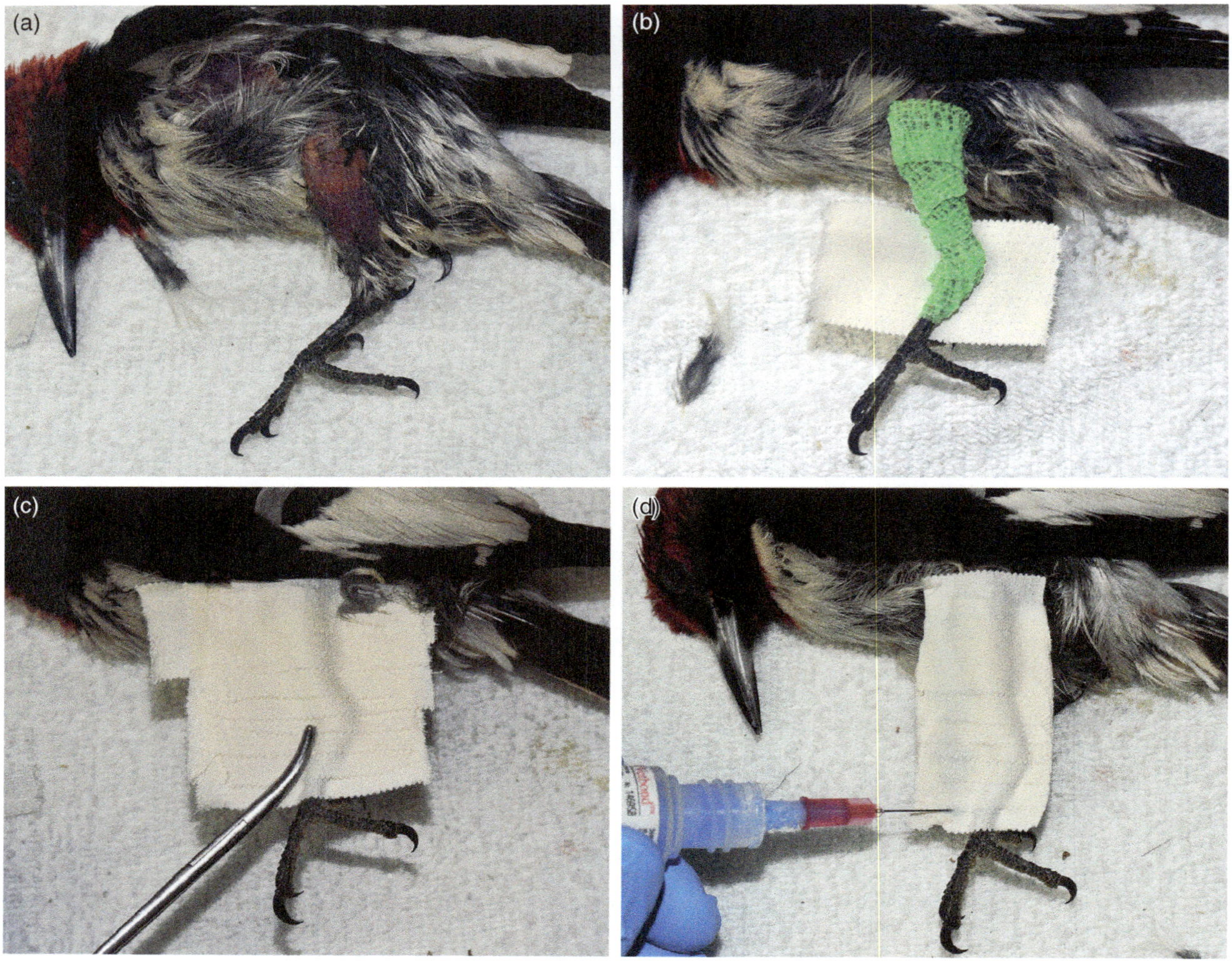

Figure 26.5 Tape splint (Altman splint) for treatment of tibiotarsal fractures. (a) The feathers should be carefully removed and a layer of elastic bandage applied (b). (c) White medical tape is placed in layers medially and laterally on the leg. Care should be taken to cover the joints above and below the fractured bone. A hemostat is used to compress the tape strips and conform them to the leg. (d) Superglue or tissue glue can be used to reinforce the splint and to seal the cut edge of the splint after trimming.

providing pressure relief for the diseased tissue. This type of bandage is most often used in birds of prey, poultry, and waterfowl, which frequently present with pododermatitis. In some circumstances (central pododermatitis lesions), a raised donut-shaped bandage may help decrease pressure on the bottom of the foot.

E-Collars

Immediately after applying any bandage or splint, the bird should be closely monitored to determine whether an e-collar is necessary. It may take some time for the bird to become accustomed to the bandage. Damage to the bandage or splint caused by the bird may lead to delayed healing or other complications of the wound or fracture. The bird should not be discharged until after becoming accustomed to the bandage and before the need for an e-collar is determined. More often than not, an e-collar is necessary to prevent birds from removing the splint or bandage.

E-collars are best applied under sedation, in order to minimize the stress to the bird. Sedation should not or only be partially reversed, in order for birds to get used to the e-collar gradually. There are commercial e-collars that may be purchased or one may fashion their own device (Figure 26.8). Old radiography films, plastic folders, foam tubes, and other materials may be used to create a lightweight e-collar to prevent bandage removal or self-mutilation. Old radiography films or plastic folders may be cut into a circle, with a circle in the middle for the neck and a single cut from the outer

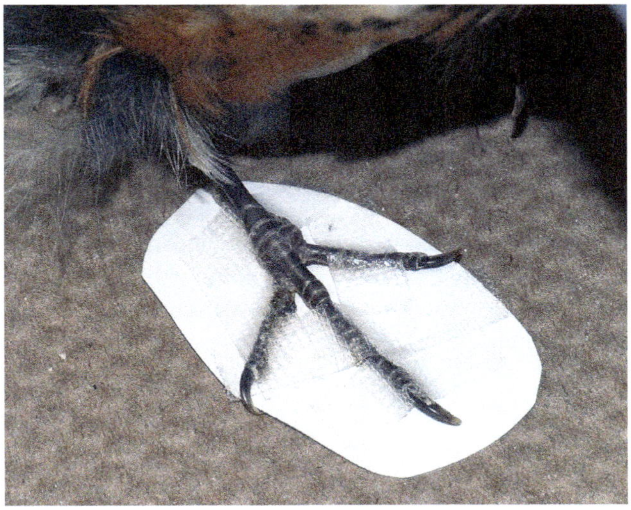

Figure 26.6 Shoe splint for immobilization of toes following traumatic injuries.

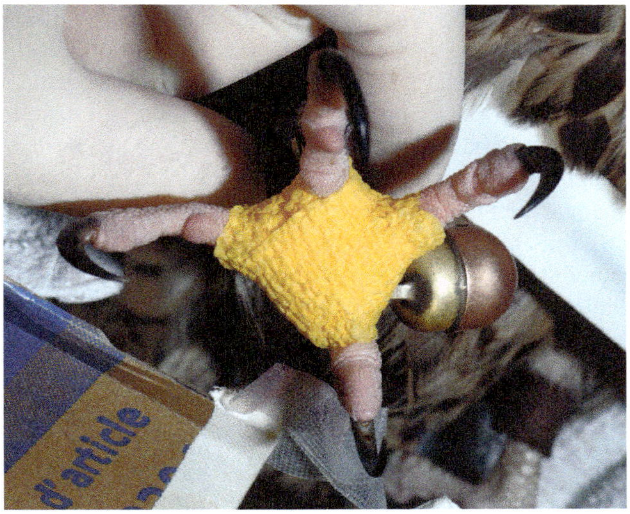

Figure 26.7 Interdigitating bandage is used to treat pododermatitis (i.e. bumblefoot) lesions affecting the foot pads in a variety of bird species.

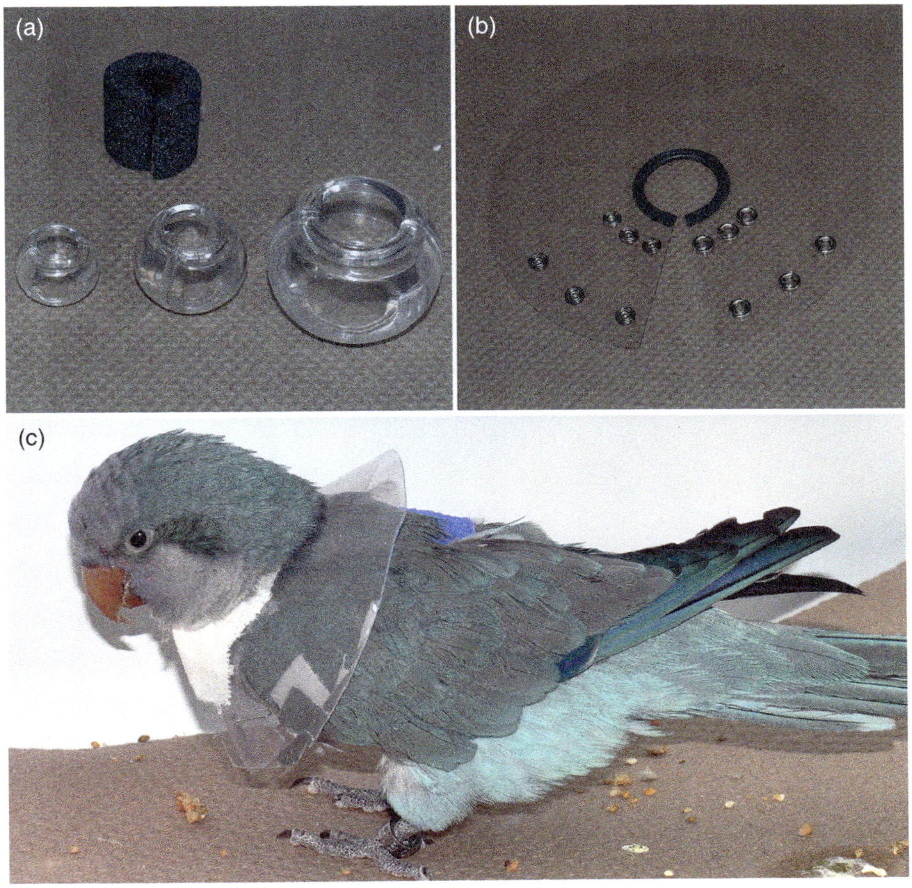

Figure 26.8 E-collars for birds. (a) Commercial plastic e-collars and foam tubing. (b) Commercial plastic film e-collar. (c) Quaker parrot with e-collar in place.

circle to the inner circle for application. Elastic tape can be used around the diameter of the inner circle to protect the neck from any sharp edge. The collar is fixed to the patient using self-stick velcro tabs or other packing type tape to overlap the ends. An alternative to this is using hollow foam tubing. The proper length is cut, and a vertical slit is made along the length to form an opening. The foam is wrapped in a self-adhesive wrap and fixed to the bird using elastic or other secure tape. The collar should be assessed to make sure the length is adequate to prevent any access to the bandage. Prior to discharge, ensure that the collar is not too tight and that the bird is able to eat and drink adequately. The most common sign noted with an e-collar that has been applied too tightly is regurgitation.

Ensuring proper adjustment to the e-collar prior to discharge from the hospital is critical. Sufficient food and water intake should be witnessed while the e-collar is in place. Birds wearing e-collars should be prevented from climbing, due to the risk of falling and inflicting further injury. Therefore, maintaining birds with e-collars in smooth-walled enclosures (e.g. plastic tubs, and boxes) is recommended.

Further Reading

Mickelson, M., Mans, C., and Colopy, S. (2016). Principles of wound management and wound healing in exotic pets. *Vet. Clin. Exot. Anim.* 19: 33–53.

Speer, B. (ed.) (2016). *Current Therapy in Avian Medicine and Surgery*, 1e. St. Louis: Elsevier.

27

CPR and Euthanasia

Claudia Kabakchiev[1] *and Hugues Beaufrère*[2]

[1] *404 Veterinary Emergency and Referral Hospital, Ontario, Canada*
[2] *Department of Medicine and Epidemiology, School of Veterinary Medicine, University of California Davis, Davis, USA*

CONTENTS

Introduction

Avian patients may present in cardiopulmonary arrest (CPA) or in critical condition necessitating a conversation with the owner about resuscitation or humane euthanasia. It is important to be knowledgeable about cardiopulmonary resuscitation (CPR) techniques, and this chapter will outline the basic steps of life support and post-resuscitation management. A brief discussion on euthanasia techniques is also included.

Cardiopulmonary Resuscitation (CPR)

Indications

Cardiopulmonary cerebral resuscitation (CPCR) should be performed immediately after CPA has been ascertained. CPCR is an active attempt to maintain perfusion and oxygenation of the vital organs until spontaneous circulation and respiration can be restored. CPA can be secondary to many processes, including hypovolemia, cardiac disease, metabolic, or electrolyte disturbances, anesthetic or sedative drugs, systemic inflammatory response, and respiratory depression. The type of precipitating event or underlying disease process will determine the probability of success when performing CPCR. The prognosis of the patient needs to be considered when determining whether to pursue CPR.

There has been limited scientific research on CPCR techniques and outcomes in avian patients. In the authors' experience, the 24-hour outcome is rarely positive after CPCR in birds, except perhaps when CPCR is performed following acute fluid and blood loss or CPA during an anesthetic procedure. The lack of effectiveness of CPCR in birds is probably related to several factors: their extreme metabolic demand and cardiopulmonary physiology when compared to mammals; the ineffectiveness of the application of mammalian CPCR techniques to birds; and the inciting causes of CPA which are often the end-result of undiagnosed long-standing severe diseases.

The only contraindication to performing CPCR is a "do not resuscitate" (DNR) order by the owner. This should be discussed in detail with every critically ill patient that presents to a veterinary hospital. In some cases, the underlying disease process contributing to the CPA is known and may suggest a poor prognosis for the patient in the short to long term. If that is the case, the chances of successful

Exotic Animal Emergency and Critical Care Medicine, First Edition. Edited by Jennifer E. Graham, Grayson A. Doss and Hugues Beaufrère.

resuscitation and later survival should be considered and CPCR may not be deemed appropriate.

Out-of-Hospital Arrest

There is currently no information available on the prognosis or survival of birds after CPA occurring outside of the hospital. In humans, the published survival rate for out-of-hospital cardiac arrest (OHCA) treated by trained personnel ranges from 3% to 16% [1, 2]; however, this number is largely influenced by the time until initiating CPCR and the type of rhythm abnormality and its response to defibrillation. A study identified 18 canine and feline patients, out of 204 CPA cases, that developed CPA prior to arriving at the hospital [3]. The median estimated interval between cardiac arrest and arrival at the hospital was five minutes, and none of the 18 patients survived to be discharged. These outcomes are suspected to be even poorer for birds, since CPR is difficult in these patients and death may happen quickly after CPA.

In-Hospital Arrest

CPA that occurs while the patient is in hospital can be addressed in a timely manner. There may be pre-arrest indicators that make it possible to intervene early and discuss the owner's wishes if CPA were to ensue. If evidence of circulatory shock is identified, the patient may be managed as described below. According to one study, survival to discharge was about 4.1% in dogs and 9.6% in cats that developed in-hospital CPA [4]. A single, yet unpublished study investigated survival rate post-CPCR in hospitalized birds (Crawford et al. personal communication, Tufts University). In that study, all CPA were during an anesthetic or peri-anesthetic period. Survival rate following CPCR was only 1 bird out of 41 cases. This study outlined or confirmed the perceived low success rate in birds because of the difficulty in delivering good chest compressions, obtaining intravenous (IV) access quickly, performing defibrillation, and because of inherent physiological peculiarities. While it is not uncommon to have short term success in reestablishing circulatory and pulmonary function (3/41 in the previously mentioned study), patients rarely survived to be discharged from the hospital. Therefore, it is important to anticipate CPA, confirm diagnoses, and intervene with intravenous fluids, medications, and ventilatory support prior to cardiac arrest whenever possible.

Anesthesia-Related Arrest

In mammals, CPA due to anesthetic or sedative drugs may have the best chance of resuscitation (about 45–50% survival to discharge vs. <10%) [3–5]. In a study, 55% of canine and feline patients that were successfully resuscitated to be discharged had anesthesia-related arrest [6]. In another retrospective study, only 2.8% of the feline and canine patients receiving CPCR survived to be discharged from the hospital and all of these patients developed CPA due to anesthesia or drug reactions [7]. Inhalant anesthetic agents and sedatives lead to more profound respiratory depression in birds than in mammals. Other common adverse effects are hypotension and cardiac arrhythmias (see "Chapter 28: Analgesia, Anesthesia, and Monitoring"). Therefore, anesthesia may lead to decompensation of clinical or subclinical conditions in birds.

Since there are limited data on the success of CPCR after anesthesia-related arrest in birds, the data obtained from mammalian patients may be extrapolated to birds. If the patient develops respiratory arrest or bradycardia during anesthesia, mechanical ventilation, fluid therapy, and drug intervention (e.g. epinephrine, atropine, glycopyrrolate, vasopressors, and doxapram) should be initiated. Successful resuscitation is most likely when CPCR attempts are performed immediately, effectively, and with appropriate post-resuscitation management. The higher success of CPCR on anesthetized birds may be explained by the ability to quickly reverse sedatives and stop inhalant anesthetic drugs, as well as the fact that most birds are already intubated and with intravenous access.

General Principles

The basic principles of CPCR are the same across species. As mentioned, there are few studies on the efficacy of CPCR techniques in avian patients specifically, so we must extrapolate from the evidence obtained in mammals.

Circulatory shock is a condition that commonly precedes CPA and the general principles of shock must be well understood in order to treat the bird presenting in shock or with CPA. Shock is a life-threatening state of poor perfusion that can be difficult to diagnose with certainty.

Clinical findings in birds with shock include [8]:

- depressed mentation
- elevated heart rate initially, up to double the normal rate
- respiratory difficulty (tachypnea, dyspnea, raised wings, tail-bobbing, and open-mouth breathing)
- bounding pulses initially, then weak pulses as patient decompensate; systolic blood pressure < 90 mmHg
- poor peripheral perfusion (low body temperature, pale, or cyanotic mucous membranes, increased refill time at the ulnar vein, and weak or absent pulse)
- hypothermia

Shock may be due to many possible causes, including hypovolemia, sepsis, anaphylaxis, toxins, and cardiac disease. The decreased perfusion can result in cellular hypoxia and organ dysfunction. In mammals, the identified stages of shock include an early compensatory phase, an early decompensatory phase, and a decompensatory phase at which point the cellular injury caused by the shock state becomes irreversible [9]. The exact mechanism in birds is unclear, but believed to be similar in its physiology and effects on the body [8].

In the *early compensatory phase*, hypotension results in stimulation of the sympathetic nervous system and release of catecholamines and renin. Renin activates the renin–angiotensin–aldosterone system and the heart rate, cardiac output, and systemic vascular resistance increase as a result [10].

In the *early decompensatory phase,* the compensatory mechanisms become ineffective and there is a loss of perfusion to organs such as the kidneys, gastrointestinal tract, and muscles. Bacterial translocation from the intestines may lead to endotoxemia.

In the *decompensatory phase*, organ failure occurs and is irreversible. It is at this stage that CPA often occurs. Birds seem to be more resistant to hypovolemic shock than mammals and may go into decompensatory shock only after more than 60% acute blood loss [11].

Two studies on the effects of experimentally induced acute hemorrhagic shock in birds have been published [11, 12]. Mallard ducks were phlebotomized under general anesthesia to induce a state of hypovolemia, and some ducks were fluid resuscitated to monitor effects on heart rate and recovery from anesthesia. All ducks became tachycardic after acute loss of 25–45% of their blood volume. The heart rate decreased again in most birds (22/28) after receiving boluses (5 ml/kg over five minutes) of a crystalloid (Plasmalyte-A; Baxter Healthcare Corp., Deerfield, IL, USA), hetastarch (Abbott Laboratories, North Chicago, IL, USA), or a (now discontinued) hemoglobin-based oxygen-carrying solution (Oxyglobin, Biopure Corporation, Cambridge, MA, USA), with the heart rate normalizing most quickly in the latter group [11]. In Leghorn chickens, acute hemorrhagic shock was again induced by removing 50% of blood volume under anesthesia. The tachycardia noted in mallard ducks was not seen with phlebotomy in chickens, which may be due to a lack of baroreceptor response during hypovolemia and hypotension. However, there was a consistently decreased arterial systolic blood pressure and increased venous lactic acid. Fluid replacement using hetastarch (HAES-steril 200/0.5, Fresenius, Bad-Homburg, Germany), a hemoglobin-based oxygen carrier (Hemospan, Sangart Inc., San Diego, CA, USA), or autotransfusion did not significantly affect the heart rate or respiratory rate, as compared to the controls; nevertheless, the fluid replacement did allow blood pressure to normalize [12]. There are immediate benefits of using fluid therapy during hypovolemic shock; however, the long-term advantages of various fluid types in birds still need to be investigated in more detail.

Treatment for circulatory shock includes basic supportive care, such as warmth, removing stress, and oxygen therapy. Intravenous or intraosseous (IO) fluid resuscitation therapy with a mixture of balanced electrolyte solutions, hypertonic electrolyte solutions, blood products, and colloids needs to be initiated as soon as possible (see "Chapter 29: Nutrition and Fluid Therapy"). The primary goal of the treatment of shock is to expand the vascular space and re-establish organ perfusion. Depending on the mentation of the patient, intravenous or intraosseous catheters may be placed with mild sedation or subcutaneous administration of a local anesthetic at the site of catheter placement (e.g. 1–2 mg/kg lidocaine buffered). If fluid therapy is insufficient, vasopressors may be indicated (e.g. dopamine, dobutamine, and norepinephrine). The underlying cause of the shock condition also needs to be managed; for example, blood loss may require transfusion with blood products.

Shock must be treated aggressively otherwise circulatory collapse can lead to respiratory arrest and loss of consciousness. CPR guidelines, as outlined below, will need to be followed if either respiratory or cardiac arrest is identified. Medical intervention prior to cardiac arrest will provide the best outcome in avian patients.

Evidence-Based Literature

In an effort to improve the current success rates of CPCR in veterinary patients, the collaborators of the RECOVER (Reassessment Campaign on Veterinary Resuscitation) [13] initiative have developed specific evidence-based guidelines for practitioners to follow when performing CPR on cats and dogs. These principles and guidelines have been applied to birds in developing the basic and advanced life support recommendations outlined in this chapter. When applying these guidelines, relevant species differences for avian patients are identified in the text.

Once CPA is identified, see Figure 27.1 for general treatment guidelines. Supplies for performing CPR should be readily available and regularly examined and stocked. Emergency drug doses should be clearly posted and legible.

Basic Life Support

Basic life support is the most important component of CPCR and should be started as soon as CPA has been identified. Unresponsiveness, apnea or agonal breathing, and lack of cardiac sounds on auscultation are all signs of potential or impending CPA. Based on evidence in human clinical research, the benefits of initiating CPCR in a patient with unconfirmed CPA far outweigh the risks of waiting to perform thoracic compressions in true arrest [14].

Establishing the "ABCs" (Airway, Breathing, Circulation) of CPR is crucial, although there has been debate about using the "CAB" approach instead. Chest compressions should be initiated as soon as possible; however, the effectiveness of these compressions is lower in birds than mammals. Based on recommendations from the RECOVER project, when multiple trained rescuers are available to

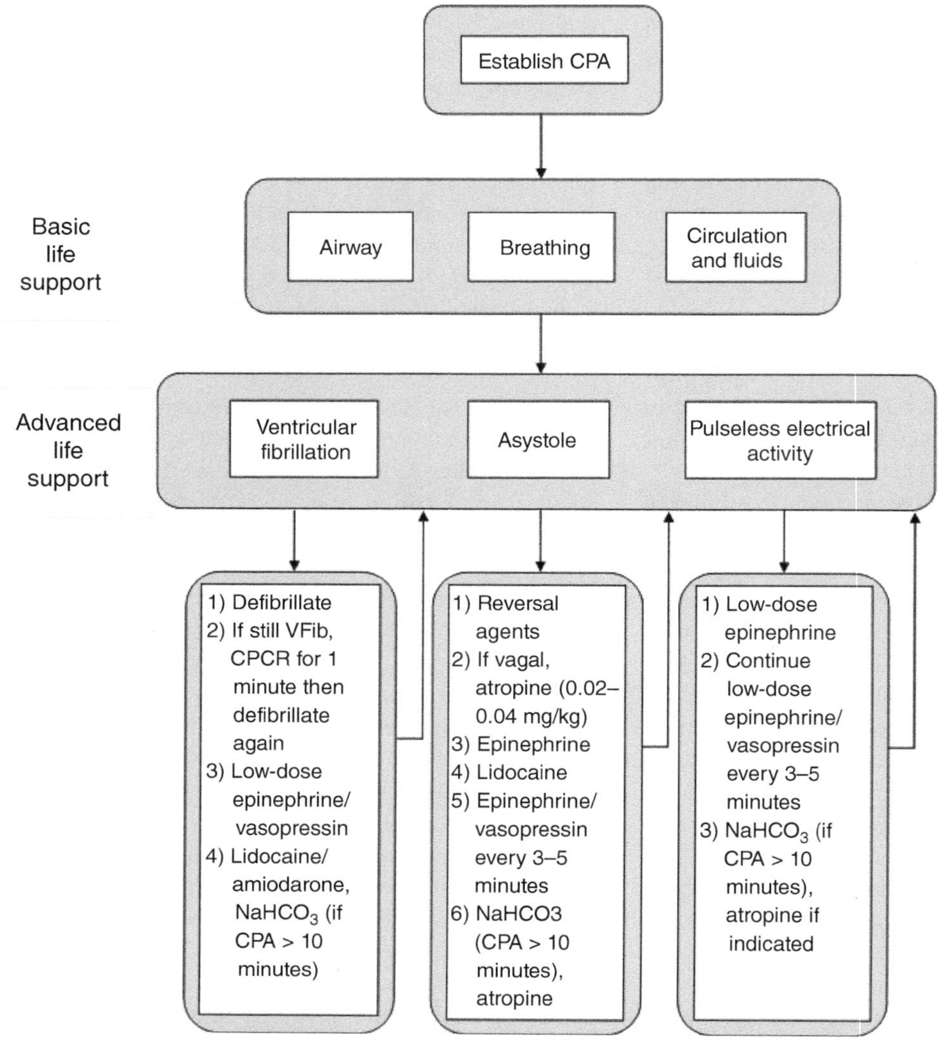

Figure 27.1 Steps for cardiopulmonary resuscitation in the critical avian patient.

provide CPR, establishing an airway should be done at the same time as thoracic compressions. If only one rescuer is present and CPA is not due to primary cardiac arrest, starting with traditional airway and ventilation is appropriate. If CPA is due to cardiac disease, initiating compressions first is recommended [14].

Chest Compressions (Cardiac)

1) If cardiac arrest is identified, start cardiac compressions.

   Note: There is limited data on the efficacy of compressions in birds, because of their large keel and the high compression rates that are probably required. Some individuals advocate the use of emergency drugs instead of compressions. Chest compressions in birds may work on the principle of a thoracic pump, increasing the intrathoracic pressure to encourage blood flow out of the heart and great vessels [15, 16]. As the heart is "shielded" by the wide sternum and the coracoids prevent depressing the cranial sternum during traditional cardiac compressions, adopting a different technique than mammals for cardiac compression may be more effective. For instance, making cardiac compressions on the lateral and dorsal aspect of the thorax rather than over the keel may be more effective as the ribs are more compliant there.

   a) >120 compressions/min; attempt to approximate normal heart rate for species.

2) Monitor cardiac activity with electrocardiography (ECG) and effectiveness of compressions with a Doppler probe.
   a) ECG leads should be attached to the skin at the base of both wings and both thighs. This can be done using hypodermic needles, paperclips, gel-soaked gauzes, or self-adhesive patches [15, 17].
   b) The Doppler probe can be placed near the proximal ulna or medial tibiotarsus, with a cuff for blood pressure monitoring placed on the humerus or

femur, respectively. The width of the cuff should be 30–40% the circumference of the limb. Indirect blood pressure measurements in birds are not very accurate; however, it can be used to monitor trends [18, 19]. See "Chapter 28: Analgesia, Anesthesia, and Monitoring" and Chapter 25 for more information on blood pressure measurements.

3) In dogs and cats, internal cardiac massage is recommended if efforts are ineffective after two to five minutes of external compressions or if a disease process would limit the effectiveness of closed-thorax compressions [20]. The different anatomy and small size of birds make this technique impractical unless performed while the patient is already in surgery [15].
4) Every one to two minutes, discontinue compressions and assess for return of spontaneous circulation via the ECG, Doppler probe, and auscultation.

Ventilation

1) Remove any obstruction in the oral cavity.
2) Intubate with an appropriately-sized *uncuffed* endotracheal (ET) tube (see Table 27.1). Secure the tube to the beak or head to prevent shifting while performing CPR (see Figure 27.2).
3) Signs of upper airway obstruction: open-mouthed breathing with neck extended, upper respiratory sounds (e.g. stridor). If suspect upper airway obstruction that cannot be relieved, place *air sac cannula* [21, 22] (ET tube or red rubber feeding tube) in caudal thoracic or abdominal air sac (also see Chapter 24):
   a) Position patient in right lateral recumbency with left leg pulled cranially or caudally.
   b) The tube can be placed in the lateral flank region caudal to the last rib. Palpate the edge of the last rib, pluck feathers, and surgically prepare the skin over this site.
   c) Make a skin incision and blunt dissect through the body wall.
   d) Place sterile tube of appropriate size (as per ET tube) in this area and ensure proper tube placement by ventilating.
   e) Secure tube to skin (Figure 27.3).
4) Start mechanical ventilation with 100% oxygen (turn off any anesthetic gases and flush the circuit).
   a) 10–20 breaths/min. A mechanical ventilator may be used for high respiratory rate.
   b) Inspiratory time: 1 second.
   c) Avoid airway pressures greater than 15–20 cm H_2O (10–15 mmHg).

Table 27.1 Approximate endotracheal (ET) tube sizes for various avian species commonly seen in practice.

Species	Average weight (g)	ET tube (mm)
Canary	15–25	1 or 20 g catheter
Budgie	30–40	1.5 or 16–18 g catheter
Cockatiel	85–95	2
Quaker Parrot	110–120	2–2.5
Pigeon	300–350	3–3.5
Grey parrot	350–550	3.5–4
Cockatoo	700–900	4–4.5
Macaw	1000–1200	5–6

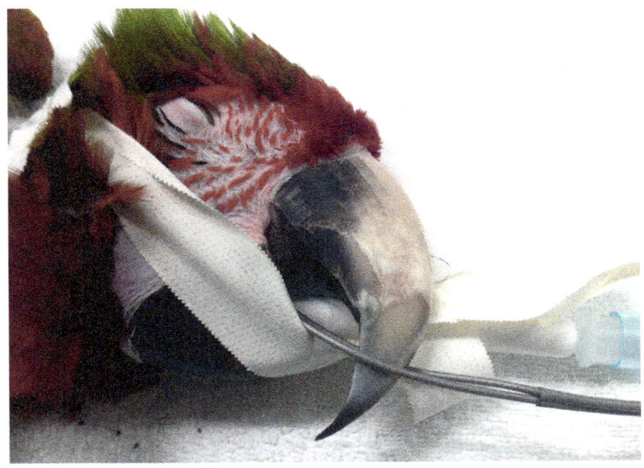

Figure 27.2 Catalina macaw intubated with an uncuffed endotracheal tube and monitored with a Doppler probe positioned over the palatine artery to monitor heart rate.

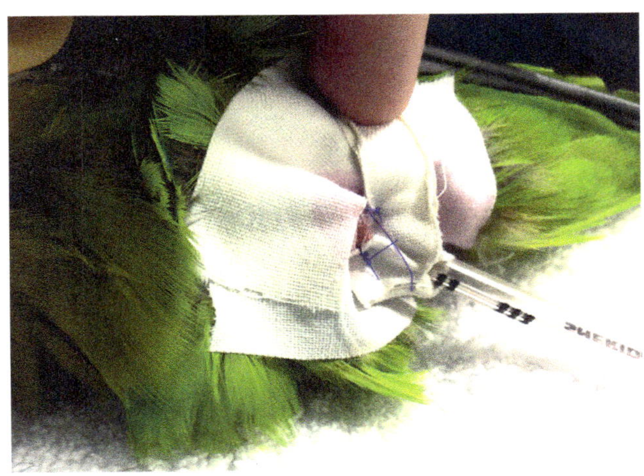

Figure 27.3 Quaker parrot with air sac cannula placed in the caudal thoracic air sac and secured to the skin for air sac ventilation.

5) Monitor end-tidal carbon dioxide (ETCO2) with a capnograph connected to the breathing circuit. Adjust the tidal volume, inspiratory time, and respiratory rate to prevent hypercapnia (<45 mmHg). $ETCO_2$ may not be measurable when an air sac cannula is placed as expiratory gas will exit through the trachea (unless the ET tube is plugged with a piece of tape for instance).
6) Doxapram (1–2 mg/kg IM/IV/IO, or 2–4 mg/kg via ET tube) may be administered to stimulate independent respiratory efforts providing the hypovolemia and tissue perfusion have been reversed.
7) If unable to place an ET tube or air sac cannula, ventilation can be encouraged by moving the wings up and down or lifting the sternum [16, 21].

Advanced Life Support

Advanced life support is performed when the ABCs have been established. It includes the use of emergency drugs, fluid therapy, and defibrillation if needed.

Vascular Access

In order to maintain appropriate circulation, intravenous or intraosseous access is necessary (see Chapter 25) [23].

Catheterization Sites:

1) Basilic/cutaneous ulnar vein: ulnar branch of this vein is easily visualized over the ulna near the elbow joint (Figure 27.4).
2) Medial metatarsal vein: useful in larger birds, chickens, pigeons, and Anseriformes (e.g. ducks, geese).
3) Right jugular vein: large vein that is easy to visualize but may be difficult to secure catheter. Risk of inadvertent administration of fluids or hemorrhage into air sac space or sinusal cervicocephalic diverticulum.
4) Intraosseous into ulna or tibiotarsus: easy to place and maintain. Use a 22 gauge spinal needle in larger birds. A standard 25–27 gauge needle may be required for small birds. Place into the distal ulna at a point just medial to the dorsal ulnar condyle. Do not use the ulna in Cathartiformes and some Pelecaniformes in which this bone is pneumatized.

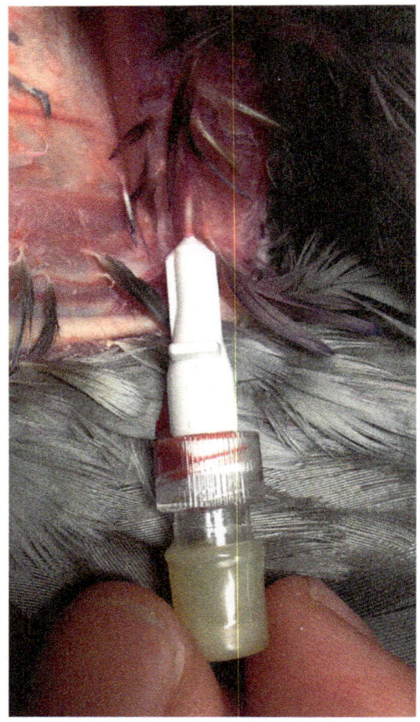

Figure 27.4 Placement of a 26 g intravenous catheter in the ulnar vein of a parrot.

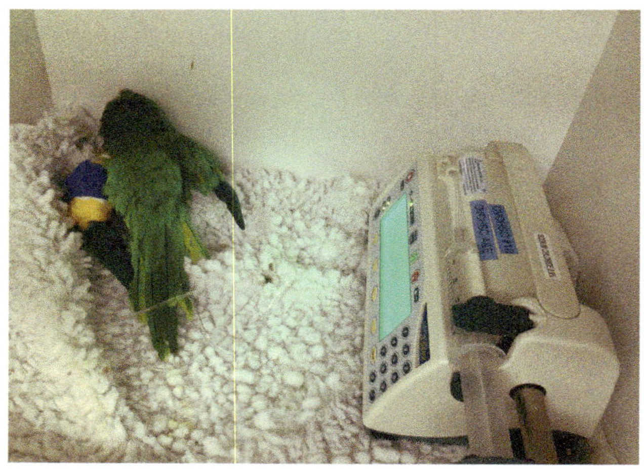

Figure 27.5 Fluid therapy provided to a critical avian patient via an intraosseous catheter and using a fluid pump.

Once intravascular or intraosseous access has been established, it is possible to administer fluids as needed for the patient (Figure 27.5) [9] See Chapter 29 for further details on this topic.

1) If *hypovolemic* or there are ongoing losses of fluid/blood, give shock rate boluses of isotonic fluids: 10–15 ml/kg of isotonic, alkalinizing crystalloid. Repeat as needed. Plasmalyte-A has an osmolarity closer to avian plasma osmolarity and is preferred over Lactated Ringer's solution for rapid intravenous administration. To rapidly expand intravascular space, use colloids at 3–10 ml/kg over 5–10 minutes, hypertonic saline at 3 ml/kg over 10 minutes, or a combination of both with or without crystalloids.
2) If there is *severe blood loss* (packed cell volume (PCV) < 15%) and blood products are available, give

Table 27.2 Emergency drug doses commonly used in avian patients.

			Amount to administer in milliliters (ml) for a given body weight						
Drug	**Indication**	**Dose**	**20 g**	**50 g**	**100 g**	**200 g**	**500 g**	**1 kg**	**2 kg**
Epinephrine low-dose (1 : 1000)	Cardiac arrest	0.01 mg/kg IV, IO, intratracheal			0.01 (once diluted 1 : 10000)	0.02 (once diluted 1 : 10000)	0.05 (once diluted 1 : 10000)	0.01	0.02
Epinephrine high-dose (1 : 1000)	Cardiac arrest, after 10 min	0.1 mg/kg IV, IO, intratracheal	0.02 (dilute 1 : 10000)	0.05 (dilute 1 : 10000)	0.01	0.02	0.05	0.1	0.2
Vasopressin (20 U/ml)[a]	Cardiac arrest	0.8 U/kg IV, IO, intratracheal[a]					0.02	0.04	0.08
Atropine (0.54 mg/ml)	Cardiac arrest, bradycardia	0.2–0.5 mg/kg IV, IO, intratracheal	0.01–0.02	0.02–0.04	0.04–0.09	0.08–0.18	0.2–0.4	0.4–0.9	0.8–1.8
Amiodarone (50 mg/ml)[a]	Arrhythmia	5–10 mg/kg[a]		0.01	0.01–0.02	0.02–0.04	0.05–0.1	0.1–0.2	0.2–0.4
Lidocaine (20 mg/ml)	Arrhythmia	1–3 mg/kg IV, IO, intratracheal			0.01	0.01–0.03	0.03–0.07	0.05–0.15	0.1–0.3
Doxapram (20 mg/m)	Respiratory depression/arrest	2–20 mg/kg IM, IV, IO, intratracheal	0.01–0.02	0.01–0.05	0.01–0.1	0.02–0.2	0.05–0.5	0.1–1	0.2–2
Naloxone (0.4 mg/ml)	Reversal of opioids	0.01–0.05 mg/kg			0.01	0.01–0.02	0.02–0.06	0.03–0.12	0.05–0.25
Flumazenil (0.1 mg/ml)	Reversal of benzodiazepines	0.05 mg/kg	0.01	0.02	0.05	0.1	0.25	0.5	1
Atipamezole (5 mg/ml)	Reversal of α2-agonists	Same volume as dex(medetomidine)							
Sodium bicarbonate (1 mEq/ml)	Acidosis or CPA for >10 min	0.5–1 mEq/kg IV, IO	0.01–0.02	0.03–0.05	0.05–0.1	0.1–0.2	0.25–0.5	0.5–1	1–2
Defibrillation[a]	Ventricular fibrillation	2–10 J/kg[a]	n/a	n/a	1	1	1	2	4

Doses administered via ET tube are doubled.
[a] Limited data on use in veterinary patients; no data in avian species.

whole blood based on PCV. If blood products are not available or there is *hypoproteinemia* (<3 g/dl), give colloids (3–5 ml/kg over 10 minutes). If available, hemoglobin-based oxygen-carrying solutions may be used as well. For transfusion of birds, homologous blood transfusions are ideal. Several donors of the same species may be needed.

3) If *euvolemic*, give a crystalloid bolus of 5–10 ml/kg then maintenance rates. Be careful not to fluid overload the small patient.

Drugs

The sequence and doses of emergency drugs used will vary depending on the case (see Table 27.2 and Figure 27.1). If there is an anesthesia-related cardiac arrest, reversal agents for any administered sedatives should be given. If there is bradycardia or a vagal arrest, administer atropine [24]. Otherwise, epinephrine is one of the first drugs to be used in CPA cases.

If ECG is available for patient monitoring, then emergency drugs can be used based on the ECG findings:

1) *Anesthetic CPA and asystole*: Administer reversal agents, then epinephrine (0.01–0.1 mg/kg), lidocaine (1–3 mg/kg), repeat epinephrine (+/− atropine, sodium bicarbonate, vasopressin).
2) *Vagally mediated CPA and asystole*: Administer atropine (0.02–0.2 mg/kg), then epinephrine (+/− sodium bicarbonate, vasopressin).
3) *Pulseless electrical activity* (PEA): Epinephrine (+/− atropine, sodium bicarbonate, vasopressin).

4) *Ventricular fibrillation (VFib)*: Defibrillate (if appropriate), re-evaluate ECG, defibrillate again, then administer epinephrine (+/− vasopressin, lidocaine, amiodarone).

High-dose epinephrine (0.1 mg/kg) is not currently recommended during CPCR [24]. Studies on humans and canines have not identified a clear benefit to resuscitation attempts when using this dose. However, if there is no response to low-dose epinephrine use or if the small patient size necessitates it, it may be warranted to try a higher dose or vasopressin.

Although vasopressin has been investigated in mammalian species, there are currently no studies on the pharmacologic properties of vasopressin in birds, especially since the avian hormone is slightly different (arginine vasotocin). It is worth considering when epinephrine is ineffective. Similarly, there is no data on the use of amiodarone in avian patients.

Atropine is commonly used in conjunction with epinephrine as part of the CPCR process. In mammals, there is limited evidence that it is more effective than use of epinephrine alone except in cases of high vagal tone and arrest (e.g. respiratory distress or severe gastrointestinal disease). On the other hand, there are no contraindications to using it so it often becomes part of the CPCR algorithm.

The use of sodium bicarbonate during resuscitation attempts is controversial due to the secondary effects of its use [24]. Sodium bicarbonate boluses can result in a transient hypotension, hypercarbia (as bicarbonate is converted into carbon dioxide), and intracellular acidosis which can depress cellular function. Sodium bicarbonate use is recommended in cases of severe hyperkalemia, pre-existing metabolic acidosis, or if CPA has been ongoing for more than 10 minutes [15, 25]. It should only be administered once other CPCR efforts have been unsuccessful and after having assessed the acid-base and electrolyte parameters of the patient.

Calcium is not generally recommended in the treatment of CPA, but may be administered in patients with known severe hyperkalemia or ionized hypocalcemia (this may be assessed with some blood gas radiometers that also measure electrolytes). Calcium gluconate may be given *slowly* at a dose of 50 mg/kg (dilute to 50 mg/ml first).

The use of dextrose is also not generally recommended during CPCR due to the fact that glucose promotes anaerobic metabolism and subsequent cellular injury. On the other hand, dextrose may be beneficial in patients with known or suspected hypoglycemia. A 50% dextrose solution can be diluted 1 : 1 with saline to produce a 25% solution and administered slowly at 50–100 mg/kg.

If intravenous or intraosseous catheterization is not possible, many emergency drugs can be given intratracheally via the ET tube. When given by this route, twice the intravascular dose is generally required (or in the case of epinephrine, give high dose). The intratracheal drug needs to be applied as deep into the trachea as possible and flushed into the airways and lungs by positive pressure ventilation. Any drugs administered intravenously or intraosseously also need to be flushed with sufficient fluid volume to deliver them to the heart.

Monitoring

Every one to two minutes during the CPR process, the patient should be assessed for return of spontaneous circulation. Direct auscultation is important; however, monitoring should also include the use of a Doppler probe, capnography, and ECG if available. These monitors will provide important information about tissue perfusion and cardiac electrical activity. Further details on monitoring during and after resuscitation may be found in Chapter 28.

ECG is used more frequently in mammals than in birds, although ECG lead placement and normal ECG parameters have been evaluated for many avian species [16, 26–33]. Leads need to be placed at the base of both wings and near both thighs. Usually, this is done with hypodermic needles through the skin, although other techniques have also been evaluated [17]. The avian ECG appears different from mammals as the mean electrical axis of most birds is negative with a prominent S wave (except in meat poultry). In medium to small-sized birds that have a high heart rate, the P waves are usually indiscernible from the T waves (P on T phenomenon), and the ST segment may be very short (ST slurring) (Figure 27.6). The interpretation of the avian ECG is otherwise similar to mammals.

In mammals, when VFib is identified by ECG, defibrillation is required. It is administered at a low dose (2 J/kg) initially, and subsequent countershocks are increased up to 10 J/kg. In avian species, there are no studies to determine the efficacy or adverse effects of using defibrillation. The

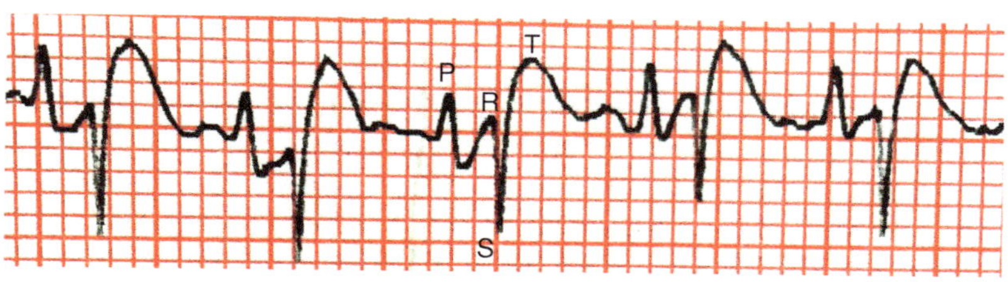

Figure 27.6 Lead II of the electrocardiogram for a normal Amazon parrot demonstrating ST slurring.

energy that can be delivered by defibrillators is too high for very small patients, and traditional defibrillator paddles are too large. If defibrillation is not available or not feasible due to patient size, administration of epinephrine or vasopressin may be of some benefit. If defibrillation is attempted in an avian patient, ensure that feathers have been plucked and that there is no alcohol or open oxygen sources in the area where the paddles are to be used. Anecdotal information suggests the use of a nine-volt battery with leads attached to a battery connector has been used to successfully defibrillate avian species (Michelle Hawkins, personal communication).

Post-arrest Care

Once there is return of spontaneous cardiac function (auscultable heart sounds and palpable pulse), continue to monitor the patient using an ECG, Doppler unit, capnograph, and pulse oximeter. The patient can be extubated once there is normal respiration, but flow-by oxygen should still be provided. It is important to prevent hypercarbia; if necessary, mechanical ventilation may be indicated. Fluids should be continued at least at a maintenance rate. Provide analgesics appropriate for the patient's needs. Hypothermia is also common and should be anticipated.

Reperfusion injury and persistent damage from ischemia and hypoxia are a major concern after a successful CPCR. Only about 16% of canine and feline patients that have a return of spontaneous circulation after CPR survive to be discharged [3]. Unfortunately, the probability of successful CPCR, and therefore survival to discharge, in birds is likely to be lower than in mammals. Monitor the patient for the following concerns [15, 34, 35]:

a) Hypotension: if hypovolemic, provide fluid therapy; otherwise, provide dopamine, dobutamine, or norepinephrine as a continuous rate infusion.
b) Hyper- or hypoglycemia, electrolyte imbalances, or changes in blood pH.
c) Hyper- or hypothermia.
d) Neurologic dysfunction or coma.
e) Increased intracranial pressure: may present with hypertension, bradycardia, and neurologic deficits.
f) Gastrointestinal ischemic damage: treat with antibiotics in case of bacterial translocation.
g) Renal failure.
h) Pulmonary edema.

Ultimately, the cause of the CPA needs to be identified and addressed. Unfortunately, for the avian patient the prognosis for survival to discharge is poor. The above-mentioned "indications for CPR" need to be frequently considered during a case of CPA.

Euthanasia

Indications

Humane euthanasia is defined by the AVMA guidelines as "ending the life of an individual animal in a way that minimizes or eliminates pain or distress" [36]. This is an important aspect of veterinary medicine that needs to be carefully considered by the primary clinician and the pet-owner. Euthanasia should be discussed whenever there is a patient suspected to have a poor prognosis or when therapeutic options are unavailable, ineffective, or financially unfeasible.

Methods

Pet owners with birds often have a very strong social bond with their pet, and many avian patients have a long lifespan and may have been with their owner for many years. Many bird owners may elect to be present for the euthanasia process, so comfort with rapid, low-stress techniques is important.

Unfortunately, there is limited evidence-based research on appropriate euthanasia methods in birds, although some recent studies have investigated this subject [37, 38]. Most of what is known and recommended in the AVMA guidelines is based on anecdotal reports, roundtable discussions in journals, and association guidelines. The methodology selected by the clinician should be based on the patient's species, size, comfort with handling, and medical condition. Methods of euthanasia, as discussed in the AVMA guidelines, are outlined in Table 27.3.

Drugs

Chemical restraint may be beneficial to decrease stress for the patient prior to euthanasia. Intramuscular (IM) sedatives (e.g. midazolam) or inhalant anesthetic agents may be administered to render a patient sedated or unconscious and facilitate intravenous administration of a euthanasia solution, such as sodium pentobarbital.

Conditional methods of euthanasia require general anesthesia prior to administration of intracoelomic, intracardiac, or intraosseous injections, administration of potassium chloride for euthanasia, or exsanguination [36]. If injecting euthanasia solution intracoelomically, injection into air sacs must be avoided. General anesthesia may be provided by mask-induction with isoflurane or sevoflurane prior to performing injections. Unfortunately, this technique may require that the owner be absent during part of the euthanasia procedure. Thoracic compression is currently considered an unacceptable method of euthanasia by the AVMA; however, in small birds it may be an effective method if performed by a skilled individual [38].

Table 27.3 Some euthanasia methods outlined in the 2020 AVMA Guidelines.

Acceptable methods	Conditionally acceptable methods	Unacceptable methods
• IV pentobarbital with or without sedation/ anesthesia	• IC, IO, ICe pentobarbital WITH anesthesia • Inhalant anesthetic agent • IC or IV KCl WITH anesthesia • Exsanguination WITH anesthesia • Decapitation in small birds (<200 g) by experienced individual	• Thoracic compression

IC, intracardiac; ICe, intracoelomic.

Oral pentobarbital is also effective in most birds. The intended process and the owner's expectations should be discussed prior to performing the euthanasia.

Necropsy

Many birds come from client-owned collections or aviaries. Necropsies are commonly discussed to help determine the presence of infectious agents that may affect other exposed birds. Injection of euthanasia solutions, such as barbiturates, will cause artifactual changes on histopathologic post-mortem evaluation. These agents may cause erythrolysis, edema, and coagulation within the lungs or other tissues [39]. If the owner has an interest in doing a necropsy, euthanasia techniques that provide minimal changes should be selected. Euthanasia by inhalant anesthetic agent may limit tissue damage. The use of potassium chloride also causes minimal artifactual changes and can be administered by intravenous or intracardiac injection only in a previously-anesthetized or unconscious individual [40].

When preparing a carcass for necropsy, the feathers should be immediately soaked in soapy water and refrigerated in order to limit any tissue damage or changes that occur with autolysis or freezing. The carcass should be shipped as soon as possible to a pathologist for detailed post-mortem examination. This kind of examination is recommended if the cause of death is unknown, infectious agents are likely, or the bird has been in contact with other individuals.

References

1 Ishikawa, S., Niwano, S., Imaki, R. et al. (2013). Usefulness of a simple prognostication score in prediction of the prognoses of patients with out-of-hospital cardiac arrests. *Int. Heart J.* 54 (6): 362–370.

2 Nichol, G., Thomas, E., Callaway, C.W. et al. (2008). Regional variation in out-of-hospital cardiac arrest incidence and outcome. *J. Am. Med. Assoc.* 300 (12): 1423–1431.

3 Hofmeister, E.H., Brainard, B.M., Egger, C.M., and Kang, S. (2009). Prognostic indicators for dogs and cats with cardiopulmonary arrest treated by cardiopulmonary cerebral resuscitation at a university teaching hospital. *J. Am. Vet. Med. Assoc.* 235 (1): 50–57.

4 Wingfield, W.E. and Van Pelt, D.R. (1992). Respiratory and cardiopulmonary arrest in dogs and cats: 265 cases (1986–1991). *J. Am. Vet. Med. Assoc.* 200 (12): 1993–1996.

5 McMichael, M., Herring, J., Fletcher, D.J. et al. (2012). RECOVER evidence and knowledge gap analysis on veterinary CPR. Part 2: preparedness and prevention. *J. Vet. Emerg. Crit. Care* 22 (S1): S13–S25.

6 Waldrop, J.E., Rozanski, E.A., Swanke, E.D. et al. (2004). Causes of cardiopulmonary arrest, resuscitation management, and functional outcome in dogs and cats surviving cardiopulmonary arrest. *J. Vet. Emerg. Crit. Care* 14 (1): 22–29.

7 Kass, P.H. and Haskins, S.C. (2007). Survival following cardiopulmonary resuscitation in dogs and cats. *J. Vet. Emerg. Crit. Care* 2 (2): 57–65.

8 Lichtenberger, M. (2004). Principles of shock and fluid therapy in special species. *Semin. Avian Exot. Pet Med.* 13 (3): 142–153.

9 Lichtenberger, M. (2007). Shock and cardiopulmonary-cerebral resuscitation in small mammals and birds. *Vet. Clin. North Am. Exot. Anim. Pract.* 10: 275–291.

10 Astiz, M.E. (2005). Pathophysiology and classification of shock states. In: *Textbook of critical care*, 5e (eds. M.P. Fink, E. Abraham, J.-L. Vincent and P.M. Kochanek). Philadelphia: Elsevier Saunders.

11 Lichtenberger, M., Orcutt, C., Cray, C. et al. (2009). Comparison of fluid types for resuscitation after acute blood loss in mallard ducks (*Anas platyrhynchos*). *J. Vet. Emerg. Crit. Care* 19 (5): 467–472.

12 Wernick, M.B., Steinmetz, H.W., Martin-Jurado, O. et al. (2013). Comparison of fluid types for resuscitation in acute hemorrhagic shock and evaluation of gastric luminal and transcutaneous P_{CO_2} in Leghorn chickens. *J. Avian Med. Surg.* 27 (2): 109–119.

13 Boller, M. and Fletcher, D.J. (2012). RECOVER evidence and knowledge gap analysis on veterinary CPR. Part 1: evidence analysis and consensus process: collaborative path toward small animal CPR guidelines. *J. Vet. Emerg. Crit. Care* 22 (Suppl 1): S4–S12.

14 Hopper, K., Epstein, S.E., Fletcher, D.J. et al. (2012). RECOVER evidence and knowledge gap analysis on veterinary CPR. Part 3: basic life support. *J. Vet. Emerg. Crit. Care* 22 (S1): S26–S43.

15 Costello, M.F. (2004). Principles of cardiopulmonary cerebral resuscitation in special species. *Semin. Avian Exot. Pet Med.* 13 (2): 132–141.

16 Curro, T.G. (1998). Anesthesia of pet birds. *Semin. Avian Exot. Pet Med.* 7 (1): 10–21.

17 Casares, M., Enders, F., and Montoya, J.A. (1999). Comparison of two techniques for attaching electrocardiographic electrodes to Psittacines. *J. Appl. Anim. Res.* 16: 59–64.

18 Acierno, M.J., da Cunha, A., Smith, J. et al. (2008). Agreement between direct and indirect blood pressure measurements obtained from anesthetized Hispaniolan Amazon parrots. *J. Am. Vet. Med. Assoc.* 233 (10): 1587–1590.

19 Lichtenberger, M. (2005). Determination of indirect blood pressure in the companion bird. *Semin. Avian Exot. Pet Med.* 14 (2): 149–152.

20 Cole, S.G., Otto, C.M., and Hughes, D. (2002). Cardiopulmonary cerebral resuscitation in small animals – a clinical practice review. Part I. *J. Vet. Emerg. Crit. Care.* 12 (4): 261–267.

21 Briscoe, J.A. and Syring, R. (2004). Techniques for emergency airway and vascular access in special species. *Semin. Avian Exot. Pet Med.* 13 (3): 118–131.

22 Brown, C. and Pilny, A.A. (2006). Air sac cannula placement in birds. *Lab Anim.* 35 (7): 23–24.

23 Bowles, H., Lichtenberger, M., and Lennox, A. (2007). Emergency and critical care of pet birds. *Vet. Clin. North Am. Exot. Anim. Pract.* 10 (2): 345–394.

24 Rozanski, E.A., Rush, J.E., Buckley, G.J. et al. (2012). RECOVER evidence and knowledge gap analysis on veterinary CPR. Part 4: advanced life support. *J. Vet. Emerg. Crit. Care* 22 (Suppl 1): S44–S64.

25 Cole, S.G., Otto, C.M., and Hughes, D. (2003). Cardiopulmonary cerebral resuscitation in small animals – a clinical practice review. Part II. *J. Vet. Emerg. Crit. Care* 13 (1): 13–23.

26 Nap, A.M., Lumeij, J.T., and Stokhof, A.A. (1992). Electrocardiogram of the African grey (*Psittacus erithacus*) and Amazon (*Amazona* spp.) parrot. *Avian Pathol.* 21 (1): 45–53.

27 Rodriguez, R., Prieto-Montana, F., Montes, A.M. et al. (2004). The normal electrocardiogram of the unanesthetized peregrine falcon (*Falco peregrinus brookei*). *Avian Dis.* 48 (2): 405–409.

28 Talavera, J., Guzman, M.J., del Palacio, M.J. et al. (2008). The normal electrocardiogram of four species of conscious raptors. *Res. Vet. Sci.* 84 (1): 119–125.

29 Hassanpour, H. and Khadem, P. (2013). Normal electrocardiogram patterns and values in Muscovy ducks (*Cairina moschata*). *J. Avian Med. Surg.* 27 (4): 280–284.

30 Hassanpour, H., Moghaddam, A.K.Z., and Bashi, M.C. (2010). The normal electrocardiogram of conscious golden eagles (*Aquila chrysaetos*). *J. Zoo Wildl. Med.* 41 (3): 426–431.

31 Papahn, A.A., Naddaf, H., Rezakhani, A., and Mayahi, M. (2006). Electrocardiogram of homing pigeon. *J. Appl. Anim. Res.* 30: 129–132.

32 Oglesbee, B.L., Hamlin, R.L., Klingaman, H. et al. (2001). Electrocardiographic reference values for macaws (*Ara* species) and cockatoos (*Cacatua* species). *J. Avian Med. Surg.* 15 (1): 17–22.

33 Fitzgerald, B.C. and Beaufrere, H. (2016). Chapter 6: Cardiology. In: *Current Therapy in Avian Medicine and Surgery* (ed. B.L. Speer). St. Louis, MO, USA: Elsevier.

34 Boller, M., Boller, E.M., Oodegard, S., and Otto, C.M. (2012). Small animal cardiopulmonary resuscitation requires a continuum of care: proposal for a chain of survival for veterinary patients. *J. Am. Vet. Med. Assoc.* 240 (5): 540–554.

35 Plunkett, S.J. and McMichael, M. (2008). Cardiopulmonary resuscitation in small animal medicine: an update. *J. Vet. Intern. Med.* 22 (1): 9–25.

36 AVMA (2020). *AVMA Guidelines for the Euthanasia of Animals: 2020 Edition*. Schaumburg, IL: American Veterinary Medical Association https://www.avma.org/sites/default/files/2020-01/2020-Euthanasia-Final-1-17-20.pdf.

37 Kirk, N.W., Greenacre, C., and McCleery, B. (eds.) (2015). Comparison of various avian euthanasia methods. *ExoticsCon Conference Proceedings*, San Antonio, TX, USA.

38 Paul-Murphy, J., Engilis, A., Pascoe, P. et al. (eds.) (2016). Comparison of pentobarbital and thoracic (cardiac) compression to euthanize anesthetized sparrows (*Passer domesticus*) and starlings (*Sturnus vulgaris*). *ExoticsCon Conference Proceedings*, Portland, OR, USA.

39 Latimer, K.S. and Rakich, P.M. (1994). Necropsy examination. In: *Avian Medicine: Principles and Application* (eds. B.W. Ritchie, G. Harrison and L. Harrison), 355–379. Lake Worth, FL: Wingers Publishing.

40 Raghav, R., Taylor, M., Guincho, M., and Smith, D. (2011). Potassium chloride as a euthanasia agent in psittacine birds: clinical aspects and consequences for histopathologic assessment. *Can. Vet. J.* 52: 303–306.

28

Avian Pain Management and Anesthesia

David Sanchez-Migallon Guzman and Hugues Beaufrère

Department of Medicine and Epidemiology, School of Veterinary Medicine, University of California–Davis, Davis, California, USA

CONTENTS

Analgesia

Indications

Pain management is primordial in the treatment of traumatized and critical patients. While pain and nociception are physiologic processes, they can be associated with deleterious effects in critical patients such as anorexia, decreased mobility and standing, increased stress and sympathetic tone, abnormal or maladaptive behaviors, and slower healing. Consequently, inadequate pain management may worsen overall prognosis and slow down surgical recovery.

Pain Assessment/Scoring

Pain recognition may be challenging in birds and can be based on pain scales, score sheets, species-specific ethogram, subjective assessments, and extrapolation from what is considered painful in other species such as humans and domestic mammals (Figure 28.1) [1]. In critical patients, the accurate recognition and quantification of pain may be confounded by any disease processes or emergency presentations that may cause neurological disorders, dehydration, hypovolemia, metabolic disturbances, lethargy, and anorexia.

Principles of Analgesia

If a painful event can be anticipated, it is best to treat it pre-emptively to limit noxious sensitization. Pre-emptive analgesia with opioid drugs, non-steroidal anti-inflammatory drugs (NSAIDs), and/or local anesthetics can block sensory noxious stimuli from onward transmission to the central nervous system (CNS), thus reducing the overall potential for pain and inflammation and potentially improving the patient's short-term and long-term recovery.

In addition, multimodal or balanced analgesia increases the analgesic efficacy and reduces the adverse effects through combination of different analgesics with different pharmacologic profiles and mechanisms. Drugs for which measurable analgesia has been demonstrated in some bird species are reported in Table 28.1.

Exotic Animal Emergency and Critical Care Medicine, First Edition. Edited by Jennifer E. Graham, Grayson A. Doss and Hugues Beaufrère.

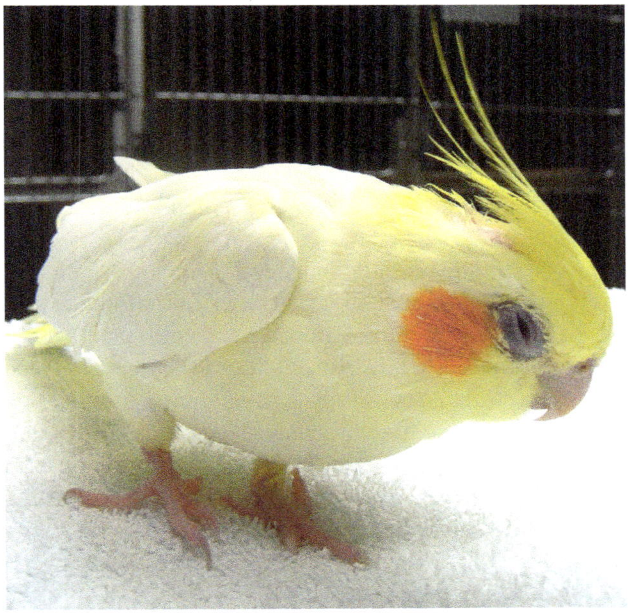

Figure 28.1 Cockatiel showing typical behavior associated with pain and discomfort such as hunched posture and closed eyelids.

Drug Classes

Opioid Drugs

Opioid drugs provide analgesia by their actions on specific opiate receptors on cell membranes (μ, κ, δ, and nociception), mimicking the effects of endogenous opioids (endorphins, enkephalins, and dynorphins). The analgesic effects of the different opioid drugs seem to vary depending on avian species. This may be due to differences in the proportion and localization of opioid receptors within the CNS of different bird species. For instance, pigeons tend to have more κ receptors while falcons more μ receptors in the brain [17, 18]. In general, doses are also much higher than in mammals.

Butorphanol, a κ-opioid receptor agonist and μ-opioid receptor antagonist, has historically been considered the opioid drug of choice for management of acute pain in Psittaciformes although recent studies are currently challenging this notion and tend to suggest that opioid drugs have more species-specific effects within bird orders than previously thought. Several studies have evaluated the analgesic effects of opioids, particularly those with κ opioid receptor affinities, as well as their effects on anesthetic requirements in psittacine birds. The accepted dose for butorphanol tartrate in psittacines of 1–3 mg of butorphanol/kg IM requires repeated administration every two to three hours [2, 3]. However, species-specific doses may vary depending on intrinsic factors. For instance, Hispaniolan Amazon parrots (*Amazona ventralis*) require a butorphanol dose of 5 mg/kg IV or IM q2–3h to achieve plasma concentrations considered therapeutic [2]. The oral bioavailability of butorphanol has also been reported to be low in parrots, at about 6%, precluding the use of this route for clinical purposes. Pre-operative butorphanol administration (2 mg/kg IM) was not associated with deleterious anesthetic or cardiopulmonary effects in the same species, suggesting that it is safe to use as part of a pre-emptive analgesic protocol [4]. However, the same analgesic effects of butorphanol could not be demonstrated in the American kestrel, used as a representative member of another group of birds, the Falconiformes. In this species, butorphanol tartrate at 1–6 mg/kg did not produce any significant antinociception, as measured using a thermal foot withdrawal model [19]. Neither resulted in sedative effects in American kestrels, but instead caused hyperaesthesia or hyperalgesia and agitation in males receiving 6 mg/kg. This study shows that it is important to use species-specific or at least order-specific information when using analgesics in birds. Further studies with different analgesiometry models,

Table 28.1 Recommended evidence-based doses of selected analgesics in birds.

Family	Drug	Dose	References
Psittacidae	Butorphanol	2–5 mg/kg q2–3h IM 1–2 mg/kg/h CRI	[2–4]
	Tramadol	30 mg/kg q6–12h PO	[5, 6]
	Meloxicam	1–1.5 mg/kg q12h IM, PO	[7–9]
Falconidae	Hydromorphone	0.1–0.3 mg/kg q3–6h IM	[10]
	Buprenorphine	0.1–0.6 mg/kg q6h IM	[13]
	Tramadol	5 mg/kg q2–12h	[14]
Accipitridae	Fentanyl	10–30 μg/kg	[15]
Columbidae	Buprenorphine	0.25–0.5 mg/kg IM q2–5h	[16]

Note: Only commercially available analgesics are shown. Doses are based on studies in a representative member of each family. Studies on drugs that have not shown a demonstrable analgesic effect are not shown. There are no published analgesiometry studies on bird families or drugs not mentioned.

Birds

formulations, dosages, routes of administration, and experimental designs are needed to further evaluate the antinociceptive and adverse effects of butorphanol in American kestrels and other species. Since the duration of action of butorphanol is short in parrots, several studies have investigated different means of prolonging its effects in birds. In a study in Amazon parrots, liposomal-encapsulated butorphanol provided analgesia for up to five days [20]. Unfortunately, this formulation is currently not commercially available. The use of an osmotic pump to deliver butorphanol chronically has also been investigated in peafowl [21]. Combining butorphanol with poloxamer 407 hydrogel in a sustained-release formulation was also reported in Amazon parrots [22].

Nalbuphine is a κ-opioid receptor agonist and μ-opioid receptor antagonist opioid drug, with a similar mechanism of action to butorphanol. Nalbuphine hydrochloride produced measurable antinociception in Hispaniolan Amazon parrots at 12.5 mg/kg for up to three hours, while higher dosages of 25 and 50 mg/kg did not result in better or longer effect [23]. Because of its low abuse potential, this opioid is currently not a Drug Enforcement Administration scheduled substance in the United States. Nalbuphine decanoate, a long acting formulation of nalbuphine, has also been shown to maintain potentially analgesic plasma concentrations for 24 hours in parrots [24].

Morphine, a pure μ-opioid agonist, is not commonly used in avian medicine because studies with domestic fowl had confusing and conflicting results [25–27]. More recent studies in adult chickens using the isoflurane sparing technique found that increasing doses of morphine at 0.1, 1, and 3 mg/kg had a significant isoflurane sparing effect [28].

Hydromorphone, a pure μ-opioid agonist drug, has shown a dose-responsive antinociceptive effect when administered intramuscular (IM) at 0.1, 0.3, and 0.6 mg/kg in American kestrels, suggesting that hydromorphone hydrochloride could produce analgesia in this species for up to six hours [10]. No significant sedative effect was detected except at the higher dose of 0.6 mg/kg. In cockatiels, hydromorphone, at the same dosages evaluated in kestrels, did not result in increased thermal antinociception [11], while 1 and 2 mg/kg IM in orange-winged Amazon parrots result in significant thermal antinociception. Interestingly, the 2 mg/kg was not superior to 1 mg/kg in the antinociceptive effects, and agitation and nausea-like behavior was significant in the birds receiving the highest dose [12].

Fentanyl is a pure μ-opioid agonist. A study in umbrella cockatoos (*Cacatua alba*) showed a short antinociceptive effect of fentanyl at high doses (0.2 mg/kg IM), and the birds appeared hyperactive [29]. Another study in Amazon parrots showed an isoflurane sparing effect, but at clinically impractical doses that would also result in a significant decrease of heart rate and indirect blood pressure [30]. However, in a recent study in red-tailed hawks (*Buteo jamaicensis*), fentanyl constant rate infusion (CRI) at 10–30 μg/kg/h significantly decreased isoflurane minimum anesthetic concentration (MAC) with no observable cardiopulmonary adverse effects [15]. The study concluded that fentanyl produced a dose-related decrease of isoflurane MAC with minimal effects on measured cardiovascular parameters in red-tailed hawks.

Buprenorphine is μ-opioid receptor agonist, but its κ-receptor activities are less well defined. Several studies suggest that buprenorphine demonstrates κ-receptor agonist activity but other evidence in mammals and pigeons (*Columba livia*) suggests that it also displays some κ antagonistic activities. Buprenorphine has unusual receptor-binding characteristics that seem to be the result of slow drug dissociation from opioid receptors. Few studies have been published evaluating the use of buprenorphine in birds. Buprenorphine hydrochloride at 0.1 mg/kg IM in grey parrots (*Psittacus erithacus*) did not produce antinociception using electrical noxious stimuli [3]. This is despite the fact that buprenorphine plasma levels considered therapeutic in humans were reached in this species at this dose [31]. In cockatiels, buprenorphine at 0.6, 1.2, and 1.8 mg/kg IM did not result in increased thermal antinociception and is currently not recommended in psittacine species for pain management [32]. In American kestrels, buprenorphine hydrochloride caused a significant thermal antinociceptive response at 0.1, 0.3, and 0.6 mg/kg for up to and over six hours [13]. At 0.6 mg/kg, a mild sedative effect was appreciated. A commercially available sustained-release formulation of buprenorphine has recently shown to have thermal antinociceptive effects for at least 24 hours in the same species. In cockatiels, buprenorphine at 0.6, 1.2, and 1.8 mg/kg IM did not result in increased thermal antinociception and is currently not recommended in psittacine species for pain management.

Tramadol, a centrally acting μ-opioid receptor agonist drug that binds weakly to κ- and δ-opioid receptors, also inhibits the reuptake of norepinephrine and serotonin. Tramadol at a dose of 30 mg/kg orally was shown to have antinociceptive properties in Hispaniolan Amazon parrots for up to six hours. Lower dosages of 10 and 20 mg/kg failed to achieve a comparable effect [5]. Antinociception was also demonstrated in American kestrels at 5 mg/kg for 1.5 hours compared to control and nine hours compared to baseline values, while higher doses resulted in less antinociceptive effects [14]. The pharmacokinetics of tramadol have been evaluated in several avian species, including bald eagles (*Haliaeetus leucocephalus*), red-tailed hawks, peafowl (*Pavo cristatus*), African penguins (*Spheniscus demersus*), and, recently, Hispaniolan Amazon parrots and American kestrels [6, 14, 33–37]. The results of these studies detected differences in pharmacokinetics between Hispaniolan Amazon parrots and other species of birds. Oral bioavailability varied from low in parrots at only 23.48% to high in eagles at 97.94% [36].

Non-steroidal Anti-inflammatory Drugs

Meloxicam is a COX-2 selective oxicam NSAID. Higher doses are required in birds to produce analgesia. Indeed, it was demonstrated in Hispaniolan Amazon parrots that 1 mg/kg meloxicam q12h IM (equivalent to 1.6 mg/kg PO considering oral bioavailability) was needed to produce detectable analgesia in an experimental chronic pain model [7]. Likewise, in pigeons, administration of meloxicam at 0.5 mg/kg q12h PO was ineffective at minimizing post-operative pain with an experimental osteotomy model, but 2.0 mg/kg was required to detect an analgesic effect [38]. Instead, in grey parrots, 1 mg/kg PO maintains above target plasma concentration for 24 hours [39]. In birds of prey species, a pharmacokinetic study also confirmed the high doses required by most birds and showed that species-specific differences in pharmacologic behavior can be high [40]. Consequently, it may be difficult to extrapolate meloxicam dosages in birds from known pharmacologic studies. Meloxicam appears to be safe in birds in general. Studies in Hispaniolan Amazon parrots, American kestrels, and Japanese quail failed to show any deleterious effects of meloxicam on renal, gastrointestinal, and hemostatic functions, even at high doses and chronic administration [8, 41, 42].

Carprofen can be administered parenterally or orally and is well absorbed through the gastrointestinal tract in mammals. The mechanism of action of carprofen has not been fully elucidated. It is a weak inhibitor of COX at therapeutic doses and yet exhibits good anti-inflammatory activity. In chickens, carprofen improved lameness in a dose-dependent manner [43]. An analgesia study with Hispaniolan Amazon parrots with experimental arthritis noted that 3 mg/kg intramuscularly q12h carprofen did not significantly improve the weight-bearing load of the arthritic limb for the 30-hour study period [44]. In pigeons, IM administration of carprofen was associated with increased aspartate aminotransferase and alanine aminotransferase enzyme concentrations, gross lesions in muscle injection sites and liver, and histologic lesions in liver and muscle [45].

Other Drugs

Gabapentin is a *gamma*-aminobutyric acid (GABA) analog. It was originally developed to treat epilepsy and currently is also used to relieve neuropathic pain. Gabapentin decreases release of excitatory neurotransmitters by binding to α 2-delta subunit of voltage-gated Ca channels. There have been a few reports of use in clinical cases in avian species. Recently, pharmacokinetic studies in Hispaniolan Amazon parrots and great horned owls were completed; based on plasma concentrations a dosage of 5–15 mg/kg q8h and 11 mg/kg q8h, respectively, were recommended [46, 47]. No pharmacodynamic studies are available to evaluate the analgesic properties of gabapentin in birds.

Local Anesthesia

Local anesthetics block ion channels to prevent pain impulse generation and conduction, and they should be combined with general anesthesia when used in birds. Lidocaine can be used preoperatively (maximum recommended dose: ≤4 mg/kg to prevent toxicosis) by local infiltration [48]. Bupivacaine (2 mg/kg) at the site of incision or as a ring block may provide post-operative analgesia. Brachial plexus block using palpation, ultrasound, or nerve locator have been used with variable degrees of success in avian species [49–51]. Sciatic and femoral nerve block in raptors have been described but not evaluated for efficacy in birds.

Sedation

Sedation facilitates common clinical procedures, such as physical examination, blood collection, or radiography. Sedation provides immobilization, reduces vocalization, and attenuates the stress response caused by manual restraint. Midazolam and midazolam/butorphanol are the most commonly used drugs for sedation of pet birds, and they provide dose-dependent sedation with no significant adverse effects for most species at the published dosages. The intranasal route of administration is a non-invasive alternative to IM administration and has been shown to be a safe and effective technique to rapidly induce sedation in birds. Reversal of midazolam with flumazenil can be performed when needed. (https://pubmed.ncbi.nlm.nih.gov/30457900/) (https://pubmed.ncbi.nlm.nih.gov/23156974/)

General Anesthesia

Pre-anesthetic Assessment

The pre-anesthetic evaluation should include a history and a physical examination. In case of a long anesthesia, general health screening using a complete blood count and a biochemistry panel is recommended. If a complete blood count and biochemistry cannot be obtained, a limited database including packed cell volume (PCV), total solid (TS), and blood glucose can alternatively be performed. Any detected abnormalities (e.g. dehydration) should be corrected with appropriate therapy (e.g. fluid therapy) before the procedure. The fasting period is variable, ranging from two to four hours in most psittacine species to 24 hours in most raptor species.

Premedication

Premedication drugs should be given to facilitate induction and reduce the requirement for inhalants as most inhalants cause hypotension and result in significant respiratory depression.

Parasympatholytics (e.g. atropine, glycopyrrolate) are not routinely administered to birds because of the concern that an increase in viscosity of the respiratory tract secretions may promote airway or endotracheal tube obstruction [52, 53]. Benzodiazepines (e.g. diazepam, midazolam) are increasingly used in birds and produce sedation, hypnosis, anxiolysis, presumed anterograde amnesia, centrally mediated muscle relaxation, and anti-convulsion. Midazolam (0.5–2 mg/kg) is preferred over diazepam because it can be administered IM or intranasal [54]. Midazolam also decreases the MAC of inhalants and has minimal adverse cardiopulmonary effects [55].

Midazolam is often combined with an opioid drug for premedication prior to induction of general anesthesia. Opioid drugs have also the potential of decreasing the MAC of inhalants. The authors frequently use butorphanol (2–3 mg/kg) for parrots and fentanyl (2–5 μg/kg) or hydromorphone (0.1–0.3 mg/kg) for birds of prey. Opioid premedication should also take into consideration the later use of other opioids in intraoperative CRI. Opioids have minimal cardiopulmonary adverse effects in birds.

Induction

Mask

Commercially available masks designed for dogs and cats can be used for induction of avian anesthesia. A properly sized mask allows the entire head and beak to be inserted while minimizing dead space. Masks can be modified to accommodate the widely diverse beak and head anatomic variations of birds. For example, for budgerigars and finches, a cut down 35- or 60-ml syringe case can be used, with a hole drilled at the closed end to facilitate insertion of the adapter piece for the circuit. At the other extreme, a 1- to 2-l soft drink bottle can be cut down to facilitate masking a large toucan.

During induction for general anesthesia, the bird is manually restrained until immobilized and then placed in sternal or lateral recumbency position on a padded surface. Birds are pre-oxygenated for two to three minutes before induction. Preferably, they can be induced at low and increasing (e.g. 0.5% for a minute, then 1% for a minute, then 1.5%) concentrations of inhalation agents, taking usually one to five minutes. Alternatively, induce at 3–5% isoflurane or 5–7% sevoflurane over one to three minutes. This may vary depending on the premedication given or the health of the bird. However, induction of anesthesia in large waterfowl and Galliformes by a propofol (4–6 mg/kg) intravenous (IV) injection in the medial metatarsal vein followed by intubation and isoflurane maintenance is the preferred method by some clinicians as these species may either breath-hold, struggle, or have a delayed induction using isoflurane mask induction. It is still recommended to oxygenate the bird via a facemask during propofol induction.

Intubation

Endotracheal uncuffed tubes are used in birds, since the use of cuff should be avoided because of the presence of complete tracheal rings. However, in large birds a cuffed tube may be used with low inflation of the cuff. The endotracheal tube used in birds varies from 1.5 to 6 mm diameter. Cole tubes provide a good seal of the glottis. Endotracheal tubes for birds weighing less than 100 g are not commercially available and red rubber feeding tubes are a good alternative. Great caution should be exercised with endotracheal tubes smaller than 2.0 mm diameter since they can get obstructed easily and dramatically increase ventilatory efforts. The dead space should be minimal, especially in small birds where CO_2 rebreathing may occur.

Intubation is performed after the patient is induced into a medium plane of anesthesia, and care should be taken to prevent tracheal trauma (see Chapter 24: Oxygen Therapy for in depth information on avian endotracheal intubation). The endotracheal tube is secured with umbilical cord tape or regular tape. An oxygen flow rate of 150–200 ml/kg/min is reported, but 1 l/min in most medium and large birds (approximately >300 g) is commonly used. Air sac anesthesia is also possible in birds when an upper respiratory obstruction is present or for surgery of the head and trachea (see Chapter 24: Oxygen Therapy).

Maintenance

Injectable Anesthesia

Injectable anesthetics, such as propofol, alfaxalone, or medetomidine–ketamine or xylazine–ketamine (followed by reversal with atipamezole or yohimbine), may be useful for remote field locations where commercial shipment of hazardous gases and anesthetic agents is logistically complicated or prohibited or for use in large birds for which mask induction may be challenging or prolonged (i.e. large waterfowls, large Galliformes, ratites). Propofol [56–65] and ketamine–medetomidine or xylazine combinations [61, 62, 66–70] have been evaluated in several avian species. Injectable anesthetics might be preferred also in surgeries involving the beak, mouth, glottis, coelomic cavity, respiratory system, or pneumatic bones. The need for ventilatory support, the challenge of maintaining a constant plane of anesthesia, and the potential for excitatory and/or prolonged recoveries limit their use in companion birds as a sole agent. Anesthetic maintenance using a propofol CRI at 1 mg/kg/min was studied in Amazon parrots and resulted in a light to surgical plane of anesthesia [58]. Neuromuscular blocking drugs such as atracurium have also been used in birds, most commonly in cataract surgery in addition to other anesthetic agents, but the use of neuromuscular blocking drugs require ventilation and close monitoring.

Inhalation Agents

Inhalation anesthesia is more commonly used than injectable anesthesia in clinical avian practice. Isoflurane is currently the anesthetic agent of choice, although sevoflurane is also an excellent, but more expensive, option. Both isoflurane and sevoflurane are considered dose-dependent respiratory and cardiovascular depressants. Isoflurane results in rapid inductions, allows rapid alterations in anesthetic plane, has a small margin between respiratory and cardiac arrest, and provides rapid and smooth recoveries. Sevoflurane, due to lower solubility than isoflurane, allows for faster induction and recovery, as well as more rapid changes in anesthetic depth, but this difference has proven to be small or non-existent in some studies in different avian species [71]. Sevoflurane also appears to be less pungent to the airways in comparison to isoflurane.

The MAC of sevoflurane and isoflurane have been determined in only a few species (Table 28.2). MAC values may differ between studies and techniques for the same species [73]. Birds are commonly maintained at 1–2.5% isoflurane and 3–4% sevoflurane for most procedures.

A variety of drugs can be administered to lower the MAC of isoflurane during an anesthetic event such as midazolam and opioids given as repeated injections or as CRI. Specifically, fentanyl CRI has been shown to significantly decrease the MAC in a dose-dependent manner by as much as 50% in red-tailed hawk at doses ranging from 10 to 30 μg/kg/h [15]. A similar study found a similar MAC reduction effect in Amazon parrots but at much higher dosages (180–380 μg/kg/h), which may not be practical in this species [30]. Isoflurane MAC reduction with fentanyl could also not be achieved in cockatoos [29]. Butorphanol as repeated injections or CRI administration (1–2 mg/kg/h) are routinely used in parrots for peri-operative analgesia and MAC reduction. Butorphanol at 1 mg/kg has been shown to decrease the isoflurane MAC in cockatoos by 25% [81]. In guineafowl, a single dose of butorphanol at 2 mg/kg IM reduced the MAC by 10–20% [76]. Midazolam at 1 and 2 mg/kg reduced isoflurane MAC in Quaker parrots by 19% and 28%, respectively [54]. Midazolam at a high dose (15 mg/kg IM) resulted in a isoflurane MAC reduction of 38% in pigeons [80]. Ketamine can also be used as a bolus dose or CRI for pain and to decrease the MAC. In a study in blue-fronted Amazon parrots, premedication with ketamine 10 mg/kg IM and a combination ketamine 10 mg/kg – diazepam 0.5 mg/kg IM reduced the sevoflurane MAC by 29% and 46%, respectively [79].

Table 28.2 Reported mean ± SD of the minimum anesthetic concentration of selected avian species.

Isoflurane			Sevoflurane		
Species	**MAC**	**References**	**Species**	**MAC**	**References**
Thick-billed parrot	1.07 ± 0.1	[72]	Thick-billed parrot	2.35	[73]
Chicken	1.24 ± 0.05	[28]	Chicken	2.21 ± 0.32	[74]
Sandhill crane	1.34 ± 0.14	[75]	Guineafowl	2.9 ± 0.1	[76]
Pekin duck	1.30 ± 0.23	[77]	Crested serpent eagle	2.03 ± 0.32	[78]
Cinereous vulture	1.06 ± 0.07	[28]	Blue-fronted Amazon parrot	2.4 ± 0.37	[79]
Quaker parrot	2.52 ± 0.41	[55]			
Red-tailed hawk	2.05 ± 0.45	[15]			
Crested serpent eagle	1.46 ± 0.3	[78]			
Pigeon	1.45 ± 0.11	[80]			
Cockatoos	1.44 ± 0.07	[81]			

Halogenated inhalants produce significant respiratory depression, hypotension, and cardiac arrhythmias in some species. Slight benefits of sevoflurane over isoflurane have been demonstrated regarding the frequency and degree of cardiorespiratory adverse effects [71, 82, 83]. The respiratory depression of isoflurane tends to be more profound in birds than in mammals, especially at a surgical plane of anesthesia [48, 52]. For instance, a study in Amazon parrots showed progressive hypercapnia and hypoventilation under isoflurane anesthesia [58]. Similar results were found in other species, such as pigeons, bald eagles, red-tailed hawks, and crested caracaras [71, 82–85]. As a consequence, intermittent positive pressure ventilation (IPVV) is always required in anesthetized birds to prevent hypercapnia. Hypotension and arrhythmias have been reported consistently in various studies in different bird species. Cardiac arrhythmias seem subjectively more common in anesthetized birds of prey than other species. In pigeons, isoflurane anesthesia resulted in significant hypotension and second- and third-degree atrioventricular blocks [84]. Hypertensive effects rather than hypotensive effects were witnessed in bald eagles as well as arrhythmias [71]. Sevoflurane had less adverse effects in this species. In crested caracaras, isoflurane and sevoflurane led to significant hypotension but no cardiac arrhythmias [82, 85].

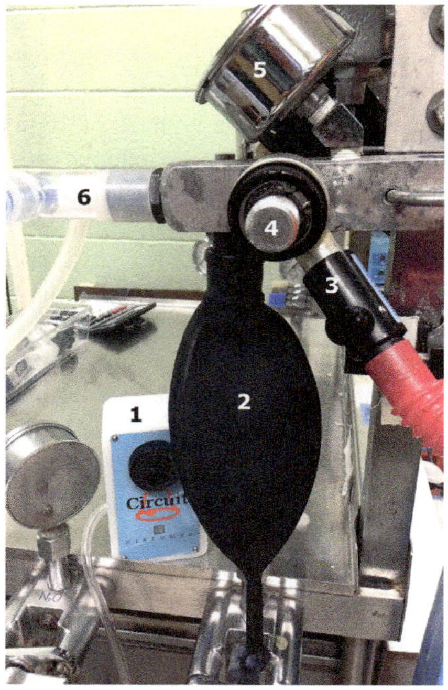

Figure 28.2 Standard Bain circuit with safety measures recommended for use in avian anesthesia. 1, high-pressure alarm; 2, breathing bag; 3, pop-off occlusion valve; 4, pop-off valve; 5, manometer; and 6, breathing tube.

Inhalation Equipment

Non-rebreathing circuits, such as the Bain circuit, are recommended for anesthesia in birds weighting less than 4 kg. The advantages of these circuits include decreased resistance to breathing by the patient and rapid responses to changes in the vaporizer setting. A 0.5- to 1.0-l bag is used for most birds. To limit the risk of volutrauma when the pop-off valve is inadvertently left closed, a pop-off occlusion valve and a high-pressure alarm may be installed on the anesthetic machine (Figure 28.2).

The weight and position of the anesthetic tube, capnograph connecting piece, and endotracheal tube may inadvertently cause extubation. As such, the tube should be well secured in place, for instance, using a dedicated piece of equipment (RES520 Circuit Secure) or tape.

As inhalants induce profound respiratory depression and basal respiratory rate of small birds can be high, it is recommended to use a small ventilator for IPVV. Avian tidal volumes tend to be larger than mammals. Cardiovascular side effects such as hypotension commonly encountered in artificially ventilated mammals are not observed in birds due to their different ventilation physiology [86]. The Vetronics small animal ventilator is a simple pressure-controlled ventilator that is easy to set up and can be used to ventilate most bird species, even passerines (Figure 28.3). The pressure is

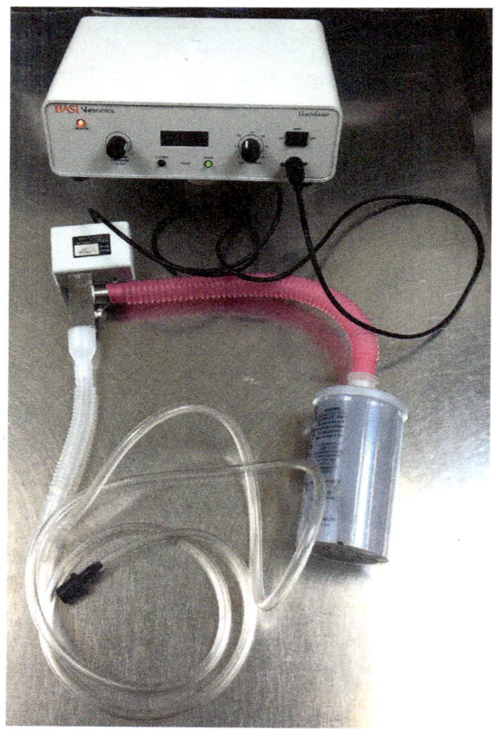

Figure 28.3 Vetronics small animal pressure-controlled ventilator. This ventilator is easy to use and can be used to ventilate birds as small as passerines.

set to the lowest pressure needed to cause keel excursions, and the respiratory rate is set based on capnography. As ventilation performed by the Vetronics is passive, a higher oxygen rate than for spontaneous ventilation is recommended (which can in turn artificially decrease $ETCO_2$) and this ventilator may not perform well on large birds. The Hallowell EMC Anesthesia Workstation is another ventilator designed for very small animals and is more technical to use, but has been studied in Amazon parrots [86]. Regular ventilators such as Hallowell EMC Multiflow ventilators work well in medium to large birds.

Monitoring and Supportive Care

Due to the rapid rate at which birds may decompensate under anesthesia, monitoring is the most important aspect of avian anesthesia. This means that having one person dedicated to consistent, hands-on monitoring and ensuring that the anesthetist has a clear view of the patient are critically important. All parameters should be recorded in a dedicated anesthesia chart. Monitoring techniques are also used in critically ill birds to assess the results of cardiopulmonary resuscitation (CPR), fluid therapy, oxygen therapy, and other treatments. Whenever available, multiparameter anesthetic monitors should be used. When not available, a combination of different monitoring instruments is recommended (Figure 28.4). At the very minimum, a Doppler unit in combination with capnography should be used for all anesthetic events to monitor cardiorespiratory parameters.

Central Nervous System Monitoring

The loss of muscle tone in the legs or wings can be useful for assessing transition from a light to a medium plane of anesthesia. The withdrawal reflexes (i.e. toe pinch) are lost when the bird is in a medium (surgical) plane of anesthesia. The palpebral reflexes are usually lost by a medium plane of anesthesia, but corneal reflexes persist until the deep plane of anesthesia. The heart and respiratory rates increase when the bird is experiencing pain or when the depth of anesthesia is too low; conversely, these rates may decrease in the deep plane of anesthesia, signaling the need to adjust the concentration of anesthetic gases accordingly. As the palpebral and corneal reflexes are suppressed and the tear production is decreased under anesthesia, the regular application of tear gel is recommended.

Cardiovascular Monitoring and Support

A stethoscope can be used to monitor heart rate and rhythm, and the use of an esophageal stethoscope can facilitate this job. The esophageal stethoscope should be placed into the thoracic esophagus bypassing the crop with digital manipulation. The ultrasonic Doppler flow detector can be used for the same function. The sensor is commonly placed over the cranial tibial artery, palpable on the cranial aspect of the hock joint; the superficial ulnar artery, palpable on the ventral surface of the elbow joint; the deep radial artery, palpable on the ventral surface of the distal radius near the carpal joint or the palatal artery in the dorsal oropharynx. The electrocardiogram (ECG) can be used as well for monitoring of the heart rate

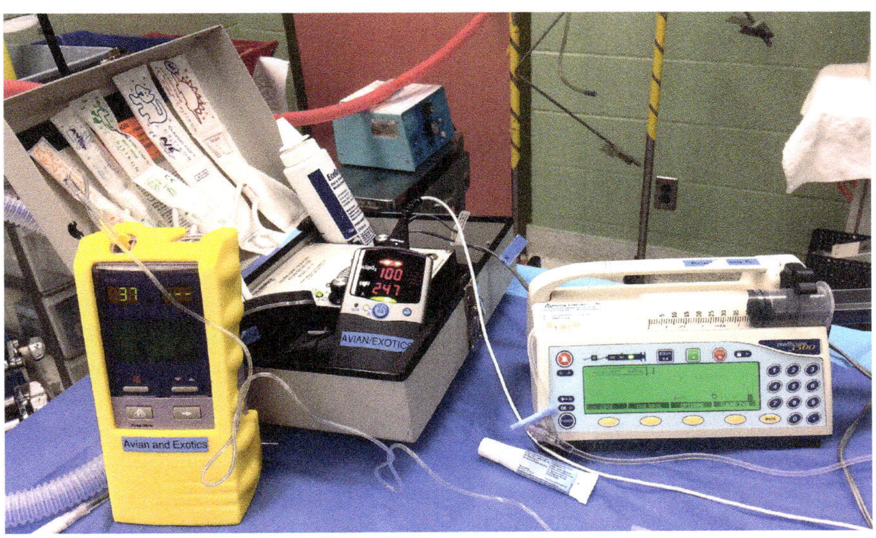

Figure 28.4 Anesthetic monitoring equipment in a bird anesthesia. Alternatively, a multiparameter monitor can be used. On the figure, from left to right, are the microstream capnography, the Doppler unit, the pulse oximeter, the tear gel, and the fluid pump.

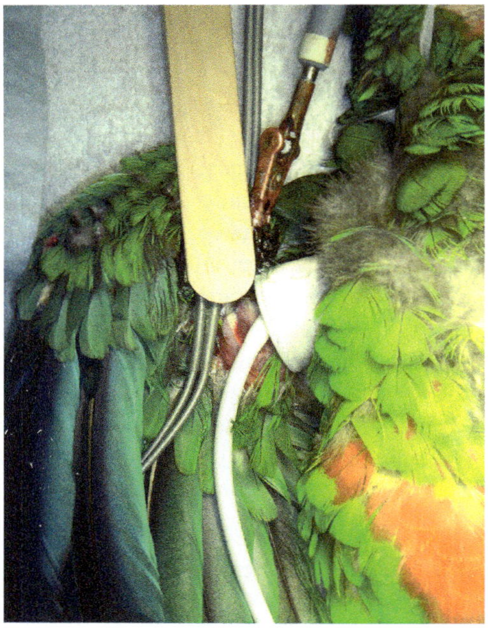

Figure 28.5 Cardiovascular monitoring in an anesthetized Amazon parrot consisting of indirect blood pressure monitoring using a cuff and a Doppler unit and electrocardiography [87].

and rhythm, and the electrodes are positioned at the patagium and inguinal skin web locations using flattened alligator clips, or small hypodermic needles are passed through the skin and attached to alligator clips (Figure 28.5). The avian ECG presents differences from mammals that should be known such as a negative mean electrical axis.

Direct arterial pressure monitoring is the gold standard for measuring blood pressure. The most common sites include the superficial ulnar artery, the deep radial artery, the cranial tibial artery, and the carotid artery (see Chapter 25: Catheterization). Indirect blood pressure monitoring is performed using a Doppler ultrasonic probe to detect arterial flow, a pressure cuff for occlusion, and a sphygmomanometer to measure pressure. Based on different studies in avian species, indirect blood pressure measurements do not have good agreement with direct systolic arterial measurements [88, 89] and are very variable between repeated measurements when cuffs are applied multiple times to the same limb [90]. In larger birds, results may be more accurate and closer to the mean than systolic arterial blood pressure [88]. Since most of the variability of the technique is attributable to cuff placement and individuals, monitoring trends in blood pressure during a single cuff placement in the same individual as during anesthetic monitoring is probably valid [90]. Oscillometric indirect blood pressure measurements have consistently been shown to be inaccurate and should not be used in birds other than very large birds [88, 89]. Indirect mean arterial pressures reported in anesthetized Hispaniolan Amazon in the wing were 140 ± 25 mmHg, while in the leg were 145 ± 28 mmHg, with a cuff width of 30–40% of the diameter [67]. In red-tailed hawks, mean arterial pressures were 155 ± 27 mmHg from both wing and leg with a cuff width of 40–50% of the diameter and under anesthesia.

Fluid therapy is a critical component of avian anesthesia, particularly for procedures lasting longer than 20 minutes (see Chapters 29: Fluid Therapy and 25: Catheterization). It is used to: treat pre-existing dehydration; counteract the hypotensive effects of inhalants which are more profound in hypovolemic patients and with other anesthetic drugs; prevent dehydration caused by the inhaled gas and surgical field; and as a vehicle for CRI medications and emergency drugs. Ideally, an intravenous or intraosseous (IO) catheter is placed to facilitate fluid administration at 10 ml/kg/h; however, subcutaneous fluid administration may be adequate for routine or relatively short procedures in otherwise stable patients. Dobutamine CRI at 5–15 μg/kg/min and dopamine CRI at 5–10 μg/kg/min have shown to help correct severe hypotension in Hispaniolan Amazon parrots caused by 2.5% isoflurane anesthesia [91]. The use of colloids may also help increase blood pressure (e.g. pentastarch or hetastarch 5–10 ml/kg/bolus).

Respiratory Monitoring and Support

Respiratory rate and character should be closely monitored throughout anesthesia. Ventilation is assessed by observing the frequency and range of sternal motion and reservoir bag movement. A change in respiratory pattern involving increased respiratory effort may indicate obstruction of the endotracheal tube, a concern in very small patients. Normal ventilation is associated with little to no respiratory tract noise. In the few species that have been studied, it appears that hypercapnia is associated with cardiovascular depression in birds and so the support of ventilation may be more routine in avian anesthesia. Inhalants have stronger respiratory depressant effects in birds than in mammals, which further justify assisted ventilation in anesthetized birds. In addition, any drugs causing myorelaxation (e.g. midazolam) may depress ventilatory muscles. Assisted ventilation can be provided through manual ventilation ("bagging") or with a ventilator (see above).

While body position during anesthesia seems to affect air sac volume in birds, these variations do not seem to be associated with clinically significant hypoxemia or ventilatory compromise [92, 93].

The capnograph is used to monitor end-tidal carbon dioxide ($PETCO_2$) and provides information regarding ventilatory status. A microstream capnography with a low sampling volume and a connecting piece that minimizes dead space is recommended. There is good correlation between $PETCO_2$ and $PaCO_2$, with $PETCO_2$ slightly exceeding $PaCO_2$ because of the avian cross-current pulmonary gaseous exchange [94, 95]. An $ETCO_2$ of 30–45 mmHg indicates adequate ventilation during inhalation anesthesia in most birds and approximates a normal physiologic range of 25–40 mmHg for $PaCO_2$ for awake birds. IPPV is recommended at a rate that depends on the $ETCO_2$; typically, 2 breaths/min in spontaneously ventilating birds, and 10–20 breaths/min in apneic birds. A maximum pressure of 10–20 cm H_2O is recommended. If used in combination with a capnograph, IPPV rate should be adjusted to maintain $ETCO_2$ between 30 and 45 mmHg.

Pulse oximetry has not been validated in birds [87]. The absorption characteristics of oxygenated and deoxygenated avian and human hemoglobin are different resulting in underestimation of hemoglobin saturation [87]. However, these monitors are often used reliably to provide a trend in the oxygen saturation and a pulse rate.

Temperature Monitoring and Support

The avian core body temperature should be monitored throughout anesthesia via a cloacal or esophageal temperature probe. It is higher than most mammals at 38–40 °C on average [96, 97]. Avian esophageal and cloacal temperatures are well correlated in studies that compared the two sites; however, cloacal temperature probes are prone to being dislodged or recording a cooler temperature if they are not secured appropriately within the cloaca [98]. Thus, the temperature is best monitored using esophageal probes.

Thermal support is necessary to prevent hypothermia in birds under general anesthesia. Radiant heat sources, water blankets, fluid warmer, and forced-air warmer systems (e.g. Bair Hugger Warming System) are routinely used to maintain core body temperature. The most effective method for maintaining the temperature has been found to be the forced-air warming device while covering the bird with a transparent drape, when compared to water blanket or radiant heat source with a drape [99]. Another study in pigeons comparing a newer conductive thermal blanket (HotDog, Augustine Biomedical and Design) with a Bair Hugger concluded that the HotDog resulted in a lower decrease in core body temperature [100]. The type of anesthetic delivery system, with or without heated air, does not appear to affect the core body temperature [101]. On the other hand, certain arctic birds can become hyperthermic under anesthesia and overzealous heat support may be deleterious in these species.

Other precautions to limit heat loss may be undertaken. Incoming oxygen and anesthetic gases may be warmed by expiratory gas in tube-within-tube design of anesthetic circuits or other systems, care should be taken to pluck the minimum area needed for surgery, asepsis should avoid the use of alcohol-based antiseptics in small birds, plastic draping may be used to more efficiently conserve heat (VSP surgical drapes, Veterinary Specialty Products, Shawnee, KS, USA), and surgical time should be kept to a minimum.

Post-anesthesia

During recovery, the bird is gently restrained in a towel and extubated once it starts to resist the presence of the tube, but oxygen is administered via an open mask through the recovery from anesthesia. A quiet, warm (approximately 25–30 °C, heated incubator), and light-reduced environment should be selected, which allows for visual control of the patient. If an IV catheter is in place, it may be removed once the bird has recovered in order to prevent the bird from biting at it and potentially bleeding. Often, birds have an excitatory phase during initial recovery manifested by wing flapping, particularly when the inhalants are the sole anesthetic agents. Minimal stimulus during this period may reduce the occurrence and length of wing flapping. If the bird is stable, extubated, has a corneal reflex, but still recumbent, it may be placed in a warmed incubator and supervised during recovery. This often prevents wing flapping completely. Some species, especially macaws, are also prone to regurgitation upon anesthetic recovery. In the experience of the authors, no drugs (including metoclopramide or maropitant) have been proven effective in reducing the rate of regurgitation in macaws.

Anesthetic Emergencies

Respiratory emergencies involving apnea are not uncommon during inhalation anesthesia. If an endotracheal tube is not already in place, one should be inserted, and manual or mechanical ventilation initiated at a rate of 10–12 breaths/min or as indicated using capnographic monitoring. The level of gas anesthesia may be reduced or stopped.

Cardiac emergencies involving bradycardia are common. If bradycardia develops, the anesthetist must assess whether it represents a true emergency. The level of inhalant anesthesia should be reduced, and IV fluids and/or anticholinergic agents such as atropine can be used to increase the heart rate. If cardiac arrest occurs, attempts should be made to compress the sternum, or lateral compressions across the thorax in small birds, at a rate of a normal heart rate/min (see Chapter 27: CPR and Euthanasia). A set of emergency drugs should be available during anesthesia or surgery. If hypotension develops, the level of anesthesia should be reduced, the rate of fluid administration increased, and core body temperature assessed and addressed as needed. Fluid therapy, colloids, and vasopressors are indicated in hypotension [102]. Blood transfusion is needed if hemorrhage is severe during surgery (see Chapter 29: Fluid Therapy).

References

1 Hawkins, M., Paul-Murphy, J., and Sanchez Migallon-Guzman, D. (2016). Recognition, assessment, and management of pain in birds. In: *Current Therapy in Avian Medicine and Surgery* (ed. B. Speer), 616–630. St Louis, MO: Elsevier.

2 Guzman, D.S.-M., Flammer, K., Paul-Murphy, J.R. et al. (2011). Pharmacokinetics of butorphanol after intravenous, intramuscular, and oral administration in Hispaniolan Amazon parrots (*Amazona ventralis*). *J. Avian Med. Surg.* 25 (3): 185–191.

3 Paul-Murphy, J.R., Brunson, D.B., and Miletic, V. (1999). Analgesic effects of butorphanol and buprenorphine in conscious African grey parrots (*Psittacus erithacus erithacus* and *Psittacus erithacus timneh*). *Am. J. Vet. Res.* 60 (10): 1218–1221.

4 Klaphake, E., Schumacher, J., Greenacre, C. et al. (2006). Comparative anesthetic and cardiopulmonary effects of pre- versus postoperative butorphanol administration in Hispaniolan Amazon parrots (*Amazona ventralis*) anesthetized with sevoflurane. *J. Avian Med. Surg.* 20 (1): 2–7.

5 Sanchez-Migallon Guzman, D., Souza, M.J., Braun, J.M. et al. (2012). Antinociceptive effects after oral administration of tramadol hydrochloride in Hispaniolan Amazon parrots (*Amazona ventralis*). *Am. J. Vet. Res.* 73 (8): 1148–1152.

6 Souza, M.J., Sanchez-Migallon Guzman, D., Paul-Murphy, J.R., and Cox, S.K. (2012). Pharmacokinetics after oral and intravenous administration of a single dose of tramadol hydrochloride to Hispaniolan Amazon parrots (*Amazona ventralis*). *Am. J. Vet. Res.* 73 (8): 1142–1147.

7 Cole, G.A., Paul-Murphy, J., Krugner-Higby, L. et al. (2009). Analgesic effects of intramuscular administration of meloxicam in Hispaniolan parrots (*Amazona ventralis*) with experimentally induced arthritis. *Am. J. Vet. Res.* 70 (12): 1471–1476.

8 Dijkstra, B., Guzman, D.S.-M., Gustavsen, K. et al. (2015). Renal, gastrointestinal, and hemostatic effects of oral administration of meloxicam to Hispaniolan Amazon parrots (*Amazona ventralis*). *Am. J. Vet. Res.* 76 (4): 308–317.

9 Molter, C.M., Court, M.H., Cole, G.A. et al. (2013). Pharmacokinetics of meloxicam after intravenous, intramuscular, and oral administration of a single dose to Hispaniolan Amazon parrots (*Amazona ventralis*). *Am. J. Vet. Res.* 74 (3): 375–380.

10 Guzman, D.S.-M., Drazenovich, T.L., Olsen, G.H. et al. (2013). Evaluation of thermal antinociceptive effects after intramuscular administration of hydromorphone hydrochloride to American kestrels (*Falco sparverius*). *Am. J. Vet. Res.* 74 (6): 817–822.

11 Houck, E.L., Guzman, D.S., Beaufrere, H. et al. (2018). Evaluation of the thermal antinociceptive effects and pharmacokinetics of hydromorphone hydrochloride after intramuscular administration to cockatiels (*Nymphicus hollandicus*). *Am. J. Vet. Res.* 79: 820–827.

12 Guzman, D., Douglas, J., Beaufrère, H. et al. (2017). Thermal antinociceptive and agitation-sedation effects after intramuscular administration of hydromorphone hydrochloride in orange-winged Amazon parrots (*Amazona amazonica*). *Vet. Anaesth. Analg.* 44: 1262–e1213.

13 Ceulemans, S.M., Guzman, D.S.-M., Olsen, G.H. et al. (2014). Evaluation of thermal antinociceptive effects after intramuscular administration of buprenorphine hydrochloride to American kestrels (*Falco sparverius*). *Am. J. Vet. Res.* 75 (8): 705–710.

14 Guzman, D.S.-M., Drazenovich, T.L., Olsen, G.H. et al. (2014). Evaluation of thermal antinociceptive effects after oral administration of tramadol hydrochloride to American kestrels (*Falco sparverius*). *Am. J. Vet. Res.* 75 (2): 117–123.

15 Pavez, J.C., Hawkins, M.G., Pascoe, P.J. et al. (2011). Effect of fentanyl target-controlled infusions on isoflurane minimum anaesthetic concentration and cardiovascular function in red-tailed hawks (*Buteo jamaicensis*). *Vet. Anaesth. Analg.* 38 (4): 344–351.

16 Gaggermeier, B., Henke, J., and Schatzmann, U (2003). Investigations on analgesia in domestic pigeons (*C. livia*) using buprenorphine and butorphanol. *Proceedings of the European Association of Avian Veterinarians*, Tenerife, 2003, pp. 70–73.

17 Reiner, A., Brauth, S.E., Kitt, C.A., and Quirion, R. (1989). Distribution of mu, delta, and kappa opiate receptor types in the forebrain and midbrain of pigeons. *J. Comp. Neurol.* 280 (3): 359–382.

18 Duhamelle, A., Raiwet, D., Langlois, I. et al. (2018). Preliminary findings of structure and expression of opioid receptor genes in a peregrine falcon (*Falco peregrinus*), a snowy owl (*Bubo scandiacus*), and a blue fronted Amazon parrot (*Amazona aestiva*). *J. Avian Med. Surg.* 32 (3): 173–184.

19 Guzman, D.S.-M., Drazenovich, T.L., KuKanich, B. et al. (2014). Evaluation of thermal antinociceptive effects and pharmacokinetics after intramuscular administration of butorphanol tartrate to American kestrels (*Falco sparverius*). *Am. J. Vet. Res.* 75 (1): 11–18.

20 Sladky, K.K., Krugner-Higby, L., Meek-Walker, E. et al. (2006). Serum concentrations and analgesic effects of liposome-encapsulated and standard butorphanol tartrate in parrots. *Am. J. Vet. Res.* 67 (5): 775–781.

21 Clancy, M.M., KuKanich, B., and Sykes, J.M. (2015). Pharmacokinetics of butorphanol delivered with an osmotic pump during a seven-day period in common peafowl (*Pavo cristatus*). *Am. J. Vet. Res.* 76 (12): 1070–1076.

22 Laniesse, D., Sanchez Migallon-Guzman, D., Smith, D. et al. (2015). Rheological properties of a sustained-release formulation of butorphanol in a poloxamer 407 base and pharmacokinetics in Amazon parrots (*Amazona ventralis*). *Proceedings of the Annual conference of the Association of Avian veterinarians*, San Antonio, 2015, pp. 19–20.

23 Sanchez-Migallon Guzman, D., KuKanich, B., Keuler, N.S. et al. (2011). Antinociceptive effects of nalbuphine hydrochloride in Hispaniolan Amazon parrots (*Amazona ventralis*). *Am. J. Vet. Res.* 72 (6): 736–740.

24 Sanchez-Migallon Guzman, D., Braun, J.M., Steagall, P.V.M. et al. (2013). Antinociceptive effects of long-acting nalbuphine decanoate after intramuscular administration to Hispaniolan Amazon parrots (*Amazona ventralis*). *Am. J. Vet. Res.* 74 (2): 196–200.

25 Schneider, C. (1961). Effects of morphine-like drugs in chicks. *Nature* 191: 607–608.

26 Bardo, M.T. and Hughes, R.A. (1978). Brief communication. Shock-elicited flight response in chickens as an index of morphine analgesia. *Pharmacol. Biochem. Behav.* 9 (1): 147–149.

27 Fan, S.G., Shutt, A.J., and Vogt, M. (1981). The importance of 5-hydroxytryptamine turnover for the analgesic effect of morphine in the chicken. *Neuroscience* 6 (11): 2223–2227.

28 Concannon, K.T., Dodam, J.R., and Hellyer, P.W. (1995). Influence of a mu- and kappa-opioid agonist on isoflurane minimal anesthetic concentration in chickens. *Am. J. Vet. Res.* 56 (6): 806–811.

29 Hoppes, S., Flammer, K., Hoersch, K. et al. (2003). Disposition and analgesic effects of fentanyl in white cockatoos (*Cacatua alba*). *J. Avian Med. Surg.* 17 (3): 124–130.

30 Hawkins, M., Pascoe, P., Knych, H. et al. (2014). Effect of fentanyl citrate target-controlled infusions on isoflurane MAC in Hispaniolan Amazon parrots (*Amazona ventralis*). *Proceedings of the Annual conference of the Association of Avian veterinarians*, 2014, New Orleans, p. 15.

31 Paul-Murphy, J., Hess, J.C., and Fialkowski, J.P. (2004). Pharmacokinetic properties of a single intramuscular dose of buprenorphine in African grey parrots (*Psittacus erithacus erithacus*). *J. Avian Med. Surg.* 18 (4): 224–228.

32 Guzman, D.S., Houck, E.L., Knych, H.K.D. et al. (2018). Evaluation of the thermal antinociceptive effects and pharmacokinetics after intramuscular administration of buprenorphine hydrochloride to cockatiels (*Nymphicus hollandicus*). *Am. J. Vet. Res.* 79: 1239–1245.

33 Kilburn, J.J., Cox, S.K., Kottyan, J. et al. (2014). Pharmacokinetics of tramadol and its primary metabolite *O*-desmethyltramadol in African penguins (*Spheniscus demersus*). *J. Zoo Wildl. Med.* 45 (1): 93–99.

34 Souza, M.J., Gerhardt, L., and Cox, S. (2013). Pharmacokinetics of repeated oral administration of tramadol hydrochloride in Hispaniolan Amazon parrots (*Amazona ventralis*). *Am. J. Vet. Res.* 74 (7): 957–962.

35 Black, P.A., Cox, S.K., Macek, M. et al. (2010). Pharmacokinetics of tramadol hydrochloride and its metabolite *O*-desmethyltramadol in peafowl (*Pavo cristatus*). *J. Zoo Wildl. Med.* 41 (4): 671–676.

36 Souza, M.J., Martin-Jimenez, T., Jones, M.P., and Cox, S.K. (2009). Pharmacokinetics of intravenous and oral tramadol in the bald eagle (*Haliaeetus leucocephalus*). *J. Avian Med. Surg.* 23 (4): 247–252.

37 Souza, M.J., Martin-Jimenez, T., Jones, M.P., and Cox, S.K. (2011). Pharmacokinetics of oral tramadol in red-tailed hawks (*Buteo jamaicensis*). *J. Vet. Pharmacol. Ther.* 34 (1): 86–88.

38 (a) Desmarchelier, M., Troncy, E., Fitzgerald, G., and Lair, S. (2012). Analgesic effects of meloxicam administration on postoperative orthopedic pain in domestic pigeons (*Columba livia*). *Am. J. Vet. Res.* 73 (3): 361–367.

39 Montesinos, A., Encinas, T., Ardiaca, M. et al. (2019). Pharmacokinetics of meloxicam during multiple oral or intramuscular dose administration to African grey parrots (*Psittacus erithacus*). *Am. J. Vet. Res.* 80: 201–220.

40 Lacasse, C., Gamble, K.C., and Boothe, D.M. (2013). Pharmacokinetics of a single dose of intravenous and oral meloxicam in red-tailed hawks (*Buteo jamaicensis*) and great horned owls (*Bubo virginianus*). *J. Avian Med. Surg.* 27 (3): 204–210.

41 Summa, N., Fitzgerald, G., Larrat, S. et al. (2015). Evaluation of toxicity of meloxicam in American kestrels (*Falco sparverius*). *Proceedings of the Annual conference of the Association of Avian veterinarians*, 2015, Paris, France, p. 335.

42 Sinclair, K.M., Church, M.E., Farver, T.B. et al. (2012). Effects of meloxicam on hematologic and plasma biochemical analysis variables and results of histologic examination of tissue specimens of Japanese quail (*Coturnix japonica*). *Am. J. Vet. Res.* 73 (11): 1720–1727.

43 McGeown, D., Danbury, T.C., Waterman-Pearson, A.E., and Kestin, S.C. (1999). Effect of carprofen on lameness in broiler chickens. *Vet. Rec.* 144 (24): 668–671.

44 Paul-Murphy, J.R., Sladky, K.K., Krugner-Higby, L.A. et al. (2009). Analgesic effects of carprofen and liposome-encapsulated butorphanol tartrate in Hispaniolan parrots (*Amazona ventralis*) with experimentally induced arthritis. *Am. J. Vet. Res.* 70 (10): 1201–1210.

45 Zollinger, T.J., Hoover, J.P., Payton, M.E., and Schiller, C.A. (2011). Clinicopathologic, gross necropsy, and histologic findings after intramuscular injection of carprofen in a pigeon (*Columba livia*) model. *J. Avian Med. Surg.* 25 (3): 173–184.

46 Baine, K., Jones, M.P., Cox, S., and Martín-Jiménez, T. (2015). Pharmacokinetics of compounded intravenous and oral gabapentin in Hispaniolan Amazon parrots (*Amazona ventralis*). *J. Avian Med. Surg.* 29 (3): 165–173.

47 Yaw, T.J., Zaffarano, B.A., Gall, A. et al. (2015). Pharmacokinetic properties of a single administration of oral gabapentin in the great horned owl (*Bubo virginianus*). *J. Zoo Wildl. Med.* 46 (3): 547–552.

48 Ludders, J. and Matthews, N. (2007). Birds. In: *Lumb & Jones' Veterinary Anesthesia and Analgesia*, 4e (eds. W. Tranquilli, J. Thurmon and K. Grimm), 841–868. Ames, IA: Blackwell Publishing.

49 Brenner, D.J., Larsen, R.S., Dickinson, P.J. et al. (2010). Development of an avian brachial plexus nerve block technique for perioperative analgesia in mallard ducks (*Anas platyrhynchos*). *J. Avian Med. Surg.* 24 (1): 24–34.

50 Figueiredo, J.P., Cruz, M.L., Mendes, G.M. et al. (2008). Assessment of brachial plexus blockade in chickens by an axillary approach. *Vet. Anaesth. Analg.* 35 (6): 511–518.

51 da Cunha, A.F., Strain, G.M., Rademacher, N. et al. (2013). Palpation- and ultrasound-guided brachial plexus blockade in Hispaniolan Amazon parrots (*Amazona ventralis*). *Vet. Anaesth. Analg.* 40 (1): 96–102.

52 Hawkins, M., Zehnder, A., and Pascoe, P. (2014). Cagebirds. In: *Zoo Animal and Wildlife Immobilization and Anesthesia*, 2e (eds. G. West, D. Heard and N. Caulkett), 399–433. Ames, IA: Wiley-Blackwell.

53 Edling, T. (2006). Updates on anesthesia and monitoring. In: *Clinical Avian Medicine* (eds. G. Harrison and T. Lightfoot), 747–760. Palm Beach, FL: Spix Publishing.

54 Mans, C., Guzman, D.S.-M., Lahner, L.L. et al. (2012). Sedation and physiologic response to manual restraint after intranasal administration of midazolam in Hispaniolan Amazon parrots (*Amazona ventralis*). *J. Avian Med. Surg.* 26 (3): 130–139.

55 Zaheer O, Sanchez A, Beaufrere H. Minimum anesthetic concentration of isoflurane and sparing effect of midazolam in Quaker parrots (*Myiopsitta monachus*). *Vet. Anaesth. Analg.*, 2020. 47 (3): 341–346.

56 Müller, K., Holzapfel, J., and Brunnberg, L. (2011). Total intravenous anaesthesia by boluses or by continuous rate infusion of propofol in mute swans (*Cygnus olor*). *Vet. Anaesth. Analg.* 38 (4): 286–291.

57 Mulcahy, D.M., Tuomi, P., and Larsen, R.S. (2003). Differential mortality of male spectacled eiders (*Somateria fischeri*) and king eiders (*Somateria spectabilis*) subsequent to anesthesia with propofol, bupivacaine, and ketoprofen. *J. Avian Med. Surg.* 17 (3): 117–123.

58 Langlois, I., Harvey, R., Jones, M., and Schumacher, J. (2003). Cardiopulmonary and anesthetic effects of isoflurane and propofol in Hispaniolan Amazon parrots (*Amazona ventralis*). *J. Avian Med. Surg.* 17 (1): 4–10.

59 Hawkins, M.G., Wright, B.D., Pascoe, P.J. et al. (2003). Pharmacokinetics and anesthetic and cardiopulmonary effects of propofol in red-tailed hawks (*Buteo jamaicensis*) and great horned owls (*Bubo virginianus*). *Am. J. Vet. Res.* 64 (6): 677–683.

60 Machin, K.L. and Caulkett, N.A. (2000). Evaluation of isoflurane and propofol anesthesia for intraabdominal transmitter placement in nesting female canvasback ducks. *J. Wildl. Dis.* 36 (2): 324–334.

61 Langan, J., Ramsay, E., Blackford, J., and Schumacher, J. (2000). Cardiopulmonary and sedative effects of intramuscular medetomidine-ketamine and intravenous propofol in ostriches (*Struthio camelus*). *J. Avian Med. Surg.* 14 (1): 2–7.

62 Machin, K.L. and Caulkett, N.A. (1998). Cardiopulmonary effects of propofol and a medetomidine-midazolam-ketamine combination in mallard ducks. *Am. J. Vet. Res.* 59 (5): 598–602.

63 Schumacher, J., Citino, S.B., Hernandez, K. et al. (1997). Cardiopulmonary and anesthetic effects of propofol in wild turkeys. *Am. J. Vet. Res.* 58 (9): 1014–1017.

64 Lukasik, V., Gentz, E., Erb, H. et al. (1997). Cardiopulmonary effects of propofol anesthesia in chickens (*Gallus gallus domesticus*). *J. Avian Med. Surg.* 11 (2): 93–97.

65 Fitzgerald, G. and Cooper, J.E. (1990). Preliminary studies on the use of propofol in the domestic pigeon (*Columba livia*). *Res. Vet. Sci.* 49 (3): 334–338.

66 Kamiloglu, A., Atalan, G., and Kamiloglu, N.N. (2008). Comparison of intraosseous and intramuscular drug administration for induction of anaesthesia in domestic pigeons. *Res. Vet. Sci.* 85 (1): 171–175.

67 Varner, J., Clifton, K.R., Poulos, S. et al. (2004). Lack of efficacy of injectable ketamine with xylazine or diazepam for anesthesia in chickens. *Lab. Anim.*. 33 (5): 36–39.

68 Atalan, G., Uzun, M., Demirkan, I. et al. (2002). Effect of medetomidine-butorphanol-ketamine anaesthesia and atipamezole on heart and respiratory rate and cloacal temperature of domestic pigeons. *J. Vet. Med. A Physiol. Pathol. Clin. Med.* 49 (6): 281–285.

69 Raffe, M., Mammel, M., and Gordon, M. (1993). Cardiorespiratory effects of ketamine-xylazine in the great horned owl. In: *Raptor Biomedicine* (eds. P. Redig, J. Cooper, D. Remple, et al.), 150–153. Minneapolis, USA: University of Minnesota Press.

70 Ludders, J.W., Rode, J., Mitchell, G.S., and Nordheim, E.V. (1989). Effects of ketamine, xylazine, and a combination of ketamine and xylazine in Pekin ducks. *Am. J. Vet. Res.* 50 (2): 245–249.

71 Joyner, P.H., Jones, M.P., Ward, D. et al. (2008). Induction and recovery characteristics and cardiopulmonary effects of sevoflurane and isoflurane in bald eagles. *Am. J. Vet. Res.* 69 (1): 13–22.

72 Mercado, J.A., Larsen, R.S., Wack, R.F., and Pypendop, B.H. (2008). Minimum anesthetic concentration of isoflurane in captive thick-billed parrots (*Rhynchopsitta pachyrhyncha*). *Am. J. Vet. Res.* 69 (2): 189–194.

73 Phair, K.A., Larsen, R.S., Wack, R.F. et al. (2012). Determination of the minimum anesthetic concentration of sevoflurane in thick-billed parrots (*Rhynchopsitta pachyrhyncha*). *Am. J. Vet. Res.* 73 (9): 1350–1355.

74 Naganobu, K., Fujisawa, Y., Ohde, H. et al. Determination of the minimum anesthetic concentration and cardiovascular dose response for sevoflurane in chickens during controlled ventilation. *Vet. Surg.* 29 (1): 102–105.

75 Ludders, J.W., Rode, J., and Mitchell, G.S. (1989). Isoflurane anesthesia in sandhill cranes (*Grus canadensis*): minimal anesthetic concentration and cardiopulmonary dose-response during spontaneous and controlled breathing. *Anesth. Analg.* 68 (4): 511–516.

76 Escobar, A., Valadão, C.A.A., Brosnan, R.J. et al. (2012). Effects of butorphanol on the minimum anesthetic concentration for sevoflurane in guineafowl (*Numida meleagris*). *Am. J. Vet. Res.* 73 (2): 183–188.

77 Ludders, J.W., Mitchell, G.S., and Rode, J. (1990). Minimal anesthetic concentration and cardiopulmonary dose response of isoflurane in ducks. *Vet. Surg.* 19 (4): 304–307.

78 Chan, F.-T., Chang, G.-R., Wang, H.-C., and Hsu, T.-H. (2013). Anesthesia with isoflurane and sevoflurane in the crested serpent eagle (*Spilornis cheela hoya*): minimum anesthetic concentration, physiological effects, hematocrit, plasma chemistry and behavioral effects. *J. Vet. Med. Sci.* 75 (12): 1591–1600.

79 Paula, V.V., Otsuki, D.A., Auler Júnior, J.O.C. et al. (2013). The effect of premedication with ketamine, alone or with diazepam, on anaesthesia with sevoflurane in parrots (*Amazona aestiva*). *BMC Vet. Res.* 9 (1): 142.

80 Smith, J., Mason, D., and Muir, W (1993). The influence of midazolam on the minimum anesthetic concentration of isoflurane in racing pigeons. *9th Annual Veterinary Midwest Anaesthesia Conference*.

81 Curro, T.G., Brunson, D.B., and Paul-Murphy, J. (1994). Determination of the ED50 of isoflurane and evaluation of the isoflurane-sparing effect of butorphanol in cockatoos (*Cacatua* spp.). *Vet. Surg.* 23 (5): 429–433.

82 Escobar, A., Thiesen, R., Vitaliano, S.N. et al. (2009). Some cardiopulmonary effects of sevoflurane in crested caracara (*Caracara plancus*). *Vet. Anaesth. Analg.* 36 (5): 436–441.

83 Granone, T.D., de Francisco, O.N., Killos, M.B. et al. (2012). Comparison of three different inhalant anesthetic agents (isoflurane, sevoflurane, desflurane) in red-tailed hawks (*Buteo jamaicensis*). *Vet. Anaesth. Analg.* 39 (1): 29–37.

84 Botman, J., Dugdale, A., Gabriel, F., and Vandeweerd, J.-M. (2016). Cardiorespiratory parameters in the awake pigeon and during anaesthesia with isoflurane. *Vet. Anaesth. Analg.* 43 (1): 63–71.

85 Escobar, A., Thiesen, R., Vitaliano, S.N. et al. (2011). Cardiorespiratory effects of isoflurane anesthesia in crested caracaras (*Caracara plancus*). *J. Zoo Wildl. Med.* 42 (1): 12–17.

86 Pettifer, G.R., Cornick-Seahorn, J., Smith, J.A. et al. (2002). The comparative cardiopulmonary effects of spontaneous and controlled ventilation by using the Hallowell EMC Anesthesia WorkStation in Hispaniolan Amazon parrots (*Amazona ventralis*). *J. Avian Med. Surg.* 16 (4): 268–276.

87 Schmitt, P., Gobel, T., and Trautvetter, E. (1998). Evaluation of pulse oximetry as a monitoring method in avian anesthesia. *J. Avian Med. Surg.* 12 (2): 91–99.

88 Zehnder, A.M., Hawkins, M.G., Pascoe, P.J., and Kass, P.H. (2009). Evaluation of indirect blood pressure monitoring in awake and anesthetized red-tailed hawks (*Buteo jamaicensis*): effects of cuff size, cuff placement, and monitoring equipment. *Vet. Anaesth. Analg.* 36 (5): 464–479.

89 Acierno, M.J., da Cunha, A., Smith, J. et al. (2008). Agreement between direct and indirect blood pressure measurements obtained from anesthetized Hispaniolan Amazon parrots. *J. Am. Vet. Med. Assoc.* 233 (10): 1587–1590.

90 Johnston, M.S., Davidowski, L.A., Rao, S., and Hill, A.E. (2011). Precision of repeated, Doppler-derived indirect blood pressure measurements in conscious psittacine birds. *J. Avian Med. Surg.* 25 (2): 83–90.

91 Schnellbacher, R.W., da Cunha, A.F., Beaufrère, H. et al. (2012). Effects of dopamine and dobutamine on isoflurane-induced hypotension in Hispaniolan Amazon parrots (*Amazona ventralis*). *Am. J. Vet. Res.* 73 (7): 952–958.

92 Hawkins, M.G., Malka, S., Pascoe, P.J. et al. (2013). Evaluation of the effects of dorsal versus lateral recumbency on the cardiopulmonary system during anesthesia with isoflurane in red-tailed hawks (*Buteo jamaicensis*). *Am. J. Vet. Res.* 74 (1): 136–143.

93 Malka, S., Hawkins, M.G., Jones, J.H. et al. (2009). Effect of body position on respiratory system volumes in anesthetized red-tailed hawks (*Buteo jamaicensis*) as measured via computed tomography. *Am. J. Vet. Res.* 70 (9): 1155–1160.

94 Edling, T.M., Degernes, L.A., Flammer, K., and Horne, W.A. (2001). Capnographic monitoring of anesthetized African grey parrots receiving intermittent positive pressure ventilation. *J. Am. Vet. Med. Assoc.* 219 (12): 1714–1718.

95 Desmarchelier, M., Rondenay, Y., Fitzgerald, G., and Lair, S. (2007). Monitoring of the ventilatory status of anesthetized birds of prey by using end-tidal carbon dioxide measured with a microstream capnometer. *J. Zoo Wildl. Dis.* 38 (1): 1–6.

96 Prinzinger, R., Preßmar, A., and Schleucher, E. (1991). Body temperature in birds. *Comp. Biochem. Physiol. A: Physiol.* 99 (4): 499–506.

97 Dawson, W.R. and Whittow, G.C. (2000). Regulation of body temperature. In: *Sturkie's Avian Physiology*, 5e (ed. G.C. Whittow), 343–390. San Diego, CA: Academic Press.

98 Phalen, D., Mitchell, M., and Cavazos-Martinez, M. (1996). Evaluation of three heat sources for their ability to maintain core body temperature in the anesthetized avian patient. *J. Avian Med. Surg.* 10 (3): 174–178.

99 Rembert, M., Smith, J., Hosgood, G. et al. (2001). Comparison of traditional thermal support devices with the forced-air warmer system in anesthetized Hispaniolan Amazon parrots (*Amazona ventralis*). *J. Avian Med. Surg.* 15 (3): 187–193.

100 van Zeeland, Y.R.A., Cardona, T., and Schoemaker, N.J. (2012). Maintenance of core body temperature in anaesthetised pigeons (*Columba livia domestica*): a comparison of two thermal devices. *Vet. J.* 194 (3): 429–432.

101 Boedeker, N.C., Carpenter, J.W., and Mason, D.E. (2005). Comparison of body temperatures of pigeons (*Columba livia*) anesthetized by three different anesthetic delivery systems. *J. Avian Med. Surg.* 19 (1): 1–6.

102 Costello, M.F. (2004). Principles of cardiopulmonary cerebral resuscitation in special species. *Semin. Avian Exot. Pet Med.* 13 (3): 132–141.

29

Nutrition and Fluid Therapy

Hugues Beaufrère

Department of Medicine and Epidemiology, School of Veterinary Medicine, University of California-Davis, Davis, California, USA

CONTENTS

Nutrition in Birds

Estimation of Daily Energy Requirement

Anorexia, weight loss, nutritional deficiencies, and challenges to oral alimentation are commonly encountered in critical avian patients. As such, nutritional support is part of the standard supportive care administered to any sick bird. In order to stabilize patients, optimize medical outcome, and prevent further weight loss, the first step to the nutritional support plan is to estimate the daily energy requirement of hospitalized avian patients.

As birds have a relatively high metabolism and are not as tolerant to manual restraint as domestic mammals, it may be challenging to meet metabolic requirements in completely anorexic birds, especially in small birds, by crop feeding alone. Supportive enteral nutrition requires repeat handling in most instances; therefore, a balance must be managed between the frequency of feeding, the volume of administered food, and the tolerance of the patient. The frequency and volumes will depend on the patient's condition and supportive enteral nutrition may cover all or only parts of the metabolic requirements.

In order to plan a supportive feeding regimen, the daily metabolic requirement must first be approximated. It is based on the basal metabolic rate (BMR), which is the rate of energy that is needed in a non-growing animal at rest in a thermoneutral zone and with basal digestive and excretive physiology. Different equations have been proposed to estimate the BMR in birds [1–6]. The most popular among avian veterinarians is an equation based on the metabolic scaling principles outlined by Sedwick (Eq. (29.1)) [2, 3, 7]. As the BMR is the minimum amount of energy necessary to sustain basal physiology in birds at rest and within their thermal neutral zone, additional energy is needed to account for activity and thermoregulation. Uricotelism requires about 3.25 more energy that ureotelism [4]. Thus, the BMR is multiplied by a factor, typically 1.5–2, to obtain the maintenance energy requirement (MER). Other authors recommend a higher factor such as 2–2.5 [8]. Higher factors are also typically used to better approximate the normal daily energy expenditure of normally active birds.

To adjust for pathological processes, the MER is also multiplied by another factor to obtain the daily energy requirement in a hospitalized patient (e.g. 0.7 for starvation, 1.5 for sepsis) [2, 7]. In addition, birds that are sick or experiencing stress are more likely to be in a hypermetabolic state.

$$\begin{aligned}&\mathrm{BMR}\left(\mathrm{kcal/d}\right)=K\times W_{\mathrm{kg}}^{0.75}\ \text{with}\\&K=129\ \text{for Passeriformes and}\\&K=78\ \text{for other orders of birds;}\\&\mathrm{MER}=2\times\mathrm{BMR}\left[2,3,7\right]\end{aligned}\qquad(29.1)$$

The BMR is more difficult to measure for practicality reasons, and a large number of other studies have measured

Exotic Animal Emergency and Critical Care Medicine, First Edition. Edited by Jennifer E. Graham, Grayson A. Doss and Hugues Beaufrère.

the MER of birds. Thus, simpler equations, roughly equivalent to Eq. (29.1) for non-passerine birds, are as follow:

$$\text{MER}(\text{kcal/d}) = 160.6 \times W_{\text{kg}}^{0.715} [8] \quad (29.2)$$

$$\text{MER}(\text{kcal/d}) = 154.6 \times W_{\text{kg}}^{0.73} [1,6] \quad (29.3)$$

It is expected that similar coefficient factors must be applied to adjust for increased metabolic demands of various pathological processes (see above).

The MER is also called the field metabolic rate (FMR) when obtained on free-living wild birds in field studies, [5] which is expected to be much higher than the MER of captive birds or pet birds. Examples of such equations are as follow:

$$\text{FMR}(\text{kcal/d}) = 278 \times W_{\text{kg}}^{0.681} [5] \quad (29.4)$$

$$\text{FMR}(\text{kcal/d}) = 229.2 \times W_{\text{kg}}^{0.73} [1,6] \quad (29.5)$$

In addition, these equations only provide an estimate of the energy requirements and critical birds must be weighed daily with feeding volumes and schedule adjustments to minimize weight loss not associated with dehydration. Furthermore, the accuracy of these equations depends on a number of factors and they are far from being universal and without controversy [9]. Whichever equation is used for the MER of resting or hospitalized birds, the end results are roughly equivalent among equations with variability of less than 10%, which is negligible for clinical use. Therefore, the simplest equation should be used in clinics such as Eq. (29.2).

For instance, the MER using the different equations for a healthy 500 g parrot would be:

1) $\text{MER} = \text{BMR} \times 2 = 78 \times 0.5^{0.75} \times 2 \approx 93\,\text{kcal/d}$
2) $\text{MER} = 160.6 \times 0.5^{0.715} \approx 98\,\text{kcal/d}$
3) $\text{MER} = 154.6 \times 0.5^{0.73} \approx 93\,\text{kcal/d}$
4) $\text{FMR} = 278 \times 0.5^{0.681} \approx 173\,\text{kcal/d}$
5) $\text{FMR} = 229.2 \times 0.5^{0.73} \approx 138\,\text{kcal/d}$

Treating underlying infections and other conditions, limiting stress, and maintaining the bird within its thermal neutral zone (e.g. in an incubator at about 29–31 °C, 84–88 °F) will decrease in-hospital weight loss and overall daily food volume needed by attempting to closely approximate the bird's BMR.

Once the daily energy requirements are calculated, the metabolizable energy (ME) of the food used to syringe feed or force feed needs to be known. The ME is the net energy that the bird will be able to generate from the food it ingests, which accounts for the energy lost digesting the food and in the urofeces. Most powdered handfeeding and recovery formulas have an approximate caloric density of 1 kcal/ml once reconstituted. The ME is generally indicated on the label or packaging of some commercial products, and it is known for selected prey items. However, only the nutritional analysis and composition are available for some other products and the ME needs to be approximated using an equation that has been determined for poultry: [8]

$$\text{ME}(\text{kcal}/100\,\text{g}) = 4.4 \times \text{Protein} + 8.7 \times \text{Fat} + 4 \times \text{NFE},$$
$$\text{with NFE being the nitrogen-free extract}$$
$$[\text{NFE} = 100 - (\text{Protein} + \text{Fat} + \text{water} + \text{ash} + \text{fiber})] \quad (29.6)$$

For instance, an enteral diet with 20% protein, 10% fat, and 55% nitrogen-free extract (NFE) would lead to:

6) $\text{ME} = 4.4 \times 21 + 8.7 \times 10 + 4 \times 55 \approx 399\,\text{kcal/100 g}$

As most handfeeding diets are in a powder form, they need to be mixed with water to be liquid in a typical ratio of 1-part powder to 2-parts water. Using the example above, it would lead to a diet with $399 \times 0.7 \times 1/3/100 = 0.93\,\text{kcal/ml}$ with 0.7 being the density of a powder similar to flour or corn starch.

Supportive Enteral Nutrition

Non-invasive Methods

There are several indications for supportive enteral nutrition in birds (Table 29.1). In most cases, the overall objectives are to meet or exceed metabolic requirements (see above) and supply a nutritionally balanced and highly digestible food to the sick avian patient. Supportive enteral nutrition may thus assist in reversing negative energy balance and correcting previous nutritional imbalances such as diets high in lipid and low in essential micronutrients. The author recommends crop-feeding psittacine birds that are hospitalized and that have been on an inadequate diet as it may be difficult to pinpoint nutritional deficiencies and which part they play in the overall clinical presentation. Crop feeding can also be used as a vehicle to enteral medications, supplements, and radiographic contrast media.

There are different means of providing enteral nutrition and repeated crop or proventriculus feedings are the most common. Other techniques include pharyngo- or esophagostomy tubes, or intestinal feeding tubes. Non-invasive supportive enteral feeding involves administering liquid or

Table 29.1 Indications for supportive enteral nutrition.

Anorexia/dysorexia
Emaciation
Diseases of the beak, head, and crop/cranial esophagus
Nutritional disorders
Hypermetabolic state (cancer)
Administration of specific nutritional formulation

Birds

solid food (birds of prey) directly into the crop for most species or in the proventriculus for species lacking a crop (e.g. Anseriformes and Strigiformes). Depending on the anatomy of the upper gastrointestinal system and the beak, different non-invasive techniques can be used. If it is needed to bypass the crop because of disease or trauma, the feeding is given directly into the proventriculus.

General contraindications of crop and proventricular feeding include various diseases of the crop/proventriculus (depending on the disease), gastrointestinal obstructions, gastrointestinal perforations, regurgitation, and vomiting (relative contraindication), inability to hold the head in an upright position, seizuring, and some head trauma (which could prevent opening the beak).

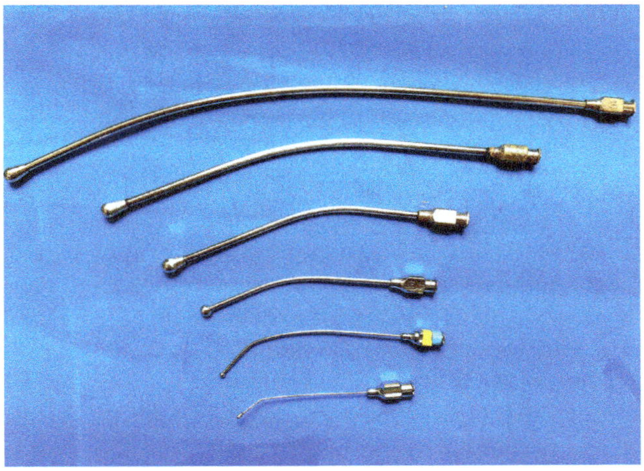

Figure 29.1 Ball-tip curved metal cannulas commonly used to gavage-feed parrots.

In Psittaciformes, in which the strong beak prevents clinicians from using soft tubes or any administering device that could be easily transected, a metal cannula is typically used (Figure 29.1). Cannulas need to be sterilized between patients. Different diameters and lengths of metal cannulas can be used and should be chosen based on the patient size and anatomy. A small diameter tube significantly increases the manual pressure necessary to inject the liquid through the cannula and injecting viscous formula may prove to be difficult. It is recommended to use a curved ball-tip metallic cannula to avoid gastroenteral trauma upon insertion. Lubricating the cannula may also reduce the occurrence of such trauma. Using luer-lock syringes also prevents disconnection of the syringe from the cannula causing leakage and splatter upon increased manual pressure on the plunger. The crop should be palpated before each feeding to assess crop emptying. In order to facilitate the insertion of the feeding cannula into the crop, the beak can be opened using a metal speculum. However, this requires two operators and may result in beak damage with frequent feedings. Except in large macaws, in which it can be challenging to open the beak, the author favors opening the beak using the cannula (Figure 29.2). The use of a beak speculum is rarely needed in small to medium-sized psittacine birds (Figure 29.3). Most birds will attempt to bite the tip of the cannula, and this allows opening of the beak using the

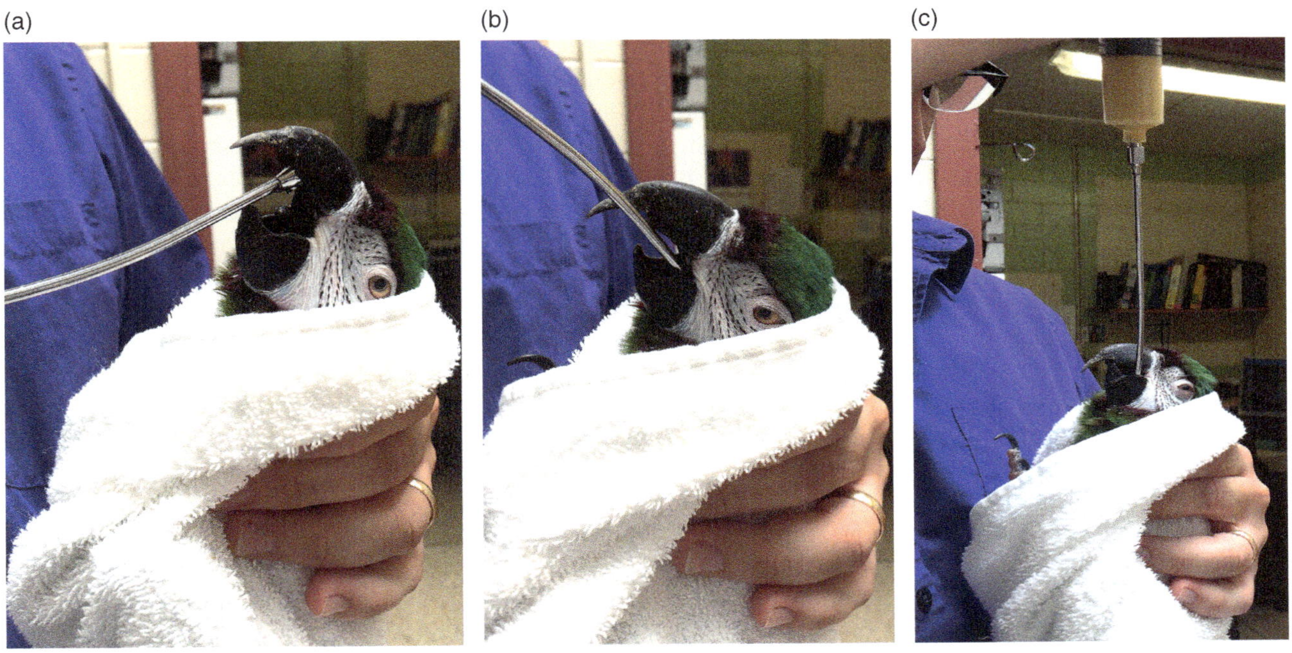

Figure 29.2 Crop-feeding in a severe macaw. The upper beak is slightly lifted using the cannula (a), then redirected at the back of the oropharyngeal cavity (b), and advanced in the crop going slightly left (right to left) of midline (c).

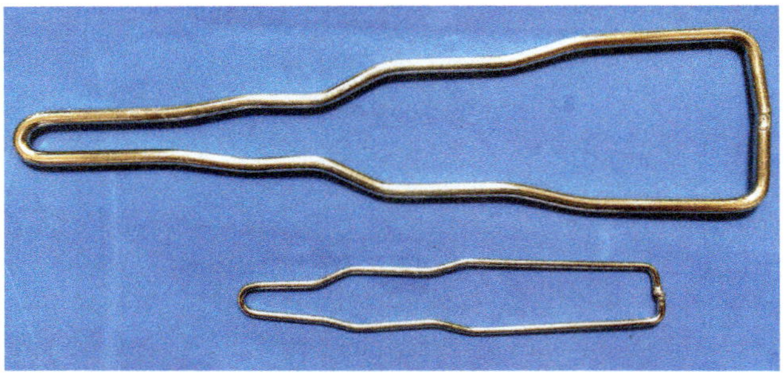

Figure 29.3 Metal speculums commonly used to open a parrot's beak.

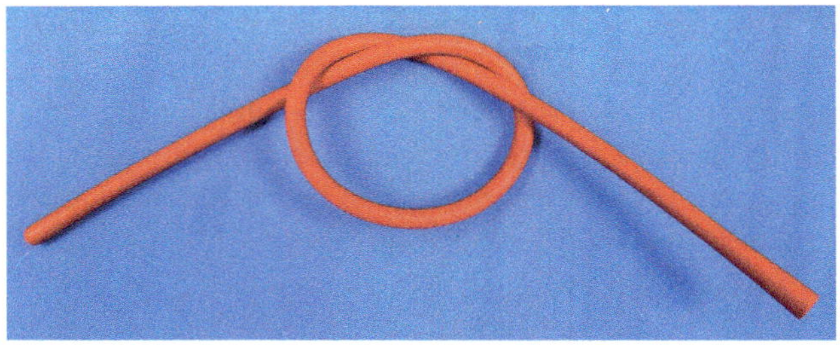

Figure 29.4 Rubber force-feeding catheter commonly used to force-feed birds of prey.

ball-tip end of the cannula by putting mild upward pressure on the underside of the rhinotheca. Alternatively, tape stirrups can be used to hold the beak open. Once the parrot has opened its beak, the cannula is carefully redirected at the back of the oropharynx, into the esophagus going slightly to the right of midline (left side for the individual passing the tube) as the cervical esophagus curves to the right in most birds, and ending into the crop (Figure 29.2). It is important to correctly restrain the bird by extending the neck vertically and preventing the bird from flexing its head when struggling, which may promote regurgitation and backflow. A slight compression just below the skull may also prevent regurgitation by occluding the proximal esophagus during the feeding. Force-feeding parrots, except in large species or when using a beak speculum, can be a one-person procedure. The cannula needs to be long enough that the bird cannot grab the extremity of it with its upper beak once inserted into the crop. If the correct size of the cannula is selected and the operator takes care to insert the cannula at the back of the throat, it is very unlikely to insert the cannula into the trachea. If it happens regardless, the bird will cough. If this is a concern, a separate handler is needed so the operator can verify the location of the cannula in the crop on palpation and that the trachea is palpated separately from the feeding cannula. In a one-person technique, the curved cannula can be slightly pushed ventrally so it is visible in the crop. It is imperative in a two-person technique to prevent up-and-down movements of the bird in relation to the cannula to prevent ingluvial perforation. In a one-person technique with an experienced handler, as the operator can control the depth of the tube and the head of the parrot at the same time, ingluvial trauma is less likely. Once in the crop, the formula is administered reasonably quickly while inspecting the oropharyngeal cavity for reflux. If the bird is regurgitating or if reflux of the formula is observed during administration, the cannula needs to be immediately removed and the bird placed back in its enclosure as soon as possible to allow self-clearing of the formula from the oropharyngeal cavity. Continuing restraint may promote further struggling and aspiration into the trachea. Syringe-feeding needs to be the last treatment performed on a bird if other medications or treatments need to be given in order to prevent regurgitations. The volume of liquid food that can safely be administered into the crop is about 30 ml/kg but up to 40–50 ml/kg can be tolerated in some individuals. Increasing the volume increases the probability of regurgitation. In neonates, a much larger volume can be used of about 100–120 ml/kg. When the crop needs to be by-passed, the cannula needs to be passed down to the proventriculus. In parrots, a similar technique to crop feeding can be used by selecting a longer metallic cannula. The cannula needs to be passed through the ingluvial sphincter dorsally. It is at the level of the thoracic inlet and can be probed by gentle up and down motions until the cannula enters freely into the thoracic esophagus.

In other species, particularly birds of prey, soft rubber tubes can be used for syringe feeding (Figure 29.4). In most birds, the beak can easily be opened by hand and the beak held open by inserting a finger at the commissures of the beak. The tube is then inserted into the crop and the food is administered. Two people are usually needed to syringe-feed raptors to avoid injury from the talons. Strigiformes and Anseriformes lack a crop and proventricular feeding must be performed. Force-feeding solid food is also possible in birds of prey and usually recommended for maintenance supportive enteral feeding as it is relatively easy, does not necessitate any specialized equipment, and whole prey is more calorie-dense. The prey is typically chopped up and fed piece by piece using a forceps. It is necessary to regularly let the bird swallow with its head unrestrained. If the bird is not swallowing, pieces may be pushed down the cervical esophagus using a long forceps or by external gentle pressure on the ventral neck. As owls mostly eat small prey whole, much larger pieces may be force-fed or whole mice/small prey items. Most piscivorous species (except accipitrid piscivorous species) also eat their prey whole and so fish can be force-fed whole. The skin, tail, and legs of prey may be removed to improve digestibility and limit casting.

A number of commercial supportive enteral products are available for Psittaciformes, omnivorous, and carnivorous birds. Baby bird handfeeding formulas are also suitable for supportive enteral feeding of adult parrots or omnivorous birds and have a caloric density similar to dedicated recovery formulas. Table 29.2 presents selected commercial products, and Table 29.3 lists prey commonly used for supportive enteral feeding. Table 29.4 presents calculated frequencies and volumes of feeding formula administration based on MER in birds of various sizes. It is clear from this table that meeting the MER in small birds may not be practically achievable with syringe-feeding. Also, the higher feeding volume necessary in small birds may lead to regurgitations upon feeding. Consequently, supportive enteral nutrition is partial in most cases and weight loss should be anticipated except in birds with partial anorexia.

Potential complications of crop and proventricular feedings include ingluvial or esophageal perforation,

Table 29.2 Caloric density of selected handfeeding and recovery formula in birds (expressed in metabolizable energy).

Product	Ratio of reconstitution (part product: part water)[a]	Caloric density (kcal/ml)
Omnivore and granivore		
Oxbow critical care omnivore[b]	1:1	2.03
Hagen tropican mash handfeeding formula[b]	1:2	0.9
Kaytee exact handfeeding formula[c]	1:2	0.9
Emeraid omnivore[b]	3:2	1.4
Zupreem embrace handfeeding formula[c]	1:2	0.9
Mazuri high energy handfeeding formula[b]	1:2	0.9
Mazuri handfeeding formula[b]	1:2	0.8
Harrison recovery formula[c]	1:2	1.0
Roudybush acute care formula	1:2	0.8
Carnivore, piscivore, and insectivore		
Hills a/d[b]	NA	1.1
Virbac rebound liquid diet[b]	NA	0.8
Virbac nutri-plus gel[b]	NA	5.9
CliniCare liquid diet	NA	1.0
Emeraid carnivore[b]	1:2	0.6
Emeraid piscivore[b]	1:2+10.5% fish oil	0.9
Oxbow critical care carnivore[b]	2:1	1.1
Mazuri nestling handfeeding formula[b]	1:2	0.8

[a] Recommended by the manufacturer or arbitrarily determined.
[b] According to manufacturers (usually expressed as kcal/weight of powder).
[c] ME calculated using Eq. (29.6).

Table 29.3 Caloric density of selected prey items for carnivorous birds.

Prey	Caloric density (kcal/100 g)
Day-old chick	600–616
Quail	556
Mouse	584–690
Rat	575–630

Source: Based on Chitty [10].

Table 29.4 Calculated frequencies and volumes of administration of a standard hand-feeding formula at 1 kcal/ml in anorexic birds fed 50 ml/kg (maximum tolerated amount).

Weight (g)	MER (kcal/d) (Eq. (29.2))	Frequency of administration	Volume of administration (ml)
30	14	9–10	1.5
50	18.9	7–8	2.5
100	31.0	6–7	5
200	50.8	5–6	10
300	67.9	4–5	15
500	97.8	3–4	25
1000	160.6	3–4	50

oropharyngeal trauma, tracheal aspiration of food, aspiration of food into the nasal cavity, and swallowing of the tube or a piece of it. Some of these complications are particularly prevalent in neonates of parrots probably because of the frequency of feeding or crop feeding by untrained people. Consequently, aspiration pneumonia is one of the most common respiratory diseases of neonatal parrots. Swallowing of the tube is possible when parrot breeders crop feed. Ingluvial perforation is uncommon, but potentially life-threatening. In the experience of the authors, it happens more frequently in large parrots. Possible scenarios leading to ingluvial perforation include when using a two-person approach to crop feeding with a bird struggling and pushing up on the metal cannula or when excessive force is used to pass the cannula down the esophagus. Subcutaneous (SC) deposition of food causes cellulitis and subsequent sepsis and can remain unrecognized until the bird is septic. The bird is typically lethargic, anorexic, and in some instances dysphagic. Inspection of the neck may reveal local swelling, erythema, and subcutaneous food. Imaging with non-barium radiographic contrast media may be needed to identify the puncture.

Invasive Methods

Invasive methods of supportive enteral nutrition in birds include pharyngostomy/ingluviotomy/esophagostomy tubes and intestinal feeding tubes.

Pharyngostomy, ingluviotomy, and esophagostomy tubes are indicated to by-pass the upper gastrointestinal system including the oropharyngeal cavity, the esophagus, or the crop (Table 29.5). In birds, examples of diseases requiring feeding tubes include beak and orofacial trauma, esophageal perforation, crop fistula, and esophagitis. Another indication is to reduce handling and the frequency of cannulation through the mouth [11, 12]. Esophagostomy tubes may maximize daily caloric intake with total daily volumes that would be impractical to give by repeated crop feeding (see Table 29.4). Consequently, it may be an effective means of providing nutrition in emaciated birds. It is particularly well tolerated in trained falconry birds, in which feeding may be performed without restraining the birds [11].

Table 29.5 Indications for esophagostomy tube placement.

Beak and maxillofacial trauma
Diseases of oropharynx
Diseases of esophagus and crop
Frequent regurgitation upon handling
Reduction of handling frequency
Long duration of nutritional support
Optimization of total daily caloric intake
Neoplasia of upper alimentary tract

Finally, when it is anticipated that the duration of supportive enteral duration will be long, it may be more practical and less stressful to administer the food through an esophagostomy tube during the recovery period.

Esophageal tube placement is fairly straightforward [11, 13, 14]. The bird should be under general anesthesia with the right area of the cranial neck surgically prepared. The esophagostomy tube length is predetermined to end roughly at the cranial end of the proventriculus. Small forceps are introduced into the oropharynx and pushed against the right lateral wall. A small incision is made with a scalpel blade until the tip of the forceps can easily be forced out through the incision. The incision can be made anywhere over the right aspect of the cranial neck or just under the mandible in parrots to prevent beak access. As the jugular vein is visible through the skin, it is easy to avoid. A small feeding tube is then grasped by the forceps and pulled inside the esophagus and out through the mouth. It is then redirected toward the distal esophagus and proventriculus. The tube is then secured to the skin using a finger trap suture pattern or other suture pattern and a bandage may be applied. The tube should be capped to prevent aerophagia and flushed after each feeding to avoid clogging of the tube. Smaller volumes but more frequent than for crop-feeding should be administered through this route. Continuous infusion using a syringe pump can also be implemented if bolus administration is not tolerated. When indicated, the tube can be removed and the wound left to heal by secondary intention.

Intestinal feeding tubes include duodenostomy or jejunostomy tubes. The indications are few, and it is rarely done in birds. The goal is to bypass the proventriculus and ventriculus in case of gastric diseases and to provide nutrition pending the resolution of these disorders. As retroperistalsis in the proventriculus and ventriculus is physiologic in various species including parrots, enteral tubes may not be completely effective at bypassing the proventriculus and ventriculus. Also, since the digestive action of the proventriculus and ventriculus is by-passed, specifically formulated diet may be indicated, whenever available (CliniCare in carnivore birds).

A technique has been described for duodenostomy tube placement in birds employing a jugular catheter [13, 15]. A midline coeliotomy is performed, and the duodenum is identified. The duodenum is relatively easy to identify, as it is right under the coelomic wall on the cranial right aspect and is closely associated with the pancreas. The through-the-needle jugular catheter is then inserted through the skin and body wall descending loop of the duodenum. The catheter is then advanced a few centimeters down the duodenum, and the duodenum is sutured to the coelomic wall at the point of entrance to seal the duodenostomy site. A finger trap suture is placed on the skin side to keep the catheter in place and the coelomic wall and skin are closed. Small and frequent feeding should be administered and it is best to use a syringe pump for a continuous infusion of liquid food (in patients that cannot handle bolus feeding). The tube should be left in place for a minimum of one week to allow a seal to form at the coelom–duodenal interface. The technique was studied in pigeons, in which a needle catheter duodenostomy was used for 14 days without adverse effects [15]. Removal of the tube before this time period may lead to intestinal content leakage into the coelomic cavity and septic coelomitis. When indicated, the tube can be removed and the wound left to heal by secondary intention.

Parenteral Nutrition

The indications of parenteral nutrition are relatively few in avian medicine, and it is still a rare procedure. Scientific publications on the subject are also scarce, and it is recommended to consult with a critical care specialist, veterinary nutritionist, or refer to a small animal reference textbook on the subject prior to its implementation in an avian patient. The main indication would be an inability for the gastrointestinal system to digest and absorb nutrients because of severe gastrointestinal diseases such as severe gastroenteritis. Malabsorptive diseases such as proventricular dilation disease and gastric neoplasia are also potential indications, but it also depends on the overall prognosis for the bird. Other indications in mammals include severe pancreatitis, intestinal obstruction, ischemic bowel, intractable vomiting, some maldigestion/malabsorption problems, and selected surgical procedures of the intestines [16]. Patients receiving parenteral nutrition should not be dehydrated.

Parenteral nutrition could be partial or total, meaning that it could partially or totally cover the MER of the patient. Partial parenteral nutrition (PPN) can be used as a supplement to enteral feeding. The parenteral alimentation is composed of essential nutrients such as dextrose, amino acids, lipids, electrolytes, and vitamins. It is 100% bioavailable. The formulation of total parenteral nutrition (TPN) is typically extrapolated from what is done in mammals.

PPN can be given at 30–50% of the MER and can help minimize weight loss in birds that have intravenous (IV) access and do not tolerate frequent crop feeding. PPN is likely more feasible in birds than TPN. PPN can be given through a peripheral or central catheter. Using a peripheral catheter to administer PPN can commonly cause phlebitis [16]. A general formulation for 1 l of PPN solution is 170–340 ml of 10% amino-acid solution (Travasol, Baxter), 660–830 ml of maintenance electrolyte solution ("Plasmalyte M and Dextrose 5%," see Table 29.7). Lipid (10% or 20% solution, Intralipid, Baxter) can be added, based on requirements, just before administration [16]. Other already formulated PPN commercial products may be used such as Clinimix (Baxter). The rate of administration is typically maintenance to twice maintenance rate of fluids.

For TPN, central venous access is necessary due to its hypertonicity [2, 16, 17]. The formulation of a TPN solution is similar to PPN except that it contains more calories and is supplemented with vitamins. In birds, it is typically achieved using a vascular access port, necessitating surgical placement. Due to the extreme physiology of birds, devising a TPN plan is challenging and potential complications are numerous including sepsis, electrolytic, and metabolic disorders. TPN has been reported in geese and pigeons [2, 17]. Continuous infusion using a syringe pump is the preferred method of TPN administration. However, intermittent administration of TPN is possible to avoid the presence of IV tubing that can be destroyed by parrots. A study on pigeons was aimed at evaluating the feasibility of TPN administered in an intermittent manner in birds through vascular access ports [17]. During a five-day trial with four times a day administration, pigeons lost about 9% of their body weight and developed hyperglycemia and glycosuria after bolus infusions. Five pigeons also developed venous thrombosis of the cranial vena cava due to the vascular access port. The authors concluded that the methodology needed to be refined as well as getting a better approximation of pigeon daily energy expenditure when receiving TPN. In another trial in two geese, marked hematologic changes were observed and one bird died [2]. In mammals, it is also known that the absence of enteral feeding has deleterious effects on the intestinal mucosa and increases bacterial translocation [18]. Thus, malabsorption and diarrhea may develop as enteral feeding resumes.

Fluid Therapy in Birds

Applied Physiology of Avian Body Fluids

The distribution of fluids in the avian body is similar to mammals [19]. About 60–70% of a bird's body weight is made of water with a third being extracellular and two-thirds intracellular [20]. The extracellular fluid is composed of interstitial and intravascular fluid (plasma). Plasma represents about 3.5–6.5% of the total avian body weight (hence blood is about 10%) [20]. In fact, blood volume varies by bird species (e.g. 5% of body weight in pheasants, 7.5% in quails, 10.5% in galahs). Body fluids contain a variety of solutes that get exchanged between fluid compartments through biological membranes with different permeability to solutes and electrolytic transport pumps. The extracellular fluid predominantly contains sodium and chloride, while the intracellular fluid mainly contains potassium, phosphorus, and magnesium [19]. Other solutes are in low concentrations in both compartments. A variety of osmoregulatory mechanisms come into play to keep body fluid composition within tight limits as part of the overall homeostasis of the avian organism. The vascular system serves to perfuse all cells of the body as a transport mechanism for fluids, dissolved respiratory gases, metabolites, proteins, and blood cells. Avian plasma has a slightly higher osmolality than mammals at about 300–340 mOsm/kg depending on the species and hydration status [20, 21]. Large molecules such as proteins in bird's plasma are responsible for 5% of plasma osmolality and for retaining fluids in the intravascular space (colloidal pressure), especially at capillary beds according to Starling mechanism. Reported avian colloid osmotic pressures range from 9 to 20 mmHg depending on species and reports [22–24].

The main osmoregulatory organs of birds include the kidneys, lower gastrointestinal system (coprodeum, colon, ceca), and salt glands (species dependent) [25]. The kidneys are typically composed of the cranial, middle, and caudal renal lobes, which contain about 30% looped nephrons and 70% loopless nephrons. A renal portal system made of a vascular circle of veins containing a renal portal valve is present ventral to the kidneys. It perfuses the tubules directly from venous blood draining from the lower part of the body. Birds are uricotelic, meaning that the end-product of protein catabolism is uric acid, produced by the liver. Uric acid is of low toxicity compared to urea and does not diffuse through biological membranes. Uric acid is excreted predominantly by tubular secretion at 90%. The low toxicity of uric acid combined with its excretion by tubular means results in the fact that birds do not need to maintain a constant glomerular filtration rate (GFR) like mammals do to eliminate toxic nitrogenous waste. Indeed, birds modulate their GFR depending on hydration status but preserve tubular perfusion through the renal portal system [25]. Once uric acid is excreted into the tubules, it combines with mucopolysaccharides and electrolytes to form microspheres that allow its existence in supersaturated suspension without precipitation and binding electrolytes [25]. Avian kidneys have a moderate ability to concentrate urine but post-renal handling of urine in the coprodeum and colon allows for further reabsorption of water and electrolytes and further concentration of the urine. Salt glands are very effective osmoregulatory organs and are present in most marine birds, some desert-dwelling birds, and other birds [25]. They may be the primary osmoregulatory organ in these bird species, thus their function should not be overlooked. While avian kidneys typically concentrate less than mammals, it is only one aspect of avian osmoregulation and birds' overall water conservation mechanisms tend to be equivalent to or superior to most mammals.

The avian water requirement in species commonly seen in clinics has been poorly investigated but is roughly estimated to be 50–100 ml/kg/d. Neonates tend to have higher maintenance requirements as well as passerine birds [2, 26].

Table 29.6 Selected routes of fluid administration in birds.

Routes	Sites	Advantages	Disadvantages	Fluid type
Per os (PO)	Crop, proventriculus	Least invasive	Contraindicated with concurrent gastrointestinal diseases (GI), neurological diseases, and in debilitated birds	Hypotonic
SC	Inguinal web Interscapular Axillary area	Non-invasive Well tolerated	Only for mild dehydration Limited volume (10 ml/kg/site)	Isotonic Hypotonic
IV	Ulnar vein Medial metatarsal vein Jugular vein	IV access for drugs Intravascular fluid Rapid dissemination More precise dosing	Low tolerance Significant bleeding if removed by bird	Isotonic Hypotonic Hypertonic Colloid Blood
IO	Ulna Tibiotarsus	See IV No bleeding if removed by bird Ideal when veins are too small or collapsed	Low tolerance Painful Potential for osteomyelitis Fluid extravasation with high rates	Isotonic Hypotonic Hypertonic Colloid Blood

Technical Aspects of Fluid Therapy in Birds

Fluids may be given through the oral, subcutaneous, intravenous, and intraosseous (IO) routes. Other routes are described but are less practical and not typically employed in practice. The choice of route of fluid administration and the type of fluid will depend on several criteria such as the degree of dehydration, the inciting cause of dehydration, the species, the demeanor of the bird, the degree of depression, and clinical, hematologic, and biochemical endpoints. Table 29.6 gives an overview of the advantages and disadvantages of different routes.

The oral route may be advantageous in low resource settings, when treating a large number of birds (e.g. rehabilitation, oil spill response), or in certain species where large volumes can be given easily. However, this route has numerous disadvantages that preclude its use in most situations for critical patients. Concurrent neurological and gastrointestinal disease, or any conditions precluding the bird from standing and holding its head upright may potentially result in regurgitation and aspiration. Also, gastrointestinal diseases may decrease the enteral absorption of water and electrolytes. In addition, oral fluids do not address hypovolemic states, may not lead to a precise and timely corrections of electrolytic and acid–base imbalances, and the choice of fluids that can be given orally are limited. In general, hypotonic enteral fluids (osmolality is typically between 250 and 300 mOsm/l) are selected such as Pedialyte or similar products or the "oral rehydration salts" formulated by the World Health Organization. Fluids with higher osmolality tend to decrease water absorption.

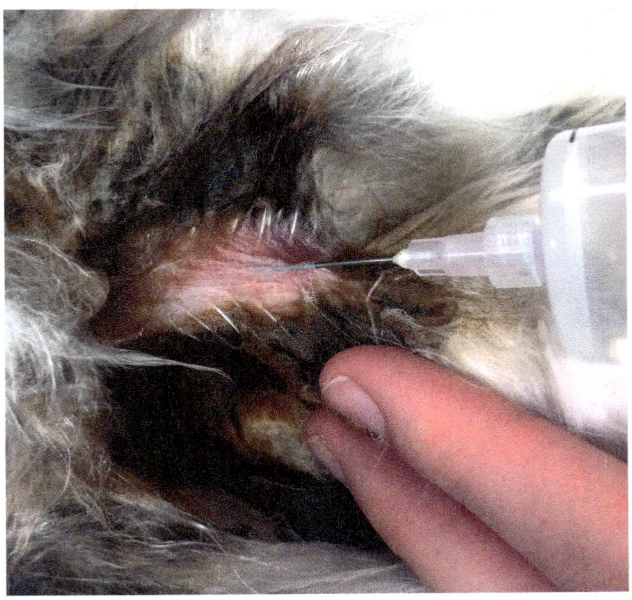

Figure 29.5 Subcutaneous fluid administration in the inguinal area in a great horned owl.

The subcutaneous route is typically used in birds for maintenance therapy, as a vehicle for tissue-irritating drugs (e.g. enrofloxacin), or for replacement therapy in mildly dehydrated birds (Figure 29.5). Peripheral vasoconstriction occurring during more severe dehydration or hypovolemia precludes the use of subcutaneous fluids. In addition, hypertonic, colloid fluids, and dextrose higher than 2.5% cannot be administered. Subcutaneous fluid is typically administered in the inguinal, axillary, or interscapular area using large needles for quickness of administration. No more than 10–30 ml/kg/site should be administered. Care should be taken to ensure fluids are placed subcutaneously, as confirmed by visualization of a "fluid bleb" just under the skin, to ensure the fluids do not enter the coelomic cavity.

The IV route is the route of choice as replacement therapy can be fine-tuned to the various electrolytic and acid–base disorders and permit rapid dissemination throughout the body. All types of fluids can be given intravenously. When IV access is available, all therapeutics may be given intravenously and constant rate infusion of drugs is also possible. The main disadvantage associated with IV catheterization is its low acceptance from birds resulting in difficulties in maintaining access, especially in Psittaciformes. However, it is well-tolerated in most Galliformes, Anseriformes, hooded Falconiformes, and many others. Significant bleeding may occur if the bird bites the IV line. Small anti-siphon valves (NP Medical Inc.) may be placed proximally so bleeding does not occur in case the line is transected by the bird. The most common sites for IV catheters include the ulnar vein, the medial metatarsal vein, and the jugular vein (see Chapter 25). Administration requires the use of fluid pumps or syringe pumps in smaller

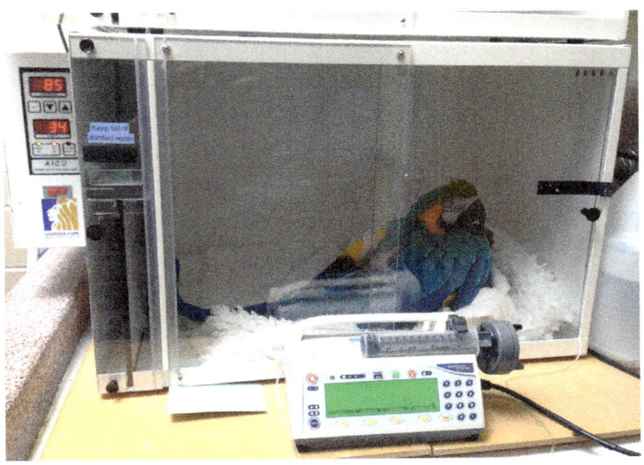

Figure 29.6 Blue and gold macaw receiving replacement fluid therapy through an IV catheter placed in ulnar vein and delivered using a syringe pump.

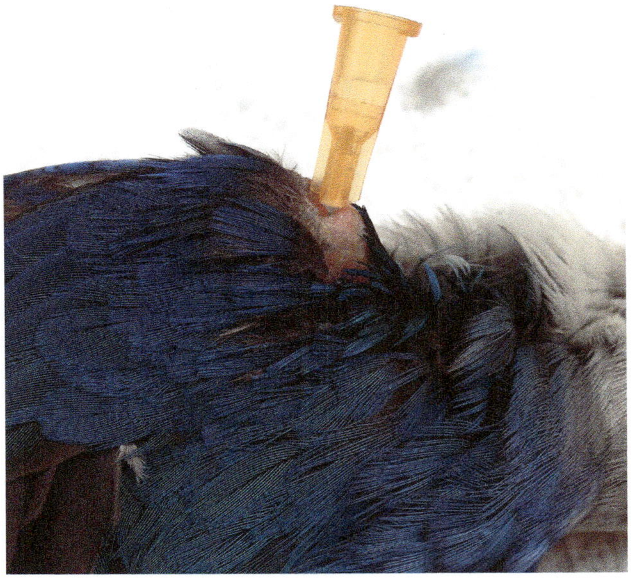

Figure 29.7 (See also Figure 25.8) Intraosseous catheter placed in the ulna of a lovebird using a 26 g needle.

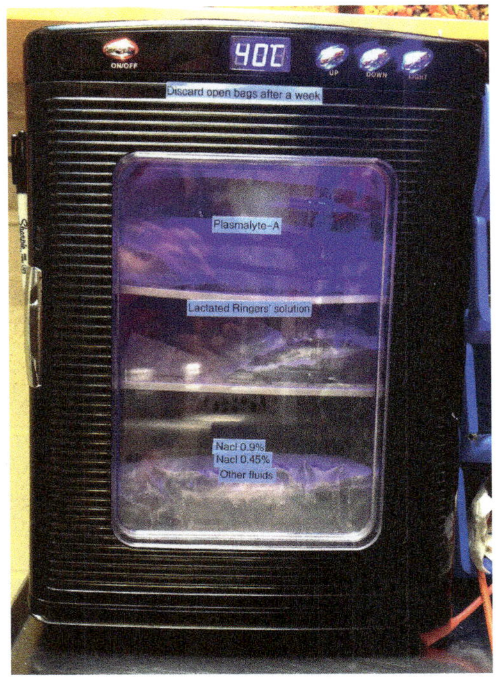

Figure 29.8 Exoterra® egg incubator used as a fluid warmer at avian body temperature.

species in order to give a precise rate (Figure 29.6). In low resource settings or in field situations, spring loaded syringe infusers (e.g. Springfusor, Admedus) may be used but the rate is predetermined. IV fluid administration is recommended for moderate-to-severe dehydration and during surgery. It is routinely performed in birds down to 100 g of body weight. Except in moribund or cooperative birds, sedation is required and the author typically uses a combination of midazolam 1–3 mg/kg and butorphanol 2 mg/kg for this purpose in Psittaciformes. The midazolam can be reversed with flumazenil 0.05 mg/kg.

The IO route is similar to the IV route and is easier and faster to secure. It can be placed in birds of all sizes. Studies have shown that it is almost identical to IV access [27, 28]. It is typically placed either in the distal ulna or proximal tibiotarsus (see Chapter 25). Pneumatic bones should be avoided. In some birds such as Cathartiformes, the ulna is pneumatized, which precludes the placement of an IO catheter at that location [29]. Placement in the ulna is favored by the author as the correctness of the placement can be verified by injecting a small fluid bolus or a bubble of air and observing it flowing in the ulnar vein. Also, birds are bipedal, and pain induced to the leg may cause lameness and discomfort while standing. Local lidocaine infusion may be used prior to placement. For the ulnar placement, a dorsal approach may be used where the manus is slightly pronated, then a small number of feathers are plucked in the area, and a 22 g 1.5 in. long spinal needle is inserted just distal to the dorsal condyle (Figure 29.7). In smaller birds, 25G or 26G hypodermic needles can be used, but a core of bone may obstruct the needle, which will need to be replaced. Alternatively, a small wire stylet may be used during placement. For tibiotarsal placement, the knee is flexed, the patellar tendon is pushed medially, and the spinal needle is inserted into the bone. In the author's experience, radiographs are not needed to confirm placement but may still be performed if unsure. Fluid accumulation in soft tissue indicates misplacement. Once in place, antiseptic ointment should be applied to the site, it should be bandaged and treated like an IV catheter. Sedation is required except in lethargic birds. The author does not routinely anesthetize birds for IO catheterization as they tend to be poor anesthetic candidates. All types of fluids may be infused; hypertonic solutions and colloids tend to cause painful reactions and are best diluted.

All administered fluids must be warmed to avian body temperature (38–40 °C, 100–104 °F). This requires storing fluid packages in incubators and using in-line fluid warmers if available (Figure 29.8).

Types of Fluids and Indications

Fluids are classified as crystalloids or colloids. Crystalloids are further divided into hypotonic, isotonic, and hypertonic. Table 29.7 gives the composition of common crystalloid fluids used in avian medicine and

Table 29.7 Selected crystalloid fluids and their characteristics.

Crystalloids	pH	mOsm/l	Na	Cl	K	Ca	Buffer	Tonicity
LRS	6.5	272	130	109	4	3	Lactate	Isotonic, slightly hypotonic for birds
Plasmalyte-A	5.5	312	140	103	10	5	Acetate	Isotonic
Plasmalyte-A 7.4	7.4	294	140	98	5	0	Acetate	Isotonic
Plasmalyte M in 5% dextrose	5.5	377	40	40	16	5	Acetate and lactate	Isotonic
Normosol-R	6.4	296	140	98	5	0	Acetate	Isotonic
Hartmann's	6.3	279	131	112	5	2	Lactate	Isotonic, slightly hypotonic for birds
0.9% NaCl	5.0	308	154	154	0	0	None	Isotonic
0.45% NaCl	5.0	154	77	77	0	0	None	Hypotonic
3% NaCl	5.0	1026	513	513	0	0	None	Hypertonic
7.5% NaCl	5.0	2566	1283	1283	0	0	None	Hypertonic
5% dextrose	4.0	252	0	0	0	0	None	Hypotonic

Table 29.8 Selected colloidal fluids and their characteristics.

Colloids	MW (kDa)	mOsm/l	Half-life	Dose
6% Hetastarch	670	310	25 h	20 ml/kg/d 5 ml/kg bolus can be repeated twice
10% Pentastarch	200	326	2.5 h	Idem as above
Avian blood	NA	300–340	8–10 d	Full volume administered over 1–4 h

MW, molecular weight.

their characteristics. Prepackaged fluids have been developed for mammals, which have lower plasma osmolality than birds. As a consequence, fluids classified as isotonic may be slightly hypotonic for birds (e.g. Lactated Ringer's solution[LRS]). Crystalloid fluids may or may not be buffered. Depending on their composition and characteristics, crystalloids are either maintenance or replacement fluids. Maintenance fluids are seldom used in avian medicine and they approximate the normal daily requirements of fluids and electrolytes for animals unable to drink. Replacement fluids approximate the extracellular fluid composition in electrolytes and are used for correcting losses of water and electrolytes. Crystalloids should be considered as interstitial rehydrators as only 25% of fluids remain in the circulation after a short period of time. LRS, Normosol-R, and Plasmalyte-A are balanced buffered solutions that more closely approximate the extracellular fluid composition and therefore can be used in most situations. 0.9% saline is not buffered and unbalanced and is typically restricted for patients with metabolic alkalosis. LRS is hypo-osmolar to avian plasma and should not be used at high IV rate (e.g. resuscitation) but is well suited for subcutaneous administration as it may be absorbed more readily than isotonic solutions. Plasmalyte-A 7.4 is the closest fluid to avian plasma composition in terms of pH, osmolality, and electrolyte concentrations. Hypertonic saline can be considered as an intravascular expander because it leads to rapid intravascular expansion equivalent to that of colloids at one-fourth the volume. It is used in resuscitation and in combination with crystalloids and colloids. Dextrose 5% is primarily used as a carrier for constant rate infusion of drugs or as a source of pure water.

Colloids are large molecules that do not readily diffuse across membranes (Table 29.8). They increase the plasma colloidal pressure attracting interstitial fluids into the intravascular space. As such, they can be considered intravascular expanders and are typically used when the colloidal pressure is low, in hypotension and hypovolemia, in hypoproteinemia, in significant hemorrhage, and in fluid resuscitation. Contraindications for colloids include coag-

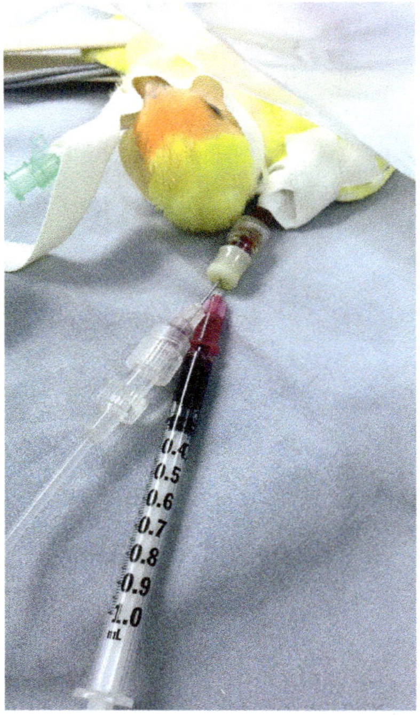

Figure 29.9 Homologous blood transfusion in a lovebird administered through an IO catheter in conjunction with fluid therapy.

ulopathy, pneumonia, congestive heart failure, and renal failure. Blood is also considered a colloid with the added benefit of providing blood cells and coagulation factors. Blood is typically transfused whole in birds and ideally collected from the same species of birds (Figure 29.9). The half-life of infused blood is about a week. Transfusing from other bird species is not indicated as transfused blood cells are rapidly destroyed [30, 31]. Oxyglobin, a hemoglobin-based oxygen carrier colloid, has been discontinued.

In case of IV or IO catheters, various additives may be added to the fluids or in separate IV lines with a dedicated syringe pump (Table 29.9). Most replacement fluids are deficient in potassium and should be supplemented after initial stabilization or hypokalemia may develop after a few days.

The Fluid Therapy Plan

The objectives of fluid replacement therapy are to replace fluid deficits in order to correct perfusion and hydration without inducing fluid overload, to anticipate fluid loss and provide maintenance needs, and to correct electrolytes and acid–base abnormalities. In addition, the fluid therapy plan must be monitored and reassessed while underlying conditions must be diagnosed and treated.

Table 29.9 Selected fluid additives commonly used in birds.

	Dose	Comments
Additives		
Dextrose 50%	Dilute to 2.5–5% 0.5 ml/kg bolus over 15 min	Treatment hypoglycemia and metabolic support
KCl	Maintenance: total dose of 15–20 mEq/l	Correct fluid deficiency
	Moderate hypokalemia: 40 mEq/l	Treatment of hypokalemia
	Severe hypokalemia: 60 mEq/l	Do not exceed 0.5 mEq/kg/h
$NaHCO_3$	0.3*W_{kg}*base excess over 30–60 min may give half initially	Metabolic acidosis
Calcium gluconate 10%	0.5–1.5 ml/kg bolus over 15–20 min	Treatment of ionized hypocalcemia or hyperkalemia
	1–5 mg elemental calcium/kg/h	Use NaCl 0.9% as fluid or precipitation may occur
Insulin	0.5 U/kg + 2 g of dextrose/insulin units	Hyperkalemia
Constant rate infusion		
Hydromorphone	0.1 mg/kg/h	Pain management (various)
Butorphanol	1 mg/kg/h	Pain management (parrots)
Fentanyl	10–20 µg/kg/h	Pain management (hawks)
Dopamine	5–15 µg/kg/min	Hypotension

Table 29.10 Signs of dehydration in birds.

	Clinical endpoints
Clinical signs of dehydration (interstitial loss)	
5%	Subclinical dehydration
	History of fluid loss
	Skin slow to return when tenting of skin over keel or eyelids
7–8%	Lethargy
	Dry and tacky mucous membranes
	Strings of thick mucus in oral cavity
10–12%	Skin very slow to return when tenting skin over keel and eyelids
	Sunken eyes
15%	Comatose, marked weakness
Clinical signs of hypovolemia (intravascular loss)	Altered consciousness
	Tachycardia
	Low ulnar vein refilling time (>1–2 s)
	Poorly palpable pulse
	Hypothermia
	Hypotension
Common laboratory findings with dehydration (depending on comorbid conditions, laboratory changes may be inconsistent)	Increased packed cell volume (PCV)
	Increased total solids (TS) and total protein (TP)
	Increased urea
	Increased uric acid
	Increased electrolyte concentrations
	Increased plasma osmolality
	Increased blood lactate (from hypoperfusion)
	Increased blood glucose (from increased sympathetic tone)
	Altered plasma pH

The first step is to determine the presence and estimate the degree of dehydration and other homeostatic abnormalities. Overall dehydration is harder to assess in birds than in mammals [26]. Typical clinical signs encountered with dehydration in birds are presented in Table 29.10. Unfortunately, indirect blood pressure measurements are unreliable in small to medium-sized birds so hypotension may have to be estimated based on physical examination in these species [32, 33]. However, arterial pressure may be monitored using an arterial catheter in larger birds [34]. If available, blood gases and electrolyte measurements are important and critical in fluid selection.

Fluid therapy is classically divided into three stages: resuscitation, rehydration, and maintenance. If the bird is unstable and has signs of hypoperfusion, shock, or active hemorrhage, then emergency fluid resuscitation is required. Fortunately, birds are more resistant to hypovolemic shock than mammals and do not go into decompensated shock until more than 60% of intravascular volume loss [35–38]. Fluids classically used in resuscitation include isotonic balanced crystalloids such as Plasmalyte-A 7.4 and/or a combination of hypertonic saline (7.5% NaCl), crystalloids, and colloids. Recommendations in order to use the least amount of fluids to reach the desired effect and to achieve fast intravascular volume expansion and reverse the hypotensive state is to use 3 ml/kg of 7.5% NaCl mixed with 5 ml/kg of colloid given over 10 minutes followed by crystalloids bolused at 10 ml/kg [35]. Crystalloid boluses may be repeated every 10–15 minutes until improvement of clinical markers is seen. If treating large birds, indirect blood pressure may be measured using a Doppler unit. Atropine (0.2 mg/kg IV) and epinephrine (0.02 mg/kg IV) may also be used if non-responsive. At this stage, blood work, electrolytes, and blood gas analysis may help assess other causes of non-responsive shock (e.g. hypoglycemia, hypocalcemia). If severe hemorrhage occurred or severe anemia is present, birds may benefit from homologous blood transfusions. The transfusion (usually 10% of body weight taken from a donor bird, as higher volume is generally not feasible unless several donors are available) is typically administered over one to four hours and the use of a pediatric microfilter is recommended [39].

For the rehydration phase of the fluid therapy plan, once perfusion has been restored and the degree of dehydration estimated, the rate of fluids should be calculated. Usually, 50–100% of estimated loss may be replenished within the first 24 hours. To this, maintenance requirements and anticipated losses should be added. In general, the more rapid the fluid loss, the more rapid the replacement should be, especially when pre-renal azotemia has been identified. Consequently, total fluid deficit may be replenished in 4–10 hours if acute dehydration is suspected. The choice of fluid type is usually guided by the acid–base and electrolytic abnormalities. Most avian patients are in metabolic acidosis with dehydration or various illness which makes plasmalyte-A 7.4 the fluid of choice. Alternatively, LRS may be used but is slightly hypotonic to avian plasma. Except for rapid rates, potassium may be supplemented to the fluids (Table 29.9). Other additives may be added to the infusion depending on identified abnormalities (Table 29.9). It should be noted that potassium artifacts are common on avian biochemistry analysis so one should exert caution before treating hypokalemia. For vomiting and loss of HCl and metabolic alkalosis, 0.9% NaCl is the fluid of choice. Calculations are just rough estimates and monitoring of the response to fluid therapy is important. Body weight gives a good estimate of the amount of rehydration. Since fluid deficits and requirements are difficult to estimate and clinical endpoints challenging to assess in birds, rehydration may continue for another 24–48 hours using a lower rate. Due to the low tolerance of avian patients for IV and IO catheters, the maintenance phase is typically performed subcutaneously and the catheters removed.

The fluid rate under anesthesia ("surgical rate") is typically 10 ml/kg/h to treat the isoflurane-induced hypotension and anticipated fluid loss due to oxygen flow and evaporation through the surgical sites.

Birds

References

1 Koutsos, E. (2016). Foundations in avian nutrition. In: *Current Therapy in Avian Medicine and Surgery* (ed. B. Speer), 142–150. St Louis, MO: Elsevier.

2 Quesenberry, K. and Hillyer, E. (1994). Supportive care and emergency therapy. In: *Avian Medicine: Principles and Applications* (eds. B. Ritchie, L. Harrison and G. Harrison), 382–415. Lake Worth, FL: Wingers Publishing.

3 Sedgwick, C. (1991). Allometrically scaling the data base for vital sign assessment used in general anesthesia of zoological species. *American Association of Zoo Veterinarians*, Calgary, Canada, 1991, p. 360–369.

4 Sales, J. and Janssens, G. (2003). Energy and protein nutrition of companion birds. *Vlaams Diergeneeskindig Tijdschr* 72: 51–58.

5 Nagy, K.A. (2005). Field metabolic rate and body size. *J. Exp. Biol.* 208 (Pt 9): 1621–1625.

6 Koutsos, E.A., Matson, K.D., and Klasing, K.C. (2001). Nutrition of birds in the order psittaciformes: a review. *J Avian Med. Surg.* 15 (4): 257–275.

7 Pokras, M., Karas, A., Kirwood, J., and Sedgwick, C. (1993). An introduction to allometric scaling and its uses in raptor medicine. In: *Raptor Biomedicine* (eds. P. Redig, J. Cooper, J. Remple and D. Hunter), 211–228. St Paul, MN: University of Minnesota Press.

8 EJ, H. (2000). Estimating the energy needs of pet birds. *J. Avian Med. Surg.* 14 (2): 95–102.

9 Glazier, D.S. (2008). Effects of metabolic level on the body size scaling of metabolic rate in birds and mammals. *Proc. Biol. Sci.* 275 (1641): 1405–1410.

10 Chitty, J. (2008). Raptors: nutrition. In: *BSAVA Manual of Raptors, Pigeons and Passerine Birds* (eds. J. Chitty and M. Lierz), 190–201. Gloucester, UK: BSAVA.

11 Huynh, M., Sabater, M., Brandão, J., and Forbes, N.A. (2014). Use of an esophagostomy tube as a method of nutritional management in raptors: a case series. *J. Avian Med. Surg.* 28 (1): 24–30.

12 Aguilar, R.F., Yoshicedo, J.N., and Parish, C.N. (2012). Ingluviotomy tube placement for lead-induced crop stasis in the California condor (*Gymnogyps californianus*). *J. Avian Med. Surg.* 26 (3): 176–181.

13 Bennett, R.A. (1994). Soft tissue surgery. In: *Avian Medicine: Principles and Applications* (eds. B. Ritchie, G. Harrison and L. Harrison), 1996–1136. Lake Worth, FL: Wingers Publishing.

14 Forbes, N. (2016). Soft tissue surgery. In: *Avian Medicine*, 3e (ed. J. Samour), 294–311. St Louis, MO: Elsevier.

15 Goring, R.L., Goldman, A., Kaufman, K.J. et al. (1986). Needle catheter duodenostomy: a technique for duodenal

alimentation of birds. *J. Am. Vet. Med. Assoc.* 189 (9): 1017–1019.

16 Mathews, K. (2006). Partial parenteral nutrition. In: *Veterinary Emergency and Critical Care*, 2e (ed. K. Mathews), 511–514. Guelph, Canada: Lifelearn.

17 Degernes, L., Davidson, G., Flammer, K. et al. (1994). Administration of total parenteral nutrition in pigeons. *Am. J. Vet. Res.* 55 (5): 660–665.

18 Mathews, K. (2006). Nutritional support. In: *Veterinary Emergency and Critical Care*, 2e (ed. K. Mathews), 499–510. Guelph, Canada: Lifelearn.

19 DiBartola, S.P., Wellman, M.L., and Kohn, C.W. (2012). Applied physiology of body fluids in dogs and cats. In: *Fluid, Electrolyte, and Acid-Base Disorders in Small Animal Practice*, 4e (ed. S. DiBartola), 2–25. St Louis, MO: Elsevier.

20 Goldstein, D. and Skadhauge, E. (2000). Renal and extrarenal regulation of body fluid composition. In: *Sturkie's Avian Physiology*, 5e (ed. G. Whittow), 265–297. San Diego, CA: Academic Press.

21 Beaufrère, H., Acierno, M., Mitchell, M. et al. (2011). Plasma osmolality reference values in African grey parrots (*Psittacus erithacus erithacus*), Hispaniolan Amazon parrots (*Amazona ventralis*), and red-fronted macaws (*Ara rubrogenys*). *J. Avian Med. Surg.* 25 (2): 91–96.

22 Keil, R., Gerstberger, R., and Simon, E. (1991). Effects of changes in intravascular oncotic pressure on renal responses to volume loading in the saltwater-acclimated Pekin duck (*Anas platyrhynchos*). *J. Comp. Physiol. B* 161 (2): 179–187.

23 Cornelius, S.T., Klugman, K.P., and Hattingh, J. (1982). Effects of haemorrhage on colloid osmotic pressure in the pigeon. *Comp. Biochem. Physiol. A: Physiol.* 71 (2): 337–339.

24 Peltonen, L.M. and Sankari, S. (2011). Ott's protein osmotic pressure of serum and interstitial fluid in chickens (*Gallus gallus*): effect of age and gender. *J. Exp. Biol.* 214 (Pt 4): 599–606.

25 Braun, E. (2015). Osmoregulatory systems of birds. In: *Sturkie's Avian Physiology*, 6e (ed. C. Scanes), 285–300. San Diego, CA: Academic Press.

26 Steinohrt, L. (1999). Avian fluid therapy. *J. Avian Med. Surg.* 13 (2): 83–91.

27 Lamberski, N. and Daniel, G. (1992). Fluid dynamics of intraosseous fluid administration in birds. *J. Zoo Wild. Med.* 23 (1): 47–54.

28 Aguilar, R., Johnston, G., Callfos, C. et al. (1993). Osseuous-venous and central circulatory transit times of Technetium-99m pertechnetate in anesthetized raptors following intraosseous administration. *J. Zoo Wildl. Med.* 24 (4): 488–497.

29 Stringfield, C. (2012). The California condor (*Gymnogyps californianus*) veterinary program: 1997–2000. In: *Fowler's Zoo and Wild Animal Medicine Current Therapy*, vol. 7 (eds. R. Miller and M. Fowler), 286–296. St Louis, MO: Elsevier Saunders.

30 Degernes, L., Harrison, L., Smith, D. et al. (1999). Autologous, homologous, and heterologous red blood cell transfusions in conures of the genus Aratinga. *J. Avian Med. Surg.* 13 (1): 10–14.

31 Sandmeier, P., Stauber, E.H., Wardrop, K.J., and Washizuka, A. (1994). Survival of pigeon red blood cells after transfusion into selected raptors. *J. Am. Vet. Med. Assoc.* 204 (3): 427–429.

32 Acierno, M.J., da Cunha, A., Smith, J. et al. (2008). Agreement between direct and indirect blood pressure measurements obtained from anesthetized Hispaniolan Amazon parrots. *J. Am. Vet. Med. Assoc.* 233 (10): 1587–1590.

33 Johnston, M.S., Davidowski, L.A., Rao, S., and Hill, A.E. (2011). Precision of repeated, Doppler-derived indirect blood pressure measurements in conscious psittacine birds. *J. Avian Med. Surg.* 25 (2): 83–90.

34 Schnellbacher, R., da Cunha, A., Olson, E.E., and Mayer, J. (2014). Arterial catheterization, interpretation, and treatment of arterial blood pressures and blood gases in birds. *J. Exot. Pet. Med.* 23 (2): 129–141.

35 Lichtenberger, M. (2007). Shock and cardiopulmonary-cerebral resuscitation in small mammals and birds. *Vet. Clin. North Am. Exot. Anim. Pract.* 10 (2): 275–291.

36 Djojosugito, A.M., Folkow, B., and Kovách, A.G. (2014). The mechanisms behind the rapid blood volume restoration after hemorrhage in birds. *Acta Physiol. Scand.* 74 (1): 114–122.

37 Lichtenberger, M., Orcutt, C., and DeBehnke, D. (2002). Mortality and response to fluid resuscitation after acute blood loss in mallard ducks (*Anas platyrhinchos*). *Proc. Annu. Conf. Assoc. Avian. Vet.* 23: 65–70.

38 Lichtenberger, M., Orcutt, C., Cray, C. et al. (2009). Comparison of fluid types for resuscitation after acute blood loss in mallard ducks (*Anas platyrhynchos*). *J. Vet. Emerg. Crit. Care.* 19 (5): 467–472.

39 Jankowski, G. and Nevarez, J. (2010). Evaluation of a pediatric blood filter for whole blood transfusions in domestic chickens (*Gallus gallus*). *J. Avian Med. Surg.* 24 (4): 272–278.

Section 2

Diagnostics

30

STAT Diagnostics

Claudia Kabakchiev[1] *and Hugues Beaufrère*[2]

[1] *404 Veterinary Emergency and Referral Hospital, Ontario, Canada*
[2] *Department of Medicine and Epidemiology, School of Veterinary Medicine, University of California Davis, Davis, USA*

CONTENTS

Point-Of-Care Blood Sampling

As with mammalian patients, blood testing is an important component of a diagnostic database in the critical avian patient. However, when collecting the sample, it is important to be mindful of the patient's size, potential sources of blood loss before presentation, and cardiovascular status. If anemia or hypovolemia are suspected, it may be necessary to take a smaller amount of blood than would normally be considered appropriate. As a general rule, in a healthy bird, a blood volume of 1% of the bird's body weight can be safely collected (ex. 0.9 ml for a 90 g cockatiel). The amount of blood you obtain will determine the number of point-of-care (POC) or laboratory tests that can be pursued; appropriate selection of tests based on the history and physical examination findings is crucial. POC blood testing aims at rapidly detecting key metabolic and homeostatic disturbances that require immediate attention and correction. The required minimum database on a critical patient that necessitates fluid therapy would include blood gas (if available) and electrolytes, packed cell volume (PCV) (or hemoglobin), total solids (TS), and blood glucose. POC blood analysis should not replace a more comprehensive blood count and biochemistry profile that should be performed whenever possible or indicated. See "Chapter 25: Catheterization and venipuncture" for further details on blood collection techniques.

Exotic Animal Emergency and Critical Care Medicine, First Edition. Edited by Jennifer E. Graham, Grayson A. Doss and Hugues Beaufrère.

Packed Cell Volume and Total Solids

PCV and TS are easy to obtain from a small blood sample in a microhematocrit capillary tube.

Indications

Assessment of the PCV is recommended if there is evidence for or a suspicion of blood loss, anemia, or erythrocytosis. A blood smear may be examined at the same time, in order to look for changes in red blood cell morphology or polychromasia which may help determine whether an anemia is regenerative.

Whenever a manual PCV is determined using a microhematocrit tube, the serum or plasma should be evaluated for TS. TS are primarily indicative of the total protein (TP) in the blood; however, TS is also influenced by glucose, electrolyte, and lipid levels. Thus, in birds, the correlation between TS and TP is low [1]. Therefore, determining the TS is indicated whenever an abnormality in these analytes is suspected. It may help determine the level of hydration when interpreted in combination with the PCV.

Manual PCV

Using the same technique as in mammals, the PCV can be easily obtained from a microhematocrit tube. For most avian species, a normal PCV ranges from 40% to 55%. An elevated PCV may be indicative of dehydration, hemoconcentration, and erythrocytosis secondary to chronic respiratory disease. A decreased PCV may occur with chronic disease, blood loss, red blood cell lysis, or bone marrow disease. A transfusion may be required if the PCV is acutely decreased (to less than 15%), the patient is clinically weak from anemia, and blood donors from the same species are available. Birds can tolerate lower PCVs if the loss occurs chronically.

Refractometer TS

The refraction of light within a plasma or serum sample is correlated to the concentration of total solutes in the liquid, what we call "TS." These solutes consist of mainly protein, but also glucose, electrolytes, and lipids, as mentioned above. When the TS is outside of the reference range (about 3–5 g/l for most birds), it is important to differentiate between these factors using a biochemical profile.

The accuracy of estimating TP from TS obtained by refractometry varies by avian species, but is generally weak. A study on chickens and turkeys found that the refractometer TS was well correlated with the TP determined by the biuret method, which is commonly used in biochemical profiles [2]. Another study in pigeons did not identify a good correlation and accuracy when interpreting TP from the refractometer TS [3]. Lipemia will interfere with the accurate determination of TP. Caution is recommended when attempting to interpret values obtained by refractometry in avian patients.

Plasma Appearance

The plasma from the microhematocrit tube or heparinized blood collection tube should be examined for color change. The normal plasma color is clear or pale yellow (from carotenoids in the diet). If it is cloudy or white in color, there is likely significant lipemia which will interfere with evaluation of the refractometer TS and other biochemical analytes. If the plasma is pink in color, hemolysis is likely present. Hemolysis may occur with sample collection, but can also be seen with septicemia, toxicosis (ex. heavy metal toxicity, aflatoxicosis, etc.), or certain blood parasites.

Glucose

The glucose can be readily determined from a plasma, serum, or whole blood sample. Commonly used POC tests for assessing blood glucose include glucometers, blood gas analyzers, or POC biochemistry analyzers.

Glucometers

The results obtained from a human or veterinary glucometer often underestimate the actual blood glucose in birds [4, 5]. A study performed with pigeons found that there was a strong linear relationship between the glucometer readings and the blood glucose measured by a biochemistry analyzer, despite the fact that glucometer readings were consistently lower [6]. Due to this consistent association, the authors were able to develop linear equations for pigeons to help predict the true blood glucose after reading with a glucometer. In psittacine birds, however, studies have not been able to demonstrate a good agreement; the use of glucometers may be limited in many avian species [7].

Normal blood glucose, when measured by laboratory biochemistry analyzers, ranges from about 10–20 mmol/l (180–360 mg/dL) in most avian patients. An elevated glucose reading may be reflective of stress, diabetes mellitus, or endogenous or exogenous corticosteroids. Hypoglycemia needs to be interpreted carefully since it may be artifactual if mild. If it is significant, the hypoglycemia may be reflective of septicemia, severe hepatic insufficiency, or starvation.

Lactate

Lactate measurements are often used to evaluate tissue perfusion and oxygenation, as well as the origin of a patient's acid–base status. Lactate may be measured as part of a blood gas/electrolyte panel or using POC lactate meters. Lactate exists as two stereoisomers, D-lactate and L-lactate; the latter is most common in humans as a product of anaerobic metabolism and the isomer that is measured by POC tests [8]. D-lactate is produced due to bacterial glucose metabolism in the gastrointestinal tract of mammals. Studies on the clinical use of lactate in birds and normal reference ranges are lacking. Blood lactate has been used to identify the immediate impact of capturing and restraining wild or zoo birds [9, 10]. It has also been used to determine the efficacy of rehabilitation programs for certain wild raptors and their readiness for release [11]. Blood lactate levels that have been reported for unstressed birds range significantly across species (from 1 to 17 mmol/l) making this a difficult analyte to interpret without well-developed species-specific reference intervals. Further research into this area is required. In general, a high lactate level in an otherwise calm and depressed bird without prior struggling may be indicative of tissue hypoperfusion.

Blood Smear: Quick Assessment

Blood smears are important to evaluate cell morphology and look for blood parasites. If anemia is identified by the PCV, the smear should be examined for polychromatophils which correlate well with the presence of reticulocytes and a regenerative response [12]. When making smears with avian blood, a squash or coverslip technique is preferred over the wedge technique used in mammals because of the fragility of avian blood cells. A more detailed discussion of blood cytology and interpretation of the hemogram can be found in "Chapter 32: Clinical Pathology."

WBC/Platelet Estimates

From the blood smear, it may be possible to estimate the white blood cell (WBC) and thrombocyte counts. See "Chapter 32: Clinical Pathology" for a detailed explanation about blood smear estimation techniques and limitations. Briefly, to estimate the WBC count with the 40× objective lens on the microscope, count all leukocytes seen in 10 microscopic fields over a monolayer region of the blood smear. To obtain the WBC count (10^9/l), the counted leukocytes are used as "*N*" in the formula

$$\frac{N}{10} \times 1.5$$

To correct for abnormalities in the PCV and therefore cellular density, the WBC count obtained is multiplied by

$$\frac{\text{PCV}}{\text{PCV expected for species}}$$

This is only an approximation and does not have high reliability. However, from this information, a differential WBC count can be obtained. Be aware that in stressed birds a mild leukocytosis (with mild heterophilia and lymphopenia) may be noted. A normal WBC count for most birds is between 5 and 15×10^9/l. Some avian species can normally have higher levels as well (ex. macaws, chickens, and some raptors). When a severe leukocytosis is identified, chlamydiosis, aspergillosis, mycobacteriosis, and sepsis should be considered as differential diagnoses.

Thrombocyte counts can also be determined as the number of thrombocytes noted per 100 leukocytes, or as a qualitative determination from examination of the blood smear. Elevated thrombocyte counts may be seen with inflammatory disease.

Coagulation Testing

Coagulation disorders are uncommon in birds (an exception is rodenticide ingestion in raptors); therefore, tests to evaluate coagulability are infrequently used. Platelet counts and clotting times of whole blood may be measured. Prothrombin time (PT) has been developed as a test in some avian species [13]. Thromboelastography (TEG) has also recently been investigated [14, 15]. A more detailed discussion of coagulation testing may be found in "Chapter 32: Clinical Pathology" and "Chapter 34: Ancillary Diagnostics."

To evaluate PT, blood should be collected on sodium citrate then centrifuged to separate the plasma. A control sample should also be submitted. There are few published reference intervals; however, there are intervals for use with both avian and mammalian thromboplastin. Due to the small size of many birds, the clinical applications of performing coagulation tests in a patient that may already be anemic are limited.

Blood Gas and Acid–Base Evaluation

Blood gas analysis and interpretation of acid–base status are important components of assessing a critical avian patient and can readily be performed as POC blood tests in medium to large-sized birds. It is essential to devising an efficient fluid therapy plan. The blood sample is ideally collected from an arterial site for blood gas analysis, although venous samples are more commonly used for acid–base evaluation because they are easier to acquire. Only arterial blood samples may be used to assess blood oxygenation and lung efficiency. Reference intervals need to be based on the sample type. The partial pressure of carbon dioxide (pCO_2) will be slightly higher in venous samples than in arterial samples, whereas the pH will be slightly lower. Reference values for avian blood gas analysis are included in Table 30.1 [9, 16–22].

Blood gas samples are collected in airtight heparinized syringes and should be analyzed within 15 minutes of collection at avian body temperature (around 100.4–105.8 °F;

Table 30.1 Reference values for blood gas analytes in various avian species without anesthesia.

Sample site	Arterial	Arterial	Venous	Venous	Venous	Venous	Venous	Venous
Species	Blue-fronted amazon[a]	Pekin duck[b]	Quaker parrot[c]	African grey parrot[d]	Mourning dove[e]	Pigeon[f]	Red-tailed hawk[g]	Budgies[h]
pH	7.452 ± 0.048	7.458 ± 0.011	7.43 ± 0.07	7.353 ± 0.075	7.453, 7.285–7.558	7.43 ± 0.05	7.43 ± 0.07	7.334–7.489
pCO_2 (mmHg)	22.1 ± 4	32.5 ± 0.8	28.6 ± 3.7	31 ± 6.1	28.6, 21–45.9	41.4 ± 4.8	26.78 ± 4.6	30.6–43.2
pO_2 (mmHg)	98.1 ± 7.6	101.3 ± 2			49, 22–63			85–99
HCO_3^- (mmol/l)	14.8 ± 2.8	21.8 ± 0.6	19.2 ± 4.3	17.4 ± 4.2	21.2, 14.4–30.1	26 ± 3.6	18.1 ± 4.25	21–26
BE	−7.9 ± 3.1		−5.1 ± 5.2	Range: −15 to +1			−6.36 ± 5.22	

Notes: Many results are presented as mean ± SD (standard deviation) or SEM (standard error of the mean), rather than reference intervals. In order to get rough estimates of the reference intervals from these values, one would have to use the mean ± 2 × SD or mean ± 2 SEM/√(sample size).

[a] Mean ± SD as measured on i-STAT (Abbott, Princeton); *Source:* Paula et al. [16].

[b] Mean ± SEM as measured on ABL2 (Radiometer Medical, Bronshoj, Denmark); *Source:* Ludders et al. [17]. (Note: $n = 9$ ducks).

[c] Mean ± SD of values that did not differ significantly with reference lab as measured on i-STAT (Abbott, Princeton); *Source:* Rettenmund et al. [18].

[d] Mean ± SD as measured on i-STAT (Abbott, Princeton); *Source:* Montesinos and Ardiaca [19].

[e] Median and range as measured on i-STAT (Heska Corp, Loveland, Colorado); *Source:* Harms and Harms [9].

[f] Mean ± SD as measured on Statprofile M (NOVA Biomedical, Mississauga, Canada); *Source:* Stampfli et al. [20].

[g] Mean ± SD as measured on Heska i-STAT (Heska Corp, Loveland, Colorado); *Source:* Heatley et al. [21].

[h] Reference range provided in "Avian Medicine: Principles and Application," Chapter 11: Biochemistries by Manfred Hochleithner [22].

38–41 °C). Reference blood gas analyzers such as radiometer analyzers provide a complete blood gas-electrolyte panel in addition to PCV, lactates, and glucose. The ABL90 FLEX PLUS (Radiometer Medical, Bronshoj, Denmark) uses only 45 ul for a complete panel. Portable POC blood gas analyzers (ex. I-STAT, Abbott Laboratories, Princeton) may be more limited in the analytes available and therefore in the ability to correctly interpret a blood gas panel.

Indications

Blood gas analysis is most important when suspecting a deficiency in tissue oxygenation or respiratory disease, and can be used for both diagnosis and monitoring of response to treatment. Blood gas and acid–base evaluation are also frequently used when evaluating disease processes that cause decreased tissue perfusion, electrolyte imbalances, homeostatic disturbances, or abnormal fluid balance. These patients require appropriate fluid therapy protocols which should be established based on the blood gas and acid–base values. See "Chapter 29: Nutrition and fluid therapy" for a further discussion on implementing fluid therapy plans.

Respiratory and Non-Respiratory

The first step to assessing the acid–base status of the avian patient is to assess the pH of the sample in order to identify acidemia or alkalemia. There is significant species variation, but on average venous blood pH ranges around 7.35–7.5 in birds. Next, non-respiratory (i.e. metabolic) or respiratory causes of the pH imbalance need to be evaluated. See Figure 30.1 for a simplified algorithm to use when assessing information from blood gas analysis.

Respiratory acidosis is present if pCO_2 is elevated. This may be accompanied by a normal or elevated bicarbonate, the latter indicating the body's attempts to compensate for the blood pH imbalance. Respiratory acidosis is seen with hypoventilation, obstructive respiratory disease, pneumonia, respiratory toxins, and manual restraint (especially of passerine birds).

Respiratory alkalosis presents with a decreased pCO_2, with or without evidence of metabolic compensation. This is seen less commonly, but can occur with hyperventilation (ex. mechanical ventilation during anesthesia), anemia, or congestive heart failure.

Metabolic acidosis is identified by a decrease in the bicarbonate. Depending on the cause of the acidosis, there may also be a normal (high anion gap normochloremic metabolic acidosis) or elevated chloride level (normal anion gap hyperchloremic metabolic acidosis). Respiratory compensation results in hyperventilation and a resultant decrease in the pCO_2 in an attempt to lower the acidifying carbon dioxide levels. Metabolic acidosis may be seen with

Birds

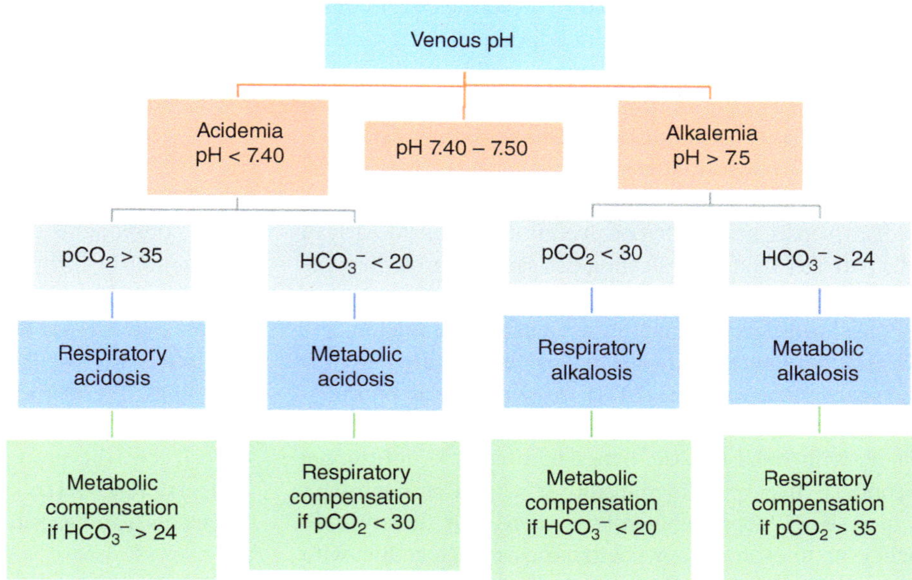

Figure 30.1 A simplified algorithm for assessing the acid–base status of an avian patient.

dehydration, renal disease, diarrhea, lactic acidosis (ex. hypoperfusion, manual restraint), or diabetic ketoacidosis.

Metabolic alkalosis presents with elevated bicarbonates and usually a hypochloremia. Hypoventilation (increased pCO_2) is a compensatory response. Causes of metabolic alkalosis include vomiting, regurgitation, gastrointestinal third spacing of fluids, and functional or mechanical ileus.

Acidemia and Alkalemia (SID, AG, BE)

Once the type of acid–base disorder is identified, further information about the patient's condition and cause of the acidemia or alkalemia can be obtained by calculating the strong ion difference (SID), anion gap (AG), and base excess (BE).

$$\mathrm{SID}(\mathrm{simplified}) = \mathrm{Na}^+ - \mathrm{Cl}^-$$

or

$$\mathrm{SID} = \left(\mathrm{Na}^+ + \mathrm{K}^+ + \mathrm{Ca}^{2+}\right) - \left(\mathrm{Cl}^- + \mathrm{lactate}\right)$$

The normal SID range in birds is about 30–40 mmol/l and is roughly similar to mammals [16]. The simplified SID is a convenient way to determine the underlying electrolytic changes associated with acid–base disorders that need to be corrected. A high SID means that chloride ions are lost compared to sodium (e.g. indicative of vomiting and gastrointestinal obstruction), or that other causes of hypernatremia are present (e.g. diabetes insipidus). A low SID means that chloride ions are increased comparatively to sodium (hyperchloremic metabolic acidosis) or that sodium levels are decreased comparatively to chloride (diarrhea, other causes of hyponatremia).

$$\mathrm{AG} = \left(\mathrm{Na}^+ + \mathrm{K}^+\right) - \left(\mathrm{Cl}^- + \mathrm{HCO}_3^-\right)$$

The normal anion gap in mammals is about 12–24 mmol/l. The anion gap in birds is slightly lower, around 10–15 mmol/l, but can be increased during restraint due to lactate levels [20, 23]. The AG is used to further characterize metabolic acidosis. When metabolic acidosis is present, the anion gap can be normal or increased depending on how the chloride level is being affected. For example, with an elevated chloride and a loss of bicarbonate (ex. diarrhea or polyuria), the AG may be normal. On the other hand, if the chloride is normal but there are unmeasured anions (ex. lactate, urate, phosphate, ketones, etc.), the AG will be elevated.

The base excess is a calculated quantity that ranges from −4 to 4 in most mammals. Based on studies in avian species, the base excess seems to normally be lower than in mammals (about −10 to 0) indicating that there is usually a base deficit.

Electrolytes (Na/Cl, K, Ca, Phos)

As described above, some electrolytes may be measured on a POC blood-gas or chemistry analyzer. Obtaining sodium, potassium, and chloride levels can be beneficial when trying to develop more information about a patient's acid–base status (ex. SID, AG) and any electrolyte disorders that may require correction during fluid therapy.

The measurement of total or ionized calcium and phosphorus is also important diagnostic parameters to help with developing the treatment plan. Some blood-gas analyzers measure ionized calcium, the active fraction in the plasma. Species-specific reference intervals should be examined when evaluating ionized calcium; nevertheless, in most birds, the normal ionized calcium is around 0.8–1.2 mmol/l.

Possible causes of ionized hypercalcemia include hypervitaminosis D, nutritional secondary hyperparathyroidism, osteolytic lesions, rodenticides, and artifactual causes (ex. lipemia). Differential diagnoses for ionized hypocalcemia include low dietary calcium or vitamin D_3, hypoparathyroidism, sepsis, and the hypocalcemic syndrome of African gray parrots [22]. Hypocalcemia can cause neurologic signs and require immediate attention.

Phosphorus levels are closely associated with calcium levels since both are directly affected by changes in vitamin D and parathyroid hormone (PTH). In general, avian phosphorus levels range around 0.9–2 mmol/l. Hyperphosphatemia occurs with renal disease, hypervitaminosis D, nutritional secondary hyperparathyroidism, or as an artifact with hemolysis. Hypophosphatemia is seen with dietary deficiency of phosphorus, hypovitaminosis D (together with hypocalcemia), or chronic glucocorticoid therapy [22].

Biochemistry (Point-Of-Care)

Comprehensive biochemical profiles are an important part of the diagnostic work-up for critical avian patients; however, these tests usually require sample submission to a reference laboratory and cannot be obtained as POC blood tests. If available, POC biochemical analyzers, such as the Vetscan (Abaxis, Union City, CA), can be used for immediate evaluation. Consideration must be made for the small volume of blood that can be obtained from a sick bird; the benefit of measuring various biochemical analytes needs to be carefully evaluated. In some cases, it may be more useful to submit the entire blood sample for a comprehensive biochemistry with a reference lab instead of doing a POC test first.

When prioritizing analytes to be tested, it is important to take into account the patient's history and physical examination findings to determine the most likely differential diagnoses. A basic screen should include at minimum: glucose, TP, electrolytes (sodium, potassium, chloride, calcium, phosphorus), aspartate aminotransferase (AST), creatine kinase (CK), uric acid, and bile acids. For a detailed discussion on biochemical analytes and their interpretation, see "Chapter 32: Clinical Patholoacgy." Briefly, the Vetscan may give valuable information quickly, but the panel is limited and reliability varies depending on the biochemical analytes.

Evaluation of Droppings

A bird's droppings should always be closely examined to assess the feces and urates/urine for changes that may suggest abnormalities of the digestive or urinary tracts. There are non-invasive tests that are easy to perform for any critical patient and may help direct their diagnostic and therapeutic plan.

General for Birds

Examine the color and consistency of both the fecal and liquid components of the droppings. In a healthy bird, the feces should be formed and brown to green in color. Various food pigments (from fruits, vegetables, or artificially colored pellets) may temporarily alter the color of the feces. The urates are usually white. The liquid component of the droppings, the urine, should be clear. The urine volume may normally differ based on the diet (ex. liquid nectar diet of lorikeets, the proportion of fruits in the diet), species, and anxiety-level (i.e. can get temporary stress polyuria). If consistently increased, then polyuria needs to be ruled out.

Evaluation of Urine

Due to the limited availability of reference data and the normal avian physiology, urine and urates in birds are not evaluated in as much detail as we are accustomed to in mammals. The urine sample is usually small and contaminated by the feces in the droppings. Cloacal cannulation to collect a urine sample has been described [24]; however, in most cases, the collection of urine from a clean surface is clinically more applicable. The urine sample should be centrifuged, and analyses should be performed on the supernatant.

Volume/Appearance

If the urates are green in color, it may be due to biliverdin. Usually, this is an indicator that there is decreased liver function and bile stasis, although it can also be seen with hemolysis [25]. When biliverdinuria is suspected, assessment of plasma bile acids, liver enzymes, and hematology is recommended.

A pink or red coloration of the urates likely indicates blood, hemoglobin, porphyrin pigments, or dietary pigments. A complete urinalysis and hematologic and renal evaluation are warranted. Hemoglobinuria can be seen with lead toxicity (especially in Amazon parrots) and hemolysis [26]. Frank blood usually indicates diseases of the cloaca, oviduct, or distal intestinal system.

Polyuria is a consistently increased volume of liquid urine in the droppings. It may often be perceived by the owner as diarrhea since the entire droppings tend to be loose and watery. Polyuria may be due to renal disease, diabetes mellitus, diabetes insipidus (especially African gray parrots), heavy metal toxicity, severe hepatic disease, gastrointestinal diseases, psychogenic polydipsia, or pituitary adenomas (most commonly in budgerigars or cockatiels) [26].

Urine-specific Gravity

The urine-specific gravity (USG) is normally calculated using a refractometer; however, commercial refractometer scales are developed for mammalian urine refractivity and may not be accurate in birds. Reference scales for most avian species have not been developed; an exception is Hispaniolan Amazon parrots [27]. Some studies using refractometry to determine the USG identified a range of about 1.005–1.020 as normal [25, 26].

USG is usually used as an indicator of renal concentrating ability; however, in birds, gastrointestinal disease can also influence the reabsorption of water from the cloaca and the colorectum, and therefore, can influence the concentration of the urine output as significant post-renal handling of urine occurs.

Urinalysis

When performing urinalysis in birds on the separated supernatant, trace glucose or protein can be normally identified possibly due to fecal contamination [28]. Stress hyperglycemia can also cause glucosuria to be noted. There is often evidence of blood in avian urine on a chemistry strip. Normal urine pH in birds is acidic (about 6–7) although this likely varies based on species and diet. Glucose should be negative. Most of the other dry reagents on the chemistry strip are of limited use in birds. As most birds do not produce aceto-acetate as the main ketone acid, the ketone strip is not useful.

On urine sediment evaluation, urate precipitates or crystals can be seen, as well as small numbers of bacteria from intestinal contamination. The urate precipitates will often contain protein from the urine if not reabsorbed in the proximal tubules of the kidneys. For more information, please see the detailed discussion on urinalysis in "Chapter 32: Clinical Pathology." (Table 30.2).

Table 30.2 General expected urinalysis results for avian patients.

USG	1.005–1.020
pH	6–7
Protein	Negative or trace
Glucose	Negative or trace
Ketones	N/A
Bilirubin	Negative
Blood	Negative or trace
Casts	Negative
Crystals	Urate crystals or precipitate
Bacteria	Small amount

Evaluation of Feces

Since it is easily obtained, the fecal component of the droppings should always be examined for evidence of gastrointestinal disease or infection. Assessment of a bird's droppings is a non-invasive way to obtain more information about gastrointestinal, urinary, or metabolic disease processes. These tests are recommended for immediate evaluation of any avian patient in order to help identify all underlying abnormalities and establish the optimal therapeutic plan.

Volume/Appearance

When assessing the appearance of a bird's droppings, diarrhea is seen as unformed fecal components (as opposed to polyuria which is an increased volume of urine). Diarrhea may be caused by bacterial or fungal infection, metabolic disorders, or gastrointestinal parasites. Undigested food, especially seeds, may be seen in the feces with any disease of the ventriculus or proventriculus including avian bornavirus infection. Melena can be seen as dark tarry feces, as in mammals, and is an indicator of hemorrhage into the upper gastrointestinal tract. A fecal occult blood test is beneficial in confirming the presence of blood if this appearance is noted. Increased fecal volume may be indicative of maldigestion or malabsorption, reproductive activity in females, obstruction of the cloaca (feces build up prior to expulsion), or may be seen with some pelleted diets. Exocrine pancreatic insufficiency (e.g. in pigeons, birds with pancreatitis) may manifest with voluminous feces with bubbles. Malodorous feces or droppings may be noted with bacterial or fungal overgrowth and is an indicator that cytology should be examined.

Cytology

Fecal wet mounts should be made up and examined as soon as possible after defecation, as some organisms will die quickly in the environment. Feces are mixed with a drop of saline and a coverslip applied. This sample is examined for motile organisms including *Trichomonas* spp. (ex. pigeons, birds of prey, more likely found in crop samples), *Spironucleus* spp. (ex. ducks, pigeons, cockatiels), and *Cochlosoma* spp. (ex. passerines, society finch). Other organisms that can be identified on a fresh smear include *Macrorhabdus ornithogaster* (finches, lovebirds, parrotlets, Eclectus parrots), coccidian oocysts, and helminth eggs.

A direct fecal smear and Gram's stain may be examined in more details for bacterial and fungal organisms. Usually, in psittacines, a healthy fecal microbial flora consists of mostly Gram-positive cocci; however, differences in diet or husbandry may alter this composition without being a concern for gastrointestinal disease. In the case of passerines (ex. finches, canaries), only a small amount of bacteria may be seen as microbial flora is believed to be less than in other birds [29]. It is important to interpret the presence of Gram-negative bacteria with caution and consider bacterial culture if there is a potential for abnormal bacterial overgrowth [30]. The presence of budding yeast (especially *Candida* spp.), coccidia, or spore-forming bacteria is considered abnormal. Examples of *Candida* spp. and *M. ornithogaster* identified on fecal smears are seen in Figures 30.2 and 30.3, from a cockatiel and an Eclectus parrot, respectively. Further information on fecal cytology is available in "Chapter 33: Cytology."

Other Tests

A fecal flotation is indicated if looking specifically for parasitic infections.

Finally, a fecal occult blood test is recommended for any avian patient with melena, anorexia, weight loss (i.e. evidence of malabsorption), or clinical signs of gastroenteritis (ex. diarrhea, undigested seed in feces). Figure 30.4 shows a positive Hemoccult® test result, with the positive and negative control regions seen toward the bottom.

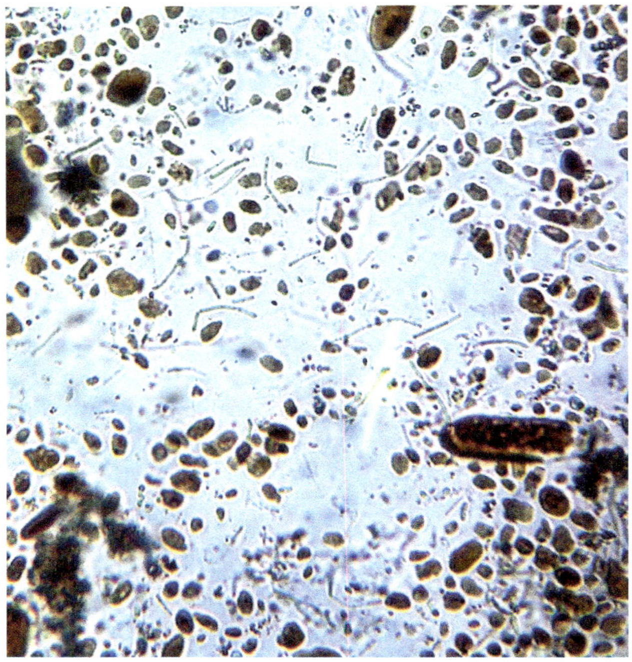

Figure 30.3 Fresh wet mount in an Eclectus parrot showing a large number of *Macrorhabdus ornithogaster* organisms. See Figure 33.7C for a higher magnification view of this organism.

Evaluation of Crop Contents

Assessment of the crop contents can be easily performed on a patient; however, the critical avian patient must be handled carefully and with consideration for the stress that might be incited by sampling the crop contents. Mindful selection of the patients to evaluate further should be based on the history and basic physical exam findings.

Indications

Further evaluation of the crop contents should be considered when presented with a history or physical examination suggestive of disease in the upper digestive tract. This may include a history of regurgitation (usually multiple episodes), dysphagia, altered appetite, or weight loss. On examination, there may be evidence of regurgitation, a fetid or sour odor from the mouth, or abnormal plaques or appearance in the

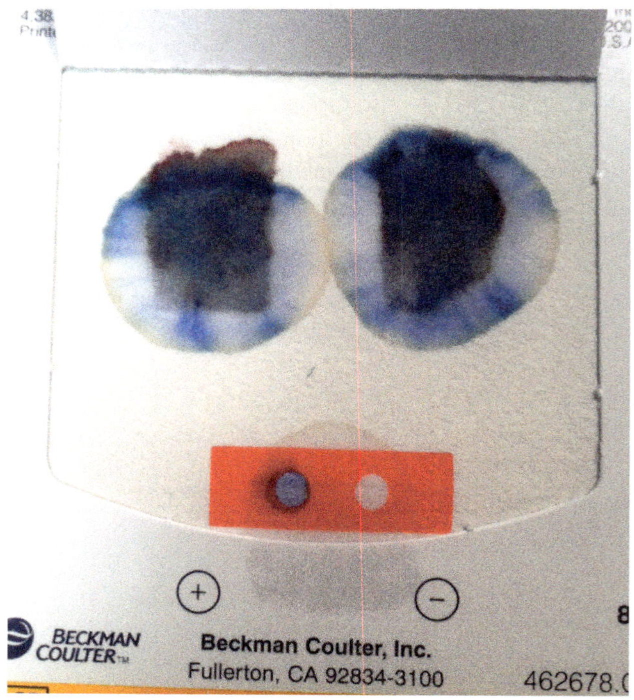

Figure 30.4 Positive hemoccult on a parrot with melena.

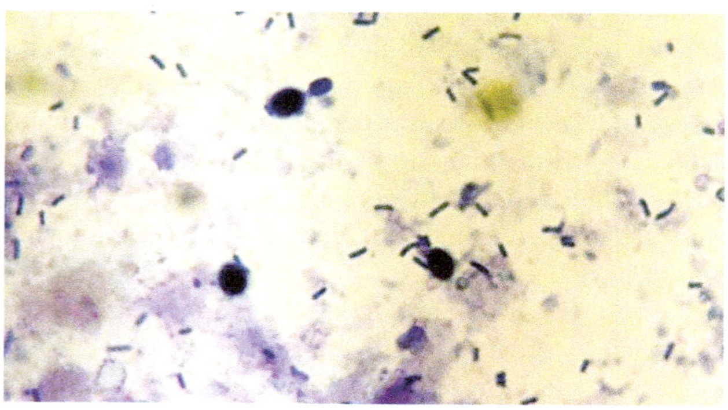

Figure 30.2 Fecal Gram's stain in a cockatiel showing budding *Candida* spp. yeasts.

oropharynx. If aspiration has occurred from regurgitation, then abnormal respiratory effort may be noted.

Crop Palpation/Direct Assessment

Palpating the crop is a routine component of any physical examination. If there is disease of the crop, one might note distension or thickened tissue. A foreign body or mass may be palpable if present. Burns or fistulae caused by feeding overheated food to baby birds may be visible or easily palpable.

Crop Cytology

As with fecal samples, crop swabs can be readily obtained and examined as direct smears, with or without Gram's stain. With a speculum placed in the mouth or tape stirrups to open the beak, a sterile swab can be passed into the crop to collect a sample. Crop lavages can also be performed using sterile saline. These samples should be assessed microscopically for organisms such as *Trichomonas* spp. (on wet mount), *Candida* spp., *Capillaria* spp., various bacterial pathogens, and *M. ornithogaster* (although this organism is more commonly found in the proventriculus and ventriculus). Budding yeast organisms in a crop sample are suggestive of infection, usually with *Candida albicans*. Spirochetes may also be found in the oral and choanal cavities of cockatiels. For further evaluation of bacterial agents, a culture may be indicated. For more detailed information on crop cytology, please see "Chapter 33: Cytology."

Cardiovascular Assessment

Evaluation of a bird's cardiovascular system is important when they are in critical condition; nevertheless, it can be difficult to obtain a thorough assessment due to the size, physiologic characteristics of some birds, and limitations of monitoring equipment on non-mammalian species. Further information about cardiovascular monitoring equipment can be found in "Chapter 28: Avian pain management and anesthesia." POC ultrasound (see later) may also be used for a quick assessment of cardiac function, chamber dilation, and the presence of cardiogenic effusion.

Clinical Assessment

A patient with cardiovascular compromise may have a history of lethargy, weakness, decreased appetite, or exercise intolerance. On physical examination, thoracic auscultation should be performed to assess the heart rate, rhythm, and note any abnormal cardiac or respiratory sounds. It can be difficult to evaluate a pulse even in healthy birds, but this should be attempted at the superficial ulnar artery or femoral artery. The venous refill time of the ulnar vein, the color of mucous membranes (pallor or cyanosis), body temperature, and skin turgor can be used to evaluate the patient's overall hydration and perfusion status. If in heart failure, coelomic distension, tachypnea, or dyspnea may be noted. If respiratory compromise is suspected, the patient should be offered supplemental oxygen in a low-stress environment prior to and during examination.

Doppler

Doppler probes may be beneficial in order to assess the heart rate and rhythm. These can be placed on the superficial ulnar artery (wing) or on the cranial tibial artery (leg). A clamp can be formed out of two taped together tongue depressors in order to keep the probe on the ulnar artery. In larger birds, the Doppler probe may also be placed in the oropharynx and directed at the dorsal arteries.

Blood Pressure

Blood pressure monitoring in birds is relatively imprecise, unless assessing a direct arterial blood pressure. A sphygmomanometer and blood pressure cuff (30–40% of limb circumference) may be placed proximal to a Doppler probe; however, the accuracy of this method is limited [31, 32]. This indirect measuring technique may be of use when assessing trends in an individual bird, but not for determining the accurate blood pressure of a critically ill patient on arrival to the hospital [33]. Oscillometric blood pressure measurement has been found to be unreliable in all birds studied [31].

Avian blood pressure is generally higher than mammalian blood pressure, with a systolic pressure ranging from about 90–200 mmHg depending on species. As in mammals, a patient is considered hypotensive if the direct arterial systolic blood pressure decreases below 90 mmHg or the mean blood pressure below 60 mmHg [32].

ECG

Electrocardiography (ECG) is an excellent tool for assessment of cardiac rate, rhythm, and electrical conductivity. It can also help to identify certain disorders of the myocardium [34]. Unfortunately, it can be difficult to place the leads and establish a good ECG assessment on an unsedated or unanesthetized patient.

Normal ECG parameters have been developed for some avian species [35–41]. The usual mammalian leads are placed proximally on both wing webs (propatagia) and near both thighs (see Figure 30.5 of ECG placement on a sun conure). This can be done using hypodermic needles, adhesives, or paperclips with the electrodes attached [42]. In one

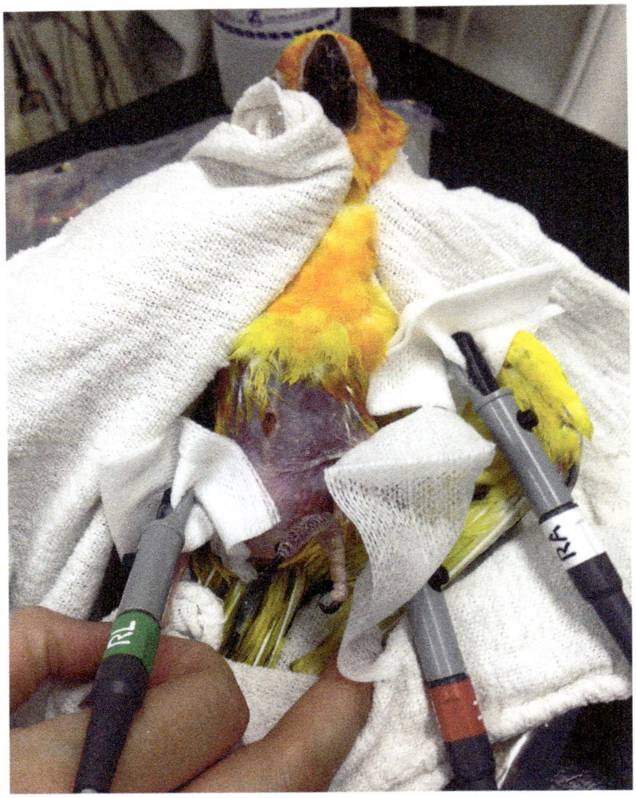

Figure 30.5 Electrocardiogram being performed on a sun conure.

study on grey and Amazon parrots, it was noted that about 16% of partially anesthetized birds (i.e. not yet at a deep plane) had arrhythmias; about 11% being sinus arrhythmias and the other 5% being due to ventricular premature contractions [35]. Other studies also identified sinus arrhythmias in various healthy avian species [37, 40, 41]. Sinus arrhythmias, wandering pacemaker, and occasional sinoatrial block or first and second-degree atrioventricular block are caused by vagal tone and are considered physiologic in birds. Pathologic arrhythmias, on the other hand, may be caused by cardiac chamber enlargement, myocarditis, nutritional or electrolyte imbalances, toxicoses, or anesthetic agents.

Respiratory Assessment

Respiratory assessment should be made together with cardiovascular assessment. If necessary, oxygen supplementation should be provided prior to stressful handling and treatments. Respiratory assessment is discussed in more detail in "Chapter 28: Avian pain management and anesthesia."

Clinical Assessment

The respiratory rate and quality should be examined on every critical avian patient, and can be performed prior to handling and without causing stress. If dyspnea is appreciated, the patient should be handled with care and for only short periods of time between providing oxygen in an incubator.

History and physical examination findings may help differentiate upper vs. lower respiratory tract disease. A history of exposure to airborne toxins or infectious agents will help with developing a list of differential diagnoses. Evidence of rhinitis or sinusitis (sneezing, discharge, periorbital swelling) is indicative of upper airway disease. Inspiratory dyspnea usually indicates upper respiratory disorders; expiratory dyspnea usually indicates disease of the lower respiratory tract. Compression of the air sacs by fluid or an intracoelomic mass can also manifest itself as respiratory disease, so coelomic palpation is important.

Pulse Oximeter

Pulse oximetry is commonly used in avian patients, but with limited information about its accuracy. Pulse oximeters are supposed to provide indirect measurements of hemoglobin oxygen saturation; however, the calibration curves used to calculate this saturation are based on human/mammalian hemoglobin. In one study, spectral photometric analyses were used to assess the behavior of avian vs. human blood [43]. This identified differences that are likely to cause pulse oximeters to underestimate the actual saturation value in birds. Pulse oximetry may also be of limited use in a critical avian patient (without anesthesia) due to inevitable motion artifacts. Pulse oximeters may provide valuable information on heart rate and can be placed on unpigmented regions of skin (ex. feet).

Capnograph

Capnography can be used in an anesthetized or obtunded patient that is intubated. Measurement of the end-tidal carbon dioxide concentration ($EtCO_2$) is used to reflect the arterial concentration of carbon dioxide ($PaCO_2$), although it was found to overestimate the $PaCO_2$ by 5 mmHg in anesthetized African grey parrots receiving intermittent positive pressure ventilation [44]. In another study on raptors, the $EtCO_2$ correlated well with the $PaCO_2$; however, the level of agreement between these parameters varied. The agreement was closest when the $EtCO_2$ was maintained around 30–49 mmHg using positive pressure ventilation [45]. The capnograph wave is useful for assessing ventilation and perfusion to the lungs (if $EtCO_2$ reads low), but must be evaluated cautiously in avian patients when requiring an accurate assessment of $PaCO_2$.

Point-Of-Care Ultrasound (POCUS)

Ultrasound assessment of avian patients is discussed in more detail in "Chapter 31: Diagnostic Imaging." A brief discussion on the use of POC ultrasonographic evaluation follows. POCUS generally uses a portable ultrasound machine. Portable ultrasound machines are, in general, of lower quality and resolution than standard ultrasound machines. In case of abnormalities, it is recommended to perform a more thorough ultrasound examination once the patient is more stable or during normal working hours. POCUS is also a dynamic technique and can be used for monitoring.

Indications

Ultrasound evaluation in birds is more limited than in mammals due to the inability of ultrasound waves to penetrate the air sacs. Nevertheless, it has some important applications as a POC test. It is useful in patients with coelomic distension where evaluation for intracoelomic masses or fluid is required. It is also beneficial in patients with suspected egg-binding; a mineralized egg may be visualized as a round to oval structure with layers [46]. Evaluation of the heart (echocardiography) and screening for pericardial effusion can be performed when signs of cardiovascular disease are noted.

Coelomic (CFAST)

Three approaches may be used: cranioventral (just caudal to sternum on midline), caudoventral (between pubic bones), and lateral (flank behind last ribs) [46]. The patient should be restrained or sedated/anesthetized with the head elevated. Feathers can be wetted with a small amount of alcohol. The ventriculus, liver, enlarged kidneys (if effusion is present), ascites, soft-shelled eggs, and active or enlarged reproductive organs may be apparent when examining the coelomic cavity.

Thoracic/Cardiovascular (TFAST)

A cranioventral approach is required for thoracic ultrasound, and this is primarily used to evaluate cardiac function. Echocardiography is usually performed by a cardiologist or ultrasonographer rather than as a POC test; this is discussed in more detail elsewhere. However, grossly enlarged cardiac chambers and pericardial fluid may be easily observed.

Limitations

As previously mentioned, ultrasonography in birds is limited by the presence of air sacs as well as the small size of the patient. The detail offered by the image may be less than in mammals, and certain organs (gastrointestinal tract, normal kidneys, spleen, etc.) are difficult to evaluate in detail. In some cases, more advanced imaging such as radiographs, computed tomography, or coelioscopy may provide more in-depth information about various organs.

References

1 Lumeij, J.T. (2008). Chapter 28: Avian clinical biochemistry. In: *Clinical Biochemistry of Domestic Animals* (eds. J.J. Kaneko, J.W. Harvey and M.L. Bruss), 839–872. Burlington, MA: Elsevier Inc.

2 Andreasen, C.B., Latimer, K.S., Kircher, I.M., and Brown, J. (1989). Determination of chicken and turkey plasma and serum protein concentrations by refractometry and the biuret method. *Avian Dis.* 33 (1): 93–96.

3 Lumeij, J.T. and Maclean, B. (1996). Total protein determination in pigeon plasma and serum: comparison of refractometric methods with the biuret method. *J. Avian Med. Surg.* 10 (3): 150–152.

4 Acierno, M.J., Mitchell, M.A., Schuster, P.J. et al. (2009). Evaluation of the agreement among three handheld blood glucose meters and a laboratory blood analyzer for measurement of blood glucose concentration in Hispaniolan Amazon parrots (*Amazona ventralis*). *Am. J. Vet. Res.* 70 (2): 172–175.

5 Lieske, C.L., Ziccardi, M.H., Mazet, J.A.K. et al. (2002). Evaluation of 4 handheld blood glucose monitors for use in seabird rehabilitation. *J. Avian Med. Surg.* 16 (4): 277–285.

6 Mohsenzadeh, M.S., Zaeemi, M., Razmyar, J., and Azizzadeh, M. (2015). Comparison of a point-of-care glucometer and a laboratory autoanalyzer for measurement of blood glucose concentrations in domestic pigeons (Columba livia domestica). *J. Avian Med. Surg.* 29 (3): 181–186.

7 Acierno, M.J., Schnellbacher, R., and Tully, T.N. (2012). Measuring the level of agreement between a veterinary and a human point-of-care glucometer and a laboratory blood analyzer in Hispaniolan amazon parrots (*Amazona ventralis*). *J. Avian Med. Surg.* 26 (4): 221–224.

8 Allen, S.E. and Holm, J.L. (2008). Lactate: physiology and clinical utility. *J. Vet. Emerg. Crit. Care* 18 (2): 123–132.

9 Harms, C.A. and Harms, R.V. (2012). Venous blood gas and lactate values of mourning doves (*Zenaida macroura*), boat-tailed grackles (*Quiscalus major*), and house sparrows (*Passer domesticus*) after capture by mist net, banding, and venipuncture. *J. Zoo Wildl. Med.* 43 (1): 77–84.

10 Burgdorf-Moisuk, A., Wack, R., Ziccardi, M. et al. (2012). Validation of lactate measurement in American flamingo (*Phoenicopterus ruber*) plasma and correlation with duration and difficulty of capture. *J. Zoo Wildl. Med.* 43 (3): 450–458.

11 Holz, P.H., Naisbitt, R., and Mansell, P. (2006). Fitness level as a determining factor in the survival of rehabilitated peregrine falcons (*Falco peregrinus*) and brown goshawks (*Accipiter fasciatus*) released back into the wild. *J. Avian Med. Surg.* 20 (1): 15–20.

12 Johns, J.L., Shooshtari, M.P., and Christopher, M.M. (2008). Development of a technique for quantification of reticulocytes and assessment of erythrocyte regenerative capacity in birds. *Am. J. Vet. Res.* 69 (8): 1067–1072.

13 Morrisey, J.K., Paul-Murphy, J., Fialkowski, J.P. et al. (2003). Estimation of prothrombin times of Hispaniolan amazon parrots (*Amazona ventralis*) and umarella cockatoos (*Cacatua alba*). *J. Avian Med. Surg.* 17 (2): 72–77.

14 Keller, K.A., Sanchez-Migallon, G.D., Acierno, M.J. et al. (2015). Thromboelastography values in Hispaniolan amazon parrots (*Amazona ventralis*): a pilot study. *J. Avian Med. Surg.* 29 (3): 174–180.

15 Strindberg, S., Nielsen, T.W., Ribeiro, A.M. et al. (2015). Thromboelastography in selected avian species. *J. Avian Med. Surg.* 29 (4): 282–289.

16 Paula, V.V., Fantoni, D.T., Otsuki, D.A., and Auler, J.O.C. Jr. (2008). Blood-gas and electrolyte values for Amazon parrots (*Amazona aestiva*). *Pesqui. Vet. Bras.* 28 (2): 108–112.

17 Ludders, J.W., Mitchell, G.S., and Rode, J. (1990). Minimal anesthetic concentration and cardiopulmonary dose response of isoflurane in ducks. *Vet. Surg.* 19 (4): 304–307.

18 Rettenmund, C.L., Heatley, J.J., and Russell, K.E. (2014). Comparison of two analyzers to determine selected venous blood analytes of Quaker parrots (*Myiopsitta monachus*). *J. Zoo Wildl. Med.* 45 (2): 256–262.

19 Montesinos, A. and Ardiaca, M. (2013). Acid–base status in the avian patient using a portable point-of-care analyzer. *Vet. Clin. North Am. Exot. Anim. Pract.* 16 (1): 47–69.

20 Stampfli, H., Taylor, M., McNicoll, C. et al. (2006). Experimental determination of net protein charge, [A]tot, and Ka of nonvolatile buffers in bird plasma. *J. Appl. Phys.* 100 (6): 1831–1836.

21 Heatley, J.J., Demirjian, S.E., and Wright, J.C. (2005). Electrolytes of the critically ill raptor. *Proc. Assoc. Avian Vet.*: 23–24.

22 Hochleithner, M. (1994). Chapter 11: Biochemistries. In: *Avian Medicine: Principles and Application* (eds. B.W. Ritchie, G.J. Harrison and L.R. Harrison), 223–227. Lake Worth, FL: Wingers Publishing Inc.

23 Heatley, J.J., Cary, J., Kingsley, L. et al. (2015). Midazolam sedates Passeriformes for field sampling but affects multiple venous blood analytes. *Vet. Med.: Res. Rep.* 6: 61–69.

24 Halsema, W.B., Alberts, H., de Bruijne, J.J., and Lumeij, J.T. (1988). Collection and analysis of urine from racing pigeons (*Columba livia domestica*). *Avian Pathol.* 17 (1): 221–225.

25 Harr, K.E. (2002). Clinical chemistry of companion avian species: a review. *Vet. Clin. Pathol.* 31 (3): 140–151.

26 Styles, D.K. and Phalen, D.N. (1998). Clinical avian urology. *Semi. Avian Exot. Pet. Med.* 7 (2): 104–113.

27 Brock, A.P., Grunkemeyer, V.L., Fry, M.M. et al. (2013). Comparison of osmolality and refractometric readings of Hispaniolan Amazon parrot (*Amazona ventralis*) urine. *J. Avian Med. Surg.* 27 (4): 264–268.

28 Tschopp, R., Bailey, T., Di Somma, A., and Silvanose, C. (2007). Urinalysis as a noninvasive health screening procedure in Falconidae. *J. Avian Med. Surg.* 21 (1): 8–12.

29 Dorrestein, G.M. (2003). Diagnostic approaches and management of diseases in captive passerines. *Semi. Avian Exot. Pet. Med.* 12 (1): 11–20.

30 Evans, E.E., Mitchell, M.A., Whittington, J.K. et al. (2014). Measuring the level of agreement between cloacal gram's stains and bacterial cultures in Hispaniolan amazon parrots (*Amazona ventralis*). *J. Avian Med. Surg.* 28 (4): 290–296.

31 Acierno, M.J., da Cunha, A., Smith, J. et al. (2008). Agreement between direct and indirect blood pressure measurements obtained from anesthetized Hispaniolan amazon parrots. *J. Am. Vet. Med. Assoc.* 233 (10): 1587–1590.

32 Lichtenberger, M. (2005). Determination of indirect blood pressure in the companion bird. *Semi. Avian Exot. Pet. Med.* 14 (2): 149–152.

33 Johnston, M.S., Davidowski, L.A., Rao, S., and Hill, A.E. (2011). Precision of repeated, Doppler-derived indirect blood pressure measurements in conscious psittacine birds. *J. Avian Med. Surg.* 25 (2): 83–90.

34 Curro, T.G. (1998). Anesthesia of pet birds. *Semi. Avian Exot. Pet. Med.* 7 (1): 10–21.

35 Nap, A.M., Lumeij, J.T., and Stokhof, A.A. (1992). Electrocardiogram of the African grey (*Psittacus erithacus*) and Amazon (*Amazona* spp.) parrot. *Avian Pathol.* 21 (1): 45–53.

36 Zandvliet, M.J.M. (2005). Electrocardiography in psittacine birds and ferrets. *Semi. Avian Exot. Pet. Med.* 14 (1): 34–51.

37 Talavera, J., Guzman, M.J., del Palacio, M.J. et al. (2008). The normal electrocardiogram of four species of conscious raptors. *Res. Vet. Sci.* 84 (1): 119–125.

38 Rodriguez, R., Prieto-Montana, F., Montes, A.M. et al. (2004). The normal electrocardiogram of the unanesthetized peregrine falcon (*Falco peregrinus brookei*). *Avian Dis.* 48 (2): 405–409.

39 Casares, M., Enders, F., and Montoya, J.A. (2000). Comparative electrocardiography in four species of macaws (genera *Anodorhynchus* and *Ara*). *J. Vet. Med. A Physiol. Pathol. Clin. Med.* 47 (5): 277–281.

40 Papahn, A.A., Naddaf, H., Rezakhani, A., and Mayahi, M. (2006). Electrocardiogram of homing pigeon. *J. Appl. Anim. Res.* 30: 129–132.

41 Oglesbee, B.L., Hamlin, R.L., Klingaman, H. et al. (2001). Electrocardiographic reference values for Macaws (*Ara* species) and cockatoos (*Cacatua* species). *J. Avian Med. Surg.* 15 (1): 17–22.

42 Casares, M., Enders, F., and Montoya, J.A. (1999). Comparison of two techniques for attaching electrocardiographic electrodes to psittacines. *J. Appl. Anim. Res.* 16: 59–64.

43 Schmitt, P.M., Göbel, T., and Trautvetter, E. (1998). Evaluation of pulse oximetry as a monitoring method in avian anesthesia. *J. Avian Med. Surg.* 12 (2): 91–99.

44 Edling, T.M., Degernes, L.A., Flammer, K., and Horne, W.A. (2001). Capnographic monitoring of anesthetized African grey parrots receiving intermittent positive pressure ventilation. *J. Am. Vet. Med. Assoc.* 219 (12): 1714–1718.

45 Desmarchelier, M., Rondenay, Y., Fitzgerald, G., and Lair, S. (2007). Monitoring of the ventilatory status of anesthetized birds of prey by using end-tidal carbon dioxide measured with a microstream capnometer. *J. Zoo Wildl. Med.* 38 (1): 1–6.

46 Helmer, P. (2006). Advances in diagnostic imaging. In: *Clinical Avian Medicine* (eds. G.J. Harrison and T.L. Lightfoot), 657–658. Palm Beach, FL: Spix Publishing Inc.

31

Diagnostic Imaging

Claire Vergneau-Grosset[1] and Hugues Beaufrère[2]

[1] *Faculté de médecine vétérinaire, Université de Montréal, Saint-Hyacinthe, Quebec, Canada*
[2] *Department of Medicine and Epidemiology, School of Veterinary Medicine, University of California-Davis, Davis, California, USA*

CONTENTS

Some avian emergency presentations require diagnostic imaging, which may include radiographs, coelomic ultrasound and, when available, cardiac ultrasound, computerized tomography-scan (CT-scan), and/or magnetic resonance imaging (MRI). This chapter will mainly focus on avian radiographs as radiographic equipment is most commonly available in emergency settings. Handling the bird, even with sedation or anesthesia, may be stressful and it is critical to assess whether the patient should be stabilized before performing imaging tests.

Image Acquisition and Normal Anatomy

Radiographs

Positioning

Whole body radiographs may be obtained either in anesthetized patients, with the use of sedation, or may be possible without sedation in select patients. Non-anesthetized birds may also be placed in a box for quick metal or calcified egg screening. Good positioning may not be achievable without sedation or anesthesia in most birds. In addition, care should be taken to palpate the crop before positioning. If the crop is full, positioned radiographs should be delayed or the content should be emptied with a feeding tube. If the crop is not empty, the head of the patient should be elevated compared to the rest of the body to decrease the risk of regurgitation and aspiration. In case of coelomic fluid, it is also important to elevate the front half of the patient by placing foam under the plastic board supporting the body, preventing compression of air sacs leading to dyspnea. To achieve patient sedation, midazolam 1–2 mg/kg may be administered intramuscularly (IM) or intranasally [1] and may be combined with an opioid, such as butorphanol 1–2 mg/kg IM. Other protocols can be found in "Chapter 28: Avian Pain Management and Anesthesia". If the patient suffers from a painful condition, other opioid agents may be preferable [2, 3]. Sedation protocol should be adapted depending on the patient's condition.

Radiographic equipment used for domestic carnivores can be used in birds. Due to rapid avian respiratory rates, short exposure times, ranging between 0.01 and 0.05 seconds, are recommended to avoid motion artifact [4]. Lower kV will increase contrast. Placing the cassette on tabletop maximizes detail by

Exotic Animal Emergency and Critical Care Medicine, First Edition. Edited by Jennifer E. Graham, Grayson A. Doss and Hugues Beaufrère.

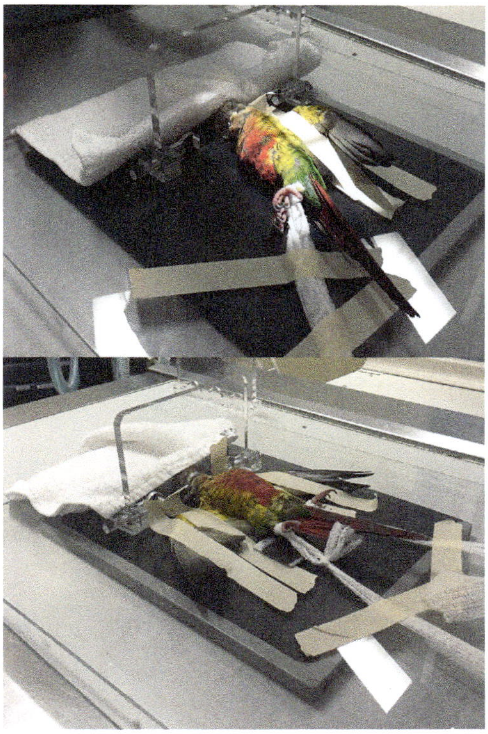

Figure 31.1 Radiographic positioning of a green-cheeked conure (*Pyrrhura molinae*) sedated with midazolam and butorphanol: right lateral view on top, ventro-dorsal view below.

decreasing the distance between the bird and cassette and is recommended for patients thinner than 10cm [4]. Scatter radiation adversely affects the detail of radiographs and close collimation is recommended [4]. While using conventional radiographs, mammography cassettes improve definition; these cassettes require higher exposure setting due to the single intensifying screen [4]. Digital radiographs allow post-acquisition post-processing, including zooming on details, contrast variations, and negative images. While using digital radiographs, a DICOM viewer (such as Osirix 64 bit v. 5.8.2, Pixmeo, Bernex, Switzerland) is used for image post-processing.

Whole body ventro–dorsal and lateral views are typically obtained for complete radiographic assessment. The keel and vertebral column should be superimposed on dorso–ventral views and hind limbs should be extended caudally with a parallel pelvis. Wings should be extended from the body to evaluate lateral thoracic areas or placed alongside the body to include bilateral distal wings on a single ventro–dorsal view. In optimally positioned lateral views, bilateral coracoids, and femoral heads should be overlapping, respectively. This can be achieved placing a foam pad between the legs in large birds and lightly taping the superior wing to the table to prevent dorsal rotation of the bird's body (Figure 31.1). Depending on the area of interest (coelomic cavity or legs), both legs may be extended caudally and superimposed, or the right leg may be extended more cranially than the left leg. The cranial cervical area at the level of the mandible can be secured with a Plexiglas radiolucent board or masking tape; masking tape can be used to secure the wings and legs, (Figure 31.1) [4] or a twisted sand bag in larger birds. Do not prevent chest excursion during restraint. Legs may be extended with a slipknot made of cling bandage attached to the board or table. A distance marker should be placed close to any fracture site to allow calibration of measurement programs, and thus allow accurate measurement of osseous structures to choose orthopedic devices.

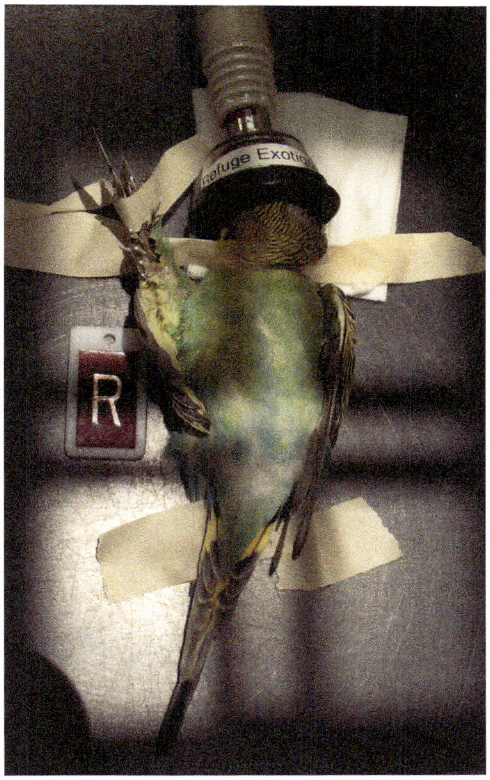

Figure 31.2 Radiographic positioning of an anesthetized budgerigar (*Melopsittacus undulatus*) to obtain a caudo-cranial view of the right carpometacarpus: the distal extremity of the wing is taped cranially.

When positioning the bird under minimal sedation, wings should be secured at the level of the elbow and wrist to prevent flapping and subsequent iatrogenic fractures, especially if metabolic bone disease is suspected. Alternatively, appropriately gowned personnel may restrain the bird during radiograph acquisition with proper radioprotection measures. Additional views, including cranio-caudal views, are required in case of wing lesions (Figure 31.2), as only ventro-dorsal views of the wings are obtained with the ventro-dorsal and lateral coelomic radiographs. In addition, an oblique view (H view) may be used to confirm thoracic inlet lesions [5]. This view is obtained by rotating the X-ray collimator 45° while keeping the same focal distance; it prevents superimposition

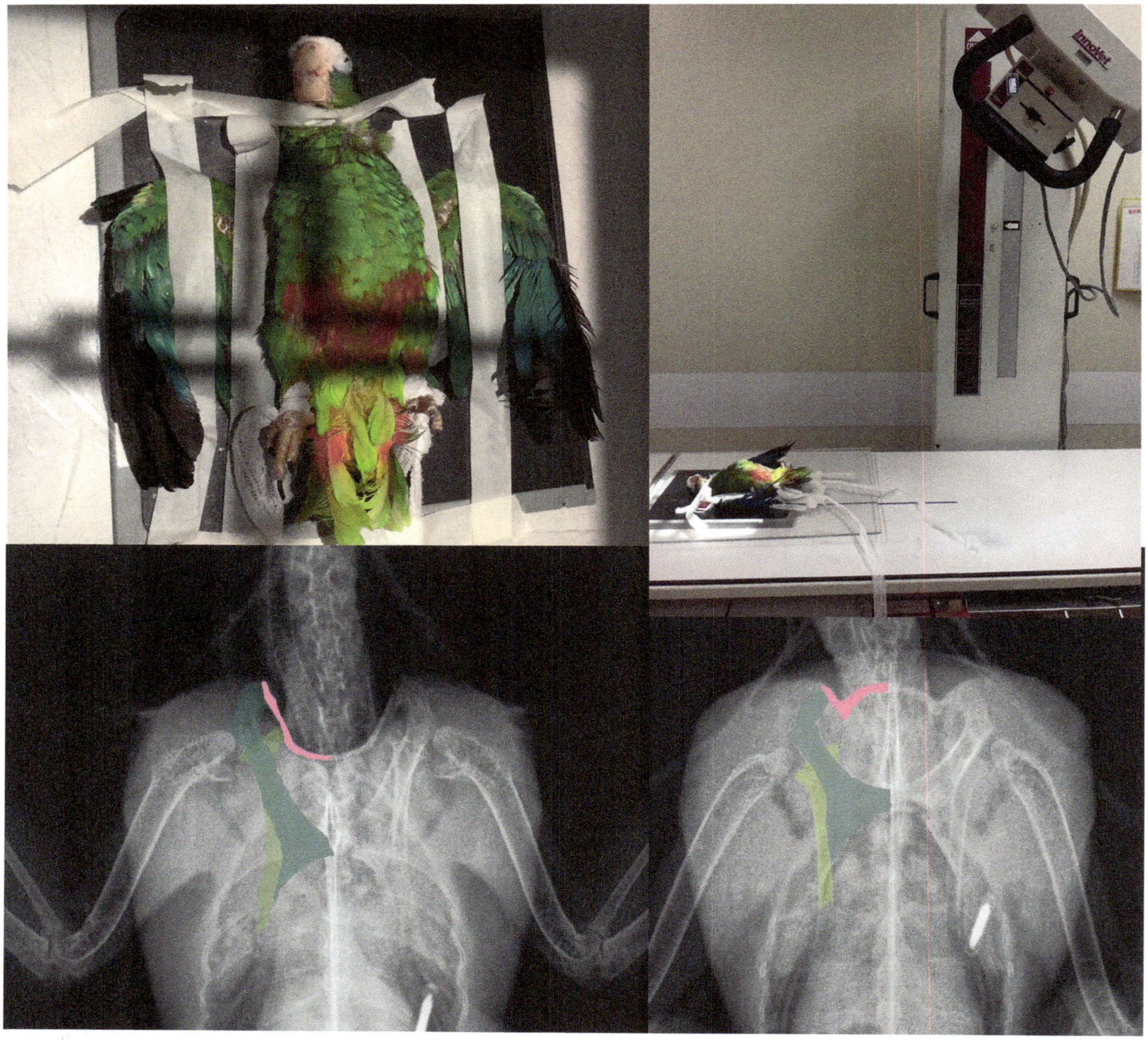

Figure 31.3 Radiographic positioning and radiographs obtained from a Hispaniolan Amazon parrot (*Amazona ventralis*) sedated with midazolam and butorphanol: H view on the right and ventro-dorsal views on the left (pink: clavicle, light green: scapula, dark green: coracoid).

of clavicular and coracoid bones (Figure 31.3) [5]. Other views of the skull may also be recommended but CT-scan is the best technique to assess skull lesions.

Complications/Contraindications

Birds positioned for radiographs are restrained, this carries risks of aspiration in case of regurgitation. Therefore, it is contraindicated to perform positioned radiographs on birds with a full crop. In this case, standing radiographs may be obtained or the crop may be emptied with a feeding tube prior to radiograph acquisition. Other contraindications are similar to those of general anesthesia or sedation. Standing radiographs can be obtained by placing the bird in a cardboard box, in a Plexiglas induction chamber or in a radiotransparent bag for smaller species. Appropriate ventilation of the box or bag is an important consideration if multiple views are to be obtained. Dorso-ventral views can be acquired with a vertical beam while lateral or cranio-caudal views can be obtained with a horizontal beam. If the bird is not completely motionless, focusing its attention with a sound may be useful to reduce motion artifact.

In case of coelomic effusion, positioning the bird on its dorsum may also affect its respiration by compressing the air sacs. Clinicians should be aware of this potential complication and stop the procedure if the bird becomes dyspneic. Horizontal beam standing radiographs or a flash coelomic ultrasound may be performed first to screen for coelomic fluid. Moreover, it may be preferable to perform radiographs before coelomic fluid aspiration: anecdotally, in case of disruption of the air sac membranes' integrity, fluid would enter the respiratory system in rare cases, resulting in death. After coelomic fluid aspiration with a fine needle, it is recommended to maintain the bird in physiological standing position for a few hours.

Contrast Studies

Contrast studies of the upper gastrointestinal tract are indicated to investigate altered digestive transit, subtraction images associated with intraluminal lesions, coelomic space-occupying masses, or body wall abnormalities [4]. Although these procedures can be delayed most of the time, some situations such as foreign body ingestion may require early removal before small elements can reach more distal segments of the digestive tract. If endoscopy or surgical assistance is foreseen, for instance in case of proventricular foreign bodies, iodinated contrast should be administered rather than barium sulfate [5]. A 1:1 mixture of barium 60% and feeding formula or water is prepared and thoroughly homogenized [6]. A volume of 15–25 ml/kg is administered by gavage into the crop [4, 6]. Normal digestive transit has been established in a few avian species, including Hispaniolan Amazon parrots (*Amazona ventralis*) [6], blue-fronted Amazon parrots (*Amazona aestiva*) [7], grey parrots [8], and others [9]. In birds with delayed crop emptying, it is preferable to obtain upright preliminary views in a box to assess whether a large amount of contrast medium is still in the crop before positioning the bird horizontally on the table. Once the crop is empty, the risk of regurgitation and aspiration is decreased, and the bird may be sedated and positioned on the table. Of note, anesthesia and sedation have been reported to affect gastrointestinal transit time [7] and some clinicians prefer to perform positioned radiographs without sedation in these cases. This implies staff exposure to radiation and the use of sedation does not result in clinically significant increase of gastrointestinal transit time in our experience. In birds presented with delayed crop emptying and regurgitation, an alternative is to administer the contrast media directly into the proventriculus or ventriculus (see "Chapter 29: Nutrition and Fluid Therapy") (Figure 31.4).

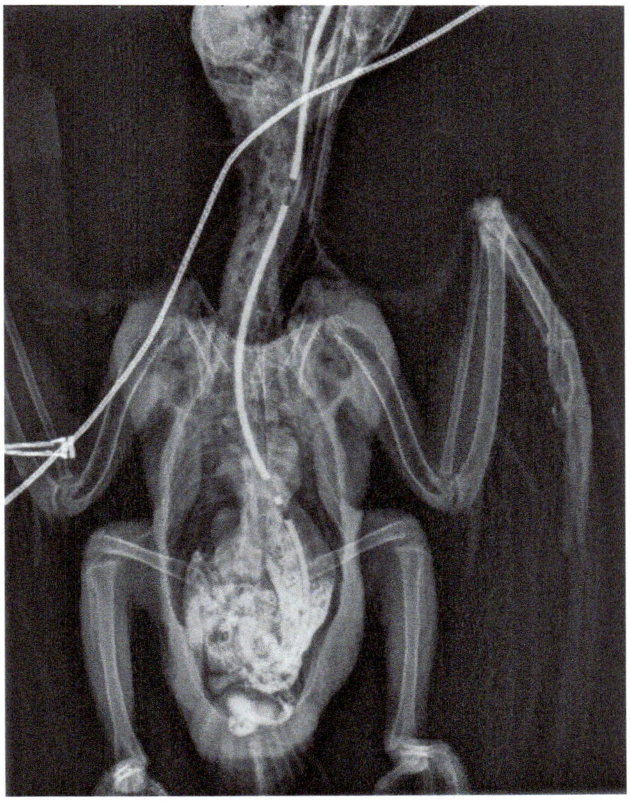

Figure 31.4 Ventro-dorsal view of an anesthetized blue and gold macaw (*Ara ararauna*). The Doppler is visible on the right wing and a red-rubber tube filled with barium 30% w/v is placed in the caudal proventriculus, for administration of contrast media. By convention, the right side of the bird is on the left side of the radiographic image throughout this chapter.

Normals

Skeletal elements are evaluated radiographically, including bone quality and integrity. Normal skeletal anatomy is shown in Figure 31.5. The vertebral column can be divided into cervical vertebrae, notarium, thoracic vertebrae, synsacrum, coccygeal vertebrae, and pygostyle. The free mobile thoracic vertebra is a frequent site of spinal disease in birds (Figure 31.6). Normal angulation of the intertarsal joint has been described in views obtained in perched birds with a horizontal beam [10].

Species-specific organ measurements have been established in a few avian species [11, 12].

In addition, as female birds are usually larger than males of the same species, it is pertinent to establish reference intervals for organ measurement in each sex [12]. In optimally positioned lateral radiographs, the proventriculus to keel ratio should be below 0.48 in parrots (except Eclectus parrots), regardless of the stage of digestion and this ratio is unaffected by anesthesia [13, 14]. This ratio has been shown to have a high sensitivity for detecting proventricular enlargement (Figure 31.7) [15]. However, appropriate positioning is needed for accurate measurement as rotation of the bird on the lateral view makes this ratio inaccurate [14]. A proventricular diameter of 3.6–4.7 femoral diameter has also been described in Hispaniolan Amazon parrots [6]. The ventriculus should be superimposed ventral to the left hip joint, and may be more visible if filled with mineral particles, for example in Columbiformes, poultry, or psittacine species with grit.

The spleen is sometimes visible, and is physiologically located dorsal to the isthmus, at the junction between the

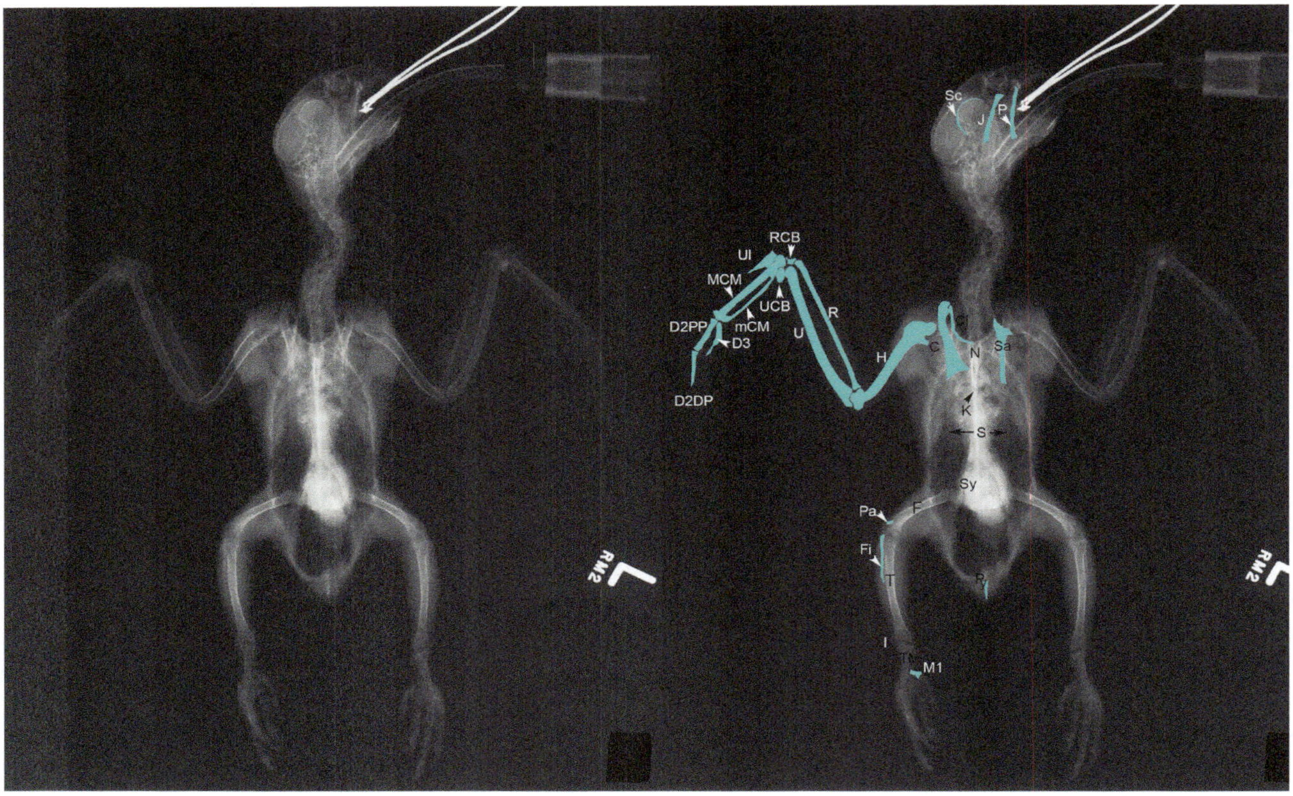

Figure 31.5 Normal skeletal anatomy of the grey parrot (*Psittacus erithacus*). The bird is intubated, and a Doppler is placed on the palatal artery. C: coracoid, Cl: clavicle, D2PP: digit two proximal phalanx, D2DP: digit 2 distal phalanx, D3: digit three, F: femur, Fi: fibula, H: humerus, I: intertarsal joint, J: jugal arch, K: keel, M1: metatarsal bone 1, MCM: major part of the carpometacarpal bone, mCM: minor part of the carpometacarpal bone, N: notarium, P: palatal bone, Pa: patella, Py: pygostyle, R: radius, RCB: radius carpal bone, S: sternum, Sa: scapula, Sc: sclera, Sy: synsacrum, T: tibiotarsus, TM: tarsometatarsus, U: ulna, UCB: ulnar carpal bone, Ul: alula.

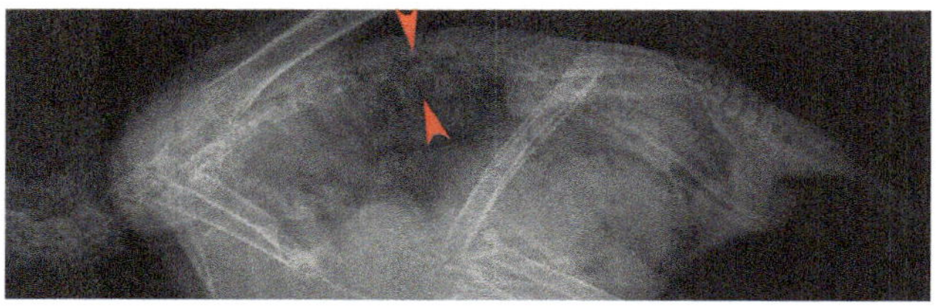

Figure 31.6 Position of the free thoracic vertebra (red arrowheads) in a Hispaniolan Amazon parrot (*Amazona ventralis*).

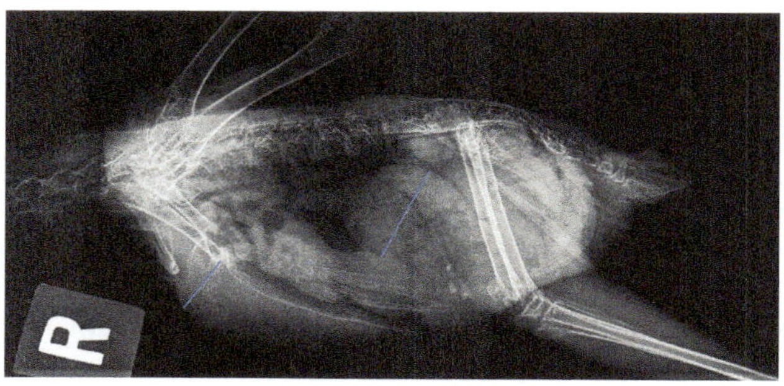

Figure 31.7 Right lateral view: severe proventricular dilatation in an Umbrella cockatoo (*Cacatua alba*): the proventriculus to keel ratio (blue lines) is 1.7 in this bird. *Source:* Courtesy of the Zoological Medicine Service, Université de Montréal.

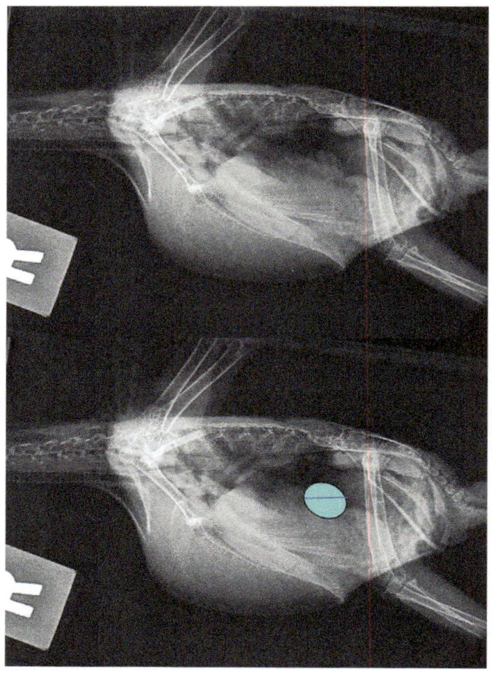

Figure 31.8 Splenomegaly in a blue and gold macaw (*Ara arowana*): the spleen diameter to femoral width ratio is 3.2, which is higher than the 1.5 limit. *Source:* Courtesy of the Zoological Medicine Service, Université de Montréal.

proventriculus and ventriculus [12]. Normal spleen diameter has been defined in a few species [12, 16] and should be less than 1.5 times the femoral diameter in Psittaciformes [17, 18]. A higher ratio may be indicative of splenomegaly (Figure 31.8) although no peer-reviewed study has correlated this finding with postmortem findings. Differential diagnoses for splenomegaly include sepsis, bacterial infections including chlamydiosis and mycobacteriosis, and fungal infections, iron storage disease and neoplastic diseases. However, these ratios are affected by the size of the bird as peripheral beams are more diffracted which distorts the image at the periphery of the radiograph. Hence, strictly speaking, measurements taken in peripheral regions of radiographs are not comparable with the central region of the view.

Many avian species display a hourglass-like cardio-hepatic silhouette with a distinct waist [12]. A crude way to evaluate the cardio-hepatic silhouette is to draw lines from the shoulder to the hip on each side of the bird; a normal hourglass-like shape should not pass these lines. A larger hourglass-like silhouette may be an indication of cardiomegaly, hepatomegaly (Figure 31.9), coelomic effusion,

(a)

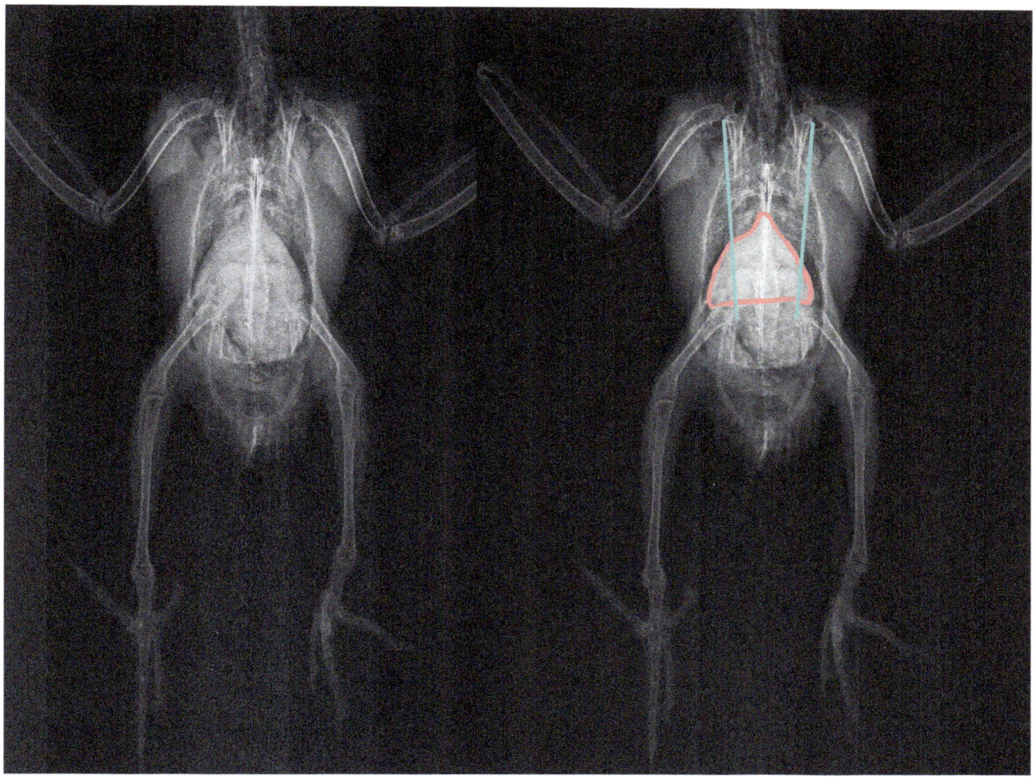

(b)

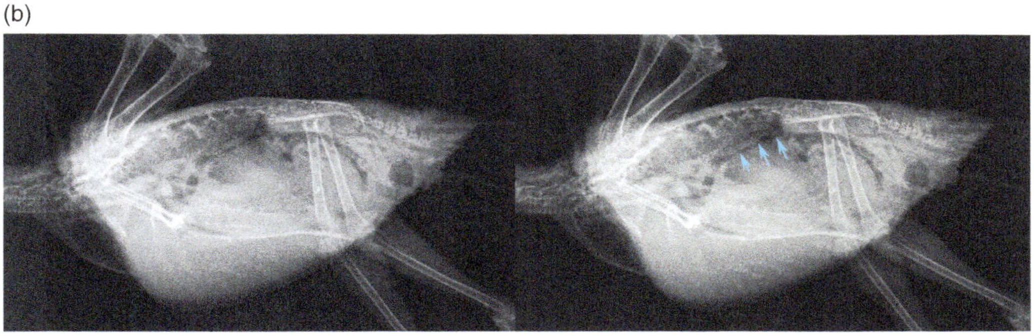

Figure 31.9 Hepatomegaly in a cockatiel (*Nymphicus hollandicus*). On the ventro-dorsal view, the hepatic silhouette (outlined in pink) is wider than the bilateral lines (in blue) connecting the shoulder to the ipsilateral hip. On the right lateral view, the dorsal proventricular wall (delineated by arrows) is displaced dorsally by a ventral coelomic mass effect: this is compatible with hepatomegaly among other mass effects (distension of the proventriculus, mass localized in the wall of the proventriculus, etc.).

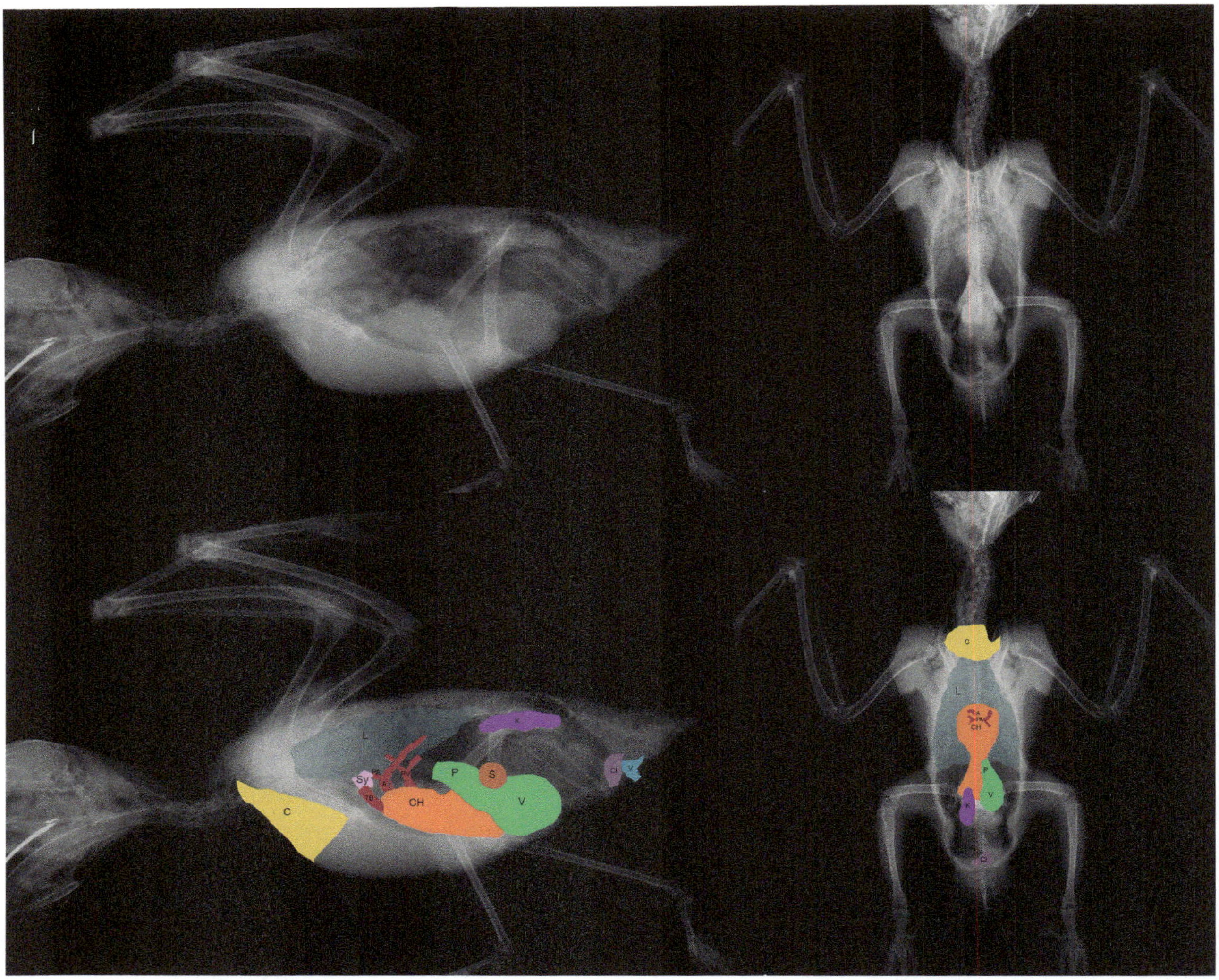

Figure 31.10 Right lateral and ventrodorsal radiographic views of a healthy green-winged macaw (*Ara chloropterus*). *Source:* Courtesy of the University of Guelph. Labels: A: aortic arch, BT: brachiocephalic trunk, C: crop, CH: cardio-hepatic silhouette, Cl: cloaca, K: right kidney, L: lung field, PA: pulmonary arteries, P: proventriculus, PV: pulmonary veins, S: spleen, Sy: syrinx, V: ventriculus, Ve: vent.

proventricular dilatation if it is larger on the left side, or may be associated with a recent meal in birds of prey [19]. On the ventro-dorsal view, the maximum heart width to thoracic width ratio should be below 63% in psittacine species but species-specific reference intervals provide a better sensitivity for cardiomegaly detection [11]. In peregrine falcons, sternal width was shown to have a stronger correlation with cardiac width than thoracic width (TW), which is influenced by respiratory movement [20]. Numerous reference intervals have been developed for cardiac measurements in birds [11, 12, 20, 22]. In budgerigars (*Melopsittacus undulatus*), cardiac width and thoracic width have been shown to be significantly correlated as opposed to cardiac width and respectively, coracoid width, clavicular distance, synsacrum width and the distance between the third and fourth rib [11]. Although insensitive, detection of radiopaque lines along vascular structures, representing calcifications of large vessels, is a fairly specific indication of atherosclerosis in birds (see section "Investigation of dyspnea") [23]. Large vessels, such as the brachiocephalic trunk, aorta, pulmonary arteries, pulmonary veins, and caudal vena cava are typically visible (Figures 31.10–31.17). Major differential diagnoses for common radiographic lesions are indicated in Table 31.1.

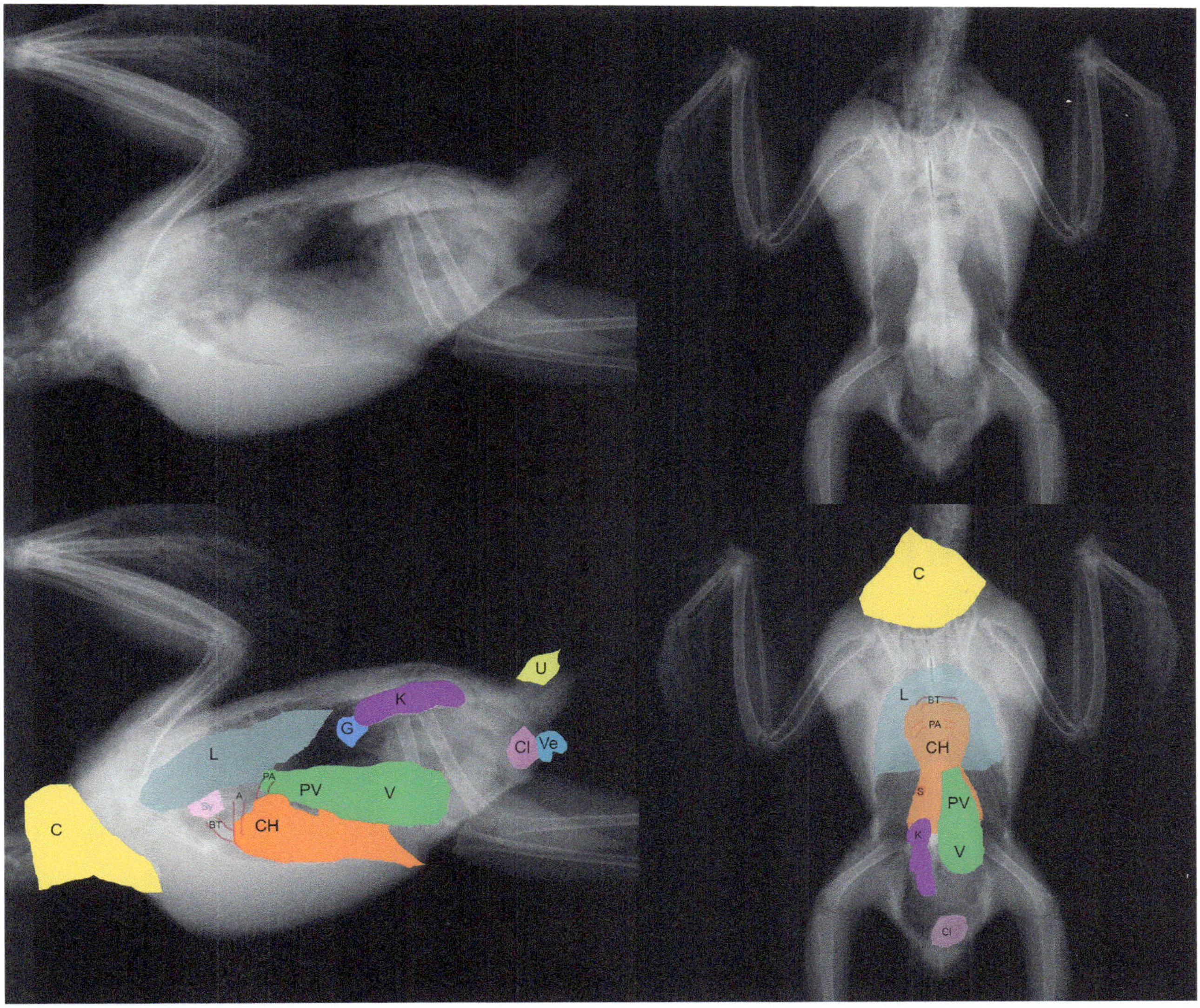

Figure 31.11 Right lateral and ventrodorsal radiographic views of a healthy grey parrot (*Psittacus erithacus*). *Source:* Courtesy of the University of Guelph. Labels: A: aortic arch, BT: brachiocephalic trunk, C: crop, CH: cardio-hepatic silhouette, Cl: cloaca, G: gonad, K: right kidney, L: lung field, PA: pulmonary arteries, PV: proventriculus, S: spleen, Sy: syrinx, U: uropygial gland, V: ventriculus, Ve: vent.

Kidneys can be visualized ventral to the pelvis, and typically show three divisions, with a few exceptions [24, 25]. In most species, a diverticulum from the abdominal air sac runs between the kidneys and the synsacrum. Obliteration of this radiolucent area may indicate renomegaly.

Lungs are positioned dorsally in the cranial coelom and show a typical honeycomb pattern. Air sac lines should not be radiographically visible in healthy birds (Figure 31.18). Considerable anatomical diversity may be seen in the trachea. Examples of extreme tracheal anatomy seen on radiographs are trumpeter swans.

In some instances, it is possible to radiographically determine the sex of avian patients. It may be as obvious as the presence of an egg, or gonad, located cranially to the kidney; dimorphic characteristics may also be visualized, such as the drum in the syrinx of male ducks (Figure 31.19); or physiological processes such as polyostotic hyperostosis in female birds. In most females, only the left gonad is developed with notable exceptions being some female Passeriformes. Testes may be very prominent during the breeding season, especially in Anseriformes and Columbiformes and should not be mistaken for pathologic masses.

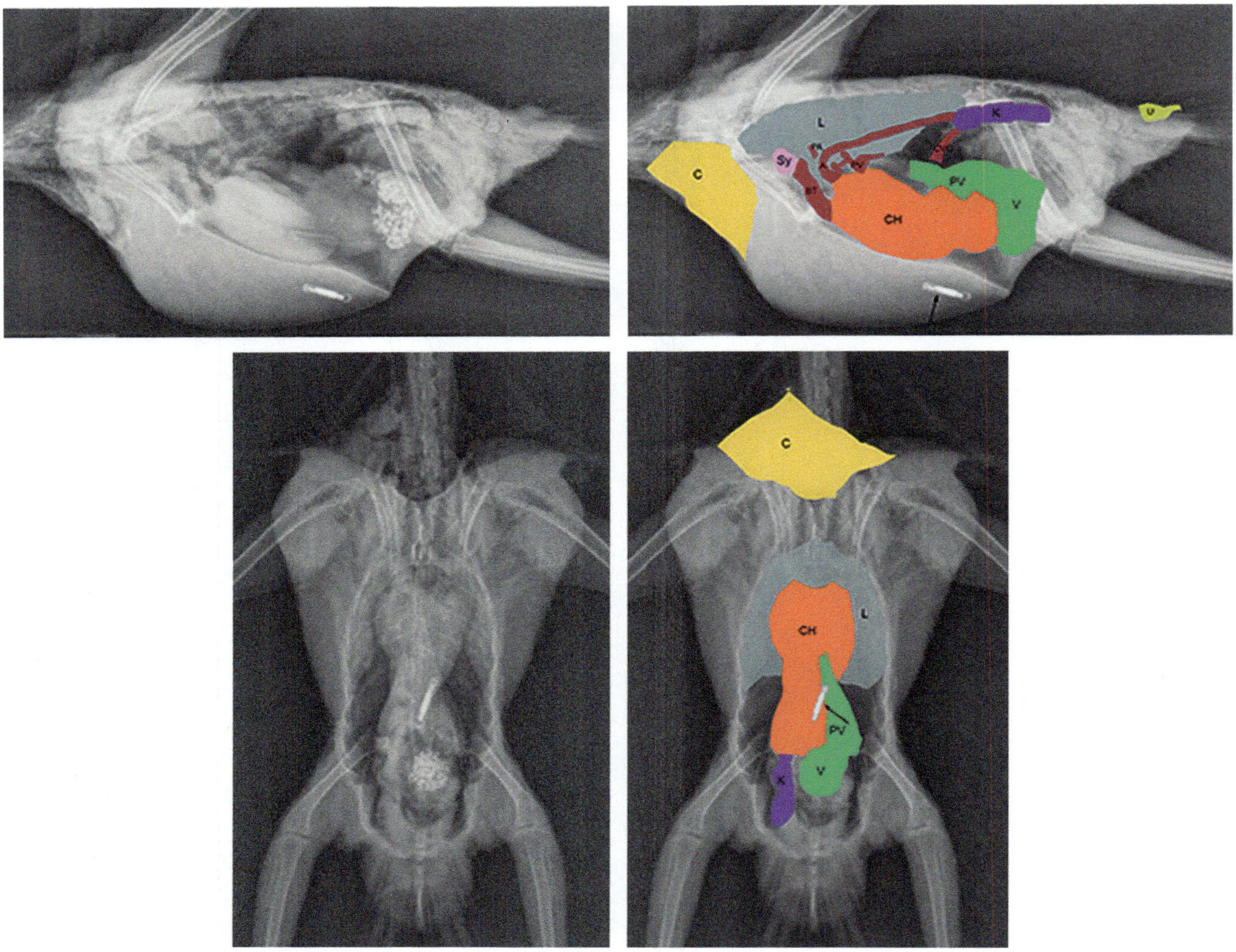

Figure 31.12 Right lateral and ventrodorsal radiographic views of a healthy rose-breasted cockatoo (*Eolophus roseicapilla*). *Source:* Courtesy of the Companion Avian and Exotic Pet Medicine Service, University of California, Davis. A microchip is visible in the left pectoral muscle (arrow). Labels: A: aortic arch, BT: brachiocephalic trunk, C: crop, CH: cardiohepatic silhouette, Cl: cloaca, CVC: caudal vena cava, G: gonad, K: right kidney, L: lung field, PA: pulmonary arteries, PV: proventriculus, S: spleen, Sy: syrinx, U: uropygial gland, V: ventriculus, Ve: vent.

Blood feathers in molting birds have a radiopaque shaft. The uropygial gland is also visible dorsal to the pygostyle except in species that do not possess this gland.

Ultrasound

Indications

Coelomic ultrasound is particularly indicated in birds with coelomic effusion, improving visualization of coelomic organs. A limitation of coelomic ultrasound in healthy birds is the presence of air sacs and the long and wide sternum, but birds with coelomic effusion have a larger acoustic window. Indications include investigation of any soft-tissue lesion in the coelom (Figure 31.20), digestive foreign body localization, localization of eggs (in the salpinx or ectopic egg) and ultrasound-guided fine needle aspirates, among others. Please see the Advanced Imaging Diagnosis section for information regarding echocardiography.

General Information

Coelomic ultrasound may be performed in standing position with a parasternal acoustic window located on the mid-coelom caudally to the sternum [25, 26], or in lateral

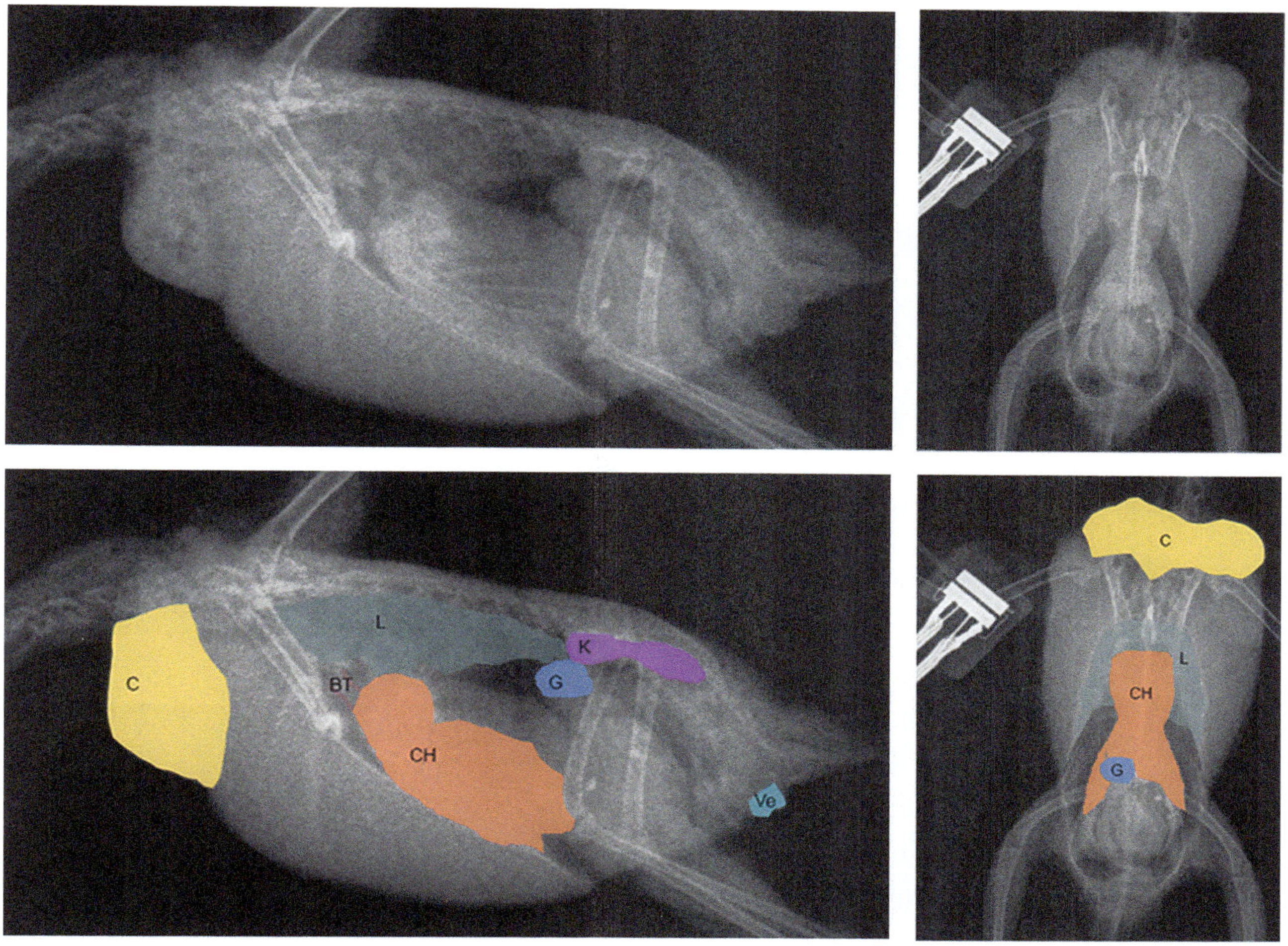

Figure 31.13 Right lateral and ventrodorsal radiographic views of a healthy budgerigar (*Melopsittacus undulatus*). *Source:* Courtesy of the Zoological Medicine Service, Université de Montréal. Labels: BT: brachiocephalic trunk, C: crop, CH: cardio-hepatic silhouette, K: right kidney, L: lung field, G: gonad (testis), Ve: vent.

recumbency with the upper leg extended forward with an acoustic window just caudal to the last rib (Figure 31.21), allowing visualization of the reproductive tract [27].

Species-specific Information

References have been published for ultrasonographic images of certain coelomic organs in Amazon parrots [21], and chicken (*Gallus domesticus*) [28], among others.

Normals

The liver is visualized on midline (Figure 31.22). Ultrasound-guided fine needle aspiration of the liver has been described in healthy Amazon parrots and may be performed under general anesthesia [21].

The digestive tract is partially visible and should not contain air in flying birds. Similar to fluoroscopy, retrograde peristaltic contractions are physiologically present in most parts of the gastrointestinal system and are not an indication of digestive obstruction (Figures 31.23 and 31.24) [7]. The cloaca may be visualized if it is filled. To differentiate the cloaca from a cystic mass, it is possible to introduce a cotton-tip applicator in the cloaca.

Normal kidneys are not always visible via ultrasound due to their intrapelvic position surrounded by air sacs [27], but may be distinguished in certain birds (Figure 31.25). Inactive gonads are not generally identified [27]. In contrast, active testes and ovaries may be visualized, and eggs may be identified in the salpinx, on the left side [27].

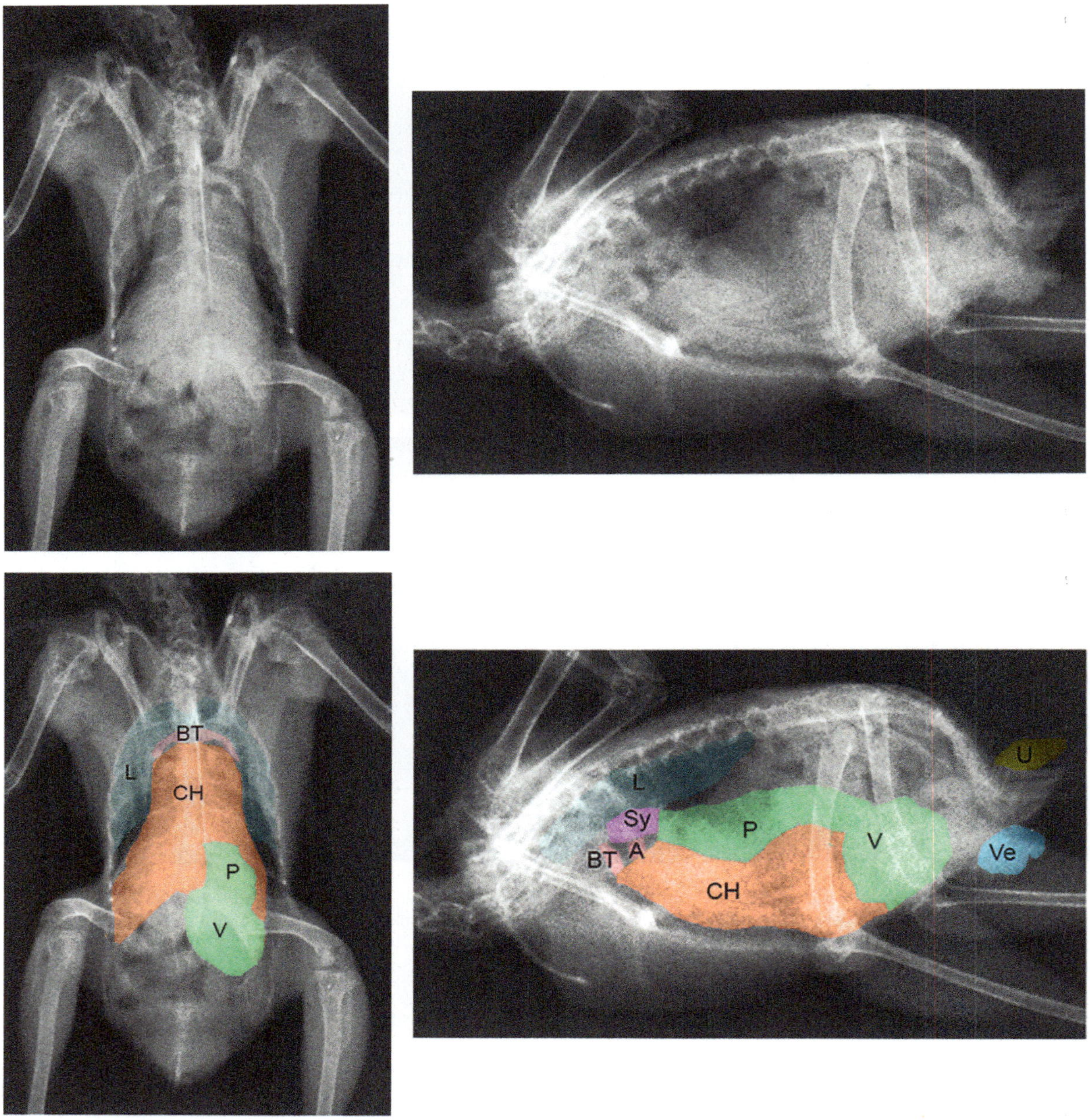

Figure 31.14 Left lateral and ventro-dorsal radiographic views of a superb starling (*Lamprotornis superbus*). *Source:* Courtesy of Granby Zoo, Canada. Labels: A: aorta, BT: brachiocephalic trunk, CH: cardiohepatic silhouette, L: lung field, P: proventriculus, Sy: syrinx, V: ventriculus, Ve: vent, U: Uropygial gland.

Testicular parenchyma displays a medium echogenicity and is surrounded by a hyperechoic serosa [27]. Ovarian follicles appear as round structures with anechoic or hypoechoic content and are heterogenous in size (Figure 31.26) [27]. At more advanced stages of development, the content becomes more echoic, corresponding to yolk [27]. In contrast, eggs are formed of concentric layers with the central yolk being echogenic, surrounded by a poorly echoic perimeter of albumin (Figure 31.27). A hyperechoic shell is added in the uterus [27]. Normal ovarian structures in chickens may be differentiated from ovarian lesions including neoplasms (Figure 31.28) using the following criteria: presence of septations, papillary projections, cystic areas associated with prominent central blood flow visualized by Doppler mode, other than at the periphery of large follicles [28].

Other Diagnostic Imaging Modalities

Echocardiography

Brief cardiac ultrasound may be performed in emergency settings to detect pericardial effusion requiring aspiration.

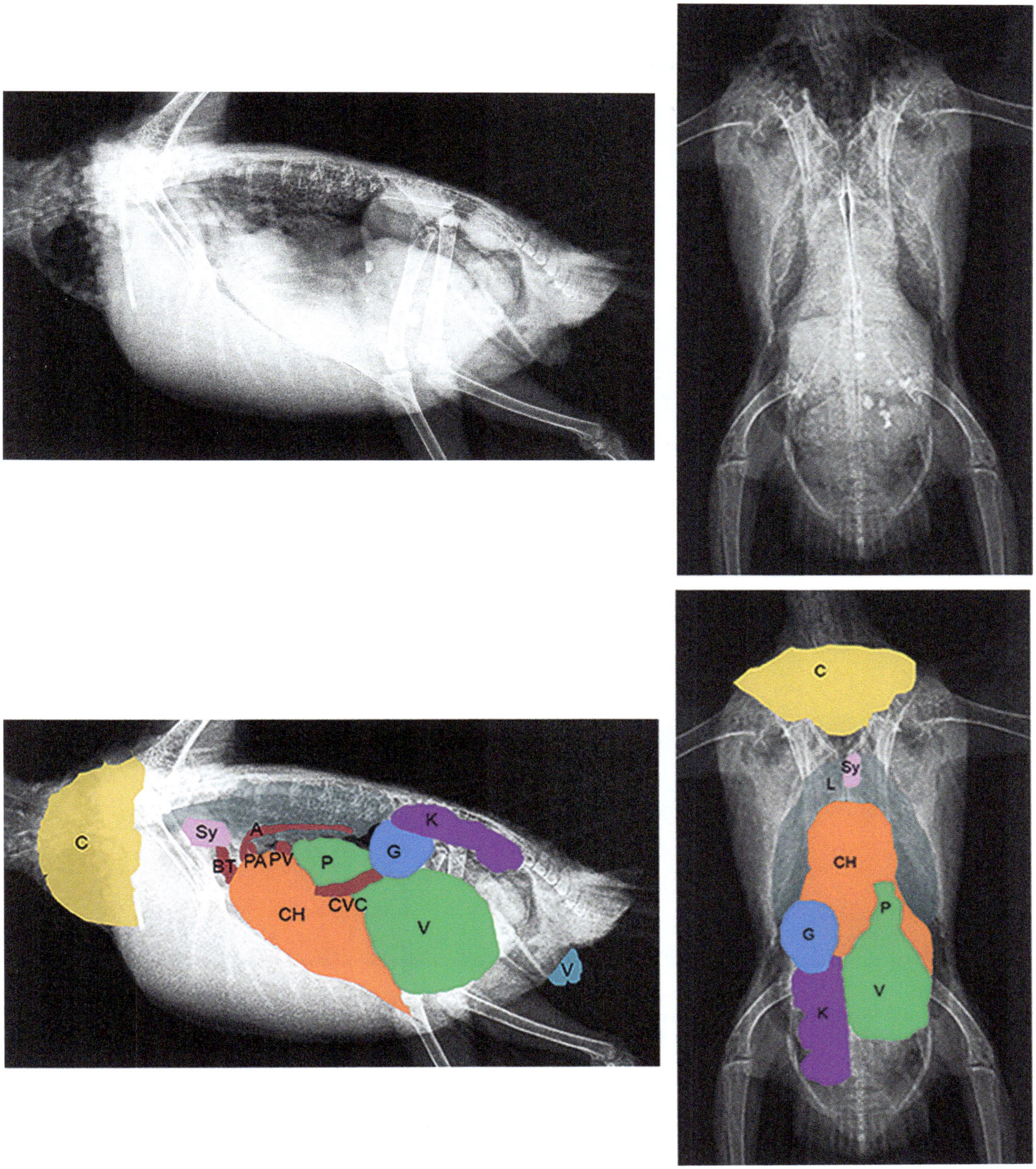

Figure 31.15 Right lateral and ventro-dorsal radiographic views of a male ring-necked dove (*Streptopelia capicola*). *Source:* Courtesy of the Zoological Medicine Service, Université de Montréal. A pulse oximeter is place on the left foot. Labels: A: aortic arch, BT: brachiocephalic trunk, C: crop, CH: cardiohepatic silhouette, CVC: caudal vena cava, G: right gonad (testis), K: right kidney, L: lung field, P: proventriculus, PA: pulmonary arteries, PV: pulmonary veins, Sy: syrinx, V: ventriculus, Ve: vent.

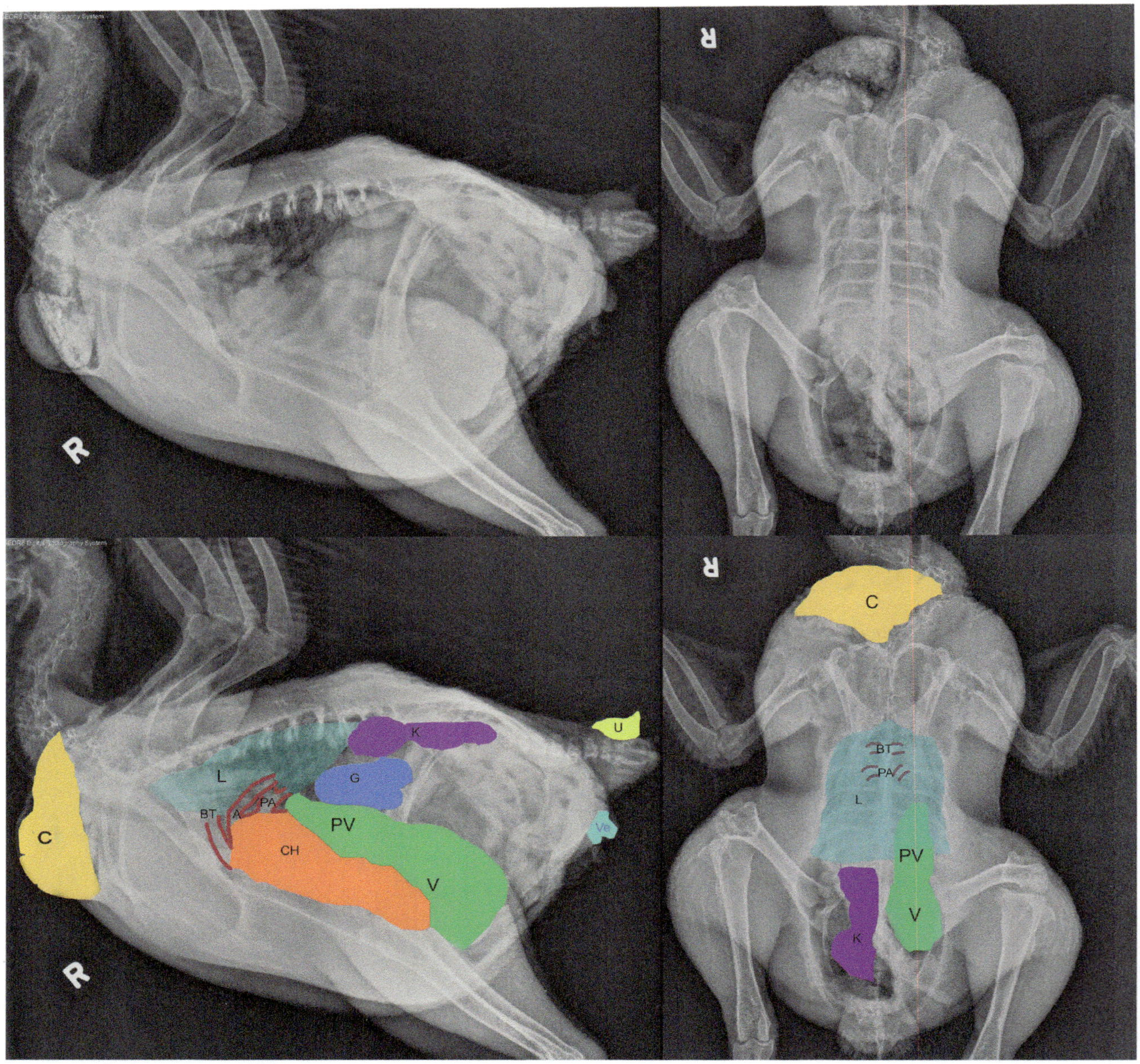

Figure 31.16 Right lateral and ventrodorsal radiographic views of a healthy chicken (*Gallus domesticus*). *Source:* Courtesy of the Companion Avian and Exotic Pet Medicine Service, University of California, Davis. Labels: A: aortic arch, BT: brachiocephalic trunk, C: crop, CH: cardiohepatic silhouette, G: gonad (ovary), K: right kidney, L: lung field, PA: pulmonary arteries, PV: proventriculus, U: uropygial gland, V: ventriculus, Ve: vent.

Complete cardiac ultrasound is more often performed after initial stabilization of the patient [29]. Description of techniques to perform avian echocardiography [30, 31] and reference intervals for cardiac ultrasound have been published in pigeons (*Columba livia*) [32], chickens [33], and certain psittacine species including the grey parrot [34], sulfur-crested cockatoo (*Cacatua galerita*) and *Ara* spp. [35]

Fluoroscopy

Fluoroscopy can be useful in an emergency, especially to investigate digestive intraluminal lesions or foreign bodies in unstable birds, or to characterize ileus or dilation of segments of the digestive tract, such as the proventriculus. Reference intervals for digestive fluoroscopy has been described in blue-fronted [7] and Hispaniolan Amazon parrots [6]. In healthy birds, 3–6.6 gastric cycles

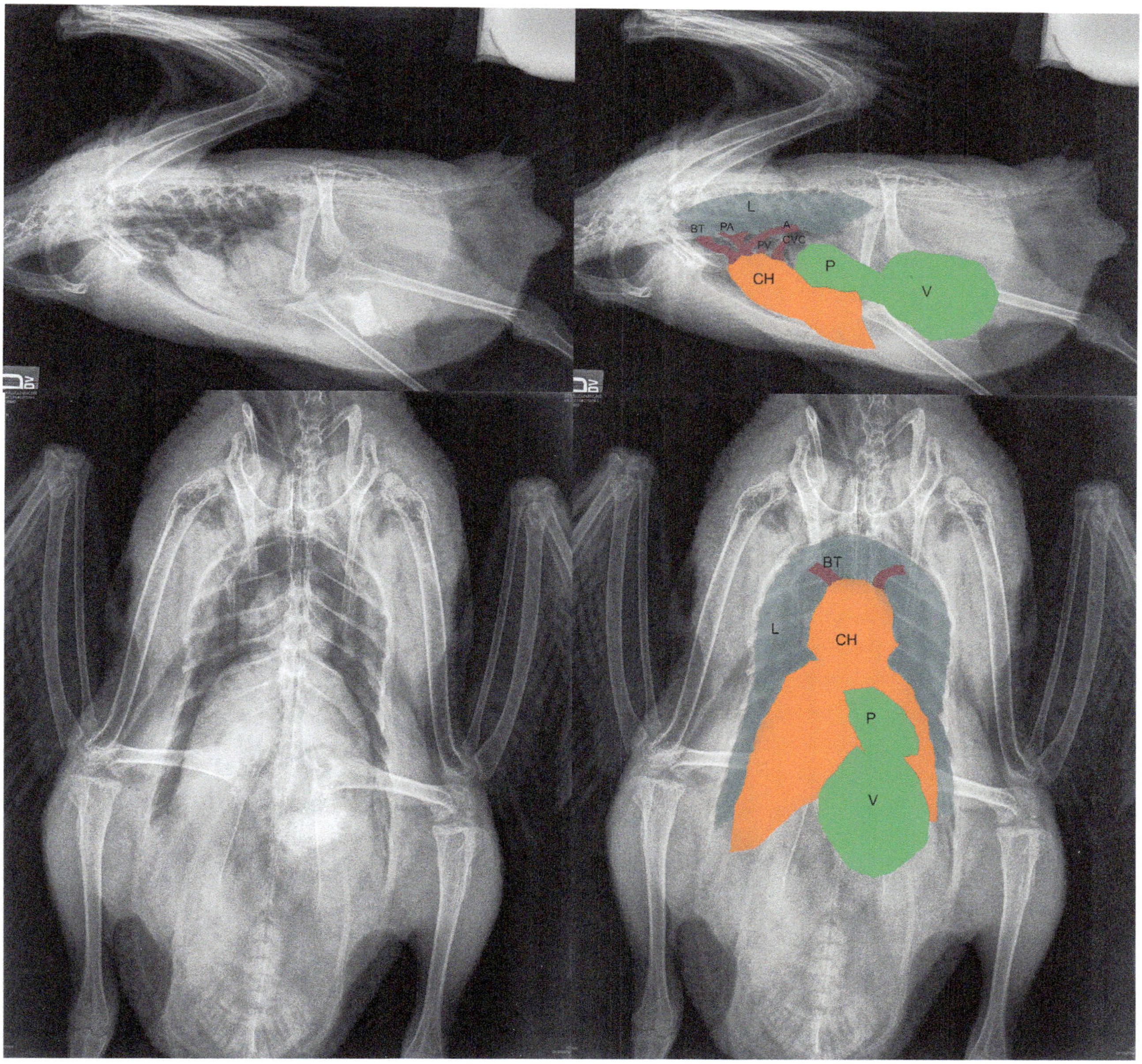

Figure 31.17 Right lateral and ventro-dorsal radiographic views of a goose. *Source:* Courtesy of the Zoological Medicine Service, Université de Montréal. Labels: A: aortic arch, BT: brachiocephalic trunk, CH: cardio-hepatic silhouette, CVC: caudal vena cava, L: lung field, P: proventriculus, PA: pulmonary arteries, PV: pulmonary veins, V: ventriculus.

are observed per minute, with each cycle being divided into six phases: anterograde peristaltic wave of the proventriculus with ejection into the ventriculus, closure of the isthmus, horizontal contraction of the ventriculus, vertical contraction of the ventriculus, and ejection into the duodenum and opening of the isthmus [6]. Of note, retrograde peristaltic contractions are physiologic in the small intestine, from the ventriculus to the proventriculus, from the proventriculus to the esophagus, and from the esophagus to the crop, and are not an indication of digestive obstruction [7].

Computed Tomography and Magnetic Resonance Imaging

Due to the limited time window for successful therapeutic interventions and low sensitivity of radiographs to assess degree of medullary and skull trauma, advanced

Table 31.1 Differential diagnoses for common radiographic lesions.

Radiographic lesions	Main differential diagnoses
Splenomegaly, hepatomegaly	• Bacterial infection: Chlamydiosis, mycobacteriosis, other bacterial infectious diseases (colibacillosis, salmonellosis, Coxiella-like organisms, clostridiosis in chicken, riemerellosis in geese) • Viral infection (polyomavirus, adenovirus, reovirus, herpesvirus) • Parasitic infection • Neoplasms (including viral-induced neoplasm: Marek's disease, avian leukosis, reticuloendotheliosis in poultry)
Proventricular dilatation	• Proventriculitis (fungal (i.e. mostly candidiasis or macrorhabdosis), bacterial, parasitic (i.e. *Spiruridae*, *Cryptosporidium* in lovebirds) etiologies) • Heavy metal intoxication (lead, zinc) • Digestive tract obstruction (mass, foreign body) • Coelomitis • Bornavirus infection (proventricular dilatation disease) • Proventricular neoplasm
Digestive intraluminal filling defect	• Foreign body (with local reaction if chronic) • Granuloma (mycobacteriosis, parasitic) • Digestive neoplasm
Enlarged cardiac silhouette	Cardiomegaly and/or pericardial effusion, may be: • Infectious (West Nile virus, toxoplasmosis, duck parvovirus), or • Nutritional (atherosclerosis, vitamin E deficiency) in origin
Increased bone opacity	• Physiologic (egg-laying hen, high blood regeneration) • Inflammatory (trauma) • Infectious (aspergillosis, mycobacteriosis, avian leukosis) • Neoplastic
Tracheal intraluminal opacity	• Granuloma (aspergillosis) • Foreign body • Tracheal hemorrhage • Tracheal stenosis • Parasites (*Syngamus trachea* in waterfowl, poultry, *Cyathostoma* spp., *Sternostoma tracheacolum* mites in Passeriformes) • Tracheal neoplasm
Increased pulmonary opacity	• Pneumonia • Cardiogenic edema • Pulmonary hemorrhage (trauma) • Neoplasm • Artifacts (superimposed large vessels, molting feathers, skin folds) • Airborne toxins
Air sac line	• Air sacculitis (aspergillosis, bacterial, or parasitic (*Serratospiculum*, *Serratospiculoides*) etiology) • Respiratory neoplasm

Source: Data from Evans [17].

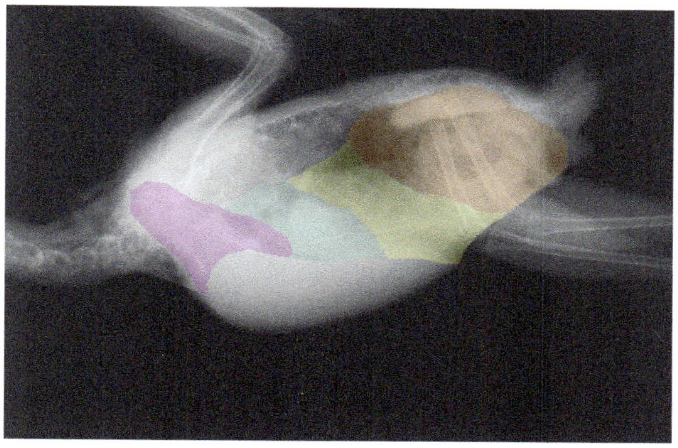

Figure 31.18 Anatomic position of intracoelomic air sacs and potential position of air sac lines in psittacine birds with air sacculitis: in purple: clavicular air sac (intrathoracic and extrathoracic diverticula), in green: cranial thoracic air sacs, in yellow: caudal thoracic air sacs, in orange: abdominal air sacs.

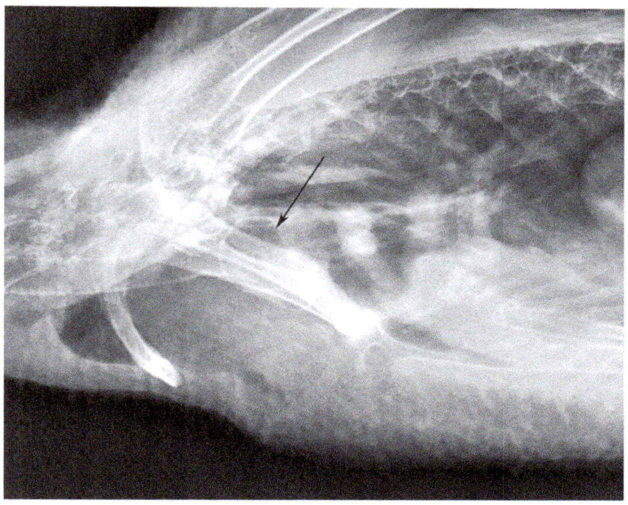

Figure 31.19 Lateral view of the thoracic inlet of a male duck (*Anas platyrhynchos domesticus*) illustrating a syringeal drum (arrow). *Source:* Courtesy of the University of Guelph.

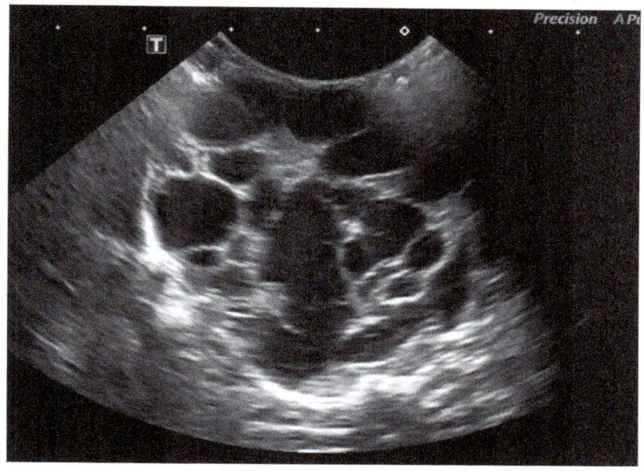

Figure 31.20 Coelomic ultrasound of a polycystic hepatic neoplasm in a budgerigar (*Melopsittacus erithacus*).

imaging techniques such as CT-scan and MRI are occasionally required with emergency neurologic presentations including stroke [36], and cerebral and medullary trauma (Figure 31.29) [37].

In addition, these modalities may be helpful when increased definition is needed to detect small foreign bodies or skull lesions (Figure 31.30) [38], although resolution limitations should be acknowledged in very small birds. In passerines and small psittacine birds, micro-CT-scan and micro-MRI may be required for appropriate definition. Similar to radiographs, CT-scan can be performed under sedation in birds [39], especially since straight positioning is not absolutely required. Positive pressure ventilation may be needed for optimal visualization of thoracic structures (Figure 31.31). If the bird is not ventilated, sternal recumbency is preferred over lateral recumbency to evaluate intracoelomic respiratory structures [40]. Administration of IV radiographic or MRI contrast is also performed routinely in birds for advanced imaging. Atlas of normal brain anatomy [41] and coelomic anatomy [42] is available for some avian species. Of note, the glycogen body in the caudal part of the medullary canal [43] should not be mistaken for a lesion. For more details about advanced imaging techniques, including nuclear-imaging techniques, the reader can refer to other reviews [23, 37].

Clinical Presentations Requiring Emergent Imaging

Investigation of Intestinal Foreign Bodies

Suspicion of foreign body ingestion or inhalation should prompt rapid imaging tests to dislodge the foreign body before complications occur. This is especially true for crop foreign bodies, which can be retrieved under anesthesia with or without endoscopic assistance when quickly detected before they progress further in the digestive tract. Radiolucent foreign bodies may be particularly challenging to detect and gastrointestinal contrast study with fluoroscopy may be needed to detect subtraction images. If a surgery is expected, iohexol 20–25 ml/kg [44] should be used as a contrast media, rather than barium.

Metallic foreign bodies may be detected radiographically on standard radiographs (Figures 31.32 and 31.33) or with

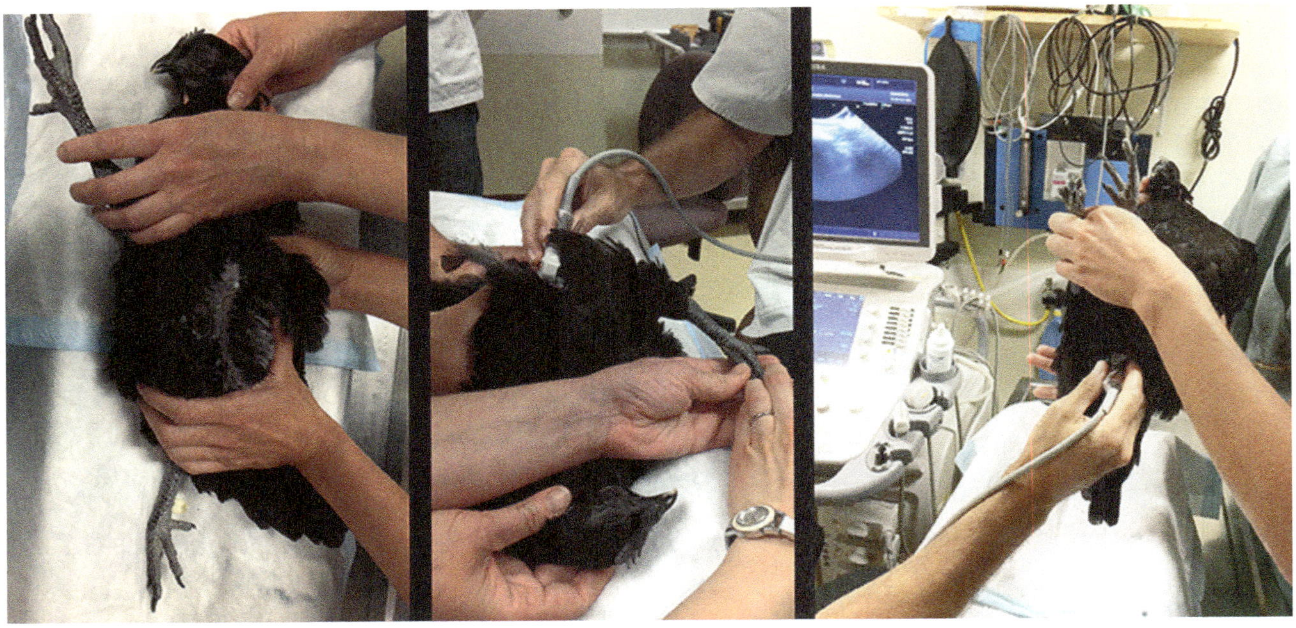

Figure 31.21 Coelomic ultrasound in standing position in a chicken (Gallus domesticus). *Source:* Courtesy of the Zoological Medicine Service, Université de Montréal.

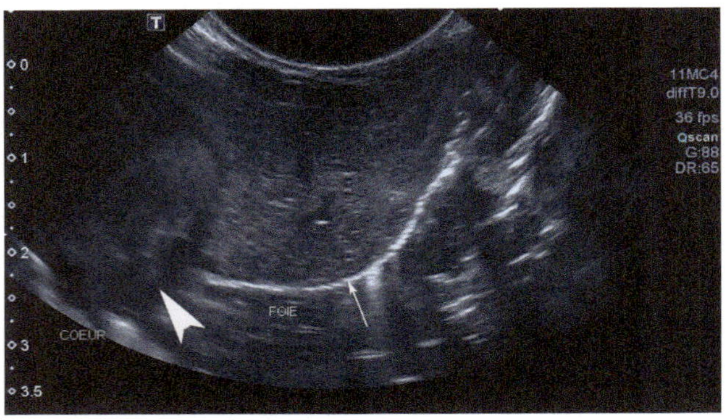

Figure 31.22 Normal ultrasonographic appearance of the heart (arrowhead) and liver (arrow) in a sulfur-crested cockatoo (*Cacatua galerita*). *Source:* Courtesy of the Zoological Medicine Service, Université de Montréal.

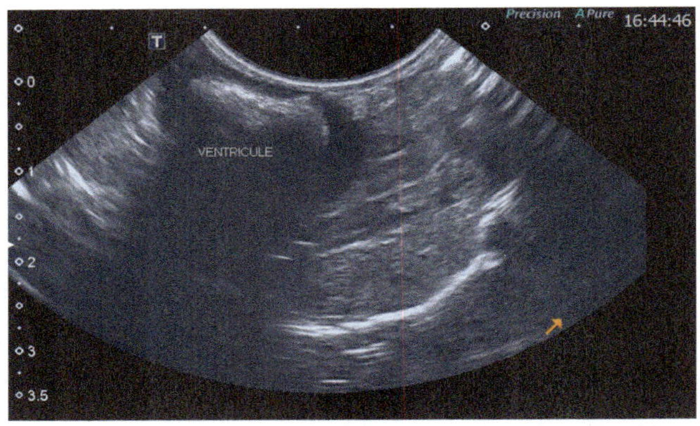

Figure 31.24 Normal ultrasonographic appearance of the ventriculus in a blue and gold macaw (*Ara ararauna*). *Source:* Courtesy of the Companion Avian and Exotic Pet Medicine Service, University of California, Davis.

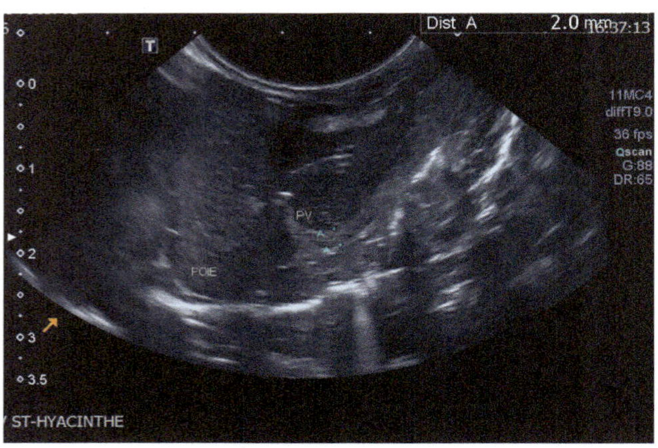

Figure 31.23 Normal ultrasonographic appearance of the proventriculus in a sulfur-crested cockatoo (*Cacatua galerita*). *Source:* Courtesy of the Zoological Medicine Service, Université de Montréal.

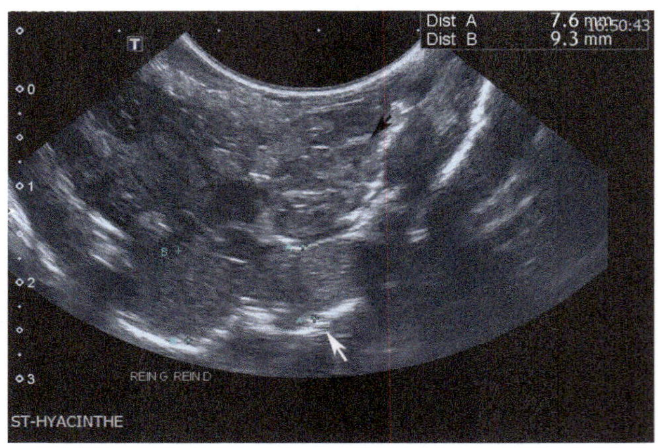

Figure 31.25 Normal ultrasonographic appearance of the kidneys, with bilateral cranial divisions visualized in transverse section (A and B markers) in a sulfur-crested cockatoo (*Cacatua galerita*). Small intestinal loops are visible ventral to the kidneys (black arrow) and the synsacrum (white arrow) lies just dorsal to the kidneys. *Source:* Courtesy of the Zoological Medicine Service, Université de Montréal.

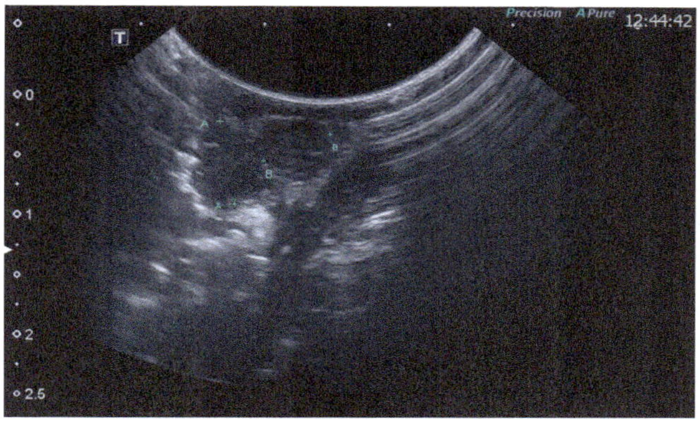

Figure 31.26 Normal ultrasonographic appearance of ovarian follicles in a sun conure (*Aratinga solstitialis*). *Source:* Courtesy of the Zoological Medicine Service, Université de Montréal.

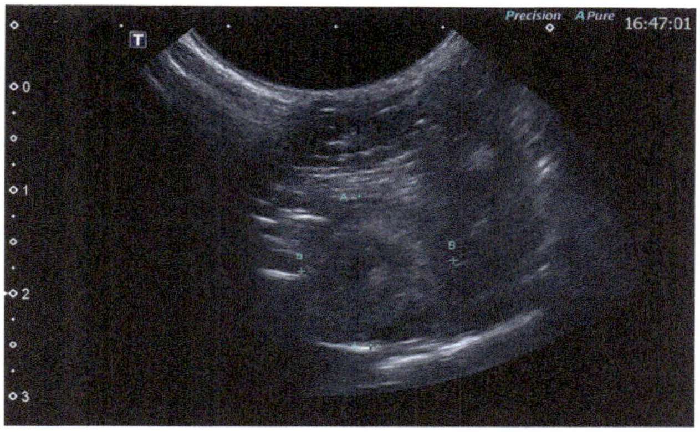

Figure 31.27 Normal ultrasonographic appearance of an egg in a sun conure (*Aratinga solstitialis*). *Source:* Courtesy of the Zoological Medicine Service, Université de Montréal.

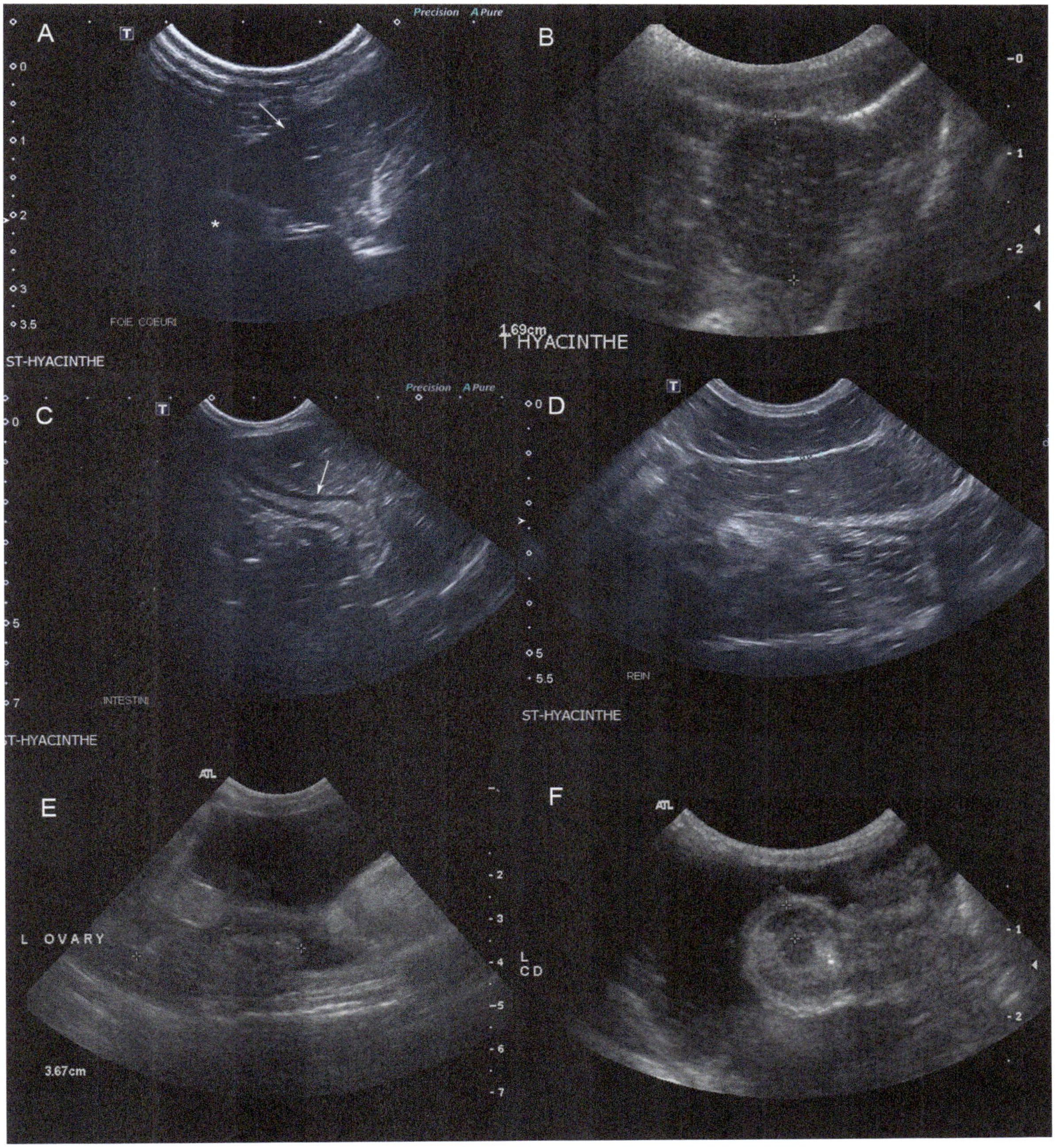

Figure 31.28 Chicken coelomic ultrasound: A: heart (*) and liver (arrow), B: gallbladder (line), C: intestine (arrow), D: kidneys (a and b labels), E: left ovary, and F: egg in the salpinx. *Source:* Courtesy of the Zoological Medicine Service, Université de Montréal.

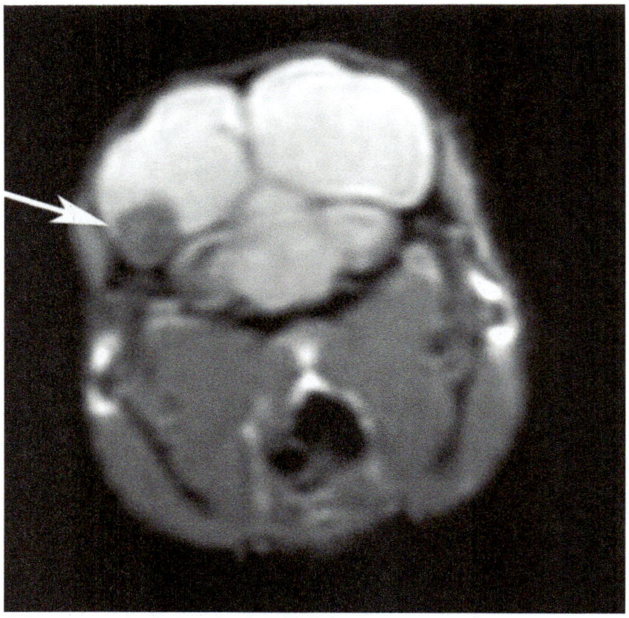

Figure 31.29 MRI transverse section of the skull of a white-capped Pionus (*Pionus seniloides*) presented for convulsions after a trauma (the right side of the patient on the left of the picture): a ventrolateral T1-hypointense lesion is noted in the right hemisphere (arrow). *Source:* Courtesy of the University of Guelph.

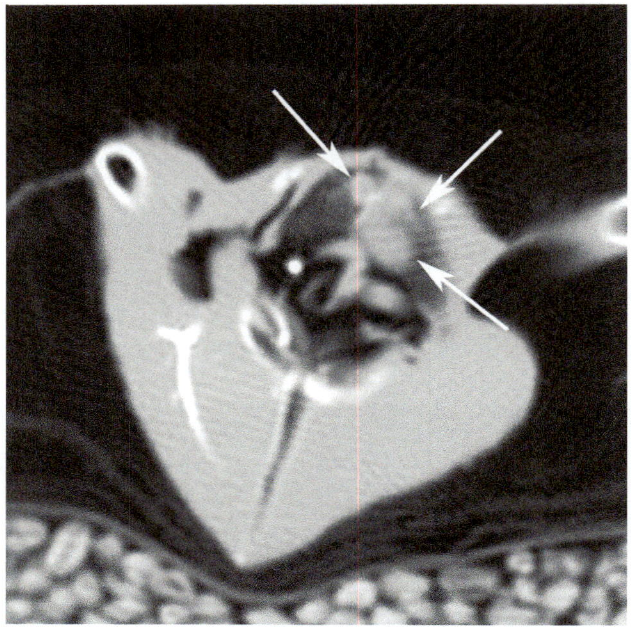

Figure 31.31 Transverse section of the thorax of a cockatiel (*Nymphicus hollandicus*) obtained with CT (the right side of the patient on the left of the picture): a pulmonary radiopaque lesion is noted and was confirmed to be a pulmonary neoplasm. *Source:* Courtesy of the University of Guelph.

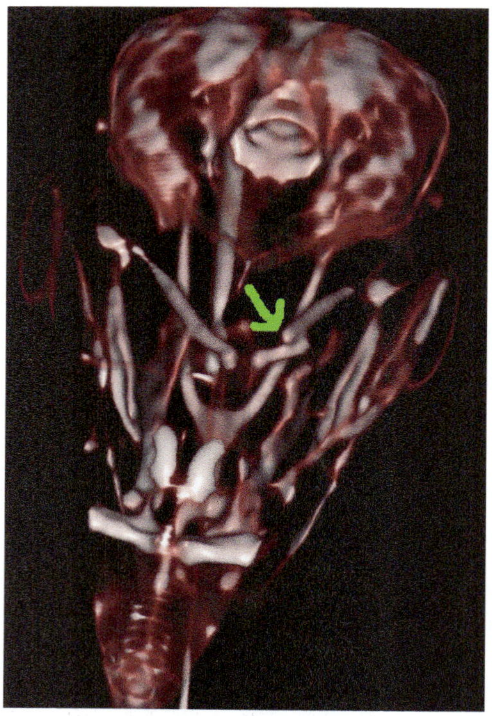

Figure 31.30 Ventral view of the skull of a hawk-headed parrot (*Deroptyus accipitrinus*) obtained by CT and three-dimension reconstruction: fracture of the right pterygoid bone is noted (green arrow). *Source:* Courtesy of the University of Guelph.

the avian patient standing in a box or bag. Of note, radiographs have been reported to be very insensitive to screen for heavy metal intoxication [45, 46] since lead can be stored in bone following digestive absorption and zinc can be found in nonmetallic objects such as rubber or pliable plastics [47]. Thus, normal radiographs do not rule out heavy metal intoxication.

Investigation of Dyspnea

Avian patients displaying dyspnea on emergency presentation often require radiographic assessment. Radiographs enable discrimination between respiratory and non-respiratory causes of dyspnea, such as coelomic masses or effusion compressing the air sacs. Among respiratory causes of dyspnea, lower respiratory tract lesions such as cardiogenic edema (Figure 31.34), pneumonia, pulmonary hemorrhage, air sacculitis (Figure 31.35), respiratory neoplasms, and respiratory toxins should be differentiated from upper airway obstructions, because emergency placement of an air sac cannula would be indicated in the latter category only. Upper airway obstruction causes include food aspiration, tracheal stenosis (Figure 31.36) that may be secondary to tracheal intubation, and tracheal or syringeal fungal granuloma. Whole body radiographs should be obtained under oxygen in patients with dyspnea. CT-scan and MRI are more sensitive modalities

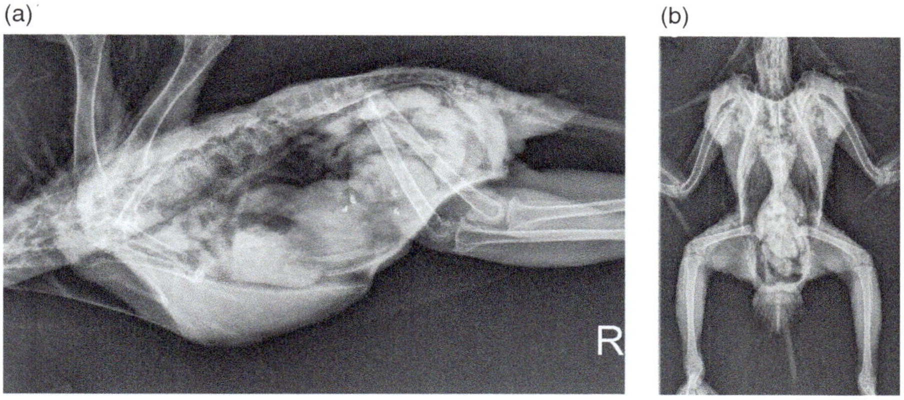

Figure 31.32 Metallic foreign bodies in the proventriculus and ventriculus of a male sulfur-crested cockatoo (*Cacatua galerita*), associated with proventricular dilatation suggesting possible heavy metal intoxication. Zinc intoxication was confirmed by plasmatic measurement. *Source:* Courtesy of the Companion Avian and Exotic Pet Medicine Service, University of California, Davis.

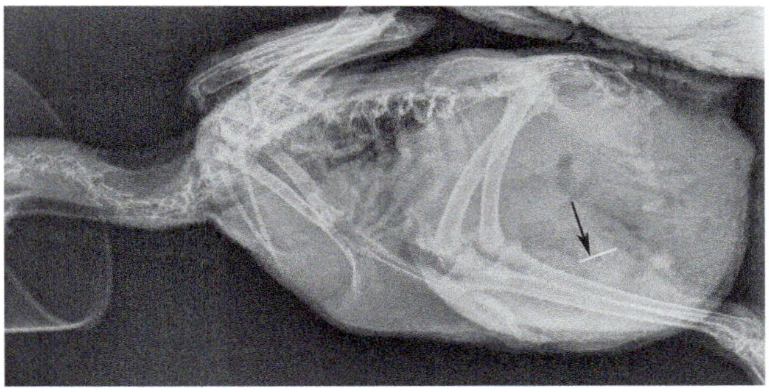

Figure 31.33 Egg-laying chicken presented for coelomic pain diagnosed with a nail in the ventriculus and an ovarian mass. *Source:* Courtesy of the Companion Avian and Exotic Pet Medicine Service, University of California, Davis.

for imaging of avian nasal cavities and infraorbital sinuses [38]. The trachea should be followed throughout its length if an upper airway obstruction is suspected. Tracheal and syringeal cartilages calcify with age and may make the syrinx more conspicuous on lateral radiographic views. Fungal and mycobacterial lesions tend to be focal to multifocal while bacterial lesions tend to be more diffuse (Figure 31.37). A "parabronchial" pattern may be seen with diffuse pneumonitis such as the macaw chronic obstructive pulmonary disease or air borne toxicosis. Clinicians should look for air sac lines based on species-specific normal anatomy and differentiate them from skin folds. To assess pulmonary opacity, it is key to pull both humeri forward to prevent superimposition over the lung field. In case of cardiomegaly

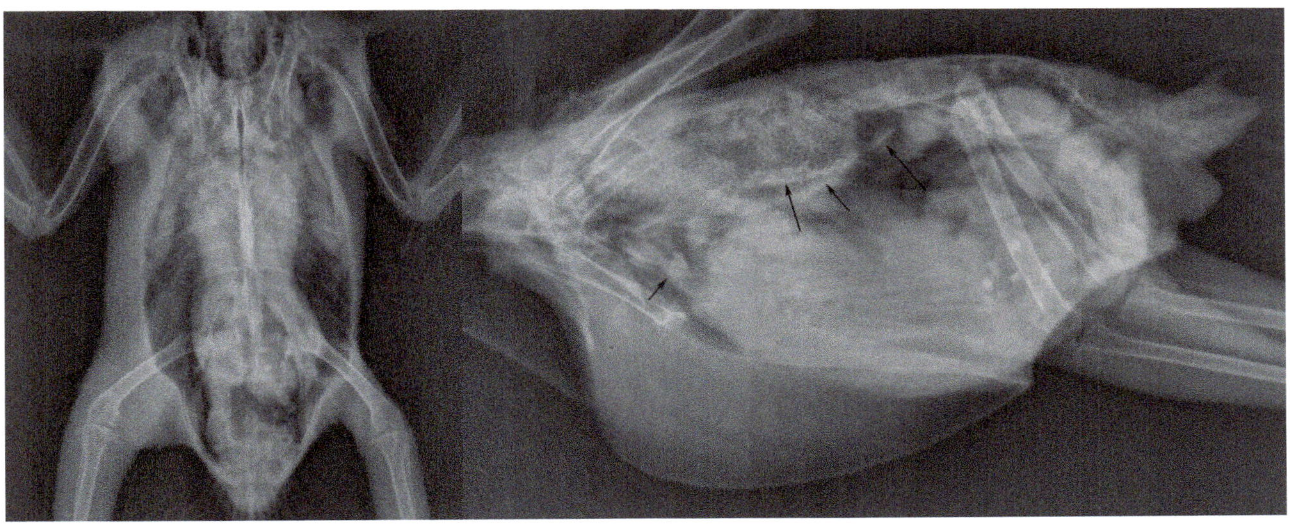

Figure 31.34 Ventro-dorsal and lateral view of an Grey parrot presented with dyspnea: cardiomegaly, increased pulmonary opacity and calcifications of the brachiocephalic trunk, aorta and pulmonary arteries (arrows). *Source:* Courtesy of the Companion Avian and Exotic Pet Medicine Service, University of California, Davis.

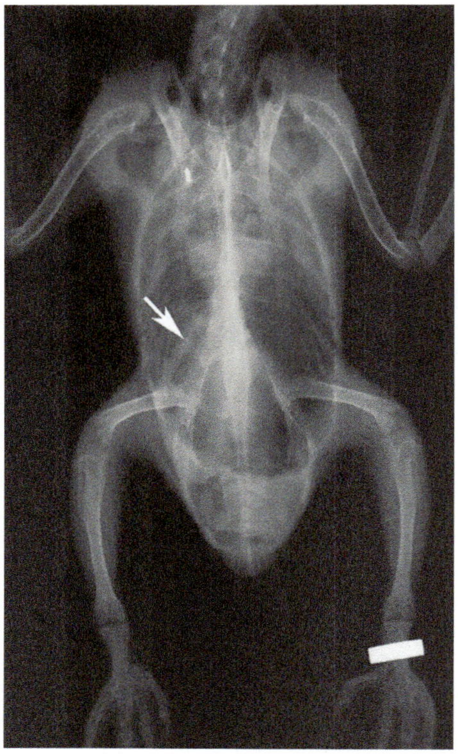

Figure 31.35 Ventro-dorsal view of a psittacine bird with right caudal thoracic air sac opacity (arrow) association with air sacculitis. *Source:* Courtesy of the University of Guelph.

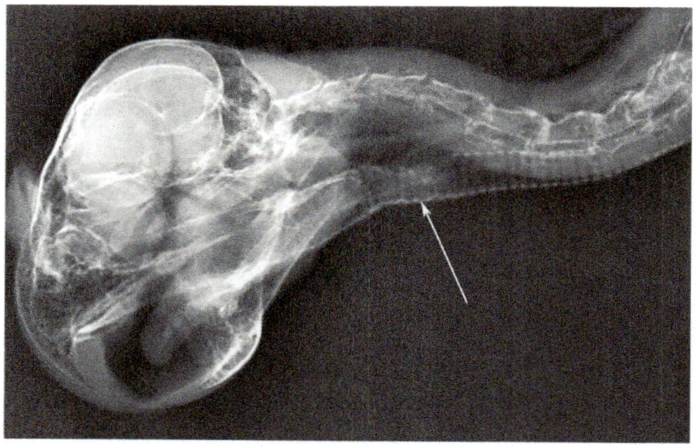

Figure 31.36 Right lateral view of the skull and cranial cervical area of a blue and gold macaw (*Ara ararauna*) presenting with tracheal stenosis. *Source:* Courtesy of the University of Guelph.

and increased pulmonary opacity, suggesting cardiac disease, handling should be minimized, and treatment of pulmonary edema should be instituted. Overinflation of the caudal air sacs may be seen with sub-obstructive tracheal and syringeal diseases and overinflation of the axillary diverticulae of the interclavicular air sac may be seen with caudal coelomic expansion and pulmonary and caudal air sac diseases.

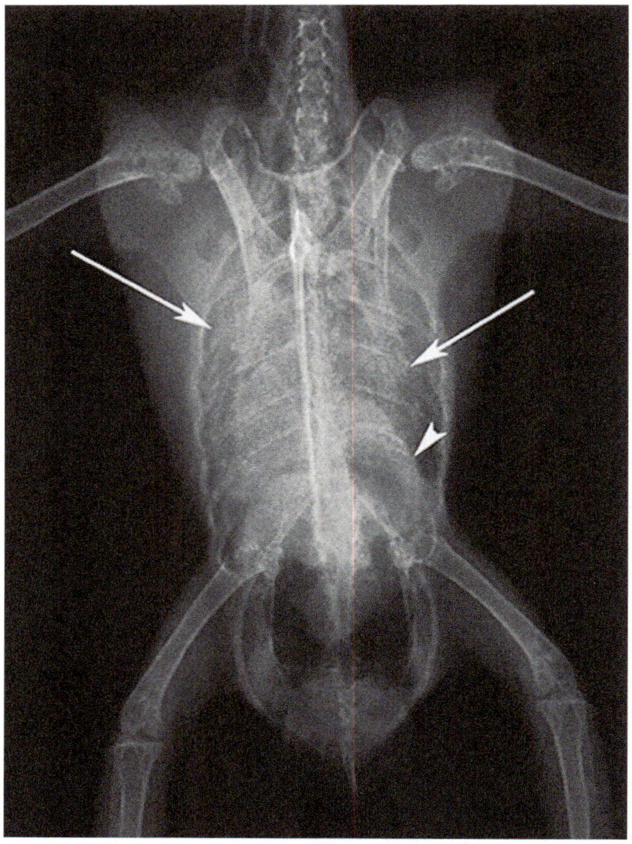

Figure 31.37 Ventro-dorsal view of a Pionus parrot with multifocal to diffuse pulmonary opacities (arrows) and left caudal thoracic air sac line (arrowhead). *Source:* Courtesy of the University of Guelph.

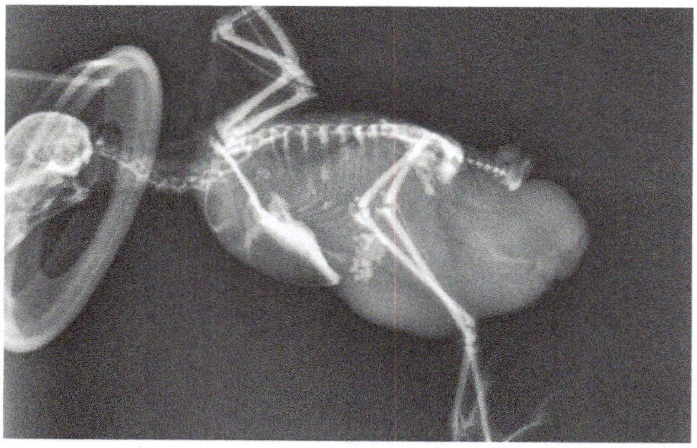

Figure 31.38 Female canary presented with a cloacal prolapse: coelomic effusion and polyostotic hyperostosis are noted. Polyostotic hyperostosis indicates a reproductively active female; reproductive tract lesions should be further investigated with coelomic ultrasound.

Investigation of Cloacal Prolapses

Cloacal prolapse is an emergency in birds and investigating the cause of the problem is important to prevent recurrence. Radiographs and/or coelomic ultrasound are indicated.

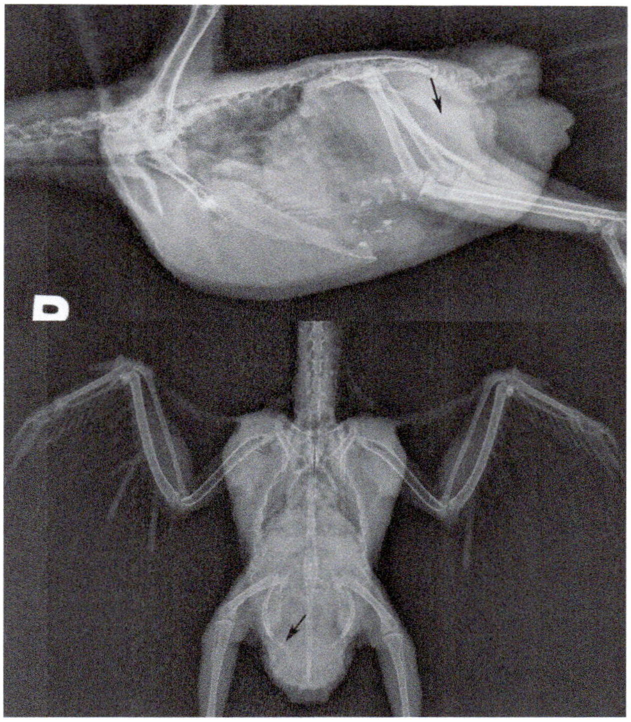

Figure 31.39 Ventro-dorsal and lateral radiographic views of a female Eclectus parrot (*Eclectus roratus*) presented for tenesmus. A poorly calcified egg is noted in the caudal coelom. *Source:* Courtesy of the Companion Avian and Exotic Pet Medicine Service, University of California, Davis.

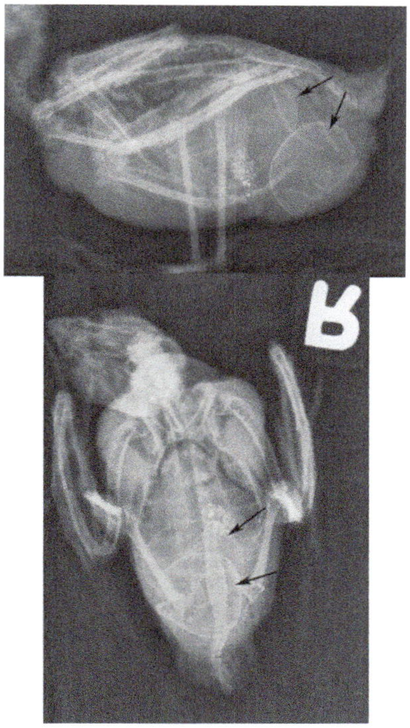

Figure 31.41 Standing radiographs of a female cockatiel (*Nymphicus hollandicus*) presented with dystocia: the lateral view was obtained with a horizontal beam. Two shelled eggs are visible in the coelom, which is unusual. This exemplifies the need for radiographic assessment before attempting an emergency procedure. *Source:* Courtesy of the Companion Avian and Exotic Pet Medicine Service, University of California, Davis.

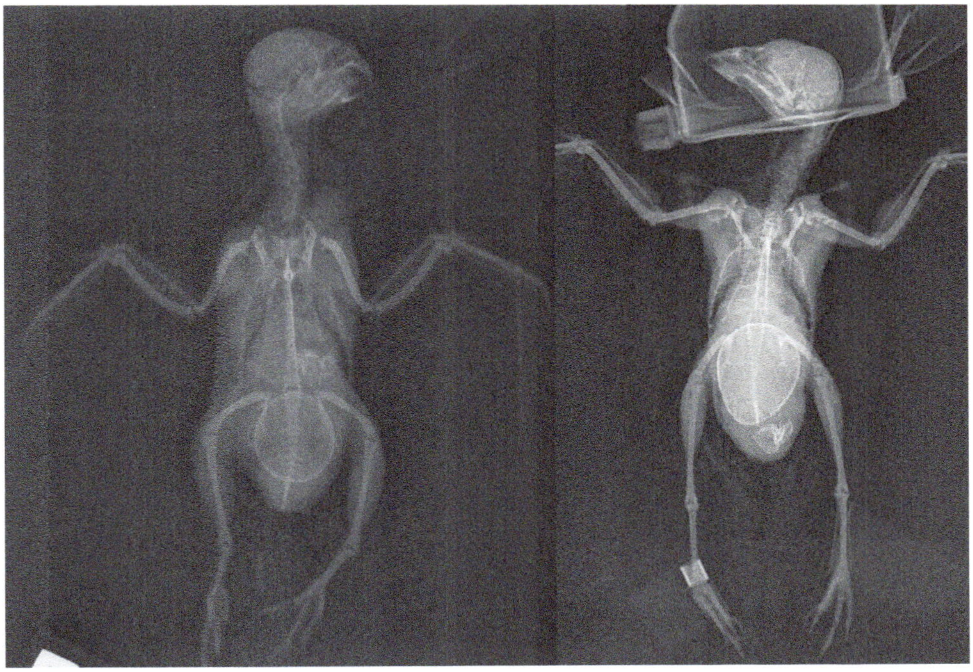

Figure 31.40 Ventro-dorsal radiographic views obtained respectively from a female budgerigar (*Melopsittacus undulatus*), on the left, and a female canary (*Serinus canaria*), on the right. Note the calcified egg in the caudal coelom, polyostotic hyperostosis in both birds, and the cranial displacement of the ventriculus containing elements of mineral density in the budgerigar. *Source:* Courtesy of the Zoological Medicine Service, Université de Montréal, and of the Companion Avian and Exotic Pet Medicine Service, University of California, Davis.

Differentials include tenesmus from digestive obstruction or inflammation, reproductive disorders (Figure 31.38) such as dystocia, ovarian cyst or neoplasm, salpingitis or hypersexual behavior [48], urolithiasis including cloacoliths [49], cloacal masses [50], coelomic effusion, and any coelomic mass causing a mass effect or idiopathic (cockatoos). Recurrent cloacal prolapses may be complicated by cloacal inflammation creating a vicious cycle. Therefore, the cause of the problem needs to be addressed as soon as possible during an emergency presentation. In case of coelomic effusion, coelomic ultrasound provides better visualization of coelomic organs due to decreased radiographic contrast [51]. Evidence of reproductive disease may also be evident on radiographs including polyostotic hyperostosis, egg binding, or oviductal impaction. For more information regarding digestive foreign bodies, see paragraph under 'Investigation of Intestinal Foreign Bodies'.

Investigation of Reproductive Disease

Female birds may present with dystocia. Owners may not be aware of the sex of their bird or may not be aware that female birds may lay eggs in the absence of fertilization. Therefore, the reason of presentation may be vague, such as dyspnea, coelomic distension, tenesmus or hematochezia. Retained eggs may have an uncalcified (Figure 31.39) or calcified shell (Figure 31.40). Usually a single egg is present but multiple eggs have been observed in rare cases (Figure 31.41). In some cases, intracoelomic yolk or ectopic eggs may be present. This may occur following a rupture or retroperistalsis of the salpinx or intracoelomic ovulation. Presence of coelomic effusion associated with coelomitis may complicate radiographic diagnosis (Figure 31.42) but is an indication for coelomic ultrasound (Figure 31.43).

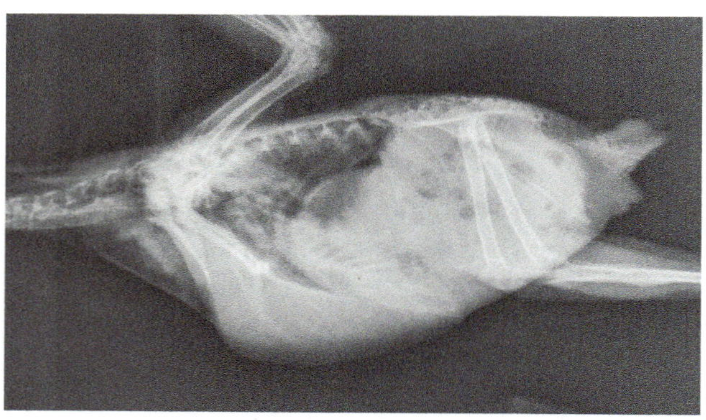

Figure 31.42 Lateral radiographic view of a female Senegal parrot (*Poicephalus senegalensis*) presented with coelomic distension and melena: decreased coelomic contrast is compatible with coelomic effusion and coelomic GI opacities are compatible with enteritis or digestive perforation. Differential diagnoses for coelomitis should also include reproductive tract disorders. *Source:* Courtesy of the Zoological Medicine Service, Université de Montréal.

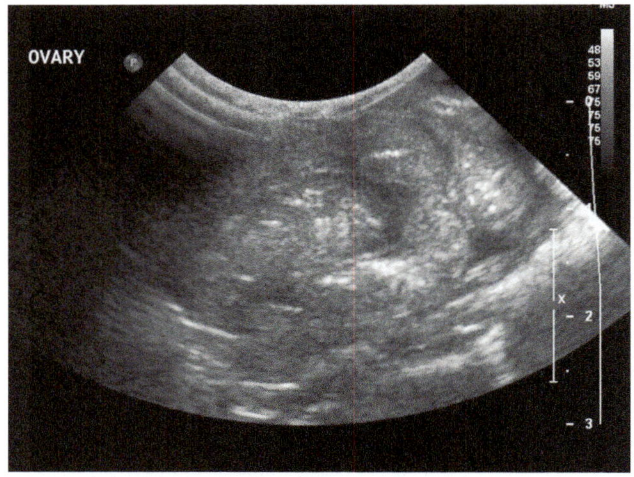

Figure 31.43 Coelomic ultrasound of the bird radiographed in Figure 31.42: multiple follicles are visible on the ovary.

Eggs are easier to visualize when intracoelomic fluid provides an acoustic window.

When evaluating birds in dystocia, the examiner should assess the quality and integrity of the shell (Figure 31.39), the presence of concurrent lesions, and whether the egg is in oviposition (caudal in coelom with small end pointing caudally). The absence of polyostotic hyperostosis (Figure 31.40) in an egg-laying bird may indicate a hypocalcemic state. An egg that is cranial in the coelom or far from a normal oviposition location may indicate an ectopic egg. An egg that shows fluid lines on fluoroscopic examination (the bird needs to be standing to visualize fluid lines), indicates chronicity and putrefaction of the egg.

Coelomic ultrasound is valuable to diagnose reproductive disorders and may allow the assessment of the oviduct, an unshelled egg, the presence of coelomic fluid, ovarian cysts, and follicles.

Investigation of Osteomyelosclerosis

One indication of female reproductive activity is the presence of polyostotic hyperostosis. Polyostotic hyperostosis is characterized by increased opacity of long bones, especially pneumatized bone medulla, and occasionally vertebrae (Figure 31.40). The increased opacity is usually bilateral but may be asymmetrical in some cases. This should be differentiated from osteomyelosclerosis, which is an increased bone opacity associated with pathologic conditions in non-laying birds (Figure 31.44) [52].

Investigation of Lameness

Orthopedic lesions require emergency treatment including reduction and immobilization with a bandage, or cage rest

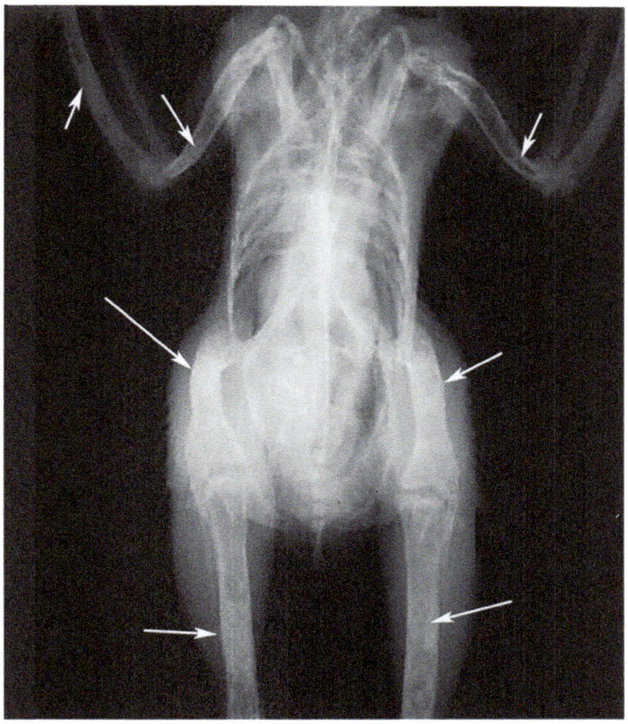

Figure 31.44 Ventro-dorsal view of a domestic chicken presented with avian leukosis: osteomyelosclerosis is noted on the long bones (white arrows). *Source:* Courtesy of the University of Guelph.

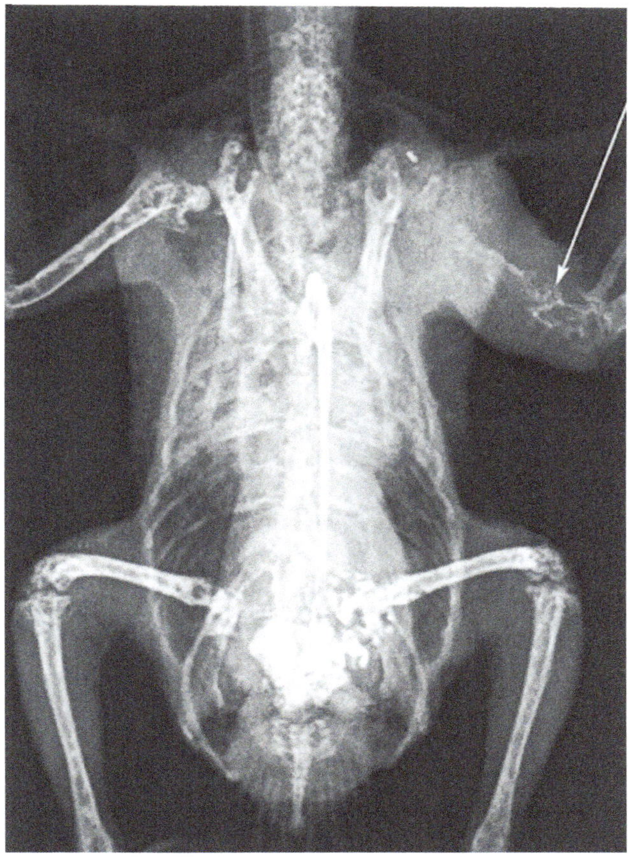

Figure 31.45 Pathologic fracture of the humerus (white arrow) in a lovebird (*Agapornis roseicollis*). *Source:* Courtesy of the Zoological Medicine Service, Université de Montréal.

and appropriate analgesia. Traumatic musculoskeletal injuries are discussed in the following paragraph. Lameness may also be associated with pathologic fractures (Figure 31.45) and soft tissue lesions. Diagnosis of orthopedic injuries through imaging techniques is a prerequisite for appropriate therapy. If no trauma is reported and abnormal bone density is suspected or if nutritional disease is expected based on history, great care is recommended during bird handling to avoid iatrogenic fractures; general anesthesia may be preferable during radiographic acquisition (Figure 31.46).

In birds, differential diagnoses for pelvic limb lameness include musculoskeletal lesions (Figures 31.47 and 31.48), tendinous and ligamentous lesions, and any cause of compression of the ischiatic nerve, including a renal or gonadal mass. Gonadal masses are particularly common in chickens. Renal masses are also very common in budgerigars [53]. These conditions associated with mass effects affecting nerves can also be investigated via radiographs.

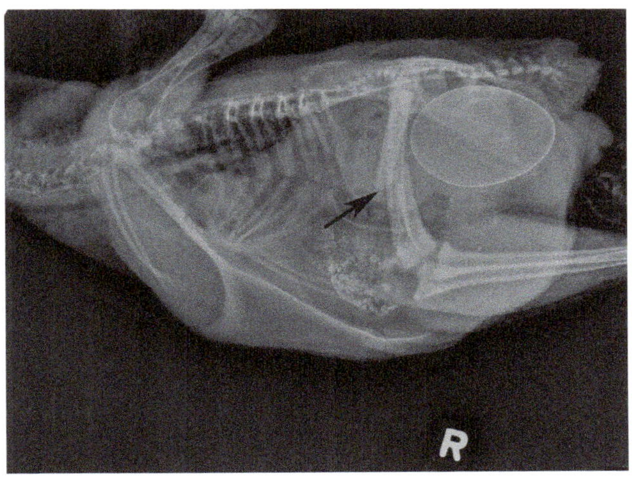

Figure 31.46 Femoral fracture (arrow) associated with chronic hypocalcemia in an egg-laying chicken. Note the abnormally radiolucent bone density of pneumatized bones in a reproductive female.

Investigation of Trauma and Self-Trauma

Polytraumatized patients require whole body radiographs (Figure 31.49) to enable appropriate therapy, including analgesia and prognosis determination. For instance, ver-

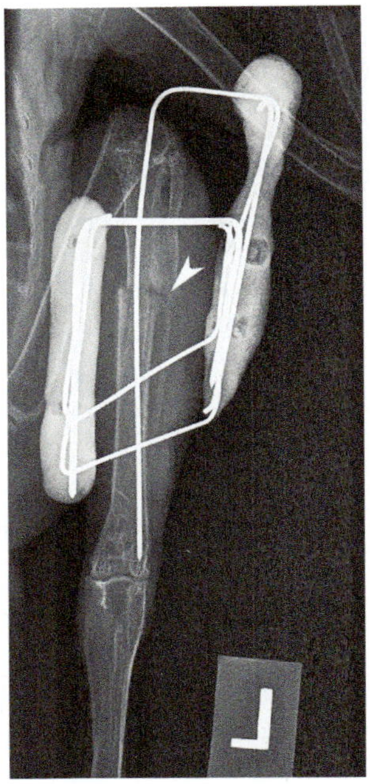

Figure 31.47 Dorso-plantar view of the left tibiotarsus in an grey parrot (*Psittacus erithacus*): a tie-in has been placed to stabilize a closed transverse fracture of the proximal third of the left tibiotarsus and fibula (arrowhead). Epoxy putty has been used to stabilize K-wire pins of the type 2 external fixator (Fast-fix, Kaohsiung City, Taiwan). *Source:* Courtesy of the Zoological Medicine Service, Université de Montréal.

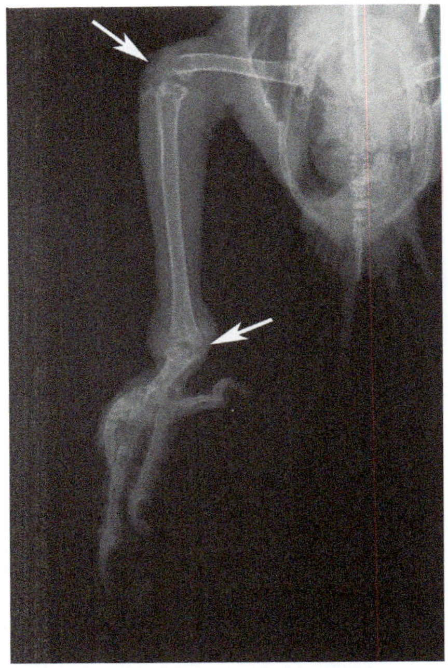

Figure 31.48 Dorso-plantar view of the left hindlimb in a Hispaniolan Amazon parrot (*Amazona ventralis*): chronic severe osteoarthritis of the stifle and intertarsal joints (arrows).

tebral fractures require prompt immobilization. Coracoid fractures are rarely diagnosed without radiographs, except in thin birds, and may be managed with cage rest [54]. It is important to add a marker to the radiographs to allow accurate measurement of implants prior to orthopedic surgery. Fracture of the ocular sclera may be treated conservatively or may require enucleation. Neurologic lesions secondary to trauma may also be detected radiographically: in case of brachial plexus avulsion, pectoral muscles will be asymmetric after a few days.

Feather destructive behavior and self-mutilation can be a manifestation of pain. In this context, investigation of the etiology of the problem should be performed to best determine the treatment plan (Figures 31.50 and 31.51).

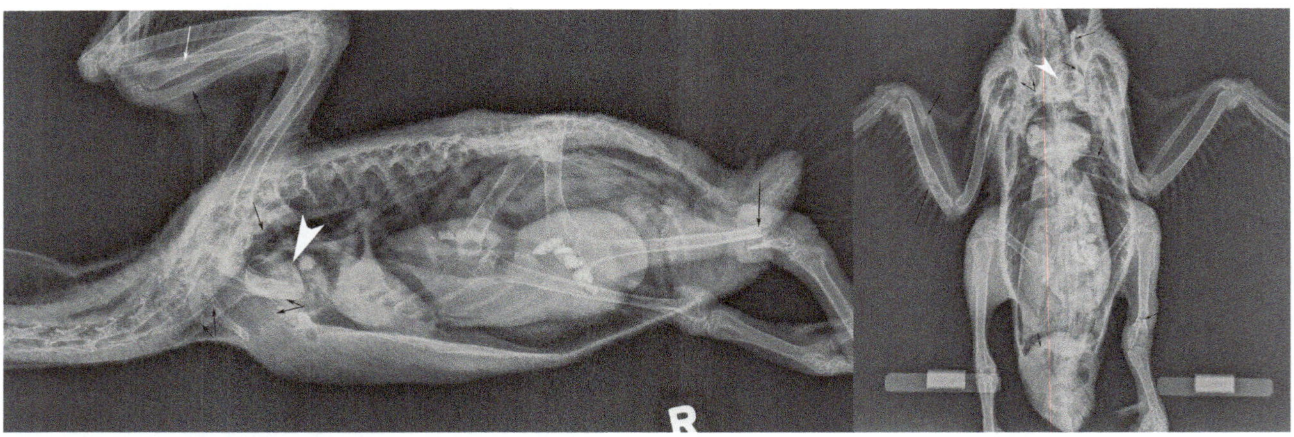

Figure 31.49 Polytraumatized male Pekin duck (*Anas platyrhynchos domesticus*) presented for open distal left tibiotarsal fracture. On radiographs, closed fractures of the left clavicle, left coracoid, right scapula, right distal radius, right proximal ulna, right pelvic bone, and ribs are also detected (black arrows). The syringeal drum is characteristic of male ducks (white arrowhead). All fractures healed successfully. *Source:* Courtesy of the Companion Avian and Exotic Pet Medicine Service, University of California, Davis.

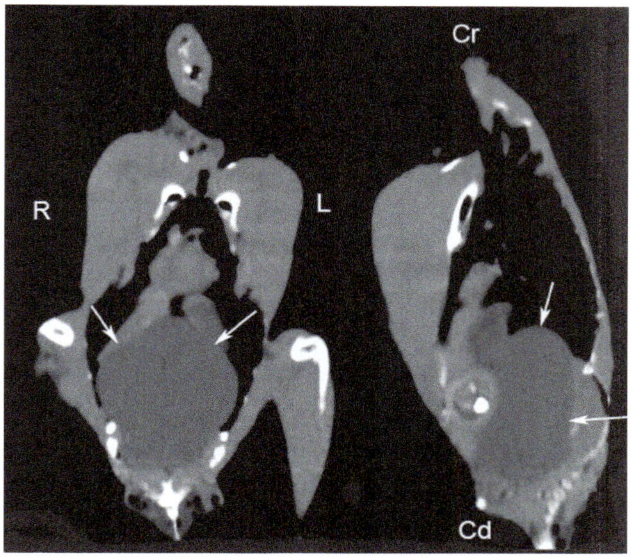

Figure 31.50 Sagittal CT-scan view (left part of the figure) and longitudinal CT-scan view (right part of the figure) (Cr: cranial, Cd: caudal, R: right, L: left) in a mitred parakeet (*Psittacara mitrata*) presented with feather destructive behavior dorsally to the synsacrum (arrowhead) associated with a large coelomic mass (arrows). *Source:* Courtesy of the Zoological Medicine Service, Université de Montréal.

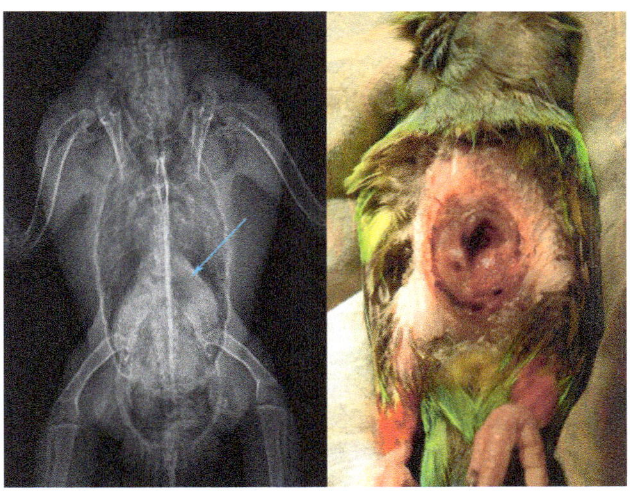

Figure 31.51 Self-mutilation mutilation of the pectoral muscles in a Nanday conure (*Aratinga nenday*) associated with a proventriculitis. Auto mutilation ventral to the area of the proventriculus is noted on radiographs (air visible in the wound). *Source:* Courtesy of the Zoological Medicine Service, Université de Montréal.

Investigation of Contagious Diseases

In some instances, radiographs may be obtained to determine whether a bird is likely to be a contagion risk for other patients and should therefore be isolated with special

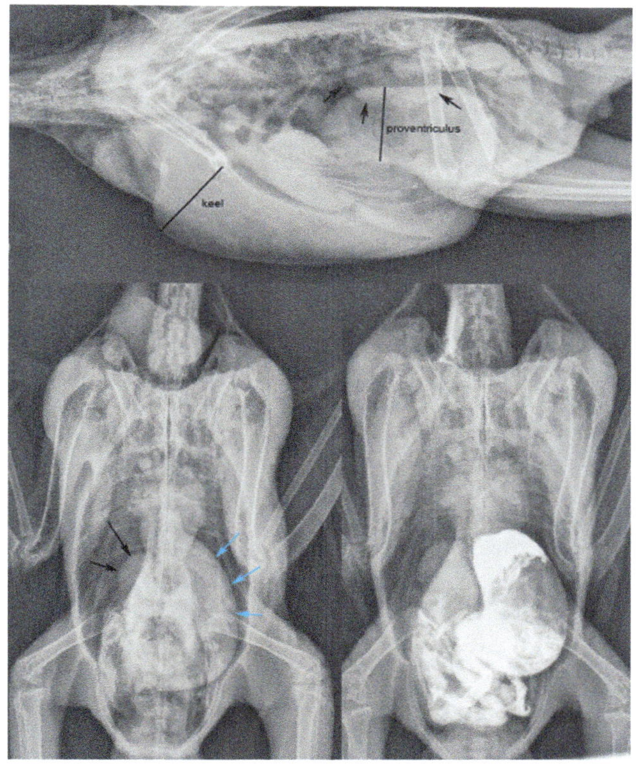

Figure 31.52 Right lateral and ventro-dorsal radiographic views of a blue and gold macaw (*Ara ararauna*) presenting for regurgitation. The ventro-dorsal view on the right was obtained after administration of 15 ml/kg of barium sulphate mixed 1:1 with feeding formula. The proventriclus to keel ratio is severely increased on the lateral view, at 0.95. Birds presenting with proventricular dilatation should be kept isolated as differential diagnoses include bornavirus infection. In this case, the cause of proventricular distension (blue arrows) was a coelomitis associated with a neoplasm of the cranial division of the right kidney (black arrows). *Source:* Courtesy of the Companion Avian and Exotic Pet Medicine Service, University of California, Davis.

biosecurity measures pending more specific tests, such as polymerase chain reaction (PCR) or histopathology available during regular hours. This is the case for patients presenting with maldigestion and potentially infected with avian bornavirus: radiographs typically allow screening for proventricular dilatation. In case of proventricular dilatation characterized by a proventriculus:keel ratio above 0.48 (Figure 31.52), differential diagnoses include proventricular dilatation disease, but also heavy metal intoxication, coelomitis, fungal, bacterial, or parasitic proventriculitis, gastrointestinal obstruction or narrowing, digestive neoplasm, diffuse inflammatory disease, or hypocalcemia. Therefore, patients presented with proventricular dilatation are not necessarily contagious, but they should be isolated from other birds while awaiting additional test results. Similarly, suspicion of chlamydiosis may be increased if hepatomegaly, splenomegaly and air sac lines are detected

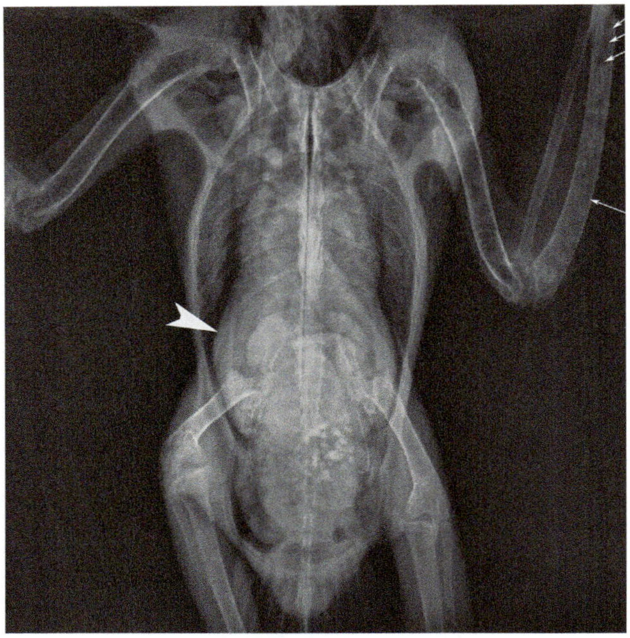

Figure 31.53 Hepatomegaly (arrowhead) and osteolytic lesions (white arrows), suggestive of mycobacteriosis in a blue and gold macaw (*Ara ararauna*).

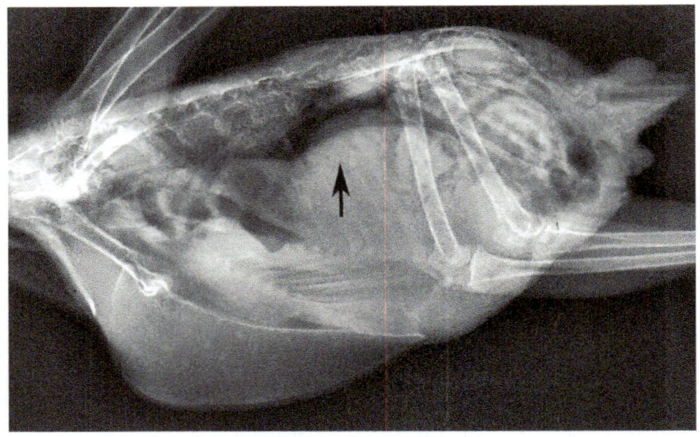

Figure 31.54 Splenomegaly (arrow) in an Eclectus parrot (*Eclectus roratus*) with coxiellosis. Note the large proventriculus that is considered within normal limits for this species. *Source:* Courtesy of the University of Guelph.

radiographically [55, 56]. Birds affected by other infectious diseases, such as mycobacteriosis or coxiellosis, may also present with splenomegaly (Figures 31.53 and 31.54) [57]. These birds should be isolated from conspecifics and biosecurity measures should be taken to decrease zoonotic potential.

Conclusion

Diagnostic imaging techniques are an important management tool for evaluating avian emergency presentations. All attempts should be made to minimize patient stress during image acquisition, especially in unstable patients.

Acknowledgments

We would like to thank the faculty, residents, interns and technicians who contributed to these cases, especially Drs. Marion Desmarchelier, Noémie Summa, and Molly Gleeson.

References

1 Mans, C., Sanchez-Migallon Guzman, D., Lahner, L. et al. (2012). Sedation and physiologic response to manual restraint after intranasal administration of midazolam in Hispaniolan Amazon parrots (*Amazona ventralis*). *J. Avian Med. Surg.* 26 (3): 130–139.

2 Guzman, D.S., Drazenovich, T.L., Olsen, G.H. et al. (2013). Evaluation of thermal antinociceptive effects after intramuscular administration of hydromorphone hydrochloride to American kestrels (*Falco sparverius*). *Am. J. Vet. Res.* 74 (6): 817–822.

3 Gustavsen, K.A., Guzman, D.S., Knych, H.K. et al. (2014). Pharmacokinetics of buprenorphine hydrochloride following intramuscular and intravenous administration to American kestrels (*Falco sparverius*). *Am. J. Vet. Res.* 75 (8): 711–715.

4 Helmer, P. (2006). Chapter 25: Advances in diagnostic imaging. In: *Clinical Avian Medicine*, 2e (eds. G. Harrison and T. Lightfoot), 653–659. Palm Beach, FL: Spix Publishing.

5 Herpel A-M, Visser M, de Swarte M, Bellah J. Radiographic evaluation of the thoracic girdle in raptors using a novel caudoventral 45° craniodorsal radiographic view. In: ExoticsCon conference. 2015. p. 25.

6 Beaufrère, H., Nevarez, J., Taylor, W.M. et al. (2010). Fluoroscopic study of the normal gastrointestinal motility and measurements in the Hispaniolan Amazon parrot (*Amazona ventralis*). *Vet. Radiol. Ultrasound* 51 (4): 441–446.

7 Vink-Nooteboom, M., Lumeij, J.T., and Wolvekamp, W.T.C. (2003). Passage through the gastrointestinal tract in six healthy amazon parrots (*Amazona aestiva*). *Vet. Radiol.* 44 (1): 43–48.

8 Kubiak, M. and Forbes, N.A. (2012). Fluoroscopic evaluation of gastrointestinal transit time in African Grey parrots. *Vet. Rec.* 171 (22): 563–564.

9 Silverman S, Tell LA. Radiology of Birds. An Atlas of Normal Anatomy and Positioning. 2010. 299 p.

10 Bonin, G., Lauer, S.K., Guzman, D. et al. (2009). Radiographic evaluation of perching-joint angles in cockatiels (*Nymphicus hollandicus*), Hispaniolan Amazon parrots (*Amazona ventralis*), and barred owls (*Strix varia*). *J. Avian Med. Surg.* 23 (2): 91–100.

11 Velayati, M., Mirshahi, A., Razmyar, J., and Azizzadeh, M. (2015). Radiographic reference limits for cardiac width of budgerigars (*Melopsittacus undulatus*). *J. Zoo Wildl. Med.* 46 (1): 34–38.

12 Caliendo, V., Middelton, R., and Raghav, R. (2016). Radiographic measurement of internal organs in gyr falcons (*Falco rusticolus*) and gyr peregrine hybrids (*Falco rusticolus* × *Falco peregrinus*). J. Exot. Pet Med. 25 (1): 13–17.

13 Dennison, S.E., Paul-Murphy, J.R., and Adams, W.M. (2008). Radiographic determination of proventricular diameter in psittacine birds. *J. Am. Vet. Med. Assoc.* 232 (5): 709–714.

14 Dennison, S.E., Paul-Murphy, J.R., Yandell, B.S., and Adams, W.M. (2010). Effect of anesthesia, positioning, time, and feeding on the proventriculus: keel ratio of clinically healthy parrots. *Vet. Radiol. Ultrasound* 51 (2): 141–144.

15 Dennison, S.E., Adams, W.M., Johnson, P.J. et al. (2009). Prognostic accuracy of the proventriculus: keel ratio for short-term survival in psittacines with proventricular disease. *Vet. Radiol. Ultrasound* 50 (5): 483–486.

16 McMillan, M. (1994). Chapter 12: Imaging techniques. In: *Avian Medicine: Principles and Application* (eds. B.W. Ritchie and G.J.H. Harrison), 246–326. Lake Worth, FL: Wingers Publishing, Inc.

17 Evans M. Avian radiography. In: British small animal veterinary congress proceedings. Birmingham; 2008.

18 Boyer CM. Etude rétrospective de la taille de la rate sur des radiographies chez le Gris du Gabon (*Psittacus erithacus*) [Internet]. Faculté de médecine de Créteil; 2013. Available from: theses.vet-alfort.fr/telecharger.php?id=1672

19 Samour, J. and Naldo, J. (2007). *Anatomical and Clinical Radiology of Birds of Prey*. Abu Dhabi, United Arab Emirates: Saunders Elsevier. 279p.

20 Lumeij, J.T., Shaik, M.A.S., and Ali, M. (2011). Radiographic reference limits for cardiac width in peregrine falcons (*Falco peregrinus*). *J. Am. Vet. Med. Assoc.* 238 (11): 1459–1463.

21 Nordberg, C., O'Brien, R.T., Paul-Murphy, J., and Hawley, B. (2000). Ultrasound examination and guided fine-needle aspiration of the liver in Amazon parrots (*Amazona* species). *J. Avian Med. Surg.* 14 (3): 180–184.

22 Locke, S., Shimp, J., Johnson, D., and Pridgen, T.J. (2020). Radiographic reference intervals of cardiac silhouette width in the bald eagle (*Haliaeetus leucocephalus*). *J. Av. Med. Surg.* 34 (3): 260–267.

23 Beaufrère, H., Pariaut, R., Rodriguez, D., and Tully, T.N. (2010). Avian vascular imaging: a review. *J. Avian Med. Surg.* 24 (3): 174–184.

24 King, A. and McLelland, J. (1984). Chapter 10: Urinary system. In: *Birds, Their Structure and Function*, 2e (eds. A. King and J. McLelland), 175–186. Philadelphia, PA: Baillière Tindall.

25 Dutton, C. (2003). Chapter 30: Coraciiformes. In: *Zoo and Wild Animal Medicine*, 5e (eds. M. Fowler and R. Miller), 254–260. St. Louis, MO: Saunders.

26 Krautwald-Junghanns, M.-E. and Pees, M. (2011). Ultrasonographic examination. In: *Diagnostic Imaging of Exotic Pets: Birds, Small Mammals, Reptiles* (eds. M.-E. Krautwald-Junghanns, M. Pees, S. Reese and T.N. Tully), 36–53. Vet S. Hannover.

27 Hofbauer, H. and Krautwald-Junghanns, M.E. (1998). Transcutaneous ultrasonography of the avian urogenital tract. *Vet. Radiol. Ultrasound* 40 (1): 58–64.

28 Barua, A., Bitterman, P., Bahr, J.M. et al. (2010). Detection of tumor associated neoangiogenesis by Doppler ultrasound during early stage ovarian cancer in laying hens: a preclinical model of human spontaneous ovarian cancer. *J. Ultrasound Med.* 29 (2): 173–182.

29 Pees, M., Straub, J., and Krautwald-Junghanns, M.-E. (2004). Echocardiographic examinations of 60 African grey parrots and 30 other psittacines. *Vet. Rec.* 155: 73–77.

30 Pees, M. and Krautwald-Junghanns, M.E. (2005). Avian echocardiography. *Semin. Avian Exot. Pet Med.* 14: 14–21.

31 Beaufrère, H., Pariaut, R., Rodriguez, D. et al. (2012). Comparison of transcoelomic, contrast transcoelomic, and transesophageal echocardiography in anesthetized red-tailed hawks (*Buteo jamaicensis*). *Am. J. Vet. Res.* 73 (10): 1560–1568.

32 Schulz M. Morphologische und funktionelle Messungen am Herzen von Brieftauben (*Columba livia* forma *domestica*) mit Hilfe der Schnittbildechokardiographie. [Internet] Vet Med Dissertation, 1995.

33 Martinez-Lemus, L.A., Miller, M.W., Jeffrey, J.S., and Odom, T.W. (1998). Echocardiographic evaluation of cardiac structure and function in broiler and leghorn chickens. *Poult. Sci.* 77: 1045–1050.

34 Pees, M., Straub, J., and Krautwald-Junghanns, M.-E. (2004). Echocardiographic examinations of 60 African grey parrots and 30 other psittacine birds. *Vet. Rec.* 155: 73–76.

35 Carrani, F., Gelli, D., and Salvadori, M. (2003). A preliminary echocardiographic initial approach to diastolic and systolic function in medium and large

parrots. In: *European Association of Avian Veterinarians Proceedings*, 145–149.

36 Grosset, C., Guzman, D., Keating, M.K. et al. (2014). Central vestibular disease in a blue and gold macaw (*Ara ararauna*) with cerebral infarction and hemorrhage. *J. Avian Med. Surg.* 28 (2): 132–142.

37 van Zeeland, Y., Schoemaker, N., and Hsu, E. (2016). Advances in diagnostic imaging. In: *Current Therapy in Avian Medicine and Surgery* (ed. B. Speer), 531–549. St. Louis, MO: Elsevier.

38 Pye, G.W., Bennett, R.A., Newell, S.M. et al. (2000). Magnetic resonance imaging in psittacine birds with chronic sinusitis. *J. Avian Med. Surg.* 14 (4): 243–256.

39 Kusmierczyk, J., Wall, C.R., Hoppes, S. et al. (2013). Comparison of computed tomographic images of birds obtained with sedation versus general anesthesia. *J. Exot. Pet Med.* 22 (3): 251–257.

40 Malka, S., Hawkins, M.G., Jones, J.H. et al. (2009). Effect of body position on respiratory system volumes in anesthetized red-tailed hawks (*Buteo jamaicensis*) as measured via computed tomography. *Am. J. Vet. Res.* 70 (9): 1155–1160.

41 Jarvis E. Avian Brain [Internet]. 2012 [cited 2016 Feb 7]. Available from: http://www.avianbrain.org/atlases.html

42 Petnehazy, O., Benczik, J., Takacs, I. et al. (2012). Computed tomographical (CT) anatomy of the thoracoabdominal cavity of the male Turkey (*Meleagris gallopavo*). *J. Vet. Med. Ser. C Anat. Histol. Embryol.* 41 (1): 12–20.

43 King, A. and McLelland, J. (1984). Chapter 15: Nervous system. In: *Birds, Their Structure and Function*, 2e (eds. A. King and J. McLelland), 237–283. Philadelphia, PA: Baillière Tindall.

44 Ernst, S., Goggin, J.M., Biller, D.S. et al. (1998). Comparison of iohexol and barium sulfate as gastrointestinal contrast media in mid-sized psittacine birds. *J. Avian Med. Surg.* 12 (1): 16–20.

45 Redig, P. and Arent, L. (2008). Raptor toxicology. *Vet. Clin. North Am. Exot. Anim. Pract.* 11 (2): 261–282.

46 DeFrancisco, N., Ruiz Troya, J., and Agüera, E. (2003). Lead and lead toxicity in domestic and free-living birds. *Avian Pathol.* 32 (1): 3–13.

47 Wismer, T. (2016). Chapter 18: Advancements in diagnosis and management of toxicologic problems. In: *Current Therapy in Avian Medicine and Surgery* (ed. B. Speer), 589–599. Elsevier.

48 Van Zeeland, Y.R.A., Schoemaker, N.J., and Van Sluijs, F.J. (2014). Incisional colopexy for treatment of chronic, recurrent colocloacal prolapse in a sulphur-crested cockatoo (*Cacatua galerita*). *Vet. Surg.* 43 (7): 882–887.

49 Beaufrère, H., Nevarez, J., and Tully, T.N. (2010). Cloacolith in a blue-fronted Amazon parrot (*Amazona aestiva*). *J. Avian Med. Surg.* 24 (2): 142–145.

50 Curtiss, J.B., Leone, A.M., Wellehan, J.F.X. et al. (2015). Renal and cloacal cryptosporidiosis (*Cryptosporidium* avian genotype V) in a Major Mitchell's cockatoo (*Lophochroa leadbeateri*). *J. Zoo Wildl. Med.* 46 (4): 934–937.

51 de Matos, R. (2015). Ultrasound examination of the reproductive tract of domestic chickens in health and disease. In: *2nd ICARE (International conference on avian herpetological and exotic mammal medicine) Proceedings*. Paris, 272.

52 Bowles, H.L. (2006). Chapter 18: Evaluating and treating the reproductive system. In: *Clinical Avian Medicine: Principles and Applications*, 2e (eds. G. Harrison and T. Lightfoot), 519–539. Palm Beach, FL: Spix Publishing.

53 Simova-Curd, S., Nitzl, D., Mayer, J., and Hatt, J.-M. (2006). Clinical approach to renal neoplasia in budgerigars (*Melopsittacus undulatus*). *J. Small Anim. Pract.* 47: 504–511.

54 Scheelings, T.F. (2014). Conservative treatment coracoid fractures in wild birds: a comparison of surgical repair versus conservative treatment. *J. Avian Med. Surg.* 28 (4): 304–308.

55 Fowler, M.E., Schulz, T., Ardans, A. et al. (1990). Chlamydiosis in captive raptors. *Avian Dis.* 34 (3): 657–662.

56 Johns, J.L., Luff, J.A., Shooshtari, M.P. et al. (2009). What is your diagnosis? Blood smear from an injured red-tailed hawk. *Vet. Clin. Pathol.* 38 (2): 247–252.

57 Woc-colburn, A.M., Garner, M.M., Bradway, D. et al. (2008). Fatal coxiellosis in Swainson's blue mountain rainbow lorikeets (*Trichoglossus haematodus moluccanus*). *Vet. Pathol.* 45: 247–254.

32

Clinical Pathology

Hugues Beaufrère[1] and Claire Vergneau-Grosset[2]

[1]*Department of Medicine and Epidemiology, School of Veterinary Medicine, University of California-Davis, Davis, California, USA*
[2]*Faculté de médecine vétérinaire, Université de Montréal, Saint-Hyacinthe, Quebec, Canada*

CONTENTS

Hematology

Preliminary Concepts

The complete blood cell count (CBC) is often the first line of diagnostic tests performed in clinical situations and is regularly used for health assessment and in quarantine protocols in many bird species. Indeed, the CBC has been shown to be one of the most sensitive tests to detect illnesses in avian patients [1].

To minimize artifacts, blood collection should be performed quickly after the initiation of manual restraint and using adequate techniques. Venipuncture is described in detail in "Chapter 25: Catheterization and Venipuncture". The anticoagulant EDTA is recommended in birds for the CBC as it results in less artifacts, better temporal effect, and does not lead to thrombocyte aggregations on blood smear evaluation [2, 3]. In addition, heparin may lead to staining and cytological artifacts and does not prevent thrombocyte aggregation [4, 5]. Heparin anticoagulant should be used in species reported to hemolyze in EDTA such as ostriches, crowned cranes, and some species of the family Corvidae, Coracidae, Anatidae, Rallidae, Cracidae, Gruidae, Struthionidae, Sturnidae, and Megapodidae [4, 5]. Overall, blood cell counts have been shown to be similar between heparin and EDTA in Amazon parrots [6]. The CBC should be performed within 12–24 hours of blood collection to minimize hemolysis [2].

Since all avian blood cells are nucleated, most of the techniques employed to perform an avian CBC are manual, which introduces a significant amount of analytical variability and uncertainty to, notably, white blood cell (WBC) counts [3]. While some advanced flow cytometry protocols have shown promise in birds to automatize the hemogram, they are far from being applicable to a wider use in clinics [7–10]. No commercially available automated blood analyzers have shown to produce reliable CBC in birds (other than chickens) to date to the authors' knowledge. Other limitations in avian hematology include the scarcity of published and correctly determined reference intervals, the lack of automation and standardization, the significant biological variability that can be encountered, and the variability of the hematologic response to disease in the diverse avian species [3]. In order to minimize laboratory errors, one is encouraged to submit to reputable veterinary laboratories performing avian CBC and decrease the generation of in-house avian hematology, whenever practical. To minimize interpretation errors, one is encouraged to keep in mind the high variability inherent to manual cell count, multiple sources of biological variability, extrapolation, and carefully consider published species-specific reference intervals.

Exotic Animal Emergency and Critical Care Medicine, First Edition. Edited by Jennifer E. Graham, Grayson A. Doss and Hugues Beaufrère.

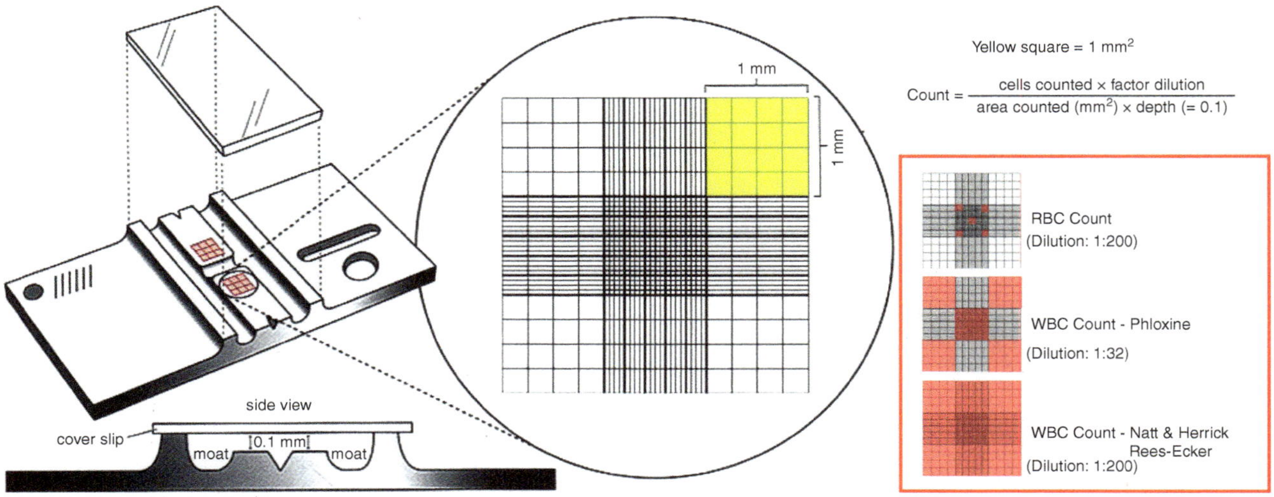

Figure 32.1 Hemacytometer and a close-up view of the counting areas as seen under the microscope. The red insert box shows the different counting areas depending on the technique with the dilution factor. The general formula for hemocytometer-based cell count is also given. (*Source:* Adapted from Hippel [13]. © 2007, Elsevier.)

RBC Assessment

The packed cell volume (PCV) and hemoglobin concentration are obtained using similar techniques as in other companion animals. The PCV is performed using a microhematocrit tube and centrifugation. Hemoglobin concentration can be obtained using either the cyanmethemoglobin method or using a hemoglobinometer such as the HemoCue Hb® using a spectrophotometric azide-methemoglobin method [11]. A study in birds has shown that there was a linear relationship between the hemoglobin and the PCV in most birds of $Hb = 0.3 \times PCV$. Only flamingos departed from this general relationship [12].

For the red blood cell count (RBC), different techniques are available. Since RBC outnumber WBCs by a factor 1000, the RBC count can be obtained using standard automated laboratory instruments. Manual RBC is more commonly performed in birds and consists of counting stained or unstained RBCs in a hemocytometer (Figure 32.1). The blood is typically diluted by a factor of 200. The Natt and Herrick solution is the most commonly employed stain for the RBC. The technique is described below [3]:

Using a micropipette, mix 10 µl of blood with 2 ml of Natt and Herrick solution (Vetlab supply, Palmetto Bay, FL, USA) to obtain a 1:200 dilution. The stain is based on methyl violet 2B. Incubate for five minutes at room temperature on a rocker. Transfer on hemocytometer and allow five minutes for cell settling in chambers. Read at the 40× objective (Figure 32.2). All erythrocytes are counted in five small squares (four corner and the central small square = 5/25 small squares) of the central square millimeter of one chamber using the L rule (of all the cells touching the border of a square, only the cells touching the left and bottom borders are included).

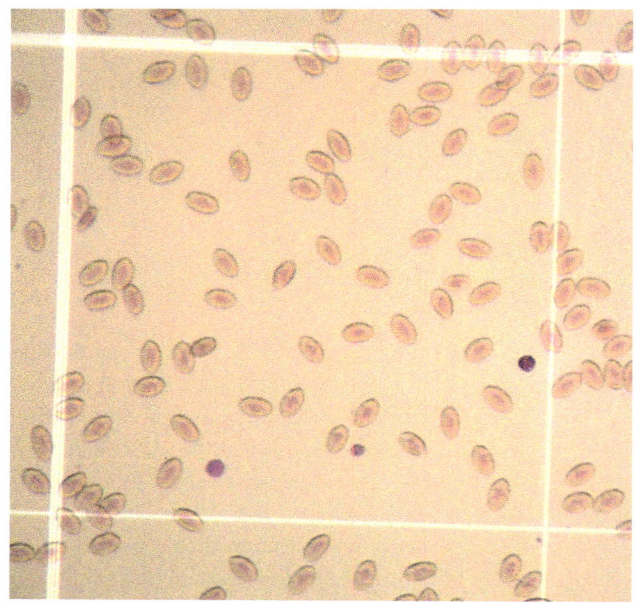

Figure 32.2 Natt and Herrick method. The red blood cells are easily visualized and counted. The two dark purple staining cells are white blood cells. The smaller lighter cell is a thrombocyte and should not be counted as a WBC. It may be difficult to differentiate small lymphocytes from thrombocytes with this technique. (*Source:* Beaufrere and Ammersbach [3], 2016. Reproduced with permission of Elsevier.)

$$\text{Formula}: \text{RBC}\left(\times 10^{12} / \text{l or} \times 10^{6} / \mu l\right) = \text{N} * 200 * 5 / \left(0.1 * 1000000\right)$$

$$\text{Simplified formula: RBC } \left(\times 10^{12}/\text{l or} \times 10^{6}/\mu l\right) = N/100$$

RBC indices may then be calculated and may assist in the characterization of anemia. The formulas are the same as in mammals:

$$\text{MCV}(\text{fl}) = \text{PCV} * 10/\text{RBC}$$

$$\text{MCH}(\text{pg}) = \text{Hb} * 10/\text{RBC}$$

$$\text{MCHC}(\text{g/l}) = \text{Hb} * 100/\text{PCV}$$

While the PCV is quite homogeneous among avian species, RBC and RBC indices tend to vary significantly from one species to another.

Polychromasia and the amount of polychromatophils are usually reported qualitatively or semi-quantitatively (number per high power fields). Reticulocytes may be obtained using new methylene blue stain and their numbers are highly correlated to polychromatophil numbers [14].

WBC Assessment

The avian white blood cell count (WBC) is manually determined. Since all avian blood cells are nucleated, automated analyzers designed for mammalian cells cannot reliably distinguish leukocytes from erythrocytes and thrombocytes for various reasons [3]. Overall, specific cellular differences and species variation make the development of species-specific protocols applicable to the majority of patients difficult.

As a result, the hematologic techniques used in birds to obtain a WBC have changed minimally for over 50 years [3, 15, 16]. Indeed, the WBC is still obtained using hemocytometers and various stains including phloxine B, Natt and Herrick solution, Rees-Ecker solution, eosin, or other colorants; and the differential count is still obtained using a microscope and a human observer [3, 15–19]. Studies have shown that there may be significant disagreement between manual blood cell count techniques in birds [3].

First, blood smears should be performed using fresh blood (see following section). One of the easiest methods to obtain a WBC is the estimate from the smear. It may be particularly useful in an emergency to have a quick glance at the cellular inflammation. At 400 magnification (40× objective and 10× eyepiece), all leukocytes in 10 fields are counted in the monolayer area. Then the following formula is applied [3]:

$$\text{WBC}\left(\times 10^{9}/\text{l or} \times 10^{3}/\mu l\right) = N/10 * 1.5$$

The fields of view that are examined vary with the microscope, and formulas may have to be adapted to the specific microscope used. This may be accomplished by performing a small in-house study comparing with a quantitative method. The WBC count obtained from the smear is heavily influenced by blood smear technique and can only provide an estimate, as the leukocytes are not quantitated in a set volume of blood. In addition, since most leukocytes are present near the feather edge, the WBC obtained from the smear may be artificially altered. If many cells are lysed during the blood smear preparation, the WBC may be artificially decreased. Consequently, WBC estimates from the smear are likely the least reproducible and accurate techniques and may be subject to large intra and interobserver variability. Nevertheless, the differential count is performed on a stained blood smear. It is usually calculated based on 100 cells, but hematologic studies in various species have shown that by increasing the number of counted cells, there is an increase in the precision and accuracy of the technique [3, 20]. As the WBC is obtained from a monolayer area with a certain spread of the RBCs, it needs to be corrected in case of erythrocytosis or anemia using the following formula:

$$\text{WBC}_{\text{corrected}}: \text{WBC} * \text{PCV}/\text{PCV}_{\text{expected mean for the species}}$$

For more accurate counting methods, the indirect phloxine technique or the direct Natt and Herrick's method are most commonly employed. In an emergency situation, the eosin method (using the eosin stain diluted at 1:10 using distilled water, from a classically used quick stain such as J-322-3, Jorgensen Laboratories Inc. Loveland, Colorado, USA), which is almost identical to the phloxine-based method, may prove to be useful without access to phloxine B [17]. To obtain the WBC using the phloxine technique, 25 µl of blood is sampled using a micropipette and mixed with 775 µl of 0.1% phloxine B (Vetlab supply, Palmetto Bay, FL, USA) to obtain a 1:32 dilution. Incubate for five minutes at room temperature on a rocker. Transfer on hemocytometer and allow five minutes for cell settling in chambers. Read at the 10× objective. All red-staining cells are counted in five square millimeters (four corner and the central large squares) of both chambers using the L rule (see above). The phloxine only stains heterophils and eosinophils (Figure 32.3). The following formula, based on the differential cell count, is then applied [3]:

$$\text{Formula: WBC}\left(\times 10^{9}/\text{l or} \times 10^{3}/\mu l\right) = N * 32 * 100/\left(10 * 0.1 * 1000 * \text{Percentage}_{\text{heterophils+eosinophils}}\right)$$

$$\text{Simplified formula: WBC}\left(\times 10^{9}/\text{l or} \times 10^{3}/\mu l\right) = N * 3.2/\text{Percentage}_{\text{heterophils+eosinophils}}$$

Birds

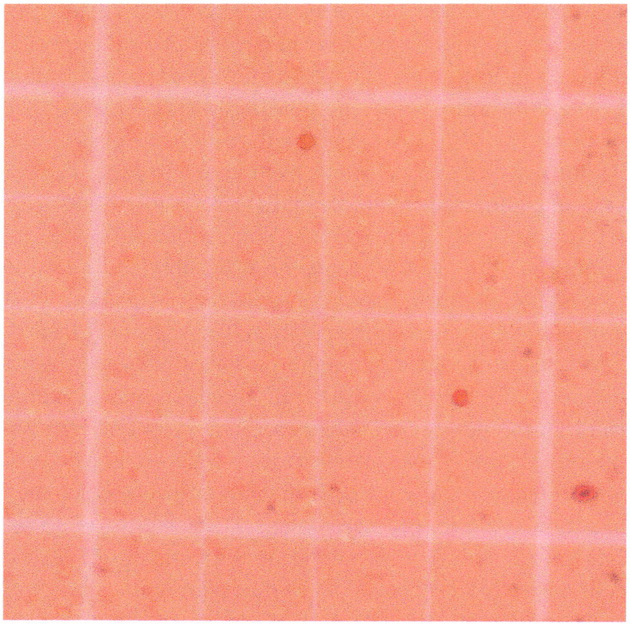

Figure 32.3 Phloxine B method for WBC determination. Three red-staining cells are positive. (*Source:* Beaufrere and Ammersbach [3], 2016. Reproduced with permission of Elsevier.)

To obtain the WBC using the Natt and Herrick's method, 10 μl of blood is sampled using a micropipette and mixed with 2 ml of Natt and Herrick solution (Vetlab supply, Palmetto Bay, FL, USA) to obtain a 1:200 dilution. Incubate for five minutes at room temperature on a rocker. Transfer to hemocytometer and allow five minutes for cell settling in chambers. Read at the 10× objective. All dark purple-staining cells are counted in 9 mm^2 (all large squares) of one chamber using the L rule (Figure 32.2). Caution must be taken not to count thrombocytes (they should not be larger than the RBC nucleus width unlike leukocytes). The following formula is then applied [3]:

$$\text{Formula}: \text{WBC}\left(\times 10^9 / \text{l or} \times 10^3 / \mu l\right) = N * 200 / \left(9 * 0.1 * 1000\right)$$

$$\text{Simplified Formula}: \text{WBC}\left(\times 10^9 / \text{l or} \times 10^3 / \mu l\right) = N / 4.5$$

Thrombocyte Assessment

Since thrombocytes tend to clump together, thrombocyte count is typically estimated from the blood smear in birds. The estimation is usually performed by comparison with the distribution of other cells and given for instance as the number of thrombocytes per 100 leukocytes or as a qualitative assessment (decreased, normal, and increased) [16]. An absolute count may also be obtained using the Natt and Herrick's method using the same dilution as for the leukocyte count.

Blood Smear and Differential Count

Blood smears are made to produce a monolayer of blood cells that is used for calculating estimated cell counts, providing differential cell counts, and assessing cell morphology. Blood smears are subject to numerous potential artifacts, depending on the techniques employed [3, 4, 16, 20–22]. Therefore care should be taken to perform good quality blood smears on a consistent basis. Avian cells are particularly prone to lysis (smudged cells), and this is more common in Psittaciformes than in other taxonomic orders [3, 4]. In order to decrease the percentage of smudged cells, different procedures have been implemented such as performing a squash preparation instead of a smear using the wedge technique, using the coverslip method with two coverslips, and adding bovine albumin to the blood prior to performing the smear [3, 4, 16]. Depending on the technique used, a large degree of variation may be seen between techniques, which may add additional uncertainty to the CBC or subsequently affect comparisons between labs using different techniques. The stains used, and the staining process may also affect cytologic assessment of the hemogram. Quick in-house stains are typically not as consistent and frequently result in low quality staining. They are also frequently contaminated with debris. Manual staining methods result in much variability, and automatic slide stainers are recommended (e.g. Hema-tek). Smears made with the coverslip techniques cannot be stained using an automated slide stainer, requiring manual staining methods instead. The experience and qualification of the observer (trained clinical pathologists) are also of paramount importance, and more experience and skill may decrease the variability in interpretation and the accuracy of hematologic diagnostics.

All avian blood cells are nucleated. Representative avian blood cells are depicted in Figure 32.4. Avian erythrocytes are elliptical, larger than mammalian erythrocytes, and have a lifespan of about one month. Polychromatophils are immature erythrocytes and correspond to reticulocytes. They appear more basophilic with a less condensed nucleus. In deeply regenerative anemia, earlier erythrocyte precursors may be seen in circulation such as rubricytes.

Thrombocytes are small with a condensed nucleus and colorless cytoplasm. One or several eosinophilic granules may be present in the cytoplasm. Thrombocytes are frequently differentiated from small lymphocytes based on their colorless cytoplasm. Erythrocytes lacking a nucleus are called erythroplastids.

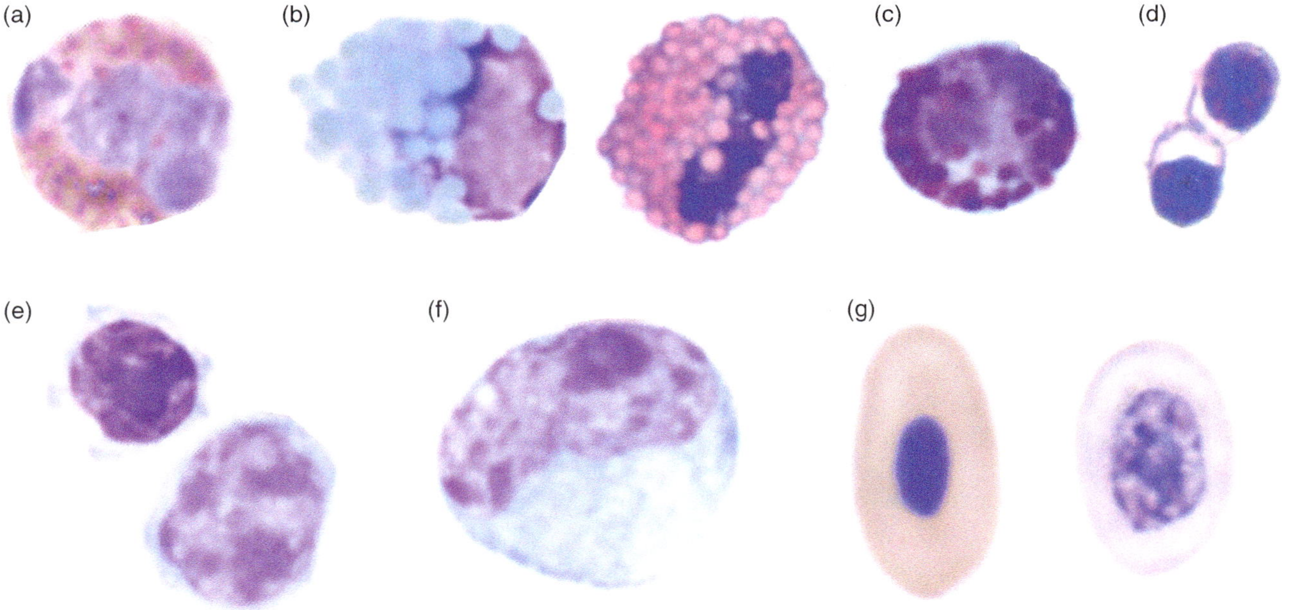

Figure 32.4 Morphology of white blood cells, representative cells stained with a modified Wright stain in an automated slide stainer. (a) heterophil; (b) blue eosinophil (parrot) and red eosinophil (raptors); (c) basophil; (d) 2 thrombocytes; (e) a small and a large lymphocyte; (f) monocyte; (g) erythrocyte and polychromatophil. (*Source:* Adapted from Beaufrere and Ammersbach [3], 2016. Reproduced with permission of Elsevier.)

Regarding WBCs, heterophils usually predominate (heterophilic species) but lymphocytes may also constitute most of the cells in lymphocytic species (ex: Passeriformes). Heterophils are equivalent to mammalian neutrophils but lack several enzymes including myeloperoxidase. Heterophils are large leukocytes with a colorless cytoplasm and numerous rod-shaped eosinophilic granules with a refractile center. The nucleus is usually segmented but the segmentation may be difficult to assess. Toxic heterophils may be encountered in inflammation and sepsis. Toxicity is usually graded from 1 to 3 (+ to +++) and is characterized by degranulation, the presence of primary granules, a more basophilic cytoplasm, and vacuolation of the cytoplasm. Band heterophils are immature heterophils characterized by a decreased degree of segmentation of the nucleus, which classically has a horse-shoe shape. The granules can partially obscure the nucleus; therefore, it can become difficult to identify mature from immature heterophils in birds. Eosinophils are characterized by multiple large round deeply eosinophilic granules and a basophilic cytoplasm. In some species, such as parrots, eosinophils can have basophilic granules instead. Basophils have deeply dark granules that frequently obscure the nucleus. Different sizes of lymphocytes may be seen on the blood smear. Lymphocytes have a weakly to moderately basophilic cytoplasm with a high nucleus-to-cytoplasm ratio and a round nucleus. The nuclear chromatin is usually heavily clumped. Reactive lymphocytes may be seen when antigenic stimulation occurs and are characterized by deeply basophilic cytoplasm and can occasionally have a pale perinuclear Golgi zone. Monocytes are typically the largest WBCs and have a bean-shaped nucleus with abundant lightly basophilic cytoplasm. A light-staining perinuclear zone is frequently present.

It may be difficult to differentiate some cells from others such as large lymphocytes from monocytes, or small lymphocytes from thrombocytes. Circulating abnormal cells are uncommonly seen but lymphocytic leukemia or leukemic lymphosarcoma would be the most common diagnosed neoplastic processes [23–27]. In chicken infected with retroviruses (avian leukosis, avian reticuloendotheliosis), a variety of leukemia types may been diagnosed. Blood parasites may be present depending on the species. They are commonly seen in wild birds, especially birds of prey and passerines. Most are non-pathogenic but an increase in parasitemia may be associated with certain disease states or an overall decline in general health status. The most commonly identified hematozoans are *Haemoproteus* spp., *Plasmodium* spp., and *Leucocytozoon* spp.. They are transmitted by blood-sucking insects. They all infect erythrocytes with *Leucocytozoon* gametocytes also infecting thrombocytes [16, 28]. *Haemoproteus* spp. and *Plasmodium* spp. look similar except that *Plasmodium* spp. tend to displace the nucleus, schizogony may be seen, other blood cells may be parasitized, and extra-erythrocytic stages may be observed [16]. *Leucocytozoon* spp. are large, basophilic, and completely distort the cells. In specific cases, hematozoans may be highly pathogenic such as *Plasmodium* spp. in penguins and Northern birds of prey species or *Leucocytozoon* spp. in Anatidae and Columbidae. Pathogenicity may also be witnessed in baby birds. Microfilariae may occasionally be seen on blood smears of wild birds and pathogenicity has been questioned in boreal owls (*Aegolius funereus*) [29].

Interpretation of the Hemogram

A substantial part of most clinical decisions is based on the interpretation of the hemogram. The magnitude of hematologic changes observed must be weighed against the multiple sources of variability inherent to avian hematologic techniques including biological variability (interindividual and intraindividual) and laboratory variability (preanalytical, analytical, and post-analytical). If these sources of variability are not considered, gross misinterpretation may ensue and confound diagnostic, therapeutic, and follow up assessments of patients. A high variability coupled with a low magnitude of changes in cell counts may substantially decrease the sensitivity and value of hematology in many circumstances.

When interpreting the avian hemogram, it is also important to compare to reference values. Reference intervals are the intervals including 95% of values in a healthy population. They are typically established using a sample of healthy representative birds and gold standard hematological techniques. However, significant flaws and imprecision have been identified in the generation of avian reference intervals [3, 30]. In addition, even properly determined reference intervals are dependent on laboratory and methodology. For this reason, reference intervals should be established by each laboratory, which is most often not available in avian species. Consequently, the avian clinicians must acknowledge that published reference intervals only constitute rough estimates of hematological values and that their sensitivity to detect abnormalities may be low. When reference intervals are not available for a given species, extrapolation must be performed carefully taking into consideration phylogenetic and ecologic relationships to the target species [3]. Common physiological effects must also be taken into consideration. Stress may induce a mild lymphopenia, heterophilia, and increased H : L ratio [3]. A mild leukocytosis (most birds) or mild leukopenia (passerines) may also be seen. Reproductively active female birds may show a mild anemia and leukocytosis [3, 31]. Typical reference values for birds are given in Table 32.1.

Serial sampling to obtain consecutive hematological values may also be performed to identify trends toward pathophysiological states, dynamic hematological responses to disease, or response to treatment. In the absence of reference values, this strategy may prove to be clinically valuable. Significant changes between consecutive measurements are called reference change value or critical differences. Considering the high biological and laboratory variability associated with avian hematology, critical differences of 50–100% have been proposed [3]. These differences may appear large, but some hematological variables such as the WBC appear to show greater variation in birds than other analytes such as the PCV (with critical differences expected to be around 14% in birds). It is also true that these variations may mask changes attributed to disease effects and dynamics and in turn lower the sensitivity of the avian CBC. Therefore, blood counts must differ greatly from reference limits to have diagnostic significance.

Also, while the numbers are useful, it must be realized that cell morphology on the blood smear may provide tremendous information such as the presence of a left shift, erythrocyte regeneration, cell toxicity, the presence of blood parasites, and other cytological changes. In any case, once a diagnosis is obtained, initial hematologic values can be used for follow-up. It should also be recognized that, by definition, 2.5% of the normal population will have higher values and 2.5% lower values than the reference intervals.

Selected differential diagnoses for common hematological abnormalities are given in Table 32.2.

Anemias are common in birds. Regeneration may be assessed based on polychromatophil or reticulocyte numbers. The diagnostic approach is similar than in mammals. Some birds such as chickens have a lower PCV than most other birds. In case of a regenerative anemia, causes of hemorrhage and hemolysis should be investigated through a complete diagnostic work up including diagnostic imaging, fecal occult blood test, screening for hematuria (using a urinary dipstick), and a biochemistry profile. Once regeneration is underway, its rate can be astonishing in birds and they can regenerate to reach a normal PCV in just a few days [38]. Anemia of chronic disease is fairly common in birds and is characterized by a mild to moderate non-regenerative anemia. Nutritional deficiencies may also cause chronic non-regenerative anemia [39]. Lead and zinc poisoning may cause non-regenerative anemia by dyserythropoiesis [40]. While lead toxicosis is common in birds, basophilic stippling of the erythrocyte cytoplasm is not, unlike mammals [40]. Due to the shorter lifespan of avian RBCs, depression anemia and anemia of chronic disease develop more quickly than in mammals [16]. Immune-mediated hemolytic anemia is rare in birds and only one case has been reported in the peer-reviewed literature in an Eclectus parrot (*Eclectus roratus*) [41]. In this bird, autoagglutination and large numbers of erythroplastids were observed. Severe anemia in conjunction with pancytopenia is a hallmark of viral diseases, in particular psittacine circovirus in susceptible species, especially grey parrots

Table 32.1 Typical reference values for selected clinical pathologic analytes in birds.[a]

Analytes	Typical reference values (SI units)	Typical reference values (American units)	Comments
CBC			
PCV	0.4–0.55 l/l	40–55%	25–40 in chickens
RBC	$2.5–4.5 \times 10^{12}$/l		
Polychromatophils	5–10/HPF	5–10/HPF	
TS	3–5 g/l	30–50 g/dl	
WBC	$5–15 \times 10^{9}$/l	$5–15 \times 10^{6}$/µl	5–20 in macaws 10–30 in chickens and some raptors
Monocytes	$<1 \times 10^{9}$/l	$<1 \times 10^{6}$/µl	
Biochemistry			
Glucose	10–20 mmol/l	180–360 mg/dl	
Uric acid	<700 µmol/l	12 mg/dl	Can go as high as 1500 µmol/l in non-fasted raptors
Urea	<0.8–1 mmol/l	2.2–2.8 mg/dl	Higher in raptors
Total protein	3–5 g/l	30–50 g/dl	
AST	<400 IU/l	<400 IU/l	
GLDH	<10 IU/l	<10 IU/l	<20 in owls
GGT	<10 IU/l	<10 IU/l	
LDH	<400–800 IU/l	<400–800 IU/l	Subject to frequent artifacts
Bile acids	<70 µmol/l	<29 µg/ml	Fasted samples, can go as high as 100–120 µmol/l (41–49 µmol/l) in non-fasted birds
CK	<400–800 IU/l	<400–800 IU/l	
Cholesterol	<8–9 mmol/l	308–386 mg/dl	Can go as high as 10–20 in reproductively active females
Amylase	<1000 IU/l	<1000 IU/l	
Lipase	<500 IU/l	<500 IU/l	
Sodium	130–150 mmol/l	130–150 mmol/l	
Potassium	3–5 mmol/l	3–5 mmol/l	
Chloride	100–125 mmol/l	100–125 mmol/l	
Calcium	2.5–4.5 mmol/l	10–18 mg/dl	
Carbon dioxide	20–25 mmol/l	20–25 mmol/l	
Plasma osmolarity	300–320 mOsm/l	300–320 mOsm/l	

[a] These numbers are intended to be used as rough guidelines only and veterinarians should consult species-specific reference intervals whenever possible. Substantial departures from these values may be observed in some avian species. All values for biochemical analytes are reported for commonly used reference laboratory analyzers (e.g. Cobas, Hitachi). HPF, high-power field.

(*Psittacus erithacus*) [16, 42]. A bone marrow aspirate may be necessary to characterize non-regenerative anemia further (see Chapter 33: Cytology).

Erythrocytosis may be caused by dehydration (relative erythrocytosis) or secondary to cardiopulmonary diseases (secondary erythrocytosis). Secondary erythrocytosis is not uncommon with chronic respiratory diseases such as chronic aspergillosis, pneumonia, or respiratory neoplasia. Primary erythrocytosis (polycythemia vera) has not been reported in birds.

Thrombocytosis may be observed in birds with inflammation. Thrombocytopenia is uncommon in birds and is typically caused by iatrogenic toxicities such as chlorambucil [25], or disseminated intravascular coagulation (DIC) and bone marrow disease [16].

Table 32.2 Selected common differential diagnoses for selected clinicopathologic abnormalities in birds.

Abnormalities	Differential diagnoses
Hematologic abnormalities	
Anemia	
Regenerative	• Hemolysis • Heavy metal toxicosis • Other toxicosis (mycotoxins, oil) • Septicemia • Blood parasites • Hemorrhages • Gastrointestinal ulcers, gastroenteritis • Cloacal diseases • Bleeding tumors • Blood-sucking parasites • Wounds • Anticoagulant toxicosis
Non-regenerative	• Anemia of chronic disease • Heavy metal toxicosis • Viral infection • Nutritional deficiencies • Neoplasia
Erythrocytosis	• Dehydration • Respiratory diseases • Cardiac diseases
Leukocytosis	
Mild to moderate	• Stress • Microbial and parasitic infection • Neoplastic diseases • Trauma • Toxicosis
Moderate to marked	• Microbial infection (usually systemic) • Aspergillosis • Avian mycobacteriosis • Avian chlamydiosis • Large wounds
Severe	• Leukemia • Avian mycobacteriosis • Sepsis
Monocytosis	• Chronic inflammation/infection
Leukopenia	• Viral infection (circovirus) • Inbreeding • Toxicosis (fenbendazole, chorambucil) • Laboratory error
Biochemical abnormalities	
High AST, LDH, CK[a]	• Nonspecific tissue damage (also see below)
High AST, LDH; low CK	• Hepatic tissue damage
High AST; low LDH, CK	• Nonspecific tissue damage • Hepatic tissue damage

Table 32.2 (Continued)

Abnormalities	Differential diagnoses
High CK	• Nonspecific tissue damage • Muscle damage • Capture myopathy (marked elevations) • Chronic tissue damage (neoplasia) • Seizures • Intramuscular injections
High GLDH	• Hepatic tissue necrosis/damage
Hyperglycemia	• Stress • Shock/hypovolemia • Diabetes mellitus
Hyperuricemia	• Dehydration (assess urea) • Renal disease, gout, urate nephrosis • Stage 3 starvation • Post-prandial (raptors)
High bile acids	• Post-prandial (mild increase) • Hepatic disease
Hypercholesterolemia	• Post-prandial • Cholestasis/hepatic disease • Reproductively active female • Metabolic dyslipidemia • (obesity, atherosclerosis, hepatic lipidosis)
High pancreatic enzymes	• Gastrointestinal disease • Pancreatic disease
Hypercalcemia	• Hyperproteinemia • Reproductive activity in females • Hypervitaminosis D/ calciferol rodenticides • Osteolytic lesions • Metabolic bone disease
Hyperosmolar plasma	• Dehydration (moderate increase) • Diabetes insipidus (marked increase) • Diabetes mellitus

[a] Cytosolic enzymes are considered high when three- to fourfold increase is seen.*Source:* Lumeij [32]; de Matos [33]; Vergneau-Grosset et al. [34]; Tarrant and Westlake [35]; Phalen et al. [36]; Fudge [37].

Leukocytosis is a common finding in birds and can be marked. Before making a diagnosis of leukocytosis, it is important to acknowledge that several bird species have a relatively high upper reference limit, sometimes higher than 30 × 10^9/l, such as chickens, owls, ducks, and wild birds [3, 43, 44]. However, most commonly seen birds in practice have an approximate WBC of 5–15 × 10^9/l. Within parrots, macaws tend to show slightly higher WBC than other species. Only absolute leukocyte values should be used for interpretation. The magnitude of leukocytosis depends on the disease but also on species-specific response to diseases. A variety of inflammatory and infectious disorders may cause mild to marked leukocytosis (Table 32.2). Toxicity of heterophils and the presence of a left shift may give indications regarding severity of the disease and prognosis. Monocytosis are usually interpreted as evidence of chronic inflammation. Basophilia and eosinophilia are further evidence of inflammation and do not have any specific interpretation. Unlike mammals, eosinophilia is not a reliable indicator of parasite infestation or hypersensitivity.

Leukopenia is uncommon in birds and sampling or laboratory artifacts should be ruled out as artefactual cell lysis is common. Inbreeding such as observed in specific color mutations (e.g. lutino cockatiels) may be associated with low WBC and decreased magnitude of hematologic inflammatory reactions. Viral diseases, particularly infection with circoviruses (psittacid or columbid circovirus), are common causes of leukopenia and pancytopenia in young birds. Toxicosis with fenbendazole, chlorambucil, or other chemotherapeutic drugs may lead to leukopenia [26, 45, 46]. Other diseases of the bone marrow such as neoplasia and severe chronic diseases may also cause leukopenia (Table 32.2).

Coagulation

Coagulation disorders are not well characterized in birds. Anticoagulant intoxications are probably the most common coagulation disorder seen in birds. It is particularly prevalent in wild birds of prey, especially great horned owls (*Bubo virginianus*), as a secondary poisoning from rodent prey [47–49]. The most commonly incriminated rodenticide is brodifacoum. Other less commonly seen causes of coagulation disorders in birds include hypocalcemia, nutritional deficiencies, hepatic insufficiency, aflatoxicosis, DIC, and the conure bleeding syndrome (rare) [50].

Published studies on avian coagulation are scarce. Avian coagulation is reported to be mainly initiated through the extrinsic pathway [32, 50]. Laboratory assays that can be performed to assess avian coagulation include whole blood clotting time, thrombocyte counts, prothrombin time, modified Russels' viper venom test, and fibrinogen estimation [32]. The prothrombin time is reported as the most useful test in birds and reference intervals have been reported for a few species [32, 50–52]. Prothrombin time values may vary depending on the use of mammalian thromboplastin, bird thromboplastin, or Russels's viper venom [32]. Regardless of the method used, blood should be collected on citrate and control samples on the same bird species should be submitted for comparison. Recently, the use of thromboelastography (TEG), a nonspecific method assessing "whole coagulation," has been investigated and reference values reported in birds [51, 53]. TEG values tend to be lower in birds and show relative hypocoagulability when compared to mammals [51, 53]. Reference intervals for other techniques using viscoelastometry have also been established in chickens.

Clinical Biochemistry

Preliminary Concepts

Biochemistry is one of the diagnostic tools available to evaluate avian patients. Understanding the limitations of avian biochemistry analysis and the differences in interpretation from mammals are important for an appropriate interpretation. The same precautions regarding biological variability and the use of reference intervals for avian hematology should be taken with biochemistry (see above). However, analytical variability tends to be low with most modern instrumentation.

Typical reference values for biochemical analytes are given in Table 32.1 and common differential diagnoses for selected biochemical abnormalities are given in Table 32.2.

Most of the biochemical artifacts are related to sample collection, storage, and processing (pre-analytic variability). Studies comparing the use of serum and plasma for biochemistry have been published in various avian species, but plasma is typically used as a larger volume can be obtained [54–56]. When the volume of the blood sample is limited by the size of the patient, dilution of plasma with sterile water, or ultracentrifugation in microhematocrit tubes has been reported [57, 58]. While ultracentrifugation does not appear to alter biochemical results, dilution with sterile water tends to alter results for most analytes.

Suboptimal blood samples are sometimes obtained from small patients and it is important to prioritize selected biochemical parameters, especially if the patient's size precludes repeated venipuncture. Similar to mammals, hemolysis increases the value of analytes present in RBCs, and may also artifactually decrease or increase biochemical values, depending on analytical techniques [59, 60]. Likewise, lipemic samples can mimic an increase of liver enzymes, bile acids, calcium, phosphorus, glucose, and some proteins when analytes are determined via refractometry and via many spectrophotometric methods [33, 59]. Previous intramuscular injections may increase the AST and CK for several days [32]. Clotting may artificially decrease total and ionized calcium.

Various biochemical analyzers are available, and it needs to be acknowledged that most of them, specifically point-of-care or in-house biochemical analyzers, have not been validated for use in all the various species of birds. Several tabletop analyzers, such as the VetScan VS2 Chemistry Analyzer (Abaxis Inc., Union City, CA) and IDEXX VetTest 8008 Chemistry Analyzer (IDEXX Laboratories Inc. Westbrook, ME) among others, are available to veterinary clinics [34]. Many require a low volume of blood; for instance only 0.1 ml of serum, plasma, or whole blood needed to perform a reduced biochemistry panel on an avian/reptile rotor (Avian/Reptilian Profile Plus, Abaxis Inc., Union City, CA) (Table 32.3). However, a larger biochemistry panel is needed in many clinical situations. Most reference analyzers can perform a full biochemical profile on a small quantity of blood (about 0.2 ml of plasma) [34]. It may be important to know the accuracy, precision, overall reliability, and species-specific interference (e.g. flamingos) of these analyzers before interpretation of the output. For instance, while the Vetscan has shown fair general agreement with reference analyzers for clinical use, there were still significant disagreements demonstrated in

Table 32.3 Suggested biochemistry panels in birds.

Comprehensive avian biochemistry panel	VetScan avian/reptile panel
• Glucose • Uric acid • Urea • Total protein • (Albumin and globulin)[a] • AST • GLDH • GGT • LDH • Bile acids • CK • Cholesterol • Triglycerides • Amylase • Lipase • Sodium • Potassium • Chloride • Phosphorus • Calcium • Carbon dioxide	• Glucose • Uric acid • Total protein • (Albumin and globulin)[a] • AST • Bile acids • CK • Sodium • Potassium • Phosphorus • Calcium

[a] Not reliable in birds by methods other than protein electrophoresis.

different studies [61, 62]. Point-of-care single analyte meters such as glucometers have also shown significant discrepancies in birds [63, 64].

The Avian Biochemistry Panel

Selected avian biochemistry panels should maximize information in a reasonable volume of plasma and include a variety of analytes related to various organs and metabolic processes. The panel should take into consideration the sensitivity and specificity of each analyte as well as their temporal changes in the plasma in accordance with disease dynamics. The goals are to screen for major homeostatic abnormalities, metabolic disturbances, organ damage, and dysfunction. We recommend that the standard panel includes at least electrolytes, total proteins, analytes associated with major organs such as liver, pancreas, kidneys, muscles, and metabolic parameters such as glucose, cholesterol, and uric acid (Table 32.3). Reduced panels may also be offered such as liver or renal panels. Furthermore, some biochemical values of clinical significance may be calculated such as anion gap, strong-ion difference, Na : K ratio, and calculated osmolality. A rough guideline to interpretation of the biochemical panel is given in Table 32.2 for selected parameters.

Once the standard panel is performed and differential diagnostic list has been narrowed or upon strong clinical suspicion, other analytes may be subsequently obtained to further assess organ and metabolic functions. These include blood gases analysis, other electrolytes such as ionized calcium and magnesium, glucose metabolism parameters such as BHBA and fructosamine, toxicological tests, other hepatic enzymes such as sorbitol dehydrogenase, lipid metabolism parameters such as lipoproteins, triglycerides, and fatty acids, myocardial injury markers such as troponins, or inflammatory markers such as protein electrophoresis and fibrinogen.

There is a trade-off in using point-of-care biochemical analyzers in that they are typically less accurate, and the panel is limited when compared to reference laboratories. They should be reserved for situations of low sample volume or limited access to reference laboratories with avian biochemical panels.

Protein Characterization

For protein measurement techniques, protein electrophoresis and the Biuret method can be used. Refractometry enables determination of total solids, which is consistently higher than total protein value in birds, and should not be used to evaluate total proteins as the correlation between the two is weak [32]. Albumin cannot be reliably determined in birds using traditional albumin assays developed for mammals such as bromcresol dye binding assays [32, 65]. Albumin and globulin have to be obtained using protein electrophoresis. Total proteins tend to be slightly lower in birds than in mammals. Similar causes for hyperproteinemia and hypoproteinemia as mammals are found in birds. Reproductively active female birds may show relatively high total proteins and total solids.

Protein electrophoresis is typically used to obtain the albumin level, monitor inflammatory patterns, and characterize dysproteinemia [66–69]. Changes in the protein electrophoretogram are nonspecific and should not be used to make specific diagnosis such as certain bacterial or fungal infections. Because inflammatory patterns are similar in numerous diseases, electrophoresis can strengthen a clinical suspicion, but confirmation of the type of lesion through other testing modalities is needed for accurate diagnosis. While protein electrophoresis has limited usefulness in individual medicine other than specific dysproteinemia, it can be useful as an additional test to assess general health in quarantined birds. Protein migration patterns vary among avian species therefore specific reference intervals are necessary [34, 67]. Often a prealbumin fraction is observed in birds [32]. Proteins included in the alpha and beta-globulins fractions are usually acute phase proteins, whereas gamma-globulins are typically raised in case of chronic inflammation [32, 67]. The albumin to globulin (A/G) ratio is typically greater than one in healthy birds and inflammation may raise the globulin fractions with or without hypoalbuminemia, resulting in a decrease of the A/G ratio [32]. Monoclonal gammopathy has been described in a limited number of psittacine birds with lymphoproliferative diseases [70].

Recently, acute phase proteins have been investigated in birds [71]. Overall, acute phase proteins are a promising tool in avian medicine but studies are needed to establish their clinical and prognostic significance in a variety of diseases. In falcons, serum amyloid A may be used to monitor response to pododermatitis therapy [72].

Renal Values

Avian renal function can be evaluated by measuring plasmatic uric acid, urea, and N-acetyl-beta-D-glucosaminidase (NAG) concentrations and via urinalysis (see later). Unlike mammals, creatinine is not a relevant parameter of the biochemistry panel for clinical evaluation of renal function [32, 34]. When interpreting the biochemical panel, one needs to be aware of basic concepts in avian osmoregulation and renal physiology. Specifically, relevant clinical differences from mammals include the fact that the avian kidneys are composed of a combination of looped nephrons (as in mammals) and loopless nephrons (as in other sauropsids), all birds are uricotelic, birds do not maintain a constant glomerular filtration rate, significant post-renal handling of urine occurs in the cloaca and distal colon, birds have a renal portal system that supplies blood to the renal tubules, and some birds use the salt glands as their main osmoregulatory organs. In addition, the biochemistry panel is relatively insensitive to detect renal diseases in birds, until the disease becomes advanced.

The main end-product of protein catabolism in birds is uric acid with minimal urea production. Uric acid is relatively nontoxic but can precipitate in super saturated solutions and cause gout and urate nephrosis. Urea is excreted by glomerular filtration while 90% of uric acid is secreted at the level of the tubules and only 10% is filtered [32, 73]. Hyperuricemia may not be observed until more than 70% of the kidneys are nonfunctional. In case of dehydration, urea demonstrates a more pronounced increase than uric acid due to the decreased glomerular filtration rate while tubular secretion is maintained somewhat by the renal portal system. Therefore, urea is a sensitive and reliable marker of pre-renal azotemia in birds. Uric acid will also significantly increase with dehydration. Controversies exist on the degree of dehydration necessary to see an increase in uric acid. While numerous references state that uric acid is only increased in severe dehydration once tubular secretion gets impaired, uric acid seems to be frequently elevated with moderate dehydration in birds seen in clinical practice [34]. Uric acid frequently increases post-prandially in carnivorous and piscivorous birds with levels similar to those observed in renal diseases. Thus, these bird species should ideally be fasted for 24 hours to reduce this effect [32, 74, 75]. Gastrointestinal bleeding has not been shown to result in an increase in uric acid or urea in pigeons at a single timepoint [76]. However more studies are needed to state whether this applies to other granivorous birds and to later digestion stages. Phase 3 starvation may also lead to an increased uric acid level [32].

Exogenous creatinine by intramuscular injection has been used to evaluate glomerular filtration rate in healthy pigeons, although the technique remains to be validated in patients with decreased renal function [77]. Recently, serum and urinary NAG concentrations have been evaluated as markers of tubular dysfunction in birds [78, 79].

Electrolytes

Total calcium includes ionized calcium, protein-bound calcium, and complexed calcium [33]. Evaluation of both total calcium and ionized calcium is recommended to obtain the most accurate assessment, as ionized calcium is the active calcium fraction, and does not tend to increase during the egg-laying process, in contrary to total calcium [33]. The ionized calcium can be estimated from adjusted calcium formula determined in various species of birds, but it is usually not reliable [32]. Therefore, direct measurement of ionized calcium is recommended whenever possible.

Differential diagnoses for hypercalcemia include physiological, pathological, and artifactual causes (see Table 32.2) [32–36]. Primary hyperparathyroidism has yet to be reported in birds. The occurrence of paraneoplastic hypercalcemia in birds is controversial and has not been thoroughly demonstrated [32, 33, 80]. Hypocalcemia can be due to nutritional causes including low dietary calcium or vitamin D, increased consumption associated with chronic egg laying, and has been commonly reported in grey parrots, manifesting by seizures despite appropriate bone structure [32]. Magnesium should also be measured in case of hypocalcemia in grey parrots, as magnesium complexes with parathyroid hormone receptors and hypomagnesaemia results in impaired response to parathyroid hormone [81]. A significant association between renal disease and hypocalcemia has not been demonstrated in birds, and renal secondary hyperparathyroidism has also not been confirmed in birds [33].

Potassium, chloride, sodium, and bicarbonate (=carbon dioxide on biochemistry panel) concentrations are also important, and mostly pertains to critical patients with fluid and electrolyte losses and acid–base disturbances. The carbon dioxide parameter of the biochemistry panel is an indirect measure of bicarbonate. Results of electrolyte measurement should guide the choice of fluid therapy and may lead to specific measures to re-establish electrolyte balance in case of potassium or ionized calcium abnormalities, due to the potential risks for cardiac malfunction. The pattern of electrolytic disorders should be interpreted with acid–base disorders using standard approach and/or strong ion difference approach (see Chapter 30).

Plasma Osmolality

Plasma osmolality tends to be slightly greater in birds than in mammals [82, 83]. Plasma Osmolality can be estimated using equations with a fair agreement [84]. Unlike mammals, birds gradually increase their plasma osmolality in response to water deprivation to conserve water as protein catabolic wastes are eliminated through tubular secretion [34, 85]. Plasma osmolality is particularly useful when investigating marked polyuro-polydypsia. For instance, marked polydipsia associated with high plasma osmolality is almost pathognomonic for diabetes insipidus while a low plasma osmolality is typical of psychogenic polydipsia. Specifically, both disorders have been diagnosed in grey parrots [86, 87].

Clinical Enzymology

Avian tissue enzyme activities have been determined in a variety of species [32, 78, 88–90]. Presence of an enzyme in a tissue does not necessarily mean an increase of this enzyme in case of tissue damage. For instance, renal cytosolic enzymes tend to get excreted in the urine and may not lead to significant plasma increase [37, 91]. Also some enzymes of low cytosolic concentrations such as GGT may have increased expression during certain states. Normal enzyme levels in avian patients tend to be higher than in mammals and specific reference intervals established with the same methodology are critical for confident interpretation of a panel [77]. Because of the variable half-lives of hepatic enzymes, the degree of enzyme elevation does not correlate to the severity of the lesions or the degree of liver function impairment if any [37]. Values of hepatic enzymes must be much greater than the upper reference limit (at least three to fourfold) to be considered clinically significant.

Hepatocellular leakage is associated with AST, LDH, and alanine aminotransferase (ALT) increase, while hepatic necrosis can cause GLDH elevation and biliary tract damage can cause GGT and ALP increase [32, 37, 59, 92]. ALP is of limited use in birds as plasma activity is generally low and marked elevations have not been documented with liver disease. Increased ALP activity has been reported with enhanced osteoblastic activity and egg laying [59, 93]. Likewise, ALT is of limited use and is typically not included in avian biochemistry panel [37, 59]. In pigeons, GLDH declines most rapidly, followed in order by LDH, CK, AST, and ALT [88]. A common recommendation to interpret increased enzymes is to compare CK to values obtained for AST; however CK has a shorter half-life than AST, therefore chronic muscle damage can result in elevated AST, with a normal CK after return to baseline [32]. This situation should be kept in mind when analyzing elevated hepatic enzymes. The main advantage of including LDH into an avian biochemistry panel is to differentiate muscle from liver damage: as LDH half-life is shorter than CK half-life, a persistently elevated LDH concomitant with a decreasing CK and increased AST points toward hepatic disease (Table 32.2) [32, 37]. However, hemolysis leads to LDH elevation. Overall, these enzymes are considered sensitive but poorly specific and their interpretation can be complicated.

Recently, SDH has been shown to be a potentially sensitive and specific marker for liver hepatocellular damage [92]. GLDH is a mitochondrial enzyme that is considered liver-specific, but sensitivity is low [32, 34, 94]. Since the enzyme is mitochondrial, significant cell lysis must occur before plasmatic elevation is observed such as with hepatic necrosis and hepatic tumors.

The CK is frequently elevated with a variety of factors including intramuscular injections, striated and smooth muscle lesions, seizures, and struggle during transport and restraint [34]. The magnitude of change is also meaningful. For instance, injections usually cause a mild increase in CK around a few thousand U/L while capture myopathy induces changed of a few hundred thousand U/L. The magnitude of CK elevation may also have prognostic indications in certain situations. In addition, nonspecific tissue necrosis such as caused by neoplasia may lead to moderate to large chronic elevations in CK [34].

No specific marker for evaluation of the exocrine pancreas has been described in birds. Both plasma amylase and lipase can increase in case of pancreatitis, enteritis, and renal disease causing a decrease in their excretion [59]. However, the value of these tests to diagnose pancreas disease is unknown.

Hepatic Function

In case of liver disease, bile acids plasmatic concentration can be increased due to impaired entero-hepatic cycle, or alternatively can be decreased if the liver is not producing bile acids, in case of impaired intestinal absorption [59, 95]. Decreased bile acid concentration is not a specific indicator of liver disease and can also be observed in physiologic situations. Clinicians should also be aware that bile acid values obtained via radioimmunoassay are typically lower than via colorimetry [59]. Bile acids, measured by radioimmunoassay, is both a sensitive and specific marker to diagnose hepatic disease [32, 96]. Bile acids also slightly increase post-prandially in many species of birds, including parrots and birds of prey, and it is recommended to obtain fasted plasma samples in these species [32, 97, 98]. In psittacine birds, bile acids also increase post-prandially but reference intervals combining pre- and post-prandial values have been established and a single sample may be obtained to assess liver function. Typical reference values for bile acids are lower than 70 µmol/l when fasted using a colorimetric reference laboratory analyzer.

Bilirubin occurs in scant quantities in avian plasma due to the lack of biliverdin reductase [37]. Therefore, bilirubin assays have been reported to provide limited clinical information, although increased bilirubin can be seen in advanced liver disease and viral necrotizing hepatitis [34, 37].

Currently, plasmatic ammonia measurements do not have common applications in avian medicine, as hepatic encephalopathy has not been conclusively documented in birds yet. Fasted ammonemia in healthy psittacine birds is much higher than in dogs and could be mistaken for an increased value [32].

Evaluation of hepatic function also includes the assessment of metabolites produced by the liver such as proteins, glucose, cholesterol, and uric acid. In case of late-stage liver disease, one or several of these metabolites can be lowered in the blood.

Carbohydrate Metabolism

Glycemia values are typically higher in birds than in mammals, at about 180–360 mg/dl (10–20 mmol/l) [32]. Glucometers have not been shown to be reliable in birds [64, 99]. Regulation mechanisms are similar to mammals although glucagon concentration is typically higher and insulin concentration typically lower in granivorous birds' pancreas in comparison to mammalian pancreas [32]. Hyperglycemia can be associated with stress, pancreatitis, steroid administration, and diabetes mellitus, reported in numerous avian species [100–102]. Diabetes mellitus in pet birds is usually associated with significant polyuria and glycosuria and mostly respond to insulin therapy. Mild increase in glucose is typically due to stress.

Hypoglycemia can be associated with septicemia, liver failure, neoplasia and rarely, starvation.

Fructosamine has been used in birds to confirm the chronicity of hyperglycemia [101]. However, it is unknown if its interpretation is similar to mammals and it is likely that increased fructosamine is associated with a shorter duration of hyperglycemia. Beta-hydroxyl-butyric acid is the main ketone acid found in most birds.

Lipid Metabolism

Dyslipidemia are frequent in pet birds and in female reproductive diseases. Dyslipidemia in birds are presumably caused by disturbances in normal lipid metabolism associated with inadequate nutrition, captive lifestyle and possibly other species and individual factors [103]. Therefore, birds are prone to a variety of lipid-related diseases such as obesity, hepatic lipidosis, lipoma, xanthomatosis, egg yolk coelomitis, and atherosclerosis where the assessment of blood lipid may be of interest. Some species have higher blood cholesterol than others such as Quaker parrots and Amazon parrots. Female birds undergoing physiological or pathological reproductive activity have high blood cholesterol, triglycerides, and VLDL levels.

Various lipoprotein assays are used in mammals to measure the different lipoprotein fractions, but most have not been properly validated in the different avian species. Some laboratory tests may not be accurate for measuring cholesterol fractions in birds. It is recommended that birds are fasted prior to measurement as some lipid fractions may greatly increase after a meal. Standard laboratory analyzers with specific reagents are most commonly used to measure cholesterol/lipoprotein fractions in birds. Other methods include ultracentrifugation, electrophoresis, and magnetic resonance spectroscopy. HDL is typically measured directly, but VLDL and LDL concentration are usually calculated using the Friedewald formula although this formula has not been thoroughly validated in most birds [104–107].

$$\text{LDL}\left(\text{mmol/l}\right) = \text{Total cholesterol} - \text{HDL} - \text{Tryglycerides}/2.18\left(\text{or 5 for American unit}\right)$$

HDL are the predominant lipoproteins in most birds, as opposed to humans and most companion mammals [107, 108]. An association between atherosclerosis and hypercholesterolemia is most likely in pet psittacine birds, but it has not been conclusively demonstrated yet [105, 106, 109, 110]. Hypercholesterolemia and dyslipidemia has been shown in some species of birds of prey with inappropriate diet [110–112]. Associations between various dyslipidemic patterns and specific diseases need to be further investigated.

Urine Evaluation

Urinalysis is not routinely performed in birds in typical clinical practice. Urine collection is typically made from the cage floor. More invasive urine collection using ureter cannulation within the urodeum is possible [113], but is invasive and only assesses part of the avian osmoregulation as post-renal handling of urine is an important process. Therefore, reference intervals obtained on cannulated urine may be different from normally voided urine. As urine is excreted via the urodeum, then back-flows into the coprodeum and colon, and the oviduct and rectum also empty in the cloaca, an abnormality detected in urine may be related to other organ systems than just the kidneys. Urine volume may vary depending on bird species and a variety of diseases may cause polyuria such as renal, hepatic, gastrointestinal, cloacal diseases, diabetes mellitus, diabetes insipidus, hypercalcemia, and psychogenic polydipsia. Therefore, like mammals, polyuria is not specific for renal disease in birds.

Urine color is typically translucent and uric acid is white. Yellowish or greenish urine coloration may be seen with liver disease (biliverdinuria). Red urine may be an indication of hematuria, hemoglobinuria, myoglobinuria, or porphyrin excretion. Lead poisoning may lead to red urine and porphyrinuria [113]. Pigments in the diet and vitamin supplements may also lead to color changes in the urine.

Urinary dipsticks may be employed to screen for glycosuria or hematuria. As stated above, hematuria may also originate from the reproductive and gastrointestinal system. However, true hematuria tends to be located within the urine portion of the urofeces. If urine is collected from the cloaca or cage floor, glycosuria may be artifactual and result from contact with digestive content (in case of malabsorption) or disinfectants, including bleach and hydrogen peroxide. Other dry reagents of the urinary sticks are not reliable or useful.

Cytosolic enzymes may also be measured and may correlate with kidney injury [91]. Proteinuria is difficult to assess because of contamination with feces and the presence of proteins surrounding uric acid microspheres. However, presence of urinary casts should be considered as an indicator of tubular disease. To examine casts, the urine sample may be centrifuged, then sediments may be resuspended and mounted with methylene blue [114].

Urine osmolarity and specific gravity is extremely variable and depends on the hydration status of the bird and concurrent diseases of the cloaca and gastrointestinal tract. It tends to be lower than in mammals in normally hydrated birds [113]. It is typically around 100–200 mOsmol/kg in normally voided urine but can go at about 400–500 in dehydrated birds [113]. Urine osmolarity can be used during water deprivation test and in the diagnostic work up of diabetes insipidus, where it is typically lower than 50 mOsmol/Kg.

The microscopic examination of urinary sediment may be useful in birds and it has been proposed that identification of casts in urinary sediment is suggestive of renal disease [113, 115]. As urine is contaminated with feces, it is usual to find bacteria upon microscopic evaluation. Uric acid is also excreted as mucopolysaccharide microspheres visible under the microscope. Some of the uric acid may also be precipitated in the form of crystals.

References

1 Briscoe, J.A., Rosenthal, K.L., and Shofer, F.S. (2010). Selected complete blood cell count and plasma protein electrophoresis parameters in pet psittacine birds evaluated for illness. *J. Avian Med. Surg.* 24 (2): 131–137.

2 Harr, K.E., Raskin, R.E., and Heard, D.J. (2005). Temporal effects of 3 commonly used anticoagulants on hematologic and biochemical variables in blood samples from macaws and Burmese pythons. *Vet. Clin. Pathol.* 34 (4): 383–388.

3 Beaufrère, H. and Ammersbach, M. (2016). Variability and limitations in clinical avian hematology. In: *Current Therapy in Avian Medicine and Surgery* (ed. B. Speer), 467–486. Saunders.

4 Fudge, A. (2000). Avian blood sampling and artifacts considerations. In: *Laboratory Medicine: Avian and Exotic Pets* (ed. A. Fudge), 1–8. Philadelphia, PA: W.B. Saunders Company.

5 Campbell, T. and Ellis, C. (2007). Hematology of birds. In: *Avian & Exotic Animal Hematology & Cytology*, 3e (eds. T. Campbell and C. Ellis), 3–50. Oxford: Wiley-Blackwell.

6 Sanchez-Migallon Guzman, D. Mitchell, M.A., Gaunt, S.D. et al. (2008). Comparison of hematologic values in blood samples with lithium heparin or dipotassium ethylenediaminetetraacetic acid anticoagulants in Hispaniolan Amazon parrots (*Amazona ventralis*). *J. Avian Med. Surg.* 22 (2): 108–113.

7 Seliger, C., Schaerer, B., Kohn, M. et al. (2012). A rapid high-precision flow cytometry based technique for total white blood cell counting in chickens. *Vet. Immunol. Immunopathol.* 145 (1–2): 86–99.

8 De Boever, S., Croubels, S., Demeyere, K. et al. (2010). Flow cytometric differentiation of avian leukocytes and analysis of their intracellular cytokine expression. *Avain Pathol.* 39 (1): 41–46.

9 Burgess, S. and Davison, T. (1999). Counting absolute numbers of specific leukocyte subpopulations in avian whole blood using a single-step flow cytometric

technique: comparison of two inbred lines of chickens. *J. Immunol. Methods* 227 (1–2): 169–176.

10 Moritomo, T., Minami, A., Inoue, Y., and Nakanishi, T. (2002). A new method for counting of quail leukocytes by flow cytometry. *J. Vet. Med. Sci.* 64 (12): 1149–1151.

11 Pendl, H. and Samour, J. (2016). Hematology analyses. In: *Avian Medicine*, 3e (ed. J. Samour), 77–100. St Louis, MO: Elsevier.

12 Velguth, K.E., Payton, M.E., and Hoover, J.P. (2010). Relationship of hemoglobin concentration to packed cell volume in avian blood samples. *J. Avian Med. Surg.* 24 (2): 115–121.

13 Hippel, T. (2007). Routine testing in hematology. In: *Hematology: Clinical Principles and Applications*, 3e (eds. B. Rodak, G. Fritsma and K. Doig), 160–174. St Louis, MO: Saunders Elsevier.

14 Johns, J.L., Shooshtari, M.P., and Christopher, M.M. (2008). Development of a technique for quantification of reticulocytes and assessment of erythrocyte regenerative capacity in birds. *Am. J. Vet. Res.* 69 (8): 1067–1072.

15 Lucas, A. and Jamroz, C. (1961). *Atlas of Avian Hematology*, Agriculture Monograph 25, 271. Washington, DC: United States Department of Agriculture.

16 Campbell, T. (2015). *Exotic Animal Hematology and Cytology*, 4e (ed. T. Campbell), 402. Ames, IA: Wiley-Blackwell.

17 Aroch, I., Targan, N., and Gancz, A. (2013). A novel modified semi-direct method for total leukocyte count in birds. *Isr. J. Vet. Med.* 68 (2): 111–118.

18 Natt, M.P. and Herrick, C.A. (1952). A new blood diluent for counting the erythrocytes and leucocytes of the chicken. *Poult. Sci.* 31 (4): 735–738.

19 Wiseman, B.K. (1931). An improved direct method for obtaining the total white cell count in avian blood. *Exp. Biol. Med.* 28 (9): 1030–1033.

20 Latimer, K. and Bienzle, D. (2010). Determination and interpretation of the avian leukogram. In: *Schalm's Veterinary Hematology*, 6e (eds. D. Weiss and K. Wardrop), 345–357. Ames, IA: Wiley-Blackwell.

21 Maedel, L. and Doig, K. (2007). Examination of the peripheral blood smear and correlation with the complete blood count. In: *Hematology: Clinical Principles and Applications*, 3e (eds. B. Rodak, G. Fritsma and K. Doig), 175–192. St Louis, MO: Saunders Elsevier.

22 Houwen, B. (2002). Blood film preparation and staining procedures. *Clin. Lab. Med.* 22 (1): 1–14.

23 Gaharan, S., Gupta, A., Boudreaux, B., and Beaufrère, H. (2012). What is your diagnosis? Chronic lymphocytic leukemia. *J. Avian Med. Surg.* 26 (1): 45–48.

24 Osofsky, A., Hawkins, M.G., Foreman, O. et al. (2011). T-cell chronic lymphocytic leukemia in a double yellow-headed Amazon parrot (*Amazona ochrocephala oratrix*). *J. Avian Med. Surg.* 25 (4): 286–294.

25 Hammond, E.E., Guzman, D.S.-M., Garner, M.M. et al. (2010). Long-term treatment of chronic lymphocytic leukemia in a green-winged macaw (*Ara chloroptera*) *J. Avian Med. Surg.* 24 (4): 330–338.

26 Wiley, J.L.J., Whittington, J.K.J., Wilmes, C.M. et al. (2009). Chronic myelogenous leukemia in a great horned owl (*Bubo virginianus*). *J. Avian Med. Surg.* 23 (1): 36–43.

27 Rivera, S., McClearen, J.R., and Reavill, D.R. (2009). Treatment of nonepitheliotropic cutaneous B-cell lymphoma in an umbrella cockatoo (*Cacatua alba*). *J. Avian Med. Surg.* 23 (4): 294–302.

28 Zhao, W., Liu, J., Xu, R. et al. (2015). The gametocytes of leucocytozoon sabrazesi infect chicken thrombocytes, not other blood cells. *PLoS One* 10 (7): e0133478.

29 Larrat, S., Locke, S., Dallaire, A.D. et al. (2012). Fatal aerosacculitis and pneumonia associated with *Eucoleus* sp. (Nematoda: Capillaridae) in the lungs of a Peregrine Falcon (*Falco peregrinus*). *J. Wildl. Dis.* 48 (3): 832–834.

30 Beaufrère, H., Kearney, M.T., and Tully, T.N. (2015). Can we trust the avian medical literature: survey and critical appraisal of the use of statistics in avian medicine from 2007 to 2011. *J. Exot. Pet Med.* 24 (4): 415–426.

31 Joyner, K.L. (1994). Theriogenology. In: *Avian Medicine: Principles and Applications* (eds. B.W. Ritchie, G.J. Harrison and L.R. Harrison), 748–804. Lake Worth, FL: Wingers Publishing.

32 Lumeij, J.T. (2008). Avian clinical biochemistry. In: *Clinical Biochemistry of Domestic Animals*, 6e (eds. J.J. Kaneko, J.W. Harvey and M.L. Bruss), 839–872. New York;, NY: Academic Press.

33 de Matos, R. (2008). Calcium metabolism in birds. *Vet. Clin. North Am. Exot. Anim. Pract.* 11(1): 59–82, vi.

34 Vergneau-Grosset, C., Beaufrère, H., and Ammersbach, M. (2016). Clinical biochemistry. In: *Current Therapy in Avian Medicine and Surgery* (ed. B. Speer), 486–500. Saint Louis, MI: Elsevier.

35 Tarrant, K.A. and Westlake, G.E. (1984). Histological technique for the identification of poisoning in wildlife by the rodenticide calciferol. *Bull. Environ. Contam. Toxicol.* 32 (2): 175–178.

36 Phalen, D.N., Drew, M.L., Contreras, C. et al. (2005). Naturally occurring secondary nutritional hyperparathyroidism in cattle egrets (*Bubulcus ibis*) from central Texas. *J. Wildl Dis.* 41 (2): 401–415.

37 Fudge, A. (2000). Avian liver and gastrointestinal testing. In: *Laboratory Animal Medicine* (ed. A. Fudge), 47–55. Philadelphia, PA: Saunders.

38 Finnegan, M., Daniel, G., and Ramsay, E. (1997). Evaluation of whole blood transfusions in domestic pigeons (*Columba livia*). *J. Avian Med. Surg.* 11 (1): 7–14.

39 Gupta, A., Tully, T.N., Beaufrère, H. et al. (2011). What is your diagnosis? Bone marrow aspirate from a hyacinth macaw (*Anodorhynchus hyacinthinus*). *Vet. Clin. Pathol.* 40 (4): 565–566.

40 Dumonceaux, G. and Harrison, G. (1994). Toxins. In: *Avian Medicine: Principles and Applications* (eds. B. Ritchie, G. Harrison and L. Harrison), 1030–1052. Lake Worth, FL: Wingers Publishing.

41 Johnston, M.S., Son, T.T., and Rosenthal, K.L. (2007). Immune-mediated hemolytic anemia in an eclectus parrot. *J. Am. Vet. Med. Assoc.* 230 (7): 1028–1031.

42 Schoemaker, N.J., Dorrestein, G.M., Latimer, K.S. et al. Severe leukopenia and liver necrosis in young African grey parrots (*Psittacus erithacus erithacus*) infected with psittacine circovirus. *Avian Dis.* 44 (2): 470–478.

43 Ammersbach, M., Beaufrère, H., Gionet Rollick, A., and Tully, T. (2015). Laboratory blood analysis in Strigiformes—Part I: hematologic reference intervals and agreement between manual blood cell counting techniques. *Vet. Clin. Pathol.* 44 (1): 94–108.

44 Wakenell, P. (2011). Hematology of chickens and turkeys. In: *Schalm's Veterinary Hematology*, 6e (eds. D. Weiss and K. Wardrop), 958–967. Ames, IA: Wiley-Blackwell.

45 Bonar, C.J., Lewandowski, A.H., and Schaul, J. (2003). Suspected fenbendazole toxicosis in 2 vulture species (*Gyps africanus, Torgos tracheliotus*) and Marabou Storks (*Leptoptilos crumeniferus*). *J. Avian Med. Surg.* 17 (1): 16–19.

46 Weber, M.A., Terrell, S.P., Neiffer, D.L. et al. (2002). Bone marrow hypoplasia and intestinal crypt cell necrosis associated with fenbendazole administration in five painted storks. *J. Am. Vet. Med. Assoc.* 221 (3): 417–419, 369.

47 Murray, M. (2011). Anticoagulant rodenticide exposure and toxicosis in four species of birds of prey presented to a wildlife clinic in Massachusetts, 2006–2010. *J. Zoo Wildl. Med.* 42 (1): 88–97.

48 Stansley, W., Cummings, M., Vudathala, D., and Murphy, L.A. (2014). Anticoagulant rodenticides in red-tailed hawks, *Buteo jamaicensis*, and great horned owls, *Bubo virginianus*, from New Jersey, USA, 2008–2010. *Bull. Environ. Contam. Toxicol.* 92 (1): 6–9.

49 Thomas, P.J., Mineau, P., Shore, R.F. et al. (2011). Second generation anticoagulant rodenticides in predatory birds: probabilistic characterisation of toxic liver concentrations and implications for predatory bird populations in Canada. *Environ. Int.* 37 (5): 914–920.

50 Powers, L. (2000). Avian hemostasis. In: *Laboratory Animal Medicine* (ed. A. Fudge), 35–45. Philadelphia, PA: W. B. Saunders.

51 Strindberg, S., Nielsen, T.W., Ribeiro, Â.M. et al. (2015). Thromboelastography in selected avian species. *J. Avian Med. Surg.* 29 (4): 282–289.

52 Morrisey, J.K., Paul-Murphy, J., Fialkowski, J.P. et al. (2003). Estimation of Prothrombin times of hispaniolan Amazon parrots (*Amazona ventralis*) and Umbrella cockatoos (*Cacatua alba*). *J. Avian Med. Surg.* 17 (2): 72–77.

53 Keller, K.A., Sanchez-Migallon Guzman, D., Acierno, M.J. et al. (2015). Thromboelastography values in Hispaniolan Amazon parrots (*Amazona ventralis*): a pilot study. *J. Avian Med. Surg.* 29 (3): 174–180.

54 Franco, K.H., Hoover, J.P., Backues, K.A., and Payton, M.E. (2010). Comparison of biochemical values of paired serum and plasma samples from american flamingos (*Phoenicopterus ruber*), Indian runner ducks (*Anas platyrhynchos*), and Hyacinth macaws (*Anodorhynchus hyacinthinus*). *J. Exot. Pet Med.* 19 (2): 169–176.

55 Hawkins, M.G., Kass, P.H., Zinkl, J.G., and Tell, L.A. (2006). Comparison of biochemical values in serum and plasma, fresh and frozen plasma, and hemolyzed samples from orange-winged Amazon parrots (*Amazona amazonica*). *Vet. Clin. Pathol.* 35 (2): 219–225.

56 Hrubec, T., Whichard, J., Larsen, C., and Pierson, F. (2002). Plasma versus serum: specific differences in biochemical analyte values. *J. Avian Med. Surg.* 16 (2): 101–105.

57 Waldoch, J., Wack, R., and Christopher, M. (2009). Avian plasma chemistry analysis using diluted samples. *J. Zoo Wildl. Med.* 40 (4): 667–674.

58 Pond, J., Thompson, S., Hennen, M. et al. (2012). Effects of ultracentrifugation on plasma biochemical values of prefledged wild peregrine falcons (*Falco peregrinus*) in northeastern Illinois. *J. Avian Med. Surg.* 26 (3): 140–143.

59 Harr, K. (2006). Diagnostic value of biochemistry. In: *Clinical Avian Medicine* (eds. G. Harrison and T. Lightfoot), 611–630. Palm Beach, FL: Spix Publishing.

60 Roman, Y., Bomsel-Demontoy, M.-C., Levrier, J. et al. (2009). Effect of hemolysis on plasma protein levels and plasma electrophoresis in birds. *J. Wildl. Dis.* 45 (1): 73–80.

61 Greenacre, C.B., Avian, D.A., Dvm, B.F. et al. (2008). Comparison of avian biochemical test results with Abaxis Vet Scan and Hitachi 911 analyzers. *J. Avian Med. Surg.* 22 (4): 291–299.

62 Ammersbach, M., Beaufrere, H., and Tully, T. (2015). Laboratory blood analysis in Strigiformes—Part II: plasma biochemistry reference intervals and agreement between the Abaxis Vetscan V2 and the Roche Cobas c501. *Vet. Clin. Pathol.* 44 (1): 128–140.

63 Acierno, M.J., Mitchell, M.A., Schuster, P.J. et al. (2009). Evaluation of the agreement among three handheld blood glucose meters and a laboratory blood analyzer for measurement of blood glucose concentration in Hispaniolan Amazon parrots (*Amazona ventralis*). *Am. J. Vet. Res.* 70 (2): 172–175.

64 Acierno, M.J., Schnellbacher, R., and Tully, T.N. (2012). Measuring the level of agreement between a veterinary and a human point-of-care glucometer and a laboratory blood analyzer in Hispaniolan Amazon parrots (*Amazona ventralis*). *J. Avian Med. Surg.* 26 (4): 221–224.

65 Cray, C., Wack, A., and Arheart, K.L. (2011). Invalid measurement of plasma albumin using bromcresol green methodology in penguins (*Spheniscus* species). *J. Avian Med. Surg.* 25 (1): 14–22.

66 Cray, C., Reavill, D., Romagnano, A. et al. (2009). Galactomannan assay and plasma protein electrophoresis findings in psittacine birds with aspergillosis. *J. Avian Med. Surg.* 23 (2): 125–135.

67 Cray, C., Rodriguez, M., and Zaias, J. (2007). Protein electrophoresis of psittacine plasma. *Vet. Clin. Pathol.* 36 (1): 64–72.

68 Cray, C. and Tatum, L. (1998). Applications of protein electrophoresis in avian diagnostics. *J. Avian Med. Surg.* 12 (1): 4–10.

69 Tatum, L.M., Zaias, J., Mealey, B.K. et al. (2000). Protein electrophoresis as a diagnostic and prognostic tool in raptor medicine. *J. Zoo Wildl. Med.* 31 (4): 497–502.

70 Lennox, A., Clubb, S., Romagnano, A. et al. (2014). Monoclonal hyperglobulinemia in lymphosarcoma in a cockatiel (*Nymphicus hollandicus*) and a blue and gold macaw (*Ara ararauna*). *Avian Dis.* 58 (2): 326–329.

71 Cray, C. (2013). Biomarkers of inflammation in exotic pets. *J. Exot. Pet Med.* 22 (3): 245–250.

72 Caliendo, V., McKinney, P., Bailey, T. et al. (2013). Serum amyloid A as an indicator of health status in falcons. *J. Avian Med. Surg.* 27 (2): 83–89.

73 Lumeij, J.T. (1987). Plasma urea, creatinine and uric acid concentrations in response to dehydration in racing pigeons (*Columba livia domestica*). *Avian Pathol.* 16 (3): 377–382.

74 Lumeij, J.T. and Remple, J.D. (1991). Plasma urea, creatinine and uric acid concentrations in relation to feeding in peregrine falcons (*Falco peregrinus*). *Avian Pathol.* 20 (1): 79–83.

75 Cray, C., Stremme, D.W., and Arheart, K.L. (2010). Postprandial biochemistry changes in penguins (*Spheniscus demersus*) including hyperuricemia. *J. Zoo Wildl. Med.* 41 (2): 325–326.

76 Sheldon, J., Hoover, J.P., and Payton, M.E. (2007). Plasma uric acid, creatinine, and urea nitrogen concentrations after whole blood administration via the gastrointestinal tract in domestic pigeons (*Columba livia*). *J. Avian Med. Surg.* 21 (2): 130–134.

77 Scope, A., Schwendenwein, I., and Schauberger, G. (2013). Plasma exogenous creatinine excretion for the assessment of renal function in avian medicine—pharmacokinetic modeling in racing pigeons (*Columba livia*). *J. Avian Med. Surg.* 27 (3): 173–179.

78 Wimsatt, J., Canon, N., Pearce, R.D. et al. (2009). Assessment of novel avian renal disease markers for the detection of experimental nephrotoxicosis in pigeons (*Columba livia*). *J. Zoo Wildl. Med.* 40 (3): 487–494.

79 Dijkstra, B., Sanchez-Migallon Guzman, D., Gustavsen, K. et al. (2015). Renal, gastrointestinal, and hemostatic effects of oral administration of meloxicam to Hispaniolan Amazon parrots (*Amazona ventralis*). *Am. J. Vet. Res.* 76 (4): 308–317.

80 de Wit, M., Schoemaker, N.J., Kik, M.J.L., and Westerhof, I. (2003). Hypercalcemia in two Amazon parrots with malignant lymphoma. *Avian Dis.* 47 (1): 223–228.

81 Kirchgessner, M.S., Tully, T.N., Nevarez, J. et al. (2012). Magnesium therapy in a hypocalcemic African grey parrot (*Psittacus erithacus*). *J. Avian Med. Surg.* 26 (1): 17–21.

82 Beaufrère, H., Acierno, M., Mitchell, M.A. et al. (2011). Plasma osmolality reference values in African Grey parrots (*Psittacus erithacus erithacus*), Hispaniolan Amazon parrots (*Amazona ventralis*), and red-fronted macaws (*Ara rubrogenys*). *J. Avian Med. Surg.* 25 (2): 91–96.

83 Acierno, M.J., Mitchell, M.A., Freeman, D.M. et al. (2009). Determinination of plasma osmolality and agreement between measured and calculated values in healthy adult Hispaniolan Amazon parrots (*Amazona ventralis*). *Am. J. Vet. Res.* 70 (9): 1151–1154.

84 Nevarez, J.G., Acierno, M.J., Angel, M., and Beaufrere, H. (2012). Determination of agreement between measured and calculated plasma osmolality values in captive-reared american alligators (*Alligator mississippiensis*). *J. Herpetol. Med. Surg.* 22 (1–2): 36–41.

85 Saito, N. and Grossmann, R. (1998). Effects of short-term dehydration on plasma osmolality, levels of arginine vasotocin and its hypothalamic gene expression in the laying hen. *Comp. Biochem. Physiol. A: Mol. Integr. Physiol.* 121 (3): 235–239.

86 Lumeij, J.T. and Westerhof, I. (1988). The use of the water deprivation test for the diagnosis of apparent psychogenic polydipsia in a socially deprived African grey parrot (*Psittacus erithacus erithacus*). *Avian Pathol.* 17 (4): 875–878.

87 Starkey, S.R., Wood, C., de Matos, R. et al. (2010). Central diabetes insipidus in an African Grey parrot. *J. Am. Vet. Med. Assoc.* 237 (4): 415–419.

88 Lumeij, J.T., De Bruijne, J.J., Slob, A. et al. (1988). Enzyme activities in tissues and elimination half-lives of homologous muscle and liver enzymes in the racing pigeon (*Columba livia domestica*). *Avian Pathol.* 17 (4): 851–864.

89 Battison, A.L., Buczkowski, S., and Archer, F.J. (1996). The potential use of plasma glutamate dehydrogenase activity for the evaluation of hepatic disease in the

cockatiel (*Nymphicus hollandicus*). *Vet. Clin. Pathol.* 25 (2): 43–47.

90 Sulakhe, S.J. and Lautt, W.W. (1985). The activity of hepatic gamma-glutamyltranspeptidase in various animal species. *Comp. Biochem. Physiol. Part B: Comp. Biochem.* 82 (2): 263–264.

91 Tschopp, R., Bailey, T., Di Somma, A., and Silvanose, C. (2007). Urinalysis as a noninvasive health screening procedure in Falconidae. *J. Avian Med. Surg.* 21 (1): 8–12.

92 Williams, S.M., Holthaus, L., Barron, H.W. et al. (2012). Improved clinicopathologic assessments of acute liver damage due to trauma in Indian ring-necked parakeets (*Psittacula krameri manillensis*). *J. Avian Med. Surg.* 26 (2): 67–75.

93 Harr, K.E. (2002). Clinical chemistry of companion avian species: a review. *Vet. Clin. Pathol.* 31 (3): 140–151.

94 Lumeij, J.T., Meidam, M., Wolfswinkel, J. et al. (1988). Changes in plasma chemistry after drug-induced liver disease or muscle necrosis in racing pigeons (*Columba livia domestica*). *Avian Pathol.* 17 (4): 865–874.

95 Tennant, B. (2008). Hepatic function. In: *Clinical Biochemistry of Domestic Animals* (eds. J. Kaneko and M. Bruss), 379–412. San Diego, CA: Academic Press.

96 Cray, C., Gautier, D., Harris, D. et al. (2008). Changes in clinical enzyme activity and bile acid levels in psittacine birds with altered liver function and disease. *J. Avian Med. Surg.* 22 (1): 17–24.

97 Lumeij, J.T. and Remple, J.D. (1992). Plasma bile acid concentrations in response to feeding in peregrine falcons (*Falco peregrinus*). *Avian Dis.* 36 (4): 1060–1062.

98 Lumeij, J. (1991). Fasting and postprandial plasma bile acid concentrations in racing pigeons (*Columba livia domestica*) and Mallards (*Anas platyrhynchos*). *J. Assoc. Avian Vet.* 5 (4): 197–200.

99 Burdick, S., Mitchell, M.A., Neil, J. et al. (2012). Evaluation of two point-of-care meters and a portable chemistry analyzer for measurement of blood glucose concentrations in juvenile white-tailed deer (*Odocoileus virginianus*). *J. Am. Vet. Med. Assoc.* 240 (5): 596–599.

100 Desmarchelier, M. and Langlois, I. (2008). Diabetes mellitus in a nanday conure (*Nandayus nenday*). *J. Avian Med. Surg.* 22 (3): 246–254.

101 Gancz, A.Y., Wellehan, J.F.X., Boutette, J. et al. (2007). Diabetes mellitus concurrent with hepatic haemosiderosis in two macaws (*Ara severa, Ara militaris*). *Avian Pathol.* 36 (4): 331–336.

102 Pilny, A.A. and Luong, R. (2005). Diabetes mellitus in a chestnut-fronted macaw (*Ara severa*). *J. Avian Med. Surg.* 19 (4): 297–302.

103 Beaufrere, H. (2016). Dyslipidemia/hyperlipidemia. In: *5-Minute Veterinary Consult : Avian* (ed. J. Graham), 98–100. Ames, IA: Blackwell Publishing.

104 Friedewald, W.T., Levy, R.I., and Fredrickson, D.S. (1972). Estimation of the concentration of low-density lipoprotein cholesterol in plasma, without use of the preparative ultracentrifuge. *Clin. Chem.* 18 (6): 499–502.

105 Beaufrère, H., Nevarez, J., Clubb, S., and Tully, T. (2013). Diet-induced experimental atherosclerosis in Quaker parrots (*Myiopsitta monachus*). *Vet. Pathol.* 50 (6): 1116–1126.

106 Beaufrère, H., Vet, D.M., Cray, C. et al. (2014). Association of plasma lipid levels with atherosclerosis prevalence in psittaciformes. *J. Avian Med. Surg.* 28 (3): 225–231.

107 Beaufrère, H. (2013). Atherosclerosis: comparative pathogenesis, lipoprotein metabolism and avian and exotic companion mammal models. *J. Exot. Pet Med.* 22 (4): 320–335.

108 Petzinger, C., Heatley, J.J., Cornejo, J. et al. (2010). Dietary modification of omega-3 fatty acids for birds with atherosclerosis. *J. Am. Vet. Med. Assoc.* 236 (5): 523–528.

109 Pilny, A.A., Quesenberry, K.E., Bartick-Sedrish, T.E. et al. (2012). Evaluation of *Chlamydophila psittaci* infection and other risk factors for atherosclerosis in pet psittacine birds. *J. Am. Vet. Med. Assoc.* 240 (12): 1474–1480.

110 Beaufrère, H. (2013). Avian atherosclerosis: parrots and beyond. *J. Exot. Pet Med.* 22 (4): 336–347.

111 Potier, R. (2013). Lipid blood profile in captive Brahminy kite (*Haliastur indus*) as a possible indication of increased susceptibility to atherosclerosis. *J. Zoo Wildl. Med.* 44 (3): 549–554.

112 Facon, C., Beaufrère, H., Gaborit, C. et al. (2014). Cluster of atherosclerosis in a captive population of black kites (*Milvus migrans* subsp.) in France and effect of nutrition on the plasma lipidogram. *Avain Dis.* 58 (1): 176–182.

113 Lumeij, J. (1994). Nephrology. In: *Avian Medicine: Principles and Applications* (eds. B. Ritchie, G. Harrison and L. Harrison), 538–555. Lake Worth, FL: Wingers Publishing.

114 Echols, M. (2006). Evaluating and treating the kidneys. In: *Clinical Avian Medicine* (eds. T. Lightfoot and G. Harrison), 451–484. Palm Beach, FL: Spix Publishing.

115 Phalen, D. (2000). Avian renal disorders. In: *Laboratory Animal Medicine* (ed. A. Fudge), 61–67. Philadelphia, PA: W. B. Saunders.

33

Cytology

Helene Pendl[1], Peter M. Wencel[2], and Hugues Beaufrère[3]

[1]Pendl Lab, Hematology, Cytology, and Histopathology in Birds and Reptiles, Zug, Switzerland
[2]Al Aseefa Falcon Hospital, Dubai, United Arab Emirates
[3]Department of Medicine and Epidemiology, School of Veterinary Medicine, University of California-Davis, Davis, California, USA

CONTENTS

Introduction

Cytology is a simple, rapid, low-risk, and cost-effective diagnostic tool, ideal to be applied in critical care patients. Common applications include fine needle aspirates (FNAs) from solid masses, cysts, joints, sinuses, bone marrow, and the coelomic cavity. Swabs and scrapings are taken from skin, conjunctiva, oropharynx, air sacs, crop, cloaca, feces, and freshly cut organ surfaces during necropsy. Successful implementation of cytology will stand or fall with time- and cost-effective sample collection and preparation, proper equipment, good archiving of results for comparison, and *last but not least* the expertise of the examiner [1]. Investment into a good quality microscope is of utmost importance. Only high standard equipment will allow for a rapid and unequivocal recognition of cytologic features necessary to achieve meaningful results in a timely manner. Minimum requirements for a good microscope include a powerful Köhler's transmission light source with a continuous brightness control. Eyepieces together with 4×, 10×, 40×, and 100× objectives should allow for a total magnification from 40× to 1000×. Polarized light and phase contrast are helpful additional features. Evaluation of cytologic specimens has its limitations when done by personnel other than experienced cytopathologists [2]. To avoid erroneous results, examination under emergency conditions should be restricted to easy-to-detect changes such as parasitic, microbial, or crystalline agents and the presence of inflammation. Samples with findings beyond this scope should be referred to a specialist for full evaluation.

Sampling and Processing

Sampling and processing techniques depend on tissue type and accessibility. Surface tissues are more easily accessed than internal tissues. Firm connective tissue requires more aggressive methods of collection than epithelial or round cell tissues, where cells are less tightly connected and isolation of single cells is easier. Immediate processing of the sample is of vital importance for proper evaluation.

Fluids from joints, sinuses, cystic structures, coelomic effusions are best aspirated by using a 1–5 ml syringe armed with a hypodermic needle of 25–20 gauge. Coating with 4% disodium ethylenediamine tetraacetic acid (EDTA) prior to use will diminish the risk of clotting [3]. Any fluid aspirate should be evaluated macroscopically prior to analysis. Determination of specific gravity, total protein content,

Exotic Animal Emergency and Critical Care Medicine, First Edition. Edited by Jennifer E. Graham, Grayson A. Doss and Hugues Beaufrère.

Table 33.1 Differentiation of fluids into transudates and exudates.

Type	Color	Specific Gravity	Cellularity (cells/µl)	Total Protein (g/dl)	Pathogenesis
Transudate	Clear to straw colored	<1.017	<1000	<2.5	Low oncotic or high hydrostatic intravascular pressure
Modified transudates	Clear to straw colored	<1.025	1000–5000 macrophages, reactive mesothelial cells	2.5–3.0	Like transudate, but more chronic stage
Exudates	Variable color and turbidity, foul odor possible; tendency to clot	>1.025	>5000, type depending on pathogenic agent, intensity, and duration of process – see types of inflammation	>3.0	Inflammatory processes, increase of capillary permeability

Source: Adapted from Campbell [3].

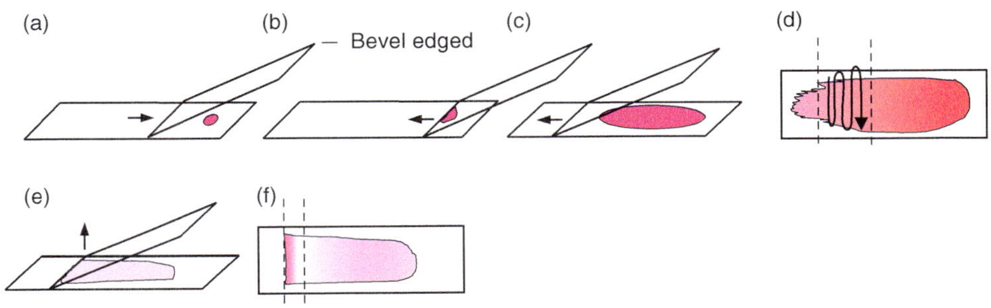

Figure 33.1 Preparation of fluid samples: (a–d) Blood film technique for opaque fluids; full, even spread onto the slide; evaluation in the monolayer area marked with the dotted lines; e, f line smear concentration technique for translucent fluids; lifting of the spreader slide before the sample is fully spread; evaluation in the area of concentration marked with the dotted lines. *Source:* Adapted from Stacy and Pendl [1].

and cellularity will allow for differentiation into transudates, modified transudates, and exudates (Table 33.1).

If sample volume allows, aliquots can be submitted for microbiology, clinical chemistry, and viscosity tests in joint aspirates. The remainder of the harvested fluid should be put into EDTA, which not only reduces clot formation but also calcium dependent phagocytic activity of leukocytes [4, 5]. Opaque hypercellular samples are best processed with the blood film technique (Figure 33.1a–d). The use of a bevel edged spreader slide will reduce cell destruction. In contrast, hypocellular, transparent fluids should be processed with the line concentration technique (Figure 33.1e,f). The cells within the fluid will concentrate at the end of the film, where the glass slide is lifted. In very hypocellular samples, cytospin centrifugation may be necessary to achieve sufficient cellularity of the sample.

FNAs are performed with the same equipment as outlined for fluids and are the preferred method for sampling solid masses. Except for highly hyperemic tissues, delicate negative pressure should be maintained during cell collection. Aspiration from several sites within the lesion will enhance the probability of a representative sample. Ultrasound guided aspiration is recommended for sampling of internal masses. In birds with hepatomegaly, the liver may also be readily visible under the skin and a FNA may be performed without ultrasound guidance. Retrieval from the lesion is always performed without vacuum to avoid aspiration of the material from the needle lumen into the syringe. After being expelled onto a slide, the sample is squashed and spread gently with a second slide (Figure 33.2). The pressure applied should be as low as possible to ensure sufficient cell separation with minimal cell destruction [6].

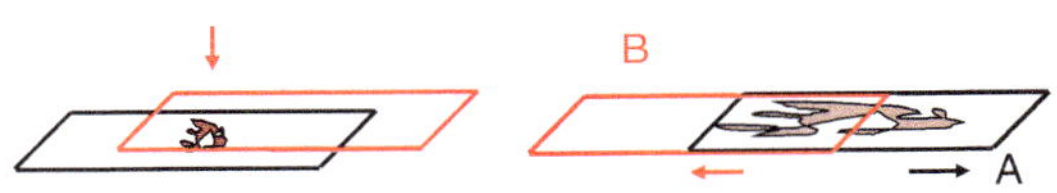

Figure 33.2 Squash preparation technique: the pressure applied should be as low as possible to ensure sufficient cell separation with minimal cell destruction. Usually slide A contains more diagnostic material than slide B.

Cytology performed during necropsy represents an invaluable tool in flock emergency cases, such as an outbreak of atoxoplasmosis or the septicemic form of pox in canaries. Samples taken from a freshly deceased bird with clinical symptoms will give initial information upon which to guide therapy while awaiting results from more in-depth and time consuming diagnostic procedures.

Birds

Table 33.2 Features and limitations of the three most commonly used stains in avian cytology.

Stain	Features	Limitations
Romanowsky	Good overview – stains most cellular and noncellular structures in the sample	Acid fast organisms remain unstained
Acid fast	Stains acid fast organisms red such as mycobacteria, mature crypto- and microsporidia	Poor delineation of cellular structures, not suitable for general evaluation; false negative results due to improper technique; commercially available quality control slides recommended for comparison
Gram	Allows to classify bacteria present in the sample as G+ or G–	Poor delineation of cellular structures, not suitable for general evaluation; acid fast organisms remain unstained; knowledge of normal flora required for interpretation; unreliable results due to improper technique; commercially available quality control slides containing mixture of G+ and G– bacteria recommended for comparison

Fixation and Staining

After air drying, fixation of slides is best achieved by placing them into high quality, acetone-free, absolute methanol for five minutes. As for staining, a Romanowsky-type-based stain together with an acid-fast stain, and a gram stain is the most common combination used in avian practice for staining cytology specimens. Their characteristics and limitations are summarized in Table 33.2. Romanowsky stains such as Diff Quik®, Wright's, Wright–Giemsa, or similar will give a good overview of the sample, as they stain all cellular structures and most of the microbial agents. They do not allow differentiation between Gram-positive and Gram-negative bacteria. Some structures such as sporulated oocysts, mature microsporidium spores, and mycobacteria will stay stainless and appear as negative images against colored background. Quick stains such as Diff Quik® and Hemacolor® are easy and rapid to perform. A Wright–Giemsa staining (WGS) protocol has been demonstrated to be of superior value in terms of quality and delineation of subcellular details in hematology (Table 33.3). However, longer staining time is often required for cytologic specimens [7]. Acid fast staining techniques like Ziehl–Neelsen will selectively stain acid-fast organisms such as mycobacteria, crypto- and microsporidia, and can also be

Table 33.3 Wright–Giemsa staining protocol for avian hematology and cytology samples.

Colorant	Staining protocol
• 3 g Wright – Powder[a] • 0.3 g Giemsa – Powder[b] • 5 ml glycerine • 1000 ml absolute methanol (acetone free)[c] • Filter and store in a dark vial • Stable for several weeks	Use air-dried native blood films Flood blood film 3 min with colorant Add equal amount of buffer pH 6.8[d] Mix gently by blowing with a pipette or a straw until metallic green sheen appears on the surface Allow to stand for 6 min Rinse and flood with buffer for 1 min Wash copiously with buffer Wipe the back of the blood film to remove excess stain Prop in rack until dry or use hair dryer Mount with Entellan®[e] and cover glass

[a] Merck® No. 1.09278.0025.
[b] Merck® No 1.09203.0025.
[c] Merck® No 1.06009.1000.
[d] Merck® No 1.11374.0100.
[e] e.g. Entellan Neu, Merck® No 1.07961.0100.

performed on samples previously stained with Romanowsky and Gram stains. Gram stain will allow for classification of bacteria as Gram-positive or -negative. Cytologic features are poorly depicted in both stains making them unsuitable for general assessment of the sample. Special stains may be obtained from specialized laboratories but are seldom used in practice [1].

Evaluation

Evaluation of Wet Mounts and Native Samples

Wet mounts are ideally prepared with a drop of warm sterile saline to maintain motility of certain parasites [1, 3]. Common applications on emergency include fecal samples and crop swabs to quickly screen for motile flagellates, coccidial oocysts, nematode eggs, and yeasts. Mounting with a coverslip should result in a static image without flow movement. Examination starts under 100× magnification to search for parasitic structures and areas of interest such as cell clusters and mucus aggregates. Specific areas of interest are scanned under higher magnification. Although the preparation technique should aim for the creation of a layer as thin as possible, a wet mount will always comprise more layers than a dried, stained sample. This is important to keep in mind, when switching to higher magnifications, as different pathogens may appear in different layers and changing of the focus plane will be necessary to assess all layers correctly.

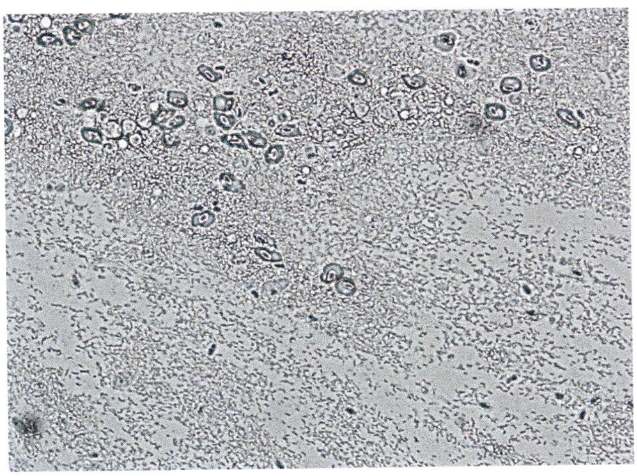

Figure 33.3 Mycobacteriosis: masses of uniform rods in the background. Correct settings of light, diaphragm, and condenser will make the rods visible due to increased light refraction around the edges of the bacilli; final confirmation by acid fast stain. Spleen imprint, Lesser Goldfinch (*Carduelis psaltria*), native, dry, non-mounted slide, 400×.

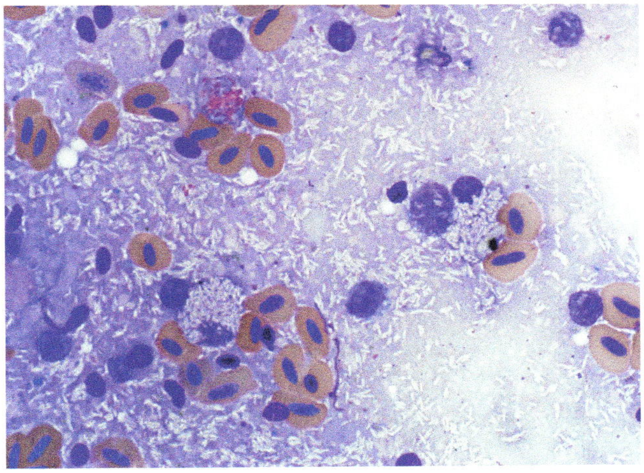

Figure 33.4 Mycobacteriosis: negative staining mycobacterial rods visible against basophilic background coloration and within macrophages. Liver imprint, Macaw (*Ara* sp.), modified Wright's stain, 400x.

Rapid evaluation of native, fresh, not yet dried samples under 100×–400× magnification allows for quick assessment of the cellularity and the presence of artifacts. In case of poor results, repetition of the sampling can be performed in a timely manner. High light settings with a partially closed diaphragm or a condenser pulled downward will result in increased light refraction at the edges of translucent structures such as bacterial rods. For example *Mycobacterium spp.* bacilli are often easy to spot in drying serosal or organ touch preparations if present in considerable amounts (Figure 33.3). In Romanowsky stained preparations mycobacteria do not take up the dye and will soon become invisible in mounted slides or when covered with immersion oil unless piled up in clusters or seen as *ghost rods* against contrasting background and inside cells (Figure 33.4). Examination of stained, but still wet samples under 100×–400× magnification will allow viewing of details in crisp, clear, smooth, and bright colored appearance comparable to properly mounted slides, which are difficult to view in dried and non-mounted specimens due to dulling of the colors and uneven roughening of the sample surface. Mounting the wet slide temporarily with an appropriately sized coverslip furthermore allows a switch to the oil immersion objective and examination of the slide as it was sealed with proper mounting medium. The underside of the slide should be wiped clean to avoid sticking onto the stage of the microscope. After examination, the coverslip is removed and the slide left to air-dry.

Evaluation of Stained Samples

As mentioned previously, evaluation of cytologic specimens under emergency conditions should be restricted to the detection of easily recognizable features with the aim to start initial

EVALUATION PROTOCOL CYTOLOGY

Name/ID: Date: ______________________________

History: ______________________________

____

1. DOES THE SLIDE CONTAIN INTACT CELLS OF THE TISSUE INTENDED TO BE SAMPLED?

(LOW MAGNIFICATION 40x -100x)

a) Technical aspects and quality (sample location, preparation technique, staining, semiquantitative scale from 1=inacceptable to 5=excellent)______________
b) Cellularity (low, moderate, high)______________
c) Cell Distribution (% individual cells, % clusters)______________
d) Representative cell flecks (yes/no)______________
e) Percentage of cell types present (% ery, % round cell, %epithelial, % mesenchymal)______________

____

2. DOES THE SLIDE CONTAIN MICROBIAL OR NON-VITAL STRUCTURES?

(HIGH MAGNIFICATION, 400x -1000x)

a) Microbial structures (bacterial, fungal, viral, parasitic, other)______________

____

b) Non-vital structures (esp. urate/cholesterol crystals from joint/skin swellings, other)______________

____

3. ARE THERE SIGNS OF INFLAMMATION, HEMORRHAGE, DEGENERATION, NEOPLASIA?

(HIGH MAGNIFICATION, 400x -1000x)

a) inflammation (heterophil – mixed cell – granulomatous – eosinophilic – lymphoplasmacytic)______________

____

b) acute/chronic hemorrhage______________

____

c) degeneration/necrosis (atypic cytoplasmic vacuolation, cytolysis, karyorrhexis, -pyknosis, -lysis)______________

____

d) signs of malignancy (mild/moderate/severe, cellular/cytoplasmic/nuclear signs, > 3 signs per cell yes /no)_

____

4. CYTOLOGIC DIAGNOSIS AND LIST OF DIFFERENTIALS

____

DATE/SIGNATURE:______________

Figure 33.5 Evaluation protocol for cytology. *Source:* Adapted from Stacy and Pendl [1].

evaluation while awaiting the results from more time-consuming full interpretation from a specialist. The evaluation protocol outlined in Figure 33.5 has been amended from a full examination protocol [1] to meet the needs of a quick check under timely limitations. Every sample is scanned from low to high magnification to answer three main questions:

1) Does the slide contain intact cells of the tissue intended to be sampled?
2) Does the slide contain pathogenic microbial or non-vital structures?
3) Are there signs of inflammation, hemorrhage, degeneration, neoplasia?

The first two questions are usually answered within a very short time, the third always requires a more thorough examination and likely submission to a specialist, especially if question two is answered in the negative.

Representativity of the Sample

Any cytologic sample consists of a variable mixture of epithelial, mesenchymal, and hematic (*round cell*) cells typical for the tissue they were sampled from. The characteristic features in terms of cellularity, distribution pattern on the slide and cytomorphology for these three cell types are summarized in Table 33.4.

Microbial Structures

A number of microbial structures may be detected in cytologic samples. However, cytologic diagnosis should be considered tentative and confirmation should be carried out by other diagnostic means. **Bacteria** may be present in samples as natural flora, contaminants, postmortal colonisation or truly pathogenic agents. Differentiation between the four requires knowledge of physiological flora and may be challenging especially when evaluating samples from natural surfaces such as skin, conjunctiva, and gastrointestinal tract. Generally, numbers of bacteria with uniform morphology free in the background of a fecal or a gut sample are suggestive of at least an abnormal bacterial overgrowth. Presence of inflammatory cells and signs of bacterial phagocytosis suggest a bacterial infection. In histology, uniform bacterial nests in samples from internal organs without signs of inflammation strongly point to a secondary infection caused by primary immunosuppression (Figure 33.6a). However, this may be difficult to ascertain in cytologic samples. Chlamydial inclusions typically present as small, round to oval, intracytoplasmic membrane-bound microcolonies which consist of a mixture of elementary bodies, intermediate stages, and reticulate bodies [3]. They are most frequently detected in samples from the conjunctiva, sinuses, airsacs, liver, and spleen. As infected cells tend to rupture during slide preparation, chlamydial bodies are often found free in the background of the sample. Differentiation of chlamydial bodies from cellular debris, stained dust particles, and the basophilic granulation of basophils, immature heterophils, and eosinophils of certain species may be difficult. The central bodies in understained heterophilic granules may additionally pose a pitfall for unexperienced examiners, although these subgranular structures stain eosinophilic instead of basophilic (Figure 33.6b). Chlamydial bodies can be confounded with other microbial agents staining basophilic in Romanowsky-type stains,

Table 33.4 Characteristics of different tissue cell types within a cytology sample.

Type	Cellularity	Distribution on the slide	Cytomorphology
Epithelial cells	Moderate to high	Usually in clusters, acinar or tubular arrangement in secretory/excretory epithelia possible, increased number of single cells in case of irritation or neoplasia	Variable size and form (round, cuboidal, columnar, flat, and polygonal); occ. Microvilli (intestine) or cilia (trachea, caudal sinuses, and primary bronchi); distinct cytoplasmic borders in surface epithelia; poorly visible cytoplasmic borders in secretory/excretory epithelia (kidney, liver)
Mesenchymal cells	Low to moderate	Aggregates and individual cells, occ. alignment into a certain direction; increased number of single cells in case of irritation or neoplasia	Spindle form, unipolar or bipolar trailing (fibrous), roundish (osteochondral) single cells with diffuse cytoplasmic borders; eosinophilic background in osteoid/chondroid tissue samples
Round (hematic) cells	High	Evenly distributed	Small to moderately large, different types (see hematology); always clear cytoplasmic borders

Source: Adapted from Stacy and Pendl [1].

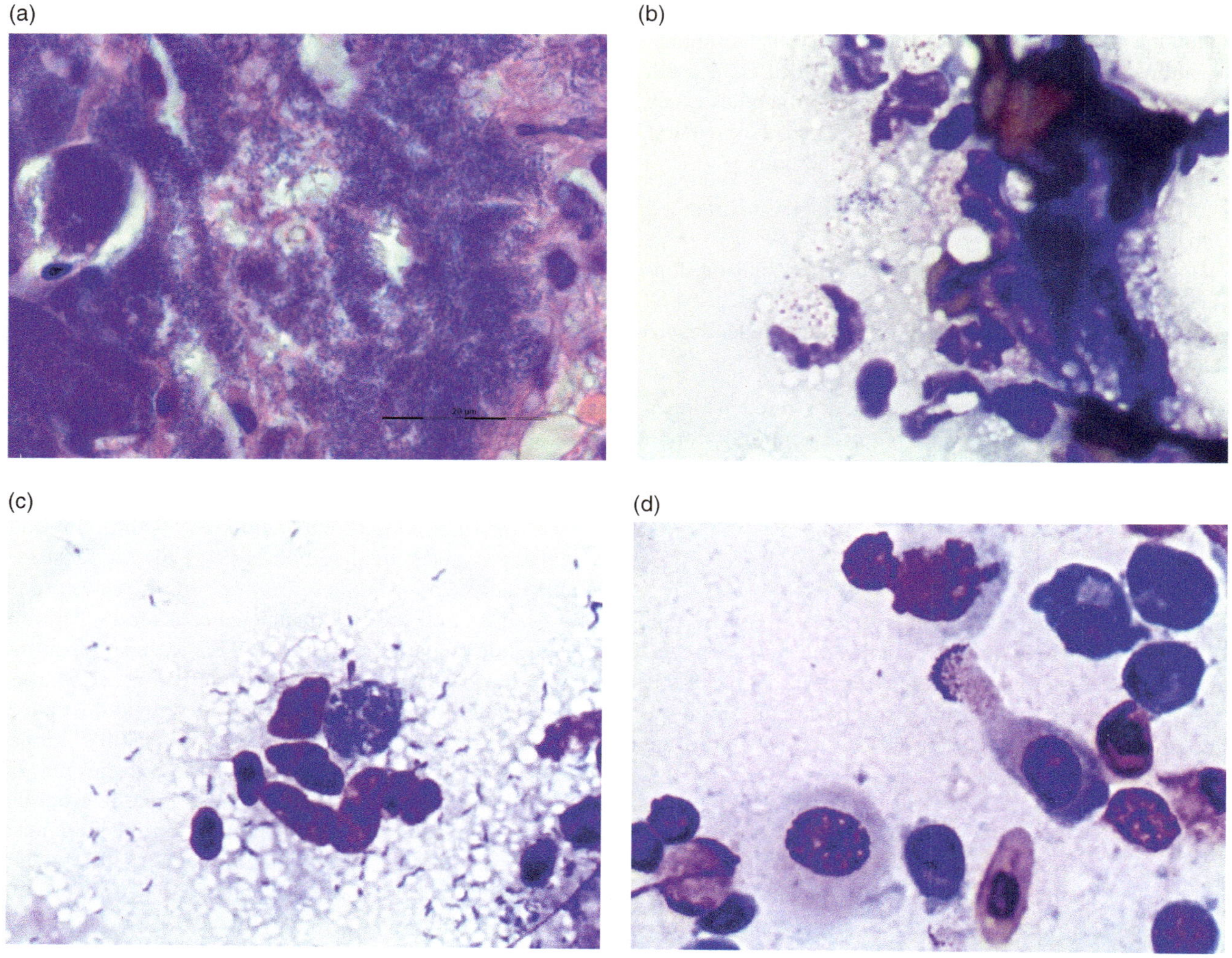

Figure 33.6 (a–d) Bacterial structures. (a) Secondary bacterial pneumonia due to circovirus infection (confirmation by PCR): massive uniform bacterial nests without signs of inflammation indicating immunosuppression; histologic section lung, Grey parrot (*Psittacus erithacus*), Histologic section Hematoxylin-Eosin, 1000×. (b) Chlamydiosis: Mixed cell inflammation with delicate, *poppy seed* like basophilic elementary bodies in the center, which must be differentiated from the eosinophilic central bodies of understained granules in the heterophils. Close inspection of the latter reveals an ellipsoid colorless granule around every central body; Airsac swab, Domestic pigeon (*Columba livia var dom*); Diff Quik®, 1000×. (c) Campylobacteriosis: In contrast to the characteristic *gull-wing*, comma shape appearance of the extracellular bacteria, the phagocytized degenerate forms in the macrophage present as coccoid structures of different sizes which may be confused with chlamydial inclusions. Pericardial swab, Domestic pigeon (*Columba livia var dom*), Diff Quik®, 1000×; (d) Mycoplasmosis: Small coccobacilli like structures attached to the apical surface of an epithelial cell in the center. Mixed cell inflammation with prominent portion of plasma cells with well visible golgi apparatus as light area in the deep basophilic cytoplasm. Conjunctival swab, Backyard chicken (*Gallus gallus var dom*), Diff Quik®, 1000×

especially phagocytized bacteria with coccoid or coccobacilloid morphology such as *Staphylococcus* sp., *Streptococcus* sp., degenerate forms of *Campylobacter* sp. (Figure 33.6c), and *Mycoplasma* sp.. *Mycoplasma* sp. presents as punctate structures attached to the apical surface of epithelial cells. When seen from the side they will be attached to the cell membrane in a *brush border* manner (Figure 33.6d). When seen from above, however, they may give a false impression of intracytoplasmic, chlamydia-like inclusions. **Fungal infections** typically occur in patients with an impaired physiologic microbial flora of natural body surfaces and under general immunosuppression [3]. *Candida* spp. may present as discrete, budding, or filamenting cells or as septated pseudohyphae with branches and lateral buds (Figure 33.7a). They are most commonly found in oropharyngeal swabs, crop swabs, and fecal samples. In severely immunocompromised patients *Candida* sp. may also occur in internal tissues such as lung, kidney, and liver. *Staining* of fungal elements in these tissues is often weak (Figure 33.7b). *Macrorhabdus ornithogaster* colonizes the isthmus between the proventriculus and ventriculus of many avian species [3] (Figure 33.7c). They are intermittently shed in feces. Proventricular scrapings collected post mortem provide the best sample for detection and quantitative analysis [3]. In Romanowsky stained samples, *Macrorhabdus ornithogaster* stains weakly basophilic to even colorless. Nuclei are visible as one to two small, purple staining, oblongate structures per cell (Figure 33.7d). *Aspergillus* sp. is the most common fungal pathogen affecting the respiratory tract of birds. Cytology is characterized by the presence of moderately thick (5–10 μm in width) septate hyphae with parallel longitudinal sides and rounded short ends. Branching typically occurs at an angle of 45° [3]. *Aspergillus* spp. spores can be differentiated into round mature spores of about 2 μm in diameter with a *shelled*, greenish-blue, *empty* appearance and smaller, immature spores, which are round and stain light basophilic with a purple content giving them a *still-viable* appearance (Figure 33.7e). Microsporidia are obligate intracellular pathogens with a unique life cycle and in birds seem to mainly infect enterocytes but have also been isolated from conjunctival, liver and kidney samples (8–11). Both immature and mature spores can be distinguished. Fully mature spores are small (1 × 1.5–2 μm) ovoid structures which remain colorless in Romanowsky-type stains (Figure 33.7f), but stain positive in acid-fast stains. Immature spores resemble immature *Aspergillus* sp. spores, but develop intracellularly. Heavily infected host cells often rupture during sampling and slide preparation releasing variably aged spores, which can be seen lying freely in the background.

Protozoal infections commonly detected from cytologic samples include flagellates from the gut and tissue stages from hematozoa and coccidia in the liver, spleen, and lungs. Motile flagellates from swabs of the crop, gastrointestinal tract, or fecal samples are best viewed in wet mounts prepared with warm saline [1, 3]. In contrast to the rather slow often circular movements of trichomonads in crop swabs, trophozoites of *Spironucleus/Hexamita columbae* in swabs of fresh fecal samples show a quick, dart-like motion with sudden twitches [1]. In stained samples, Trichomonas trophozoites are relatively large (12-20 μm in length), roundish or teardrop in shape, with four anterior flagella, posteriorly protruding axostyle, and undulated membrane. A single nucleus is located close to the anterior pole of the cell [1] (Figure 33.8a). Hexamita trophozoites are smaller and more slender (6–12 x 2–5 μm), often described as sausage shaped with eight long symmetrically arranged flagella. The nuclear complex consists of two nuclei and is situated directly at the anterior pole of the cell. It varies in shape from triangle to horseshoe or bilobed [1] (Figure 33.8b). *Cryptosporidia* infections in birds mainly affect the mucosa of the gastrointestinal tract, but have also been described in conjunctival and respiratory epithelium, the urogenital tract, *the auditory tube*, and the bursa of Fabricius. Concerning the latter, coinfection with psittacine circovirus is common [10]. Mature oocysts are characterized by their small (6–8 μm), uniform ovoid appearance and complete lack of staining in Romanowsky stains (Figure 33.8c). Similar to microsporidial spores, intact mature oocysts stain acid fast positive (Figure 33.8d). Apicomplexa such as *Toxoplasma*, *Sarcocystis, some Isospora* sp. and hematozoa such as *Leukocytozoon*, *Hemoproteus*, and *Plasmodium* sp. can cause significant systemic disease [10] especially in naive hosts, juvenile birds, and immunocompromised patients. Tissue stages are usually detected in samples from lung, liver, and spleen (Figure 33.8e,f). **Viral diseases** may be detected by the presence of inclusion bodies. Characteristic intranuclear inclusion bodies (INIBs) are known to occur in adeno-, polyoma-, and herpesvirus (Figure 33.9a–d), intracytoplasmic inclusion bodies (ICIBs) may be visible with pox- and circovirus infections (Figure 33.9e,f). Cytologic features of viral inclusion bodies (IBs) together with clinical and pathologic key findings [10] are summarized in Table 33.5.

Inflammation

Evaluation of inflammatory changes requires knowledge of the morphology of different types of immune cells (see Chapter 32: Clinical Pathology). Depending on the predominant cell type, inflammation in birds can be classified as heterophilic–suppurative, mixed cell-pyogranulomatous, macrophagic-granulomatous, eosinophilic, and lymphoplasmacytic [1, 3]. Type and degree of accumulation depends on the type of pathogen, the intensity, and the duration of the irritation. Therefore, assessment of the type of inflammation in a cytologic sample allows for certain conclusions on the pathogenesis, possible etiologies, and the duration of the process. Table 33.6 summarizes the most important characteristics of each type of inflammation, general interpretation, and the most commonly occurring etiologies. In any case, careful examination for signs of phagocytosis of microorganisms and/or signs of heterophilic degeneration is recommended. The former confirms septic inflammation, the latter raises suspicion of a septic infection with accumulation of microbial toxins in the microenvironment. Degenerative changes in heterophils, also called *toxic* changes, include nuclear swelling, karyorrhexis, karyolysis, increased cytoplasmic basophilia, vacuolation, abnormal granulation, and degranulation [3, 6, 13] (Figure 33.10). Plasma cells in lymphoplasmacytic

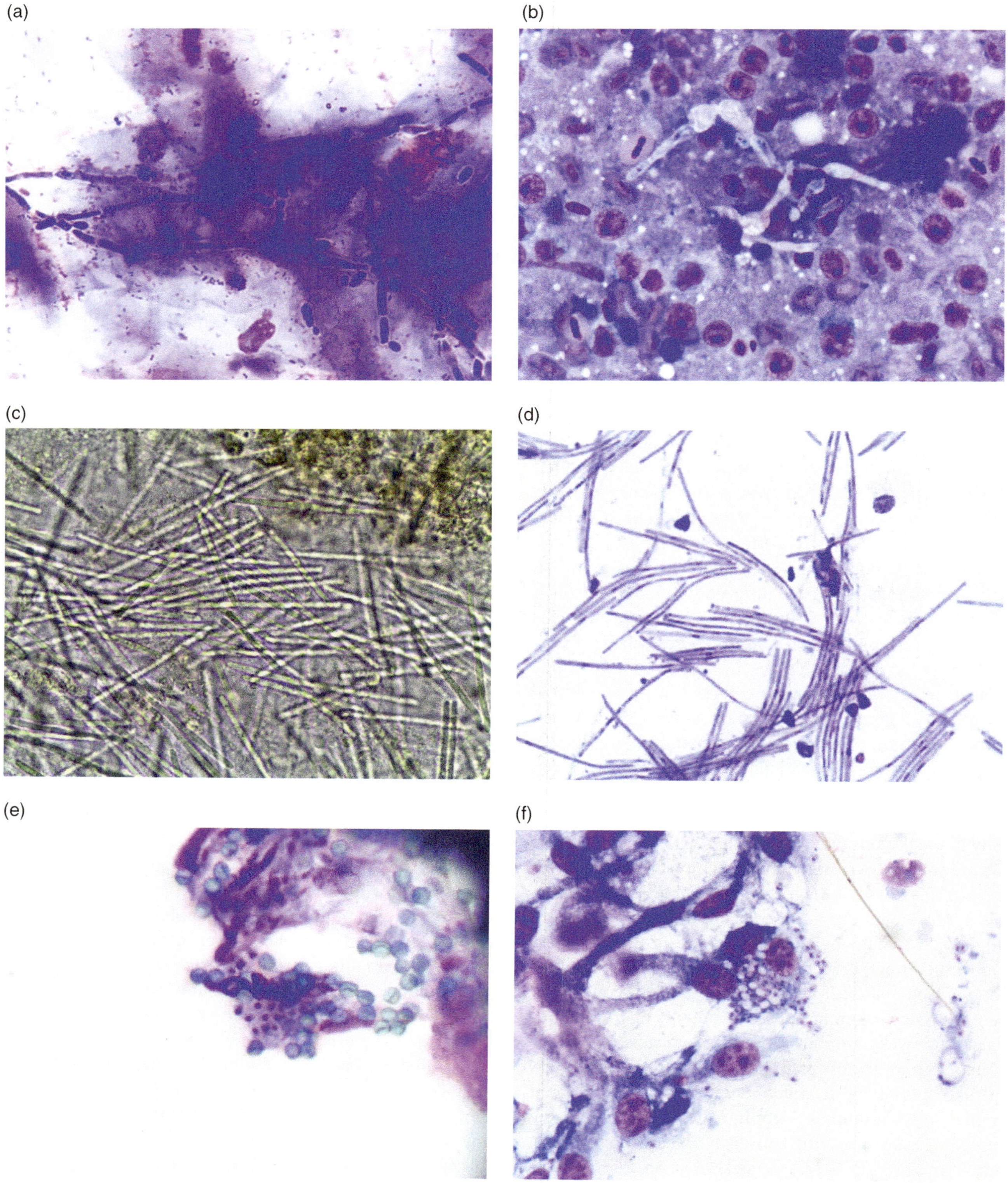

Figure 33.7 (a–e) Fungal structures. (a): Candidiasis: Pseudohyphal filaments of *Candida albicans* showing branching, septations, and lateral buds. Crop swab, Gyrfalcon (*Falco rusticolus)*, Diff-Quik® 1000×; (b) Candidiasis: pseudohyphal filaments of *Candida albicans* with weak staining of fungal structures characteristic for tissue samples. Liver granuloma squash preparation, Goldfinch (*Carduelis carduelis*), Diff-Quik® 1000×; (c) *Macrorhabdus ornithogaster*: Long (up to 70 μm in length), round ended, uniformly looking, rod shaped organisms with sparse, vacuolar intracellular structures. Proventricular mucosal scraping, Backyard chicken (*Gallus gallus var dom),* wet mount, 400×; (d) *Macrorhabdus ornithogaster*: Light basophilic, long rods in *haystack* arrangement with one to two small, purple staining, oblong nuclei per cell. Proventricular mucosal scraping, Canary finch (*Serinus canaria*), Diff-Quik® 400×; (e) Aspergillosis: Mature *Aspergillus* spp. spores with *shelled,* greenish-blue, empty appearance in contrast to smaller light basophilic, round, still *viable* looking, immature spores with purple content. Air sac biopsy squash preparation. Racing pigeon (*Columba livia*), Diff-Quik® 1000×; (f) Microsporidiosis; Mixture of mature and immature spores of *Encephalitozoon hellem*. Mature spores do not pick up the stain and are slightly bigger (up to 2.5 μm) than immature spores. Ruptured infected enterocyte from a rectal scraping. Gouldian Finch (*Chloebia gouldiae*), Diff-Quik® 1000×.

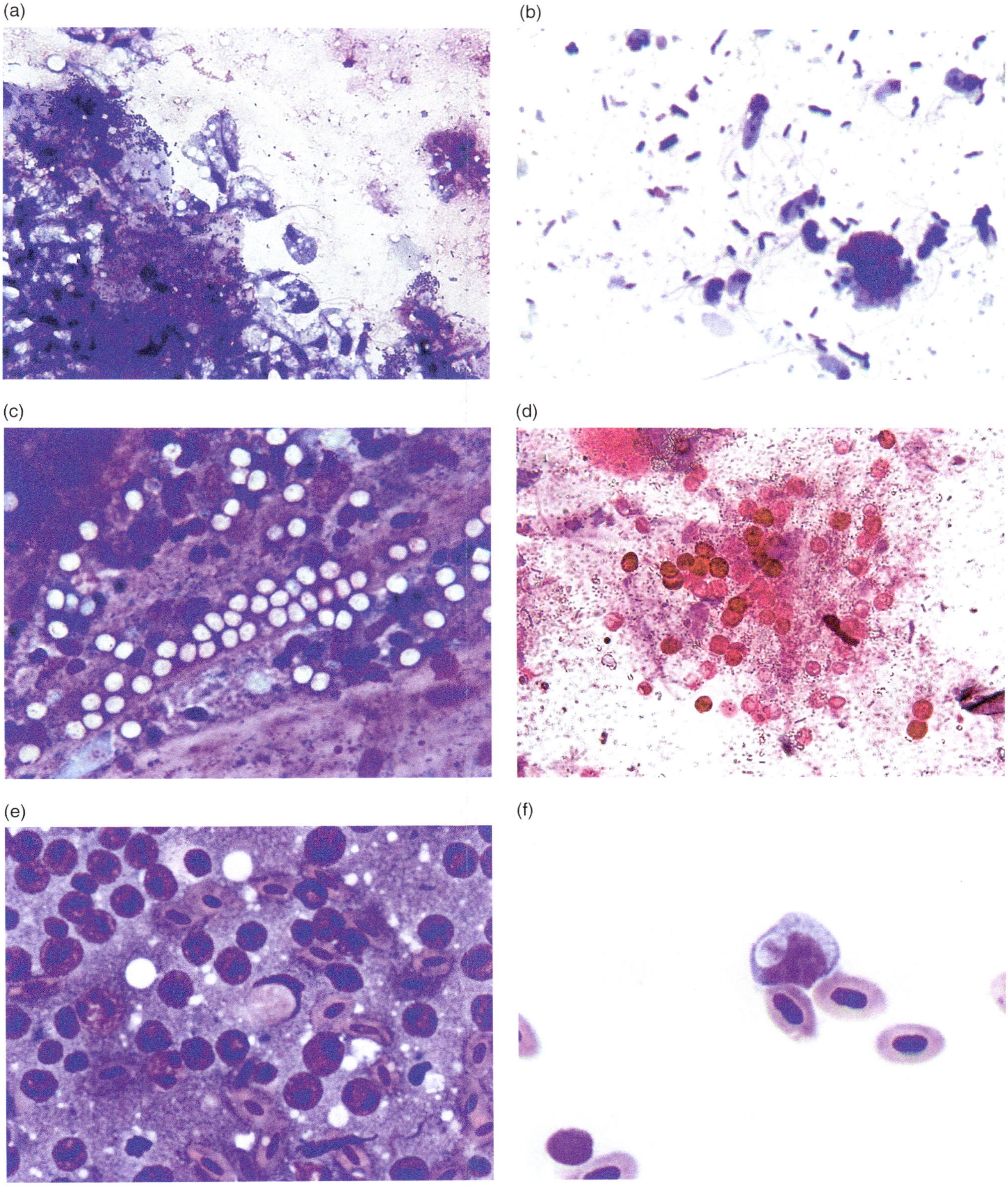

Figure 33.8 (a–e) Protozoal structures. (a) Trichomoniasis: Trophozoites with a clearly visible axostyle in the vacuolated slightly basophilic cytoplasm. A single nucleus is located close to the anterior pole, from which a tuft of four flagella is protruding. The unilateral undulated membrane is poorly visible. Crop swab, Racing Pigeon (*Columba livia var dom)*, Diff Quik® 1000×; (b) Spironucleosis/Hexamitiasis: *Spironucleus* (*Hexamita*) *columbae* trophozoites with variable size and shape and long flagella. In the large trophozoites a prominent nuclear complex at the anterior pole is visible. Intestinal scraping, Racing Pigeon (*Columba livia var dom)*, Diff Quik® 1000×; (c) Cryptosporidiosis: Mature oocysts of *Cryptosporidium baileyi* with uniform ovoid appearance and complete lack of staining. Impression smear bursa of Fabricius, Peacock (*Pavo cristatus*), Diff-Quik® 1000×, (d) Cryptosporidiosis. Acid fast positive staining of mature *Cryptosporidium galli* oocysts. Intact organisms stain intensively ruby red, distorted oocysts are colored in various shades of pink. Immature organisms and those with damaged walls will stain blue and faint red. Fecal smear, Diamond Firetail (*Stagonopleura guttata*), Ziehl–Neelsen, 1000×; (e) Leukocytozoonosis: Pinkish round intracytoplasmic gametocyte displacing and deforming the host nucleus to a lateral crescent. Liver squash preparation, Saker falcon (*Falco cherrug*) Diff Quik®, 1000×. (f) Atoxoplasmosis: Single merozoite within the cytoplasm of a mononuclear cell, note the characteristic indentation of the host cell nucleus caused by the parasite. Canary finch (*Serinus canaria*), lung imprint. Diff-Quik®, 1000×

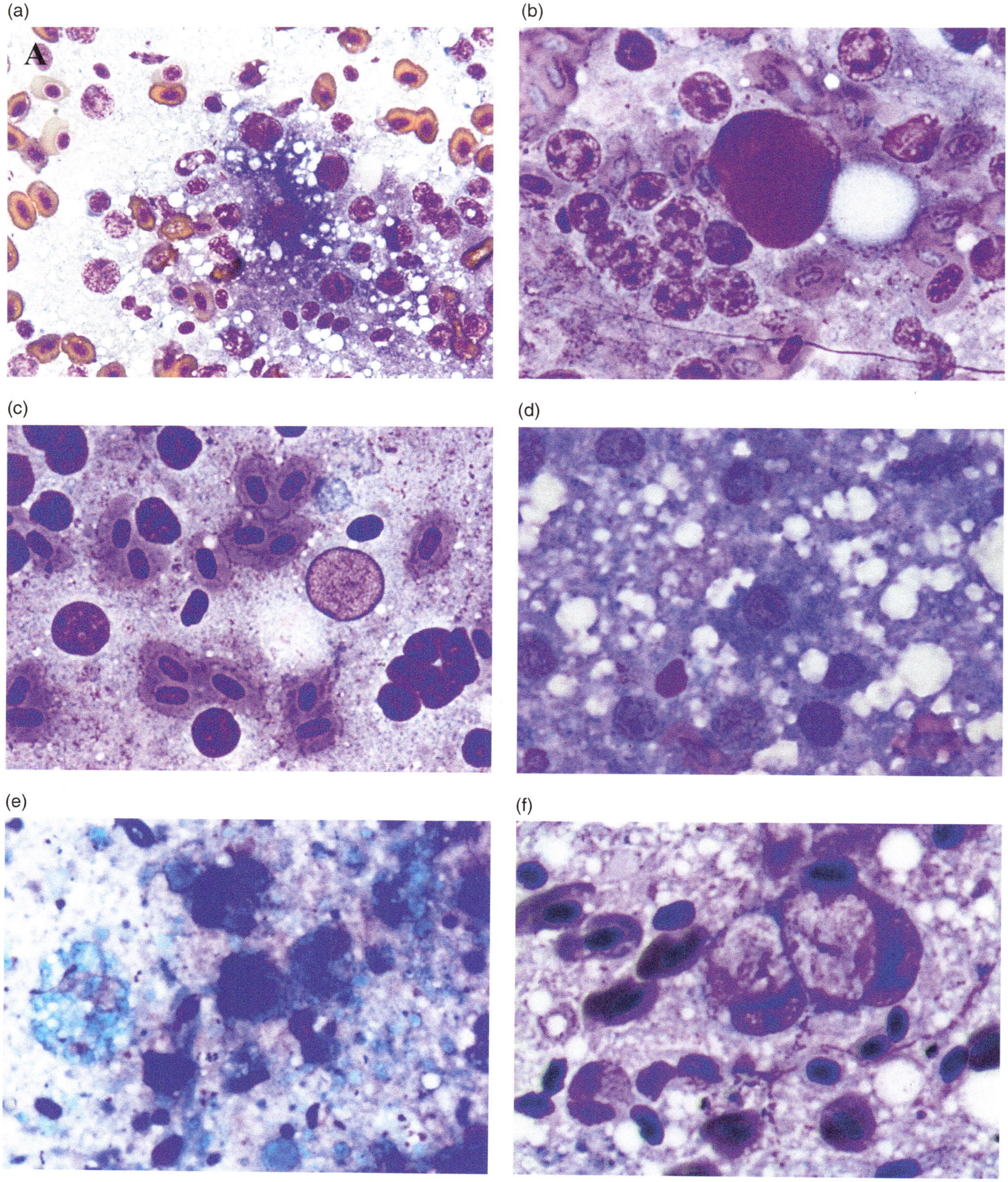

Figure 33.9 (a–f) Viral structures. Intranuclear (INIB) and intracytoplasmic (ICIB) inclusion bodies from organ squash preparations during necropsy; decisive confirmation by PCR; (a) Pigeon Adenovirus (PiAdV) inclusion body hepatitis: amphophilic, multiple small to single medium sized INIBs in enlarged nuclei with displacement of nucleoli to the nuclear membrane. The cytoplasmic vacuolation indicates moderate hepatolipidosis; Racing Pigeon (*Columba livia var dom),* May Grünwald Giemsa, 400×; (b) Adenovirosis: Very large, amphophilic INIB displacing the nucleolus to the left, normally sized nuclei of renal epithelial cells in tubular arrangement, kidney squash preparation, Canary finch (*Serinus canaria*); Diff Quik®, 1000×; (c) Polyomavirus: Karyomegaly with pale, finely granulated INIB filling the entire nucleus, delicate chromatin margination, nucleolus displaced to the nuclear membrane; kidney squash preparation, Gouldian finch (*Erythrura gouldiae)*; Diff Quik®, 1000×; (d): Strigid Herpesvirus (StrHV) inclusion body hepatitis: Small basophilic INIBs without halo in two shrunken nuclei with increased basophilia compared to unaffected hepatocyte in the center; liver squash preparation, Snowy owl (*Nyctaea scandiaca*); Diff Quik®, 1000×; (e): Pigeon circovirus (PiCV): Multiple botryoid, translucent, light basophilic ICIBs resembling crystalline structures in mononuclear cells. Free inclusions originating from ruptured cells are visible in the background; bursal squash preparation, Racing Pigeon (*Columba livia var dom*); Diff Quik® 1000×; (f): Poxvirus: Two epithelial cells with large ICIBs (*Bollinger bodies*) containing pinkish gray granular matter and displacing the nucleus aside. Centrally empty ring forms due to artificial dissolution of ICIB contents may occur. Lung squash preparation, Canary finch (*Serinus canaria*); Diff Quik® 1000×.

Table 33.5 Cytologic features of viral IBs and corresponding clinical and pathologic key findings.

Virus	Inclusion body/cytology	Clinical and pathologic key findings
Adeno	INIB, small to medium sized (liver *Columbiformes*) to extremely large (other species), basophilic to amphophilic	• Hemorrhagic necrotizing hepatosplenitis, enteritis, serofibrinous polyserositis (hydropericardium) in *Galliformes, Columbiformes, Falconiformes, Psittaciformes, Passeriformes* • Hemorrhagic necrotizing bronchitis (quail)
Herpes	INIB, small, eosinophilic to basophilic, with or without halo; nuclear pyknosis; syncytia	• Hemorrhagic necrotizing (laryngo-) tracheitis (*Galliformes, Psittaciformes, Passeriformes*) • Hemorrhagic necrotizing hepatosplenitis (*inclusion body hepatitis*) and/or gastroenteritis (*Anseriformes, Falconiformes, Gruiformes, Strigiformes, Columbiformes*)
Polyoma	INIB, medium-sized to large, colorless to light basophilic or amphophilic INIBs; *hollow nuclei*	• Budgerigar fledgling disease (*Melopsittacus undulatus; French moult, feather dusters*) • Non-budgerigar polyoma virus infection (*Psittaci-, Passeri-, Anseriformes*) • Peracute hemorrhagic-septicemic course in preweaned neonates with varying degrees of hepatorenal, neurologic, and dermal symptoms
Pox	ICIB, eosinophilic with light center, called *Bollinger bodies* in cytology, ballooning degeneration of epithelia	• ***Septicemic form** (esp. in canaries)*: marked hyperplasia of respiratory epithelium with obstruction of airways, hemorrhagic necrotizing inflammation, myocardial necrosis possible, ICIBs rather rare • ***Cutaneous form*** (many species) nodular to diffuse proliferative dermatitis/blepharitis of primarily the unfeathered skin, hemorrhagic-ulcerative bacterial superinfections common • ***Wet form***: proliferative oropharyngitis with caseous covering, hemorrhagic-ulcerative bacterial superinfections common
Circo	ICIB, botryoid, baso- to amphophilic	• Circovirus infection (many bird species) • Psittacine beak and feather disease (PBFD, *Psittaciformes*) • Hemorrhagic-necrotizing pulpitis, bursitis, myelonecrosis, immunosuppression with subsequent secondary opportunistic infections

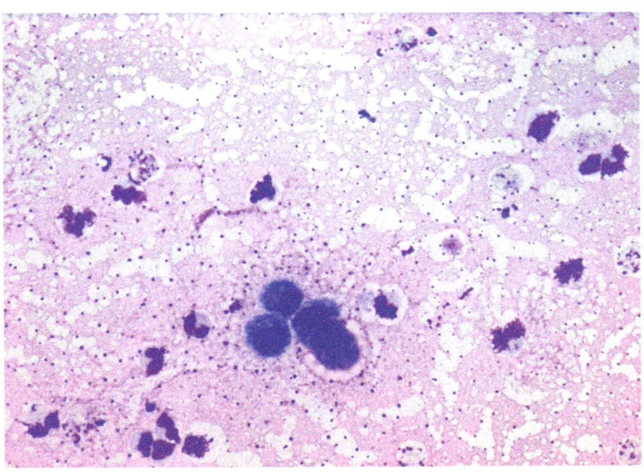

Figure 33.10 Suppurative septic arthritis: Four deeply basophilic synoviocytes, osteo- or chondroblasts indicating increased turnover of joint tissue, heterophils with signs of degeneration suggestive of septic inflammation; FNA carpal joint with radiologically confirmed osteolysis, Red-tailed black cockatoo (*Calyptorhynchus banksii*); Wright–Giemsa, 400×.

inflammation are large round to oval lymphocytes with an abundant, deeply basophilic cytoplasm, and an eccentric nucleus. A prominent golgi apparatus is frequently present (Figure 33.6d).

Hemorrhage vs. Hemodilution

Hemorrhage caused by trauma or injury needs to be differentiated from iatrogenic hemodilution during sampling. Sudden appearance of blood during aspiration indicates dilution whereas continuous red coloration raises suspicion of true hemorrhage.

In acute hemorrhages, lack of thrombocytes in the otherwise blood like aspirate speaks for true hemorrhage, as thrombocytes quickly disappear in the hemorrhagic fluid. Presence of erythrophagocytosis with still visible fully intact cells (Figure 33.11) confirms a subacute haemorrhage, with erythrocytic remnants and iron pigments a more chronic stage of hemorrhage. Hematomas in progressed organization contain many fibroblasts and may look like a neoplastic mesenchymal process [3].

Malignancy vs. Inflammatory Reactive Atypia

Tissue inflammation may cause significant cytomorphologic alterations which may resemble neoplastic changes. Therefore, the presence of inflammation together with cytologic signs of neoplasia always raises doubts of true malignancy. Criteria of malignancy are differentiated into general

Table 33.6 Types of inflammation in birds, adapted from [1, 3].

Type of inflammation	Predominant cell of the inflammatory infiltrate	Commonly associated etiologies	Interpretation
Heterophilic *suppurative*	≥80% heterophils	Esp. bacterial and fungal infections, cell death from circulatory insufficiency within the tissue	Acute phase of inflammation ≤6 h [12]; phagocytosed microorganisms indicate septic inflammation, degenerate heterophils raise suspicion of microbial toxins in the microenvironment [3, 6, 13]
Mixed cell *pyogranulomatous*	About 50% heterophils, lymphocytes, macrophages	Variable	Fully established active inflammation rather subacute ≥6 h [12], most common type of inflammation in birds; presence of giant cells and epitheloid cells may indicate necrosis, as necrotic tissue stimulates a foreign-body-like reaction in birds [3]
Macrophagic *granulomatous*	≥50% macrophages (including multinucleated giant cells and epitheloid cells), heterophils, lymphocytes	Esp. fungal (*Aspergillus sp.*), bacterial (*Mycobacterium* sp.), parasitic (*Trichomonas* sp., *Capillaria* sp.) infections, chronic tissue necrosis of noninfectious origin, fibrogranulomatous tissue repair by secondary intention	Subacute to chronic inflammation ≥24 h; epitheloid cell and multinucleated giant cell formation indicates necrosis and/or unsuccessful elimination of the pathogen with subsequent attempt of compartmentalization into granulomatous tissue; additional presence of fibroblasts indicates progressed stage of chronicity (≥7d) with deposition of collagen
Eosinophilic	≥10% eosinophils	Inflammation of natural body surfaces (skin, respiratory, gastrointestinal, urogenital tract)	Rarely diagnosed due to poor cell recognition [3]; function of eosinophils not fully understood, rather indicator for delayed than acute hypersensitivity in chicken; poor correlation with intestinal parasitism [14–19]
Lymphoplasmacytic	≥50% lymphocytes sometimes mixed with plasma cells	Immune mediated disorders of hypersensitivity type II to IV [19]; some viral, bacterial (*Mycoplasma* sp.), and protozoal (Toxo-/Atoxoplasma, Sarcocystis spp.) diseases	Rather subacute to chronic inflammation without prominent tissue necrosis or hemorrhages; adaptive response to antigen stimulus

Source: Adapted from Stacy and Pendl [1], Campbell [3].

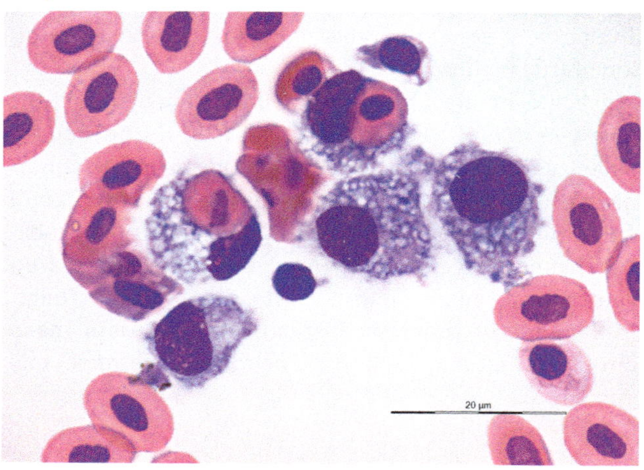

Figure 33.11 Erythrophagocytosis, coelomic effusion African grey parrot (*Psittacus erithacus*): Modified transudate with 95% hematic cells, (90% erythrocytes, 5% physiologic monocytes, and heterophils); 5% mesothelial cells with signs of erythrophagocytosis and increased cellular reactivity (increased amounts of cytoplasm with vacuolation and membrane protrusions, eccentric nucleus); Wright–Giemsa stain, 1000×.

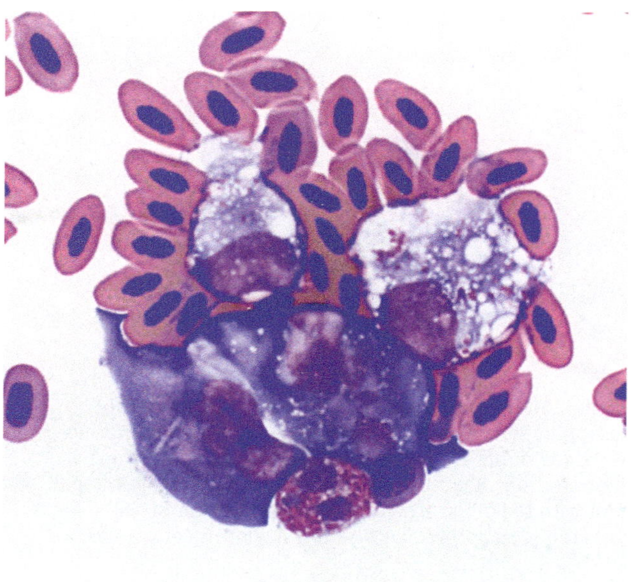

Figure 33.12 Undifferentiated round cell tumor: Mixed cell inflammation with suspicion of macrophagic phagocytosis and two round cells displaying five criteria of malignancy: macrocytosis, severe poikilonucleosis (irregular shape of nucleus), cytoplasmic basophilia, vacuolation, and delicate *hairy* membrane projections. Ultrasound-guided FNA from a cystic structure in the liver; Yellow-collared macaw (*Primolius auricollis*); Wright–Giemsa, 1000×.

cellular, cytoplasmic, and nuclear criteria. For further details, the reader is referred to comprehensive textbooks [3, 20]. Malignancy diagnosis should be performed or confirmed by a clinical pathology specialist. Concurrent signs of septic inflammation and malignancy are most frequently encountered in ulcerated superficial neoplasias and malignant effusions (Figure 33.12).

Cytology of Common Samples Obtained in Emergency Presentations

Coelomocentesis

In an emergency situation, the most common fluid sample would be fluid aspirated by coelomocentesis. Apart from its diagnostic value, coelomocentesis may also be therapeutic in birds that are dyspneic due to the coelomic fluid compressing the air sacs (Figure 33.13). Normal coelomic fluid is present in scant amounts. It is colorless, translucent and contains very few mesothelial cells, macrophages with occasionally some lymphocytes and heterophils [3]. Effusions can be of transudate and exudate type (Table 33.1). Common causes for transudates include right heart failure, atherosclerosis, chronic indurating liver disease of various causes, compression of vessels due to space occupying granulomatous or neoplastic processes and chronic emaciating diseases with catabolic protein metabolism resulting in hypalbuminemia such as mycobacteriosis. Common causes for exudative effusions include any local inflammatory process within the coelomic cavity and/or systemic reactions with increased permeability of capillary endothelia. Egg-yolk coelomitis would be an example for the former and is characterized by the presence of amorphous basophilic globules of various size and color intensity (protein bodies) in the sample often accompanied by fat droplets and variable signs of inflammation. Polyomavirus septicemia would be an example for a hemorrhagic exudative effusion due to increased vascular permeability.

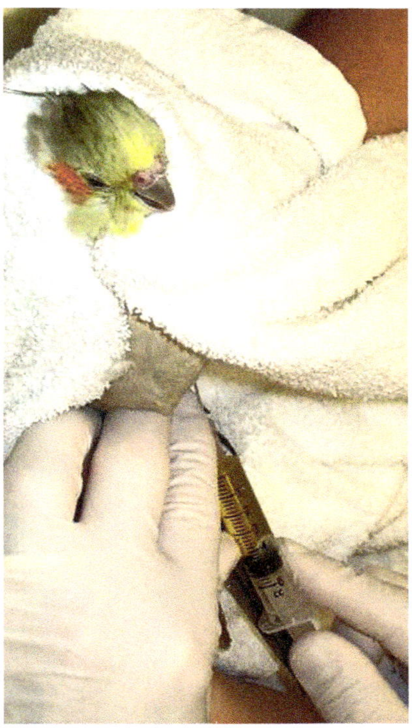

Figure 33.13 Coelomocentesis in a Cockatiel *(Nymphicus hollandicus)*. The bird is held in a slightly upright position. The needle is inserted paramedian from caudal, fluid is aspirated with gentle negative pressure. Coelomocentesis may also be therapeutic in birds that are dyspneic due to the coelomic fluid compressing the air sacs.

Joints

Stained samples of normal synovial fluid are characterized by a more or less pinkish granular pattern of the background which corresponds to the amount of mucin within the sample. Due to the high viscosity, cells in normal synovial fluid tend to align in parallel rows resulting in a line pattern of the sample. This *windrowing of cells* can be used as a rough cytologic criterion for normal viscosity [3, 20]. Viscosity is tested by measuring the length of the fluid strand before the drop breaks off when lifted perpendicular from the slide with a small stick or a fingertip [3, 20]. If the strand breaks before reaching 2 cm in length, the viscosity is considered reduced [3]. The most common cause for reduced viscosity is hemodilution and effusion due to inflammation (Figure 33.10). A normal synovial differential count is predominated by mononuclear cells (≥90%) and a few granulocytes (≤10%). The mononuclear cells consist of macrophages and synoviocytes, which usually present as large vacuolated cells with a low nuclear-cytoplasmic (N:C) ratio and an eccentric nucleus. The cytoplasm frequently contains light eosinophilic granules. In severely affected joints with osteolytic changes, the fluid sample may contain exfoliated osteoid/chondroid cells (Figure 33.10). Their characteristic pinkish cytoplasmic tinge may be almost completely camouflaged by a deep basophilia indicating increased cell metabolism. **Articular gout**, is characterized macroscopically by swollen joints with whitish tophi visible through the overlaying skin (Figure 33.14). Cytology typically reveals a mixed cell inflammation with free or phagocytized crystalloid material presenting as golden brown needles or amorphous structures positive under polarized light (Figure 33.15).

Respiratory Tract and Conjunctiva

Sinus aspirates from the infraorbital sinus may be obtained from swollen areas around the eye (Figure 33.16) by an

Birds

approach rostral or ventral to the eye (Figure 33.17). With current advances in endoscopy, nasal, tracheal, and air sac flushes may be replaced by more targeted biopsies and swabs harvested under visual control. Common infectious agents isolated from the respiratory tract and conjunctiva include various bacteria, chlamydia, mycoplasma, poxvirus, and fungi. Plaques narrowing the upper respiratory tract may consist of squamous metaplastic debris due to Vitamin A deficiency.

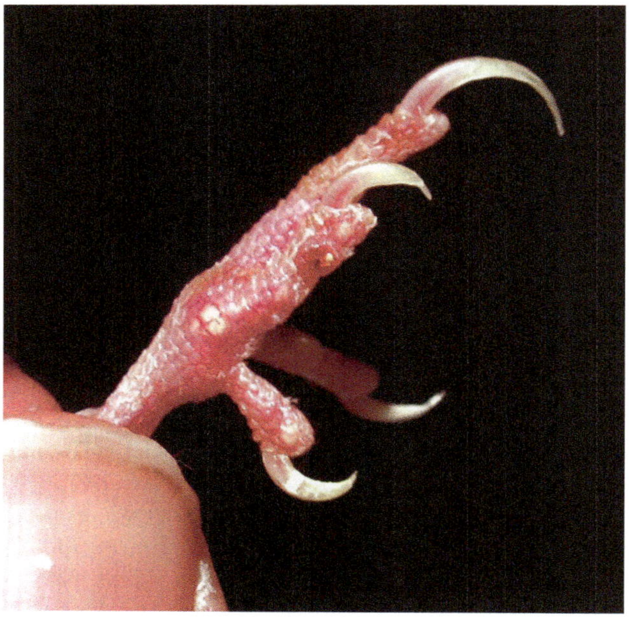

Figure 33.14 Articular gout in a budgerigar (*Melopsittacus undulatus*): Whitish tophi located at the digital joints visible through the partially ulcerated skin.

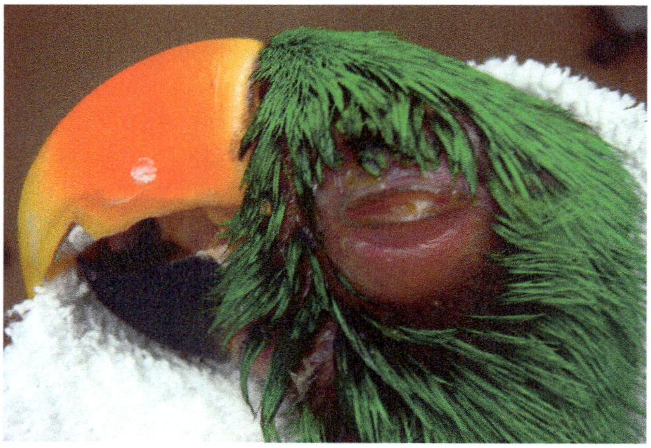

Figure 33.16 Infraorbital sinusitis in an Eclectus parrot (*Eclectus roratus*).

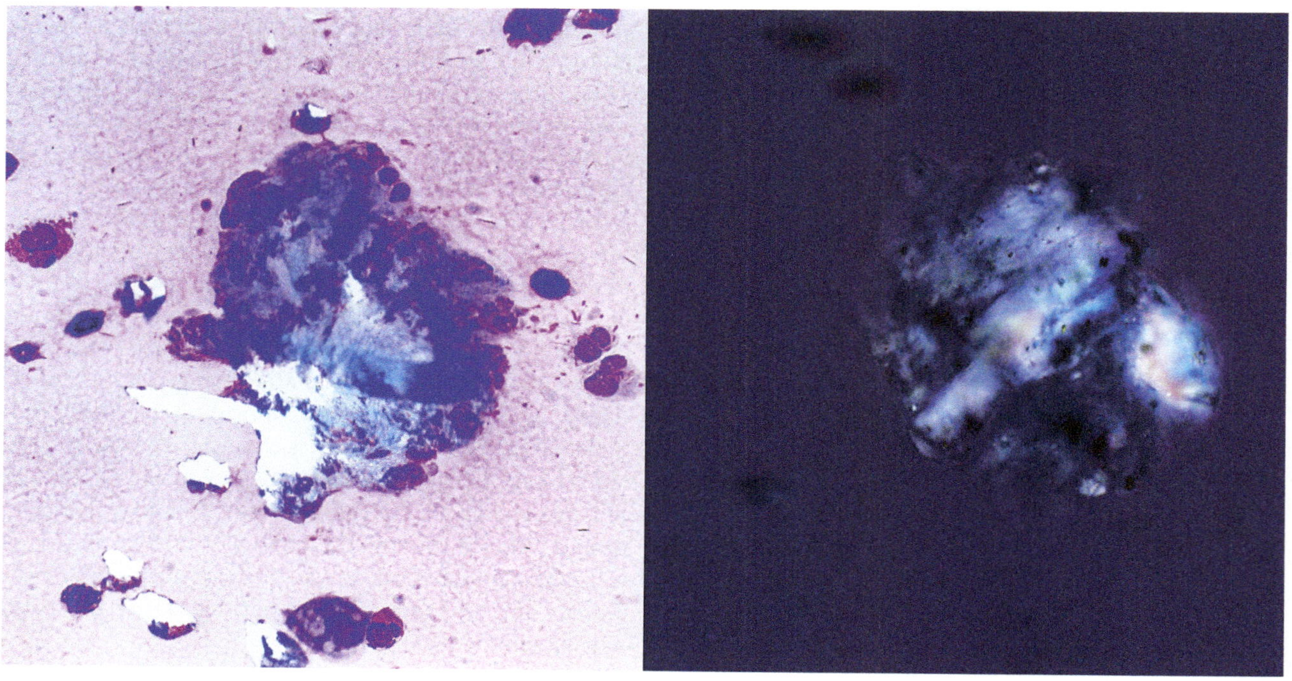

Figure 33.15 Articular gout in a budgerigar (*Melopsittacus undulatus*) with mixed cell inflammation and free or phagocytized crystalloid material, birefringence under polarized light; Wright–Giemsa stain, 400×.

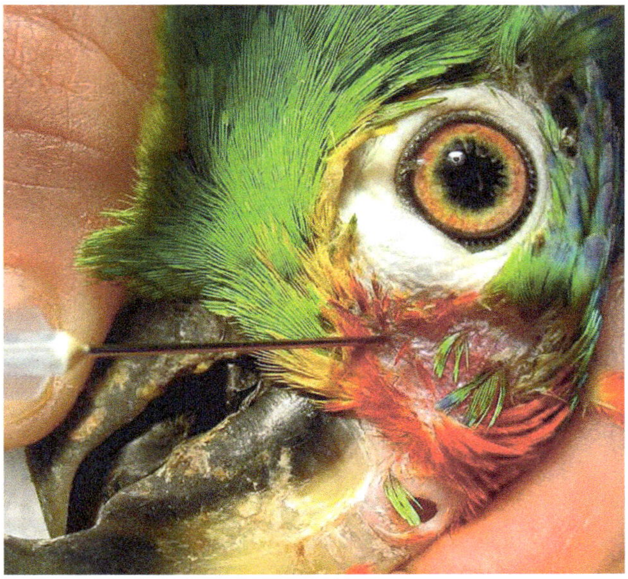

Figure 33.17 Rostral access for fluid aspiration from the right infraorbital sinus, Red-colored Amazon parrot (*Amazona autumnalis*).

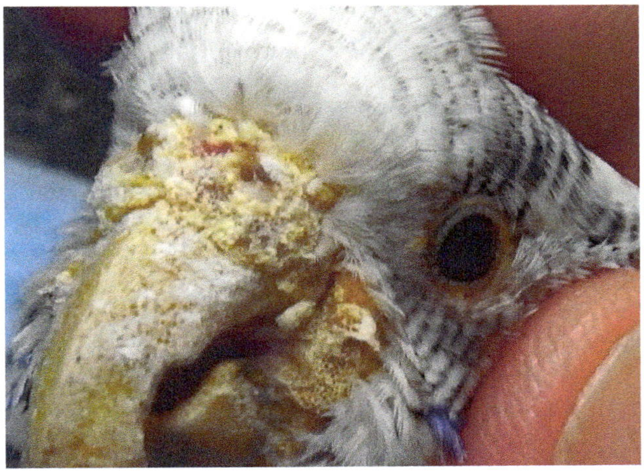

Figure 33.18 Budgerigar (*Melopsittacus undulatus*) with beak mange due to *Knemidocoptes* sp. *Source:* Photo by Neil Forbes, in Stacy and Pendl [1]. Reproduced with permission of Elsevier.

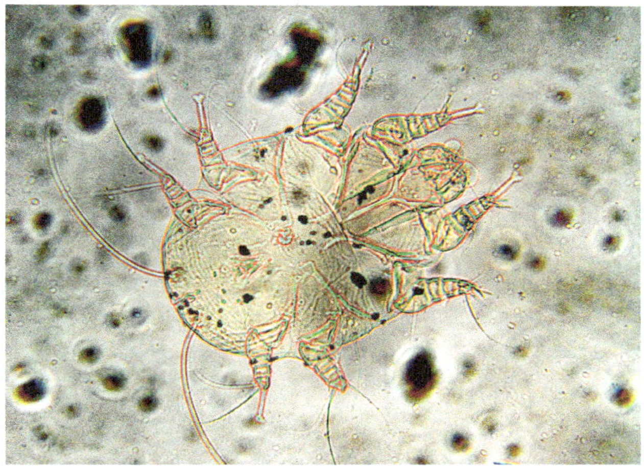

Figure 33.19 *Knemidocoptes pilae,* Macaw (*Ara* sp.), 160×. *Source:* Photo by Heather Walden, in Stacy and Pendl [1]. Reproduced with permission of Elsevier.

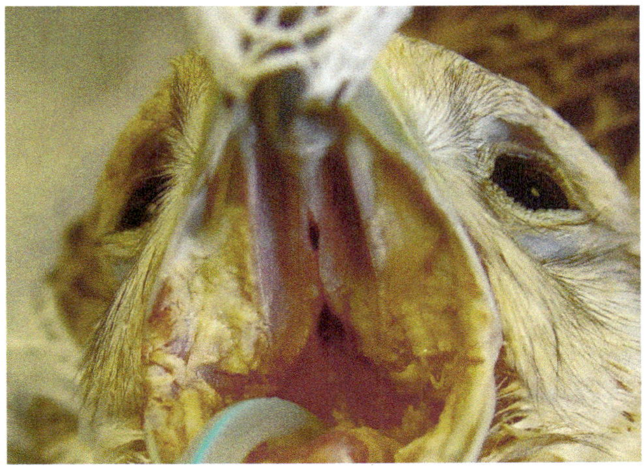

Figure 33.20 Diphtheroid-hemorrhagic, ulcerative oropharyngitis due to capillariasis with bacterial superinfection; Gyrfalcon (*Falco rusticolus*). *Source:* Photo by Neil Forbes, in Stacy and Pendl [1]. Reproduced with permission of Elsevier.

Skin and Feathers

Commonly encountered etiologies for skin masses include squamous cell carcinoma, fibroma, sarcoma, lipoma, and xanthoma. Bacterial, fungal (*Malassezia* spp., *Candida* spp., Figure 33.7a,b), and viral (*Pox-, Polyoma-, Circovirus* Figure 33.9c,e,f) structures may be detected samples from skin lesions and feather pulps. Deep skin scrapings may be necessary for detection of knemidocoptic mites in dry hyperkeratotic lesions. The affected area is held between the thumb and forefinger of one hand and bluntly scraped with a scalpel blade in the other until first petechiae occur (Figures 33.18 and 33.19).

Gastrointestinal Tract

Swabs from the oropharynx, the crop, the cloaca, and fecal samples are the most common cytologic samples for evaluation of the gastrointestinal tract in a live bird. Apart from commonly encountered bacterial infections oral or ingluvial diphtheroid lesions should be examined for Trichonomas, Capillaria, and Candida spp.. (Figure 33.20).

In addition, an infection with Herpes- or Polyomavirus or a Vitamin A deficiency may be the primary underlying cause for these lesions. Typical cytologic features for these primary pathogens are inconsistent.

Feces for microscopic analysis should preferably be freshly voided and collected from a clean surface. Pooled fecal samples taken from the bird's environment at different times of the day may be useful in the detection of intermittently shed parasite structures such as coccidial oocysts, but bear the risk of misinterpreting environmental organisms and inorganic structures as pathogens. Using a pointed tool such as a toothpick allows selection of small amounts of urate free feces suitable for microscopic evaluation.

Fecal wet mounts should be scanned for *Spironucleus/Hexamita* spp. trophozoites and cysts in pigeons, Anseriformes, and cockatiels with diarrhea/polyuria. *Macrorhabdus ornithogaster* (Figure 33.7c) may be observed in small psittacine species, Eclectus parrots, passerines, and backyard chicken. with chronic gastrointestinal disease, weight loss, and proventricular enlargement. *Eimeria, Isospora,* and *Caryospora* spp. are commonly encountered coccidia in pigeons, birds of prey, chickens, and passerines. Various nematode (e.g. *Capillaria* spp., *Ascaridia* spp.) and trematode eggs may be seen depending on the species. Stained fecal smears should be additionally scanned for small microbial structures such as Cryptosporidia (Figure 33.8c,d). *Candida* spp. causes gastroenteral infections in a variety of birds and is especially common in cockatiels, psittacine neonates, pigeons, falconry birds and nectivorous birds (Figure 33.7a). Truly pathogenic yeasts need to be differentiated from transient passengers from food items by budding propagation. Common yeast containing food items include bread, apple sauce, baby parrot formula, and brewer's yeast formulas for racing pigeons. Some microorganisms like *Campylobacter* sp. (Figure 33.6c) and microsporidia (Figure 33.7f) can only be found in stained samples under high magnification (1000×). Although largely advocated in the past, a fecal Gram's stain may not provide indications of the presence of pathogenic bacteria and their identification as long as the physiologic flora is unknown. The composition may vary dramatically under physiologic conditions with a variety of factors such as diet, species, and hormonal status. In addition, there may be poor correlation between fecal Gram's stain and bacterial culture [21]. One of the few exceptions is the presence of typically safety pin-shaped *Clostridia* spp. in conjunction with signs of acute enteritis and enterotoxemia in birds of prey, Galliformes, nectivorous birds, and many other psittacine species.

Bone Marrow

Bone marrow cytology should only be interpreted by clinical pathologists and in conjunction with a complete cell blood count (CBC) from a simultaneously taken peripheral blood sample [3, 20]. In broad terms, assessment includes

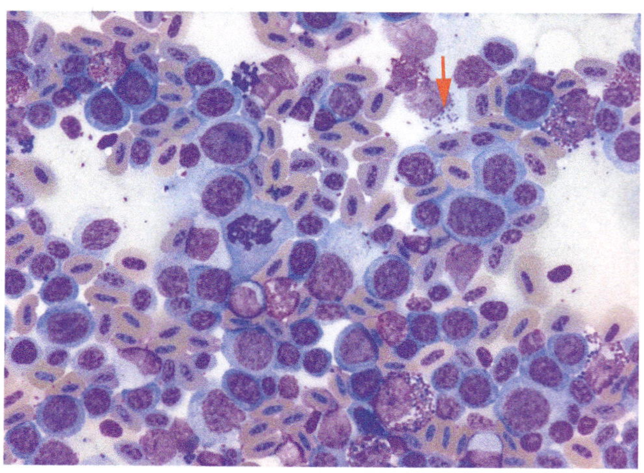

Figure 33.21 Bone marrow aspirate from a Sun conure (*Aratinga solstitialis*) with hemolytic anemia and heterophilic toxic left shift in the CBC: hypercellularity with erythroid predominance (M:E approx. 1 : 4), dyscrasia (left shift, many blast cells) indicating an increased erythropoiesis, and suspicion of phagocytized microbes (arrow), Wright–Giemsa, 400×.

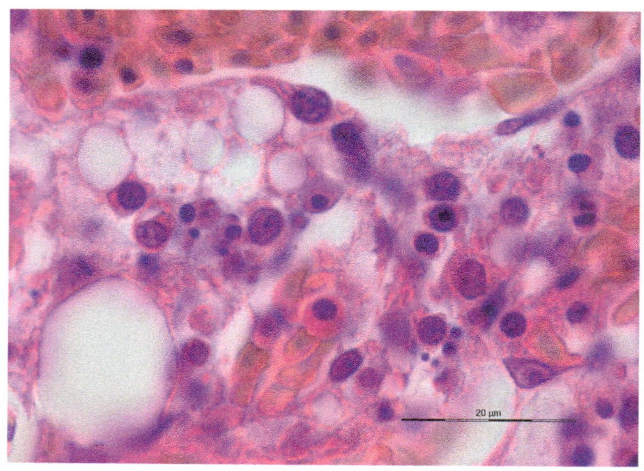

Figure 33.22 Degeneration and necrosis of myeloid cells in the bone marrow of a young Grey parrot (*Psittacus erithacus*) infected with circovirus (confirmed by PCR) characterized by pyknosis (dense shrunken nuclei), karyorrhexis (nuclear fragmentation), and overall cell shrinkage. Histologic section, Hematoxylin-Eosin, 1000×.

the estimation of cellularity, the myeloid:erythroid (M:E) ratio, and the proportions of different stages of development. For detailed information on sampling techniques and evaluation protocols the reader is referred to specialized literature [3, 6, 20, 25]. Preliminary diagnoses may be drawn in case of phagocytized microbes (Figure 33.21) and signs of degeneration and necrosis. Severe peripheral anemia and heteropenia combined with bone marrow hypoplasia, degeneration, and necrosis have been reported to be associated with circovirus infection (Figure 33.22) and benzimidazole intoxication [22–24].

References

1 Stacy, N. and Pendl, H. (2016). Cytology. In: *Current Veterinary Therapy in Avian Medicine. Current Veterinary Therapy*, 1ee (ed. B. Speer), 501–522. St. Louis: Elsevier.

2 Lanaux, T.M., Rozanski, E.A., Simoni, R.S. et al. (2011). Interpretation of canine and feline blood smears by emergency room personnel. *Vet. Clin. Pathol.* 40 (1): 18–23.

3 Campbell, T.W. (2015). *Exotic Animal Hematology and Cytology*, 4ee. Ames: Wiley.

4 Bohmer, R.H., Trinkle, L.S., and Staneck, J.L. (1992). Dose effects of LPS on neutrophils in a whole blood flow cytometric assay of phagocytosis and oxidative burst. *Cytometry* 13 (5): 525–531.

5 Rothwell, D.J. and Doumas, B.T. (1975). The effect of heparin and EDTA on the NBT test. *J. Lab. Clin. Med.* 85 (6): 950–956.

6 Mischke, R. (2005). *Zytologisches Praktikum für die Veterinärmedizin*. Hannover: Schlütersche Verlagsgesellschaft mbH & Co. KG.

7 Pendl, H. and Samour, H.J. (2016). Hematology analyses. In: *Avian Medicine*, 3ee (ed. H.J. Samour), 77–99. St. Louis: Elsevier.

8 Phalen, D.N., Logan, K.S., and Snowden, K.F. (2006). Encephalitozoon hellem infection as the cause of a unilateral chronic keratoconjunctivitis in an umbrella cockatoo (*Cacatua alba*). *Vet. Ophthalmol.* 9 (1): 59–63.

9 Pulparampil, N., Graham, D., Phalen, D., and Snowden, K. (1998). *Encephalitozoon hellem* in two eclectus parrots (*Eclectus roratus*): identification from archival tissues. *J. Eukaryot. Microbiol.* 45 (6): 651–655.

10 Schmidt, R.E., Reavill, D.R., and Phalen, D.N. (2015). *Pathology of Pet and Aviary Birds*, 2ee. Ames: Wiley.

11 Snowden, K., Daft, B., and Nordhausen, R.W. (2001). Morphological and molecular characterization of *Encephalitozoon hellem* in hummingbirds. *Avian Pathol.* 30 (3): 251–255.

12 Smits, J.E., Bortolotti, G.R., and Tella, J.L. (1999). Simplifying the phytohaemagglutinin skin-testing technique in studies of avian immunocompetence. *Funct. Ecol.* 13: 567–572.

13 Maier, K., Fischer, D., Hartmann, A. et al. (2015). Vertebral osteomyelitis and septic arthritis associated with staphylococcus hyicus in a juvenile peregrine falcon (*Falco peregrinus*). *J. Avian Med. Surg.* 29 (3): 216–223.

14 Montali, R.J. (1988). Comparative pathology of inflammation in the higher vertebrates (reptiles, birds and mammals). *J. Comp. Pathol.* 99 (1): 1–26.

15 Maxwell, M.H. (1987). The avian eosinophil – a review. *World's Poult. Sci.* 43: 190–207.

16 Seliger, C., Schaerer, B., Kohn, M. et al. (2012). A rapid high-precision flow cytometry based technique for total white blood cell counting in chickens. *Vet. Immunol. Immunopathol.* 145 (1–2): 86–99.

17 Campbell, T.W. (1995). *Avian Hematology and Cytology*, 2ee. Ames: Iowa State University Press.

18 Fudge, A.M. and Joseph, V. (2000). *Disorders of Avian Leukocytes. Laboratory Medicine Avian and Exotic Pets*, 19–25. Philadelphia: W. B. Saunders Comp.

19 Pendl, H. and Tizard, I. (2016). Immunology. In: *Current Veterinary Therapy in Avian Medicine and Surgery. Current Veterinary Therapy*, 1ee (ed. B. Speer), 400–432. St. Louis, MO: Elsevier.

20 Cowell, T.W., Tyler, D.R., Meinkoth, J.H., and DeNicola, D.B. (2008). *Diagnostic Cytology and Hematology of the Dog and the Cat*, 3ee. St. Louis: Mosby Elsevier.

21 Evans, E.E., Mitchell, M.A., Whittington, J.K. et al. (2014). Measuring the level of agreement between cloacal Gram's stains and bacterial cultures in Hispaniolan Amazon parrots (*Amazona ventralis*). *J. Avian Med. Surg.* 28 (4): 290–296.

22 Schoemaker, N.J., Dorrestein, G.M., Latimer, K.S. et al. (2000). Severe leukopenia and liver necrosis in young African grey parrots (*Psittacus erithacus*) infected with psittacine circovirus. *Avian Dis.* 44 (2): 470–478.

23 Weber, M.A., Terrell, S.P., Neiffer, D.L. et al. (2002). Bone marrow hypoplasia and intestinal crypt cell necrosis associated with fenbendazole administration in five painted storks. *J. Am. Vet. Med. Assoc.* 221: 417–419.

24 Howard, L.L., Papendick, R., Stalis, I.H. et al. (2002). Fenbendazole and albendazole toxicity in pigeons and doves. *J. Avian Med. Surg.* 16: 203–210.

25 Schwartz, D., Guzman, D. S. M., Beaufrere, H., Ammersbach, M., Paul-Murphy, J., Tully Jr, T. N., & Christopher, M. M. (2019). Morphologic and quantitative evaluation of bone marrow aspirates from Hispaniolan Amazon parrots (Amazona ventralis). *Veterinary clinical pathology, 48*(4), 645–651.

34

Ancillary Diagnostics

Delphine Laniesse[1] *and Hugues Beaufrère*[2]

[1] *Evidensia Eläinsairaala, Tammisto, Vantaa, Finland*
[2] *Department of Medicine and Epidemiology, School of Veterinary Medicine, University of California-Davis, Davis, California, USA*

CONTENTS

Infectious Disease Assessments

Culture and Sensitivity Testing

Bacterial and fungal cultures are indicated if a bacterial or fungal infection is suspected. A culture is usually performed on dedicated aerobic or anaerobic swabs collected from a lesion or a biopsy sample. Blood culture usually requires specific media and a minimum amount of blood (1–3 ml). Sometimes the lesions will be obvious and a culture of these lesions will be performed; on other occasions, cultures may be performed on organ biopsies or blood even though no specific lesion is noted, but rather a systemic infection is suspected (e.g. elevated white blood cell count, enlarged spleen, suspected sepsis). Both aerobic and anaerobic bacterial cultures may be performed, but most veterinary laboratories will only perform a sensitivity panel on aerobic bacteria. Likewise, most laboratories do not perform a sensitivity panel for fungal cultures.

If possible, the samples should be collected before the patient is given antibiotics or antifungals. Swabs, once collected (Figure 34.1), can be sent to the laboratory immediately or kept refrigerated. For blood cultures, the blood should be collected in a specific blood culture bottle, and should not be kept refrigerated. A blood culture media may also be used for synovial samples to increase sensitivity. Finally, biopsies should be kept in a sterile container, without fixative or preservative, with a drop of saline to keep it moist, and either sent to the laboratory immediately, or refrigerated.

Some bacteria may require specific culture media, enrichment, or specific microbiological techniques, so the clinician should ensure that the suspected bacterial species are mentioned to the veterinary laboratory (e.g. *Salmonella*, *Mycoplasma*, and *Mycobacterium* spp.).

Results for bacterial cultures usually take three to five days to become available. Fungal cultures usually take much longer. *Mycobacterium* sp. culture may take several months for final results.

Exotic Animal Emergency and Critical Care Medicine, First Edition. Edited by Jennifer E. Graham, Grayson A. Doss and Hugues Beaufrère.

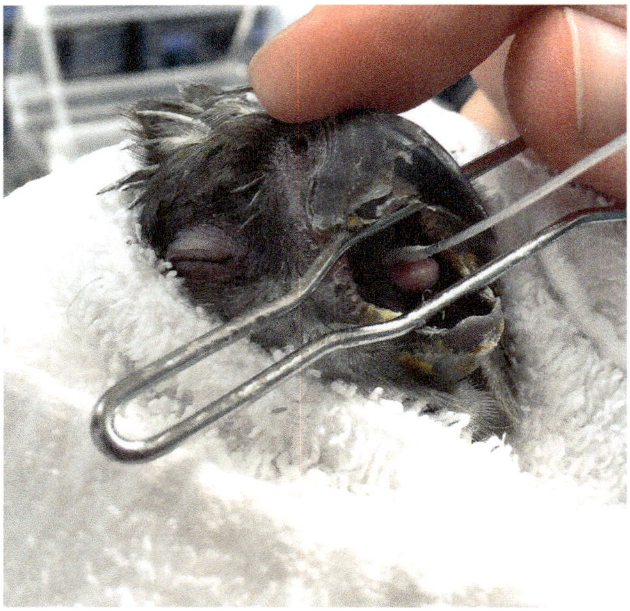

Figure 34.1 Choanal swab being collected in a Senegal parrot. This swab may be used for molecular diagnosis of avian chlamydiosis or upper respiratory infection.

Interpretation of bacterial and fungal cultures should be performed cautiously as many commensals, opportunistic pathogens, or saprophytic organisms may be isolated. A specific knowledge of the external surfaces and intestinal microbial flora and common microbial pathogens is useful. In most pet birds, Gram-negative bacteria predominantly cause a variety of infectious processes such as *Escheria coli*, *Pseudomonas* sp., *Klebsiella* sp., *Campylobacter* sp., *Pasteurella* sp., and many others. Among Gram-positive bacteria of clinical significance, one may encounter clinical disease with *Staphylococcus* sp., *Enterococcus* sp., and *Streptococcus* sp. In addition, anaerobic infections have been seen in a variety of lesions, but mainly in the gastrointestinal system with predominantly *Clostridium* sp. Some common opportunistic pathogens (*Candida* sp., *Aspergillus* sp., and *Mycobacterium* sp.) are also ubiquitous in the environment so their recovery must be associated with compatible clinical signs or lesions.

Molecular Diagnostics

Multiple PCR tests are available in various veterinary laboratories for birds (Table 34.1) [1]. As for culture results, PCR results should be interpreted in the clinical context and according to the dynamics of specific viral infections in the various bird species. For example, several bacterial and viral diseases are only associated with short viremia/bacteremia or shedding (e.g. West Nile virus), some have variable shedding routes (e.g. avian influenza, *Chlamydia psittaci*), and some have intermittent/inconsistent shedding (e.g. avian bornavirus). While PCR primers and protocols have been developed for many organisms, only a small subset of the most common diseases have commercially available PCR tests. One should also select a reputable laboratory with good laboratory standards and accreditations as inaccuracies have been demonstrated with some laboratories [2, 3].

Serology

Serology is uncommonly employed in avian medicine (except in poultry) because of the difficulties in developing tests with reagents cross-reacting with a variety of avian species. The most useful serologic tests in avian patients are those targeting *C. psittaci* infection. Infection with these bacteria typically causes a variety of lesions including respiratory and liver disease. Although PCR is the most commonly used test to detect the bacteria, serology may be used as well. The elementary body agglutination (EBA) assay is used to detect anti-chlamydia IgM and may be detected within 15 days of infection [1]. The sensitivity and specificity is good in psittacine birds displaying clinical signs of the disease. The titer usually becomes negative after treatment. Another serologic test, the complement fixation assay (CF), detects anti-chlamydia IgG. It will only become positive a few days after the EBA. It is not as commonly used as the EBA in psittacine birds, but seems to be more sensitive than the EBA for doves and pigeons. An ELISA test for anti-chlamydia IgG may also be available depending on laboratories.

Toxicology Assays

Heavy Metal Screening

Heavy metal toxicosis should be suspected in case of metallic foreign body ingestion, neurological signs, chronic anemia, and gastrointestinal signs. The two most common heavy metals responsible for toxicity are lead and zinc.

Zinc toxicosis will occur secondary to local corrosive effects on the gastro-intestinal tract, and will result in damage to the liver, kidneys, and pancreas. Clinical signs associated with zinc toxicity include lethargy, weakness, PU/PD, diarrhea, regurgitation, and less commonly, neurologic signs [4]. Excess zinc is thought to result in a functional iron deficiency leading to reduced heme synthesis and erythropoiesis [5]. Therefore, a CBC may show anemia and evidence of dyserythropoiesis. Heterophilia has also been reported. Radiographs can be useful to detect a metallic foreign body in the gastrointestinal tract, but the source of the intoxication is not always obvious, so the diagnosis is based on measurement of zinc blood levels. This test is run on plasma or serum, so the blood should be collected in an

Table 34.1 Available PCR tests for various infectious diseases in birds.

Infectious agent	Recommended sample site	Sensitivity/specificity	Comments
Psittacine Circovirus – Beak and feather disease	• Whole blood (EDTA) • Pin feather	Blood: specific but not sensitive as viremia is not permanent Pin feather: sensitive and specific for chronic infected patients	Birds become viremic 7–14 days after infection. Then virus may persist in skin and feathers. Viremia is common and usually persistent in clinical disease. Old world species mainly
Avian bornavirus	• Cloacal swab • Crop biopsies	Sensitivity: Virus is intermittently shed in the feces. Lesions may not be present in the harvested biopsy (increases sensitivity to take several biopsies) Specificity: The presence of the virus does not confirm a diagnosis of proventricular dilation disease as incubation is variable. If compatible clinical signs are noted, it suggests the disease is present	Budgerigars appear resistant
Psittacine herpesvirus 1 (Pacheco disease, internal papillomatosis)	• Oral mucosa swab • Cloacal swab		
Psittacine polyomavirus	• Choanal/cloacal swab • Whole blood	Blood: specific but not sensitive as viremia is not permanent Choanal/cloacal swab: specific but not sensitive as shedding can be intermittent	Birds are viremic within 7–14 days of infection. Viremia is not persistent but the virus can be shed in the feces for up to six months or longer
Chlamydia psittaci	• Swab of the conjunctiva/choana/cloaca • Blood • Affected tissues (biopsy)	Not 100% sensitive; may increase sensitivity by doing in conjunction with serology. Good specificity	Can be detected five days after infection in the choana, 10 days after infection in the cloaca and 15 days after infection in the blood
Coxiella-like organism	Affected tissues (biopsy)		Uncommon
Mycobacterium sp.	Affected tissues (biopsy)	Sensitivity and specificity are low in the feces and blood, but specificity is good in tissues	*Mycobacterium avium*, *Mycobacterium genavense* are most commonly the cause of mycobacteriosis in birds
Mycoplasma sp.	• Swab of a lesion • Affected tissues	Some laboratories will test for all Mycoplasma organisms: good sensitivity but poor specificity	*Mycoplasma synoviae, Mycoplasma bovis, Mycoplasma gallisepticum, Mycoplasma meleagridis, Mycoplasma iowae* Mycoplasma are most likely commensals in birds of prey and potentially other birds
Avian avulavirus 1 (Newcastle disease)	• Choanal/cloacal swab		Common in pigeons and cormorants
Avian influenza	• Choanal/tracheal/cloacal swab • Affected tissues (biopsy) • Nasal/tracheal secretions		H5, H7 subtypes are usually more likely to lead to HPAI. Anseriformes are reservoir species
Gallid herpesvirus 1 (Infectious laryngotracheitis)	• Choanal/tracheal swab • Affected tissues (biopsy)		
Gallid herpesvirus 2 (Marek's disease)	• Tissues		Not commonly available – most often diagnosed post mortem. Poor correlation between infection and disease

Source: Phalen [1]. © 2006, Spix Publishing.

all plastic or glass tube. Rubber stoppers in serum/plasma separation tubes may be a source of zinc contamination and should be avoided [6, 7]. The sample should be kept refrigerated if not processed immediately. Plasma zinc concentrations above 4 ppm are suggestive of toxicosis. A concentration less than 2 ppm is considered non-toxic. Eclectus parrots and cockatoos tend to have higher physiologic concentrations of zinc, so values up to 3.5 ppm for cockatoos and 2.5 ppm for Eclectus may be considered normal [8]. On post mortem examination, zinc toxicosis may result in ulcerations of the ventriculus, and in more severe cases necrotizing ventriculitis [4, 9]. Necrosis of the ventricular mucosa may result in koilin exfoliation and secondary impaction of the gastrointestinal tract.

Lead toxicosis leads to demyelination of the vagus and other nerves, causing decreased to absent nerve conduction, resulting in decreased gastrointestinal motility [9]. Lead also causes dyserythropoiesis and anemia. Clinical signs associated with lead toxicosis are similar to zinc toxicity, but neurological signs, such as seizures, are more common [4]. Blood work may show anemia, heterophilia, and elevation of aspartate aminotransferase (AST), lactate dehydrogenase (LDH), creatine phosphokinase (CPK) and uric acid [4]. Some authors have also noted a marked reticulocytosis and basophilic stippling of the erythrocytes [10]. However, basophilic stippling of erythrocytic cytoplasm is not common in birds. Radiographs may or may not show a gastrointestinal metallic foreign body, and signs associated with the decreased gastrointestinal motility such as dilation of the proventriculus and accumulation of food in the crop [4]. A definitive diagnosis is usually obtained from blood lead level measurement. This test should be run on whole blood as 90% of circulating lead is in the erythrocytes [6, 11]. The sample should be kept refrigerated if not processed immediately. In Hispaniolan Amazon parrots, levels less than 0.02 ppm are considered non-toxic, whereas levels above 0.2 ppm are suspicious and levels above 0.5 ppm are diagnostic for lead toxicosis [12]. In raptors, treatment is recommended if levels are above 0.2 ppm [13]. Although blood lead level is the most commonly used test to diagnose lead toxicosis, other tests are available. Lead inhibits the enzyme heme synthetase, which results in the accumulation of protoporphyrin IX in the erythrocytes [6]. When blood of a healthy animal is examined under UV light (400 nm), 75–100% of the erythrocytes show a red fluorescence. When protoporphyrin is present in the erythrocytes, the fluorescence of the erythrocytes is impaired. This test, called fluorocyte test, has been used with success to diagnose lead intoxication in waterfowl [14]. Another test measures the free erythrocyte protoporphyrin levels. In ducks, the highest value was noted eight days after ingestion of a lead object [6]. In humans, free erythrocyte protoporphyrin was shown to bind to zinc and form a fluorescent compound called zinc protoporphyrin; this compound can be measured in the blood and was found to be significantly higher in raptors with high blood levels of lead than in other species of birds with similar blood levels.

Cholinesterase-Inhibitors: Organophosphate and Carbamate Intoxication

The clinical signs associated with organophosphate or carbamate intoxication are due to inhibition of acetylcholinesterase, and include ataxia, and seizures characterized by a rigid paralysis [7]. Such intoxications can usually be suspected upon taking the history if the bird has recently been exposed to pesticide. These toxicities are common in wild birds. Organophosphate and carbamate cause acute toxicity, and the diagnosis is most often made post-mortem. Pre-mortem, plasma cholinesterase activity may be measured to help confirm the diagnosis and reference ranges have been established in many avian species [14–21].

Rodenticide

Intoxication with anti-coagulant rodenticide has been widely described in birds, and is particularly common in wild birds of prey (especially the great horned owl), which feed on intoxicated rodents. Anticoagulants inhibits coagulation synthesis by inhibiting 1,2,3-vitamin K epoxide reductase, thereby depleting active vitamin K. Antemortem suspicion of intoxication may be based on compatible clinical signs, increased prothrombin time (PT) and increased whole-blood clotting time, but limited information exists regarding reference intervals in avian patients (Table 34.2) [28]. In a study performed in Japanese quail and barn owls, exposure with brodifacoum, a common anticoagulant found in second-generation rodenticides, caused a significant increase in PT, one and three days after exposure [25]. Tissue levels are, however, necessary for a confirmatory diagnosis, which is thus generally made post mortem.

Blood samples for coagulation testing should be collected in a serum or silicone tube containing 3.8% sodium citrate, and should be processed immediately [6]. The PT assay should ideally be performed with homologous brain thromboplastin as PT will falsely increase if heterologous avian or mammalian thromboplastin is used [6]. However, most veterinary laboratories only use mammalian thromboplastin. Whole blood clotting times should be measured on a sample collected in non-siliconized glass tubes or capillary tubes [6]. Reference intervals have been established for some species of birds (Table 34.3) [29].

Botulism

Botulism is a disease caused by ingestion of *Clostridium botulinum* neurotoxin [30]. Once absorbed through the

Table 34.2 Normal values of prothrombin time for various species of birds.

	Prothrombin time (seconds)	Thromboplastin source	References
Hispaniolan Amazon parrots (*Amazona ventralis*)	7.5–13.4 (fresh plasma) 9–11.3 (frozen plasma)	Chicken	[22]
Chicken (*Gallus gallus*)	7.5–10.6 (fresh plasma) 7–11.1 (frozen plasma)	Homologous	[22]
	7.8–11.4	Homologous	[23]
	38.6 ± 16.3 (SD)	Homologous	[24]
	>600	Heterologous – sheep plasma	[24]
	>600	Heterologous – human plasma	[24]
Japanese quail (*Coturnix japonica*)	Mean: 13.2 95% CI: 12.5–13.8 Min–Max: 10.8–15.4	Chicken	[25]
	10 ± 1 (SD)	Homologous	[26]
Barn owl (*Tyto alba*)	Mean: 21.4 95% CI: 20.4–22.3 Min–Max: 12.6–30.5	Chicken	[25]
Pigeon (*Columba livia*)	Mean: 25 Min–Max: 17.2–34.4	Homologous – pigeon brain	[27]
	Mean: 11 Min–Max: 7–14	Homologous – pigeon lung	
	Mean: 85.1 Min–Max: 72–107	Heterologous – goat lung	
	Mean: 35.2 Min–Max: 32–40.5	Heterologous – rabbit lung	
	Mean: 169.7 Min–Max: 85.8–299	Heterologous – human brain	
Kite (*Milvus migrans*)	Mean: 18.2 Min–Max: 13.5–24.4	Homologous – kite brain	[27]
	Mean: 8.5 Min–Max: 5–14	Homologous – kite lung	
	Mean: 100.4 Min–Max: 40.5–194	Heterologous – human	
Vulture (*Neophron percnocterus*)	Mean: 16.2 Min–Max: 14.5–18	Homologous – vulture brain	[27]
	Mean: 13.7 Min–Max: 11.6–15.8	Homologous – vulture lung	
	Mean: 237.5 Min–Max: 150–277	Heterologous – human brain	
Ostrich (*Struthio camelus*)	73 ± 13.7 (SD)	Homologous: ostrich plasma	[24]
	90.1 ± 15.3 (SD)	Heterologous – chicken plasma	
	>600	Heterologous – sheep plasma	
	>600	Heterologous – human plasma	

Source: Ponder et al. [28]. © 2015, Elsevier.

Table 34.3 Normal values of whole blood clotting time for various species of birds.

		Whole blood clotting time (min)			
Species	**Age**	**At ambient temperature (20–22 °C)**	**At 37 °C**	**At 42 °C**	**References**
Chickens	4 months			Mean: 28 Min–Max: 8–57	[29]
	10 months			Mean: 69 Min–Max: 13–180	
	12 months (F)			Mean: 36 Min–Max: 17–83	
	12 months (M)			Mean: 26 Min–Max: 13–50	
Mallard ducks	Adult	Mean: 123 Min–Max: 55–360		Mean: 47 Min–Max: 15–105	[29]
Turkeys	6 weeks	Mean: 163 Min–Max: 20–395		Mean: 188 Min–Max: 90–310	[29]
	12 weeks	15–270		Mean: 557 Min–Max: 36–>840	
	14 weeks	Mean: 428 Min–Max: 25–720			
Pigeons	Adult	Mean: 113 Min–Max: 50–220		Mean: 144 Min–Max: 25–540	[29]
Japanese quail	Adult	Mean: 99 Min–Max: 5–360		Mean: 32 Min–Max: 3–90	[29]
	Adult		<2.5		[25]

Source: Modified from Bigland [29].

intestinal tract, the toxins ascend into the spinal cord and block the production of acetylcholine at the level of the neuromuscular junction. This causes an ascending flaccid paralysis and the death of the bird is generally caused by respiratory paralysis. Confirming a diagnosis of botulism is challenging, as it requires a mouse lethality assay to prove the presence of the neurotoxin. ELISA tests have been described to detect *C. botulinum* toxins C and D, but with a low sensitivity compared with the mouse lethality assay [31]. This test is not commonly offered in laboratories.

Tetanus

Although tetanus has only been reported once in birds, it should be part of the differential diagnosis for a patient presenting with spastic paralysis, especially if the patient also presents with a wound [32]. A swab of the wound may be sent for bacterial culture, and a tentative diagnosis of tetanus can be made if *Clostridium tetani* is identified. However, a definitive diagnosis can only be made with a mouse lethality assay.

Carbon Monoxide

Carbon monoxide (CO) competes with oxygen for binding to hemoglobin, and hemoglobin has a much higher affinity for the former [33]. Binding of CO to hemoglobin results in the production of carboxyhemoglobin (COHb), and blood concentrations higher than 30% cause acute toxicosis [34]. COHb may be measured in the blood, but the presentation of this disease is very acute, and birds die shortly after being exposed, making pre-mortem diagnosis usually irrelevant. In addition, this test is not available in most veterinary laboratories.

Ammonia

Ammonia, a commonly used substance in house cleaning products, can be inhaled by birds and be absorbed in the blood stream, thereby possibly causing intoxication. Blood levels exceeding 1 mg/dl can indicate toxicity [7]. However, measurement of ammonia is problematic as it rapidly increases with storage in whole blood (leakage from erythrocytes) and

Table 34.4 Reported values of blood 25-OH-D3 in various species of birds.

Species	25-OH-D3 (nmol/l)	Comments	References
Domestic chicken (*Gallus gallus*)	27.2–68	Unknown	[36]
Thick billed parrot (*Rhynchopsitta pachyrhyncha*)	19.04 ± 13.24 (SD)	Radioimmunoassay	[37]
Humboldt Penguins (*Spheniscus humboldti*)	3.7 ± 2.4 (SD)	Radioimmunoassay	[38]
American crows (*Corvus brachyrhynchos brachyrhynchos*)	20 ± 6.04 (SD)	Unknown	[39]
African grey parrot (*Psittacus erithacus erithacus*)	7.2–380	Enzyme immunoassay	[36]
Pigeon (*Columba livia*)	30.8–35	Radioimmunoassay	[36]
Falcon (Gyr x Peregrine)	8.1–38.4	Unknown	[40]

Table 34.5 Reported values of blood PTH in various species of birds.

Species	PTH (pmol/l)	References
Thick billed parrot (*Rhynchopsitta pachyrhyncha*)	19.77 ± 19.58 (SD)	[37]
Humboldt Penguins (*Spheniscus Humboldti*)	0.8 ± 0.3 (SD)	[38]
Ostrich (*Struthio camelus*)	203–207	[36]
Falcon (Gyr x Peregrine)	<0.01–1.1	[40]

also increases with storage in separated plasma (any ammonia in the environment, such as the air, can contribute to the ammonia in the sample). Decreased values may also occur if the blood tube is not completely filled or stoppered, through loss of ammonia gas. The sample therefore needs to be separated immediately after collection, and either processed right away or kept frozen until analysis. This test is thus rarely performed.

Metabolic/Endocrine Assessments

Metabolic Diseases

Most metabolic disorders can be assessed with a comprehensive biochemistry panel, which was already detailed in Chapter 32: Clinical Pathology. We will only discuss the disorders of calcium metabolism, a condition frequently encountered in grey parrots. Clinical signs of calcium deficiency may include bone weakness, ataxia, seizures, bone deformities, pathological fractures, egg binding, and abnormal eggs [35]. As previously mentioned in Chapters 32: Clinical Pathology and 30: STAT Diagnostics, ionized calcium may be measured if hypocalcemia is suspected. Measurement of blood levels of parathyroid hormone (PTH) and vitamin D3 may also aid in the diagnosis. Vitamin D3 can be assessed by measuring 25-OH-D3 either by radioimmunoassay or by enzyme immunoassay [36]. The blood sample should be collected in heparin or dry glass tube and the plasma or serum frozen unless immediately processed. Reference values have been described in some species of birds (Table 34.4). PTH can be measured on whole blood, serum or plasma, but the sample should be either processed immediately or frozen within one hour of sampling as PTH is very labile. PTH normal values have been reported for some species of birds (Table 34.5). Both Vitamin D3 levels and PTH should be interpreted in conjunction with the ionized calcium levels. In cases of nutritional secondary hyperparathyroidism, the PTH levels will increase, and the ionized calcium should either be normal or low. If the ionized calcium is high on the other hand, PTH levels should be low. Cases of pseudohyperparathyroidism (hypercalcemia associated with neoplasia) have also been described twice in Amazon parrots with lymphosarcoma [41].

Endocrine Diseases

Endocrine diseases are generally uncommon in birds.

Diabetes Insipidus

Diabetes insipidus (DI) has rarely been described in birds [42–46]. The main clinical sign is a marked polyuria and polydipsia (PU/PD). The authors recorded a water consumption of 2.5 l/kg/day in an grey parrot diagnosed with central DI. DI may be central (grey parrot, trauma, neoplasia), or nephrogenic (autosomal recessive disease in chickens and quails, transient DI with metabolic disorders) [42–46]. Most severe PU/PD presentations are usually due to DI or psychogenic polydipsia.

The first diagnostic test needed to differentiate diabetes insipidus from psychogenic polydipsia is a water deprivation test. The patient is placed in a cage with no substrate so that urine can be collected throughout the process. The weight of the bird as well as the plasma osmolality, urine specific gravity and urine osmolality are measured before removing water and two hours after water removal. In cases of psychogenic polydipsia, plasma osmolality is usually decreased before water removal, and increases to normal values when water is removed while urine osmolality and specific gravity increase. In DI cases, on the other hand, plasma osmolality is normal to highly elevated before water removal, and increases after water removal while urine osmolality and specific gravity stay low. The weight of the bird also significantly decreases with time and dehydration. If DI is diagnosed after two hours, an arginine vasopressin/vasotocin (antidiuretic hormone – ADH – Desmopressin) stimulation test is performed to differentiate central DI from nephrogenic DI. In mammals, in cases of central DI, urine osmolality increases after the administration of ADH and plasma osmolality stops increasing. In cases of nephrogenic DI, however, urine osmolality stays low and plasma osmolality continues to increase. Similar observations have been made in birds where mammalian ADH seemed to be effective [45]. However, the authors noted that ADH had no significant effect on an grey parrot diagnosed with central DI while the administration of arginine vasotocin (AVT), the avian antidiuretic hormone, was responsible for a significant response [47]. The use of AVT is therefore recommended to diagnose and treat central DI in birds, whenever available.

Hypothyroidism

Hypothyroidism is not commonly described in birds. Clinical signs reported include small body size, sensitivity to cold, decreased fertility, weight gain/obesity, feather loss, abnormal molts, and epidermal atrophy [48, 49]. Goiter is also reported in budgerigars and pigeons [50]. Diagnosis of hypothyroidism should be made upon noticing compatible clinical signs and lack of response to the thyroid-stimulating hormone (TSH) stimulation test. Low basal total and free thyroxine (Total T4) and response to thyroxine therapy can suggest hypothyroidism but are insufficient to confirm the diagnosis because of the possibility of a euthyroid sick syndrome. Total and free T4 values are much lower in birds than they are in mammals so low values may be difficult to detect [49, 51, 52]. The recommended method to measure T4 in avian patients is a radioimmunoassay test (RIA) [35]. The total T4 value (RIA and equilibrium dialysis) in psittacine birds is usually between 2 and 8 nmol/l [51, 52]. TSH stimulation tests were historically performed using bovine TSH, which is not available anymore, and is now performed with human synthetic TSH, which is extremely expensive [35]. Therefore, this test is rarely performed in practice.

Hyperthyroidism

This condition seems to be rare in birds. Thyroid tumors in birds do not appear to be functional, unlike in mammals [35]. One case of hyperthyroidism was diagnosed in a barred owl with elevated free T4 and total T4 [53].

Diabetes Mellitus

Although not considered common, diabetes mellitus has been described on several occasions in birds and is encountered with some frequency in practice [54–61]. The clinical signs include polyuria, polydipsia, polyphagia, lethargy, and weight loss. A presumptive diagnosis can be made if a patient presents with compatible clinical signs, hyperglycemia and glycosuria. As in mammals, birds can develop stress-associated hyperglycemia; therefore, it is recommended to recheck the blood glucose several times to get a better assessment of the true glycemia. Blood glucose levels above 800 mg/dl (44 mmol/l) are considered diagnostic [55]. Another option is to measure the fructosamine level, as this is an indicator of the glycemia over a period of several days [35]. The normal blood levels of fructosamine were reported to be between 113 and 238 μmol/l in psittacine birds [54]. Urine dip strips may be used to evaluate the patient for glycosuria; the urine sample needs to be taken as soon as passed to limit fecal contamination. Other tests have been described in birds to investigate diabetes mellitus, but are not commonly performed in practice, such as insulin plasma levels, glucagon plasma levels and β-hydroxybutyric acid blood levels [35].

Bone Marrow Assessments

Bone marrow aspiration or biopsy may be performed in order to evaluate a patient with disorders of myelo- and erythropoiesis, such as a non-regenerative anemia, heteropenia, pancytopenia, or leukemia [62]. The sample may be taken from the proximal tibiotarsus (recommended), the keel or most of the long bones, with the exception of the pneumatic bones [62]. The patient should be placed under anesthesia, or at least deep sedation, and a local infiltration with lidocaine and bupivacaine may be performed prior to sampling. The technique used is the same as described for small animals, but a smaller sample volume is collected. If an aspiration is performed, the sample should be placed on a glass slide immediately after collection, and a second glass slide is placed on top of the first, and pulled apart to allow the bone marrow sample to spread between the two slides. Extra blood should be removed prior to smear preparation. If a core biopsy is collected, it can be retrieved from the biopsy needle using a stylet, and placed in a small cassette in a formalin jar. The sample should be sent to a laboratory which is used to

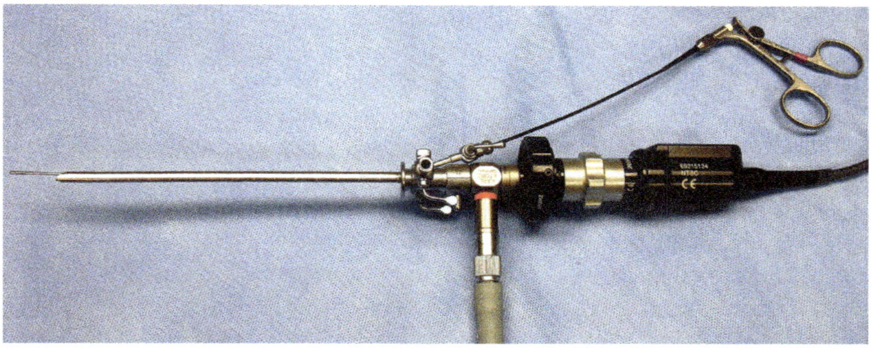

Figure 34.2 Avian endoscopic examinations are typically performed using a 2.7 mm 30° angle rigid endoscope, such as shown in this picture. The operating sheath allows for the introduction of a 5 Fr biopsy forceps, which may be used to collect targeted biopsies of lesions or organs during the procedure.

processing and reading avian samples. For more information, the reader is referred to Chapter 33: Cytology.

Endoscopy

Small diameter rigid endoscopes are used for a variety of indications in birds: examination of the trachea to look for obstructive foreign bodies or masses, examination of the gastrointestinal tract, mostly to look for foreign bodies and masses, examination of the cloaca, and examination of the coelomic cavity. In all cases, endoscopically guided biopsies may be taken during the examination and sent for histopathology, bacterial or fungal culture and/or cytology to aid in the diagnosis (Figure 34.2). The authors recommend additional training before considering performing endoscopy and endoscopically guided biopsies in live patients using endoscopic biopsy forceps. More information on biopsy techniques can be found in the literature [63, 64]. The endoscopic instrumentation most commonly used in avian medicine includes a 2.7 mm 30° angle rigid endoscope with an examination sheath, an operating sheath, 5 Fr endoscopic biopsy forceps, grasping forceps, an endoscopic injection needle, and single-action endoscopic scissors. In smaller birds (<100 g), smaller diameter endoscopes can be used such as a 1.9 mm rigid endoscope.

Tracheoscopy

Tracheoscopy is recommended to evaluate the trachea and the syrinx in patients presenting with inspiratory dyspnea, indicating an upper respiratory disease, or change/loss of voice (Figure 34.3). For birds weighing 400 g or more, a 2.7 mm rigid endoscope may be used [64]. For smaller birds, a 1 mm semi rigid endoscope or a 1.9 mm rigid endoscope will be needed. If possible, it is recommended to use the protecting sheath to prevent damage to the endoscope, but in smaller birds, the sheath may need to be removed. The patient is anesthetized and, if necessary, an air sac tube may be placed, leaving the trachea clear for the tracheoscopy; however, if the bird is stable and the procedure is fast, it may be possible to keep the bird on a mask for delivery of anaesthetic gas, and remove the mask for a few seconds during the tracheoscopy. If a biopsy needs to be performed or a foreign body removed, it is recommended to place an air sac tube to prevent asphyxia as the procedure will be significantly longer.

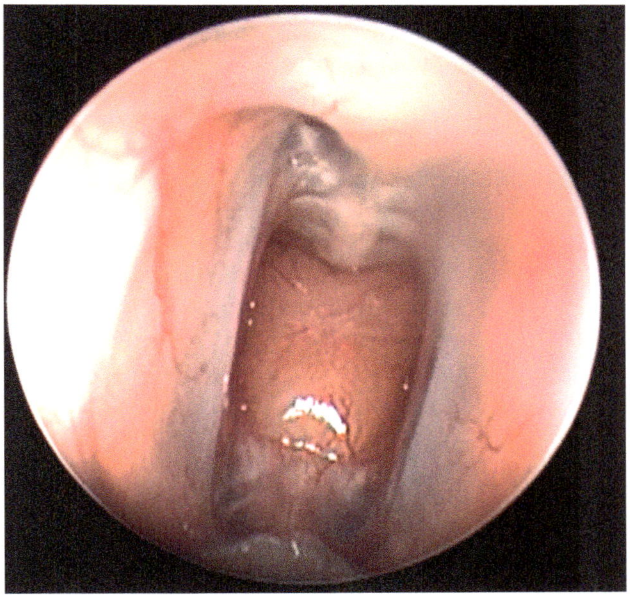

Figure 34.3 Tracheoscopy using a 2.7 mm rigid endoscope in an Amazon parrot with a syringeal mycobacterial granuloma.

Endoscopy of the Gastrointestinal Tract

Endoscopy of the gastrointestinal tract is recommended to identify and remove foreign bodies and harvest biopsy samples. The ventriculus and proventriculus may be examined with either a flexible or a rigid endoscope. In large birds, a flexible endoscope is preferred to a rigid endoscope, as it is longer and allows for the proventriculus and ventriculus to be reached. The endoscope may either be introduced through the oral cavity, or via a midline ingluviotomy incision [65]. The birds are anesthetized and intubated for the procedure, and gauze may be placed inside the throat to prevent aspiration secondary to regurgitation that may occur during the examination. The skin and crop are incised over the midline and the endoscope is introduced into the crop. Once inside the crop, the entrance to the thoracic esophagus can be visualized on the ventral, midline border of the crop. Air or saline can be infused through the endoscopic sheath to allow for better visualization. Ideally, the bird should be fasted for at least half a day before the procedure, and feeding soft food for a few days before the endoscopy will also allow a better examination. If there is still a lot of content in the proventriculus, it may be rinsed and flushed with saline. If a foreign body is visualized, it may be removed with fine or coarse grasping forceps, or a wire basket, introduced through the sheath. The proventricular mucosa, the isthmus, and the ventricular cuticle layer can also be screened for any lesion.

Cloacoscopy

Cloacoscopy is recommended to evaluate the three chambers of the cloaca (coprodeum, urodeum, and proctodeum), when the patient is presenting for cloacal prolapse, decreased or absent production of feces, hematochezia, or a mass in the cloaca. A 2.7 mm rigid endoscope may be used for this procedure in most species. The patient is usually anesthetized for this procedure, although deep sedation may also be used if the patient is not stable enough to undergo a full anaesthesia. The cloaca should be cleaned first, to remove any feces and urates, and saline can be infused through the endoscopic sheath while manually closing the vent lips to allow for better visualization. If lesions or masses are noted, biopsies may be taken using an endoscopic biopsy forceps.

Coelioscopy

Coelioscopy is recommended to evaluate internal organs such as the liver, the kidneys, the spleen, the lungs, the air sacs, and the reproductive organs. There are four commonly used approaches to the coelom: left lateral, right lateral, ventral and interclavicular [63, 64]. Lateral and ventral approaches should not be performed if the patient is obese, as the accumulation of fat will prevent visualization of the organs, or if the gastrointestinal tract is very distended, as the risk of perforating the proventriculus when entering the coelom is high. Therefore, it is highly recommended to have another type of diagnostic imaging performed before the coelioscopy, such as radiographs or CT scan. If the bird presents with ascites, one should be extremely careful not to puncture the coelomic cavity containing the effusion if performing coelioscopy; in this situation a ventral approach is recommended.

Left Approach

The left approach is the most commonly performed and allows for visualization of the liver, spleen, kidneys,

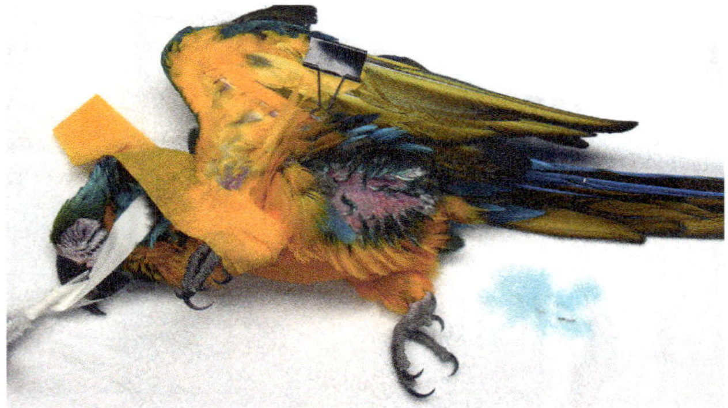

Figure 34.4 This picture illustrates the position of an avian patient for a coelioscopic procedure through a left-sided approach. The left leg is extended cranially, and the point of insertion of the endoscope is behind the last rib and just ventral to the *flexor cruris medialis* muscle. The area doesn't usually need to be plucked, but should be surgically prepared and draped before the procedure.

reproductive tract, adrenal glands, air sacs, lungs, and gastrointestinal tract. The patient is anesthetized, intubated, and placed in right lateral recumbency, with the wings extended dorsally. The left leg is either extended caudally, in which case the point of insertion of the endoscope is caudal to the last rib, cranial to the muscle mass of the femur and ventral to the synsacrum, or extended cranially, in which case the point of insertion is behind the last rib and just ventral to the *flexor cruris medialis* muscle (Figure 34.4) [63, 64]. Surgical prepping of the site should be performed, and sterile instruments and endoscope should be used. A 2.7 mm rigid endoscope, 30° angle, is recommended for this procedure. A small skin incision is made, and blunt dissection is used to reflect the *flexor cruris medialis* muscle dorsally. Hemostats are then used to puncture the body wall; this part of the procedure is facilitated by the anesthetist manually ventilating the bird at the same time. The hemostat is then replaced by the endoscope, which should enter the caudal thoracic air sac, or the abdominal air sac. Examination of the adjacent air sacs may be made by causing a breach in the air sac membrane using the endoscope beveled tip; these small puncture holes do not need to be sutured afterwards. The muscles and skin should be sutured closed at the end of the procedure.

Right Approach

The technique is the same as previously described, but performed on the right side. This approach may be useful to assess the pancreas, or if a right-sided lesion was noted on radiographs or on CT scan prior to coelioscopy [64]. Bilateral approaches are recommended for multifocal diseases or screening.

Ventral Approach

The patient is placed in dorsal recumbency, and the incision is made just ventral to the keel, on the midline. The endoscope is then introduced cranially into the left or right ventral hepatoperitoneal cavity, allowing for visualization of the left and right lobes of the liver. The post-hepatic septum will have to be incised to access these cavities. Biopsies of the liver may be performed.

Interclavicular Approach

This approach is used less commonly, but allows visualization of the external aspect of the syrinx, the heart base, great vessels, thyroid glands, and any coelomic mass which would have been identified in this region on previous radiographs or CT scan [64]. The patient is placed in dorsal recumbency, and an incision is made on the midline, just cranial the furcula. Blunt dissection is used to reflect the crop laterally, and the clavicular air sac is punctured carefully.

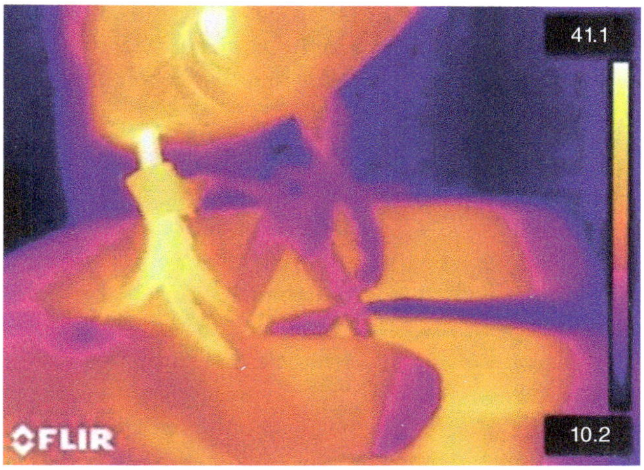

Figure 34.5 An infrared thermographic camera was used to take this picture of an American kestrel presented 24 hours following frost bite injury to the right foot. The right foot appears significantly warmer than the left, indicating increased vascularization and inflammation.

Biopsy/Histopathology Assessments

Biopsies are required to confirm most diagnoses. The most common biopsies taken in pet birds include masses, skin biopsies in case of dermal lesions or feather abnormalities, liver biopsies in case of elevated liver enzymes or hepatomegaly, crop biopsies in case of suspected avian bornavirus infection, spleen biopsies in case of splenomegaly or systemic infectious processes, and targeted organ biopsies taken during a coelioscopic examination. To increase the quality of the sample and the likelihood of achieving a diagnosis upon histopathologic examination, the sample should not be too small and it should be manipulated with care to decrease crushing artifacts. To minimize crushing artifacts during endoscopic biopsy procedures, the biopsy forceps should be open midway, and the tissue sample should be removed from the forceps cusps by gently flushing with saline or by agitating the forceps in a saline filled tube. For skin and crop biopsies, it is recommended to keep them flat in a small cassette before placing them in formalin to facilitate post-processing orientation. It may be beneficial to keep a sample frozen for other tests such as bacterial culture or PCR. If electron microscopy is required, the sample should not be placed in formalin but rather in specific fixatives (such as glutaraldehyde) and be processed as soon as possible. Submit the sample to a laboratory with veterinary staff competent with avian medicine and histopathology. Special stains, immunohistochemistry, or PCR may be required to reach a diagnosis.

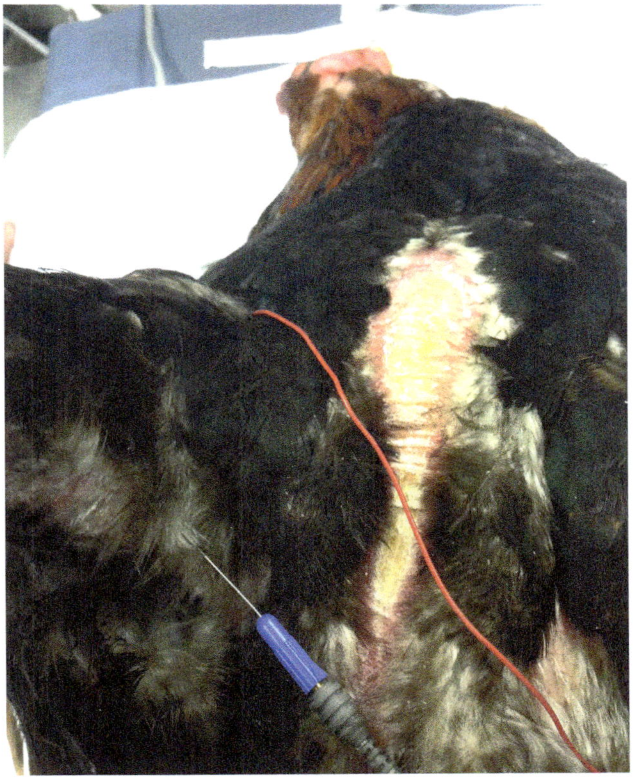

Figure 34.6 An electromyogram (EMG) is performed in a male Shamo chicken with left pelvic limb lameness. In this picture, a concentric needle electrode (Technomed Europe, Maastricht-Airport, the Netherlands) along with a subcutaneous needle electrode (Ambu Neuroline; Ambu Inc., Columbia, MD), used as a ground, are inserted in the right gastrocnemius muscle for comparison to the left side.

Infrared Thermography

Infrared cameras may be used to assess the perfusion of non-feathered areas, such as the feet, beak, and cere. It may be useful to detect inflammation associated with pododermatitis, or in contrast, a defect in perfusion associated with frost bite, trauma, or inflammation (Figure 34.5). It may also be used to monitor the progression of wound healing.

Electromyography

Electromyography is the recording of muscular electrical activity in response to a nerve stimulation using electrodes inserted into the muscle. It has been used in avian species to evaluate traumatic injuries and establish a prognosis for release of wild birds [66]. Electromyography was also used to aid in the antemortem diagnosis of Marek's disease in a chicken (Figure 34.6) [67]. Furthermore, this test was used to evaluate the neurologic lesions of a lead-induced peripheral neuropathy in a turkey vulture [68].

Ophthalmologic Tests

The eyes should be examined with a direct or indirect ophthalmoscope on each avian patient; this is particularly important if the bird is presented with a history of trauma or suspected trauma and in birds of prey. Multiple tests may be performed if an ophthalmologic lesion is noted or suspected: Schirmer tear test (Figure 34.7) or red phenol thread test to assess lacrimal production, fluorescein stain to identify corneal ulcers, and tonometry to measure the intraocular pressure. Reference intervals have been published for these tests, but in a limited number of species. If blindness is suspected or cataract surgery is considered, retinal function can be assessed with electroretinography; however, the equipment used in mammals, with contact lens, will not accommodate the small eyes of most parrots. Other types of electrodes may be used for smaller eyes but are not commonly available in veterinary hospitals. To evaluate the intraocular structures and the retro-orbital space, an ocular ultrasound or a skull CT/MRI scan can be performed. Finally, optical coherence tomography (OCT) shows cross section images of the anterior and posterior eye segments, and more specifically of the retina. It was tested in a variety of birds and enables more accurate diagnosis and prognosis of ocular diseases [69]. It may be used to evaluate retinal diseases, glaucoma, and avian bornavirus associated ocular disease. [69, 70] It is, however, rarely available in veterinary facilities.

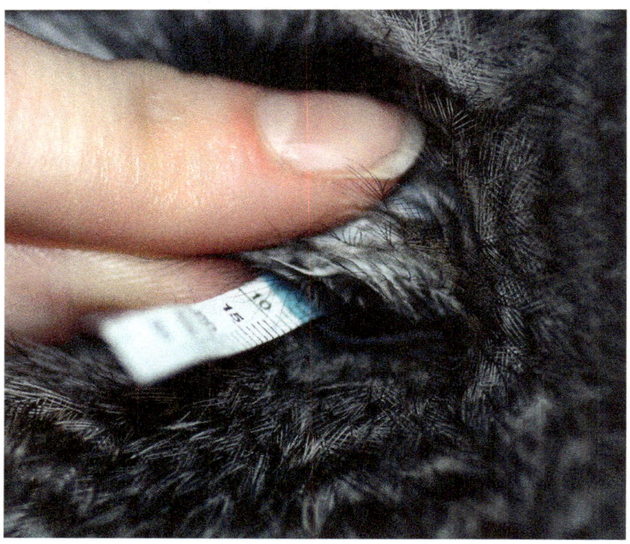

Figure 34.7 Schirmer tear test being performed in a great grey owl.

Parasitologic Tests

Tests to screen for parasites include fecal wet mount, fecal flotation, fecal sedimentation (trematodes), skin scrapings, trachea- and coelioscopy, and blood smears for hematozoans (see other chapters).

Selected parasites of high clinical significance in birds include the following:

- Oral cavity/GI tract: Trichomoniasis is a common parasitic disease of pigeons and various birds of prey, but may also be identified in other birds. It is caused by *Trichomonas gallinae*, and causes a variety of clinical signs including weight loss, poor growth, delayed gastrointestinal motility, caseous lesions in the oral cavity, sinusitis and conjunctivitis. Diagnosis is made by finding characteristic motile trophozoites in a wet mount of crop content or swabs of the oral or ocular lesions [71]. Among nematodes, capillarids and ascarids are usually the most pathogenic. A variety of coccidian parasites may be encountered in chickens, birds of prey, and passerine birds, especially in youngsters

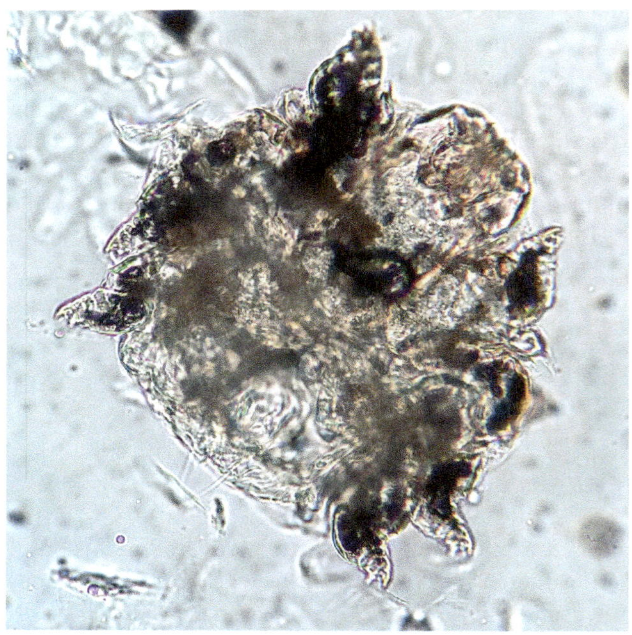

Figure 34.8 *Knemidocoptes pilae* recovered from a skin scraping in a budgerigar with hyperkeratotic cere lesions.

and juveniles. Diagnosis for nematodes and coccidia are made from a fecal flotation or a fecal wet mount.

- Trachea/lungs/air sacs: Tracheal worms are caused by strongylid nematodes such as *Syngamus trachea* and *Cyathostoma bronchialis*, and may be identified in the trachea or respiratory tract of water birds, birds of prey, Galliformes, Anseriformes, and other species kept outside. They may cause various respiratory clinical signs including dyspnea, coughing, and open mouth breathing. They may be identified by transillumination of the trachea. Characteristic eggs may also be found on a fecal floatation test or in the oral cavity [71]. The air sac mite *Sternostoma tracheacolum* is also prevalent in canaries and certain finches.
- Skin: Multiple arthropods may be found in birds including ticks, mites (such as *Dermanyssus gallinae* and *Ornithonyssus sylviarum*, *Knemidocoptes* sp., feather mites), lice (Malophaga), mosquitoes, blackflies (Simuliidae), and flat flies (Hippoboscidae). Some arthropods may cause skin disease directly (e.g. *Dermanyssus* sp., *Knemidocoptes* sp.), and others may act as a vector for systemic diseases (e.g. mosquitoes for West Nile virus, Hippoboscidae for *Hemoproteus* spp.). Diagnosis requires microscopic identification of skin scraping samples (knemidocoptic mites, [Figure 34.8]) or of the incriminated arthropod.

References

1 Phalen, D.N. (2006). Preventive medicine and screening. In: *Clinical Avian Medicine Volume II* (eds. G.J. Harrison and T.L. Lightfoot), 573–585. Palm Beach: Spix Publishing.

2 Fitzgerald, B., Olsen, G., and Speer, B. (2013). Laboratory reporting accuracy of polymerase chain reaction testing for avian polyomavirus. *J. Avian Med. Surg.* 27 (1): 32–37.

3 Olsen, G. and Speer, B. (2009). Laboratory reporting accuracy of polymerase chain reaction testing for psittacine beak and feather disease virus. *J. Avian Med. Surg.* 23 (3): 194–198.

4 Lightfoot, T.L. and Yeager, J.M. (2008). Pet bird toxicity and related environmental concerns. *Vet. Clin. North Am. Exot. Anim. Pract.* 11 (2): 229–259, vi.

5 Christopher, M.M., Shooshtari, M.P., and Levengood, J.M. (2004). Assessment of erythrocyte morphologic abnormalities in mallards with experimentally induced zinc toxicosis. *Am. J. Vet. Res.* 65 (4): 440–446.

6 Lumeij, J.T. (2008). Avian clinical biochemistry. In: *Clinical Biochemistry of Domestic Animals*, 6e (eds. J.J. Kaneko, J.W. Harvey and M.L. Bruss), 839–872. New York;, NY: Academic Press.

7 Dumonceaux, G. and Harrison, G.J. (1996). Toxins. In: *Avian Medicine: Principles and Applications* (eds. B.W. Ritchie, G.J. Harrison and L.R. Harrison), 1030–1052. Lake Worth: Winger Publishing.

8 Puschner, B., Leger, J.S., and Galey, F.D. (1999). Normal and toxic zinc concentrations in serum/plasma and liver of psittacines with respect to genus differences. *J. Vet. Diagn. Invest.* 11: 522–527.

9 Langlois, I. (2003). The anatomy, physiology, and diseases of the avian proventriculus and ventriculus. *Vet. Clin. North Am. Exot. Anim. Pract.* 6: 85–111.

10 Lumeij, J.T. (1985). Clinicopathologic aspects of lead poisoning in birds: a review. *Vet. Q.* 7 (2): 133–138.

11 Black, P.A., Macek, M., Tieber, A., and Weber, M. (2013). Reference values for hematology, plasma biochemical analysis, plasma protein electrophoresis, and Aspergillus serology in elegant-crested tinamou (*Eudromia elegans*). *J. Avian Med. Surg.* 27 (1): 1–6.

12 Osofskydvm, A., Jowettphd, P.L.H., Hosgoodbvsc, G. et al. (2001). Determination of normal blood concentrations of lead, zinc, copper, and iron in Hispaniolan Amazon parrots (*Amazona ventralis*). *J. Avian Med. Surg.* 15 (1): 31–36.

13 Redig, P.T. and Arent, L.R. (2008). Raptor toxicology. *Vet. Clin. North Am. Exot. Anim. Pract.* 11 (2): 261–282.

14 Barrett, M.W. and Karstad, L.H. (1971). A fluorescent erythrocyte test for lead poisoning in waterfowl. *J. Wildl. Manage.* 35 (1): 109–119.

15 Ludke, J.L., Hill, E.F., and Dieter, M.P. (1975). Cholinesterase (ChE) response and related mortality among birds fed ChE inhibitors. *Arch. Environ. Contam. Toxicol.* 3 (1): 1–21.

16 Hill, E.F. (1989). Sex and storage affect cholinesterase activity in blood plasma of Japanese quail. *J. Wildl. Dis.* 25 (4): 580–585.

17 Bunyan, P.J., Jennings, D.M., and Taylor, A. (1968). Organophosphorus poisoning: some properties of avian esterases. *J. Agric. Food Chem.* 16 (2): 326–331.

18 Vaughan-Higgins, R., Vitali, S., Reiss, A. et al. (2016). Development of reference ranges for plasma total cholinesterase and brain acetylcholinesterase activity in free-ranging Carnaby's black-cockatoos (*Calyptorhynchus latirostris*). *J. Wildl. Dis.* 52 (3): 592–598.

19 Zwarg, T., Prioste, F., Thijl Vanstreels, R.E. et al. (2012). Normal plasma cholinesterase activity of neotropical falconiformes and strigiformes. *J. Raptor Res.* 46 (2): 201–207.

20 Roy, C., Grolleau, G., Chamoulaud, S., and Rivière, J.-L. (2005). Plasma B-esterase activities in European raptors. *J. Wildl. Dis.* 41 (1): 184–208.

21 García-Rodríguez, T., Ferrer, M., Recio, F., and Castroviejo, J. (1987). Circadian rhythms of determined blood chemistry values in buzzards and eagle owls. *Comp. Biochem. Physiol. A* 88 (4): 663–669.

22 Morrisey, J.K., Paul-Murphy, J., Fialkowski, J.P. et al. (2003). Estimation of prothrombin times of Hispaniolan Amazon parrots (*Amazona ventralis*) and umbrella cockatoos (*Cacatua alba*). *J. Avian Med. Surg.* 17 (2): 72–77.

23 Doerr, J.A., Wyatt, R.D., and Hamilton, P.B. (1975). Investigation and standardization of prothrombin times in chickens. *Poult. Sci.* 54 (4): 969–980.

24 Frost, C.L., Naudé, R.J., Oelofsen, W., and Jacobson, B. (1999). Comparative blood coagulation studies in the ostrich. *Immunopharmacology* 45 (1): 75–81.

25 Webster, K.H. (2009). *Validation of a Prothrombin Time Assay for Assessment of Brodifacoum Exposure in Japanese Quails and Barn Owls*. Simon Fraser University.

26 Belleville, J., Cornillon, B., Paul, J. et al. (1982). Haemostasis, blood coagulation and fibrinolysis in the Japanese quail. *Comp. Biochem. Physiol. Part A Physiol.* 71 (2): 219–230.

27 Tahira, N., Dube, B., and Agrawal, G.P. (1977). Blood coagulation studies in some wild Indian birds: effect of different tissue thromboplastins. *J. Comp. Pathol.* 87 (3): 451–457.

28 Ponder, J. and Willette, M. (2015). Strigiformes. In: *Fowler's Zoo and Wild Animal Medicine Current Therapy*, vol. 8 (eds. R. Miller and M. Fowler), 189–198. St. Louis, MO: Elsevier.

29 Bigland, C.H. (1964). Blood clotting times of five avian species. *Poult. Sci.* 43 (4): 1035–1039.

30 Gerlach, H. (1994). Bacteria. In: *Avian Medicine: Principles and Applications* (eds. T.W. Campbell, B.W. Richie, G.L. Harrison and L.R. Harrison), 949–983. Wingers Publishing.

31 Thomas, R. (1991). Detection of *Clostridium botulinum* types C and D toxin by ELISA. *Aust. Vet. J.* 68 (3): 111–113.

32 Beaufrère, H., Laniesse, D., Stickings, P. et al. (2016). Generalized tetanus in a gyrfalcon (Falco rusticolus) with pododermatitis. *Avian Dis.* 60 (4): 850–855.

33 Ernst, A. and Zibrak, J.D. (1998). Carbon monoxide poisoning. *N. Engl. J. Med.* 339 (22): 1603–1608.

34 Wismer, T. (2016). Advancements in diagnosis and management of toxicologic problems. In: *Current Therapy in Avian Medicine and Surgery* (ed. B. Speer), 589–599. Saint Louis, MI: Elsevier.

35 Orosz, S.E., Monks, D.J., and De Matos, R. (2016). Clinical endocrinology of the protein hormones. In: *Current Therapy in Avian Medicine and Surgery*, 1e (ed. B.L. Speer), 378–399. China: Elsevier.

36 de Matos, R. (2008). Calcium metabolism in birds. *Vet. Clin. North Am. Exot. Anim. Pract.* 11 (1): 59–82, vi.

37 Howard, L.L., Kass, P.H., Lamberski, N., and Wack, R.F. (2004). Serum concentrations of ionized calcium, vitamin D3; and parathyroid hormone in captive thick-billed parrots (*Rhynchopsitta pachyrhyncha*). *J. Zoo Wildl. Med.* 35 (2): 147–153.

38 Adkesson, M.J. and Langan, J.N. (2007). Metabolic bone disease in juvenile Humboldt penguins (Spheniscus humboldti): investigation of ionized calcium, parathyroid hormone, and vitamin D3 as diagnostic parameters. *J. Zoo Wildl. Med.* 38 (1): 85–92.

39 Tangredi, B.P. and Krook, L.P. (1999). Nutritional secondary hyperparathyroidism in free-living fledgling American crows (*Corvus brachyrhynchos brachyrhynchos*). *J. Zoo Wildl. Med.* 30 (1): 94–99.

40 Kubiak, M. and Forbes, N. (2012). Effects of diet on total calcium, vitamin D and parathyroid hormone in falcons. *Vet. Rec.* 171 (20): 504.

41 de Wit, M., Schoemaker, N.J., Kik, M.J.L., and Westerhof, I. (2003). Hypercalcemia in two Amazon parrots with malignant lymphoma. *Avian Dis.* 47 (1): 223–228.

42 Braun, E.J. and Stallone, J.N. (1989). The occurrence of nephrogenic diabetes insipidus in domestic fowl. *Am. J. Physiol. – Ren. Physiol.* 256 (4): F639–F645.

43 Minvielle, F., Grossmann, R., and Gourichon, D. (2007). Development and performances of a Japanese quail line homozygous for the diabetes insipidus (di) mutation. *Poult. Sci.* 86 (2): 249–254.

44 Brummermann, M. and Braun, E.J. (1995). Renal response of roosters with diabetes insipidus to infusions of arginine vasotocin. *Am. J. Physiol. Regul. Integr. Comp. Physiol.* 269 (1): R57–R63.

45 Starkey, S.R., Wood, C., de Matos, R. et al. (2010). Central diabetes insipidus in an African grey parrot. *J. Am. Vet. Med. Assoc.* 237 (4): 415–419.

46 Westerhof I. Thirsty Sjaak, the African grey parrot. ECZM Symp. 2016;

47 Laniesse, D., Beaufrere, H., and Smith, D. (2016). Diabetes insipidus in a 4 year old Congo African grey parrot (*Psittacus erithacus erithacus*) concurrently infected with avian bornavirus. *Exot. Proc. Portl.* 339.

48 Oglesbee, B. (1992). Hypothyroidism in a scarlet macaw. *J. Am. Vet. Med. Assoc.* 201 (10): 1599–1601.

49 Schmidt, R.E. and Reavill, D.R. (2008). The avian thyroid gland. *Vet. Clin. North Am. Exot. Anim. Pract.* 11 (1): 15–23.

50 Lumeij, J.T. (1996). Endocrinology. In: *Avian Medicine: Principles and Applications* (eds. B.W. Ritchie, G.J.

Harrison and L.R. Harrison), 582–606. Lake Worth: Wingers Publishing.

51 Greenacre, C., Young, D.W., Behrend, E., and Wilson, H. (2001). Validation of a novel high-sensitivity radioimmunoassay procedure for measurement of total thyroxine concentration in psittacine birds and snakes. *Am. J. Vet. Res.* 62 (11): 1750–1754.

52 Brandao, J, Rick, M, Beaufrere, H, Tully, T (2014). Free and total thyroid hormones reference interval in the Hispaniolan Amazon parrot. AAV to *Proceedings of the annual meeting of the Association of Avian Veterinarians*. p. 29.

53 Brandão, J. and Manickam, B. (2012). Productive thyroid follicular carcinoma in a wild barred owl (*Strix varia*). *J. Vet. Diagn. Invest.* 24 (6): 1145–1150.

54 Gancz, A.Y., Wellehan, J.F.X., Boutette, J. et al. (2007). Diabetes mellitus concurrent with hepatic haemosiderosis in two macaws (*Ara severa, Ara militaris*). *Avian Pathol.* 36 (4): 331–336.

55 Pilny, A.A. (2008). The avian pancreas in health and disease. *Vet. Clin. North Am. Exot. Anim. Pract.* 11 (1): 25–34.

56 Desmarchelier, M. and Langlois, I. (2008). Diabetes mellitus in a nanday conure (*Nandayus nenday*). *J. Avian Med. Surg.* 22 (3): 246–254.

57 Pilny, A.A. and Luong, R. (2005). Diabetes mellitus in a chestnut-fronted macaw (*Ara severa*). *J. Avian Med. Surg.* 19 (4): 297–302.

58 Douglass, E.M. (1981). Diabetes mellitus in a Toco toucan. *Mod. Vet. Pract.* 62 (4): 293–295.

59 Candeletta, S.C., Homer, B.L., Garner, M.M., and Isaza, R. (1993). Diabetes mellitus associated with chronic lymphocytic pancreatitis in an African grey parrot (*Psittacus erithacus erithacus*). *J. Assoc. Avian Vet.* 7 (1): 39.

60 Wallner-Pendleton, E.A., Rogers, D., and Epple, A. (1993). Diabetes mellitus in a red-tailed hawk (*Buteo jamaicensis*). *Avian Pathol.* 22 (3): 631–635.

61 Appleby, R. (1984). Diabetes mellitus in a budgerigar (*Melopsittacus undulatus*). *Vet. Rec.* 115 (25–26): 652–653.

62 Campbell, T. and Ellis, C. (2007). Hematology of birds. In: *Avian & Exotic Animal Hematology & Cytology*, 3e (eds. T. Campbell and C. Ellis), 3–50. Oxford, UK: Wiley-Blackwell.

63 Taylor, M. (1994). Endoscopic examination and biopsy techniques. In: *Avian Medicine: Principles and Applications* (eds. B. Ritchie, G.J. Harrison and L.R. Harrison), 327–354. Lake Worth, FL: Wingers Publishing.

64 Divers, S.J. (2010). Avian diagnostic endoscopy. *Vet. Clin. North Am. Exot. Anim. Pract.* 13 (2): 187–202.

65 Taylor, M. and Murray, M. (1999). Endoscopic examination and therapy of the avian gastrointestinal tract. *Semin. Avian Exot. Pet Med.* 8 (3): 110–114.

66 Holland, M. and Jennings, D. (1997). Use of electromyography in seven injured wild birds. *J. Am. Vet. Med. Assoc.* 211 (5): 607–609.

67 Murthy, V., Laniesse, D., Beaufrère, H. et al. (2016). What is your diagnosis? *J. Avian Med. Surg.* 30 (2): 204–208.

68 Platt, S.R., Helmick, K.E., Graham, J. et al. (1999). Peripheral neuropathy in a Turkey vulture with lead toxicosis. *J. Am. Vet. Med. Assoc.* 214 (8): 1218–1220, 1200.

69 Azmanis, P.N., Rauscher, F.G., Werner, B. et al. (2015). The additional diagnostic value of optical coherence tomography (OCT) and its application procedure in a wide variety of avian species. *J. Clin. Exp. Ophthalmol.* 06 (03): 1000431.

70 Korbel, R., Sigg, R. (2014). Ocular coherence tomography (OCT) of the anterior eye segment – clinical findings and evaluation protocols. *Proceedings of the Annual Meeting of the Association of Avian Veterinarians*. p. 9.

71 Coutteel, P. and Wencel, P. (2016). Infectious diseases – parasitic diseases. In: *Avian Medicine*, 3e (ed. J. Samour), 507–521. St.Louis: Elsevier.

Section 3

Emergency Presentations and Management by Species

35

Psittacines

Nicole R. Wyre

Zodiac Pet and Exotic Hospital, Tin Hau, Hong Kong

CONTENTS

Common Presenting Signs

Abnormal Droppings

Introduction

- Abnormal droppings can be a problem with the feces, urates, or urine; photos from owners can be helpful in distinguishing which portion is abnormal
- Often the presenting complaint is diarrhea when in fact birds are more often polyuric
- Pigmenturia from food is commonly confused with blood in the urine or feces

Diagnosis

Clinical signs:

- Abnormal feces: no feces, diarrhea, undigested food, melena, hematochezia, pigmented feces, dark green feces (bile from hyporexia)
- Abnormal urates: blood, hemoglobin, biliverdin
- Abnormal urine: hematuria, hemoglobinuria, polyuria

Differentials:

- Absence of feces: anorexia, regurgitation, colonic obstruction

Exotic Animal Emergency and Critical Care Medicine, First Edition. Edited by Jennifer E. Graham, Grayson A. Doss, and Hugues Beaufrère.

- Diarrhea
- Polyuria: increased dietary fluid intake, renal disease, reproductive/egg bound, ABV/PDD associated ganglioneuritis (ABV/PDD), liver disease, iatrogenic hyperglycemia from steroids, behavioral, diabetes mellitus, diabetes insipidus
- Undigested food in the feces: ABV/PDD, mycobacteriosis, bacterial, or fungal gastroenteritis, intestinal neoplasia, other
- Melena/hematochezia: heavy metal toxicity, foreign body ingestion, gastric/duodenal ulceration, enteritis
- Hematuria/hemoglobinuria/hemoglobin or blood in the urates: egg bound, heavy metal toxicity, renal disease, intravascular hemolysis
- Biliverdinuria: hepatobiliary disease

STAT diagnostics:

- Diarrhea: fecal Gram's stain, fecal cytology (screen for yeast), direct exam
- Melena/hematochezia/hematuria/hemoglobinuria: PCV/TS
- Standing or whole-body radiographs if heavy metal toxicity or egg binding is suspected

Complete diagnostics:

- CBC/biochemistry
  - Hyperglycemia: iatrogenic steroids or diabetes mellitus
  - Hyperuricemia: renal disease
  - Elevated liver values: liver or infectious disease
  - Leukocytosis with respiratory signs: infectious respiratory tract disease (IRTD)
- Blood gas and electrolyte panel
- Whole body radiographs/ultrasound
- Blood lead/zinc levels
- Fecal C&S
- Urinalysis via ureteral cannulation
- Endoscopy for biopsy +/− C&S

Treatment

- Stabilization and supportive care
- Assisted feeding / crop feeding (see Chapter 29)
- Fluid replacement therapy (see Chapter 29)
- Broad-spectrum antibiotics (enrofloxacin, amoxicillin/clavulanic acid)
- Enrofloxacin: 10–20 mg/kg PO q24h [1, 2]
- Amoxicillin-clavulanate: 125 mg/kg PO q8 h [3]
- Specific therapy based on diagnosing the underlying disease

Coelomic Distention

Introduction

- Birds have an extensive air sac system, therefore, coelomic distention commonly presents with dyspnea by reducing air sac volume

Diagnosis

Clinical signs:

- Distended coelom with palpable fat, egg, fluid, organomegaly, or mass
- Dyspnea
- Exercise intolerance
- Wide based stance
- Droppings accumulated around vent
- Arrhythmia or cardiac murmur if cardiac related
- Yellow-green urates if liver related
- Widened pubic bones and pink/tumescent vent if egg laying related

Differentials:

- Obesity
- Egg (in oviduct or ectopic)
- Fluid
  - Reproductive tract: egg yolk coelomitis, ruptured ovarian cyst, reproductive-associated ascites
  - Coelomitis
  - Liver failure
  - Congestive heart failure
  - Hypoproteinemia
  - Hemorrhage (trauma or coagulopathy)
  - Iron storage disease
- Organomegaly/neoplasia
  - Reproductive: salpingitis, ovarian cyst/carcinoma, dystocia
  - Gastrointestinal: dilation (foreign body vs. ABV/PDD, other causes of proventricular dilation and ileus), neoplasia
  - Hepatomegaly: hepatic lipidosis, hepatitis, *Chlamydia psittaci*, mycobacteriosis, lymphoma, iron storage disease
  - Splenomegaly: *Chlamydia psittaci*, mycobacteriosis, bacterial splenitis
  - Neoplasia: lipoma, lymphoma, gonadal, renal, pancreatic, other
- Body wall pseudohernia (female bird)
- Granuloma

STAT diagnostics:

- PCV/TS/blood smear
  - Hyperproteinemia: inflammation, reproductive disease, neoplasia
  - Hypoproteinemia: liver failure, ABV/PDD, neoplasia, protein losing nephropathy, protein losing enteropathy
  - Leukocytosis: infectious disease, neoplasia, granuloma, coelomitis
  - Regenerative anemia: bleeding into coelom
    - Non-regenerative anemia: nonspecific

- Standing radiograph to assess for mineralized eggs
- POCUS
  - Coelomic: differentiate fluid from mass (organomegaly, neoplasia, egg, granuloma) or hernia
  - Cardiac: pericardial fluid, chamber enlargement
- Coelomocentesis if fluid is causing dyspnea
  - Fluid analysis/cytology
    - Exudate: coelomitis (i.e. GI perforation), neoplasia, granuloma, infectious disease
    - Transudate and modified transudate: reproductive tract disease, liver failure, neoplasia, congestive heart failure, hypoproteinemia, iron storage disease
    - Lipid/yolk globules: yolk coelomitis
    - Neoplastic cells
    - Hemorrhage
- C&S depending on cytology
    - Complete diagnostics
- Biochemistry
  - Liver disease: elevated liver enzymes/bile acids, hypouricemia, hypoproteinemia
  - Reproductive disease: hyperproteinemia, lipemia, hypercalcemia
- Radiographs or CT-scan
  - Assess for masses, organomegaly or egg
  - Contrast radiographs to assess for gastrointestinal displacement or dilation
- Full ultrasound with FNA for masses or organomegaly
- Endoscopic or surgical biopsies
- Infectious disease testing as warranted

Treatment

Stabilization:

- Oxygen support (most of these birds are dyspneic)
- Therapeutic coelomocentesis in case of ascites
- IV/IO fluid replacement therapy (colloid for hypoproteinemia)
- Homologous blood transfusion for severe blood loss

Continued care:

- Nutritional support (see Chapter 29)
- Antibiotics or antifungal treatment for infectious diseases
- Surgery: debridement of granulomas, remove neoplasia
- Neoplasia: chemotherapy, radiation or surgical therapy
- Obesity: conversion to commercial pelleted diet with fruits and vegetables, increased exercise
- Liver failure – targeted treatment depends on cause based on FNA or hepatic biopsy
  - Nutritional support – controversy if should feed low protein diet [4]
  - Dextrose (IV, IO) if hypoglycemic (2.5–5%)
  - Colloid support (IV, IO) if hypoalbuminemic
  - Antibiotic if bacterial hepatitis
  - Fibrosis/cirrhosis: Colchicine: 0.5–0.1 mg/kg PO q12–24h [1]
  - Low-fat diet and lifestyle changes for hepatic lipidosis
  - Therapies used in other species such as silymarin, S-adenosyl methionine, ursodiol and lactulose have not been proven to work in psittacine birds but can be considered [4]
- Iron storage disease
  - Deferoxamine mesylate: 20–100 mg/kg SC/IM q24h [1], deferiprone
  - Phlebotomy
- See "CHF"
- See "ABV/PDD"
- See "Egg binding/dystocia"
- See "Yolk coelomitis"

Egg Binding/Dystocia

Introduction

- Depending on the cause, medical or surgical therapy is warranted
- Problems with the hen [5]
  - Hypocalcemia (medical) – oviductal inertia, unmineralized egg
  - Salpingitis (can attempt medical first)
  - Oviductal torsion/rupture or neoplasia (surgical)
  - Thin body condition (can attempt medical first)
  - Musculoskeletal deformity of pelvic inlet (surgical)
- Problems with the egg [5]
  - Fractured or malformed (usually surgical)
  - Multiple eggs in oviduct (usually surgical)
  - Ectopic (surgical)

Diagnosis

Clinical signs:

- Dyspnea
- Coelomic distension +/– palpable egg
- Widened pubic bones and pink/tumescent vent
- Wide based stance
- Tenesmus
- Hematochezia
- Cloacal prolapse
- Tetany or seizure
- Wing droop or lameness
- Differentials
  - Coelomic distention
  - Dyspnea
  - Cloacal prolapse
  - Hematochezia

- Seizures
- Trauma

STAT diagnostics:

- Tetany or seizures – ionized calcium and magnesium
- Standing radiograph
  - Mineralized egg, integrity of the shell, presence of multiple eggs
  - Assess bone quality – can see medullary hyperostosis or osteopenia with chronic egg layers

Complete diagnostics:

- CBC
  - Inflammatory leukogram and non-regenerative anemia: salpingitis or egg yolk coelomitis, can be normal in reproductive females if mild
- Biochemistry
  - Hypercalcemia, hyperproteinemia, and lipemia with active egg laying
  - Hypocalcemia: inadequate diet, chronic egg laying
  - Hyperuricemia: ureteral compression, dehydration
- Radiographs
  - Egg size, shape, shell quality
  - Bone quality, pathologic fractures, pelvic deformities/fractures
- Ultrasound
  - Coelomic effusion, oviductal/ovarian disease, egg location (intra or extra-oviductal)
- Coelomocentesis when ascites present
  - Diagnostic and therapeutic (if causing dyspnea)
  - Fluid analysis, cytology, Gram stain +/− C&S

Treatment

Stabilization:

- Seizures/tetany (see "Seizures")
- Fluid therapy (see Chapter 29)
- Cloacal prolapse (see "Cloacal prolapse")
- Analgesia (see Chapter 28)
- Antibiotics: salpingitis or coelomitis (see "Yolk coelomitis")

Continued care:

- Medical management: Attempt first if not immediately surgical
- Calcium therapy
  - Calcium gluconate: 50–100 mg/kg IV (very slow using a syringe pump)/IO/SC (diluted in SC fluids)
  - Calcium glubionate or calcium carbonate: 23–150 mg/kg of elemental calcium PO q12–24h [1]
- Nutritional support (see Chapter 29)
- Oxytocin and prostaglandins can be tried ONLY after hydrated, normal ionized calcium, intact oviduct and egg, egg in oviduct and no mechanical obstruction
  - First relax vaginal sphincter: prostaglandin E2 gel (0.02–0.1 mg/kg topically) [5] or misoprostol tablet crushed, mixed with water, and applied as thin paste to cloaca
  - Then facilitate egg laying: oxytocin (5–10 IU/kg IM) or prostaglandin F2 alpha (0.02 mg/kg IM) [5]
- Hormonal therapy to prevent further laying
  - Leuprolide acetate: 700–800 μg/kg IM, may not prevent oviposition of the current clutch [5, 6]
  - Deslorelin implant: 4.7–9.5 mg implant SC
- Surgical management (under anesthesia/sedation)
  - Egg located in cloaca
    - Digital removal with a lubricated, gloved finger
    - Collapse egg via ovocentesis [5]
      - ONLY an option if the eggshell is visible in cloaca or vagina – a needle should never be passed through oviductal tissues or through the skin because iatrogenic damage to the internal organs can occur
      - Pass large gauge needle (20–22 gage) into visible eggshell, remove contents with suction or syringe (12–20 ml)
      - Collapse empty egg
      - Remove eggshell with small forceps or cotton tipped applicators
      - Radiographs ensure removal of entire shell. If shell fragments persist, they may be eliminated naturally by the hen
  - If egg is not in the cloaca/vagina – exploratory surgery to remove the egg +/− salpingohysterectomy

Neurologic Signs

Introduction

- Neurologic signs can occur from any disease which causes damage to the nervous system
- Clinical signs are based on the part of the nervous system affected
- Nonspecific signs of weakness and depression can be difficult to differentiate from true neurologic disease (see "Sick bird syndrome")

Diagnosis

Clinical signs:

- Seizures
- Ataxia
- Collapse
- Head tilt
- Paresis/paralysis
- Change in mentation or consciousness
- Blindness
- Limb weakness/tremors
- Dysphagia

Differentials:

- Head/spinal trauma, post-traumatic seizures
- Seizures
- Organomegaly or coelomic neoplasia (see "Coelomic distention")
- Cardiac disease: atherosclerosis/stroke
- Hypocalcemia (see "Nutritional deficiencies")
- Toxins: heavy metal, organophosphates, cardiac glycoside, or grayanotoxin containing plants
- Systemic infectious disease
  - Bacterial: mycobacteriosis, chlamydiosis, Gram-bacteria, listeriosis
  - Fungal: *Aspergillosis*
  - Viral: Avulavirus, bornavirus, herpesvirus
  - Parasitic: *Baylisascaris* larva migrans, *Sarcocystis* spp., *Toxoplasma gondii*
- Neoplasia (pituitary adenoma in budgerigars)
- Otitis media/interna
- Congenital: cyst, hydrocephalus

STAT diagnostics:

- PCV/TS/blood smear
  - Anemia
  - Leukocytosis: suspect infectious disease or neoplasia
- Ionized calcium and magnesium
- Blood glucose point-of-care blood lead measurements (LeadCare®)

Complete diagnostics:

- Blindness: complete ophthalmic exam, +/− ultrasound or ERG
- Head tilt/torticollis: optic exam, +/− cytology, +/− C&S
- CBC and Biochemistry
  - Depends on underlying disease
- Radiographs and/or ultrasound
  - Cardiomegaly, arterial calcification (see "Atherosclerosis" and "CHF")
  - Organomegaly, coelomic masses, GI dilation (see "Coelomic distention" and "ABV/PDD")
  - Metal density (see "Heavy metal toxicity")
  - Spinal fracture
  - EMG to differentiate disease of nerve vs. muscle
- CT or MRI (MRI being better)

Treatment

Stabilization:

- Control seizures (see "Seizures")
- Treat anemia (see "Anemia")

Continued care:

- Placement in padded cage with no perches
- Fluid therapy
- Nutritional support – patients with dysphagia may require feeding tube placement
- See "ingested intoxications"
- Organophosphate toxicity
  - Pralidoxime: 10–100 mg/kg IM q24–48 [1]
- Treatment of underlying disease

Respiratory Distress

Introduction

- Pre-oxygenate prior to exam
- Higher metabolism, a more efficient respiratory system with a larger exchange surface area makes birds more susceptible to airborne toxins
- Coelomic disease compressing air sacs causes respiratory distress
- Birds lack alveoli – cannot have pulmonary crackles
- Stress-induced physiologic tachypnea may be difficult to differentiate from distress

Diagnosis

Clinical signs:

- Dyspnea (expiratory, inspiratory, mixed, open-mouth, tail-bobbing, wheezes)
- Voice change, voice loss
- Blocked nares, nasal discharge, sneezing
- Auscultation of lungs or air sacs – dullness, rubbing, wheezes
- Coelomic distention
- Arrhythmia or cardiac murmur
- Pale/cyanotic mucous membranes

Differentials:

- Pain causing hyperventilation
- Coelomic distension (ascites, masses, organomegaly)
- Respiratory toxin (PTFE, carbon monoxide)
- Lower airway obstruction (seeds, masses, aspergilloma, post-intubation tracheal stenosis)
- Anemia
- IRTD (aspergillosis, chlamydiosis, pneumonia, air sacculitis)
- Congestive heart failure
- Aspiration pneumonia (more common in unweaned juveniles)
- Macaw pulmonary hypersensitivity
- Avocado toxicity

STAT diagnostics:

- PCV/TS/blood smear
  - Anemia

- Erythrocytosis: macaw pulmonary hypersensitivity, chronic respiratory infection, pulmonary neoplasm
- Leukocytosis: IRTD, other inflammatory disorder
- ECG if arrhythmia
- POCUS to assess for coelomic effusion, masses, cardiac chamber enlargement or pericardial effusion

Complete diagnostics:

- CBC/biochemistry: depends on underlying disease
- Radiographs/CT-scan/Ultrasound
  - Cardiomegaly, mineralization of great vessels, pulmonary effusion (see "CHF" and "Atherosclerosis")
  - Avocado (persin) toxicity: pulmonary edema and/or pericardial effusion [7] (see "Ingested intoxications")
  - Pulmonary and air sac changes (see "IRTD")
  - Organomegaly or coelomic masses (see "Coelomic distention")
  - Trauma
  - Egg (see "Dystocia")
- Echocardiogram if cardiac disease is suspected (see "CHF")
- Endoscopy/tracheoscopy for biopsy, bacterial culture and sensitivity
- Infectious disease testing (see "IRTD")

Treatment

Stabilization:

- Oxygen therapy
- Fluid therapy
- Therapeutic coelomocentesis

Continued care:

- See "Lower airway obstruction"
- See "Egg binding"
- See "Respiratory toxin"
- See "CHF"
- See "Atherosclerosis"
- See "IRTD"
- Nutritional support
- Nebulization
  - Need nebulizer with particles <20 μm to reach air sacs and < 1 μm to reach pulmonary parenchyma [8]
- Aspiration pneumonia
  - Anti-inflammatories
    - Meloxicam: 0.1–2 mg/kg PO, IM, IV/IO q12–24h [1]
  - Broad spectrum antibiotics depending on regurgitant
    - Gram negative infection - enrofloxacin (10–20 mg/kg) SC (in saline fluid pocket), IV/IO q24h [2] if IV/IO give slowly over 15 minutes and dilute at least 1:3 with saline
    - Gram positive infection - ampicillin (50–100 mg/kg IM q4–8h) [9] or cefazolin (25–50 mg/kg IM, IV q12h) [2]
    - Anaerobic bacteria - metronidazole (20–50 mg/kg PO q12h), ampicillin (50–100 mg/kg IM q4–8 h), amoxicillin (100 mg/kg PO q8-12 hour).
  - Saline or hypertonic saline nebulization

Sick Bird Syndrome

Introduction

- "Sick Bird Syndrome" is a common, nonspecific presenting complaint for many psittacine birds – obtain a thorough history before examination
- Prey species – hide signs of illness until they are extremely ill/sick
- Provide heat and oxygen before physical examination – assess patient in cage before handling

Diagnosis

Clinical signs:

- Non-specific are more common such as:
  - Fluffed at bottom of cage
  - Dehydration
  - Anorexia/hyporexia
  - Thin body condition/weak
  - Abnormal droppings
- Signs specific to a particular organ system may also be observed
  - Regurgitation/polyuria
  - Neurological signs (seizures, ataxia, head tilt)
  - Dyspnea
  - Others

Differentials:

- Any systemic disease may lead to this presentation

STAT diagnostics:

- PCV/TS/blood smear/Blood glucose
  - Anemia
  - Leukocytosis: with respiratory signs (see "IRTD"), neoplasia, bacterial, or fungal infection, toxin, trauma
  - Hyperproteinemia: reproductive, dehydration, chronic infection
  - Hypoproteinemia: blood loss, ABV/PDD, GI disease, liver disease, malnutrition
  - Hyperglycemia: stress, shock, iatrogenic steroids, diabetes mellitus
  - Hypoglycemia: sepsis, anorexia, neoplasia, liver disease
- Standing radiograph
  - Mineralized egg (see "Dystocia") or metal density
- POCUS if coelomic effusion is suspected (see "Coelomic distention")

Complete diagnostics:

- CBC and biochemistry
  - Hyperuricemia: renal disease
  - Elevated liver enzymes/bile acids: liver disease or Chlamydiosis
  - Hypocalcemia: nutritional deficiency, sepsis, hypomagnesemia
  - Hypercalcemia: reproductive disease, vitamin D toxicity
- Radiographs/CT-scan/Ultrasound
  - Organomegaly, coelomic mass (see "Coelomic distention")
  - GI gas, distention, or foreign material (see "GI foreign body" and "ABV/PDD")
  - Cardiac or pulmonary changes (see "Atherosclerosis", "CHF" and "IRTD")
- Infectious disease testing as warranted
- Heavy metal testing

Treatment

Stabilization:

- Oxygen
- Fluid replacement therapy +/− colloids or blood transfusion for anemia (see Chapter 29)

Continued care:

- Nutritional support
- Analgesia
  - Use NSAIDs once patient is hydrated, properly perfused and renal values are normal
- Broad-spectrum antibiotics (enrofloxacin, amoxicillin/clavulanic acid, TMS)
- Treatment of underlying disease

Trauma

Introduction

- Small bite wounds from carnivorous species can be deadly due to sepsis – if the owner did not witness the trauma occur and there is a dog/cat in the house, it may be advisable to treat the trauma as if it were a bite wound
- Compared to a mammal of the same size, an otherwise healthy bird can better compensate for acute blood loss [10]

Diagnosis

Clinical signs:

- Wound and feather loss
- Bleeding
- Lameness
- Wing droop
- Subcutaneous emphysema or air sac hyperinflation
- Seizures
- Change in mentation or consciousness
- Dyspnea from pain, anemia, tracheal, or beak trauma

Differentials:

- Neurologic signs
- Seizures
- Dyspnea
- Lower airway obstruction
- Heavy metal toxicity

STAT diagnostics:

- PCV/TS
  - Anemia with hypoproteinemia
  - Acute bleeding: may have normal PCV/TS, it may take up to 24 h for the PCV to reflect the degree of blood loss
- Blood smear
  - Leukocytosis: associated with the trauma itself or secondary infection
- Indirect blood pressure: not reliable in most small birds
- Thermal imaging: may help assess blood flow to apparently necrotic limbs or toes and assess the degree of inflammation

Complete diagnostics:

- CBC/Biochemistry
  - Elevated AST, LDH, CK from muscle damage
- Radiographs
  - Fractures - rule out pathologic fractures from neoplasia or poor bone quality
  - Pulmonary contusions
  - Air sac damage
- Coelomic ultrasound
  - Effusion, hemorrhage
  - Organ damage
- MRI/CT for head trauma

Treatment

Stabilization:

- Traumatic airway obstruction (air sac canula placement)
- Stop hemorrhage: digital compression, bandage, topical hemostatic agents
- Fluid therapy +/− colloids or blood transfusion
- Analgesia – opioids or NSAIDS (avoid NSAIDS in cases of hypoperfusion)
- Antibiotics

- Carnivore bite – IV/IO broad spectrum coverage against Gram negatives and anaerobes
  - Cefotaxime: 75–100 mg/kg IM, IV/IO q4–8h [1]
  - Ceftiofur: 10 mg/kg IM q4–12h [1]
  - Amoxicillin-clavulanate: 125 mg/kg PO q8h [3]
- If from another psittacine (including self-inflicted) - Gram positive coverage
  - Ampicillin: 50–100 mg/kg IM q4–8h [9]
  - Cefazolin: 25–50 mg/kg IM, IV/IO q12h [2]
  - Trimethoprim sulfamethoxazole: 10–100 mg/kg PO, IM q12–24h [1]
- Wound flushing with warm saline - CAUTION if ruptured air sacs

Continued care:

- Wet to dry, antimicrobial dressing, or medical honey bandages for contaminated wounds
- See Table 35.1 for specific long bone fracture repair and Table 35.2 for beak injury repair
- Coelomic trauma with body wall compromise – exploratory surgery
- Head trauma with suspected increased intracranial pressure (see "Seizures")
- Broken blood feathers – may require sedation; remiges are attached to periosteum
  - Warm saline to remove blood to visualize base of calamus
  - Use hemostats to grasp the entire calamus as close to the skin as possible
  - Use continuous gentle pressure to remove entire calamus – should visualize inferior umbilicus
  - If not removed entirely, use smaller hemostats to reattempt removal
  - If pulp/sheath remaining inside the follicle, the follicle will have to be incised to extract the stump
- Self-induced wounds (see "Feather destructive/mutilation behavior")

Systemic Disease

Anemia

Diagnosis

Clinical signs:

- Acute bleeding
- Dyspnea/tachypnea
- Tachycardia
- Pale mucous membranes
- Lethargy/weakness/collapse
- Melena/hematochezia
- Hemoglobinuria

Differentials:

- Regenerative anemia
  - Acute blood loss
  - Hemolysis
  - Heavy metal toxicity
  - IMHA (rare)
- Non regenerative anemia
  - Anemia of chronic disease (most common)
  - Chronic heavy metal toxicity (lead), viral disease (especially psittacine circovirus infection)
  - Neoplasia
  - Chronic hemorrhage
  - Bone marrow suppression (iatrogenic: fenbendazole, chlorambucil)

STAT diagnostics:

- PCV/TS – assess for hemolysis in serum and degree of anemia
- Blood smear – assess for polychromasia
- Agglutination
- Fecal exam – assess for RBCs, fecal occult blood test

Complete diagnostics:

- CBC
  - MCV, MCHC for further anemia classification
  - Leukocytosis: chronic infection/inflammation
- Biochemistry – depends on underlying disease
- Radiographs/CT-scan/ultrasound – depends on underlying disease
- Coelioscopy, cloacoscopy
- Zinc and lead blood test (see "Ingested intoxications")
- Bone marrow aspiration
- Infectious disease testing (See Chapter 34)

Treatment

Stabilization:

- Severe decompensated anemia (PCV <20%, tachycardia, tachypnea, collapse): IV/IO fluid therapy with colloid and/or homologous blood transfusion
- Hemostasis: digital compression, bandage, topical hemostatic agents

Continued care:

- Nutritional support, nutritional deficiency correction
- Fluid therapy
- Surgery to definitely control hemorrhage
- Treatment of underlying disease
  - Trauma
  - Melena
  - Chelation
  - Antibiotics
  - Chemotherapy

Table 35.1 Long bone fracture repair.

PELVIC LIMB		Repair method	Follow up	Average time to healing (wk)	References
Femur	Small bird <300 g	Cage rest or Spica splint	BC q1–2wk R 4–6wk	4–6	[11]
	Large bird >300 g	IM pin +/− external fixation tie-in			[12]
Tibiotarsus	Small bird <200 g	Tape splint	BC q1wk R 3–4wk	3–4	[11]
	Large bird – simple	Robert Jones bandage with orthopedic casting	BC q1–2wk R 4–6 wk	4–6	[13]
	Large bird – comminuted	IM pin +/− Type 1 or 2 external fixation tie-in			[12]
Tarsometatarsus	Small bird <200 g	Tape splint	BC q1wk R 3–4 wk	3–4	[11]
	Large bird – simple	Schroeder-Thomas splint or Robert-Jones bandage	BC w 1 wk R 4–6 wk	4–6	[13]
	Large bird – comminuted	Cross pin or type II external fixation			[12]
Phalanges		Tape splint Ball bandage	BC as needed	3–4	[11, 13]
THORACIC LIMB					[14]
Coracoid	Simple or comminuted	Body wrap	R 3 wk BC as needed to keep in place for 3 wk	3	
	Severe luxation	Internal fixation			
Scapula and clavicle	Small birds <300 g	Cage rest			
	Large birds >300 g	Body wrap	R 3 wk BC as needed to keep in place for 3 wk	3	[14]
Humerus	Proximal	Body wrap	BC q3wk R q3wk	3–6	[14]
	Midshaft	Type 1 external fixation +/− IM pin tie-in	PT 1–2 d post op R q2wk	3–6	
Radius/ulna	Simple	Figure 8 bandage × 3wk Cage rest × 1wk Internal fixation (IM pins, IM-ESF tie-in)	PT and BC 2 w post op q3d R q3wk	3–4	[14]
	Comminuted	Internal fixation	PT 10 d post op R q2wk	3–6	[14]
Carpometacarpal	Simple	Figure 8 bandage + metacarpal splint		5	[14]
	Comminuted	Type 1 external fixation	PT 10d post op R q2wk	5–6	

BC, bandage change; R, radiographs; PT, physical therapy.

- Crop or fecal cytology: assess for secondary bacterial or yeast overgrowth secondary to crop stasis
- Radiographs/CT-scan: dilated or gas filled proventriculus or ventriculus
  - Normal proventricular diameter-to-keel height ratio <0.48 [18]
- Fluoroscopy: Assess motility of crop, proventriculus and ventriculus
- Crop biopsy (PCR on tissue and IHC may also be available to confirm the diagnosis)
- PCR testing for ABV on fecal swab or tissue biopsy: positive fecal PCR with compatible clinical signs is generally interpreted as positive for avian bornaviral disease. However, due to extensive incubation period, birds may be positive and not clinical for the infection. Likewise, infected birds may be negative due to intermittent shedding.
- ECG and echocardiography for cardiac signs

Treatment

Stabilization:

- Control seizures
- IV/IO fluid support with colloid if hypoproteinemic
- Management of arrhythmia or congestive heart failure
- Correction of electrolyte imbalances

Continued care:

- Nutritional support with highly digestible diet
- Antimicrobial/antifungal for treatment of secondary infections
- NSAIDS may be helpful to reduce inflammatory cell infiltration
  - Celecoxib: 10–20 mg/kg PO q24h [1]
  - Meloxicam: Use in cockatiels with ABV/PDD may enhance severity of infection [19]
  - Robenacoxib: 2–10 mg/kg IM weekly for four weeks and then monthly [20]
- Immunosuppressive medications may be attempted to control clinical signs (as they are caused by an immune-mediated process). This may also predispose to secondary infections due to immunosuppression, therefore closely monitor the CBC and the patient for any signs of fungal or bacterial infection
  - Prednisolone: 0.1–0.2 mg/kg PO q12–24 hours
  - Cyclosporine A

Seizures

Diagnosis

Clinical signs:

- Generalized seizure: wing flapping, rhythmically kicking legs, rhythmic vocalizations
- Focal seizure: extension of one wing or leg, clenched feet, head twitching
- Postictal: altered mentation, blindness, circling, head tilt/turn, or decreased ability to grip
- Bruising on head or face

Differentials:

- Head trauma, post-traumatic seizures
- Heavy metal or chocolate toxicity
- ABV/PDD
- Hypocalcemia/hypomagnesemia
- Hypoglycemia
- Atherosclerosis
- Neoplasia
- Diseases that can mimic seizures: syncope, tremors, vestibular disease, claudication like syndrome

STAT diagnostics:

- Ionized calcium, ionized magnesium, and blood glucose

Complete diagnostics:

- CBC and biochemistry
  - Elevated CK: muscle contractions and/or injury
- Whole body radiographs/CT scan
- Blood lead and zinc levels
- ABV/PDD testing
- Lipoprotein profile if atherosclerosis is suspected
- Advanced imaging (MRI)

Treatment

Stabilization:

- Stop the seizure [21, 22]
  - Benzodiazepines: Diazepam IV/IO/cloacal (0.5–2.0 mg/kg) or midazolam administered IV/IO/IM/IN (0.1–2 mg/kg); CRI of diazepam (0.1–0.5 mg/kg/h IV or IO); if 1–2 doses fail to control seizures add phenobarbital or levetiracetam
  - Phenobarbital: no longer recommended as it is not effective in most parrots and has been shown not to be absorbed orally in African grey parrots
  - Levetiracetam: 100–150 mg/kg PO q8–12 hours, DRUG OF CHOICE
  - Still having seizures: propofol boluses (1–2 mg/kg IV/IO), ketamine boluses (5 mg/kg IV/IO) or isoflurane
- Correct the underlying condition [21]
  - Hypocalcemia: 10% calcium gluconate IV/IO (0.5–1.5 ml/kg) over 10 minutes with continuous ECG
  - Hypomagnesemia: magnesium sulfate IM (20 mg/kg PRN) [23]
  - Hypoglycemia: 50% dextrose IV/IO to effect

  - Head trauma with suspected increased intracranial pressure: hypertonic saline (7.5% NaCl:4 ml/kg, 3% NaCl:5.4 ml/kg over 15–20 minutes IV/IO) or mannitol (0.5–1.0 g/kg over 15–20 minutes IV/IO)

Continued care:

- Nutritional support
- Correct nutritional deficiencies
- Chelation therapy
- Additional drugs in combination therapy: zonisamide, gabapentin, clonazepam, topiramate

Cardiopulmonary Disease

Arrhythmias

Diagnosis

Clinical Signs:

- Arrhythmia
- Syncope
- Lethargy/weakness
- Exercise intolerance
- Respiratory distress
- Cardiac murmur
- Coelomic distention
- Sudden death

Differentials:

- Congestive heart failure (valvular insufficiency, dilated cardiomyopathy, valvular endocarditis)
- Atherosclerosis
- ABV/PDD
- Ingested toxins: avocado, chocolate, or plant cardiac glycoside
- Electrolyte imbalance
- Normal catecholamine induced arrhythmia

STAT diagnostics:

- ECG [24]
  - Can be difficult in awake birds. Isoflurane may induce mild ECG alterations
  - Use 4 leads with alligator clips attached to base of feather or subcutaneous needles
- Electrolyte evaluation
- POCUS: assess for pericardial effusion, chamber enlargement, and contractility

Complete diagnostics:

- Echocardiography (see "CHF")
- CBC/Biochemistry: to screen for electrolyte disorders, note that bile acids are frequently elevated with hepatic congestion
- Infectious disease testing: blood culture (valvular endocarditis), ABV cloacal PCR
- Radiographs – CT scan
  - Cardiomegaly, enlargement or mineralization of great vessels: CHF, atherosclerosis
  - Mass in the thorax

Treatment

Stabilization:

- Oxygen support for respiratory distress
- Atropine (0.01–0.5 mg/kg SC, IM, IV) or epinephrine (1 : 1000; 0.5–1 mg/kg IM, IV/IO, IT) for bradycardia [1]
- Propranolol (0.04–0.2 mg/kg IM, IV) for supraventricular arrhythmia, atrial flutter, fibrillation [1]

Continued Care:

- Correct electrolyte imbalance
- Atherosclerosis
- See "Ingested intoxications (avocado, chocolate or plant)"
- See "CHF"

Atherosclerosis

Diagnosis

Clinical signs:

- Depend on arteries affected and type of lesion
  - Carotid artery – neurologic signs (seizure, weakness, ataxia, cranial nerve deficits, altered consciousness)
  - Coronary artery – cardiopulmonary (dyspnea, coelomic effusion, exercise intolerance, cardiac murmur, arrhythmia)
  - Peripheral arteries – hind leg disease (permanent or intermittent limb weakness, lameness, gangrene)
  - Sudden death, fatal arrhythmias

Differentials:

- Neurologic signs: trauma, hypocalcemia, hypoglycemia, ABV/PDD, heavy metal toxicity, CNS neoplasia
- Cardiopulmonary signs: congestive heart failure, valvular disease, cardiotoxins
- Hind leg signs: trauma, lead toxicity, renal disease, gonadal disease, spinal disease

STAT diagnostics:

- ECG for arrhythmia
- Indirect blood pressure: not reliable in most small birds

Complete diagnostics:

- Biochemistry: hypercholesterolemia, dyslipidemia, elevated bile acids if concurrent hepatic lipidosis, elevated creatinine kinase from seizures or ischemic myositis
- Lipoprotein profile
- Radiographs: rarely helpful, assess for mineralization or enlargement of great vessels or cardiomegaly (see "CHF")
- CT scan: CT is more sensitive for arterial calcification as well as identification of affected arteries
- Echocardiography: hyperechogenicity at base of ascending aorta (not sensitive), evidence of congestive heart failure
- Advanced imaging: MRI, angiography

Treatment

Stabilization:

- Oxygen support for respiratory distress
- Control seizures
- Coelomocentesis for ascites causing dyspnea
- Management of congestive heart failure

Continued Care:

- Nutritional support
- Fluid therapy
- Client education – conversion to commercial pelleted diet with fruits, vegetables, and omega 3 fatty acids, increased exercise, decreased egg laying stimulation
- Statins – empirical dose
  - Rosuvastatin and atorvastatin: 10–30 mg/kg PO q12–24h
  - Hispaniolan Amazon parrots: rosuvastatin @ 10–25 mg/kg PO failed to reach therapeutic concentrations [25]
- Control hypertension
  - Enalapril: 1.25–5 mg/kg PO q12h [26]
- Peripheral arterial disease - vasodilators
  - Pentoxifylline: 15 mg/kg PO q12h [26]
  - Isoxsuprine: 5–10 mg/kg PO q24h [26]

Congestive Heart Failure (CHF)

Diagnosis

Clinical signs:

- Dyspnea
- Ascites
- Subcutaneous edema
- Arrhythmia
- Cardiac murmur
- Muffled heart sounds
- Decreased or absent over air sacs
- Exercise intolerance
- Syncope
- Cyanosis

Differentials:

- Dyspnea
- Coelomic effusion
- Weakness (see "Sick bird syndrome" and "Neurologic signs")
- Atherosclerosis
- Cardiotoxin ingestion
- Neoplasia
- Vasculitis

STAT diagnostics:

- POCUS
  - Ascites, pericardial effusion, cardiac chamber enlargement, hepatomegaly
- ECG

Complete diagnostics:

- CBC/Biochemistry
  - Leukocytosis: infectious cardiac disease
  - Hyperuricemia: acute visceral gout
- Radiographs
  - Cardiomegaly: For healthy medium sized parrots on V/D radiograph width of heart should be 51–61% of the thoracic width and 35–41% of the sternal length [27]
  - Enlarged or mineralized great vessels [28]
  - Widened hepatic silhouette: hepatic congestion or ascites
  - Displacement of air sacs: cardiomegaly or ascites
  - Increased radiodensity of lungs: pulmonary edema
- Complete transcoelomic echocardiography (four chambered and aortic outflow view): assess for contractility, fractional shortening, valvular insufficiency, pericardial effusion, thinning or thickening of cardiac muscle, chamber enlargement [28]

Treatment

Stabilization:

- Oxygen therapy
- Therapeutic coelomocentesis
- Pericardiocentesis if pericardial effusion is causing tamponade – requires full anesthesia. Easier through a midline coelioscopic approach.
- Diuretic
  - Furosemide: 0.1–10 mg/kg SC, IM IV/IO q2–12h [1]

Continued care:

- ACE inhibitor
  - Enalapril: 0.2–5 mg/kg PO q8–24 [1]

- Pimobendan – pharmacokinetics varies greatly between species and type of compounded suspension [29]
  - Empirical dose: 0.25–0.35 mg/kg PO q12h [30]
  - Hispaniolan parrots: 10 mg/kg PO single dose achieved desired plasma concentration when given in tablet suspension [29]

Infectious Respiratory Tract Disease (IRTD)

Diagnosis

Clinical signs:

- Respiratory distress
- Dyspnea (inspiratory, expiratory, mixed)
- Loss/change of voice, wheezes, coughing
- Lethargy, depression, anorexia
- Conjunctivitis, chemosis, epiphora
- Nasal discharge, sneezing
- Concomitant systemic signs:
  - Diarrhea, undigested food in feces
  - Biliverdinuria (Chlamydiosis)

Differentials:

- Respiratory distress (bacterial pneumonia, air sacculitis, fungal pneumonia and air sacculitis, respiratory neoplasm, toxin, obstruction)
- Lethargy, depression, anorexia (see "Sick bird syndrome")
- Conjunctivitis
- Other systemic diseases with respiratory lesions

STAT diagnostics:

- PCV/TS/blood smear
  - Moderate to marked leukocytosis with heterophilia and monocytosis, toxic changes to heterophils and left shift
  - Non regenerative anemia: anemia of chronic disease common
  - Erythrocytosis: chronic respiratory disease, pulmonary/thoracic neoplasia
  - Hyperproteinemia from chronic infection

Complete diagnostics:

- CBC/Biochemistry/Plasma protein electrophoresis
  - Elevated liver values
  - Hypoalbuminemia, hyperglobulinemia (gamma globulins for aspergillosis)
- Radiographs, CT scan, and ultrasound
  - Overall increased radiopacity to lungs or loss of "honeycomb" appearance; hyperinflation, consolidation or increased opacity to air sacs; pulmonary nodules (aspergillosis); tracheal stenosis or collapse
  - Hepatosplenomegaly with chlamydiosis and mycobacteriosis
  - Thickened or dilated bowel loops with mycobacteriosis
- Specific disease testing
  - Bacterial culture and sensitivity from respiratory samples
  - Aspergillus: galactomannan assay (low sensitivity), lesion cytology and biopsy
  - Chlamydia: PCR from conjunctiva, choana, and cloaca; paired serology titers; antigen detection
  - Mycoplasma: PCR from conjunctiva, serology. Isolation/identification of mycoplasma does not necessarily confirm pathogenicity as they are frequent commensals in some bird species
  - Mycobacteria: culture or molecular testing on tissue samples
- Coelioscopy/tracheoscopy for direct airway visualization, histopathology (lungs, air sacs), cytology, C&S

Treatment

Stabilization:

- Oxygen therapy
- Air sac cannula placement for syringeal aspergilloma, tracheal foreign body, tracheal stenosis (see "Tracheal obstruction")

Continued care:

- Nutritional support
- Fluid therapy
- Saline nebulization
- Aspergillosis
  - Surgical debridement of large granulomas
  - Antifungal therapy
    - Itraconazole: 2.5–10 mg/kg PO q12–24h, caution with African grey parrots [1]
    - Voriconazole: 10–40 mg/kg PO, IV q8–12 h [1]
- Bacterial pneumonia/air sacculitis
  - Enrofloxacin: 10–20 mg/kg PO q24h [1]
  - Amoxicillin/clavulanic acid: 125 mg/kg PO q8h [3]
- Chlamydiosis
  - Doxycycline (oral): 25–50 mg/kg PO q12–24h × 45d [1]; 35 mg/kg PO q24 × 21d in cockatiels [1]
  - Azithromycin: 40 mg/kg PO q48h × 21d in cockatiels [1]
  - Vibravenos (injectable doxycycline): 25–100 mg/kg IM q5–7d × 5–7 treatments; not available in the US without written permission from FDA [1]
- Mycobacteriosis
  - Combination antibiotic therapy is long term and extrapolated from human medicine, treatment not recommended

Respiratory Toxins

Diagnosis

Clinical signs:

- Dyspnea
- Burn wounds on skin, burnt feathers
- Aerosolized toxin on the feathers
- Blood tinged foam from nares/glottis

Differentials:

- Teflon (Polytetrafluoroethylene [PTFE])
- Smoke inhalation
- Volatilized household chemicals
- See respiratory distress for other common causes

STAT diagnostics:

- Stabilize before any diagnostics

Complete diagnostics:

- Whole body radiographs or CT scan
  - Increased radiodensity of lungs or loss of "honeycomb pattern": pulmonary edema or hemorrhage
  - Air sac lines: fluid or inflammation
- CBC and biochemistry
  - Usually unremarkable
- Endoscopy/tracheoscopy to examine lungs and air sacs, +/− biopsy, C&S

Treatment

Stabilization:

- Oxygen therapy
- Bronchodilator
  - Aminophylline: 4–10 mg/kg PO, IV/IO q6–12h [1] or nebulized in saline
  - Terbutaline: 0.01 mg/kg PO or nebulized in saline [1]
- Diuretic
  - Furosemide: 0.1–10 mg/kg SC, IM IV/IO q2–12h [1]
- Anti-inflammatory
  - Meloxicam: 1 mg/kg q12h [1]
  - Dexamethasone: 2 mg/kg IM once SHORT-TERM USE ONLY – secondary aspergillosis can occur [31]
- Analgesia – especially with concurrent burns (see Chapter 28)
- Antifungals (respiratory toxins and steroids are associated with aspergillosis development)
  - Itraconazole: 10 mg/kg PO q12–24 hours [1]
  - Voriconazole: 10–20 mg/kg PO q12–24 hours [1]

Continued care:

- Nebulization with saline or bronchodilator (see "Respiratory distress")
- Nutritional support
- Remove toxin from feathers with warm water +/− soap

Lower Airway Obstruction

Diagnosis

Clinical signs:

- Dyspnea (inspiratory)
- Open-mouth breathing
- High pitched wheeze on inspiration
- Extension of head and neck
- Over expansion of air sacs
- Visible obstruction of the choana, nares, glottis

Differentials:

- Aspiration of foreign material (a seed being the most common)
- Trauma, tracheal collapse
- Post-intubation tracheal stenosis
- Syringeal aspergilloma
- Neoplasia
- Other causes of respiratory distress

STAT diagnostics:

- Suction airway or physical removal of obstruction
  - May require light sedation with midazolam
- Radiographs
  - Assess air sacs and lungs before placing air sac cannula
  - Radio-opaque foreign material in air sac

Complete diagnostics:

- CBC and biochemistry
  - Severe leukocytosis with heterophilia and monocytosis: aspergillosis (Note: not all cases show severe leukocytosis)
- Radiographs/CT-scan: tracheal trauma, extraluminal compression, foreign body, neoplasia or stricture, extra-syringeal disease with secondary occlusion
- Tracheal and syringeal endoscopy for foreign body or aspergilloma removal, +/− C&S, +/− histopathology

Treatment

Stabilize:

- Oxygen therapy
- Placement of air sac cannula if the obstruction/disease is only affecting the upper airway, trachea, or syrinx

Continued care:

- Antifungal for aspergillosis
- Anti-inflammatory therapy if renal values are normal and patient is hydrated

- Meloxicam: 0.1–2 mg/kg PO, IM, IV/IO q12–24h [1]
- Tracheal resection and anastomosis for tracheal stenosis or neoplasia

Gastrointestinal Disease

Crop Burn

Diagnosis

Clinical signs:

- Acute injury (hours-days) – erythema/edema of skin overlying crop, anorexia, regurgitation
- Chronic injury (several days-week) – skin discoloration/eschar at site of burn, crop fistula with food/food leakage, crop stasis, regurgitation, weight loss

Differentials:

- Juvenile bird crop fed hot formula
- Ingluvitis
- Regurgitation

STAT diagnostics:

- PCV/TS
  - Anemia, hypoproteinemia: blood loss
  - Hemoconcentration: dehydration
- Blood smear
  - Leukocytosis: acute inflammation or secondary infection (chronic injury)
- Blood glucose
  - Hypoglycemia from decreased intake
- Cytology and Gram's stain of wound
  - Secondary bacterial or yeast infection

Complete diagnostics:

- CBC and biochemistry
- Usually nonspecific – assess general health status of juvenile bird
- C&S from wound

Treatment

Stabilization:

- Fluid therapy (see Chapter 29)
- Hypoglycemia: 50% dextrose IV/IO
  - Dilute and give slowly to effect
  - Maintenance of 2.5–5% dextrose in fluids
- Parenteral analgesia (see Chapter 28)

Continued care:

- Acute injury
  - Topical silver sulfadiazine
  - Monitor skin for discoloration, eschar formation, fistula formation
  - NSAIDs: analgesia and decrease inflammation
    - Meloxicam: 0.1–2 mg/kg PO, IM, IV/IO q12–24h [1]
  - Feed small frequent meals
- Chronic injury
  - Clean necrotic skin or eschar
  - Bandage placement with daily changes
  - Antibiotics based on cytology
  - NSAIDs (see Continued Care "Acute Injury")
  - Nutritional support
    - Small fistula or eschar: small frequent meals
    - Large fistula: placement of feeding tube
  - Surgical repair
    - Delay until a fistula is formed and the margin of necrotic and healthy tissues is known (1–2 weeks after insult)
    - Excise fistula margin and close crop and skin in separate layers

Diarrhea

Diagnosis

Clinical signs:

- Watery fecal component (as opposed to formed feces with polyuria)
- Fecal staining around vent/tail
- Lethargy
- Hematochezia
- Tenesmus
- Anorexia/hyporexia

Differentials:

- Dietary indiscretion/rapid change in diet
- ABV/PDD
- Heavy metal toxicity
- Endoparasites: *Giardia, Trichomonas*
- Gram negative or clostridial enteritis
- Yeast overgrowth in juveniles
- Intestinal mycobacteriosis

STAT diagnostics:

- Fecal Gram's stain
  - Normal flora: Gram-positive bacteria, rare candida
- Fecal cytology
  - WBCs or RBCs: inflammation
- Fecal wet mount
  - *Trichomonas, Giardia*

Complete diagnostics:

- CBC/biochemistry
  - Severe leukocytosis: mycobacteriosis
  - Anemia, hypoproteinemia: blood loss, ABV/PDD

- Radiographs/ultrasound
  - GI gas or dilation: ileus from enteritis, ABV/PDD, GI foreign body
  - Thickened intestines: neoplasia, mycobacteriosis
- Fecal C&S, Salmonella culture
- Fecal parasite testing (flotation, sedimentation tests): GI coccidia and nematodes are rare in indoor pet parrots
- Fecal occult blood: can get false positives with prior consumption of red meat, cantaloupe, and grapefruit
- Mycobacteria testing: may be positive with saprophytic mycobacterium going through the GI, therefore, it is not a confirmatory test
- Barium fluoroscopy
  - Assess motility and filling defects
- Blood lead/zinc testing

Treatment

Stabilization:

- Fluid therapy

Continued care:

- Nutritional support
- Antifungal as warranted based on Gram's stain
  - Candida overgrowth
    - Nystatin: 100 000–600 000 U/kg PO q8–12 h [1]
- Chelation therapy
- Giardia
  - Metronidazole: 25 mg/kg PO q12h, 50 mg/kg PO q24h × 5–10d [1]
- Trichomonas
  - Metronidazole: 40 mg/kg PO q24h × 7d [1]
- Mycobacteriosis
  - Combination antibiotic therapy is long term and extrapolated from human medicine, treatment not recommended
- Parasites
  - Coccidia: toltrazuril
  - Nematodes: fenbendazole (be cautious about myelosuppression in some avian species)

Gastrointestinal Foreign Body Ingestion

Diagnosis

Clinical signs:

- Regurgitation
- Anorexia
- Crop distention
- Palpable foreign material in crop
- Diarrhea, hematochezia, melena
- Dehydration
- Coelomic distention if GI perforation

Differentials:

- ABV/PDD
- Regurgitation
- Abnormal droppings

STAT diagnostics:

- Standing radiograph – may visualize radiodense foreign material such as grit or metal
- PCV/TS/blood smear
  - Anemia with normal or hypoproteinemia: acute or chronic GI hemorrhage
  - Leukocytosis/leukopenia: GI perforation, secondary infection
- POCUS if GI perforation is suspected – may see coelomic effusion

Complete diagnostics:

- Coelomocentesis if coelomic effusion
- Radiographs – CT scan
  - Gas or dilation of proventriculus, ventriculus or intestines
  - Contrast radiographs if radiolucent foreign body or obstruction is suspected
- Coelomic ultrasound
  - Assess for GI motility, perforation, coelomic effusion or presence of foreign body
  - Perforating foreign bodies may be surrounded by granuloma and/or affect the liver [32]
- Fluoroscopy to assess GI motility
- CBC and biochemistry
  - Findings depend on toxicity of ingested material
  - Hyperuricemia or elevated liver enzymes with coelomitis
- Blood lead and zinc testing

Treatment

Stabilization:

- IV/IO fluid therapy for dehydration, +/− colloid if GI perforation or anemia is suspected (see Chapter 29)
- Broad spectrum parenteral antibiotics if GI perforation is suspected
  - Cefotaxime: 75–100 mg/kg IM, IV/IO q4–8h [1]
  - Cefazolin: (25–50 mg/kg IM, IV/IO q12h) [2] or ampicillin (50–100 mg/kg IM q4–8h) [9] + enrofloxacin (10–20 mg/kg) SC (in saline fluid pocket), IV/IO q24h [2] if

IV/IO give slowly over 15 minutes and dilute at least 1:3 with saline
- Piperacillin/tazobactam: 100 mg/kg IM, IV q6–12h [1]

Continued care:

- Foreign body in crop – e.g. tip of feeding tube in hand reared juveniles
  - Digital manipulation of the foreign body from the crop to the back of the oral cavity
  - Caution if fluid in crop – may need to first remove fluid with gavage tube or suction to avoid aspiration
  - May require sedation/anesthesia with intubation and crop or proventriculus lavage with warm saline and suction
- Analgesia: parenteral opioids, avoid NSAIDs if GI ulceration is suspected
- Suspected esophageal/crop ulceration
  - Sucralfate: 25 mg/kg PO q8h – do not give with other PO medications [1]
- Antiemetic and promotility after ruling out obstruction and perforation
  - Metoclopramide: 0.2–2 mg/kg IM, IV q8–12h [1]
- Nutritional support only after ruling out obstruction and perforation and regurgitation is resolved
- Heavy metal or other toxin ingestion
- Endoscopic or surgical removal of foreign material [32]

Regurgitation/Vomiting

Diagnosis

Clinical signs:

- Dried food on beak/head
- Crop dilation
- Hematemesis
- Coelomic distention
- Abnormal droppings
- Poor body condition

Differentials:

- Dietary indiscretion
- ABV/PDD
- Heavy metal or other ingested toxin
- *Macrorhabdus ornithogaster*
- Ingluvitis or crop burn in unweaned juveniles
- Foreign body ingestion
- *Trichomonas*
- GI neoplasia/papillomatosis
- See “Coelomic distention” for other common causes
- See “Abnormal droppings” for other common causes

STAT diagnostics:

- PCV/TS/blood smear
  - Hypoproteinemia and non-regenerative anemia: chronic disease
  - Regenerative anemia: recent gastric hemorrhage, zinc toxicity
  - Hemoconcentration: dehydration
- Crop wash for cytology, saline direct examination, Gram’s stain and aerobic C&S if warranted.
  - Normal flora: Gram-positive bacteria, rare candida
- Fecal examination (stained and direct wet mount): *Macrorhabdus ornithogaster*, Trichomonas, *Candida albicans*

Complete diagnostics:

- CBC/Biochemistry: look for underlying disease
- Blood lead and zinc levels
- Radiographs/Ultrasound
  - Metallic or other radio-opaque objects in GI tract: heavy metal toxicity, GI foreign body
  - GI gas or dilation: ABV/PDD, GI foreign body, enteritis
  - Thickened intestines: neoplasia, mycobacteriosis
- Barium fluoroscopy
  - Assess: motility of GI tract, filling defects
- Endoscopy +/− biopsies of the crop, esophagus, proventriculus, ventriculus

Treatment

Stabilization:

- Fluid therapy
- NPO until regurgitation resolved

Continued care:

- Esophagitis/ingluvitis
  - Sucralfate: 25 mg/kg PO q8h – do not give with other PO medications [1]
- Antiemetic and promotility after ruling out obstruction
  - Metoclopramide: 0.2–2 mg/kg IM, IV q8–12h [1].
- Nutritional support only after ruling out obstruction and perforation and regurgitation is resolved
- Antibiotics or antifungal based on Gram’s stain
- Heavy metal or other ingested toxin (see “Ingested intoxications”)
- *Macrorhabdus ornithogaster*
  - Amphotericin B: 100 mg/kg PO q12h × 10–30d [1]
- *Trichomonas* (see “Diarrhea”)

Urogenital and Reproductive Disease

Cloacal Prolapse

Diagnosis

Clinical signs:

- Prolapsed tissue from vent: identify as either cloaca, oviduct, colon or neoplastic tissue
- Hematochezia
- Tenesmus
- Coelomic distension
- Dyspnea
- Droppings with no urates or no feces

Differentials:

- Cloacal prolapse
  - Primary cloacal disease: papillomatosis/neoplasia, severe cloacitis
  - Secondary to coelomic disease: organomegaly, neoplasia
  - Chronic: behavioral/idiopathic in cockatoos
- Oviductal prolapse: chronic egg laying, egg bound, salpingitis, oviductal tumors
- Internal papillomatosis (Psittacid herpesvirus 1)
- Colonic prolapse: severe diarrhea, colonic papillomatosis/neoplasia, intestinal mycobacteriosis
- See "Coelomic distention" for other common causes
- See "Abnormal droppings" for other common causes

STAT diagnostics:

- Standing radiograph
  - Mineralized egg
- PCV/TS/blood smear
  - Anemia and hypoproteinemia: blood loss
  - Leukocytosis: necrotic/infected cloacal tissue, neoplasia
- Diarrhea: Fecal Gram's stain, fecal wet mount, C&S (See "Diarrhea")

Complete diagnostics:

- CBC and biochemistry
  - Hypercalcemia, hyperproteinemia, and lipemia: reproductive
  - Hyperuricemia: ureteral obstruction, renal disease
- Radiographs/Ultrasound
- Coelomic effusion, organomegaly, masses, ovarian/oviductal disease
- Polyostotic hyperostosis: egg laying
  - Cloacoscopy +/− biopsy

Treatment

Stabilization:

- Oxygen therapy if dyspneic
- Fluid therapy (See Chapter 29)
- Analgesia (See Chapter 28)
  - Do not use NSAIDs until ureteral patency is confirmed
- Devitalized tissue / cloacitis: broad spectrum antibiotics
  - Amoxicillin-clavulanate: 125 mg/kg PO q8h [3]
  - Cefazolin: (25–50 mg/kg IM, IV/IO q12h) [2] or ampicillin (50–100 mg/kg IM q4–8h) [9]+ enrofloxacin (10–20 mg/kg) SC (in saline fluid pocket), IV/IO q24h [2] if IV/IO give slowly over 15 minutes and dilute at least 1:3 with saline
  - Piperacillin/tazobactam: 100 mg/kg IM, IV q6–12h [1]
- Protect prolapsed tissue and decrease edema
  - Topical sterile lubricating jelly
  - Topical 50% dextrose or mannitol

Continued care:

- Reduce prolapsed tissue ONLY if not devitalized and radiographic confirmation that there is not an egg in the coelom
  - Sedate or anesthetize patient
  - Reduce prolapsed tissue with lubricated cotton tipped applicators or lubricated, gloved finger
  - Place transverse sutures or horizontal mattress sutures with stents (IV tubing or butterfly catheter tubing) on either side of the vent – ensure there is enough space for feces and urates to pass [5]
  - Do NOT place purse string suture
- Devitalized or torn prolapsed tissue – emergency exploratory surgery
- See "Egg binding/dystocia"
- Behavioral/idiopathic chronic cloacal prolapses in cockatoos: surgical cloacopexy, ventoplasty, applied behavioral analysis
- Cloacal neoplasia or papillomas: laser therapy or surgical debulking

Renal Failure

Diagnosis

Clinical signs:

- Polyuria
- Polydipsia
- Anuria/oliguria
- Dehydration
- Hematuria
- Unilateral or bilateral lameness/paralysis
- Digital joint swelling or tophi
- Coelomic distention (fluid or soft tissue from mass or renomegaly)
- Dyspnea secondary to coelomic distention
- Feather destruction over synsacrum

Differentials:

- Urate nephrosis
- Interstitial nephritis
- Bacterial nephritis
  - Hematogenous from sepsis/ascending
  - Common pathogens: *Enterobacteriaceae, Pasteurella* spp, *Pseudomonas* spp, *Streptococcus* spp, and *Staphylococcus* spp [33]
- Neoplasia (renal carcinoma, nephroblastoma, lymphoma)
- Nephrotoxin exposure (NSAIDs, aminoglycosides, heavy metal, vitamin D, *Rheum* plant, *Allium* plants, ethylene glycol)
- Prolonged hypovitaminosis A
- Polyomavirus (young birds)
- Trauma

Diagnostics

STAT diagnostics:

- Voided urinalysis
  - Renal casts
  - Cannot evaluate for USG, protein, bacteria, WBC, RBC as they are mixed with feces
- Biochemistry
  - Hyperuricemia: mild elevation with hyperproteinemia and polycythemia could indicate dehydration; moderate to severe elevation with renal disease; false positive hyperuricemia with lipemia and blood collection from nail may occur, but depends on the analyzer used
  - Hyperphosphatemia (not sensitive in birds)
  - Hypoproteinemia: advanced tubular nephrosis or glomerular damage (rare)
- CBC
  - Non-regenerative anemia
  - Inflammatory leukogram if caused by infection or inflammation
- Acid-base status: moderate metabolic acidosis secondary to hyperuricemia and damage to proximal tubules

Complete diagnostics:

- Radiographs
  - Renomegaly or increased renal opacity
  - Rule out ureteral obstruction (egg, mass)
  - Assess joints for arthritis lesions secondary to articular gout
- Ultrasound
  - Renomegaly, cysts, masses or change in echogenicity
  - Increased echogenicity of liver or pericardium can be seen with visceral gout
  - Assess ureters and ureteral openings for obstruction
  - Rarely coelomic effusion with hypoproteinemia
- Indirect blood pressure: Not reliable in most small birds
- Urinalysis via sedated ureteral cannulation (uncommonly done)
- Endoscopy for renal biopsies and C&S
- Heavy metal testing

Treatment

Stabilization:

- IV/IO fluid therapy +/− colloids if hypoproteinemic
- Once rehydrated, consider mannitol for anuric renal failure although difficult to assess for overhydration
  - Mannitol: 0.5–1.0 g/kg over 15–20 minutes IV/IO [1]

Continued care:

- Nutritional support – do not use any diet with animal protein which may worsen hyperuricemia
- Analgesia
- Antibiotics for bacterial nephritis – usually 4–6-week course
  - Based on C&S or broad spectrum (Gram-negative and Gram-positive nephritis reported) [33]
  - Amoxicillin-clavulanate: 125 mg/kg PO q8h [3]
  - Cefotaxime: 75–100 mg/kg IM, IV/IO q4–8h [1]
  - Cefazolin (25–50 mg/kg IM, IV/IO q12h) [2] or ampicillin (50–100 mg/kg IM q4–8h) [9] + enrofloxacin (10–20 mg/kg) SC (in saline fluid pocket), IV/IO q24h [2] if IV/IO give slowly over 15 minutes and dilute at least 1:3 with saline
  - Piperacillin/tazobactam: 100 mg/kg IM, IV q6–12h [1]
- Reduce fibrosis
  - Colchicine: 0.01–0.1 mg/kg PO q12–24h – may potentiate gout formation [1]
- Decrease hyperuricemia
  - Urate oxidase: 100–200 U/kg IM q24h (doses based on pigeons and red-tailed hawks) [1]
  - Allopurinol: 10–30 mg/kg PO q4–24h [1] (controversial, reported to cause renal dysfunction in red-tailed hawks) [1]
- Vitamin A supplementation if chronic hypovitaminosis A is suspected
  - 20 000–33 000 IU/kg IM [1]
- Neoplasia: chemotherapy may be option for lymphoma and renal adenocarcinoma
- Chelation therapy
- See "Ingested intoxications"

Yolk Coelomitis

Diagnosis

Clinical signs:

- Dyspnea
- Coelomic distention with fluid +/− egg

- Egg laying behavior (building or sitting on a nest)
- Wide based stance
- Widened pubic bones and pink/tumescent vent

Differentials:

- Other causes of coelomic distention
- Other causes of respiratory distress
- Egg binding

STAT diagnostics:

- Standing radiographs to assess for mineralized egg
- POCUS to confirm presence of fluid
- Coelomocentesis if fluid is causing dyspnea
  - Fluid analysis/cytology consistent with exudate (+/− septic) and yolk/fat globules
  - C&S of fluid

Complete diagnostics:

- CBC
  - Severe leukocytosis
  - Non regenerative anemia
- Biochemistry
  - Hypercalcemia, hyperproteinemia, and lipemia with active egg laying
  - Elevated liver enzymes or hyperuricemia: coelomitis affecting liver/kidney
  - Hyperglycemia: coelomitis affecting pancreas
  - Hypoglycemia: sepsis
- Radiographs
  - Commonly see polyostotic hyperostosis
  - Widened hepatic silhouette due to coelomic fluid
  - Assess for ovarian/oviductal enlargement or egg
- Ultrasound
  - Assess ovary for cysts, follicles, and neoplasia
  - Assess liver and kidneys (if visible) if values are elevated

Treatment

Stabilization:

- Oxygen support for dyspnea
- IV/IO fluid therapy +/− colloids if septic

Continued care:

- Nutritional support
- Analgesia: NSAIDs are ideal to decrease inflammation if properly hydrated and normal renal values
- Antibiotics based on Gram's stain and C&S or broad-spectrum antibiotics if unavailable
  - Amoxicillin-clavulanate: 125 mg/kg PO q8h [3]
  - Cefazolin (25–50 mg/kg IM, IV/IO q12h) [2] or ampicillin (50–100 mg/kg IM q4–8h) [9] + enrofloxacin (10–20 mg/kg) SC (in saline fluid pocket), IV/IO q24h [2] if IV/IO give slowly over 15 minutes and dilute at least 1:3 with saline
- Therapeutic coelomocentesis as needed
- Surgery to remove septic material +/− salpingohysterectomy (unlikely to stop further ovulation)
- Hormonal therapy to control egg laying (see "Egg binding/dystocia")

Dermatologic Disease

Feather Destructive/Mutilation Behavior

Diagnosis

Clinical signs:

- Feather loss and/or damage except on head
- Bleeding/open wounds from mutilation of skin, muscle, or bone – most common on pectoral region
- Bleeding from broken blood feathers

Differentials:

- Behavioral (diagnosis of exclusion)
- Pain
- Numerous underlying diseases (skin hypersensitivity, orthopedic, endocrine, and systemic diseases, nutritional deficiencies, dermal neoplasia, bacterial, or fungal dermatitis, contact irritants, toxin exposure, endo, and ectoparasitism) [34]
- *Circovirus* (usually also affects beak and feathers on entire body including the head)

STAT diagnostics:

- If bleeding, PCV/TS/blood smear to assess for anemia
  - Non regenerative anemia: seen with underlying disease
  - Leukocytosis: chronic inflammation or secondary infection

Complete diagnostics:

- Radiographs
  - Assess for underlying disease
  - Assess for bone involvement in cases of mutilation (commonly seen with extensive/chronic trauma over keel)
- CBC and biochemistry to assess for underlying disease
- Skin and feather follicle biopsy for histopath and bacterial/fungal cultures

Treatment

Stabilization:

- Control hemorrhage with digital pressure, bandages, or hemostatic agents

- IV/IO fluid therapy with colloids or blood transfusion for severe anemia

Continued care:

- Analgesia – opioids and NSAIDs
- Open wounds: antibiotics, bandage placement and flushing (see "Trauma")
- Remove broken blood feathers (see "Trauma")
- E-collar placement in cases of mutilation - not always indicated for patients with feather destruction alone
- Client education on appropriate diet, foraging, environmental enrichment
- Hormonal intervention if warranted
- Refractory cases may need psychotropic medications (paroxetine, clomipramine) in combination with environmental enrichment and behavioral modifications

Ophthalmic Disease

Conjunctivitis

Diagnosis

Clinical signs:

- Chemosis
- Blepharospasm
- Photophobia
- Epiphora
- Periocular feather loss or swelling (sinusitis)
- Nasal discharge
- Sneezing
- Dyspnea if associated with systemic disease

Differentials:

- Trauma +/− secondary bacterial infection
- Infection: *Chlamydia psittaci, Mycoplasma gallisepticum* (rare), *Cryptosporidium* spp, *Bordetella avium*, *Mycobacterium* spp.
- Hypovitaminosis A
- Contact irritant: smoke, volatilized chemicals such as bleach
- Foreign body
- Neoplasia

STAT diagnostics:

- Swab for cytology and Gram's stain
- Use saline to remove debris to allow for complete ophthalmic examination
- Fluorescein staining to assess for corneal ulceration

Complete diagnostics:

- Testing for chlamydia or mycoplasma
- C&S if warranted
- Biochemistry, CBC and radiographs to rule out underlying disease
- Conjunctival biopsy

Treatment

Stabilization:

- Contact irritant – flush with sterile saline
- Fluid therapy if dehydrated

Continued care:

- Nutritional support
- Antibiotics as directed by Gram's stain results
  - Systemic treatment for chlamydiosis or mycoplasma
  - Topical: triple antibiotic ointment (neomycin-polymyxin B-gramicidin), tobramycin, chloramphenicol, ciprofloxacin, gentamicin (if no corneal ulcer); if using ointment preparation, the periocular feathers can become greasy causing further irritation and rubbing
- Analgesia
  - Parenteral: NSAIDs more appropriate to also decrease inflammation if patient is hydrated and normal renal values
  - Topical: flurbiprofen or diclofenac; steroids contraindicated in birds
- Hypovitaminosis A: vitamin A supplementation
  - 20 000–33 000 IU/kg IM [1]
- Topical lubricating therapy if associated with corneal ulceration
- Trauma

Birds

References

1 Hawkins, M., Guzman, D., Beaufrere, H. et al. (2018). Birds. In: *Exotic Animal Formulary*, 5e (ed. J. Carpenter), 167–375. St. Louis, MO: Elsevier.

2 Flammer, K. (2006). Antibiotic drug selection in companion birds. *J. Exot. Pet Med.* 15 (3): 166–176.

3 Orosz, S.E., Jones, M.P., Cox, S.K. et al. (2000). Pharmacokinetics of amoxicillin plus clavulanic acid in blue-fronted Amazon parrots (*Amazona aestiva aestiva*). *J. Avian Med. Surg.* 14 (2): 107–112.

4 Grunkemeyer, V.L. (2010). Advanced diagnostic approaches and current management of avian hepatic disorders. *Vet. Clin. North Am. Exot. Anim. Pract.* 13 (3): 413–427.

5 Hadley, T.L. (2010). Management of common psittacine reproductive disorders in clinical practice. *Vet. Clin. North Am. Exot. Anim. Pract.* 13 (3): 429–438.

6 Mans, C. and Pilny, A. (2014). Use of GnRH-agonists for medical management of reproductive disorders in birds. *Vet. Clin. North Am. Exot. Anim. Pract.* 17 (1): 23–33.

7 Lightfoot, T.L. and Yeager, J.M. (2008). Pet bird toxicity and related environmental concerns. *Vet. Clin. North Am. Exot. Anim. Pract.* 11 (2): 229–259.

8 Corbanie, E.A., Matthijs, M.G., Van Eck, J.H. et al. (2006). Deposition of differently sized airborne microspheres in the respiratory tract of chickens. *Avian Pathol.* 35 (6): 475–485.

9 Ensley, P.K. and Janssen, D.L. (1981). A preliminary study comparing the pharmacokinetics of ampicillin given orally and intramuscularly to psittacines: Amazon parrots (*Amazona* spp.) and blue-naped parrots (*Tanygnathus lucionensis*). *J. Zoo Anim. Med.* 12 (2): 42–47.

10 Gildersleeve, R.P., Galvin, M.J., Thaxton, J.P., and McRee, D.I. (1985). Hematological response of Japanese quail to acute hemorrhagic stress. *Comp. Biochem. Physiol. A Physiol.* 81 (2): 403–409.

11 Eshar, D. and Briscoe, J.A. (2009). External coaptation using a tape splint for treatment of distal pelvic limb fractures in small birds. *Lab Anim.* 38 (8): 262.

12 Harcourt-Brown, N.H. (2002). Orthopedic conditions that affect the avian pelvic limb. *Vet. Clin. North Am. Exot. Anim. Pract.* 5 (1): 49–81.

13 Degernes, L.A. (1994). Trauma medicine. In: Avian Medicine: Principles and Application (eds. B.W. Ritchie, G.J. Harrison and L.R. Harrison), 417–433. Lake Worth, FL: Wingers Publishing Inc.

14 Orosz, S.E. (2002). Clinical considerations of the thoracic limb. *Vet. Clin. North Am. Exot. Anim. Pract.* 5 (1): 31–48.

15 Wheler, C.L. (2002). Orthopedic conditions of the avian head. *Vet. Clin. North Am. Exot. Anim. Pract.* 5 (1): 83–95.

16 Denver, M.C., Tell, L.A., Galey, F.D. et al. (2000). Comparison of two heavy metal chelators for treatment of lead toxicosis in cockatiels. *Am. J. Vet. Res.* 61 (8): 935–940.

17 Degernes, L.A., Frank, R.K., Freeman, M.L., and Redig, P.T. (1989). Lead poisoning in trumpeter swans. In: *Proceedings of Annual Conference Association Avian Veterinarians*, 144–155.

18 Dennison, S.E., Paul-Murphy, J.R., and Adams, W.M. (2008). Radiographic determination of proventricular diameter in psittacine birds. *J. Am. Vet. Med. Assoc.* 232 (5): 709–714.

19 Hoppes, S., Heatley, J.J., Guo, J. et al. (2013). Meloxicam treatment in cockatiels (*Nymphicus hollandicus*) infected with avian bornavirus. *J. Exot. Pet Med.* 22 (3): 275–279.

20 Rossi, G., Dahlhausen, R.D., Galosi, L., and Orosz, S.E. (2018). Avian ganglioneuritis in clinical practice. *Vet. Clin.: Exot. Anim. Pract.* 21 (1): 33–67.

21 Delk, K. (2012). Clinical management of seizures in avian patients. *J. Exot. Pet Med.* 21 (2): 132–139.

22 Beaufrère, H., Nevarez, J., Gaschen, L. et al. (2011). Diagnosis of presumed acute ischemic stroke and associated seizure management in a Congo African grey parrot. *J. Am. Vet. Med. Assoc.* 239 (1): 122–128.

23 Kirchgessner, M.S., Tully, T.N. Jr., Nevarez, J. et al. (2012). Magnesium therapy in a hypocalcemic African grey parrot (*Psittacus erithacus*). *J. Avian Med. Surg.* 26 (1): 17–21.

24 Pees, M. and Krautwald-Junghanns, M.E. (2009). Cardiovascular physiology and diseases of pet birds. *Vet. Clin. North Am. Exot. Anim. Pract.* 12 (1): 81–97.

25 Beaufrere, H., Papich, M.G., Brandão, J. et al. (2015). Plasma drug concentrations of orally administered rosuvastatin in Hispaniolan Amazon parrots (*Amazona ventralis*). *J. Avian Med. Surg.* 29 (1): 18–24.

26 Beaufrere, H. (2016). Atherosclerosis. In: Blackwell's Five-Minute Veterinary Consult: Avian (ed. J. Graham), 29–32. Ames, IO: Wiley.

27 Straub, J., Pees, M., and Krautwald-Junghanns, M.E. (2002). Measurement of the cardiac silhouette in psittacines. *J. Am. Vet. Med. Assoc.* 221 (1): 76–79.

28 Beaufrere, H., Pariaut, R., Rodriguez, D. et al. (2010). Avian vascular imaging: a review. *J. Avian Med. Surg.* 24 (3): 174–184.

29 Guzman, D.S., Beaufrère, H., KuKanich, B. et al. (2014). Pharmacokinetics of single oral dose of pimobendan in Hispaniolan Amazon parrots (*Amazona ventralis*). *J. Avian Med. Surg.* 28 (2): 95–101.

30 Graham, J.E. (2016). Common dosages for birds. In: *Blackwell's Five-Minute Veterinary Consult: Avian* (ed. J. Graham), 312–317. Ames, IO: Wiley.

31 Verstappen, F.A. and Dorrestein, G.M. (2005). Aspergillosis in Amazon parrots after corticosteroid therapy for smoke-inhalation injury. *J. Avian Med. Surg.* 19 (2): 138–141.

32 Hoefer, H. and Levitan, D. (2013). Perforating foreign body in the ventriculus of an umbrella cockatoo (*Cacatua alba*). *J. Avian Med. Surg.* 27 (2): 128–135.

33 Schmidt, R.E., Reavill, D.R., and Phalen, D.N. (2003). Urinary system. In: *Pathology of Pet and Aviary Birds*, 95–107. Ames, IA: Iowa State Press.

34 Van Zeeland, Y.R., Spruit, B.M., Rodenburg, T.B. et al. (2009). Feather damaging behaviour in parrots: a review with consideration of comparative aspects. *Appl. Anim. Behav. Sci.* 121 (2): 75–95.

36

Passerines

David N. Phalen[1] *and Hamish Baron*[2]

[1] *Sydney School of Veterinary Science, University of Sydney, Camden, New South Wales, Australia*
[2] *The Unusual Pet Vets, Frankston, Victoria, Australia*

CONTENTS

Scope of the Chapter

This chapter covers emergency presentations and management of canaries and other finches.

Passerines: Common Presenting Signs

Neurologic

Introduction

Hypocalcemic tetany, trauma, viral, and parasitic diseases are the most common causes of neurological disease in canaries and finches.

Diagnosis

History:

- Inquire about recent reproductive activity
- Does the diet contain sufficient calcium?
- Is there a history of recent trauma?
- Have new birds been introduced into the collection?
- Have there been recent mortalities in the collection?

Signalment:

- Neurologic disease can occur in birds of any age. Hypocalcemic tetany would only occur in laying hens

Clinical signs:

- Seizures and tetany
- Unilateral hind limb paresis or paralysis
- Dilated cloaca
- Paralysis of the tail
- Paresis or paralysis of the wings
- Head tilt, nystagmus, rhythmic movements of the head

Differentials:

- Hypocalcemia secondary to egg laying
- Hypoglycemia
- Obtunded secondary to starvation or anorexia
- Renal disease including neoplasia
- Bornavirus disease
- Paramyxovirus (avulavirus) infection
- Bacterial, fungal, or parasitic (toxoplasmosis) infection of the central nervous system
- Trauma

Exotic Animal Emergency and Critical Care Medicine, First Edition. Edited by Jennifer E. Graham, Grayson A. Doss and Hugues Beaufrère.

STAT diagnostics:

- Response to calcium therapy
- Response to oral glucose/assist feeding
- PCV/TS, estimated white blood cell count

Complete diagnostics:

- Radiographs
- Biochemical profile
- Diagnostic necropsy: If infectious diseases are suspected and other birds are at risk

Treatment

Stabilization:

- Supportive care (all cases): Supplemental heat and oxygen
- Assist feeding: Critical care formula up to 5% of body weight PO q6h
- Calcium gluconate (hypocalcemic tetany): 100 mg/kg IM q2h repeat twice then q12h
- Oral dextrose (in emaciated birds): 5% or 50% dextrose, small drops PO q15min
- Antibiotics (suspected bacterial infection): Enrofloxacin diluted 1:3 in saline 20 mg/kg IM or SC q12h, combined with amoxicillin and clavulanic acid 175 mg/kg SC, PO q8h
- Analgesia (if trauma is suspected): Meloxicam 1 mg/kg PO q12h
- Anticonvulsants: Diazepam or midazolam 1 mg/kg IM as needed

Continued care:

- Further treatment is based on initial response to treatment and diagnostic findings

Abdominal (Coelomic) Distention

Introduction

Abdominal distention can be the result of fluid accumulation, the presence of an egg, enlargement, or distention of an organ or organs, neoplasia, or a combination of these.

Diagnosis

History:

- Inquire about recent reproductive activity, particularly egg laying

Signalment:

- Birds that are at least reproductive age

Clinical signs:

- Enlargement of the coelom (palpate the space between the vent and the end of the sternum for distention)
- The feathers covering this space may be absent or separated exposing the underlying skin
- Inspiratory dyspnea
- On palpation, the coelom may feel tense like a balloon filled with water, or a distinct mass, or an enlarged organ (typically the liver) may be palpable
- Wide based stance

Differentials:

- Fluid
  - Transudate or modified transudate secondary to heart, liver disease, or neoplasia
  - Exudate secondary to digestive or reproductive tract disease, or a systemic infectious disease
  - Massive cloacal distention secondary to a neurological deficit or cloacal obstruction (external fecal concretion or internal cloacal concretion)
- Mass
  - Upper left quadrant: Caudal displacement of the ventriculus
  - Large smooth surface hard mass in a female bird: Egg
  - Flattened structure emanating from under the sternum on the right and less likely on the left: Enlarged liver (can generally see dark color under skin with hepatomegaly)
  - Smooth or irregular shape in any location: Neoplasm or cysts
- Diffuse doughy abdomen
  - Intestinal dilation
  - Oviduct
  - Peritonitis with limited fluid

STAT diagnostics:

- Inspection of the vent – mass of dried faces, evaluate the cloaca for masses, cloacal concretions, distention with feces and urates
- Coelomocentesis and cytology of the aspirated fluid
- If an egg is suspected, attempt to express into the cloaca
- Fine needle aspiration of the mass and cytology
- Ultrasound may confirm the presence of fluid or a large mass, but is limited by the size of the probe in passerine

Complete diagnostics:

- Imaging: Radiographs or ultrasound. Complete blood count
- Culture of fluid suspected to contain bacteria

Treatment
Stabilization:

- Before proceeding with any diagnostics, provide oxygen and supplemental heat, continue these after diagnostics or treatment procedures
- If the abdominal distention is the result of fluid, remove as much fluid as you can and as much as the bird can tolerate. This may have to be done incrementally. Fluid removal will allow air sac distention and improve breathing
- If the abdominal distention is caused by an egg, see treatment for egg binding
- If aspirated fluid contains bacteria, select an antibiotic based on the Gram staining characteristics of the bacteria
- If a cloacal concretion is found, attempt to remove it with a lubricated cotton tipped applicator
- If the cloaca is distended with feces and urates, attempt to express manually or empty with a cotton tipped applicator

Continued care:

- Minimally, continued supportive care (oxygen, fluids, supplemental heat, and assist feeding if not eating)
- Additional care will depend on the underlying etiology

Abnormal Droppings

Introduction
Normal droppings contain feces, urates, and liquid urine. It is important to consider each of these components separately.

Diagnosis
History:

- The owners may recognize that the bird has abnormal droppings, but often they do not or owners do not recognize their significance

Signalment:

- Abnormal findings can be observed in any bird of any age or sex

Differentials:

- Scant feces: Anorexia
- Dark green to black feces: In most instances this is concentrated bile, death may be imminent. It may also be digested blood
- Diarrhea: This is rare and a nonspecific finding that could be associated with stress, enteritis, or a range of other diseases
- Gray or voluminous dropping: Maldigestion
- Whole seeds in the droppings: Ventricular disease
- Fresh blood in the droppings: Ulcerated cloacal lesion
- Large dropping: Female that is about to lay or has recently laid an egg
- Limited liquid urine: This is normal in many finches, but it may represent dehydration
- Excessive liquid urine: Stress, systemic illness of any kind, primary renal disease, diabetes mellitus
- Thick dry or slightly moist urates: Dehydration

STAT diagnostics:

- Fecal wet mount – *Trichomonas* spp., parasite eggs, large numbers of budding yeasts, characterize the bacteria present in the droppings
- Gram stain and quick stain of droppings – Characterize the bacteria and yeast flora of the digestive tract, evidence of bleeding, presence of white blood cells. Passerines should have limited numbers of Gram-positive rods and cocci in the droppings. Gram-negative bacteria and yeasts (*Macrorhabdus ornithogaster* and Candida-like yeasts) are abnormal
- Fecal flotation – Evaluate for parasite eggs
- Urine biochemicals – Test for blood and glucose. A one plus reading of blood is often an artifact, higher concentrations indicate hemoglobin or myoglobin is present in the urine. A fecal occult blood test may also be used

Complete diagnostics:

- Complete blood count
- Imaging

Treatment:
Stabilization and continued care:

- Fluids: SC with a balanced electrolyte solution 0.5–1.0 ml SC q6h
- Assist feeding: Critical care formula 5% of body weight, q6h
- Heat support
- Oxygen supplementation
- Nystatin (Candida-like yeasts): 0.01 ml/g PO q8h
- Amphotericin *(M. ornithogaster):* 100 mg/kg PO q24h
- Enrofloxacin (Gram-negative bacteria or evidence of enteritis): diluted 1 : 3 in saline, 20 mg/kg PO q12h
- Fenbendazole (Nematodes, Cestodes): 33 mg/kg PO q24h for 3 d
- Metronidazole (Flagellates): 50 mg/kg PO q12h
- Toltrazuril (Coccidia): 10 mg/kg PO q48 h for three treatments

Bleeding

Introduction

Blood loss in canaries and finches is quickly life threatening. At the same time, birds can lose a greater proportion of their blood volume than mammals and survive.

Diagnosis

History:

- Inquire about the possibility of the bird experiencing trauma, cage mate aggression, or exposure to a predator

Signalment:

- Birds of any age or sex

Clinical signs:

- Blood on perches or other parts of the cage
- Bloodstained feathers

Differentials:

- Blood on the perch or feet
- Laceration of the skin of the foot or a bleeding toenail
- Blood on the feathers of the wing or the body adjacent to the wing
  - Broken blood feather
  - Cutaneous wound
  - Compound fracture of a bone in the wing
  - Tumors of the wing
- Blood on the back of the head: Scalping wound
- Blood at the base of the beak and on the feathers surrounding the nares: Is most likely from the respiratory tract and could represent injury to the nasal turbinates

STAT diagnostics:

- Physical Examination – Determine the source of the bleeding

Complete diagnostics:

- PCV – Generally is not indicated as small passerines cannot afford to lose more blood

Treatment

- If bleeding has stopped
  - Stabilization with warmth, oxygen, and subcutaneous fluids first. If bleeding continues, immediate intervention is necessary
- Broken blood feather: Grasp the feather near its base at the junction with the skin with a pair of needle drivers or hemostats, pull out the feather while twisting. Put pressure on the empty feather follicle until bleeding has stopped
- Lacerations: Stop bleeding with pressure, close wound with tissue glue or sutures
- Broken toe nail: Remove any remaining attached toe nail. It may be necessary to do this with scissors. Use silver nitrate sticks to cauterize the end of the toe
- Bleeding from the cloaca or vent: This is generally secondary to prolapse of the cloaca. The most common cause of cloacal prolapse is egg laying. See treatment for cloacal prolapse
- Sneezing blood from the nares or coughing up blood: The most likely cause of these signs are trauma either to the nasal turbinates (sneezing blood) or deeper in the respiratory system (sneezing or coughing blood). If sneezing of blood continues, then it may be possible to stop it by dripping dilute 1 : 10 000 epinephrine into the nostrils. Stabilize the bird with supplemental heat, oxygen, and subcutaneous fluids
- Do a more detailed physical examination once the bird is stable

Lesions to the Unfeathered Skin of the Feet and Legs

Introduction

Lesions of the feet and lower legs are relatively common and may represent a range of disease problems

Diagnosis

History:

- Birds may present with a history of lameness, bleeding, wounds, swellings, or proliferative changes
- Inquire about the cage setup with special emphasis on the presence of a nest and type of nest material provided

Signalment:

- All ages, no sex predilection

Clinical signs and differentials:

- Proliferative or honeycombed lesions of the skin. Knemidokoptes mites
- Collapsed band on the leg. The ends of open metal bands can fold over each other resulting in the band cutting into the soft tissue over the tarso-metatarsus
- Pale slightly raised round to oblong subcutaneous periarticular masses. These are urate tophi. In most instances these birds will be in renal failure
- Crusty, often bleeding lesions around the tarsometarsus phalangeal joint. These are likely to be caused by fine threadlike nesting material wrapped around the foot

Birds

STAT diagnostics:

- Proliferative skin lesions: Skin scrape – abundant Knemidokoptes mites
- Urate tophi and other masses: Fine needle aspirate and wet mount – urate crystals; cytology - poxvirus inclusions, neoplastic cells
- Crusty, often bleeding lesions around the tarsometarsus phalangeal joint: Using magnification dislodge scabs and crusts – fine fibers enmeshed in the lesion

Treatment

Stabilization:

- Supportive care: As indicated based on diagnosis
- Ivermectin (Knemidocoptes mites): 0.4 µg/g PO q7d
- Band removal: With good restraint or under anesthesia, the ends of the bands can often be pulled apart or one end twisted up and the other end twisted down and the band removed. Because the bands are so small and it is difficult to grasp the ends, it may be necessary to cut the band. A dedicated band cutter can be used for this purpose
- Another method requires the use of a circular blade attached to a dental unit. Water should be dripped onto the band while it is being cut to prevent it heating and burning the leg. Extreme care will be necessary so as not to create additional soft tissue injury
- Removal of constricting fibers: Loops of thread can be teased free and should be cut, do not pull on them until cut ends come away without resistance. Once all threads have been removed treat it as an infected open wound
- Analgesia: Meloxicam 1 mg/kg PO q12h
- Antibiotics: Amoxicillin/clavulanic acid 150–175 mg/kg q8h SC, PO

Continued care

- Refer to an avian veterinarian for long-term care

Dead on Arrival

Introduction

Many finch owners have more than one bird, therefore finding out why one bird died may prevent additional deaths. While it would be unlikely that a postmortem examination would be done in an emergency clinic, it is essential that the carcass be preserved so that a postmortem can be done by an avian veterinarian as soon as possible.

Diagnostics

History:

- A complete history should be taken focusing on husbandry and flock history

Signalment:

- All ages and sexes

Clinical signs:

- Although dead, it is still possible to do a modified physical examination of the bird and, in some cases, determine the cause of death
- Preservation for necropsy – If the bird is to be necropsied, the plumage of the bird should be completely soaked in cold soapy water. The bird should then be wrapped in a wet paper towel, put in a sealable plastic bag with all the air removed, and immediately placed in the refrigerator. It should not be frozen. Transfer to an avian pathologist as soon as possible (within 24 hours)

Egg Binding and Post Egg Laying Complications

Introduction

Egg binding is common in canaries and finches as hens will lay multiple clutches even if they are not with a male. Even with calcium rich diets, it is difficult for these hens to replace the calcium lost with the formation of each eggshell. Repeated egg laying or difficulty with egg laying can result in egg binding and in other instances a cloacal prolapse.

Diagnosis

History:

- Inquire about the history of reproductive behavior and egg laying
- Collect a detailed description of the diet
- If there is a cloacal prolapse the owners may notice the red tissue protruding through the vent

Signalment:

- Mature hens

Clinical signs:

- Fluffed up, quiet, not eating
- Large droppings
- Coelomic distention
- Palpable egg

- Cloacal/ oviduct prolapse containing the egg or prolapsed cloaca following egg laying

Differentials:

- As these birds will show nonspecific signs of illness, differentials would include any systemic illness
- Differentials for coelomic distention are included above

STAT diagnostics:

- Coelomic Palpation – Detection of the egg
- Radiographs – Visualization of the egg

Treatment

Stabilization (egg-bound bird):

- Supportive care: Supplemental heat and oxygen
- Calcium gluconate: 100 mg/kg IM or SC (diluted in saline) q2h repeat twice then q12h

Continued care (egg-bound birds):

- Egg removal: Under isoflurane anesthesia, express the egg through the cloaca. Lubricate the cloaca and its membranes prior to and during the procedure. As the egg is expressed it will be necessary to use a cotton tipped applicator to push back the cloacal membranes allowing the release of the egg. If this is unsuccessful, a transcloacal or percutaneous ovocentesis may be attempted. Percutaneous ovocentesis may lead to fatal coelomitis. This will allow the bird to be stabilized until additional diagnostics and therapeutics can be done by an avian specialist. If the egg is already prolapsed through the cloaca, the treatment is the same. With heavy lubrication, the membranes are pushed back away from the egg allowing the opening of the oviduct to dilate and release the egg. If the membranes are dried around the egg, then euthanasia of the bird is indicated.
- Fluids: Balanced electrolyte solution 0.5 to 1 ml SC
- Antibiotics: Amoxicillin and clavulanic acid 175 mg/kg q8h SC, PO
- Leuprolide acetate: 1000 IU/kg IM repeat in two weeks

Stabilization (prolapsed cloaca):

- Supportive care: Supplemental heat and oxygen
- Fluids (Balanced electrolyte solution): 0.5-1 ml SC q4h

Continued care (prolapsed cloaca):

- Replace prolapse: If the tissue is viable, lubricate, and gently push back into its normal location with a cotton-tipped applicator. This can be done awake in some instances or under anesthesia. Dripping a hydroscopic solution such as 50% dextrose over the prolapsed tissue may reduce the swelling and make replacement easier. After the cloaca is replaced, infuse the cloaca with liquid barium (0.25 ml) to reduce swelling and irritation. Single sutures can be placed on either side of the opening of the vent to reduce the size of the opening by 50%
- Leuprolide acetate (to prevent additional egg laying)- 1000 IU/kg q14d. Owners should be warned that even with these treatments, it is likely that at least one more egg will be laid and additional consequences are likely

Musculoskeletal Signs

Introduction

Trauma in passerines occurs occasionally and can result in fractures of the wings and legs.

Diagnosis

History:

- Inquire about a history of trauma
- Birds may be unable to fly or be non-weight bearing on one or both legs
- The owners may have seen blood on the wing or the leg

Signalment:

- Any aged bird, no sex predilection

Clinical signs:

- The wing is held with a drooped posture (extension of the shoulder and the elbow)
- Non-weight bearing
- Blood on the wing or leg
- Extensive soft tissue bruising
- Skin laceration with or without a protruding bone
- Crepitus

Differentials:

- Soft tissue injury (bruising or laceration) without a fracture
- Tumor, feather cyst, xanthoma on the wing
- Constricted band on the leg
- Pododermatitis

STAT diagnostics:

- Physical examination
- Radiographs

Treatment

Stabilization:

- Supportive care: Supplemental heat and oxygen
- Fluids (Balanced electrolyte): 0.5–1 ml SC
- Analgesia: Meloxicam 1 mg/kg
- Amoxicillin/clavulanic acid: 150–175 mg/kg SC, PO q8h

Continued care:

- Immobilize wing: Figure 8 bandage on wing (ulna, radius, metacarpal bones, and phalange fractures). Body wrap (humeral fractures)
- Immobilize leg: Place overlapping tape splint on leg (tarsometarsus and tibiotarsus fractures). Femoral fracture: Cage rest

Fluffed Up on Perch or Down at the Bottom of the Cage

Introduction

As with all birds, passerines often hide signs of illness until their disease becomes advanced. Thus, many birds are very sick on presentation. They are very fragile, and handling and treatment can cause them to die. Treatments need to be prioritized and staged, with heat and oxygen provided in between, so as not to push them over the edge.

Diagnosis

History:

- A complete history, as described above and in other chapters should be taken, but this may have to wait until the bird is stabilized

Signalment:

- The bird may be of any age, there is no sex predilection

Clinical signs:

- Fluffed up
- Sleeping more than normal
- Down at the bottom of the cage
- Emaciated
- Organ specific signs may or may not be present
- Subcutaneous emphysema

Differentials:

- There is a wide range of infectious and non-infectious diseases that can cause a canary or finch to present in a critical condition
- Differentials will depend on historical and physical findings and the diagnostic findings
- If subcutaneous emphysema is present, this is most likely to be secondary to trauma in finches

STAT diagnostics:

- Fecal wet mount and crop aspirate – Check for flagellates, parasite eggs, yeasts, motile bacteria
- Fecal and crop aspirate Gram's stain and quick stain – Check for yeasts, large numbers of Gram-positive or Gram-negative bacteria, bacterial spores, red, and white blood cells
- Blood smear – Leukocytosis suggesting an inflammatory disease (most passerines have relatively low white blood cell counts [2000–6000 cells/μl]), monocytosis suggesting a chronic inflammatory disease, intracellular blood parasites, *Plasmodium* would be the most likely, polychromasia suggesting an appropriate response to blood loss

Complete diagnostics:

- Biochemistry profile
- Radiographs

Treatment

Stabilization:

- Supplemental heat and oxygen
- Fluids: Balanced electrolytes 0.5 to 1 ml SC q6h
- Assist feeding: Critical care formula up to 5% of body weight PO q4h

Continued care:

- Antibiotics, antifungals, and anthelmintics as indicated by the results of the diagnostic testing

Increased Respiratory Effort

Introduction

As with all species, increased respiratory effort can be associated with either or both upper respiratory and lower respiratory disease. Increased respiratory effort can also be caused by systemic disease, cardiac disease, and stress.

Diagnosis

History:

- Owners may have noted open mouth breathing, a tail bob, or a respiratory click or squeak

Signalment:

- Any aged bird, no sex predilection

Clinical signs:

- Tail bob, open mouth breathing, respiratory click or squeak
- Nasal discharge on feathers surrounding the nares
- Coelomic distention resulting in air sac compression

Differentials:

- Bacterial infections of the upper or lower respiratory tract
- Tracheal/air sac mites (*Sternostoma tracheocolum*)
- Trichomonas lesion in the esophagus putting pressure on the trachea
- Squamous metaplasia of the respiratory epithelium (vitamin A deficiency)
- Space occupying mass or fluid in the coelomic cavity

STAT diagnostics:

- Gram's stain of oral swabs or nasal secretions – For bacteria and yeasts
- Crop wash – For trichomonads
- Tracheal transillumination – For tracheal mites
- Estimated white blood cell count, differential – If blood can be safely obtained
- See diagnostics for abdominal distention

Complete diagnostics:

- Radiograph

Treatment

Stabilization:

- Supportive care: Oxygen and supplemental heat
- Antimicrobials, antifungals, anthelmentics: Based on cytology
- Vitamin A: 200 IU/kg repeat in two weeks
- Remove abdominal fluid if present
- Treat for egg binding if an egg is present
- Nebulization (respiratory bacterial disease suspected): Enrofloxacin 10 mg/ml 10 min q12h
- Nebulization (fungal bacterial infection suspected): With F10 disinfectant diluted as per the manufacturer's recommendation 10 min q12h
- Assist feed: Critical care formula up to 5% of body weight PO q6 h

Continued Care:

- As above, maintain in hospital until stable, eating, and gaining weight

Ocular and Periocular Disease

Introduction

The causes of ocular and periocular disease in birds are like those in other species and in most instances, should be worked up with the same approaches. However, because of the small size of passerines some diagnostic approaches are limited. An additional difference is that birds have an infraorbital sinus that may distend as the result of upper respiratory disorders and in some cases lesions of the infraorbital sinus can result in protrusion of the eyeball.

Diagnosis

History:

- Owners report that their bird is keeping one or both of its eyes closed
- Owners report matting of feathers around the eye
- Owners report swelling around the eye

Signalment:

- All ages, no sex predilection

Clinical signs:

- Periocular edema or infraorbital sinus distention
- Crusting of the lids or feathers around the lids
- Ocular lesions: Blepharitis, reddening of the conjunctiva, corneal edema, corneal ulceration, corneal neovascularization, corneal perforation, fibrin in the anterior chamber, cataract, hemorrhage in the anterior or posterior chamber, pigmentation of the retina, retinal detachment

Differentials:

- Periocular edema: Poxvirus in canaries
- Periocular proliferative often crusted lesions: Poxvirus in all species
- Infraorbital sinus distention: Vitamin A deficiency, bacterial sinusitis including mycoplasmosis and mycobacteriosis, mycotic sinusitis
- Conjunctival granuloma: Mycobacteriosis in canaries
- Conjunctivitis: Bacterial infection (local or systemic), herpesvirus infection, cryptosporidiosis, exposure to noxious gases or fine particulate matter
- Keratitis: Trauma, bacterial, and fungal infections
- Intraocular lesions: Differentials would be like those for other species of birds

STAT diagnostics:

- Through ophthalmological examination
- Fluorescein staining of the cornea
- Cytology – Needle aspirates of masses, the contents of distended infra-orbital sinuses, and the conjunctiva as indicated

Complete diagnostics:

- Complete cell count
- PCR assays for suspected infectious diseases
- Biopsy of masses
- Surgical exploration of distended infraorbital sinuses

Treatment

Stabilization:

- Supportive care: Supplemental heat and oxygen
- Fluids: Balanced electrolyte solution 0.5–1 ml SC q6h
- Assist feeding: Critical care formula up to 5% of body weight q6h
- Antimicrobials (topical or systemic, as indicated by the physical examination and diagnostic results)

Continued care:

- Refer to an avian veterinary specialist

Further Reading

Bowles, H., Lichtenberger, M., and Lennox, A. (2007). Emergency and critical care of pet birds. *Vet. Clin. Exot. Anim. Pract.* 10: 345–394.

De Matos, R. and Morrisey, J.K. (2005). Emergency and critical care of small psittacines and passerines. *Semin. Avian Exot. Pet Med.* 14 (2): 90–105.

Dorrestein, G.M. (2003). Diagnostic approaches and management of diseases in captive passerines. *Semin. Avian Exot. Pet Med.* 12 (1): 11–20.

Dorrestein, G.M. (2009). Bacterial and parasitic diseases of passerines. *Vet. Clin. Exot. Anim. Pract.* 12: 433–451.

37

Pigeons and Doves

Kenneth R. Welle

Zoological Medicine University of Illinois Veterinary Teaching Hospital Urbana, Illinois, USA

CONTENTS

Unique Species Considerations

- The domestic pigeon (*Columba livia*) is commonly kept for racing, exhibition, or as pets
- Ringneck doves (*Streptopelia capicola*) are commonly kept as pets
- Pigeons are relatively hardy; subclinical infectious disease is common
- Pet doves are often chronically malnourished from all seed diets
  - Calcium deficiency and vitamin A deficiency are common
  - Egg-laying exacerbates calcium deficiency
- Crop milk produced to feed the young
- Large relative liver size-caution when placing air sac tube and during left lateral coelioscopy (Figure 37.1)

Common Presenting Signs

Abnormal Droppings

- Abnormal droppings may be a result of alterations of the feces, urates, or urine
- Interpretation of the meaning depends on which component(s) are altered

Signalment:

- All birds susceptible
  - Individual problems may be more common in certain ages

Clinical signs:

- Abnormal stools are a clinical sign

Exotic Animal Emergency and Critical Care Medicine, First Edition. Edited by Jennifer E. Graham, Grayson A. Doss and Hugues Beaufrère.

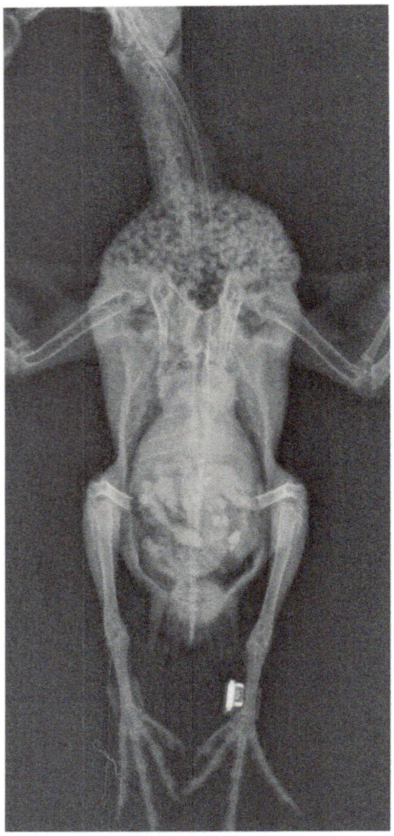

Figure 37.1 Whole body radiograph of a pigeon showing the well-developed crop and the large hepatic shadow typical of this order of birds.

Differentials:

- Loose feces suggest digestive tract disease
  - Bacterial: Gram-negative bacteria, *Salmonella* spp., *Clostridium* spp.
  - Viral: Herpes virus, adenovirus
  - Parasites: Nematodes (*Capillaria* spp.), coccidia (*Eimeria* spp.), *Trichomonas gallinae*
  - Fungal: *Candida* spp.
- Increased urine volume suggests lower GI, renal, endocrine, hepatic disease, or polydipsia
- Polyuria is common with several systemic viral diseases in pigeons
- Reduced feces suggests inanition or GI obstruction
- Increased urates suggests catabolism
- Green or yellow urine or urates (biliverdinuria) suggests hepatic disease or rarely hemolysis
- Hemoglobinuria is rare but usually indicates hemolysis from lead poisoning
- Whole seeds in feces indicate gastric (proventricular or ventricular, in particular traumatic gastritis) disease
- Melena suggests upper GI bleeding

STAT diagnostics:

- Oropharyngeal and crop fresh smear to screen for *Trichomonas*
- Visual evaluation of droppings to categorize
- Fecal Cytology if diarrhea to screen for yeasts (see Chapter 33: Cytology)
- Urine specific gravity and glucose if polyuria
- Chemistry if biliverdinuria
- Radiographs if hemoglobinuria or whole seeds

Complete diagnostics:

- CBC
- Chemistry
- Radiographs
- PCR for viral disease
- Blood lead

Treatment:

- Highly dependent on cause; some may require no treatment
- Treat the underlying cause
- Supportive care
  - Fluid therapy if there is fluid loss (see Chapter 29: Nutrition and fluid therapy)
  - Nutritional support if there is malabsorption
  - Sucralfate (25 mg/kg PO q8h) if melena is present
  - Antibiotics/antiparasitics if warranted

Bleeding from Vent

- The cloaca is the common exit for the gastrointestinal, urinary, and reproductive systems
- Hemorrhage of any of these systems, or the cloaca itself can cause bleeding from the vent

Signalment:

- All birds can develop this sign. Mature females may be overrepresented

Clinical signs:

- Bleeding from the vent is usually visually evident
- Occasionally it will be intermittent and blood will be noted on cage bottom
- Depending on the severity of the hemorrhage, anemia, and weakness may occur

Differentials:

- Cloacal bleeding can occur from trauma or passage of large/abrasive droppings or eggs
- Reproductive tract bleeding may occur following traumatic egg passage or neoplasia
- Urinary tract bleeding is rare but could occur from urate concretions

- Gastrointestinal bleeding may occur from necrotizing enteritis
- Coagulopathies from rodenticides or other causes

STAT diagnostics:

- Physical examination
- Cloacal examination, possibly under anesthesia
- PCV, total solids
- Radiographs may be indicated
- Fecal cytology

Complete diagnostics:

- Radiographs
- Cloacal endoscopy may be helpful
- CBC, chemistries
- Fecal cultures or PCR if GI bleeding is present
- Clotting time (*in vitro* clotting profiles generally not available for birds)

Therapy:

- Hemorrhage should be controlled
  - A gauze tampon can be made and inserted into cloaca
  - A vasoconstrictor such as epinephrine can be applied
  - Barium suspension will often staunch bleeding of the cloaca
- If known, the underlying cause should be treated

Bleeding

- Bleeding is a somewhat self-explanatory clinical sign

Signalment:

- All birds are susceptible; some causes may be more common in specific ages or sexes

Clinical signs:

- Blood may be found on the bird, in the cage, elsewhere in the environment, or on the owner
- It may or may not be evident where the blood is coming from

Differentials:

- Blood feather trauma and breakage is far less common than in psittacine birds
- Flying injuries
  - Open fractures
  - Scalping injuries are common
- Attacks from other animals may also result in punctures
- Bleeding from the vent (see previous section)
- Coagulopathies

STAT diagnostics:

- Thorough examination to determine source of bleeding PCV, total solids

Complete diagnostics:

- Depending on circumstances a more complete workup may be warranted
- CBC, chemistry
- Radiographs
- Clotting time if coagulopathy is suspected

Therapy:

- Direct pressure to the site of bleeding
  - Blood feathers can be pinched closed to stop bleeding or pulled
  - Toes can be held firmly on the sides to stop toe bleeding
  - Pressure bandages can be used to exert pressure longer
- Indirect pressure from a tourniquet can be briefly used if needed
- Absorbable cellulose sponges or other clotting aids can be used
- Surgical ligation may be required in severe cases
- Homologous blood transfusion, colloids, fluid support, or other support measures may be needed depending on the severity of hemorrhage
- Analgesics should be used; butorphanol (1–2 mg/kg) for more severe injuries, meloxicam (0.5–1 mg/kg) for comparatively minor injuries

Intoxications

- Accidental intoxications are less common than in psittacine birds but pigeons are sometimes intentionally poisoned

Signalment:

- There are no breed, sex, or age predilections for most toxicoses
- Aminopyridine (Avitrol) is a bird poison that is sometimes used to kill feral pigeons or other birds [1]
  - Free lofted birds may become exposed unintentionally

Clinical signs:

- Signs are dependent on the toxin
  - Heavy metals and aminopyridine show neurologic signs
  - Heavy metals (lead) also show biliverdinuria or hemoglobinuria
  - Airborne toxins often result in sudden death

Differentials:

- Heavy metals in particulate form may be ingested but columbids do not chew
- Airborne toxins are a concern for any indoor bird
  - Polytetrafluoroethylene (PTFE) gas produced from overheated non-stick surfaces may result in acute death following dyspnea
  - Methane also results in acute death, although no premonitory signs are usually noted

STAT diagnostics:

- CBC often shows anemia, hemolysis, poikilocytosis, and other toxic changes with heavy metal intoxication
- Chemistries show variable signs, depending on the toxin ingested
- Radiographs may show metal particles in heavy metal intoxication or grain filled crops in birds poisoned with aminopyridine

Complete Diagnostics:

- Blood lead or zinc
- Blood or tissue toxin analysis

Therapy:

- Heavy metals
  - Chelation with CaEDTA 20 mg/kg IM q12h
  - Supportive care
  - Particles can be removed from digestive tract conservatively, but will often be ground down and excreted over time (birds should receive chelation therapy during that time)
- Aminopyridine
  - Decontamination
  - Crop lavage, proventricular lavage, activated charcoal Supportive care
- Airborne toxins
  - Remove bird from contaminated area
  - Oxygen cage
  - Meloxicam 0.5 mg/kg
  - Diuresis with furosemide may be helpful

Lameness/Wing Injuries

- Lameness may occur with problems in the pelvic limbs while difficulties with flight may occur due to pectoral limb disorders

Signalment:

- All birds would be susceptible to these problems
- Certain conditions may occur more commonly in specific groups
  - Nutritional disorders more common in very young or old birds
  - Egg laying increases risk of pathologic fractures
  - Degenerative arthritis and gout more common in older birds
  - Neoplasia more common in older birds

Clinical signs:

- Lameness involves any alteration of the gait, perching, or carrying a leg
- May be weight bearing or non-weight bearing

Differentials:

- Traumatic injuries
- Pathologic fractures
  - Nutritional deficiencies (Figure 37.2)
    - Nutritional secondary hyperparathyroidism (NSHP)
  - Neoplasia
- Arthritis
  - Degenerative
- *Salmonella typhimurium* (var Copenhagen) often causes septic arthritis, especially in elbow joints in pigeons
- Articular gout

STAT diagnostics:

- Examination
- Radiography

Complete diagnostics:

- CBC
- Chemistry
- Joint aspiration and cytology if indicated

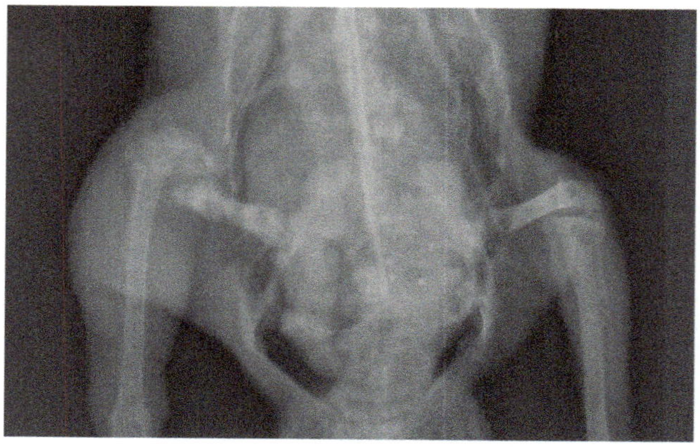

Figure 37.2 Ringneck dove with a pathologic fracture of the right femur secondary to poor nutrition and chronic egg laying.

- Thermal imaging of the limbs
- CT or MRI in rare cases

Therapy:

- Definitive therapy for specific condition
  - Splinting, surgery, or other fracture or luxation repair
  - Vitamin D, calcium supplementation for NSHP
  - Allopurinol (10 mg/kg q12h) for gout
- Analgesia
  - Butorphanol (1–2 mg/kg prn) for severe acute pain
  - NSAIDs such as meloxicam (0.5 mg/kg q12h) for chronic pain
  - Gabapentin (10 mg/kg q8–12h) for neurogenic pain

Neurologic Signs

- Ataxia and incoordination are common neurologic signs in columbids. Seizures may occur with some conditions

Signalment:

- No age or sex predilection appears to exist for neurologic signs in general although specific disorders may affect young or old birds more commonly

Clinical signs:

- Incoordination
- Torticollis or rolling of the head may occur
- Ataxia
- Seizures

Differentials:

- Viral diseases
  - Paramyxovirus (avian avulavirus 1 [AAvV] – pigeon variant) is very common in pigeons and exhibits neurologic and polyuria as primary signs
- Parasitic disease
  - *Sarcocystis calchasi* also may cause polyuria along with neurologic signs (columbids are the natural intermediate hosts) [2]
- Toxicoses
  - Aminopyridine as discussed above
  - Heavy metals as discussed above
- Head trauma may result in increased intracranial pressure
- Metabolic disorders
  - Hypocalcemia and hypoglycemia are uncommon causes in columbids
  - Hepatic disease is possible but is an uncommon cause of neurologic signs
- Vascular disease such as atherosclerosis is less common than in psittacids but could be considered in aged and inactive birds with neurologic signs

STAT diagnostics:

- CBC may indicate whether an inflammatory response is involved
- Chemistries could help rule out metabolic disorders
- Radiographs may show signs of trauma or heavy metal ingestion

Complete diagnostics:

- Heavy metal levels may be helpful if clinical signs are suggestive
- Other toxin screens may be performed if needed
- PCR or serologic tests for specific infectious diseases may be valuable

Therapy:

- Treatment of the primary disorder, if known, is ideal
- Control seizures with midazolam (0.5–2 mg/kg) as needed and levetiracetam 100 mg/kg PO
- Neurologic birds often cannot eat or drink so fluid therapy and nutritional support is often needed
- NSAIDs such as meloxicam (0.5 mg/kg q12h) are helpful for head trauma and any inflammatory etiology
- Mannitol may be useful in acute head trauma
- Vasodilators such as isoxsuprine may be helpful if atherosclerosis is suspected

Polyuria/Polydipsia

- Polyuria is a common finding but is often presented by owners as diarrhea since urine and feces are mixed

Signalment:

- There does not appear to be an age or sex predilection for polyuria, although specific causes may have such tendencies

Clinical signs:

- Polyuria is recognized as an increase in the clear urine component of the droppings
- Pigeon and dove droppings typically have little notable liquid urine
- Excessive water consumption may be noted by astute owners

Differentials:

- Common initial sign with avian avulavirus and *S. calchasi* in pigeons
- Renal disease commonly results in polyuria
- Diabetes mellitus appears to be rare in columbids
- Some healthy birds overconsume water and become polyuric
- Polyuria is also non-specific and may occur in a variety of other systemic disorders

STAT diagnostics:

- Chemistries may be the most useful diagnostic test
  - Elevated uric acid or phosphorus may suggest renal disease
  - Elevated glucose could suggest diabetes mellitus
- Urinalysis is difficult to interpret but specific gravity, glucose, and sediment alternations may be of significant help
- CBC may help detect signs of infection

Complete diagnostics:

- Radiographs/CT-scan may be useful for identifying renal changes or other contributing factors
- A water deprivation test can help determine if the bird can concentrate urine when needed
- Coelioscopy with targeted biopsies may also be considered

Therapy:

- Treatment of primary disorders is warranted
  - Treatment of renal disease depends on the etiology
    - Diuresis will have a relatively low impact on uric acid levels and will not resolve polyuria
    - Omega-3 fatty acids may minimize continued inflammatory damage to the renal tissue [3]
    - Vitamin A supplementation if squamous metaplasia from a deficiency is suspected
    - Eliminate excessive vitamin D and calcium supplementation
- Treatment of diabetes mellitus is difficult and is rarely reported in columbids
  - Treatment with dietary management, glipizide, or insulin may be useful
- Prevention of medullary washout or re-establishment of an osmotic gradient surrounding the Loop of Henle can be accomplished by substituting the water with a balanced electrolyte solution

Respiratory Distress

- Birds are often presented in real or perceived respiratory distress
- True dyspnea should be distinguished from panting and tachypnea

Signalment:

- Respiratory distress shows no age or sex predilections
- Individual conditions may have age or sex predilections

Clinical signs:

- Open mouth breathing is often serious
  - Gular flutter or panting may result from overheating
- Excessive excursion of the body with each breath
- Tail bobbing with each breath may occur
- Cyanosis may occur if the patient is hypoxic
- Wheezing or other respiratory signs may accompany respiratory distress

Differentials:

- Tracheal or pulmonary disease may result in the most severe dyspnea
- Upper respiratory disease may cause open mouth breathing but adequate oxygenation occurs
- No gas exchange occurs in the air sacs, so there may be no respiratory signs unless the volume is greatly reduced (reduced ventilation)
- Cardiac disease may result in left or right sided failure which may affect lungs or cause coelomic distension respectively
- Coelomic distension may compress the air sacs resulting in respiratory distress
  - Cardiac disease
  - Hepatic disease
  - Neoplasia or other masses
  - Reproductive diseases such as egg binding, egg coelomitis, cystic, or neoplastic ovary

STAT diagnostics:

- Physical examination to categorize/localize the disease
  - Upper respiratory disease
    - Cytology of nasal/sinusal flush or choanal swabs
  - Middle or lower airway disease
    - These are often the most severe cases of dyspnea and diagnostics should be done rapidly and carefully
    - Induce with isoflurane and rapidly intubate to control airway
      - If possible, briefly examine trachea for foreign bodies, strictures, or masses with endoscope during intubation by using an endoscope as "stylet" for endotracheal tube
    - Whole body radiographs – CT-scan
    - Blood collection for CBC and chemistry
    - Tracheal wash for cytology and/or culture
  - Coelomic distention
    - Radiographs may be unrewarding in these cases
      - Positioning is inherently risky with coelomic distention
    - Ultrasound may provide more value in identifying the problem in this case
    - Aspiration of free fluid or masses for cytologic evaluation
- Diagnostics may have to wait until patient is stabilized

Complete diagnostics:

- This is dependent on the STAT diagnostics
  - Cultures from any samples that indicate infection
  - CBC and chemistries if not done STAT
  - ECG, echocardiography
  - Endoscopy, lung or air sac sampling if needed

Therapy:

- Oxygen supplementation should be started prior to examination, continue during/between all diagnostic tests, and until breathing returns to normal
  - Chamber administration of oxygen is generally best tolerated
  - Mask or flow by administration may be helpful during procedures
- Sedation seems to benefit most dyspneic patients
  - Midazolam (0.5 mg/kg) and Butorphanol (1.0 mg/kg)
- Patients with tracheal foreign bodies, strictures, or masses should have an air sac tube placed
- Patients with coelomic effusion should have fluid removed via coeliocentesis
- Removing large volumes of fluid does not appear to have deleterious effects
- Patients with lung disease may benefit from bronchodilators such as terbutaline (IM, nebulized) or albuterol (nebulized)
- Nebulization with isotonic or hypertonic saline will enhance removal of exudate from the airways
- Nasal flushing with saline may benefit patients with upper respiratory disease
- Diuresis with furosemide (2 mg/kg q12h) for patients with ascites
- NSAIDs such as meloxicam (0.5 mg/kg q12h) for respiratory inflammation
- Treatment for the primary disorder, if identified

SBS: Sick Bird Syndrome

- Many birds present with vague, generalized, or poorly defined clinical signs. This is often referred to as Sick bird syndrome (SBS)

Signalment:

- These signs may occur in any age or sex

Clinical signs:

- Signs vary substantially but may not be specific
  - Lethargy, apathy, somnolence, or changes in behavior may be reported
  - Closing the eyes or sleeping during the visit should be considered serious
  - Feather carriage may be seen to be ruffled or "fluffed" although the stress of the veterinary exam may cause this to temporarily improve
  - The head, tail, or wings may droop somewhat
  - Variable changes to appetite, water consumption, and droppings
    - See "Abnormal Droppings" section regarding abnormal droppings

Differentials:

- Systemic disease should be suspected in such cases
- Pigeon circovirus may also predispose young pigeons to several other infectious diseases
- Pain may result in some of these changes
- Cold environmental temperatures can result in ruffling of feathers
- Orthopedic disorders may result in postural changes

STAT diagnostics:

- Physical examination to identify any more specific indicators of disease
- CBC to identify systemic response to inflammation
- Chemistries may help identify the organ system involved
- Radiographs may help identify the anatomic source of the problem

Complete diagnostics:

- Further diagnostics are often determined based on suspicions raised by the initial diagnostics
- Cultures, serology, or PCR for specific infectious diseases

Therapy:

- Initial therapy should include fluid and nutritional support
- Heat supplementation (80 °F) may help maintain body temperature and improve feather carriage
- If indicated based on initial diagnostics, antimicrobial therapy should be initiated pending results of other diagnostic tests
  - Enrofloxacin (10 mg/kg q12h) is a good initial choice for several of the bacterial diseases of columbids
  - Enrofloxacin particularly, and antibiotics in general, are widely abused by pigeon racing hobbyists; so resistance is common in these birds

Trauma

- Trauma is a common reason for emergency presentation. Columbids are frequently kept with full wings so injuries related to flying accidents are common. Injuries caused by attacks from other pets are also common

Signalment:

- No specific age or sex predilection seems to exist

Clinical signs:

- Clinical signs vary, depending on the types of injuries present
- Some birds will have no signs, but were seen to have a traumatic event
- Hemorrhage, lacerations, open wounds or other overt traumatic injuries may be seen
- Scalping injuries appear to be particularly common in columbids
- Air sac rupture may result in a large air filled swelling
- Lameness, difficulty in perching, wing drooping, or inability to fly may occur with orthopedic or spinal injuries
- Neurologic signs may occur with head trauma
  - Hemorrhage may be noted

Differentials:

- Trauma is the etiology, so the differentials include any number of injuries that could have occurred

STAT diagnostics:

- A thorough physical examination is needed to find any injuries
- Radiography is needed to identify or better define many injuries
- CBC may help identify anemia or infection in more chronic cases

Complete diagnostics:

- No further diagnostics are usually required unless complications arise

Therapy:

- Highly dependent on the injuries
- Hemostasis (see "Bleeding" section above)
- Therapy for shock if indicated
- Analgesia
  - Butorphanol (1–2 mg/kg prn) for severe acute pain
  - NSAIDs such as meloxicam (0.5 mg/kg q12h) for chronic pain
  - Gabapentin (10 mg/kg q8–12h) for neurogenic pain
  - Drugs can be used concurrently to achieve balanced analgesia
- Stabilization of fractures or luxations
  - Figure of 8 bandages, body bandages for wing injuries
  - Tape splints for leg injuries distal to the stifle
  - Surgical repair may be required for some fractures
- Mannitol can be given IV to acute head trauma patients
- Surgical repair of lacerations and scalping injuries
  - Advancement flaps often needed for scalping wounds
- Subcutaneous air can be removed by aspiration until the air sac repairs

Vomiting/Regurgitation

- Vomiting and regurgitation both occur in birds. Unlike in mammals, both processes are active in birds. Vomiting occurs from the proventriculus, ventriculus, or intestine, while regurgitation comes from the crop and esophagus. A distinguishing characteristic between them is usually the pH of the material produced (acidic with vomiting, neutral with regurgitation)

Signalment:

- No age or sex predilection for this clinical sign seems to exist

Clinical signs:

- Vomiting/regurgitation is a clinical sign

Differentials:

- Trichomoniasis is a common cause of regurgitation
- Candidiasis and bacterial ingluvitis may occasionally occur
- Pigeon herpesvirus and adenovirus may result in vomiting
- Adults regurgitate crop milk and food to the offspring; this is a normal process
- Obstruction of the gastrointestinal tract is rare
- Neoplasia is possible but rare in the gastrointestinal tract of columbids

STAT diagnostics:

- Cytologic examination of the vomited/regurgitated material or a crop wash
- CBC may reveal any systemic response to infection
- Radiographs may show problems aboral to the crop

Complete diagnostics:

- Radiographs with gastrointestinal contrast administration
- Fluoroscopy may be helpful if available

Therapy:

- Treatment of the underlying disease is most helpful
  - Metronidazole (25 mg/kg q12h) for trichomoniasis
  - Fluconazole (10 mg/kg q12h) for candidiasis
- Fluid therapy may be required in severe cases
- Metoclopramide (0.5 mg/kg q8h) may help

Systemic Disease

Salmonellosis

- Salmonellosis or paratyphoid is one of the most important diseases of pigeons
- Caused by *Salmonella typhimurium var Copenhagen*
- Systemic disease including anorexia, refusal to fly, reproductive problems, and diarrhea

Signalment:

- Most common in pigeons, occasionally doves

Clinical signs:

- Vague signs of lethargy and weight loss
- Most recognizable sign is swollen joints, especially the elbows

Diagnosis:

- Identification of the organism from live or dead birds
  - Culture or PCR from blood, joint tap, necropsy tissues

Treatment:

- Antibiotic therapy based on sensitivities possible but may not eliminate the bacteria
- Vaccine is available for this disease but its efficacy is questionable

Ornithosis Complex

- Disease complex related to *Chlamydia psittaci*, combined with various Gram-negative bacteria or mycoplasma
- Zoonotic potential present with this disease

Signalment:

- All birds are susceptible

Clinical signs:

- Referred to as "one-eye cold" by hobbyists because unilateral conjunctivitis often occurs (on the side toward the wind)
- Upper respiratory exudate or other signs may occur as well

Diagnosis:

- Diagnosis can be made based on PCR (conjunctiva, choana, and cloaca)

Treatment:

- Treatment is with doxycycline (25 mg/kg q24h) for 45 days

Circovirus

- Disease is often referred to as "young bird disease"

Signalment:

- Young birds (1–6 months)

Clinical signs:

- Circovirus suppresses the immune system and other pathogens may follow
- Rapid course of disease (3–5 days) [4]
- Anorexia, lethargy, diarrhea, weight loss, inability to fly, sneezing, and respiratory distress

Diagnosis:

- Molecular test when available
- Biopsy of the cloacal bursa (or on necropsy)

Treatment:

- No treatment is available for this disease

Herpesvirus

- Many pigeons are subclinically infected with columbid herpesvirus 1

Signalment:

- No age or sex predilection

Clinical signs:

- Affected birds may show mild to diphtheritic pharyngitis or esophagitis
- Vomiting or inclusion body hepatitis also occur

Diagnosis:

- PCR, endoscopic liver biopsy and histopathology

Treatments:

- No treatments are reported, although acyclovir could be tried

Neurologic and Musculoskeletal Disease

Avian Avulavirus 1

- Avian avulavirus is a very common disease of domestic pigeons [4]
- Caused by Pigeon AAvV-1 which is distinct from Newcastle disease virus (the velogenic viscerotropic form in chickens)

Signalment:

- All pigeons are susceptible but younger birds are more severely affected

Clinical signs:

- Polyuria and polydipsia
- Neurologic signs

- Ataxia, torticollis, poor landing, cannot prehend food
- Bloody diarrhea occasionally occurs

Diagnosis:

- Serologic antibody testing

Therapy:

- Many birds survive if supportive care is provided
  - Nutritional support is required since these birds often cannot eat
- Vaccination is helpful in prevention

Pigeon Protozoal Encephalitis

- *S. calchasi* is the causative agent
- The northern goshawk is the definitive host
- The incubation is very long with polyuria occurring over 10 days post infection and neurologic signs occurring 50 days post infection [5]
- Treatment not known; toltrazuril did not affect the disease [6]

Cardiopulmonary Disease

- Cardiac disease appears to be less common in columbids than in other pet birds
  - Left, right, or bilateral heart failure may occur
  - Respiratory distress, coelomic distention, and organ congestion
  - Diagnosis based on radiography, ECG
  - Therapy as for other birds (see Chapter 35: Psittacines)
- Infectious pneumonia/air sacculitis
  - Aspergillosis may occur in columbids but does not appear to be particularly common
  - Other causes of pneumonia and air sacculitis include aspiration and bacterial infection
- Upper respiratory infection/inflammation–ornithosis complex see above

Gastrointestinal Disease

- Endoparasites including nematodes, cestodes, and coccidia are common in pigeons, but uncommon in doves kept indoors
  - Fecal screening and treatment according to the parasites found
    - Ivermectin (0.5 mg/kg), pyrantel pamoate (20 mg/kg), and fenbendazole (10–20 mg/kg q24 × 3) for nematodes
    - Praziquantel (10 mg/kg) for cestodes
    - Coccidia may be treated but usually cannot be eliminated
      - Trimethoprim/Sulfamethoxazole (25 mg/kg q12h)
      - Ponazuril (20 mg/kg q24h × 7d)
- Diphtheric mucous membranes, oral plaques
  - Common clinical finding in columbids
  - Trichomonas, herpesvirus, candidiasis
  - Diagnosis based on wet mount and cytology
  - Treat according to findings
- Trichomoniasis
  - Commonly a subclinical problem
  - Subclinical disease may protect from more virulent disease
  - Treatment with carnidazole will reduce disease
  - Neither likely nor desirable to eliminate infection

Urogenital and Reproductive Disease

- Abnormal droppings – urine and urates: see above

- Reproductive emergencies:
  - Egg binding
  - Straining without producing an egg
- Diagnosis based on palpation and radiography
- Therapy
  - Stable patients
    - Fluids, calcium
  - Unstable patients
    - Analgesia
    - Ovocentesis under isoflurane
      - Via cloaca if possible; remove egg after collapsing
      - Percutaneous if cervix closed; give 48–72 hours to pass shell
  - Antibiotics, meloxicam, oxytocin

- Polyuria: see above

Dermatologic Disease

- Ectoparasites are not an emergency, but owners may panic when discovering them and may present the bird for treatment
  - Lice chew on feathers and are not highly pathogenic
    - Heavy infestation may suggest debilitation since healthy birds will remove most lice with preening
  - Pigeon louse flies are blood sucking flies that may transmit *Hemoproteus* blood parasites
- Molting/Feather disturbances are relatively uncommon
- Dove feathers epilate easily as a defense mechanism similar to tail autotomy in reptiles

Ophthalmic Disease

- Trauma
  - Corneal ulcers
    - Topical antibiotics (e.g. tobramycin three to four times a day) and artificial tears (three to four times a day)

- Traumatic uveitis
  - Topical (flurbiprofen, note that diclofenac is toxic in pigeons and should be avoided, even as eye drops) or systemic NSAID therapy
- Masses
  - Granuloma from numerous etiologies (esp. *Mycobacterium* spp.)
- Conjunctivitis may occur due to a number of agents but ornithosis complex should be considered: see above

References

1 McLean, M.K. and Khan, S. (2013). A review of 29 incidents involving 4-aminopyridine in non-target species reported to the ASPCA animal poison control Center. *J. Med. Toxicol.* 9: 418–421.

2 Wunschmann, A., Armien, A.G., Reed, L. et al. (2011). Sarcocystis calchasi-associated neurologic disease in a domestic pigeon in North America. *Transbound Emerg. Dis.* 58: 526–530.

3 Pollock, C. (2006). Diagnosis and treatment of avian renal disease. *Vet. Clin. North Am. Exot. Anim. Pract.* 9: 107–128.

4 Harlin, R.W. (2013). Practical pigeon medicine. In: *Proceedings Annual Conference Association of Avian Veterinarians*, 111–124.

5 Olias, P., Gruber, A.D., Heydorn, A.O. et al. (2010). Unusual biphasic disease in domestic pigeons (*Columba livia* f. domestica) following experimental infection with sarcocystis calchasi. *Avian Dis.* 54: 1032–1037.

6 Maier, K., Olias, P., Gruber, A.D. et al. (2015). Toltrazuril does not show an effect against pigeon protozoal encephalitis. *Parasit. Res.* 114: 1603–1606.

38

Backyard Poultry and Waterfowl

Vanessa Grunkemeyer[1] and Samantha Swisher[2]

[1] Department of Agriculture, Nutrition, and Food Systems, University of New Hampshire Durham, New Hampshire, USA
[2] Department of Veterinary Preventive Medicine, College of Veterinary Medicine, The Ohio State University, Columbus, Ohio, USA

CONTENTS

Exotic Animal Emergency and Critical Care Medicine, First Edition. Edited by Jennifer E. Graham, Grayson A. Doss and Hugues Beaufrère.

Unique Species Considerations

- In the United States, the Animal Medicinal Drug Use Clarification Act (AMDUCA) food animal regulations apply to all chickens, turkeys, ducks, and game birds (quail, guinea fowl, etc.)
  - *Forbidden or severely restricted drugs include:* Fluoroquinolones, cephalosporins, chloramphenicol, metronidazole. See Table 38.1
  - Most other drugs used in non-production animals are off-label and withdrawal times are unknown. Eggs and meat may not be consumed or sold if no published withdrawal period is available (most antibiotics). Veterinarians should document that withdrawal times have been discussed with the owner
  - Contact the Food Animal Residue Avoidance Databank (FARAD) or visit www.farad.org for more detailed information
- Avoid delivering medications via food or water if possible, as this results in inconsistent dosing and will not reach severely ill animals that are not eating or drinking
- Contact your local veterinary regulatory authorities for a list of poultry diseases that are reportable in your area. Diseases that are reportable in many states in the United States are listed in Tables 38.2–38.5
- Become familiar with laboratories in your area that are comfortable performing urgent necropsies with full infectious disease testing on food animals (typically state-sponsored labs or veterinary school pathology departments)

Common Presenting Signs

Nonspecific Signs

Introduction

Poultry are often presented to veterinarians for evaluation of nonspecific signs of illness. In some cases, subtle clinical signs and disease progression may be missed by the owners because the birds are housed outside with limited monitoring. However, in many cases, there are no specific clinical signs or physical exam findings; in these cases, the clinician should start with a minimum database of diagnostics, as would be performed in other species.

Table 38.1 Drugs prohibited for use in poultry in the United States.

• Antiviral medications
• Cephalosporins (e.g. ceftazidime, ceftiofur, cephalexin)
• Chloramphenicol
• Fluoroquinolones (e.g. ciprofloxacin, marbofloxacin, enrofloxacin)
• Nitroimidazoles (e.g. metronidazole)

Diagnosis

History:

- Single or multiple birds affected?
- Description of how birds are kept, including any recent changes in husbandry
- Changes in egg production?
- New animals introduced recently?

Signalment:

- Birds of any age may be affected

Clinical Signs:

- Lethargy, weakness, failure to move with flock
- Anorexia or decreased appetite
- Fluffed feathers, eyes closed, decreased/changed vocalizations
- Changes in comb color
- Accumulation of droppings around vent

Differentials:

- Nonspecific signs, by definition, can be caused by a wide variety of diseases. Some of the more common causes include:
  - Reproductive disease
  - Unwitnessed trauma
  - Bacterial infections
- Less common differentials:
  - Aspergillosis (most common in adult waterfowl)
  - Lead toxicosis (prevalence varies by region)
  - Lymphoid leukosis (young birds)
  - Marek's disease (MD) lymphoma
  - Mycobacteriosis
  - Pullorum (Salmonella)
  - Renal failure
  - Intestinal parasitism (coccidiosis, helminthiasis)

STAT Diagnostics:

- CBC/chemistry
- Radiographs
- Fecal floatation
- A-FAST ultrasound

Complete Diagnostics

- Will depend on results of baseline diagnostics and progression of clinical signs

Table 38.2 Infectious diseases causing **multisystemic** signs in poultry.

Common name	Causative agent	Reportable?[a]	Zoonotic?	Species affected	Clinical signs	Specific testing
Avian influenza	Avian influenza virus, many strains of both high and low pathogenicity	Yes	Yes	All, waterfowl often asymptomatic	Respiratory Diarrhea CNS signs Sudden death	AGID ELISA RT-PCR
Colibacillosis	*Escherichia coli*	No	Yes	All	Diarrhea Respiratory Salpingitis Septicemia	Culture Necropsy
Erysipelas	*Erysipelas rhusiopathiae*	Yes	Yes	All Galliformes, turkeys more susceptible	Diarrhea Endocarditis Sudden death	Cytology of liver/bone marrow PCR
Gumboro disease, infectious bursal disease	Birnavirus	Yes	No	Chickens, turkeys may be asymptomatic carriers. Affects young birds.	Neuro, diarrhea, vent-picking	RT-PCR Necropsy
Mycobacteriosis	*Mycobacterium* spp.	No	Yes, depending on species	Most common in waterfowl. Galliformes occasionally affected.	Chronic weight loss	Acid-fast stain PCR Necropsy
Newcastle disease	Newcastle disease virus, virulence varies by strain	Yes	Rare	All, chickens most susceptible	CNS, respiratory, hemorrhage, sudden death	RT-PCR Necropsy
Ornithosis	*Chlamydia psittaci*	Yes	Yes	Rare, but all poultry potentially affected	Respiratory, GI. Often asymptomatic.	Elementary body agglutination (EBA)/immunofluorescent antibody (IFA) ELISA PCR
Pox, fowl pox	Poxvirus	No	No	All	Cutaneous/oral lesions, respiratory signs if wet form of pox	Exam Virus isolation Necropsy

[a] Note that which infectious diseases are reportable varies by state and by country. This is intended as a general indication of diseases that are reportable in many areas of the United States, but local regulations should always be consulted.

Treatment

Stabilization:

- *Fluid therapy:* At least maintenance at 50 ml/kg/d SC, IO, IV as indicated + correct fluid deficits and anticipate fluid loss (especially for GI disease)
- *Thermal support* as necessary (using caution, as poultry are more susceptible to hyperthermia than parrots)
- *Gavage feeding* when rehydrated and at an appropriate body temperature. 30 ml/kg per feeding initially with a recovery formula. If no poultry specific option is available, an avian omnivore recovery or neonatal formula is appropriate
- *Analgesics* if there is evidence of discomfort

Continued Care:

- Will depend on specific diagnosis

Abnormal Droppings

Introduction

Clinicians should be familiar with the appearance of the normal fecal, urate, and urine components of the droppings in each species, as they can vary significantly. It is important to be aware that Galliformes periodically produce cecal

Table 38.3 Infectious diseases causing primarily **gastrointestinal** signs in poultry.

Common name	Causative agent	Reportable?[a]	Zoonotic?	Species affected	Clinical signs	Specific testing
Blackhead disease	*Histomonas meleagridis*	No	No	Galliformes, primarily turkeys	GI signs Cyanotic head (rare)	Culture Histopathology
Campylobacteriosis	*Campylobacter jejuni*	No	Yes	All	GI signs Often asymptomatic	Culture PCR
Coccidiosis	*Eimeria* spp. (all) *Tyzzeria* spp. (waterfowl)	No	No	All (by different species of coccidia)	Diarrhea Renal failure (waterfowl)	Fecal float (GI form) Necropsy
Cryptosporidiosis	*Cryptosporidium* spp.	No	Unknown – likely depends on species	Galliformes. Turkeys most commonly affected	Diarrhea	PCR
Duck viral enteritis "Duck plaque"	Anatid alphaherpesvirus[a]	No	No	Waterfowl	Bloody diarrhea Photophobia Sudden death	PCR Virus isolation Necropsy
Fowl typhoid	*Salmonella gallinarum*	Yes	Yes	Mostly galliformes, waterfowl resistant	Diarrhea, dyspnea, septicemia, sudden death	Serology Culture
Hemorrhagic enteritis	Adenovirus	No	No	Primarily affects young turkeys	Hemorrhagic diarrhea	Serology Virus isolation Necropsy
Necrotic enteritis	*Clostridium perfringens*	No	No	Young chickens, turkeys	Diarrhea Sudden death	Necropsy Culture
Paratyphoid	*Salmonella* spp.	Yes (depending on strain)	Yes	All	Diarrhea, weakness, death	Culture PCR
Pullorum disease	*Salmonella pullorum*	Yes	Yes	All Galliformes, most commonly chickens	Juveniles – white diarrhea, death Adults – asymptomatic	Necropsy, culture, serology
Transmissible enteritis, blue comb, mud fever	Coronavirus	No	No	Turkeys	Diarrhea	Serology Virus isolation Necropsy
Ulcerative enteritis	*Clostridium colinum*	No	No	Game birds	Diarrhea Sudden death	Necropsy

[a] Note that which infectious diseases are reportable varies by state and by country. This is intended as a general indication of diseases that are reportable in many areas of the United States, but local regulations should always be consulted.

droppings, which are typically less formed and darker in color. Changes in droppings may be an indicator of systemic disease, rather than a specific sign of GI disease.

Diagnosis

History:

- Determine which component(s) of the dropping is (are) affected
- Diet history
- Single/multiple animals affected?

Signalment:

- Diarrhea is a common presenting sign in young chicks, but can occur in adults as well

Clinical Signs:

- *Fecal component:* May be loose, discolored, or reduced in volume
- *Urine/urate components:* May be discolored or altered from normal volume
- *Blood in the droppings:* Often challenging to determine source (urinary, reproductive, GI)

Table 38.4 Infectious diseases causing primarily **neurologic** signs in poultry.

Common name	Causative agent	Reportable?[a]	Zoonotic?	Species affected	Clinical signs	Specific testing
Avian encephalomyelitis/ "Endemic tremor"	Picornavirus	Yes	No	Galliformes, ducks	Ataxia, tremors, adults that recover can develop cataracts	Serology Virus isolation Necropsy
Duck viral hepatitis	Duck hepatitis A virus type[a]	Yes	No	Young ducklings	Neurologic Sudden death	PCR Virus isolation Necropsy
Eastern/Western Equine encephalitis	Togaviruses	Yes	Yes (via insect vector)	Galliformes. Chickens resistant.	Ataxia, tremors, sudden death	Virus isolation Necropsy
Listeriosis	*Listeria monocytogenes*	Yes	Yes	All	Encephalitis Diarrhea Septicemia	Culture Necropsy
Marek's disease	Herpesvirus	No	No	Chickens	Unilateral paralysis, visceral tumors	Serology Necropsy
West Nile virus	West Nile virus	Yes	Yes (via insect vector)	Most asymptomatic, ducks more susceptible	Tremors, ataxia, torticollis	Serology Virus isolation

[a] Note that which infectious diseases are reportable varies by state and by country. This is intended as a general indication of diseases that are reportable in many areas of the United States, but local regulations should always be consulted.

Differentials:

- Bacterial: *Salmonella* spp., *Escherichia coli*, *Campylobacter jejuni*, *Clostridium* spp., *Mycobacterium* spp., *Chlamydia psittaci* (rare in poultry)
- Viral: Infectious bursal disease (birnavirus), Newcastle disease, avian influenza, duck viral enteritis, duck viral hepatitis
- Parasitic/protozoal: Coccidia (common), nematodes (*Ascaridia* spp., *Capillaria* spp., *Heterakis* spp., other nematodes), protozoa (*Histomonas meleagridis* [primarily turkeys, occasionally chickens]), *Trichomonas* spp., *Cryptosporidium* spp. (primarily game birds)
- Dietary: Significant variation can be seen in dropping color and consistency in animals that forage or receive table scraps
- Toxins
- Heat or cold stress (particularly in chicks)
- Neoplasia

STAT Diagnostics:

- *CBC/biochemistry*
- *Blood gases/electrolyte panel:* To guide fluid replacement therapy
- *Fecal floatation and direct smear +/− Gram stain:* Some parasites intermittently shed

Complete Diagnostics:

- *Fecal culture:* Primarily to rule out *Salmonella* spp. (shed intermittently, so serial cultures usually required)
- *Diagnostic imaging*
  - Whole body radiographs/computed tomography (CT)-scan
  - Coelomic ultrasound
- *Histopathology:* If multiple birds are severely affected

Treatment

Stabilization:

- *Supportive care:* See Section "Nonspecific Signs"
- *Antibiotics:* As indicated based on fecal Gram stain and culture
- *Antiparasitics:* As indicated based on fecal floatation

Continued Care:

- Many causes of diarrhea are of infectious origin and may affect multiple animals, so environmental management

Table 38.5 Infectious diseases causing primarily **respiratory** signs in poultry.

Common name	Causative agent	Reportable?[a]	Zoonotic?	Species affected	Clinical signs	Specific testing
Aspergillosis/ "Brooder pneumonia"	*Aspergillus fumigatus* and *A. flavus*	No	No	All. Waterfowl, turkeys, and young chicks most commonly affected	Chicks – dyspnea, increased mortality Adults – weight loss, sudden death	Serology Galactomannan Necropsy
Fowl cholera	*Pasteurella multocida*	No	Yes	All. Chickens most susceptible.	Respiratory, swollen wattle/comb and joints, septicemia	Culture Necropsy
Gapeworm	*Syngamus trachea*	No	No	Galliformes	Dyspnea, sudden death	Fecal floatation Necropsy
Infectious bronchitis	*Coronavirus*	Yes	No	Primarily chickens	Upper respiratory, reproductive	Serology Virus isolation Necropsy
Infectious coryza	*Avibacterium* (chickens) *Bordetella* (turkeys)	No	No	Galliformes – causative agent varies by species	Upper respiratory	Culture Necropsy
Infectious laryngotracheitis	Herpesvirus	Yes	No	Galliformes (mostly chickens, peafowl)	Upper respiratory Sudden death	PCR Virus isolation Necropsy
Mycoplasmosis	*M. gallisepticum, M. synoviae, Mycoplasma meleagridis*	Yes	No	All	Upper respiratory signs, periorbital sinus swelling, arthritis	PCR Culture Serology Necropsy
Turkey rhinotracheitis	Avian metapneumovirus	Yes	No	Turkeys, chickens, Muscovy ducks, guinea fowl	Upper respiratory signs "Swollen head syndrome"	Serology Virus isolation RT-PCR Necropsy

[a] Note that which infectious diseases are reportable varies by state and by country. by state and by country. This is intended as a general indication of diseases that are reportable in many areas of the United States, but l regulations should always be consulted.

and flock health recommendations should be given as indicated

- Some causes of diarrhea (e.g. paratyphoid Salmonella) are zoonotic and reportable (see Table 38.3). Owners should be counseled accordingly, and all local regulations should be followed

Acute Flock Die-Off

Introduction

Acute flock mortality events are often the result of infectious diseases, and antemortem clinical signs are similar across a wide variety of diseases. For this reason, necropsy with histopathology and infectious disease testing are often critical to reach a diagnosis. In most cases, veterinary regulatory authorities should be contacted, as many reportable diseases in poultry can cause acute mortality events without other, more specific clinical signs.

Diagnosis

History:

- Which age-groups are affected?
- Are there multiple species affected?
- Were any new birds introduced recently?
- Exposure to wildlife?
- Recent changes in diet and/or housing?

Signalment:

- Varies depending on underlying disease

Clinical Signs:

- Acute death of multiple birds without premonitory signs

Differentials:

- *Infectious:*
  - Bacterial: *Pasteurella multocida* (fowl cholera), *Avibacterium paragallinarum/Bordetella avium* (infectious coryza), *Salmonella* spp., *Clostridium enteritis, Erysipelas* (most common in turkeys)
  - Viral: Highly pathogenic avian influenza, virulent (exotic) Newcastle disease, herpesvirus (infectious laryngotracheitis), hemorrhagic enteritis (in young turkeys), duck viral hepatitis, duck viral enteritis
  - Protozoal: *H. meleagridis* (in turkeys)
  - Other: Botulism (in waterfowl), aflatoxin
- *Noninfectious causes:* Predation events (usually apparent on exam), environmental toxins, food-borne toxins

STAT Diagnostics:

- Local veterinary regulatory authorities will be involved in selecting appropriate diagnostics in most cases
- *Necropsy:* Diagnostic test of choice in cases of flock mortality events. Necropsy should be performed by a facility (usually a state laboratory or a veterinary school) that has the capability to test for a variety of infectious diseases
- *CBC/chemistry:* If live, affected birds are available

Complete Diagnostics:

- *Toxicology:* Performed on tissue samples, GI contents, feed, or other materials as clinically indicated

Treatment

Stabilization:

- *Supportive care* with fluids, gavage feeding, and antibiotics to prevent secondary infections can be attempted for individual birds until a diagnosis is reached
- These patients should not be admitted to the hospital unless appropriate biosecurity measures can be put into place to prevent transmission of infectious disease to other patients

Continued Care:

- Dependent on final diagnosis. As many causes of acute mortality are diseases of public health or economic concern, local regulatory authorities may require depopulation

Crop Distension

Introduction

Crop distension is often a sign of underlying systemic disease in poultry. While bacterial or fungal overgrowth may be identified on crop cytology, these are rarely the primary problem.

Diagnosis

History:

- Duration and progression
- Home therapies attempted?
- Diet history? Possible ingestion of foreign material?

Signalment:

- Birds of any age or sex may be affected

Clinical Signs:

- Distension of the crop with fluid or firm contents (see Figure 38.1)
- Appetite may be normal or decreased
- May be associated with regurgitation and halitosis

Differentials:

- *Recent meal:* Crop volume should decrease after several hours of fasting
- Foreign material (grass, fibrous plants), outflow obstruction

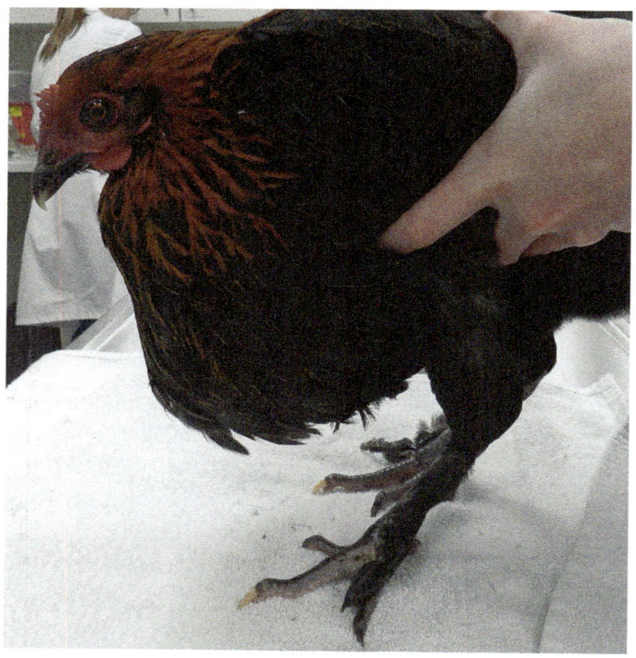

Figure 38.1 Young black copper Maran chicken (*Gallus Gallus domesticus*) with severe crop distension of undetermined etiology (see Sections "Crop Distension" and "Crop Stasis/Impaction").

- *Dehydration:* May cause impaction
- *Infectious:* Many cases of bacterial/fungal overgrowth are secondary to another underlying disease decreasing GI motility
- Coccidiosis, capillariasis, or other GI parasitism
- *Neurologic:* Lead toxicosis, Marek's disease
- Idiopathic pendulous crop (possible genetic etiology)

STAT Diagnostics:

- *Crop cytology*
- *Radiographs/CT:* Exercise caution to avoid regurgitation in sedated/anesthetized patients

Complete Diagnostics:

- *Gastrointestinal contrast radiography:* Serial films and/or fluoroscopy may help assess GI motility and potentially highlight a foreign body
- *Ultrasound*
- *Fecal flotation*
- *CBC/chemistry*
- *Blood heavy metal levels:* If radiographic or historical evidence of heavy metal toxicosis

Treatment

Stabilization:

- Handle with caution to reduce risk of aspiration
- *Fluids:* Subcutaneous (SC) +/− per os (PO) if inspissated crop contents
- *Lavage and aspiration of crop contents* via oro-esophageal tube
- *Chelation:* If heavy metal toxicosis suspected

Continued Care:

- *Supportive bandaging:* Severely distended crops are often incapable of contracting normally and will refill quickly after emptying. Placing a "crop bra" can help support the crop and prevent further distension
- *Easily digestible food*
- *Antimicrobials:* As indicated based on cytology
- *Surgery:* For removal of foreign material; partial crop resection may also be helpful in severe, refractory cases, but recurrence is possible

Lameness

Introduction

Lameness and trauma are among the most common reasons that poultry are presented for emergency care. Not all backyard flocks are closely supervised, so injuries presented as an emergency may not be acute.

Diagnosis

History:

- Duration of clinical signs?
- Single or multiple birds affected?
- Known trauma?
- How are birds housed? (Coop set-up, predator protection, etc.)

Clinical Signs:

- Lameness, reluctance to move
- *Wing droop:* May be caused by fracture, pain, or neurologic damage
- Wounds, feather loss, bruising

Differentials:

- *Trauma:* Predation event, fall, vehicular trauma, entanglement
- *Systemic disease:* Marek's disease, septic arthritis, articular gout, mycoplasma, compression of sciatic/lumbosacral plexus by intracoelomic disease
- *Congenital/nutritional:* Valgus deformities, perosis (gastrocnemius tendon dislocation), tibial dyschondroplasia, gastrocnemius tendon rupture
- *Other:* Pododermatitis, frostbite

STAT Diagnostics:

- *CBC:* If evidence of hemorrhage or infection
- *Radiographs*
- *Thermal imaging* of the leg

Complete Diagnostics:

- *Chemistry:* If gout is suspected
- *Culture:* Wounds, septic joints
- *Necropsy:* If Marek's disease is suspected
- *Electromyography:* In the absence of published normal reference values, interpretation may be limited

Treatment

Stabilization:

- *Analgesia:* Kappa agonist opiates, tramadol, or nonsteroidal anti-inflammatories; note that all of these drugs are off-label and require higher doses in birds than in mammals
- *Fluid therapy:* Intraosseous (IO), intravenous (IV), SC as indicated for shock/hypovolemia
- *Antibiotics:* As indicated for wounds or open fractures
- *Nitenpyram:* Orally or topically as indicated for myiasis
- *Wound lavage and topical therapy:* Rule out air sac involvement first

- *Bandaging:* Wing fractures, leg fractures distal to the stifle, wounds, some limb deformities, pododermatitis

Continued Care:

- Fractures
  - Poultry usually tolerate surgical fracture repair well and heal quickly with appropriate treatment
  - If surgical repair is not possible, many fractures can heal with stabilization and cage rest, but some function may be lost
- Wounds/pododermatitis (see Figure 38.2)
  - Follow standard wound care recommendations for other species (see Chapter 28: Avian pain management and anesthesia)
  - House indoors to prevent myiasis
- Congenital deformities (see Figure 38.3): Some very young animals may respond to corrective bandaging, but prognosis is poor if not treated early, especially in a heavy-bodied bird
- Marek's disease – recommend euthanasia (poor prognosis)

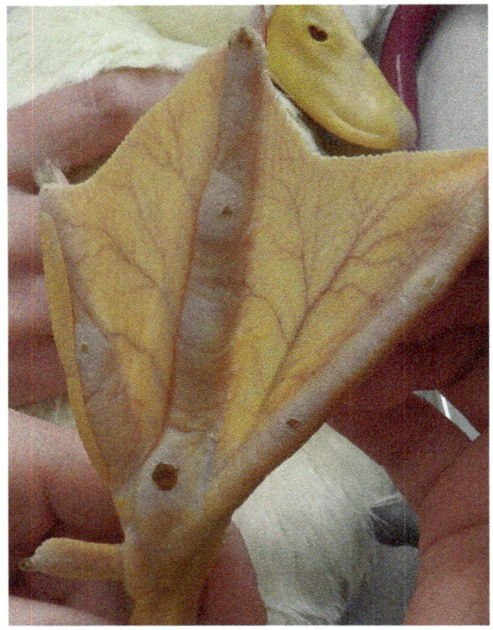

Figure 38.2 Young Pekin duck (*Anas platyrhynchos domestica*) with pododermatitis lesions secondary to septic arthritis and associated lameness (see Sections "Lameness" and "Arthritis").

Neurologic Signs

Introduction

Poultry are occasionally presented for neurologic signs, most commonly due to trauma or toxin ingestion. Infectious diseases (with the exception of Marek's disease) are relatively rare, but should be considered due to their public health significance. Many diseases that cause central nervous system (CNS) signs in poultry are reportable, and all local regulations regarding these diseases should be followed.

Diagnosis

History:

- *Dietary history:* Nutritional deficiencies are unlikely on a commercial diet that is formulated for species and life stage
- Access to toxins, including medications milled into feed
- Single or multiple birds affected?
- Exposure to wild birds

Signalment:

- Most nutritional diseases affect young chicks
- Toxins and infectious diseases can affect birds of any age

Clinical Signs:

- *Central neurologic signs:* Avian encephalomyelitis, avian influenza, Newcastle disease, Eastern/Western equine encephalitis, West Nile virus, *Toxoplasma gondii*, *Sarcocystis* spp., hypovitaminosis E, thiamine deficiency

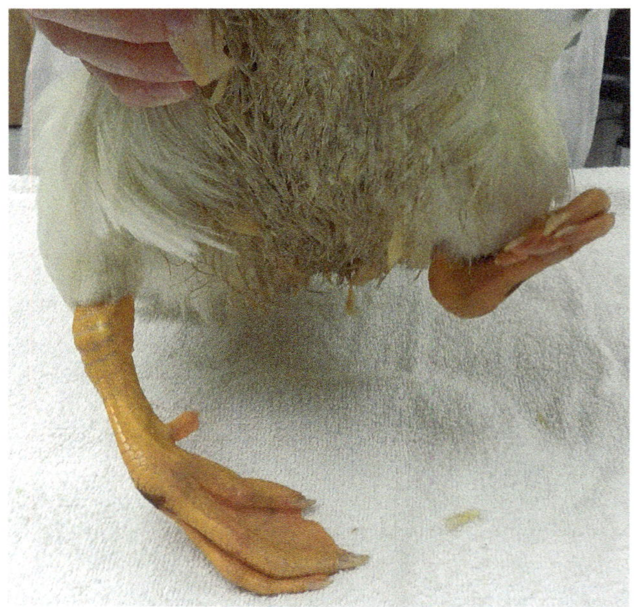

Figure 38.3 Young Pekin duck with bilateral developmental leg deformities. Due to the chronicity of the lesions and the grave prognosis for adequate correction, the duck was euthanized. No underlying etiology was determined in this case (see Sections "Lameness" and "Congenital/Developmental Limb Deformities").

- *Peripheral neurologic signs:* Sciatic compression by intracoelomic disease, Marek's disease, botulism, riboflavin deficiency, thiamine deficiency
- Note that it can be difficult to differentiate neurologic weakness/change in mentation from general systemic compromise

Differentials:

- *Young birds*
  - *Viral:* Avian encephalomyelitis (picornavirus, 1–3 weeks old)
  - *Nutritional:* Hypovitaminosis E, thiamine deficiency (>14 days of age), riboflavin deficiency (>12 days of age)
- *Any age*
  - *Viral:* Marek's disease (most common in chicks 4–20 weeks old, but can also occur in adults), West Nile virus (primarily ducks, other poultry typically asymptomatic carriers), Eastern/Western equine encephalitis, highly pathogenic avian influenza, virulent (exotic) Newcastle disease
  - *Parasitic: Toxoplasma, Baylisascaris, Sarcocystis*
  - *Toxins:* Aflatoxicosis, botulism (primarily waterfowl), heavy metal
  - Trauma
  - Neoplasia

STAT Diagnostics:

- *CBC, chemistry*
- *Radiographs:* Rule out heavy metal foreign body (evaluation of blood levels still indicated in suspected cases of lead toxicosis)

Complete Diagnostics:

- *Necropsy:* Likely the fastest and most helpful diagnostic if multiple birds affected
- *Toxicology:* Performed on GI contents (botulism), feed (aflatoxins, coccidiostats), or blood (heavy metals)
- *Advanced CNS imaging* (CT, MRI)
- Report cases to the veterinary regulatory authorities as necessary and follow all pertinent regulations and recommendations

Treatment

Stabilization:

- Most neurologic diseases carry a guarded prognosis, but some patients may survive with good supportive care
- *Fluids:* IV, IO, or SC as indicated
- *Nutritional support:* Exercise caution to prevent aspiration in patients that are not mentally appropriate
- *Antibiotics:* As indicated; trimethoprim sulfamethoxazole (TMS) 50 mg/kg PO q12h may be a good empirical choice due to activity against several parasitic organisms
- *Supportive nursing to avoid compounding injuries* (padded cages, rotating position, ocular lubrication, etc.)
- *Anti-seizure medication:* Levetiracetam 100 mg/kg PO q12h

Continued Care:

- Address underlying husbandry or biosecurity problems as needed

Reproductive Signs

Introduction

Reproductive disease is one of the most common reasons that backyard chickens are presented for veterinary care. Many chicken breeds, such as Leghorn-based strains and brown-egg strain hybrids, have been selectively bred for the relatively short periods of intense egg production that are desired in commercial operations. While backyard, dual-purpose breed chickens produce relatively fewer eggs annually, they can still maintain a high level of egg production over a longer life span than commercial layers. For these reasons, many small flock birds develop reproductive disease as they age.

Diagnosis

History:

- Laying history (including frequency of laying, last known egg production, any abnormal eggs produced, etc.). Many owners can provide this information even if they have multiple birds because individual birds have unique nesting spots or egg coloration/size
- Are the other birds in the flock affected?
- Diet being fed and quality of appetite?
- Straining to lay?
- Home remedies attempted? Owners often cause tissue trauma by attempting to assist birds with cloacal prolapse or suspected dystocia

Signalment:

- Older hens (>2–3 years old) are more affected, but reproductive disease can occur at any age

Clinical Signs:

- Lethargy, anorexia, reluctance to move, fecal accumulation around the vent
- Straining
- Coelomic distension, with or without palpable egg
- Cloacal/oviductal prolapse

- Increased respiratory effort (especially if coelomic effusion is present)
- Decrease or cessation of egg production
- Phallus prolapse in male waterfowl

Differentials:

- *Dystocia:* Underlying causes may include very young/old hen (more prone to develop eggs of abnormal shape and size), hypocalcemia, obesity, previous trauma to reproductive tract
- *Ovarian disease:* Oophoritis, ovarian adenocarcinoma (common), cystic ovaries
- *Oviductal/uterine disease:* Cystic right oviduct, salpingitis, oviductal impaction, oviductal torsion, reproductive tract rupture, oviductal adenocarcinoma, neoplasia caused by Marek's disease or avian leukosis
- *Coelomic disease:* Egg coelomitis (sterile or septic), ectopic eggs
- *Prolapse:* May be associated with dystocia; often caused by excessive mating in waterfowl (phallus in male, cloaca in female)

STAT Diagnostics:

- *Radiographs:* If patient is not stable enough for traditional positioning, consider standing radiographs to rule out the presence of a shelled egg and screen for obvious gonadal enlargement
- *A-FAST ultrasound:* Helpful to determine if coelomocentesis is indicated for birds in respiratory distress

Complete Diagnostics:

- *CBC/chemistry*
- *Coelomic ultrasound:* Interpretation of coelomic ultrasound in poultry is challenging, but can be helpful if an experienced ultrasonographer is available
- *Coelomocentesis* for cytology +/− culture

Treatment

Stabilization:

- *Dystocia:* If patient is stable, attempt medical therapy first with fluids, increased environmental humidity, parenteral calcium, thermal support, analgesia, and lubrication of cloaca. If this is not successful or patient condition is deteriorating, manual removal of a distal egg can be attempted under anesthesia
  - First, attempt gentle manual expression
  - If this is not successful, attempt to visualize the egg per-cloacally. Use of a Lonestar Retractor™ can often facilitate this
  - If the egg can be directly visualized, it can be collapsed by ovocentesis and the fragments removed (see Chapter 35: Psittacines)
  - If the egg cannot be visualized
    - Transcoelomic ovocentesis can be attempted, but risks causing coelomitis (especially if unknowingly performed on an ectopic egg)
    - Consider coelomic surgery to remove
  - Antibiotics should be considered due to prevalence of underlying infection and likelihood of tissue trauma during removal
- *Prolapse:* Cloacal/phallus prolapses should be kept clean and lubricated and replaced as soon as possible. Address dystocia first, if present, and perform radiographs to confirm that no shelled eggs remain in the reproductive tract. Temporary cloacorraphy with two laterally placed sutures may help prevent recurrence until tissue inflammation resolves. Patients should receive analgesia and antibiotics if there is any evidence of tissue compromise
- *Coelomic effusion with respiratory distress:* Coelomocentesis (see Chapter 33: Cytology)

Continued Care:

- *Palliative care for chronic disease:* Analgesics/anti-inflammatories, antibiotics, therapeutic coelomocentesis (if indicated)
- *GnRH super-agonists:* The use of GnRH super-agonists (leuprolide acetate and deslorelin) is variably effective in stopping egg production in Galliformes. At the time of this writing, use of leuprolide acetate is off-label in poultry (and typically very expensive, due to the high volume of drug required, 1000 IU/kg). While the effects of deslorelin implants have been documented in several poultry species, off-label use of commercially available deslorelin implants in food-producing animals is prohibited in the United States, due to this product's status as an Food and Drug Administration (FDA) indexed drug (personal communication, FARAD). Off-label use of other injectable products containing deslorelin may be considered, but the use of these products to prevent reproductive activity in poultry have not been documented
- *Salpingohysterectomy +/− ovariectomy*: Surgical management of reproductive disease is challenging in any species. It can be particularly difficult in deep-bodied birds like chickens, especially as many have adhesions from chronic coelomitis. These procedures should be carefully considered and should only be performed by experienced clinicians

Respiratory Signs

Introduction

Respiratory disease (especially upper respiratory disease) is very common in poultry and is often related to poor husbandry or introduction of infectious diseases through inappropriate quarantine protocols.

Diagnosis

History:

- *Review husbandry:* Poorly ventilated/unsanitary coop?
- Breach in biosecurity?
- Exposure to wild birds
- Single or multiple animals affected?

Signalment:

- Respiratory disease affects birds of all ages and both sexes

Clinical Signs:

- Oculonasal discharge, infraorbital sinus swelling (Figure 38.4)
  - Note that ducks sometimes develop serous or foaming ocular discharge without respiratory illness when stressed
- Sneezing, coughing, respiratory noise
- Open beak breathing (gaping): Also common with stress or hyperthermia, especially in turkeys
- Cyanotic comb/wattle

Differentials:

- Common in backyard flocks
  - Environmental/airborne respiratory irritants
  - Mycoplasmosis (*Mycoplasma gallisepticum, Mycoplasma synoviae*)
  - Mixed Gram-negative bacterial upper respiratory disease
  - Non-respiratory disease compressing air sacs – reproductive disease, ascites, obesity (see Figure 38.5), etc.
- Occasionally seen in backyard flocks
  - Cardiac disease (primarily meat breeds)

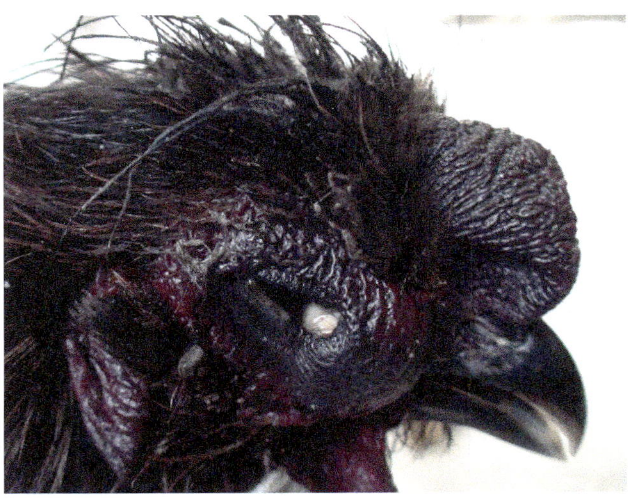

Figure 38.4 Rooster with infraorbital sinuses expanded by caseous debris.

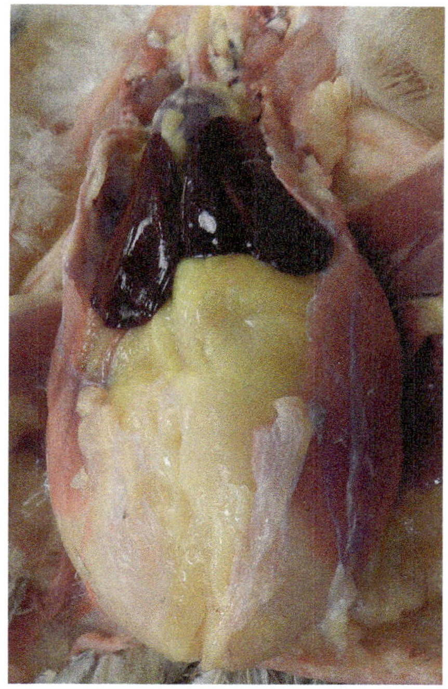

Figure 38.5 Adult Orpington chicken that died during an episode of severe, acute respiratory compromise. The bird had a short history of these episodes with no other noted clinical signs. The only significant finding on necropsy was severe obesity which is suspected to have restricted air flow through the respiratory system (see Section "Respiratory Signs").

  - Colibacillosis (*E. coli*)
  - Fowl cholera (*P. multocida*)
  - Infectious coryza (*A. paragallinarum* in chickens, *B. avium* in turkeys)
  - Infectious laryngotracheitis (herpesvirus)
  - Poxvirus (wet form)
  - Gapeworm (*Syngamus trachea*)
  - Tracheal foreign bodies/aspiration
- Rare in backyard flocks
  - Avian influenza (low pathogenicity form)
  - Aspergillosis - "brooder pneumonia" in young birds, more common in adult waterfowl
  - Infectious bronchitis (coronavirus)
  - Newcastle disease virus (low virulence endemic forms)
  - Turkey rhinotracheitis (avian metapneumovirus)

STAT Diagnostics:

- *Complete blood count/biochemistry*
- *Radiographs:* Occasionally may assist in the evaluation of severe lower respiratory disease, but primarily useful to rule out non-respiratory disease

Complete Diagnostics:

- *Culture:* Culture of discharge may be difficult to interpret due to risk of contamination. Culture of sinus aspirate/flush, or tracheal swabs may be more specific. Mycoplasma organisms require special growth conditions
- *Polymerase chain reaction* (PCR)*:* Mycoplasma can be detected in conjunctival/choanal swabs
- *Fecal floatation:* To rule out gapeworm
- *Advanced imaging:* Tracheoscopy, coelioscopy, CT
- *Necropsy:* By a facility with infectious disease testing capabilities; often the most cost-effective way to diagnose infectious diseases in a flock

Treatment

Stabilization:

- Minimalize handling to decrease stress – these patients decompensate easily
- *Oxygen therapy:* Use a large incubator with good airflow to prevent over-heating
- *Fluid therapy:* SC usually adequate except for very debilitated animals
- *Antibiotics:* Tetracyclines are a good empirical choice pending test results
- *Benzamidazoles* (off-label)*:* For gapeworm
- *Air sac cannula:* For severely dyspneic patients with suspected upper respiratory obstruction (see Chapter 24: Oxygen therapy for more detail on air sac cannula placement); as poultry have minimal air sac space compared to psittacines, this may not be helpful in poultry, particularly with coelomic pathology

Continued Care:

- Improve husbandry as indicated
- *Review infectious disease protocols:* Vaccination protocols, appropriate sources for new birds, quarantine procedures, wildlife control

Systemic Disease

Avian Influenza (AI)

Diagnosis

Clinical Signs:

- Vary by pathogenicity of viral strain
  - *Low pathogenic avian influenza* (LPAI)*:* Respiratory signs, diarrhea, lethargy, anorexia, fluffed feathers
  - *Highly pathogenic avian influenza* (HPAI)*:* CNS signs, edematous comb/wattle, cutaneous/conjunctival hemorrhage, sudden death

Differentials:

- *LPAI:* See differentials for respiratory disease, diarrhea, and nonspecific signs in Section "Common Presenting Signs"
- *HPAI:* Virulent Newcastle disease, *P. multocida*, toxin, duck viral enteritis (waterfowl only)

STAT Diagnostics:

- Contact veterinary regulatory authorities for access to rapid diagnostic methods, including agar gel immunodiffusion assay (AGID), enzyme-linked immunosorbent assays (ELISA), and reverse transcriptase polymerase chain reaction (RT-PCR) tests

Treatment:

- Not recommended. Any suspected cases of AI should be reported to veterinary regulatory authorities, and depopulation will likely be recommended

Hyperthermia

Diagnosis

Clinical Signs:

- Acute respiratory distress and/or collapse with compatible history

Differentials:

- Systemic infectious disease, reproductive disease, airborne toxin exposure

STAT Diagnostics:

- *CBC/chemistry:* To rule out other disease processes and evaluate for multi-organ dysfunction from systemic inflammatory response
- *Cloacal temperature* is generally not considered a helpful diagnostic procedure in birds

Treatment

Stabilization:

- Minimize handling to reduce stress
- *Reverse hyperthermia:* Placement in a cool, oxygen-enriched incubator is usually adequate
- *Fluid therapy:* SC, IV, IO as indicated

Continued Care:

- Assure appropriate access to water, shade, and adequately ventilated housing

Toxicoses

Diagnosis

Clinical Signs:

- *Aflatoxins:* Neurologic signs, sudden death; ducks and turkeys are more sensitive
- *Anticoagulant rodenticide:* Weakness, pallor, hemorrhage

- *Clostridium botulinum* toxin: Flaccid paralysis of wings, legs, and (most prominently) the neck; most common in waterfowl
- *Heavy metal:* Nonspecific signs, GI dysfunction, neurologic signs
- *Ionophores (e.g. monensin):* Drop in egg production (mild cases), paralysis (severe cases)
- *Polytetrafluoroethylene* (PTFE) (*e.g. Teflon®*): Death of multiple animals with no antemortem signs; usually caused by overheating of heat bulbs

Differentials:

- *Aflatoxin:* AI, ND, *Salmonella* spp., duck viral hepatitis, other infectious disease
- *Anticoagulant rodenticide:* Trauma, ectoparasite-associated anemia, chronic disease, chicken anemia virus
- *Botulinum toxin:* Severe weakness due to other systemic disease
- *Heavy metals:* Other GI or neurologic disease
- *Ionophores:* Nutritional disease, infectious disease
- *PTFE toxicosis:* See Section "Acute Flock Die-Off" for other causes of acute death

STAT Diagnostics:

- *Aflatoxin:* Chemistry (liver values)
- *Anticoagulant rodenticide:* Packed cell volume (PCV)/total solids (TS), chemistry (r/o other causes of clotting deficiencies) clotting tests (limited in interpretation due to the lack of published reference values)
- *Botulinum toxin:* Presumptive diagnosis based on history/clinical signs
- *Heavy metals:* Radiographs to diagnose metal foreign body
- *Ionophores:* None

Complete Diagnostics:

- *Aflatoxin:* Feed analysis
- *Anticoagulant rodenticide:* None
- *Botulinum toxin:* Toxin analysis by mouse injection assay is available, but rarely pursued
- *Heavy metals:* Blood lead/zinc levels
- *Ionophores:* Feed analysis

Treatment

Stabilization:

- *Fluid therapy:* SC, IV, IO as indicated. Rodenticide cases may require blood transfusion.
- Decontamination
  - *Crop lavage:* To evacuate contaminated feed material if it is still present in crop, not advised for neurologic patients due to the high risk of aspiration
  - *Activated charcoal:* Recent exposure to toxins for which this compound is safe in other species
- Specific antidotes (off-label)
  - *Vitamin K:* Suspected anticoagulant rodenticide toxicosis
  - *Chelation:* Ca ethylenediamine tetraacetic acid (EDTA) or dimercaptosuccinic acid (DMSA) for heavy metal toxicosis

Continued Care:

- Address source of intoxication. For birds with suspected heavy metal foreign bodies, gastric lavage may allow removal of foreign material without coelomic surgery

Newcastle Disease (ND)

Diagnosis

Clinical Signs:

- *Lentogenic/mesogenic ND:* Mild respiratory signs, diarrhea, lethargy, anorexia, fluffed feathers
- *Neurogenic (virulent exotic) ND:* CNS signs, hemorrhages (conjunctival, tracheal, etc.), sudden death

Differentials:

- *Lentogenic/mesogenic ND:* See differentials for respiratory disease and nonspecific signs in Section "Common Presenting Signs"
- *Virulent (exotic) ND:* High path avian influenza, *P. multocida*, toxin, duck viral enteritis (waterfowl only)

STAT Diagnostics:

- Contact veterinary regulatory authorities for access to rapid diagnostic methods including RT-PCR and fusion gene detection

Treatment:

- Not recommended. Any suspected cases of ND should be reported to veterinary regulatory authorities and euthanasia will likely be recommended

Nutritional Deficiency

Diagnosis

Clinical Signs:

- *Hypocalcemia (layers):* Fractures, weakness, paralysis, reproductive problems (thinly shelled eggs, dystocia, prolapse), acute death
- *Hypovitaminosis E:* Encephalomalacia (ataxia/paresis, rapid uncontrolled movement of extremities), exudative diathesis, myopathy in young chicks
- *Riboflavin (B2) deficiency:* Opisthotonus, hock sitting in young chicks
- *Thiamine (B1) deficiency:* Curled toes, hock sitting, emaciation in young chicks

Differentials:

- *Neurologic signs:* See Section "Neurologic Signs" for other causes of neurologic signs
- *Fractures:* Trauma

STAT Diagnostics:

- *Hypocalcemia:* Ionized calcium, radiography

Complete Diagnostics:

- *Diet analysis*

Treatment

Stabilization:

- *Parenteral supplementation with appropriate vitamin/nutrient:* Cases treated early can be reversible
- *General nutritional supplementation:* If unable to eat
- *Management of sequelae* (e.g. pathologic fractures or dystocia associated with hypocalcemia)

Continued Care:

- *Address dietary deficiencies:* Nutritional deficiencies are rarely seen in flocks fed commercially available formulated diets supplemented with judicious amounts of forage or table scraps

Septicemia

Diagnosis

Clinical Signs:

- Vary depending on specific pathogen and organ systems affected
- May include weakness, anorexia, diarrhea, respiratory signs, neurologic signs, joint swelling/lameness, and sudden death

Differentials:

- Organisms that commonly cause septicemia include
  - *E. coli* (colibacillosis)
  - *Pasteurella* (fowl cholera)
  - *Enterococcus* spp., *Staphylococcus* spp.
- Less common causes of septicemia
  - *Salmonella* spp. (pullorum, typhoid, paratyphoid)
  - Listeria

STAT Diagnostics:

- *CBC/chemistry*
- *Blood gas, electrolyte panel*

Complete Diagnostics:

- *Blood culture*
- *PCR*
- *Serology*

Treatment

Stabilization:

- Many of these diseases are reportable, and in these cases, treatment is not recommended. Flock outbreaks of septicemia should be reported to veterinary regulatory authorities and euthanasia may be recommended, depending on the causative organism
- While waiting for a diagnosis, supportive care may be provided for valuable animals with fluid therapy, nutritional support, and broad-spectrum antibiotics. Good biosecurity with isolation of clinically ill birds is necessary

Continued Care:

- Sick birds should be treated based on culture and sensitivity results
- Flock serology may also be helpful for some infectious diseases to identify asymptomatic carriers

Cardiopulmonary Disease

Aspergillosis

Diagnosis

Clinical Signs:

- *Chickens ("brooder pneumonia"):* Increased mortality in young chicks with or without dyspnea
- *Waterfowl and turkeys:* Weight loss, sudden death; respiratory signs relatively uncommon

Differentials:

- *Young birds:* See Section "Acute Flock Die-Off"
- *Adults:* Any cause of chronic nonspecific signs (see Section "Nonspecific Signs")

STAT Diagnostics:

- *Radiographs:* Evidence of air sacculitis, fungal plaques in the air sacs or trachea, and fungal pneumonia may be visible in severe cases
- *CBC:* Aspergillosis classically produces marked leukocytosis

Complete Diagnostics:

- *Tracheoscopy*
- *Coelioscopy*
- *Aspergillus panels:* Typically include serology, galactomannan assay, and protein electrophoresis; these panels are neither sensitive nor specific and confirmatory testing (cytology, histopathology) is recommended for all suspect cases
- *Necropsy*

Treatment

Stabilization:

- For valuable animals
  - *Oxygen therapy*

- *Air-sac cannula* if upper respiratory obstruction is suspected (see Chapter 24: Oxygen therapy)
- *Oral antifungals:* Azole antifungals (off-label)
- *Nebulization:* Amphotericin B and/or terbinafine (off-label)

Continued Care:

- For brooder pneumonia:
  - Thoroughly disinfect hatcher and candle eggs and discard any with evidence of fungal growth
  - Maintain cleanliness and avoid hardwood shavings when housing older chicks in brooder pens
- For adult animals
  - Maintain clean, dry housing
  - Address other diseases or causes of stress that may cause immunosuppression
  - Prognosis for affected animals is guarded

Cardiac Disease

Diagnosis

Clinical Signs:

- Dyspnea
- Coelomic fluid
- Changes in comb/mucous membrane color
- Weakness, lethargy, collapse, sudden death
- Abnormalities on cardiac auscultation including murmurs, arrhythmias, and muffled heart sounds

Differentials:

- Respiratory disease (infectious, environmental)
- Coelomic disease (reproductive disease, liver disease, GI disease)

STAT Diagnostics:

- *Radiographs:* Not very sensitive, comparison to normals from same species and breed is highly recommended for accurate interpretation, visualization of atherosclerosis associated changes in great vessels (potentially obese- or Marek's disease-associated)
- *Pulse oximetry*
- *Indirect blood pressure:* See Chapter 28: Avian pain management and anesthesia for information about blood pressure measurement in birds
- *Coelomocentesis and fluid analysis*
- *T-FAST:* To screen for pericardial effusion and cardiac chamber enlargement

Complete Diagnostics:

- *Echocardiography:* Requires an experienced ultrasonographer; easier to perform if coelomic effusion is present. Midline transcoelomic and thoracic lateral approaches are both possible in the chicken, unlike in most other birds
- *Electrocardiography:* Published normal values available for production breeds of chickens
- *CT*
- *Cardiac troponin levels* (limited in interpretation due to the lack of published reference values)
- *Blood culture* for valvular endocarditis
- *Necropsy*

Treatment

Stabilization:

- *Oxygen therapy*
- *Diuretics:* Limited data on efficacy in birds
- *Coelomocentesis* if indicated

Continued Care:

- Indications for use of cardiac drugs in poultry may be extrapolated from other species, with the understanding that information about their efficacy in poultry is limited and any use is off-label
- Cardiac disease is more common in commercial chickens and turkeys bred for meat production; avoiding these breeds for pet/backyard flocks is advisable
- Some cardiac diseases of poultry are genetic and affected animals should not be bred
- In some cases, nutrition may be a contributing factor (either through deficiency or over-nutrition leading to atherosclerosis)

Environmental Respiratory Diseases

Diagnosis

Clinical Signs:

- Dyspnea, upper respiratory signs
- Cyanotic comb and wattle
- May be worst in winter when birds spend more time in poorly ventilated and/or unsanitary coops

Differentials:

- Infectious respiratory diseases
- Cardiac disease
- Space-occupying coelomic disease
- Hyperthermia
- Stress

STAT Diagnostics:

- Positive response to removal from irritant and provision of supplemental oxygen is usually adequate for presumptive diagnosis

Complete Diagnostics:

- Consider imaging (radiography and/or CT) and CBC to rule out other causes of respiratory signs

Treatment

Stabilization:

- *Removal from irritant*
- *Supplemental oxygen*
- *Antibiotics/anti-inflammatories* as indicated
- *Bronchodilators*

Continued Care:

- Mild respiratory irritation is often self-limiting
- Maintain clean, dry, well-ventilated housing and low-dust bedding
- Allow birds outdoor time whenever weather permits

Fowl Cholera (Pasteurellosis)

Diagnosis

Clinical Signs:

- Waterfowl are less susceptible than Galliformes
- Acute mortality from septicemia (more common in turkeys)
- *Chronic form:* Swelling of infraorbital sinuses or entire head, subcutaneous caseous masses

Differentials:

- *Facial swelling: Mycoplasma* spp., infectious coryza, trauma
- *Septicemia: E. coli, Salmonella* spp., other bacterial diseases

STAT Diagnostics:

- *Necropsy* any dead bird

Complete Diagnostics:

- *Culture/PCR* for *Pasteurella*

Treatment

Stabilization:

- *Antibiotics:* Doxycycline or TMS (acute cases)
- *Supportive care*

Continued Care:

- *Surgical debridement of infected sinuses:* May be required for chronic cases with caseous masses (prognosis for cure is fair to guarded)
- *Vaccination:* Vaccines are available, but are strain-specific
- *Remove carriers:* Barn cats and rats may be reservoirs
- Complete eradication may not be possible without depopulation of the flock

Gapeworm (*Syngamus trachea*)

Diagnosis

Clinical Signs:

- More common in game birds
- Open mouth breathing, head shaking, upper respiratory noise, death from tracheal obstruction
- Prevalence varies substantially by geographic location

Differentials:

- Tracheal foreign body
- Infectious respiratory disease
- Cardiac disease
- Space-occupying coelomic disease
- Hyperthermia
- Stress

STAT Diagnostics:

- *Transillumination* of the trachea may reveal worms in some cases
- *Fecal float*

Complete Diagnostics:

- If the above, less invasive methods do not produce a diagnosis, consider tracheoscopy
- Further diagnostics investigating other causes of respiratory disease may be necessary if the response to treatment is poor

Treatment

Stabilization:

- *Benzimidazoles:* Treatment may not be successful in cases with heavy worm burden
- *Tracheoscopic worm extractions* followed by medical therapy

Continued Care:

- *Limit access to invertebrates:* Earthworms are the most common source of infection
- *Isolate infected animals:* Bird-to-bird transmission also possible

Infectious Bronchitis (Coronavirus)

Diagnosis

Clinical Signs:

- Upper respiratory signs
- Reproductive signs: Abnormal eggs (soft-shelled, shell-less, wrinkled shells)
- Systemic illness if coinfected with *E. coli* (common)

Differentials:

- Mycoplasma, fowl cholera (*Pasteurella*), low pathogenic strains of AI or ND
- Note that abnormal eggs can also be normal in hens that are going into or out of lay

STAT Diagnostics:

- *CBC*

Complete Diagnostics:

- *Serology*
- *Virus isolation*
- *PCR*

Treatment:

- Stabilization
- *Antibiotics* if secondary bacterial infection is suspected
- *Supportive care*

Continued Care:

- Vaccines are available, but are not widely used in backyard flocks. Note that vaccines are serotype-specific
- Complete eradication may not be possible without depopulation of the flock

Infectious Coryza (*Avibacterium paragallinarum, Bordetella avium*)

Diagnosis

Clinical Signs:

- Avibacterium primarily causes coryza in chickens, pheasants, guinea fowl. In turkeys and quail, Bordetella is the more common cause
- Oculonasal discharge
- Infraorbital sinus swelling
- Acute death

Differentials:

- Mycoplasma, fowl cholera (*Pasteurella*), trauma

STAT Diagnostics:

- *CBC*

Complete Diagnostics:

- *Culture:* Note that both organisms are difficult to culture
- *PCR*

Treatment

Stabilization:

- *Antibiotics:* TMS, doxycycline, or erythromycin
- *Supportive care*

Continued Care:

- *Surgical debridement* and flushing of sinuses required in severe cases
- *Vaccination:* Only effective against certain serotypes
- Complete eradication may not be possible without depopulation of the flock

Infectious Laryngotracheitis (Herpesvirus)

Diagnosis

Clinical Signs:

- Cough, head shaking
- Dyspnea, with or without hemorrhagic respiratory discharge
- Sudden death

Differentials:

- *Upper respiratory signs only:* Mycoplasma, gapeworm, "wet form" of pox
- *Dyspnea, sudden death:* Infectious disease, cardiac disease, hyperthermia, stress, space-occupying coelomic disease

STAT Diagnostics:

- *CBC*
- *Necropsy*

Complete Diagnostics:

- *PCR*
- *Histopathology*
- *Virus isolation*

Treatment

Stabilization:

- Not recommended, as birds can become latent carriers

Continued Care:

- Vaccines are available and can be used in unaffected birds in the face of an outbreak. Live vaccines can result in a carrier state.
- This disease is reportable in some areas and it is recommended to follow all necessary local regulations

Mycoplasma

Diagnosis

Clinical Signs:

- Cough, sneezing
- Infraorbital sinus swelling
- Audible respiratory sounds
- Open-beak breathing/gaping (choana often completely obstructed with caseous debris in severe cases)
- Arthritis (if present, more likely *M. synoviae*)

Differentials:

- *Upper respiratory signs:* Fowl cholera (*Pasteurella*), infectious coryza, trauma

STAT Diagnostics:

- *CBC*

Complete Diagnostics:

- *PCR* of choanal/conjunctival swabs or oculonasal discharge
- *Serology*
- *Culture:* Requires specific culture conditions

Treatment

Stabilization:

- *Antibiotics:* Tetracyclines, tylosin
- *Supportive care*

Continued Care:

- *Surgical debridement* and flushing of sinuses required in severe cases
- *Vaccines:* Reduce severity of clinical signs, but do not prevent infection
- This disease is reportable in many areas and it is recommended to follow all local regulations

Pox

Diagnosis

Clinical Signs:

- "Wet form" produces diphtheritic membranes and fibrinonecrotic material along the upper respiratory tract that can obstruct the glottis and trachea
- "Dry form" produces scabbed lesions on non-feathered skin

Differentials:

- Candidiasis (for oral lesions)
- Infectious laryngotracheitis (for tracheal signs)
- Oral and cutaneous neoplasia

STAT Diagnostics:

- *Cytology:* Intracytoplasmic inclusion bodies are present with ballooning degeneration

Complete Diagnostics:

- *Histopathology*
- *PCR*
- *Virus isolation*

Treatment

Stabilization:

- *Supportive care*

Continued Care:

- *Vaccination*
- *Insect control*

Dermatologic Disease

Ectoparasites

Diagnosis

Clinical Signs:

- Pruritus
- Feather loss
- Visible parasites

Differentials:

- *Common parasites:* Lice, mites (*Dermanyssus gallinae, Ornithonyssus sylviarum, Knemidokoptes* spp.), bedbugs, chiggers, sticktight fleas, blackflies, ticks
- *Feather loss without pruritus:* Seasonal molt, conspecific aggression (usually affects the back of the head, dorsum, or tail)
- Note that animals that have other underlying illnesses are sometimes presented for ectoparasitism due to decreased grooming behavior

STAT Diagnostics:

- *PCV:* If clinical evidence of anemia
- *Microscopic parasite exam*

Complete Diagnostics:

- Skin biopsy may be considered if there is no response to treatment, but typically is not necessary

Treatment

Stabilization:

- Supportive care (fluids, blood transfusion, nutritional support) may be required for birds with severe anemia associated with ectoparasite infestation
- Treatment of any cutaneous trauma as needed with analgesics, antibiotics, topical wound therapy, etc

Continued Care:

- Access to diatomaceous earth for dust bathing – acceptable for use in birds producing eggs for sale
- Ivermectin is effective against most ectoparasites, withdrawal times not established
- Prozap® Poultry and Garden dust (permethrin) – acceptable for use in birds producing eggs for sale

Birds

- Environmental decontamination is also required for parasites whose life cycle includes time off of the host (e.g. *D. gallinae*)
- Repeated treatment may be necessary to effectively kill emerging larvae
- Predatory mites may also be used in the environment

Dermatophytosis (Favus)

Diagnosis

Clinical Signs:

- White plaques or crusts on comb, face, or earlobes
- In severe cases, skin may acquire a honeycombed appearance
- Feather loss, starting on the head and progressing caudally

Differentials:

- *Feather loss:* Conspecific bullying, mites, other ectoparasites

STAT Diagnostics:

- *Cytology* of skin scraping

Complete Diagnostics

- *Dermatophyte culture*

Treatment

Stabilization:

- Topical antifungal therapy
- Counsel owners to wear gloves, as this infection is potentially zoonotic

Continued Care:

- Separate from other birds, scales may be infective
- Avoid frequent bathing of birds, as this may increase risk

Frostbite

Diagnosis

Clinical Signs:

- Necrosis of distal extremities, including toes, combs, and wattles with compatible history

Differentials:

- Trauma/constriction injury

STAT Diagnostics:

- None if stable
- *Thermal imaging of the limbs:* To confirm functional vascular supply

Complete Diagnostics:

- History and clinical signs are typically sufficient for diagnosis

Treatment

Stabilization:

- *Antibiotics*
- *Analgesics*
- *Topical wound care:* See Chapter 26: Wound care and bandaging techniques

Continued Care:

- *Surgical amputation (severe cases):* It is recommended to wait several days for a clear line of demarcation to appear
- *Pentoxifylline* to enhance blood flow to extremities
- *Prevention:* Discuss provision of appropriate heat support to decrease likelihood of recurrence

Gangrenous Dermatitis

Diagnosis

Clinical Signs:

- Skin necrosis over wings, thighs, breast, and head
- May develop septicemia

Differentials:

- Traumatic wounds

STAT Diagnostics:

- *CBC/chemistry* to evaluate for possible sepsis

Complete Diagnostics:

- *Tissue culture*

Treatment

Stabilization:

- *Systemic antibiotics:* Ideally chosen based on culture. Penicillin may be a good empirical choice due to frequent involvement of Clostridial organisms and *Staphylococcus aureus*
- *Supportive care:* Fluid therapy and nutritional support for systemically ill birds

Continued Care:

- *Surgical debridement* (see Chapter 26: Wound care and bandaging techniques)
- *Environmental modifications:* Reduce moisture and in poultry houses, remove sharp items that might cause wounds, assure overall good flock health (through appropriate nutrition, vaccination, etc.)

Pox

Diagnosis

Clinical Signs:

- Round, raised, scabbed lesions in the mouth and on unfeathered areas of head, neck, and feet of chickens and turkeys
- Lesions in the mouth/upper airway may cause respiratory distress

Differentials:

- Cutaneous neoplasia
- Knemidocoptes infestation

STAT Diagnostics:

- Presumptive diagnosis may be reached based on appearance of lesions

Complete Diagnostics:

- *Histopathology* of lesions
- *Virus isolation*

Treatment

Stabilization:

- *Supportive care:* Fluid therapy, nutritional support, removal of lesions causing respiratory obstruction
- *Isolation* of affected animals, as scabbed material is infectious

Continued Care:

- *Flock vaccination*
- *Control of biting arthropods*

Traumatic Wounds

Diagnosis

Clinical Signs:

- Common locations for predator injuries include the head (see Figure 38.6), dorsum, and rump
- Note that feathers can easily obscure even relatively large wounds
- +/− clinical signs associated with shock
- +/− other traumatic injuries

Differentials:

- Frostbite, gangrenous dermatitis

STAT Diagnostics:

- *CBC*

Complete Diagnostics:

- *Radiographs:* If indicated to rule out other traumatic injuries

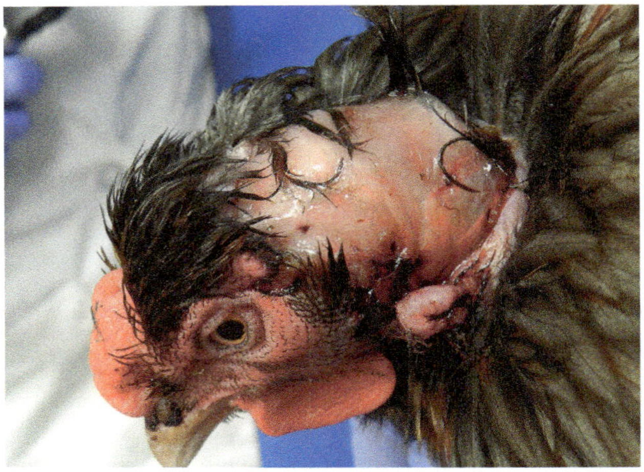

Figure 38.6 Adult domestic chicken with a severe dorsal cervical full thickness wound sustained during a hawk attack. Note the pale comb and wattle and the involvement of the left ear and earlobe.

Treatment

Stabilization:

- *Fluid therapy:* IV, IO, or SC, as indicated
- *Analgesia:* With kappa agonist opioids and/or nonsteroidal anti-inflammatories (all off-label)
- *Systemic antibiotics*: If indicated
- *Wound lavage:* First evaluating for air sac involvement to avoid aspiration

Continued Care:

- Poultry have a tremendous capacity to heal even very extensive wounds with appropriate therapy. See Chapter 26: Wound care and bandaging techniques for more detail on bandaging and wound management in avian species
- Poultry should be housed indoors until wounds are healed to prevent myiasis

Gastrointestinal Disease

Bacterial Enteritis

Diagnosis

Clinical Signs:

- Diarrhea, change in fecal color or odor, weight loss
- Nonspecific sick bird signs, septicemia, sudden death

Differentials:

- *Bacterial disease: Salmonella* spp., *E. coli*, *Clostridium* spp., *Mycobacterium* spp.
- *Viral disease:* Newcastle disease, AI, duck viral enteritis

STAT Diagnostics:

- *Fecal cytology:* Looking primarily for spore-forming organisms
- *Necropsy*

Complete Diagnostics:

- *Culture* of feces or abnormal tissue at necropsy
- *Serologic tests:* Available for *Salmonella* spp., *E. coli*
- *Fecal floatation:* Intestinal parasitism such as coccidiosis may increase risk of bacterial enteritis

Treatment

Stabilization:

- *Treatment not recommended for: Salmonella* spp. (potentially reportable and zoonotic), *Clostridium* spp. (usually unrewarding), *Mycobacterium* spp. (unrewarding, some species may be zoonotic)
- Other causes of bacterial GI disease may respond to supportive care

Continued Care:

- *Salmonella spp.:* Transmission can be vertical, so no eggs should be incubated from affected flocks
- *E. coli:* Vaccination may decrease clinical signs, but vaccine not widely available for backyard flocks
- *Clostridium spp.:* Change litter more frequently

Crop Stasis/Impaction

Diagnosis

Clinical Signs:

- Crop distended with fluid or desiccated contents (see Figure 38.1)
- Anorexia
- Regurgitation – less common than in psittacines

Differentials:

- See Section "Crop Distension"

STAT Diagnostics:

- *Crop cytology:* Note that overgrowth of yeast and bacteria is common, but may be secondary to underlying GI disease, rather than the primary problem

Complete Diagnostics:

- *CBC/chemistry*
- *Contrast radiography* to assist in diagnosing an obstruction and to evaluate GI motility
- *Ultrasound*
- *Heavy metal testing:* As indicated

Treatment

Stabilization:

- *Liquid crop contents:* Consider aspiration (though contents are often too thick), crop support (a.k.a. "crop bra")
- *Solid crop contents:* Oral and parenteral fluid therapy

Continued Care:

- Varies depending on underlying cause

GI Foreign Body

Diagnosis

Clinical Signs:

- *Nonspecific sick bird signs:* Lethargy, anorexia, weight loss
- Crop distension/delayed crop emptying
- Vomiting is rarely seen
- Potential CNS signs with heavy metal foreign body

Differentials:

- See Sections "Crop Distension" and "Nonspecific Signs"

STAT Diagnostics:

- *Radiographs* +/− contrast, as needed

Complete Diagnostics:

- *CBC/chemistry*
- *Blood lead/zinc levels*

Treatment

Stabilization:

- *Fluid therapy*
- *Chelation* if indicated

Continued Care:

- *Endoscopy* (see Figure 38.7): Often unrewarding, as visualization of foreign material is typically obscured by accumulated food material
- *Gastric lavage*
- *Surgical foreign body removal*

Hemorrhagic Enteritis (Adenovirus)

Diagnosis

Clinical Signs:

- Affects young turkeys (usually 6–12 weeks)
- Depression
- Severe intestinal hemorrhage
- Sudden death
- *Subclinical form:* Immunosuppression

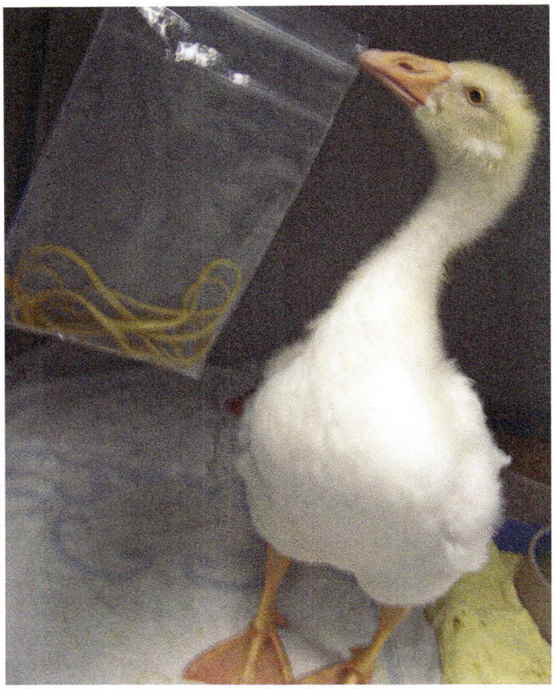

Figure 38.7 Sebastopol gosling (*Anser anser domesticus*) pictured with the large rubber band that was endoscopically retrieved from the esophagus and proventriculus. The gosling was presented for evaluation of acute anorexia and vomiting, the foreign body was confirmed with radiographs, and the bird recovered without noted complications post-procedure (see Section "GI Foreign Body").

Differentials:

- Bacterial: *Pasteurella*, *Erysipelothrix*, *Salmonella gallinarum*, paratyphoid (*Salmonella* spp.)
- Viral: Turkey coronavirus, avian influenza, Newcastle disease

STAT Diagnostics:

- *Necropsy*

Complete Diagnostics:

- *Serology*
- *Histopathology:* Spleen is preferred sample

Treatment

Stabilization:

- *Supportive care*
- *Antibiotics* for immunosuppressive form
- *Antiserum* may reduce mortality, if available

Continued Care:

- Vaccine available
- May be reportable in some areas

Histomonas meleagridis

Diagnosis

Clinical Signs:

- Primarily a disease of turkeys, but also reported in chickens (often asymptomatic)
- Diarrhea
- Nonspecific signs of illness

Differentials:

- Bacterial disease: *Salmonella* spp., *E. coli*, *Clostridium* spp., *Erysipelothrix*
- Viral diseases: Turkey coronavirus, avian influenza, Newcastle disease
- Parasitic/protozoal disease: Coccidia, ascarids, *Cryptosporidium* spp.

STAT Diagnostics:

- *Necropsy:* Necrotic liver lesions and cecal thickening. Flagellates can sometimes be identified in saline wet-mounts of necrotic hepatic lesions

Complete Diagnostics:

- *Histopathology:* Carcass must be very fresh, as Histomonads autolyze quickly
- *Culture* of cecal contents. Requires Dwyer's media, a specialized culture medium that is not widely available

Treatment

Stabilization:

- No treatment once clinical signs have developed

Continued Care:

- Do not house turkeys or game birds near chickens/pheasants, which commonly serve as reservoirs
- Nitrasone may be helpful in preventing outbreaks
- Benzamidazoles to treat for the *Heterakis* nematode that transmits *H. meleagridis* may also be helpful in prevention

Parasitic Disease

Diagnosis

Clinical Signs:

- Diarrhea, weight loss
- Often incidental finding on necropsy

Differentials:

- Bacterial enteritis

STAT Diagnostics:

- *Fecal floatation:* Common organisms seen include *Eimeria* spp. and ascarids. Cryptosporidium, cestodes, and trematodes rarely reported

Complete Diagnostics:

- *Histopathology*

Treatment

Stabilization:

- *Supportive care*
- *Coccidiostats:* Products readily available to most small animal practitioners include sulfadimethoxine and toltrazuril; amprolium has no withdrawal time and is available over the counter, but is subjectively less effective; sulfadimethoxine/toltrazuril may be more effective, but their use is off-label in the United States
- *Other anthelmintics:* As indicated. Note that most are off-label in poultry

Continued Care:

- *Environmental management* to decrease likelihood of continued infection, house adults and juveniles separately
- *Medicated feeds* for coccidia (usually contain ionophores, such as monensin)
- *Coccidia vaccines* exist and may be available through hatcheries, but typically are not used in backyard poultry

Neoplasia

Lymphoid Leukosis (Retrovirus)

Diagnosis

Clinical Signs:

- Typically chicks 14–40 weeks old
- Lack of appetite, diarrhea, emaciation, weakness
- Firm coelomic distension due to organomegaly (predominantly hepatomegaly)

Differentials:

- *Nonspecific signs:* Many differentials see Section "Nonspecific Signs"
- *Firm coelomic distension:* Organomegaly, tumors (Marek's disease lymphoma is a top consideration, but typically younger chicks), granulomas, intracoelomic eggs

STAT Diagnostics:

- *Necropsy* – multiple gray-white masses in viscera

Complete Diagnostics:

- *Serology*
- *Virus isolation* from fresh tissue

Treatment:

- No treatment – euthanasia recommended

Reproductive Neoplasia

Diagnosis

Clinical Signs:

- Lethargy, decreased appetite, weight loss
- Decreased or no egg production
- Palpable intracoelomic mass effect in some cases

Differentials:

- *Other reproductive disease:* Cystic ovaries, salpingitis, oviductal impaction, ectopic eggs

STAT Diagnostics:

- *CBC/chemistry*
- *Radiographs*
- *A-fast:* Ascites or a large mass may be visualized

Complete Diagnostics:

- *Coelomic ultrasound:* Requires experienced ultrasonographer

Treatment

Stabilization:

- *Fluid therapy:* SC, IV, or IO, as indicated
- *Antibiotics* if other concurrent reproductive diseases are suspected (common)
- *Analgesia*
- *Nutritional support*

Continued Care:

- *Salpingohysterectomy +/− ovariectomy:* Often very difficult, requires an experienced surgeon
- *Hormonal treatment* may increase survival time in early or presumptive diagnosis, see Section "Treatment" in Reproductive Signs

Neurologic/Musculoskeletal Disease

Arthritis

Diagnosis

Clinical Signs:

- Swollen, painful joint(s)

Differentials:

- Septic arthritis including that caused by *M. synoviae*
- Traumatic wounds
- Gout

STAT Diagnostics:

- *CBC*
- *Radiographs*

Complete Diagnostics:

- *Joint aspirate* for cytology, culture, Mycoplasma PCR

Treatment

Stabilization:

- *Antibiotic therapy* based on culture
- *Analgesia*

Continued Care:

- *Regional limb perfusion* with targeted antibiotics
- *Surgical intervention:* Debridement, arthrodesis, amputation (pelvic limb amputation poorly tolerated in most poultry)
- *Environmental modification* for altered mobility
- *Monitor* for development of pododermatitis (bumblefoot; see Figure 38.2) and/or keel sores

Arthropod-borne Encephalitides

Diagnosis

Clinical Signs:

- *Eastern/Western equine encephalitis:* Chickens are usually asymptomatic, game birds and turkeys may develop neurologic signs
- *West Nile virus:* Neurologic signs in ducks, most other poultry are asymptomatic carriers

Differentials:

- Neurologic signs in ducks/game birds – trauma, botulism, duck hepatitis virus, toxin, nutritional deficiencies

STAT Diagnostics:

- *Necropsy*

Complete Diagnostics:

- *Flock serology*

Treatment

Stabilization:

- *Supportive care:* No specific treatment, but some animals may survive with supportive care

Continued Care:

- All three diseases are potentially zoonotic, and this should be considered when making the decision to treat. While direct transmission is not thought to be possible, the public health ramifications of having a flock of viremic birds should be considered. These diseases may be reportable in some areas

Avian Encephalomyelitis (Picornavirus)

Diagnosis

Clinical Signs:

- Ataxia and head tremors in 1- to 3-week-old chickens and game birds
- Birds infected when >4 weeks rarely show clinical signs

Differentials:

- Nutritional deficiency
- Infectious diseases: *Pasteurella*, *Salmonella*, *Listeria*, avian influenza, Newcastle disease, eastern equine encephalitis (EEE), western equine encephalitis (WEE), west nile virus (WNV)

STAT Diagnostics:

- *Necropsy*

Complete Diagnostics:

- *Serology*

Treatment

Stabilization:

- *Supportive care:* Many birds will survive with good supportive care, but permanent neurologic deficits may remain

Continued Care:

- *Vaccinate layer hens*; vertical transmission is the most common source of infection
- This disease is reportable in many areas and it is recommended to follow all local regulations

Congenital/Developmental Limb Deformities

Diagnosis

Clinical Signs:

- Lateral deviation of one or both legs (leg can be affected at any level) (see Figure 38.3)
- *Acute dropped hock:* May indicate gastrocnemius tendon dislocation (perosis) or rupture (most common in meat birds)

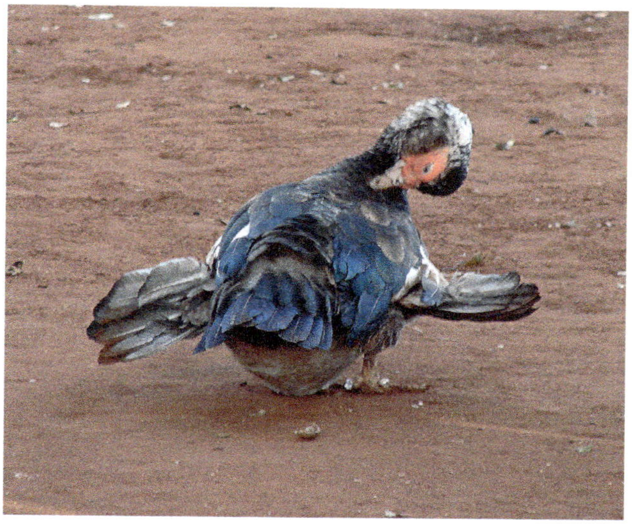

Figure 38.8 Free-range Muscovy duck in Mozambique with bilateral carpometacarpal bone deformity ("angel wing"). A nutritional etiology was suspected, as the flock primarily foraged and was not offered a formulated diet (see Section "Congenital/Developmental Limb Deformities").

- Rotation of the wings at carpometacarpal bone (angel wing; see Figure 38.8) in waterfowl

Differentials:

- Traumatic injury

STAT Diagnostics:

- *Radiographs:* To rule out fracture/luxation

Complete Diagnostics:

- None

Treatment

Stabilization:

- *Corrective bandaging* may be helpful for rotational limb deformities if started early. Owners should be aware that management can be protracted and intensive, with bandage adjustments required every 1–3 days. Corrective bandaging is unlikely to be successful in heavy-bodied birds or those in which treatment is delayed
- *Surgery:* Surgical therapy has been reported for gastrocnemius tendon dislocation, but success rates are highly variable. Prognosis worsens with chronicity. Derotation osteotomy has been reported for rotational limb deformities, but is associated with a guarded prognosis

Continued Care:

- Failure to correct the deformities could result in multiple complications (pododermatitis, arthritis, etc.) and negatively affect quality of life
- Gastrocnemius tendon dislocation has been associated with deficiencies of choline, manganese, and/or biotin. Adjust diet as indicated

Fractures

Diagnosis

Clinical Signs:

- Lameness, wing droop
- Other evidence of trauma (wounds, feather loss)

Differentials:

- *Other traumatic injury:* Soft tissue injury, nerve injury, slipped gastrocnemius tendon
- *Neurologic disease:* Marek's disease, nutritional deficiencies

STAT Diagnostics:

- *Radiographs*

Complete Diagnostics:

- None, unless other trauma is suspected

Treatment

Stabilization:

- *Supportive care:* Fluid therapy, nutritional support, analgesia
- *Wound care:* As indicated, be advised that fractures may directly communicate with the respiratory system through air sac diverticula/pneumatized bones and wound lavage could lead to aspiration
- *Bandaging:* If appropriate, based on fracture location. See Chapter 26: Wound care and bandaging techniques for more detail on bandaging in birds

Continued Care:

- *Fracture repair:* Specific techniques and prognosis depend on the location of the fracture, but chickens generally tolerate fracture repair very well. Larger-bodied or higher-stress species may be more challenging
- *Bandaging:* While return to function is generally superior with surgical fracture repair, many fractures will heal with appropriate external coaptation and cage rest
- *Other considerations:* Waterfowl should be allowed access to water as soon as possible to prevent pododermatitis. Range of motion exercises should be performed as soon as possible in birds with wing fractures to prevent patagial contracture

Marek's Disease (MD)

Diagnosis

Clinical Signs:

- *Classic form ("fowl paralysis"):* Unilateral paresis with leg extended, typically seen in 6 to 12-week-old chickens
- Torticollis, abnormal head movements
- *MD lymphoma:* Diffuse nodular lesions in viscera, occasionally with skin or ocular involvement

Differentials:

- *Classic form:* Trauma, nutritional deficiency, neurotoxin
- *MD lymphoma:* Avian leukosis virus, mycobacteriosis

STAT Diagnostics:

- *Necropsy*

Complete Diagnostics:

- *Serology:* Interpretation is difficult because many chickens are latently infected by gallid herpesvirus 2, but only a small portion will go on to develop Marek's disease
- *PCR/virus isolation:* Subject to the same limitations as serology

Treatment

Stabilization:

- No treatment

Continued Care:

- Maintaining a flock that is vaccinated for Marek's disease is strongly recommended. Most poultry distributors offer chicks that have already been vaccinated for a nominal fee. The logistics of vaccination can be challenging for chicks hatched at home

Pododermatitis

Diagnosis

Clinical Signs:

- Swelling, scabbing, or ulceration of the metatarsal pad of one or both feet. Waterfowl may also have lesions at interphalangeal joints (see Figure 38.2). Can extend to include osteomyelitis in underlying bones
- Birds typically do not display lameness until lesions are severe

Differentials:

- *Lameness:* Fracture, soft tissue injury, neurologic injury
- Note that pododermatitis is often the result of another illness, either as the result of a change in weight bearing or decreased activity

STAT Diagnostics:

- *Radiographs:* To evaluate for associated osteomyelitis

Complete Diagnostics:

- *Tissue culture: S. aureus* is the most common bacteria isolated from these lesions in chickens

Treatment

Stabilization:

- *Antibiotics, analgesia, soaks in Epsom salt:* May be adequate for mild cases
- *Surgical debridement:* Often required for advanced cases, followed by bandaging

Continued Care:

- *Wound management:* Many patients require long term bandaging, custom-made shoes, and repeat debridement. See Chapter 26: Wound care and bandaging techniques. Chickens tend to heal faster and respond better to treatment than raptors
- *Address underlying medical problems*
- *Address husbandry deficiencies*
- Provide clean, dry bedding
- Remove sharp objects that might act as penetrating foreign bodies
- Provide an accessible pond/pool for waterfowl
- Avoid over-feeding to prevent obesity

Ophthalmic Disease

Infectious Sinusitis

Diagnosis

Clinical Signs:

- While the primary disease in most of these cases is respiratory, many owners will present these patients due to concerns about ocular and periocular signs
- Severe periorbital swelling
- Oculonasal discharge
- Sneezing, increased respiratory noise, dyspnea

Differentials:

- *Oxyspiruriasis (eye worm):* Rare, typically causes conjunctivitis, responsive to ivermectin
- Ocular foreign body
- Trauma

Diagnostics:

- See Section "Respiratory Signs"

Treatment:

- See Section "Respiratory Signs"

Marek's Disease (Herpesvirus)

Diagnosis

Clinical Signs

- Blue or gray discoloration of the iris due to lymphocyte infiltration (uncommon)
- Lameness, paresis, nonspecific neurological signs
- Coelomic masses

Differentials:

- Traumatic injury
- Species/individual variation in iris color

STAT Diagnostics:

- None

Complete Diagnostics:

- See Section "Marek's Disease (MD)"

Treatment

Stabilization:

- No treatment

Continued Care:

- See Section "Marek's Disease (MD)"

Ocular Trauma

Diagnosis

Clinical Signs:

- Blepharospasm, eyelid laceration
- Discharge
- Corneal ulceration, visible ocular foreign body

Differentials:

- Mycoplasma
- Oxyspirura (eye worm, very rare)

STAT Diagnostics:

- *Fluorescein stain*

Complete Diagnostics:

- *Evaluation by ophthalmologist* – as needed

Treatment

Stabilization:

- Lubrication and analgesia, as indicated
- Note that many commonly used ophthalmic antibiotics are not approved for use in food animals in the United States. Consult the Food Animal Residue Avoidance Databank before selecting a topical antibiotic

Continued Care:

- Varies, depending on nature of injury

Urogenital and Reproductive Disease

Dystocia

Diagnosis

Clinical Signs:

- *Often nonspecific:* Anorexia, lethargy, urate accumulation around vent
- Straining to lay, coelomic distension with/without palpable egg

Differentials:

- Other intracoelomic disease

STAT Diagnostics:

- *Radiographs:* Standing radiographs may be adequate for initial imaging

Complete Diagnostics:

- *For recurrent cases:* Consider additional blood work (CBC, chemistry, ionized calcium), ultrasound, tissue biopsies, coelomic explore to determine underlying cause

Treatment

Stabilization:

- See Section "Reproductive Signs" for more detail on management of dystocia

Continued Care:

- Address underlying husbandry problems or reproductive disease that may have contributed to dystocia

Gout

Diagnosis

Clinical Signs:

- *Visceral gout:* Weakness, dehydration, anorexia
- *Articular gout:* Joint swelling (possibly affecting multiple joints)

Differentials:

- Visceral form – see Section "Nonspecific Signs"
- Articular form – septic arthritis, trauma

STAT Diagnostics:

- *Joint aspirate (articular form only):* Gout crystals are best visualized using polarized light, but can also be seen with standard microscopy

Complete Diagnostics:

- *CBC/chemistry:* Uric acid levels may fluctuate significantly, so a normal uric acid level does not rule out renal disease
- *Coelomic endoscopy:* May reveal uric acid deposits on viscera, also allows for endoscopic renal biopsy

Treatment

Stabilization:

- Visceral gout usually only occurs with acute, fulminant renal failure, so prognosis, even with aggressive fluid therapy, is guarded

Continued Care:

- Some cases of articular gout can be managed with analgesics, allopurinol, and good hydration
- Prevention
  - *Diet:* Diets very high in protein may be associated with hyperuricemia. While the levels required are so high that this is unlikely to be a contributing factor if the bird is being fed a commercial diet, exceptions could occur in cases of home-made diets or manufacturer error
  - *Genetics:* May be a contributing factor, so avoid breeding affected animals

Prolapse

Diagnosis

Clinical Signs:

- Visible prolapse of tissue from the vent, which may include cloaca, uterus/oviduct, colon, or phallus (in waterfowl)
- Seen occasionally secondary to straining with dystocia in poultry, common in waterfowl associated with excessive mating

Differentials:

- Cloacal neoplasia

STAT Diagnostics:

- *CBC*
- *Radiographs:* To rule out dystocia or other lesion causing increased coelomic pressure or straining

Complete Diagnostics:

- *For recurrent cases:* Consider additional blood work (chemistry, ionized calcium), ultrasound, tissue biopsies, coelomic explore to determine underlying cause

Treatment

Stabilization:

- *Treat dystocia*, if present
- *Replace prolapse* and *perform temporary cloacorraphy* (two to three transverse sutures)
- See Section "Reproductive Signs" for more detail

Continued Care:

- Address underlying husbandry problems or reproductive disease that may have contributed to prolapse

Other Reproductive Tract Disease:

- *Ovarian disease:* Cystic ovaries, ovarian neoplasia, oophoritis
- *Oviductal/uterine disease:* Oviductal impaction, salpingitis, uterine rupture, uterine torsion, neoplasia

Diagnosis

Clinical Signs:

- Coelomic distension
- Failure to lay, production of abnormal eggs
- Weakness, anorexia, unwillingness to stand
- Death

Differentials:

- Cardiac disease
- Other neoplasia

STAT Diagnostics:

- *Radiographs*
- *Coelomocentesis* w/fluid analysis (if coelomic effusion present)

Complete Diagnostics:

- *CBC/chemistry*
- *Coelomic ultrasound*
- *Coelomic surgical explore*
- Note that these diseases are very difficult to differentiate in a live bird and are often definitively diagnosed at surgery or necropsy. See Section "Reproductive Signs" for more detail

Treatment

Stabilization:

- *Supportive care:* Varies by underlying disease process

Continued Care:

See Section "Reproductive Signs" for more detail

Further Reading

Coles, B.H. (2000). Galliformes. In: *Handbook of Avian Medicine*, 2nde (eds. T.N. Tully, G.M. Dorrestein and A.K. Jones), 266–295. Cornwall: Butterworth-Heinemann.

Food Animal Residue Avoidance Databank [Internet] (2016). Food Animal Residue Avoidance Databank (cited 2016 June 16). www.farad.org (accessed 20 October 2020).

Greenacre, C.B. (2015). Reproductive diseases of the backyard hen. *J. Exot. Pet Med.* 24: 164–171.

Greenacre, C.B. and Morishita, T.Y. (eds.) (2015). *Backyard Poultry Medicine and Surgery*. Ames: Wiley-Blackwell.

Grunkemeyer, V.L. (2011). Zoonoses, public health, and the backyard poultry flock. *Vet. Clin. North Am. Exot. Anim. Pract.* 14: 477–490.

Marmulak, T., Tell, L.A., Gehring, R. et al. (2015). Egg residue consideration during the treatment of backyard poultry. *J. Am. Vet. Med. Assoc.* 247 (12): 1388–1395.

Merck Veterinary Manual (2016). Poultry. Kenilworth, NJ: Merck, Sharp, and Dohme Corp (cited 2016 Jun 17). http://www.merckvetmanual.com/mvm/poultry.html (accessed 20 October 2020).

Pattison, M., McMullin, P.F., Bradbury, J.M., and Alexander, D.J. (eds.) (2008). *Poultry Diseases*, 6the. Philadelphia, PA: Butterworth-Heinemann.

Routh, A. and Sanderson, S. (2000). Waterfowl. In: *Handbook of Avian Medicine*, 2nde (eds. T.N. Tully, G.M. Dorrestein and A.K. Jones), 234–265. Cornwall: Butterworth-Heinemann.

Swayne, D.E., Glisson, J.R., McDougald, L.R. et al. (eds.) (2013). *Diseases of Poultry*, 13the. Ames: Wiley-Blackwell.

Wakenell, P. (2015). Management and medicine of backyard poultry. In: *Current Therapy in Avian Medicine and Surgery* (ed. B. Speer), 550–565. Philadelphia, PA: Saunders.

Part 3

Reptile and Amphibian

Section 1

Triage and Stabilization

39

History and Clinical Exam

Grayson A. Doss and Kurt K. Sladky

Department of Surgical Sciences, School of Veterinary Medicine, University of Wisconsin-Madison, Madison, Wisconsin, USA

CONTENTS

Initial Phone Consultation

Is It an Emergency?

What constitutes a reptile or amphibian emergency? An initial phone conversation with the client allows for discernment regarding whether or not the described concerns constitute a true medical emergency. Frequently, the owner perceives decompensation of a chronic illness as an acute problem; for example, chronic preovulatory stasis in a tortoise may lead to observable, acute anorexia as described by the client. On the other hand, collapse, severe weakness, fractures or luxations, hemorrhage, dyspnea, cloacal prolapse, predator attacks, vomiting, neurologic signs, firefly ingestion, and overt lethargy constitute true emergencies in reptile and amphibian patients.

See Box 39.1 for a list of common clinical signs or abnormalities that usually warrant emergency evaluation.

Owner Instructions

See Table 39.1 for a list of first aid tips for clients regarding common emergency conditions in reptiles and amphibians.

Contacting the client before patient arrival affords the clinician the chance to provide advice regarding life-saving first aid, as well as have the owner bring relevant husbandry items, including specific information about nutrition supplements, lighting, and/or water quality. Obtaining a patient's signalment can assist the clinician in contemplating possible differentials before the patient arrives.

History

The clinical history provides important information regarding the patient and assists the clinician in making critical case management and treatment decisions. Having a second person available to obtain a history allows the clinician to focus immediate attention on the patient, while simultaneously gathering potentially useful information about the clinical presentation. For example, with traumatic injuries, the type of trauma is crucial in order to guide specific therapy. Initial fracture treatment secondary to a fall will differ from that provided to a patient who has been attacked by a dog or cat. Discussing the duration, severity, and progression of clinical signs with the owner helps guide diagnostic, treatment, and prognostic decisions. A downloadable herptile history form is available at www.wiley.com.

Husbandry

Many diseases of reptiles and amphibians are secondary to poor husbandry, therefore, developing detailed husbandry-related questions for the client is extremely important for

Exotic Animal Emergency and Critical Care Medicine, First Edition. Edited by Jennifer E. Graham, Grayson A. Doss and Hugues Beaufrère.

Box 39.1 Clinical Signs or Abnormalities Organized by Body System that Typically Warrant Immediate Evaluation in Reptiles and Amphibians

- **General**
  - Lethargy or dull mentation
  - Collapse
  - Active hemorrhage
  - Weakness
  - Prolapse of tissue from vent
  - Dehydration
  - Coelomic enlargement (unless expected, e.g. a breeding female)
  - Vocalization
  - Exposure to extreme temperatures (e.g. left in car or outside)
  - Ingestion of firefly
  - Ingestion of (suspected) toxic substance (e.g. toxic plants, rodenticides)
- **Trauma**
  - Thermal or chemical burns
  - Prey or conspecific attacks
  - Falls
  - Vehicular, lawn equipment trauma
  - Injuries from inappropriate cage furniture
- **Musculoskeletal**
  - Fractures (open and closed)
  - Lameness, limb paresis or paralysis
  - Poor body condition score
  - Masses
- **Gastrointestinal**
  - Acute-onset vomiting/regurgitation
  - Constant tenesmus
  - Oral asymmetry or discharge
- **Reproductive**
  - Dystocia
  - Phallus or hemipenal prolapse
- **Neurologic**
  - Seizures
  - Circling
  - Head tilt
  - Nystagmus
  - Abnormal posture (e.g. opisthotonus)
  - Muscle tremors or fasciculations
  - Loss of righting reflex
- **Dermatologic** (loss of skin integrity can be clinically significant for amphibians)
  - Generalized skin abnormalities
  - Skin lacerations or wounds
  - Severe mite infestation
- **Ophthalmic**
  - Blepharospasm
  - Ocular trauma
  - Foreign body
  - Proptosis
  - Corneal ulcer
- **Respiratory**
  - Abnormal respiratory noise
  - Dyspnea
  - Open-mouth breathing
  - Significant nasal discharge

case management, particularly with respect to diagnostic plans. Herptiles are often presented for clinical signs associated with nutritional secondary hyperparathyroidism, and determining diet, nutritional supplementation (e.g. calcium, phosphorus, vitamin D_3, etc.), and ultraviolet light B spectrum (UVB) exposure often reinforces a clinical impression. Having an owner fill out a prepared questionnaire regarding their pet's husbandry, while the patient is triaged, can save valuable time. A detailed overview of reptile and amphibian husbandry is beyond the scope of this chapter and an overview of important aspects will be discussed.

Enclosure

Reptiles and amphibians should be maintained in an environment that is well ventilated, yet maintains humidity and temperature levels appropriate for the natural history of the species. Enclosure temperatures should be monitored closely for fluctuations.

Use of "hot rocks" or other in-cage heating materials should be avoided due to frequent poor construction resulting in the material reaching extreme surface temperatures, which can result in severe thermal burns (Figure 39.1). Some "under-tank" heaters designed to adhere directly to the aquarium glass may also reach unsuitable temperatures, leading to thermal injuries.

Fresh water should be provided at all times, even for desert-dwelling species. For amphibians and aquatic reptiles, water quality is of utmost importance. Water should be chlorine-free and kept clean using filtration or daily water changes. Aquatic turtles produce a large amount of excreta, and, therefore, heavy filtration is typically required in order to prevent unsanitary conditions.

Table 39.1 First aid suggestions for common reptile and amphibian emergencies.

Emergency	Owner instructions
Active hemorrhage	• Apply digital pressure to the affected site using a clean object, such as gauze, paper or cloth towel, cotton ball, or cotton swab • Application of clean cornstarch, flour, or styptic powder can slow bleeding, but should be used cautiously in amphibians due to their delicate skin and percutaneous respiration and absorption • Wait 3–5 min before removing the pressure to evaluate for clotting • Create a pressure bandage to hold pressure to the area if owner is unable to maintain digital pressure (e.g. driving) • If the hemorrhage is on a distal appendage (e.g. tail or limb) and digital pressure is unsuccessful in controlling it, can apply a tourniquet – Do not use excessive tension which can result in ischemia and tissue necrosis; can loosen for several seconds every 15–20 min to support perfusion of the tissue distal to the tourniquet • Prevent contamination from substrate or other objects (e.g. wear gloves)
Cutaneous wounds	• Control hemorrhage (see above) • Prevent contamination from substrate or other objects (e.g. wear gloves)
Prolapse of tissue from vent	• Control hemorrhage (see above), if applicable • Remove animal off of substrate which can adhere to or traumatize the tissue – Place the animal in a clean enclosure lined with non-adherent substrate for transport • Remove conspecifics that can traumatize (e.g. bite) the tissue from the vicinity • Prevent contamination from substrate or other objects (e.g. wear gloves) • Can apply sterile water-based lubricant to tissue if there is a significant delay before veterinary evaluation
Exposure to extreme environmental temperatures	• Attempt to cool or warm the animal back to an environmental temperature that is within its preferred optimal temperature zone (POTZ) – Warming or cooling should be performed slowly – Can place animal on or next to a warm or ice pack wrapped in cloth ∘ Do not let the warm or ice pack directly contact the animal – Aquatic species can be placed in shallow, warm or cool water (dechlorinated for amphibians) if they are not at risk of drowning (e.g. have a dull mentation). The temperature of the water used should ideally be within the POTZ for the species. • Do not attempt to rapidly cool the animal with topical application of ice, ice water, or alcohol
Ingestion of firefly or other toxic substance	• Remove animal from the vicinity of the toxic substance to prevent further ingestion • Do not attempt to induce vomiting (e.g. administer hydrogen peroxide, ipecac syrup) • Safely collect a sample (or smartphone images) of the material (e.g. plant, insect) or product information of the substance (e.g. chemical, rodenticide) ingested, to bring to veterinary hospital
Topical exposure to harsh chemicals	• Remove animal from the vicinity of the toxic substance to prevent further exposure • Copiously rinse the area as soon as possible with tap water or with dechlorinated/enclosure water (amphibians) • Follow topical exposure recommendations for humans listed on the product label
Trauma	• Control hemorrhage (see above), if applicable • Minimize handling and place the animal in a clean enclosure lined with non-adherent substrate for transport

(*Continued*)

Table 39.1 (Continued)

Emergency	Owner instructions
Fractures	• Control hemorrhage (see above), if applicable • Minimize handling and carefully place the animal in a clean enclosure for transport – Should not contain cage furniture that can be climbed (e.g. branches) in order to prevent falls • For open fractures (e.g. shell fractures), do not touch the area except to control hemorrhage or to cover with clean material to prevent contamination from substrate or other objects • Do not attempt to splint or reduce the fracture
Neurologic signs	• Remove elevated areas or climbing structures (e.g. branches) in the enclosure to prevent inadvertent falls • Remove deep water sources to prevent drowning • Place animal in a clean enclosure padded with blankets to prevent self-injury (e.g. seizures, ataxia)
Ophthalmic abnormalities	• Control hemorrhage (see above), if applicable • Do not attempt to flush the affected eye(s) with any liquids or remove any foreign material • Attempt to prevent the animal from further traumatizing the eye(s) (e.g. rubbing eye on surfaces or with limb)

These tips can be provided to owners while they are preparing to transport the animal for veterinary evaluation. Ideally, owners should wear gloves when dealing with open wounds, exposed tissue, controlling hemorrhage, or handling potential toxic substances. These recommendations are not a replacement for veterinary medical evaluation and care.

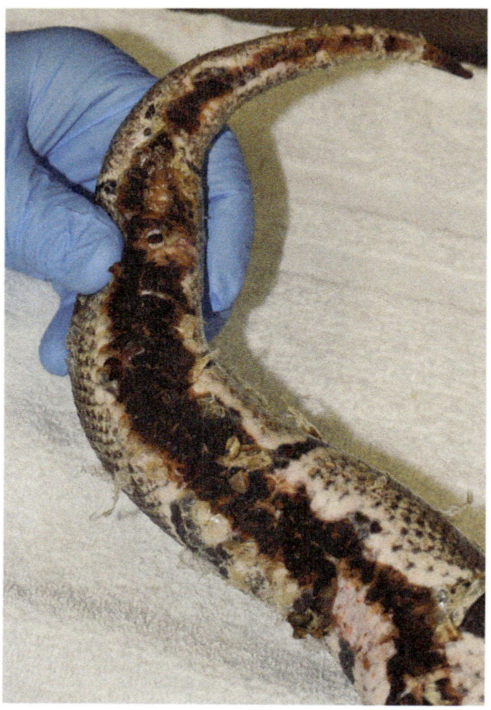

Figure 39.1 Severe thermal burns in a ball python (*Python regius*) exposed to a malfunctioning under-tank heat source.

Most common household cleaning products are unsuitable for use with amphibians, as their skin will absorb any chemical to which it is exposed, potentially causing morbidity and mortality.

UVB radiation exposure should be provided as required for the species based on natural history, and it is most critical for herbivorous reptiles. Providing UVB exposure to nocturnal and carnivorous species remains controversial, principally because there are no systematically derived, published data available. However, UVB exposure in these species may play a role in calcium homeostasis that is not currently understood. Important aspects of UVB supplementation to discuss with owners include distance of the animal from the light, presence of cage material between the animal and the light source, and manufacturer expiration of the bulb. Clients are frequently improperly educated when it comes to providing UVB supplementation for their pet reptile or amphibian, which commonly leads to inadequate exposure.

Cage furniture should be easy to clean and manufactured for safe use with reptiles and amphibians or aquatic use. Determine the cage substrate (material that covers the bottom of the enclosure) used by the client (Box 39.2). Sand and small particulate matter (e.g. wood or wood chips, smooth glass or plastic substances, etc.) should be avoided as a cage substrate, as reptiles and amphibians may inadvertently or even intentionally ingest particles over time, leading to gastrointestinal impactions and/or obstructions.

Diet

Reptiles and amphibians are characterized by diverse dietary strategies, which include herbivores, carnivores, omnivores,

Box 39.2 Substrates for Reptile and Amphibian Enclosures

- "Reptile carpet," newsprint, and recycled paper or paper fiber products are usually safe options for terrestrial reptiles and some amphibians
- Many particulate substrates (e.g. coconut byproducts, pea gravel, and sand) can cause gastrointestinal impactions
  - Are often inadvertently (if fed on substrate) or intentionally ingested (e.g. pea gravel or glass beads)
- The following options are not recommended
  - Corn cob
  - Shavings made of woods containing aromatic oils (e.g. cedar, pine)
  - Materials producing excessive amounts of dust or strong scents

and piscivores. Because of this, many clients are poorly informed about the best dietary options available for the species they own or have recently purchased. For insectivores, many readily available feeder insects have a poor calcium-to-phosphorous ratio, and it is generally recommended to "gut-load" insects prior to feeding to reptiles and amphibians; that is, provide nutritional feedstuffs for the insects to ingest prior to feeding them to a reptile or amphibian. Failure to provide appropriate calcium supplementation in the diet can lead to nutritional secondary hyperparathyroidism in many reptile and amphibian species.

Pre-killed prey items are commercially available and the best choice for feeding carnivorous species. However, live prey is still recommended by pet store employees and offered to pet herptiles by inexperienced or uneducated owners. Live insects and rodents have the potential to seriously injure pet reptiles and amphibians during the feeding process. Rodents and crickets are fully capable of preying upon the reptile or amphibian, which will not typically defend itself. Depending on the size of the herptile species, attacks from large numbers of crickets can be rapidly fatal. Rodents can remove large portions of soft tissue down to underlying bone in a matter of minutes. Bites can also occur during feeding when the rodent prey item is grabbed and it tries to defend itself; the sharp incisors easily damage mouthparts, penetrate muscle, and bites can communicate directly with the coelomic cavity. Rodent bites associated with the skull of herptiles can also be fatal. Therefore, while it is recommended that live prey items should not be fed to reptiles and amphibians in most cases, if live prey items are offered, one should never leave the reptile or amphibian unsupervised during feeding.

Clinical Exam

The clinical examination provides immediate information about the health status of the reptile and amphibian patient and is comprised of the visual and physical examinations.

Ideally, the patient should be visually examined in its home cage or aquarium, so that the clinician can get a sense of the typical environmental conditions. A visual examination of the animal in the room provides immediate information regarding patient stability. Dyspneic animals or animals that are either too weak to investigate their surroundings, or cannot adopt a defensive posture with manipulation, require immediate attention. Active hemorrhage or seizures should be addressed as soon as possible. While animals may be shy and hide in a new environment, healthy animals should have open eyes when manipulated and are expected to resist handling. Snakes will often tongue-flick readily when alert or handled, and this response can be dampened to absent in ill individuals.

Due to the chronicity of many herptile disease processes, many animals will present in a moderately to markedly dehydrated state. Examining a patient's skin tent (Figure 39.2) and viscosity of the saliva can provide information regarding hydration status. Severely dehydrated animals often have noticeably sunken eyes (Figure 39.2), and amphibians may feel tacky in hand. Evaluation of the oral or cloacal mucous membrane color or capillary refill time can provide information about patient perfusion.

All materials needed for a physical examination should be assembled prior to the procedure in order to minimize patient stress. Box 39.3 provides a list of focus areas for the reptile and amphibian examination. An inventory of helpful equipment for examinations of herptiles is outlined in Box 39.4. Prior to patient handling, powder-free gloves should be worn by the clinician.

Table 39.2 lists select biological data of some common pet reptile and amphibian species.

For detailed descriptions of neurologic, dermatologic, and ophthalmologic examinations in reptiles and amphibians, the reader is encouraged to refer to numerous, excellent exotic animal medicine texts.

Oral Cavity, Nares, Eyes, Otic

Examination of the oral cavity is facilitated by use of a pliable speculum in most amphibians, snakes, and lizards; small to medium-sized plastic kitchen spatulas, radiographic film, cotton-tipped applicators, tongue depressors, or credit cards work well for this purpose (Figure 39.3). Care must be taken when using specula made from hard

(a) (b)

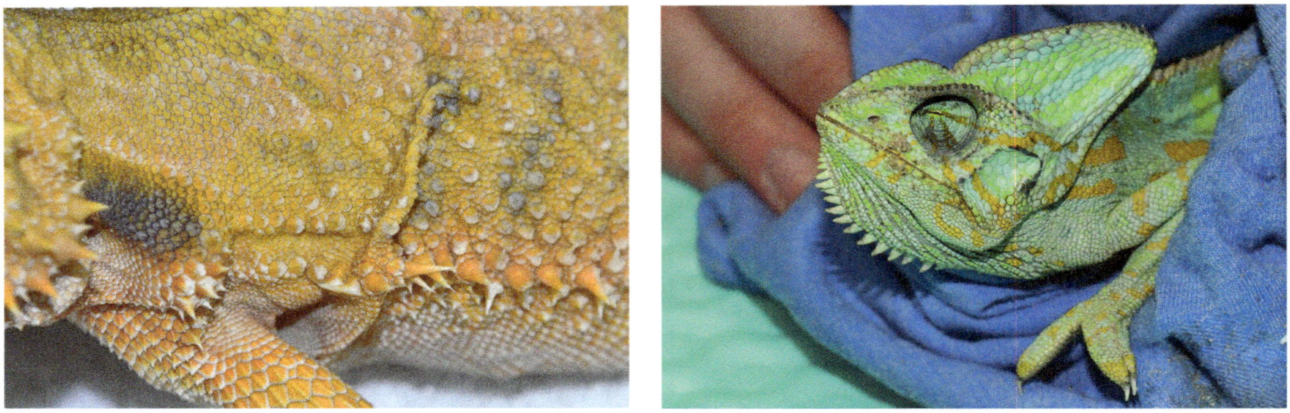

Figure 39.2 Checking skin tent in a bearded dragon (*Pogona vitticeps*) (a), and noticeably sunken eyes in a dehydrated veiled chameleon (*Chamaeleo calyptratus*) (b).

Box 39.3 Focus Areas for the Reptile and Amphibian Physical Examination

- Hydration status
- Body condition score
- Respiratory effort
- Auscultation of the heart, lungs in some species
- Heart rate using Doppler
- Symmetry of head
- Nares
- Oral cavity
- Eyes
- Tympanic membranes or ear canals
- Palpation of long bones of limbs, if present
- Skin or shell appearance and condition
- Coelomic palpation
- Coelomic transillumination in small species
- Vent

Box 39.4 Equipment List for the Detailed Reptile and Amphibian Physical Examination

- Electronic or small-sized stethoscope with moistened gauze pads or paper towel
- Doppler
- Ophthalmoscope, penlight, or transilluminator
- Soft rubber spatula, plastic card, old radiographic film, tongue depressor, cotton-tipped applicators, paperclip, or other oral speculum
- Nitrile gloves for handling amphibians
- Plastic syringe case for hinged chelonian species
- Stainless steel atraumatic probes, red-rubber, or tomcat catheter for sexing snakes

materials in species with teeth to prevent iatrogenic damage, especially those with acrodont dentition. In small snakes and lizards, gentle downward traction on the mandible usually provides a glimpse of the rostral oral cavity and teeth (Figure 39.3c). A thorough investigation of the oral cavity in chelonians and crocodilians is more challenging due to powerful jaw tone, and frequently requires sedation or anesthesia. Aquatic turtle species may attempt to bite when their head is approached, facilitating a quick glimpse of the oral cavity. In turtle species with hinged shells, using a plastic syringe case wrapped in bandage material to keep the shell from closing provides continued access to the head and forelimbs (Figure 39.4). The oral cavity should be examined for evidence of stomatitis, plaques, inflammation, or masses. Periodontal disease is a common finding in lizard species.

Serous to mucopurulent nasal discharge is common in tortoises with upper respiratory tract infections; copious amounts of discharge can lead to severe dyspnea and open-mouth breathing. The intermittent presence of bubbles stemming from the nostrils, and/or audible wheezing, is observable in some snakes with pneumonia.

Evaluation of the anterior chamber is possible using direct ophthalmoscopy or biomicroscopy, although detailed investigation of the lens may be more difficult in species with a spectacle. Snakes with severe stomatitis may present with pseudobuphthalmos or subspectacular abscesses due to obstructed nasolacrimal ducts.

Aural bacterial abscessation is common in aquatic chelonians, and is hypothesized to be related to chronic hypovitaminosis A. Penetrating injuries of the tympanum of reptiles are rarely observed, but must be considered as a differential diagnosis for tympanic membrane injuries.

Table 39.2 Selected biological data for common pet reptiles and amphibians.

Species	Heart rate (beats per min)	Respiratory rate (breaths per min)	Body weight (g)	Life span[1] (yr)
Snakes				
Corn snake (*Pantherophis guttatus*)	Female: 53 ± 17[2] Male: 65 ± 17[2]	NA	341 ± 20[3]	>20
Ball python (*Python regius*)	64 (54–80)[a] [4]	30 (25–36)[b] [5]	Female: 1300 (1100–1600)[c] [4] Male: 1100 (940–1250)[c] [4]	>30
Boa constrictor (*Boa constrictor*)	11–42[d] [6]	NA	3700 ± 2700[7]	20–30
Lizards				
Bearded dragon (*Pogona vitticeps*)	56–67[d] [8]	8–26[d] [8]	Female: 272 ± 22 [9] Male: 494 ± 21[9]	6–10
Leopard gecko (*Eublepharis macularius*)	93 (66–126)[a] [10]	24 (6–60)[a] [10]	Female: 46 ± 8[10] Male: 59 ± 11[10]	>10
Green iguana (*Iguana iguana*)	41 ± 10[11]	16 ± 6[12] 21 ± 6[12]	Female: 669 ± 231[13] Male: 1310 ± 670[14]	15–20
Chelonians				
Red-eared slider (*Trachemys scripta elegans*)	39 ± 6[15]	1.5[e] [16]	Female: 1310 (1000–2000)[c] [15] Male: 630 ± 396[17]	>20
Eastern box turtle (*Terrapene carolina*)	36–72[d] [18]	1.5[e] at 77 °F[f] [19]	276 ± 126 [20]	>20
Amphibians				
White's tree frog (*Litoria caerulea*)	77 ± 12 [21]	230[e] [21]	26 ± 4 [21]	7–10
Leopard frog	76[e] [22]	Gular: 119[e] [22] Coelomic: 84[e] [22]	31.5[e] [22]	8–12
Poison dart frog (*Dendrobates tinctorius azureus*)	95 (85–112)[b] [23]	32[e] [23]	1.1 ± 0.6[23]	5–8
Tiger salamander (*Ambystoma tigrinum*)	38–100[d] [24]	0–160[d] [24]	24 (14–27)[a] [24]	10

NA, not available; SD, standard deviation.
Heart and respiratory rates are conscious measurements. Measurements are in mean ± SD unless otherwise specified.
[a] Median (range).
[b] Median (interquartile range).
[c] Mean (range).
[d] Range.
[e] Mean.
[f] Value from the ornate box turtle (*Terrapene ornata*).

Musculoskeletal

Body condition scoring is subjective in many species but evaluation of soft tissue overlying bony prominences can be helpful. As snakes lose condition, the spinous processes of the vertebral column become more visible and palpable. In lizards, the pelvic girdle, spinal column, bones of the skull, and coccygeal vertebrae become prominent as the animal becomes cachectic (Figure 39.5). Chelonians in poor body condition often feel light when handled. Reptiles and amphibians with nutritional secondary hyperparathyroidism may present with skeletal deformities secondary to abnormal growth or bony remodeling (Figure 39.6).

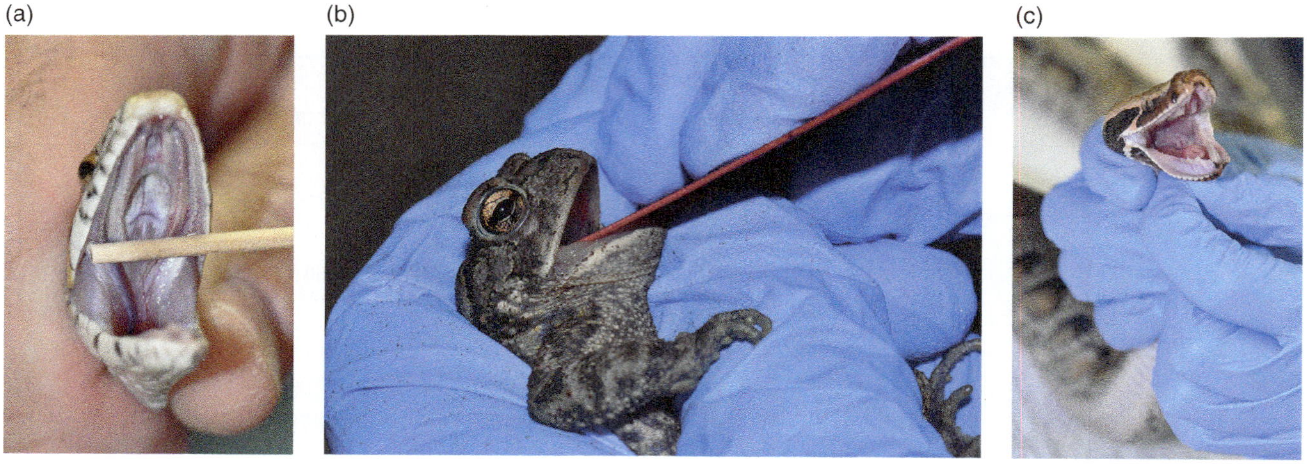

Figure 39.3 Oral examinations of a corn snake using a cotton-tipped applicator (a), a toad using a plastic credit card (b), and a python using gentle downward traction on the submandibular skin (c).

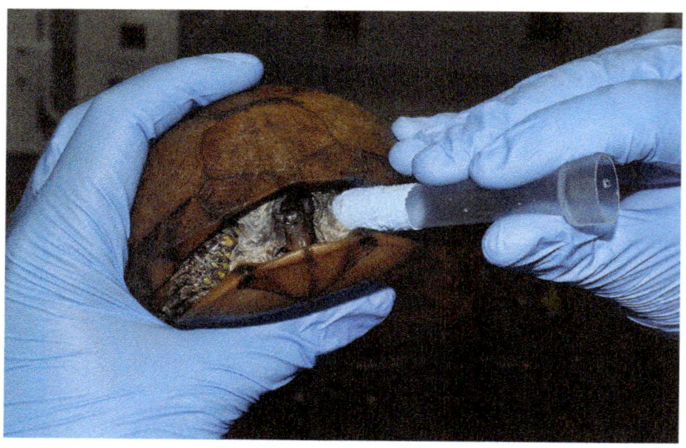

Figure 39.4 Use of a plastic syringe case to facilitate examination of a box turtle; the semi-rigid case provides a way to keep the animal's hinge from closing tight.

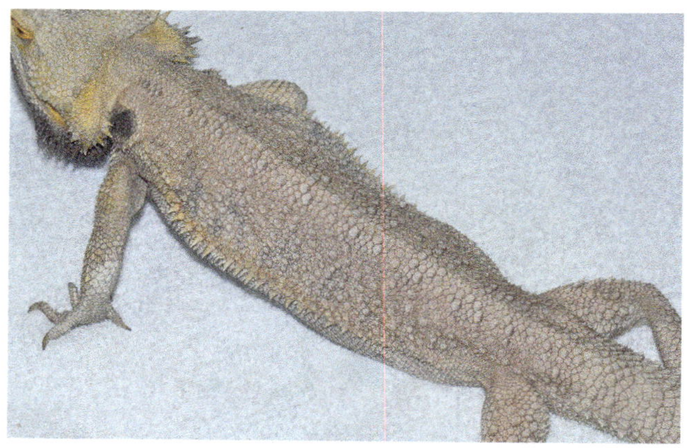

Figure 39.5 Prominent vertebral column and pelvic bones in a cachectic bearded dragon (*Pogona vitticeps*).

Cardiorespiratory

As with all physiologic processes, heart and respiratory rates are temperature dependent in reptiles and amphibians, and therefore, quantification of rates may not be particularly helpful during the exam. Qualitative parameters, such as cardiac arrhythmias, may be more beneficial than quantitative parameters. Auscultation of the heart and lungs can be difficult in reptiles and amphibians, especially small individuals. Placing a moistened gauze pad or paper towel in between the stethoscope diaphragm and the patient may result in better appreciation of sounds by limiting scale noise. Electronic stethoscopes can be useful for ausculting herptiles due to the enhanced ability to hear quieter sounds. Heart rate is quickly assessed using a Doppler probe (Figure 39.7).

Coelomic Cavity

Coelomic palpation of reptiles and amphibians is generally considered a process of determining what feels abnormal, rather than attempting to discriminate normal organ systems. In chelonians, the shell limits palpation of the coelomic cavity, and all organ systems are elongated in snakes. In chelonians, the coelomic cavity may be palpated gently using the prefemoral fossae as access points. Fat deposits, masses of follicles, eggs, or foreign bodies may be appreciated during palpation of the coelom. Hepatomegaly is possible to palpate in some herptile species. Obese carnivorous lizard and frog species frequently have marked distension of the coelomic cavity. Transillumination of the coelomic cavity can be of benefit in smaller lizard and frog species.

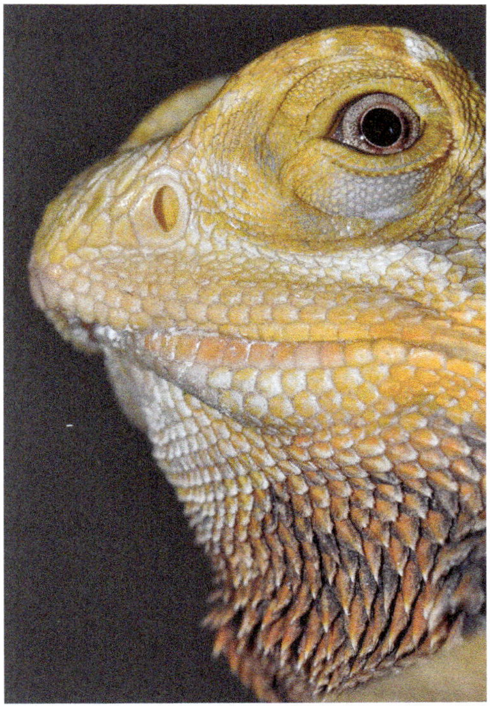

Figure 39.6 Maxillary and mandibular deformities in a bearded dragon (*Pogona vitticeps*) with nutritional secondary hyperparathyroidism.

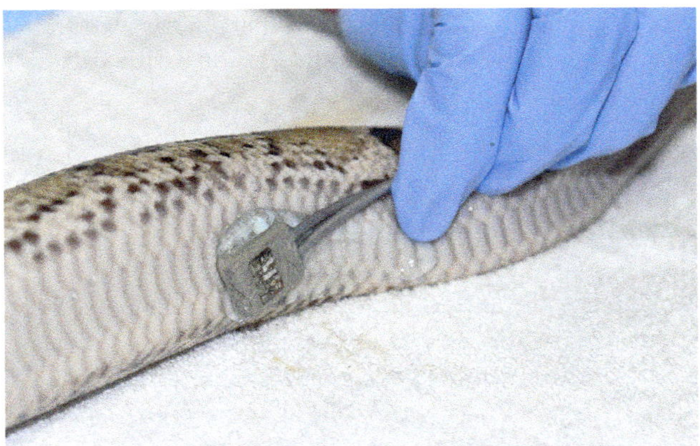

Figure 39.7 Use of Doppler to determine heart rate in a python.

Vent

The vent should be inspected for evidence of trauma or prolapse. In snakes, gentle traction of the scales cranial and caudal to the vent results in exposure of the mucocutaneous junction for inspection (Figure 39.8). Cloacal prolapse is a common presenting complaint in chelonians, lizards, frogs, and snakes. Prolapse of the phallus in male reptiles may be mistaken for other organs (Figure 39.9), such as the colon, especially if the tissue becomes desiccated secondary to chronic exposure. Determining sex in snakes is best accomplished through probing. In some

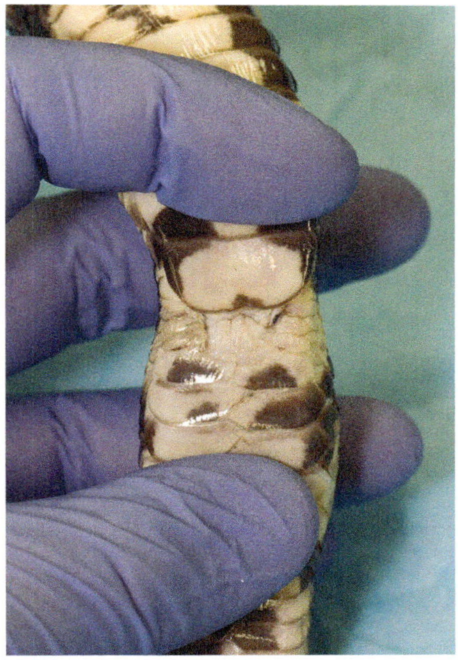

Figure 39.8 Gentle caudal traction facilitates inspection of the vent mucosa in a snake; note the large, shield-like scale normally overlying the vent opening.

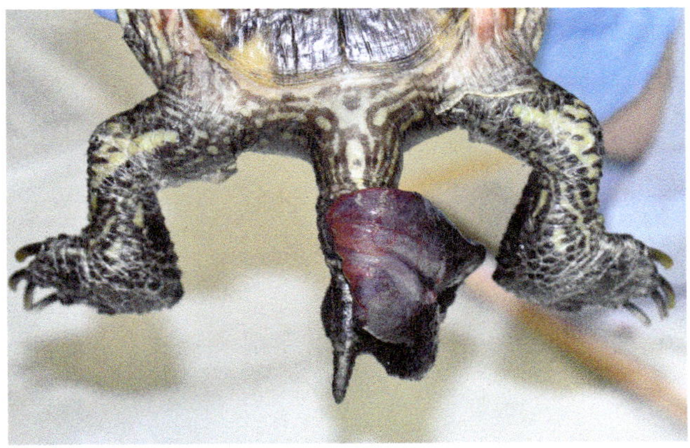

Figure 39.9 Prolapsed phallus of a slider.

lizard species, the femoral pores are more pronounced in adult males than in females (Figure 39.10). For chelonians, males may have a subtle bulge cranial to the vent indicative of the location of the phallus; additionally, males typically have longer tails with more distally located vents, some male aquatic species may have elongated claws on the forelimbs, and male tortoises often have a concave plastron to assist with copulation.

Integument

Dermatologic diseases are common in reptile and amphibian species. Dysecdysis (Figure 39.11), particularly in reptiles, is commonly associated with poor husbandry.

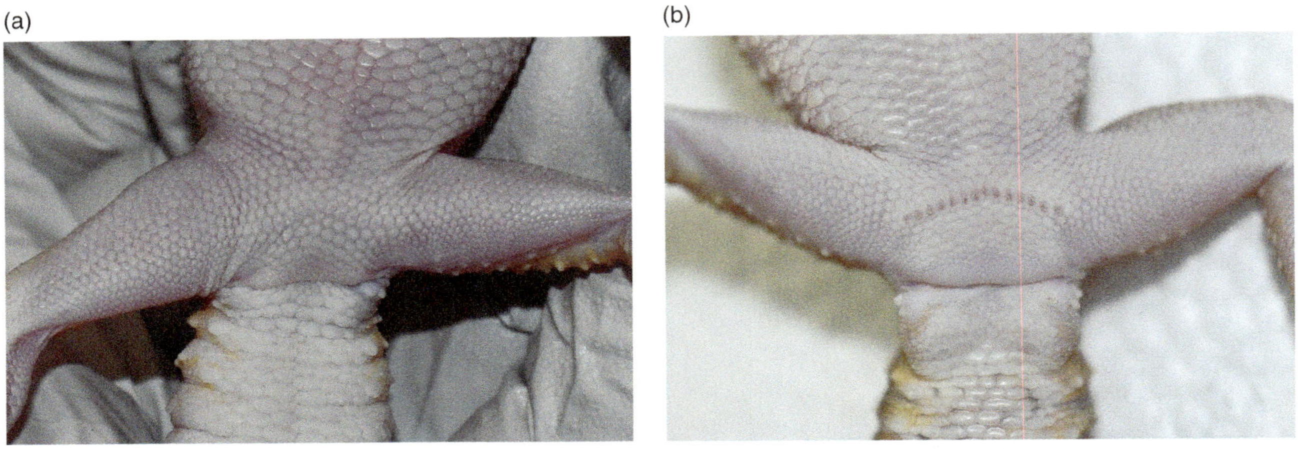

Figure 39.10 Male and female leopard geckos can be sexed by examining the prefemoral pores which are prominent in males (b) but not grossly visible in females (a); male leopard geckos also possess hemipenal bulges (b) caudal to the vent opening.

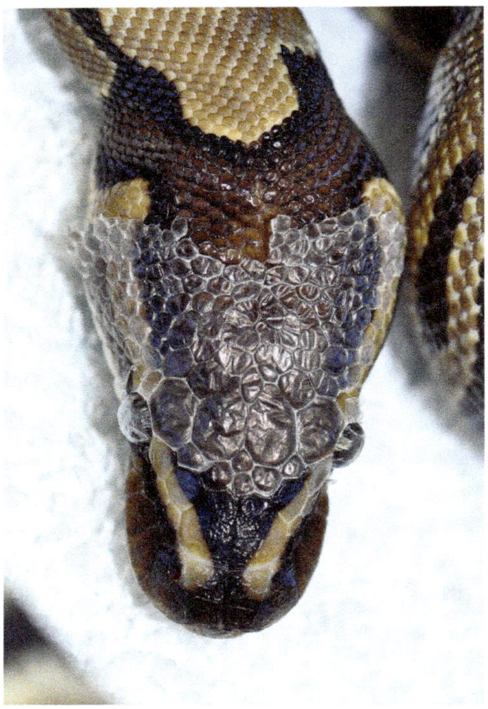

Figure 39.11 Dysecdysis in a ball python (*Python regius*).

Evaluate snakes with dysecdysis, or individuals spending large amounts of time submerged in a water dish, for ectoparasites. Common areas for snake mites (*Ophionyssus natricis*) to hide include in the fold underneath the mandible, the heat pits associated with the face in some species, and at the margins of the spectacle. Fungal dermatitis can be focal to multifocal in lizards, snakes, and amphibians, and typically appears as areas of skin discoloration, skin sloughing, and/or crusty and proliferative lesions. Amphibians may develop lumps under the skin associated with encysted cestode larvae (i.e. sparganosis), and may develop erythematous-to-ulcerative lesions with bacterial infections.

Conclusion

Excellent reptile and amphibian clinical case management should begin with a thorough patient history, a complete physical examination, appropriate diagnostic tests, and supportive care as necessary. The anamnesis enables clinicians to identify serious problems in emergent cases and helps guide conversations with clients regarding preventable and treatable problems. A comprehensive clinical examination provides a large amount of information in a short period of time. Veterinarians should approach the physical examination systematically and quickly in order not to overlook subtle abnormalities or cause undue stress to the patient.

References

1 Reptile and amphibian care sheets and species information. www.reptilesmagazine.com (accessed 24 November 2020).

2 Lewis, M., Bouvard, J., Eatwell, K., and Culshaw, G. (2020). Standardisation of electrocardiographic examination in corn snakes (*Pantherophis guttatus*). *Vet. Rec.* 186 (19): e29.

3 Acierno, M.J., Mitchell, M.A., Zachariah, T.T. et al. (2008). Effects of ultraviolet radiation on plasma 25-hydroxyvitamin D3 concentrations in corn snakes (*Elaphe guttata*). *Am. J. Vet. Res.* 69 (2): 294–297.
4 Paillusseau, C., Gandar, F., Schilliger, L., and Chetboul, V. (2020). Two-dimensional echocardiographic measurements in the ball python (*Python regius*). *J. Zoo Wildl. Med.* 50 (4): 976–982.
5 Yaw, T.J., Mans, C., Johnson, S.M. et al. (2018). Effect of injection site on alfaxalone-induced sedation in ball pythons (*Python regius*). *J. Small Anim. Pract.* 59 (12): 747–751.
6 Beaufrere, H., Schillinger, L., and Pariaut, R. (2016). Cardiovascular system. In: *Current Therapy in Exotic Pet Practice* (eds. M.A. Mitchell and T.N. Tully), 151–220. St. Louis: Elsevier Inc.
7 Banzato, T., Russo, E., Finotti, L. et al. (2012). Ultrasonographic anatomy of the coelomic organs of boid snakes (*Boa constrictor imperator, Python regius, Python molurus molurus*, and *Python curtus*). *Am. J. Vet. Res.* 73 (5): 634–645.
8 Ratliff, C., Parkinson, L.A., and Mans, C. (2019). Effects of the fraction of inspired oxygen on alfaxalone-sedated inland bearded dragons (*Pogona vitticeps*). *Am. J. Vet. Res.* 80 (2): 129–134.
9 Bucy, D.S., Guzman, D.S., and Zwingenberger, A.L. (2015). Ultrasonographic anatomy of bearded dragons (*Pogona vitticeps*). *J. Am. Vet. Med. Assoc.* 246 (8): 868–876.
10 Doss, G.A., Fink, D.M., Sladky, K.K., and Mans, C. (2017). Comparison of subcutaneous dexmedetomidine–midazolam versus alfaxalone–midazolam sedation in leopard geckos (*Eublepharis macularius*). *Vet. Anaesth. Analg.* 44 (5): 1175–1183.
11 Gustavsen, K.A., Saunders, A.B., Young, B.D. et al. (2014). Echocardiographic and radiographic findings in a cohort of healthy adult green iguanas (*Iguana iguana*). *J. Vet. Cardiol.* 16 (3): 185–196.
12 Hernandez-Divers, S.M., Schumacher, J., Stahl, S., and Hernandez-Divers, S.J. (2005). Comparison of isoflurane and sevoflurane anesthesia after premedication with butorphanol in the green iguana (*Iguana iguana*). *J. Zoo Wildl. Med.* 36 (2): 169–175.
13 Pinacho, S., Arcos-García, J.L., López-Pozos, R. et al. (2010). Reproductive parameters of green iguana (*Iguana iguana*) in captive conditions in Oaxaca, Mexico. *Revista. Cientifica. , Facultad de Ciencias Veterinarias, Universidad del Zulia.* 20 (5): 467–472.
14 Knotek, Z., Hrdá, A., Knotková, Z. et al. (2013). Alfaxalone anaesthesia in the green iguana (*Iguana iguana*). *Acta Vet. Brno* 82 (1): 109–114.
15 Poser, H., Russello, G., Zanella, A. et al. (2011). Two-dimensional and Doppler echocardiographic findings in healthy non-sedated red-eared slider terrapins (*Trachemys scripta elegans*). *Vet. Res. Commun.* 35 (8): 511–520.
16 Sladky, K.K., Miletic, V., Paul-Murphy, J. et al. (2007). Analgesic efficacy and respiratory effects of butorphanol and morphine in turtles. *J. Am. Vet. Med. Assoc.* 230 (9): 1356–1362.
17 Tucker, J.K., Dolan, C.R., Lamer, J.T., and Dustman, E.A. (2008). Climatic warming, sex ratios, and red-eared sliders (*Trachemys scripta elegans*) in Illinois. *Chelonian Conserv. Biol.* 7 (1): 60–69.
18 Raske, M., Lewbart, G.A., Dombrowski, D.S. et al. (2012). Body temperatures of selected amphibian and reptile species. *J. Zoo Wildl. Med.* 43 (3): 517–521.
19 Glass, M.L., Hicks, J.W., and Riedesel, M.L. (1979). Respiratory responses to long-term temperature exposure in the box turtle, *Terrapene ornata*. *J. Comp. Physiol.* 131 (4): 353–359.
20 Cerreta, A.J., Walker, M.E., and Harrison, T.M. (2018). Evaluation of acupuncture points governing vessels 1 and 26 on anesthetic recovery of eastern box turtles (*Terrapene carolina carolina*). *J. Zoo Wildl. Med.* 49 (4): 870–874.
21 Krisp, A.R., Hausmann, J.C., Sladky, K.K., and Mans, C. (2020). Anesthetic efficacy of MS-222 in White's tree frogs (*Litoria caerulea*). *J. Herpetol. Med. Surg.* 30 (1): 38–41.
22 Doss, G.A., Nevarez, J.G., Fowlkes, N., and Da Cunha, A.F. (2014). Evaluation of metomidate hydrochloride as an anesthetic in leopard frogs (*Rana pipiens*). *J. Zoo Wildl. Med.* 45 (1): 53–59.
23 Yaw, T.J., Mans, C., Martinelli, L., and Sladky, K.K. (2020). Comparison of subcutaneous administration of alfaxalone–midazolam–dexmedetomidine with ketamine–midazolam–dexmedetomidine for chemical restraint in juvenile blue poison dart frogs (*Dendrobates tinctorius azureus*). *J. Zoo Wildl. Med.* 50 (4): 868–873.
24 Mitchell, M.A., Riggs, S.M., Singleton, C.B. et al. (2009). Evaluating the clinical and cardiopulmonary effects of clove oil and propofol in tiger salamanders (*Ambystoma tigrinum*). *J. Exot. Pet Med.* 18 (1): 50–56.

Further Reading

Clayton, L.A. and Gore, S.R. (2007). Amphibian emergency medicine. *Vet. Clin. North Am. Exot. Anim. Pract.* 10 (2): 587–620.

Martinez-Jimenez, D. and Hernandez-Divers, S.J. (2007). Emergency care of reptiles. *Vet. Clin. North Am. Exot. Anim. Pract.* 10 (2): 557–585.

Divers, S.J. and Stahl, S.J. (eds.) (2019). *Mader's Reptile Medicine and Surgery*, 3e. St. Louis: Elsevier Inc.

Herptiles

40

Restraint and Handling

Grayson A. Doss and Kurt K. Sladky

Department of Surgical Sciences, School of Veterinary Medicine, University of Wisconsin–Madison, Madison, Wisconsin, USA

CONTENTS

Overview and Indications

Restraint refers to control of the patient, either by physical or chemical means, or a combination of both. Restraint is commonly used in veterinary medicine as a means to facilitate safe interaction with an animal, either during transport, physical examination, or a variety of other medical procedures. Proper restraint provides sufficient immobility to complete the intended task in the shortest time possible, while remaining safe for both the handler and the patient. Minimizing the restraint period is important, as it is well understood that restraint results in an acute stress response in many animal species, including reptiles [1–4]. For example, heart rate increased significantly in handled iguanas and manually restrained crocodiles [2, 5].

Manual restraint is a form of physical restraint in which a handler manually controls a conscious patient. In most pet reptile and amphibian species, manual restraint is easily accomplished and provides a means for performing a number of quick, non-invasive tasks. Chemical restraint refers to use of sedative or anesthetic drugs to facilitate safe handling of a patient. Chemical restraint may be useful for large and dangerous species, for procedures requiring a still patient (e.g. jugular blood sample collection or beak trimming in chelonians), or for more prolonged procedures (e.g. minor surgical procedures).

Transportation

Reptiles and amphibians should be transported to the hospital in escape-proof containers. Snakes can be contained in a strong cloth bag or pillowcase prior to being placed in a secondary container. Larger snakes may require a plastic container or cooler with wheels.

Aquatic amphibians should be kept moist by providing a humid environment. This can be achieved by lining the transport container with wet paper or cloth towels preferably dampened with clean water from their enclosure. Fully aquatic amphibians can be transported within plastic containers holding properly conditioned water. Unconscious or moribund animals should not be allowed to submerge in water as drowning can occur.

Reptiles and amphibians should be protected from dangerous temperature fluctuations and placement within an insulated container or supplementation with hot or cold packs may be advised for extreme ambient temperatures.

Manual Restraint

Manual restraint is commonplace in veterinary medicine. It assists the clinician in obtaining patient information both directly through the physical exam, and indirectly,

Exotic Animal Emergency and Critical Care Medicine, First Edition. Edited by Jennifer E. Graham, Grayson A. Doss and Hugues Beaufrère.

through diagnostics. Manual restraint is also used for a variety of procedures including venipuncture, lung washes, gavage feeding, ultrasound examinations, and radiographs. For most pet herptiles, manual restraint is possible using little to no specialized equipment. For aggressive animals, lightweight leather gloves, or heavy-duty products lined with penetration-resistant fabric are available to minimize the risk of injury to the handler.

A list of items required for restraint is summarized in Box 40.1. Important tips for herptile restraint are listed in Box 40.2.

Box 40.1 Checklist for Herptile Restraint by Group

Snakes

- Hooks, tongs, tubes, or light leather gloves for aggressive animals

Lizards

- Leather gloves for species prone to scratching or biting

Crocodilians

- Strong tape to secure jaw closed

Chelonians

- Circular object to balance plastron upon in order to facilitate examination or sample collection in large species

Amphibians

- Nitrile gloves
- Aquarium nets for aquatic species

Box 40.2 Important Tips During Herptile Restraint

- Compile all needed equipment prior to initiating restraint
- For chelonians, allow the patient's limbs to move unhindered for breathing to occur
- If allowed to gain traction with the cranial third of their body, snakes can easily pull their heads out of the handler's grasp
- Species like snapping turtles and softshell turtles have long necks and can bite if restrained too far forward on their bodies
- Be mindful of the tails in iguanas and crocodilians, as they can be used as weapons
- Immobilize the head of aggressive animals first to prevent injury
- Multiple handlers are required for restraining large constrictors, crocodilians, and monitor species

Snakes

Determining a handling technique for snakes depends on size and demeanor of the animal, as well as whether the snake is a venomous species. For large constrictors, several people are required to safely control and manipulate the animal. A good rule of thumb is to have at least one adult handler per four feet of patient. Supporting the length of the body with two hands and allowing the head of the patient to move and explore freely is a useful approach for smaller, docile snakes (Figure 40.1). For defensive animals, gently but firmly grasp the snake directly behind the skull in order to prevent the snake from striking (Figure 40.2); the free hand carries the weight of the patient. Be careful while restraining an aggressive animal, as snakes will often coil their bodies around a forearm in order to gain leverage to pull their heads out of the handler's grasp. If a snake is coiled tightly around the handler, removal is facilitated by grasping at the snake's tail and unwrapping slowly and gently in a caudal to cranial direction.

As snakes do not tolerate oral examinations, grasping the snake behind the skull is usually required for examining the oral cavity in even the most docile animals.

Although designed for safe manipulation of venomous species, specially designed snake restraint tubes, hooks, and tongs are also helpful for examining or handling aggressive,

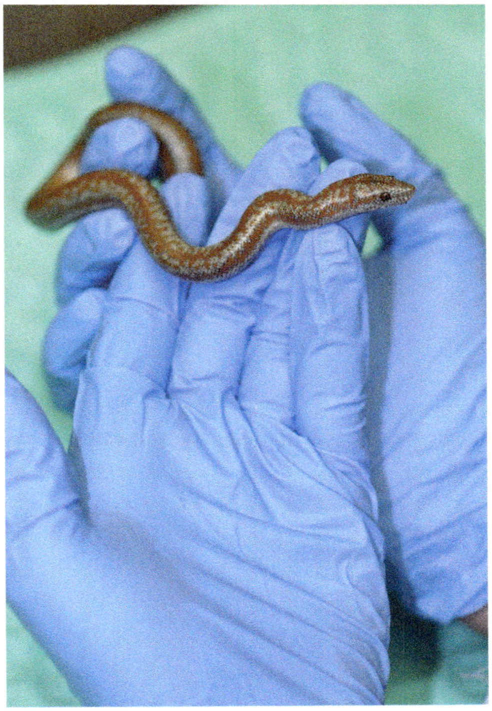

Figure 40.1 Handling a small, docile, rosy boa (*Lichanura trivirgata*) by supporting the body weight and allowing the head of the patient to investigate unrestrained.

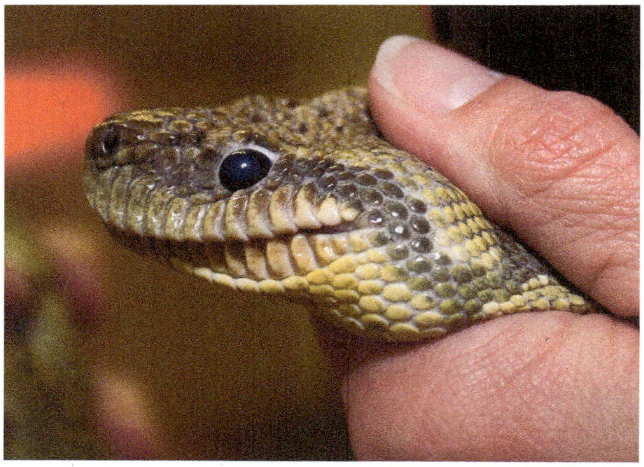

Figure 40.2 Manual restraint of an aggressive boa by maintaining a firm grip behind the skull to prevent bites to the handler.

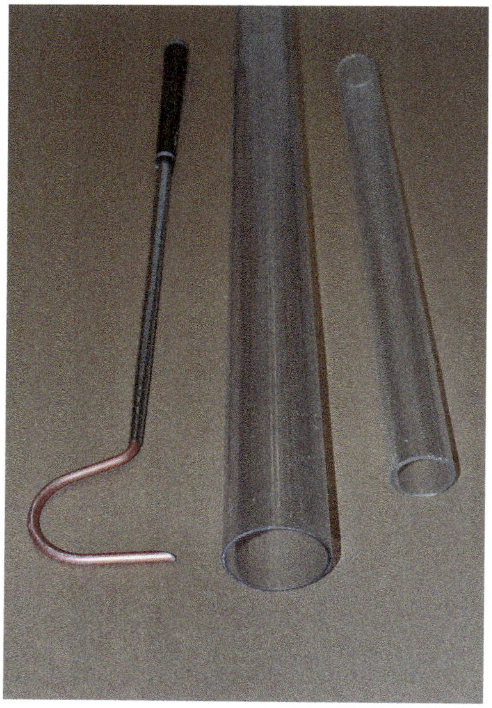

Figure 40.3 Equipment designed for handling aggressive or venomous snakes.

non-venomous snakes (Figure 40.3). Handling any venomous species is not recommended unless the institution has handlers specifically trained in venomous animal restraint.

Lizards

Medium-sized lizards like bearded dragons, water dragons, or small iguanas may be supported using two hands; one hand supports the pectoral girdle while the other secures the caudal half of the body under the pelvis. For active animals that resist restraint, holding the forelimbs and hindlimbs in extension against the body can help control an individual attempting to escape the restrainer. Grasp aggressive animals behind the head in order to prevent bites during handling attempts; the handler uses their free hand to support the remainder of the body. The handler must be careful not to grab or restrain lizards by the tail, as many species, including numerous types of geckos and skinks, exhibit tail autotomy, an anti-predator defense mechanism in which the tail fractures and is expelled as a distraction. Small, fragile, or skittish lizard species may be more amenable to handling using a small container rather than restraint by hand. Chameleons are prone to becoming stressed even with gentle handling. Minimizing the handling and restraint period or using sedation may be beneficial when working with this group of reptiles. Iguanas, tegus, frilled lizards, chuckwallas, and various monitor lizard species can cause considerable harm to handlers through biting and scratching. While usually less serious, bites from large chameleon, skink, and gecko species can be quite unpleasant. Iguanas are also known to whip their tails as a defensive maneuver, which can be very painful.

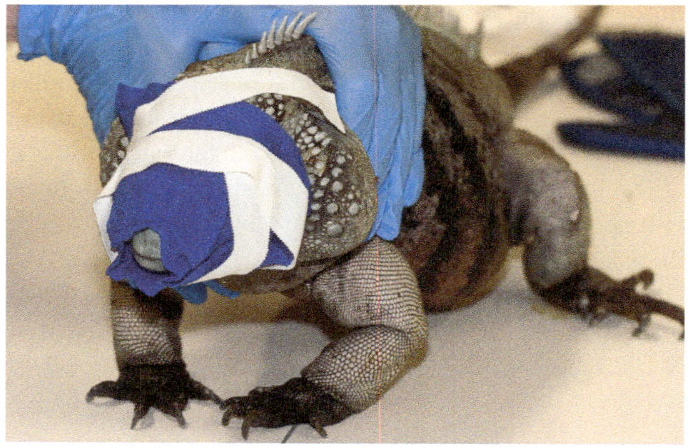

Figure 40.4 Covering the eyes of an iguanid with bandage material in order to stimulate the vasovagal response and calm the animal in order to quickly perform radiographs.

Applying gentle pressure to both eyes of some lizards and stimulating the vasovagal response for brief periods can result in a calmer animal, facilitating smooth execution of procedures like diagnostic imaging (Figure 40.4).

Chelonians

Most small to medium-sized chelonians are easily handled by grasping the shell laterally at the bridges connecting the carapace and plastron. Even the smallest chelonian species typically have sharp keratin edges to their maxilla and mandible, which can result in a painful bite. Some species, like aquatic turtles of the genera *Macroclemys*, *Chelydra*, or *Apalone*, are quite aggressive and readily defend themselves by biting strongly and rapidly. Some aquatic species can also extend their necks in a caudal direction over their carapaces when attempting to bite. Large aquatic turtles and tortoises have strong jaw power, which can result in serious injury to the handler. For many chelonians, balancing the animal's plastron on a raised object facilitates examination, blood collection, or diagnostic imaging in awake animals (Figure 40.5); while balanced, the animal should be supervised at all times so it does not fall. If the turtle or tortoise can reach the object it is balanced upon with its feet it can knock itself over, resulting in potentially serious injury. This technique is particularly useful for examining large, heavy species that are not easily restrained manually.

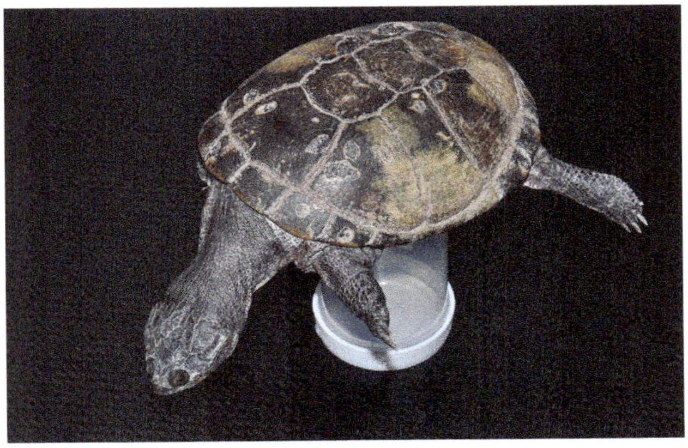

Figure 40.5 Use of an upturned specimen cup to immobilize a side-necked turtle in order to take radiographs; observe how the turtle is balanced upon the cup but is unable to contact it with its legs.

Crocodilians

Crocodilians have powerful jaw pressure and large teeth and can inflict serious bites to handlers. Opening a conscious crocodilian's mouth, once closed, is nearly impossible, although closing the mouth is quite easily performed. If an oral examination is not needed or is completed, it is advised to secure the mouth of crocodilians closed using strong tape before extensive handling; be careful not to occlude the rostrally-located nostrils. Because crocodilians can inflict serious injury with their muscular tails, it is recommended to restrain the proximal one-third of the tail during handling.

Amphibians

Before attempting to handle amphibians, make certain the exam room is escape proof, as small frogs are very quick and agile and can escape quickly under doors and into sink drains. Due to their fragile skin and potential for absorbing environmental chemicals transcutaneously, powder-free gloves should be first rinsed in the patient's own aquarium water or dechlorinated tap water before handling aquatic or semi-aquatic species. Gloves can also help protect the handler from toxins, such as those produced by various *Bufo* species. Small frogs and toads can be held in one hand by securing the head and pectoral girdle between the thumb and pointer finger (Figure 40.6); an alternative grip holds the legs in extension behind the body to prevent kicking and subsequent escape (Figure 40.6). Moistened aquarium nets are helpful for catching fast moving frogs or aquatic species (Figure 40.7). Plastic bags are also useful for restraining aquatic amphibians and can facilitate other diagnostic tests, such as imaging. Use of nets or containers is advised for handling aggressive, rounded-body frogs

(a) (b)

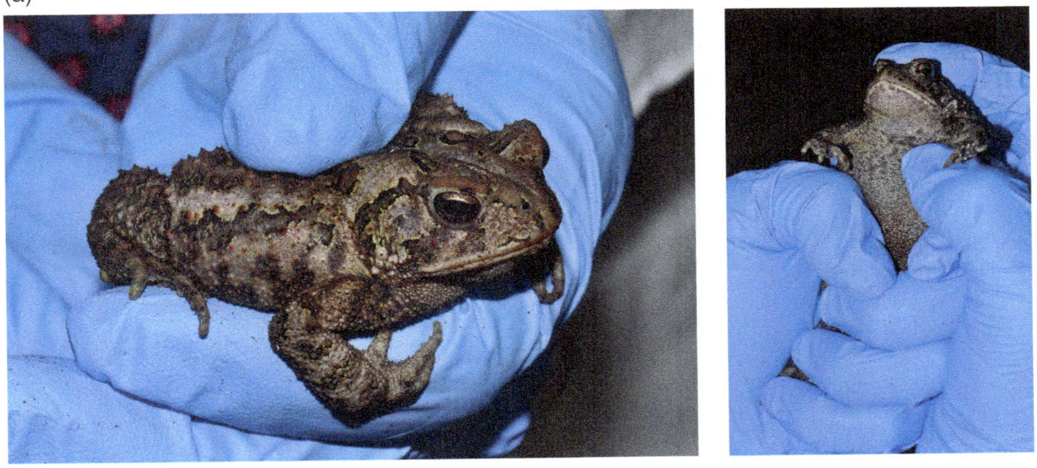

Figure 40.6 Manual restraint of a toad using a single hand applying dorsoventral pressure over the pectoral girdle (a), or holding the legs in extension to prevent kicking in flighty animals (b).

Herptiles

like African bullfrogs and horned frogs, which can inflict painful bites. Amphiumas and hellbenders can be very aggressive and inflict serious bite wounds. Use caution when handling salamanders, as some species exhibit tail autotomy.

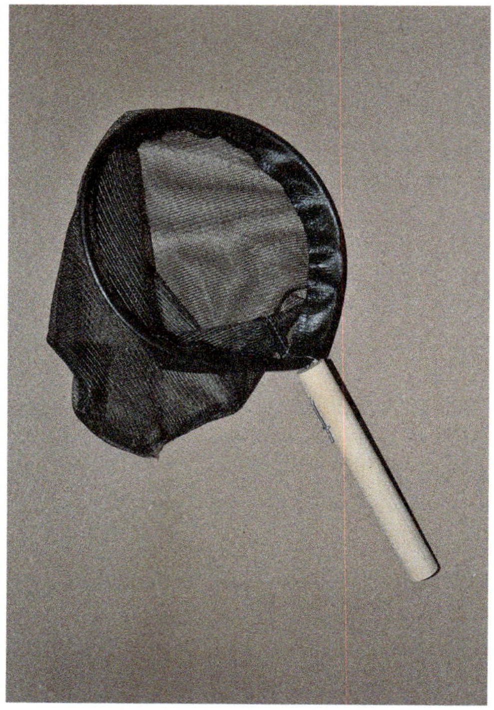

Figure 40.7 A smooth, fine-meshed net designed for use with aquatic amphibians and fish.

Chemical Restraint

Procedural sedation can allow for safe handling of aggressive animals and may result in life-saving modulation of the stress response in critical patients. Chemical restraint may also allow for hands-free diagnostic imaging, potentially decreasing personnel exposure, and can permit venipuncture in active animals or when immobility is desired, as in the case of intracardiac blood sample collection in snakes. Injectable agents can be quickly administered to severely ill animals while they remain in an oxygen cage or incubator, and breath holding is not a significant concern compared with inhalant anesthetics in herptiles.

Benzodiazepines, opioids, α2-agonists, dissociatives, and a handful of other sedative and anesthetic drugs are commonly used for chemical immobilization in reptiles. The authors routinely use various combinations of midazolam

(a)

(b)

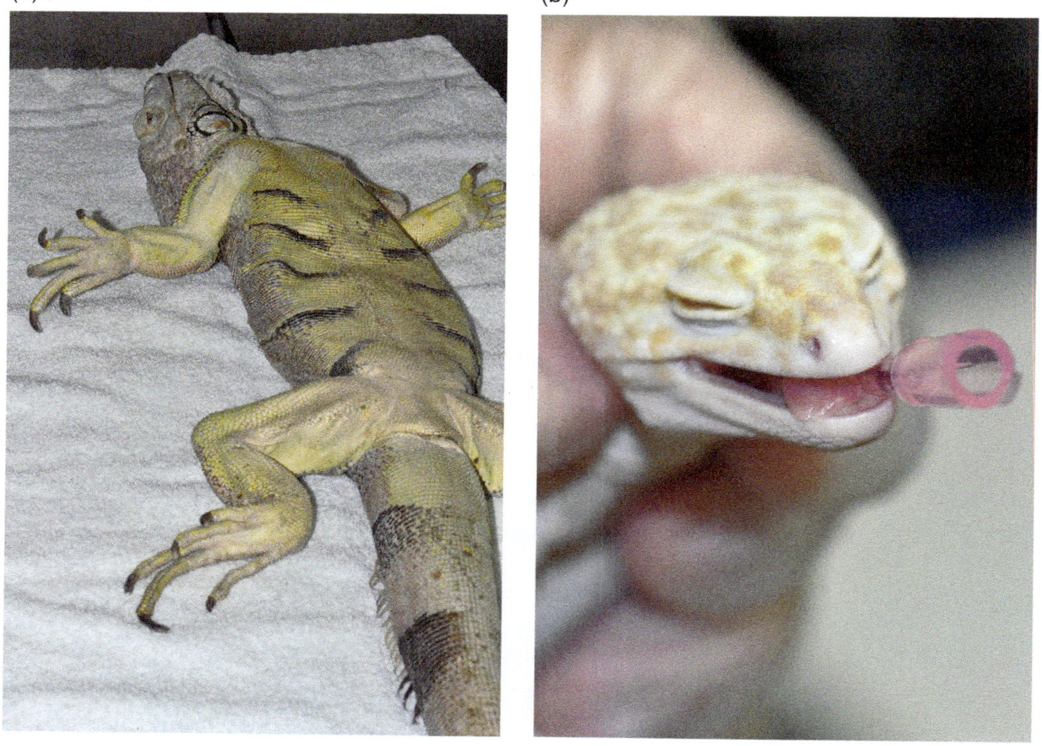

Figure 40.8 Sedated green iguana (*Iguana iguana*) with reduced righting reflex and partially closed eyes (a). Tracheal intubation was possible using sedation in this leopard gecko (*Eublepharis macularius*) (b).

and ketamine, with or without the addition of an α2-agonist, for procedural sedation in reptiles; benzodiazepine and α2-agonist combinations are completely reversible if needed, allowing for rapid recoveries. For many amphibians, topical compounds, such as tricaine methanesulfonate administered via immersion, are more commonly used for chemical restraint than injectable or inhalant anesthetics. Successful sedation often results in a relaxed patient that struggles less, and subjectively appears less stressed during restraint (Figure 40.8). In one study, sedated crocodiles returned to normal behavior more quickly, and had fewer changes to blood parameters, following a brief period of restraint, when compared to awake individuals [2].

Hospitalization and Daily Monitoring

Hospital enclosures should afford the patient a comfortable habitat while allowing for monitoring and easy cleaning. Hide boxes and thermal gradients should be provided, based on the species' natural history, so the patient can regulate its body temperature appropriately. Arboreal species should have sufficient vertical space to allow for climbing. For aquatic species, water temperature should be within the species' preferred optimum temperature zone, including an area for hauling out to dry or bask if necessary. Covering or providing a visual barrier for at least a portion of the enclosure may be warranted in order to minimize patient stress. For small frog and lizard species or snakes, make sure the enclosure is escape-proof, as even the smallest spaces can provide a route for escape. Frequently, a small patient may need to be housed in smaller, escape-proof caging, which is then placed within a larger enclosure. Ambient temperature extremes should be avoided in sick animals as this may have a negative effect on the patient's immune function. Herptiles should be housed in quiet, non-drafty areas, away from excessive audiovisual stimuli. Fresh water should be provided for all herptiles, even desert species. Moving water sources (waterfalls, drippers) are often required for chameleons. Fresh vegetable or plant matter, or prey items, should be available for patients as appropriate for each species. Live crickets should be fed under supervision in order to prevent serious injury to the patient; a food and water source should be placed within the hospital cage for the crickets if they are not consumed immediately.

Daily monitoring should include serial physical examinations in order to monitor therapeutic response. While interpretation of a single reading can be subjective, monitoring trends in pulse oximetry and non-invasive blood pressure over time is recommended for critical patients. Food and water intake, body weight, and production of feces and urine should also be monitored, if possible, to ensure the patient is receiving appropriate supportive care. Cage humidity and temperature should be constantly monitored to observe for malfunction of equipment and subsequent patient injury.

Conclusion

Both manual and chemical restraint are essential techniques when working with amphibian and reptile patients in order to prevent undue animal stress and, potentially, significant injury to the handler. Approaching restraint in a species-specific manner and utilizing chemical immobilization or specific equipment in aggressive or dangerous animals will help minimize risk for both handler and patient. Hospitalization should focus on providing the appropriate needs of the patient while minimizing undue stress.

References

1 Kreger, M.D. and Mench, J.A. (1993). Physiological and behavioral effects of handling and restraint in the ball python (*Python regius*) and the blue-tongued skink (*Tiliqua scincoides*). *Appl. Anim. Behav. Sci.* 38 (3–4): 323–336.

2 Olsson, A. and Phalen, D. (2013). Comparison of biochemical stress indicators in juvenile captive estuarine crocodiles (*Crocodylus porosus*) following physical restraint or chemical restraint by midazolam injection. *J. Wildl. Dis.* 49 (3): 560–567.

3 Guillette, L.J. Jr., Crain, D.A., Rooney, A.A., and Woodward, A.R. (1997). Effect of acute stress on plasma concentrations of sex and stress hormones in juvenile alligators living in control and contaminated lakes. *J. Herpetol.* 31 (3): 347–353.

4 Moore, M.C., Thompson, C.W., and Marler, C.A. (1991). Reciprocal changes in corticosterone and testosterone levels following acute and chronic handling stress in the tree lizard, *Urosaurus ornatus*. *Gen. Comp. Endocrinol.* 81 (2): 217–226.

5 Cabanac, A. and Cabanac, M. (2000). Heart rate response to gentle handling of frog and lizard. *Behav. Process.* 52 (2–3): 89–95.

41

Oxygen Therapy

Ian Kanda and João Brandão

Department of Veterinary Clinical Sciences, College of Veterinary Medicine, Oklahoma State University, Stillwater, Oklahoma, USA

CONTENTS

Indications for Oxygen Therapy

The decision to initiate oxygen therapy is made based on the presence of clinical signs consistent with hypoxia. Clinical signs of hypoxia include dyspnea, tachycardia, or cyanosis [1]. Increased respiratory rate, effort, neck extension, and abnormal posture or behavior can indicate dyspnea [2, 3]. In most reptiles, hypoxia leads to increased respiratory rate while hypercapnia leads to increased tidal volume. The ability to increase tidal volume may be limited by respiratory pathology such as accumulation of inflammatory debris and loss of tissue elasticity [4]. Snakes or lizards may sit with their head held up to maintain patent airways. Many reptile species exhibit thermoregulation via open mouth breathing; however in snakes, this is a sign of severe respiratory pathology. The lungs can be auscultated, although scaled skin causes difficulty. Placing a moistened gauze in between the stethoscope and the skin may reduce noise artifact [3].

Tachycardia can be difficult to assess upon intake as heart rate varies with temperature. Cyanotic membranes imply severe respiratory compromise. Knowing normal mucus membrane color for the species is important. For instance, certain python species may normally have a purple-black or even light blue oral cavity.

Confirmation of hypoxia is difficult, although a positive response to oxygen therapy should be adequate [1]. Pulse oximetry and blood gas analyzers are calibrated on the human oxygen hemoglobin dissociation curve and have not been validated in reptiles [1]. Trends in pulse oximetry can be observed and are likely to be more useful than single measurements. It is impractical to measure arterial blood gases in reptiles. Samples for blood gas analysis from cardiocentesis are unreliable as there is a mixing of arterial and venous blood within the heart. Furthermore, reptiles may regulate arterial blood gas concentrations independent of pulmonary ventilation by means of cardiac blood shunting [1]. Reptile red blood cells have a low affinity for oxygen and this allows a large amount of oxygen to be released to the tissues during times of stress [5]. Reptile blood has a maximum carrying capacity while at a temperature within the preferred optimal temperature zone [5].

Reptiles and amphibians have the ability to tolerate oxygen deprivation through metabolic suppression, and the ability to buffer increases in lactic acid and hydrogen ions during anaerobic metabolism [4, 6]. These abilities hinder observation of chronic respiratory depression until it is so severe that the animal can no longer compensate, hence emergent conditions either result from the end stages of chronic disease, or in scenarios that do not allow for metabolic suppression such as acute respiratory tract blockage or drowning.

In reptiles, respiration is stimulated by a lack of oxygen, so be prepared to provide intermittent positive pressure

Exotic Animal Emergency and Critical Care Medicine, First Edition. Edited by Jennifer E. Graham, Grayson A. Doss and Hugues Beaufrère.

ventilation when offering supplemental oxygen [3]. Oxygen therapy is increasing the fraction of inspired oxygen (FiO_2) above that of room air (21%). It is recommended to consider increasing oxygen content to only 40–50% instead of 100% to limit the deprivation of the respiratory drive [7]. However, recent studies in inland bearded dragons (*Pogona vitticeps*) and Dumeril's monitors (*Varanus dumerilii*) failed to find clinically relevant differences in recovery or physiologic variables in sedated or anesthetized lizards supplemented with either 100% oxygen or 21% oxygen [8–10]. A moistened surface is required for gas exchange, whether it is the lung tissue, skin, buccal surface, or gills [11]. Supplemented oxygen should be humidified to prevent drying of the respiratory tissues.

Oxygen Toxicity

Oxygen toxicity has been described in mammals. It is recommended to maintain oxygen levels at less than 50% for prolonged oxygen therapy to avoid oxygen toxicity (see Chapter 3: Oxygen Therapy). This aligns with the recommendation for reptiles in order to avoid potential respiratory suppression. Reptiles and amphibians have evolved to accommodate conditions of low oxygen availability. While oxygen toxicity has not been well described in reptiles or amphibians, precautions should be taken to avoid damage to respiratory surfaces.

In aquatic amphibians, dissolved gas supersaturation can cause gas bubble accumulation in the tissues. This progresses to hyperemia and petechial or ecchymotic hemorrhages. Erosion of the skin and loss of the mucous coat follows [12]. This disorder can be caused by the use of well water for enclosures, or a flaw in the filtration system which allows air to enter, become pressurized and dissolve.

Methods of Oxygen Supplementation

Noninvasive Methods

Oxygen Chamber or Cage

Oxygen cages can be used for patients in immediate respiratory distress or for long-term supplementation. The ideal oxygen chamber for reptiles is often an incubator [1]. This allows for control over supplemental heat and humidity, which need to be within the preferred optimal ranges for the species. Ideally, an air oxygen meter should be used to allow for FiO_2 monitoring and adjustment. Many commercial oxygen cages control oxygen concentration, temperature, and humidity and may also ventilate excess expired carbon dioxide. For small patients, another option is to place the entire animal into an upturned canine face mask, which serves as a miniature oxygen cage.

Flow-By Oxygen

Flow-by oxygen is easily accessible from any anesthetic machine and is a simple, initial means of oxygen supplementation (Figure 41.1). Oxygen flowing at 2–3 l/min within 2 cm of the patient's nose or mouth can provide a FiO_2 of 25–40% [13].

Face Mask Oxygen

Tight fitting face masks can provide a FiO_2 of up to 60% at an oxygen flow rate of 8–12 l/min [13] (Figure 41.2). This

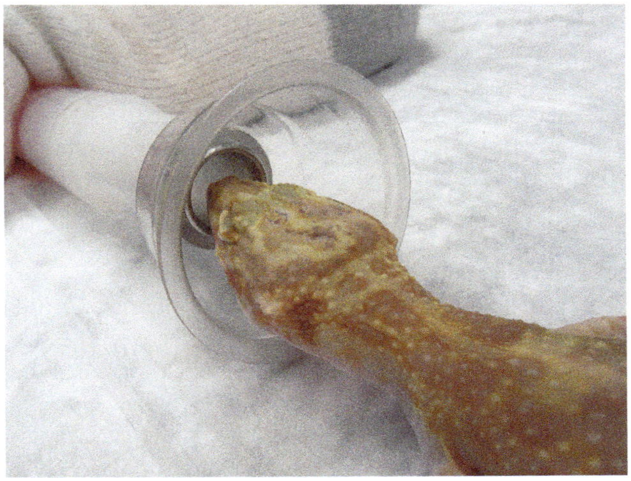

Figure 41.1 Flow-by oxygen can be a minimally stressful means for short term oxygen therapy.

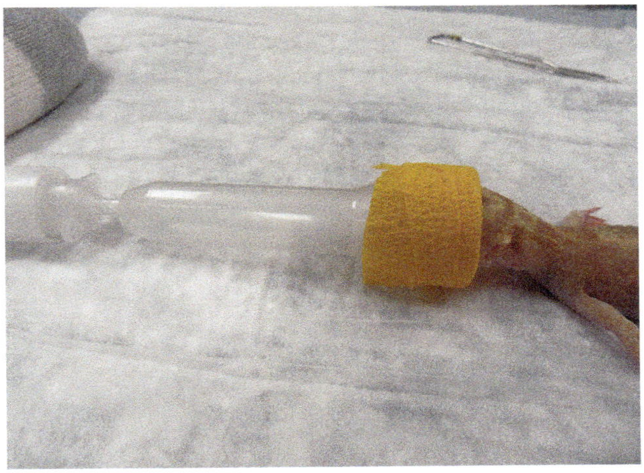

Figure 41.2 Small face masks can be made out of syringe cases and attached to anesthetic circuits for oxygen therapy. Bandage wrap can be used to create custom fit, single-use mask diaphragms. Tight fitting face masks should be periodically ventilated to remove accumulated carbon dioxide.

may be excessive for reptiles and may suppress respiratory drive. For reptiles smaller than 10 kg, an oxygen rate of 1–2 l/min is adequate. For larger reptiles, rates up to 5 l/min may be required [1]. The eyes should be lubricated if not covered by a spectacle (as in snakes) to avoid drying or damage from the mask itself. If utilized for moderate to long-term oxygen supplementation, oxygen should be humidified and the mask ventilated to avoid the accumulation of carbon dioxide [13].

Dissolved Oxygen in Water

Reptiles and amphibians utilize varying degrees of cutaneous respiration. There are hundreds of species of lungless amphibians and many salamanders, like the common mudpuppy (*Necturus m. maculosus*) have lungs, gills, and skin for respiration. Under cooler temperatures, the skin is the predominant respiratory organ, while at higher temperatures the gills predominate [14]. Many aquatic reptiles utilize cutaneous gas exchange that may be up to 50–70% of their needs [4, 11, 15–17]. Such high levels of exchange typically correspond to periods of low metabolic demands thus utilizing dissolved oxygen as a means of supplementation in reptiles is inapplicable for emergency situations.

For oxygen therapy in aquatic amphibian species, oxygen can be bubbled through the water in their enclosure. Ideally this is done with an air stone to decrease the size and increase the quantity of bubbles, which increases the surface area for osmosis into the water. Avoid air entering any filter that will pressurize the water and create conditions for supersaturation. If bubbles begin to line the enclosure sides, substrate, or the animal itself, the water may be supersaturated with gas and the patient should be removed immediately until the problem has been addressed [12]. Oxygen saturation in water is dependent on temperature and atmospheric pressure. To allow for optimal oxygen levels in water for therapy, the temperature should be kept on the cool end of the preferred optimal temperature for the species. If unknown, 20 °C (68 °F) accommodates most amphibians, or 25 °C (77 °F) for the more tropical species [12]. Water movement is necessary for ventilation of the skin as it disrupts the boundary layer [11].

Invasive Methods

Nasal Oxygen Catheters and Nasotracheal Intubation

For prolonged oxygen administration a nasal catheter can be placed [1]. A rubber catheter can be inserted into the nares and sutured to the skin. Typical pet reptiles do not have a hard palate and the airway enters into the oral cavity from the choana, making nasotracheal intubation impractical. In snakes, the glottis is positioned in a significantly rostral position and fits into the groove of the choana. The catheter used should only be long enough to secure to the nostril opening and not extend caudal past the position of the glottis. Oxygen delivery can be between 2 and 5 l/min and should be passed through a humidifier to prevent drying of the airway epithelium [7].

Oral Endotracheal Intubation

Endotracheal intubation permits the maintenance of a patent airway, reduces risk of aspiration, and allows for positive pressure ventilation. In reptile and amphibian patients, uncuffed tubes are typically used [18, 19]. This is often due to small patient size and the unavailability of appropriately-sized cuffed tubes, or to prevent tracheal trauma in chelonians who possess complete tracheal rings. Complete cartilaginous rings do not allow for significant luminal expansion, and like birds, an inflated endotracheal cuff predisposes the trachea to pressure necrosis in certain reptiles [20, 21]. Lizards and snakes have dorsally incomplete tracheal rings [11]. Commercially available 2.0, 2.5, and 3.0 mm or greater endotracheal tubes can be used in larger reptiles; however, most small species will require the use of repurposed intravenous or red-rubber catheters (Figure 41.3). With little to no modification these catheters

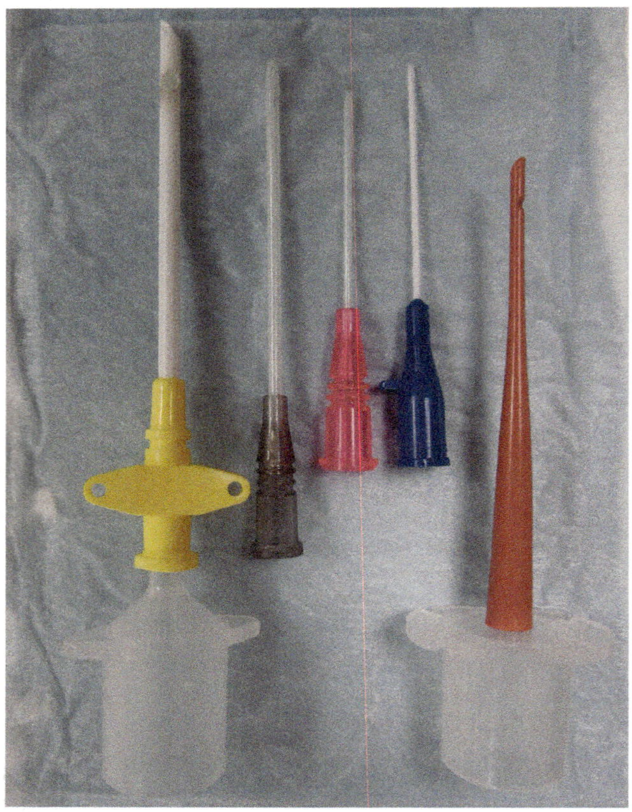

Figure 41.3 Endotracheal tubes can be custom made out of a variety of intravenous or red-rubber catheters. Murphy's eyes can be cut with a scalpel blade and edges softened with quick exposure to flame.

will attach to the connectors found on 2.5–3.5 mm endotracheal tubes. Catheters can then be shortened, and a Murphy's eye can be cut into larger gauge catheters with a scalpel. Sharp edges should be rounded with quick exposure to an open flame. Advanced preparation of several sizes of modified catheter endotracheal tubes ensures readiness for impending emergencies.

Whenever possible, use a clear endotracheal tube to allow for observation of condensation with each exhalation [18]. In small patients, this is often the only means for observing expiration as tidal volumes are insufficient for capnography [18]. Capnography has limited value in reptiles and may not correlate to PCO_2 values due to cardiac shunting of blood. Furthermore, most carbon dioxide monitors, particularly mainstream models, will increase dead space within the anesthesia circuit, which can have a significant impact on small patients.

Intubation begins with premeasurement of the endotracheal tube to avoid endobronchial intubation [18]. Some chelonian and chameleon species have a trachea that bifurcates at or cranial to the thoracic inlet, necessitating caution when intubating these species. Choose a minimum length that both secures the airway and makes dislodging of the tube unlikely. Then use a soft, atraumatic speculum to open the mouth and wipe away any visible mucus or debris from the oral cavity. In reptiles, the glottis is identified immediately caudal to the base of the tongue [18] (Figures 41.4 and 41.5). This typically allows easy intubation, although in some species like chameleons and bearded dragons the mobility of the glottis on an expandable buccal floor can cause difficulty. Once inserted into the trachea, the tube can be secured with tape to the lower jaw (Figure 41.6). In small patients, the hard, plastic hub of modified intravenous catheter endotracheal tubes can be aligned with the mandible to act as a mouth gag to prevent inadvertent damage or blockage of the tube should the animal bite down (Figure 41.7). The airway connector can be used in a similar manner for larger patients, or a mouth gag is placed to protect the tube (Figure 41.8).

Once intubated, the spontaneously breathing patient can be connected to an anesthetic machine to offer oxygen. A non-rebreathing circuit is used to minimize dead space and resistance to ventilation [18]. If the patient is not

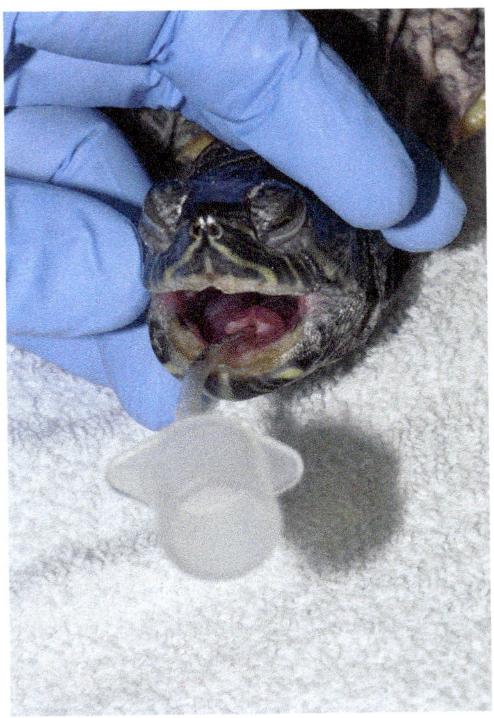

Figure 41.4 An endotracheal tube within the glottis of a red-eared slider (*Trachemys scripta elegans*). The thick, fleshy tongue can obscure visualization. *Source:* Photo courtesy of Grayson Doss.

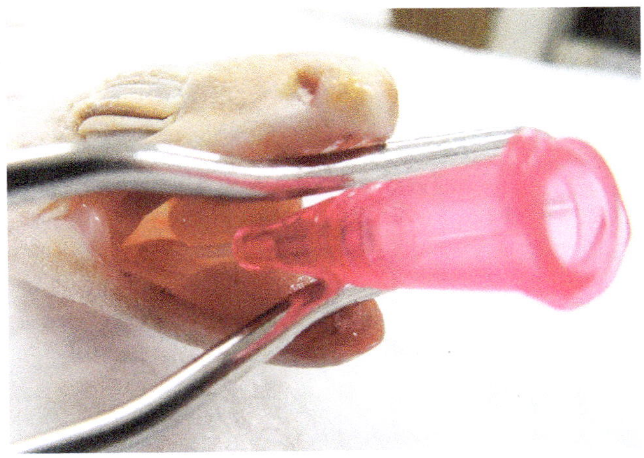

Figure 41.5 Endotracheal intubation of a leopard gecko (*Eublepharis macularius*) with a 20-gauge intravenous catheter.

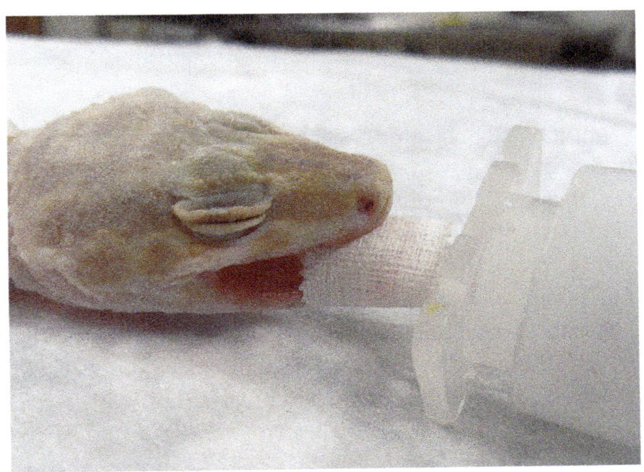

Figure 41.6 Endotracheal tubes can be secured to the bottom jaw with tape. This allows for continued access to the oral cavity.

Herptiles

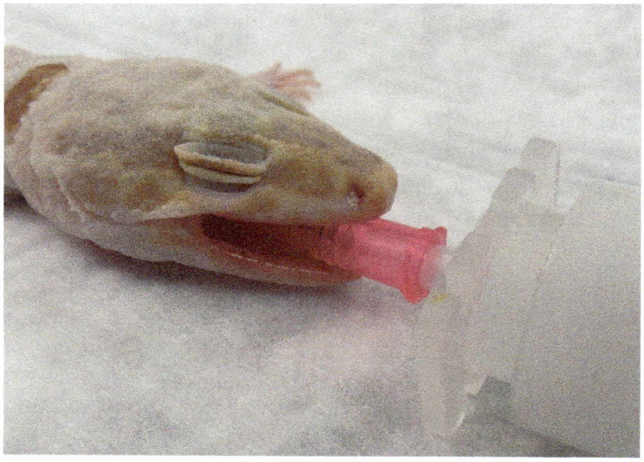

Figure 41.7 The catheter hub can be aligned to act as a mouth gag to prevent damage to the soft catheter cannula if the patient bites down on it.

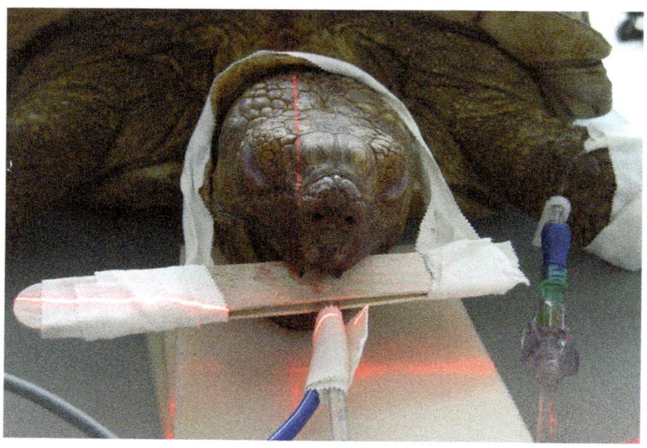

Figure 41.8 Mouth guards are necessary to protect endotracheal tubes in larger patients. Two tongue depressors have been used to protect the endotracheal tube (clear) and esophageal electrocardiogram (ECG) probe (blue) in an anesthetized sulcata tortoise during computed tomography imaging.

spontaneously breathing, begin positive pressure ventilation with a bag valve attached to the endotracheal tube, the anesthetic circuit bag, or by attaching the patient to a ventilator. Regardless of whether the ventilation is performed manually or mechanically, observe for normal coelomic expansion with each breath. Parameters for ventilation have not been thoroughly described in reptiles or amphibians; however, it has been anecdotally recommended to set ventilators to 4–6 breaths/min with a peak pressure of 12 cm H_2O, with an inspiratory time of less than one to two seconds [22, 23].

Laryngeal Masks and Supraglottic Airway Devices

Due to marked differences in laryngeal anatomy between reptile orders and the fact that the design of most commercially available laryngeal masks is based on mammalian anatomy, these airway maintenance devices are rarely, if ever, used in reptiles.

Percutaneous Emergency Airway Access

Saccular lung cannulation is an invasive emergency measure that has been described to circumvent tracheal blockage in a ball python (*Python regius*) and a boa constrictor (*Boa constrictor*) [24, 25]. With local anesthesia and aseptic preparation, create a small skin incision in the area of the right caudal lung field with the snake in left lateral recumbency. Because most snakes possess a vestigial left lung and a functional right lung, the right lung should be the planned site of placement. The target area of the lung for placement is the caudal avascular saccular lung or air sac. The vascular, gas exchange portion of the lung is cranial and should be avoided. After skin incision, bluntly dissect and gently insert small hemostats through the intercostal musculature, holding open the incision to allow visualization of the saccular lung, which is normally transparent and similar in appearance to clear cellophane. The saccular lung is entered with a stab incision. Insert an endotracheal tube through the incision into the lung. If present, inflation of the endotracheal tube cuff can prevent inadvertent removal during patient manipulation. Secure the tube to the skin with suture in a finger-trap pattern. Manual ventilation confirms placement and the tube can be attached to an anesthetic circuit for oxygen supplementation, or the end covered with sterile gauze to protect it from debris accumulation while allowing for spontaneous respiration. Inspired air needs to be humidified to prevent drying of the respiratory tissues. Saccular lung cannulas have been left in place as long as 13 days without significant deleterious side effects [24]. Surgically close the body wall musculature and skin in separate layers after cannula removal.

Tracheostomy

A tracheotomy can be performed for emergency treatment of laryngeal obstruction in reptiles. Reptilian cervical anatomy varies widely and can complicate placement of the tracheostomy tube. Some chameleons possess an accessory lung lobe cranial to the pectoral girdle [4], while many snakes have a tracheal lung extending from the dorsal opening in the tracheal rings [2, 11]. With these considerations, tracheotomies are performed as in mammals [26]. When using modified intravenous catheter endotracheal

Herptiles

tubes in small patients, the adapted endotracheal tube can be inserted without prior incision by using a removable stylet. Once in place, the tube can be temporarily held in place with a tie around the neck. After tube removal, the skin incision is left to heal by second intention. This allows the tracheal mucosa to heal prior to the skin, avoiding subcutaneous emphysema. Warm, humidified air should be provided to avoid drying of the respiratory tissues.

References

1. Schumacher, J. (2011). Respiratory medicine of reptiles. *Vet. Clin. North Am. Exot. Anim. Pract.* 14: 207–224.
2. Knotek, Z. and Divers, S.J. (2019). Pulmonology. In: *Mader's Reptile Medicine and Surgery*, 3e (eds. S.J. Divers and S.J. Stahl), 786–804. Elsevier Inc: St. Louis.
3. Music, M.K. and Strunk, A. (2016). Reptile critical care and common emergencies. *Vet. Clin. North Am. Exot. Anim. Pract.* 19: 591–612.
4. Murray, M.J. (2006). Cardiopulmonary anatomy and physiology. In: *Reptile Medicine and Surgery*, 2e (ed. D.R. Mader), 124–134. Elsevier Health Sciences.
5. Pough, F.H. (1980). Blood oxygen transport and delivery in reptiles. *Am. Zool.* 20: 173–185.
6. Bickler, P.E. and Buck, L.T. (2007). Hypoxia tolerance in reptiles, amphibians, and fishes: life with variable oxygen availability. *Annu. Rev. Physiol.* 69: 145–170.
7. Murray, M.J. (2006). Pneumonia and lower respiratory tract disease. In: *Reptile Medicine and Surgery*, 2e (ed. D.R. Mader), 865–877. Elsevier Health Sciences.
8. Bertelsen, M.F., Mosley, C., Crawshaw, G.J. et al. (2005). Inhalation anesthesia in Dumeril's monitor (*Varanus dumerilii*) with isoflurane, sevoflurane, and nitrous oxide: effects of inspired gases on induction and recovery. *J. Zoo Wildl. Med.* 36: 62–68.
9. Odette, O., Churgin, S.M., Sladky, K.K., and Smith, L.J. (2015). Anesthetic induction and recovery parameters in bearded dragons (*Pogona vitticeps*): comparison of isoflurane delivered in 100% oxygen versus 21% oxygen. *J. Zoo Wildl. Med.* 46: 534–540.
10. Ratliff, C., Parkinson, L.A., and Mans, C. (2019). Effects of the fraction of inspired oxygen on alfaxalone-sedated inland bearded dragons (*Pogona vitticeps*). *Am. J. Vet. Res.* 80: 129–134.
11. Vitt, L.J. and Caldwell, J.P. (2013). *Herpetology: An Introductory Biology of Amphibians and Reptiles*. Academic Press.
12. Wright, K.M. and Whitaker, B.R. (2001). *Amphibian Medicine and Captive Husbandry*. Krieger Publishing Company.
13. Mazzaferro, E. (2015). Oxygen therapy. In: *Small Animal Critical Care Medicine*, 2e (eds. D.C. Silverstein and H. K.). 77–80. St. Louis: Saunders.
14. Guimond, R.W. and Hutchison, V.H. (1972). Pulmonary, branchial and cutaneous gas exchange in the mud puppy, *Necturus maculosus maculosus* (Rafinesque). *Comp. Biochem. Physiol. A: Physiol.* 42: 367–392.
15. Heatwole, H. and Seymore, R. (1978). Cutaneous oxygen uptake in three groups of aquatic snakes. *Aust. J. Zool.* 26: 481–486.
16. Jammes, Y. and Grimaud, C. (1976). Ventilation, pulmonary and cutaneous gas exchange in the awake lizard *Lacerta viridis*. *Comp. Biochem. Physiol. A: Physiol.* 55: 279–285.
17. Standaert, T. and Johansen, K. (1974). Cutaneous gas exchange in snakes. *J. Comp. Physiol.* 89: 313–320.
18. Briscoe, J.A. and Syring, R. (2004). Techniques for emergency airway and vascular access in special species. *Sem. Avian Exot. Pet Med.* 13 (3): 118–131.
19. Mosley, C.A. (2005). Anesthesia and analgesia in reptiles. *Sem. Avian Exot. Pet Med.* 14 (4): 243–262.
20. Lierz, M. and Korbel, R. (2012). Anesthesia and analgesia in birds. *J. Exot. Pet Med.* 21: 44–58.
21. Nugent-Deal, J. (2016). Exotic anesthesia and analgesia. In: *Exotic Animal Medicine for the Veterinary Technician* (eds. B. Ballard and R. Cheek), 11–30. John Wiley & Sons.
22. Mans, C., Sladky, K.K., and Schumacher, J. (2019). General anesthesia. In: *Mader's Reptile Medicine and Surgery*, 3e (eds. S.J. Divers and S.J. Stahl), 447–464. St. Louis: Elsevier Inc.
23. Schumacher, J. and Yelen, T. (2006). Anesthesia and analgesia. In: *Reptile Medicine and Surgery*, 2e (ed. D.R. Mader), 442–452. Elsevier Health Sciences.
24. Myers, D.A., Wellehan, J.F., and Isaza, R. (2009). Saccular lung cannulation in a ball python (*Python regius*) to treat a tracheal obstruction. *J. Zoo Wildl. Med.* 40: 214–216.
25. Summa, N.M., Guzman, D.S.-M., Hawkins, M.G. et al. (2015). Tracheal and colonic resection and anastomosis in a boa constrictor (*Boa constrictor*) with T-cell lymphoma. *J. Herpetol. Med. Surg.* 25: 87–99.
26. Crowe, D. (2006). Emergency airway access – rapid tracheotomy. In: *Veterinary Emergency Critical Care Manual*, 2e (ed. K.A. Mathews). Guelph, ON, Canada: Lifelearn.

42

Catheterization and Venipuncture

Ian Kanda and João Brandão

Department of Veterinary Clinical Sciences, College of Veterinary Medicine, Oklahoma State University, Stillwater, Oklahoma, USA

CONTENTS

Introduction

There are unique challenges when accessing the vasculature in reptiles and amphibians. These animals are typically small, and reptiles have thick skin which limits visualization. Both classes have an extensive lymphatic system which, when penetrated, commonly causes lymphatic contamination of blood samples.

This chapter focuses on common pet reptile and amphibian species. For other species, please refer to other resources [1].

Blood Sample Collection

Venipuncture

Equipment/Materials

Most patients are small, typically requiring human pediatric venipuncture equipment. This includes needles and catheters ranging from 22- to 28-gauge (Figure 42.1). Spinal needles of 20- or 22-gauge are typically used for intraosseous (IO) catheterization; if smaller sizes are required, hypodermic needles are used.

For small patients, human pediatric blood tubes (Microtainer, Becton-Dickinson, Franklin Lakes, NJ, USA) should be used. Lithium heparin should be used as the default anticoagulant [2–6] as ethylenediamine tetraacetic acid (EDTA) may lyse the red blood cells in some species, particularly chelonians [2, 4, 7]. As heparin can cause white blood cell and thrombocyte clumping, and affect staining [2], it is advised to create blood smears as a back-up for review. Heparinized microhematocrit tubes can also be used to collect whole blood. Preheparinized syringes are commonly used to prevent sample clotting during collection but they have the potential to affect some hematology values [8].

Use moistened, powder and latex-free gloves for handling amphibians, as they have sensitive skin and some species may

Exotic Animal Emergency and Critical Care Medicine, First Edition. Edited by Jennifer E. Graham, Grayson A. Doss and Hugues Beaufrère.

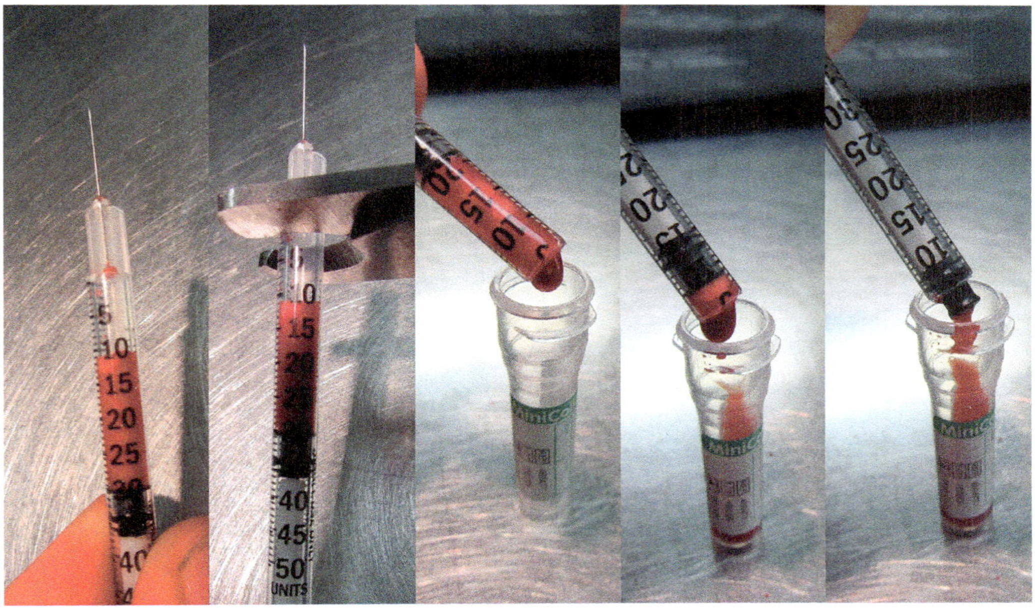

Figure 42.1 Needles are removed from syringes prior to dispensing blood to avoid cell lysis. For insulin syringes, draw back to add an airspace then cut the syringe with heavy duty nail trimmers.

also produce cutaneous toxins [2, 4, 9]. Sedation or anesthesia (see Chapter 45: Analgesia, Anesthesia and Monitoring) is often necessary for venipuncture in amphibians.

Sample Size

In healthy animals, up to 1 ml of blood/100 g body weight can be safely removed; this should be reduced to 0.5 ml/100 g body weight for debilitated animals [9, 10]. It is important to take only the minimum amount of blood necessary (Table 42.1), especially in small patients.

Venipuncture Sites

Turtles and Tortoises

Jugular Vein

The jugular vein is the ideal venipuncture site in chelonians and lymph contamination is less common at this location [10, 11]. A drawback with this site is that the head needs to be withdrawn from the shell for access, which is difficult to impossible in awake large tortoises, box turtles and aggressive aquatic species. The head is grasped between the thumb and forefinger and gently extended from the shell, which is restrained by an assistant. The turtle can be placed in lateral recumbency to assist with jugular access. The right jugular vein may be larger than the left [2] and is occluded with digital pressure at the base of the neck. While difficult to see in most species, the jugular vein may become visible or palpable after proximal occlusion. The jugular vein runs from the angle of the mandible to the carapacial inlet. Insert the needle shallowly, caudal to the tympanum, entering in a cranial-to-caudal direction (Figure 42.2).

Subcarapacial Venous Sinus

The subcarapacial venous sinus is often the most accessible venipuncture site, as it can usually be accessed even with the chelonian's head withdrawn into the shell. An exception is with some hinged-shell turtles (e.g. box turtles), where this site becomes non-accessible with the turtle retracted into a fully closed shell. The subcarapacial venous sinus is found on the dorsal midline, underneath the carapace, and dorsal to the cervical spine. For venipuncture, insert the needle on midline, underneath the carapace immediately caudal to where the skin meets the shell. Continue needle insertion in a caudodorsal direction (Figure 42.3). Since the subcarapacial sinus is caudal to large lymphatic vessels [12], lymphatic contamination is common. In large, strong tortoises, a long spinal needle with the stylet removed can be attached to an intravenous fluid extension line (Figure 42.4) to permit access. Do not redirect the needle while it is inserted to avoid vascular laceration.

Caudal Veins

Depending on the species, chelonians may possess dorsal, ventral, and/or lateral caudal veins, also known as coccygeal or tail veins [10], with the dorsal caudal vein being one of the more commonly utilized vessels. For venipuncture of the dorsal caudal vein, the needle is inserted in a cranioventral direction at an approximately 45° angle along the dorsal midline of the tail (Figure 42.5). If the needle hits a vertebra, withdraw the needle most of the way and then redirect either cranially or caudally, or improve alignment if insertion is off of midline.

Table 42.1 Common maximum blood sample sizes and collection sites in adult reptiles and amphibians.

Species	Typical adult BW (g)[a]	Typical maximum sample size (ml)[b]	Sample sites – typical order of approach	Pitfalls
Necessary sample size				
CBC/Chem: outside lab		1		
VetScan[c]		0.1		
i-STAT[d]		0.1		
CBC: in-house		0.01–0.1		
		General rule: 1 ml/100 g BW		
Boa constrictor	10 000	100	Ventral tail, IC, jugular	
Corn snake	800	8	Ventral tail, IC, jugular	
Ball python	3000	30	Ventral tail, IC, jugular	Small tail
Bearded dragon	400	4	Ventral tail, jugular	
Leopard gecko	60	0.6	Ventral tail	Tail autotomy
Crested gecko	50	0.5	Ventral tail	Tail autotomy
Green iguana	6000	60	Ventral tail, jugular	
Veiled chameleon	200	2	Ventral tail, jugular	
Green anole	4	0.04	Ventral tail vein	Small size
Box turtle	500	5	Jugular, subcarapacial	
Sulcata tortoise	45 000	450	Subcarapacial, brachial, jugular	Strong withdrawal into shell
Red eared slider	2000	20	Jugular, subcarapacial, dorsal tail	
Common snapping turtle	6000	60	Dorsal tail, jugular, subcarapacial	Dangerous bite with long neck reach
Tiger salamander	130	1.3	Ventral tail, abdominal	Delicate skin
Firebelly newt	8	0.08	Ventral tail, abdominal	Delicate skin
Red eye tree frog	10	0.1	Abdominal, lingual, femoral	Delicate skin
Bullfrog	500	5	Abdominal, lingual, femoral	Delicate skin

[a] Body weights vary by individual, age, gender, season, and captive care conditions.
[b] Only take the minimum amount of blood necessary for diagnostics or blood donation.
[c] Point of care analyzer Abaxis VetScan VS2 (Abaxis, Union City, CA, USA).
[d] Point of care analyzer Abaxis VetScan i-STAT (Abaxis, Union City, CA, USA).
BW, body weight; IC, intracardiac.

Other Sites

The brachial vein is an alternative site that can be useful for venipuncture, particularly in larger tortoises. It requires the extension of a forelimb but is otherwise easily accessible (Figure 42.6). The needle is inserted perpendicular to the humerus immediately dorsal to the palpable biceps brachii tendon [13]. The needle is advanced toward the radio-humeral joint until blood is observed [13].

Snakes

Caudal Vein

The caudal vein, also named the ventral tail or coccygeal vein is the primary venipuncture site in snakes. It can be accessed with insertion of a needle between the ventral scales of the tail (portion caudal to the vent) at a 45–90° angle (Figure 42.7). Insertion must be done on the ventral midline and a good grasp of the tail is necessary as the snake may twist away. Male snakes possess hemipenes within the tail base and both genders may have scent glands caudal to the vent opening. These structures can be avoided by utilizing the caudal 75% of the tail during caudal vein venipuncture [2].

Intra-Cardiac

Distinct from other reptile groups, the heart may be used for venipuncture in snakes. Because of the potential for cardiac damage, the authors typically reserve this venipuncture site for when caudal vein sampling has failed. The movement of the heart beating can be visually observed on the ventrum with the snake held in dorsal or lateral recumbency. An ultrasound or ultrasonic Doppler flow detector can aid in localization. The heart is located at approximately the one fourth to one third mark of the total snout to vent length [10]. Cardiocentesis can be performed

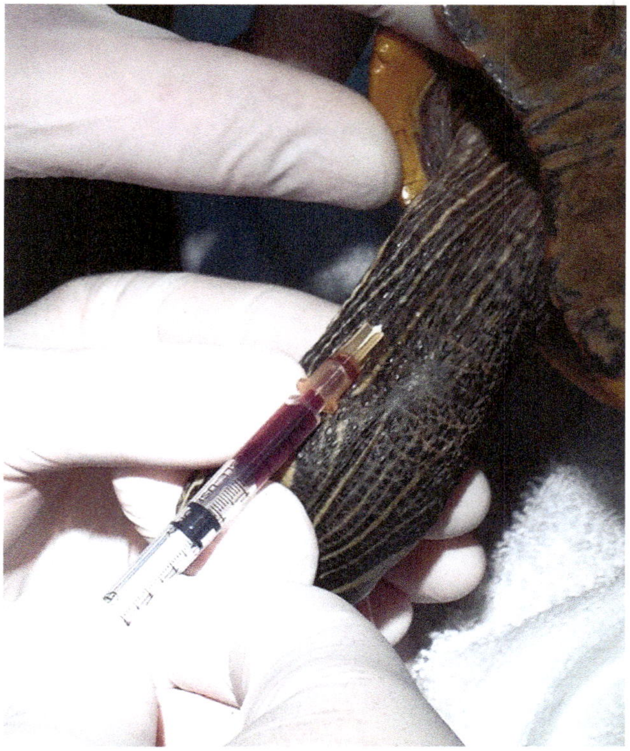

Figure 42.2 A jugular blood sample drawn from a river cooter (*Pseudemys concinna*). Note the right jugular vein is used and a shallow angle needle entry caudal to the tympanum (hidden from view). An assistant is occluding the vein at the base of the neck.

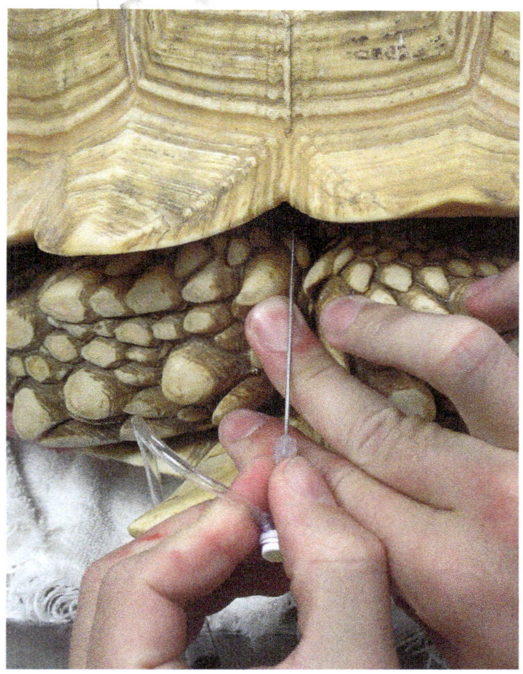

Figure 42.4 Subcarapacial sinus approach to venipuncture in a sulcata tortoise (*Centrochelys sulcata*). A 4-in. spinal needle with the stylet removed is attached to an intravenous fluid line extension to allow for an appropriate insertion angle.

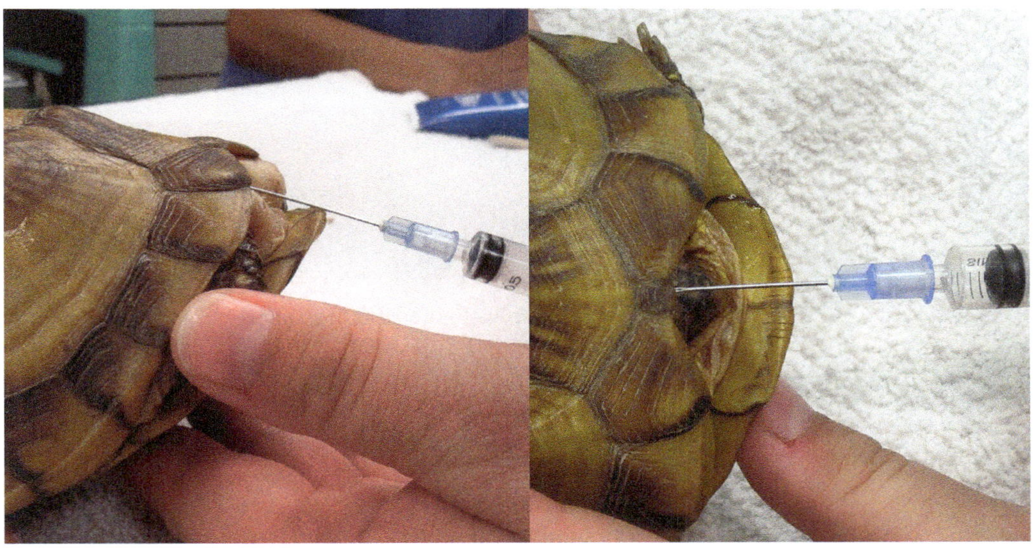

Figure 42.3 Subcarapacial sinus approach to venipuncture in a box turtle (*Terrapene carolina triunguis*). Note insertion of the needle is performed in a caudodorsal direction on midline.

in snakes without sedation; however, the authors often prefer the use of chemical immobilization to decrease patient movement during sampling. The snake is held in dorsal recumbency or upright and the heart immobilized within the coelom using digital pressure both immediately cranial and caudal to the heart (Figure 42.8). Needle insertion begins directly caudal to the heart, between two ventral scales. The needle is advanced in a craniodorsal direction

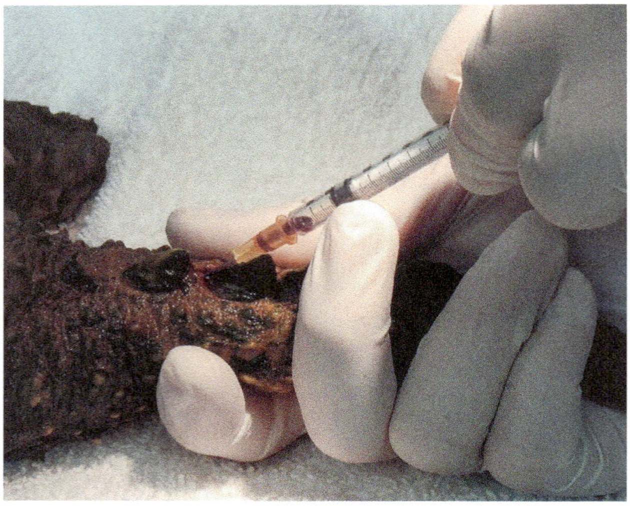

Figure 42.5 Dorsal caudal vein venipuncture in a common snapping turtle (*Chelydra serpentina*).

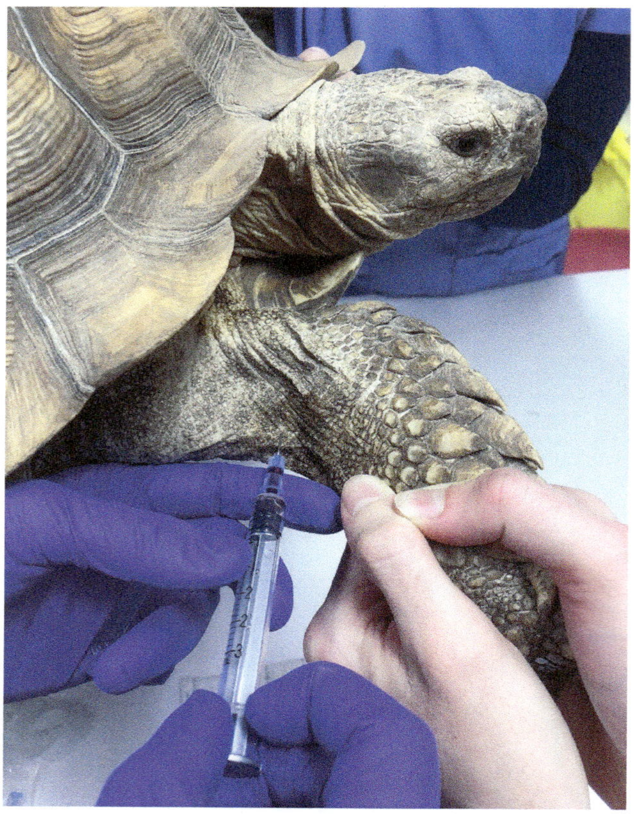

Figure 42.6 Right brachial vein venipuncture in a sulcata tortoise (*Centrochelys sulcata*). *Source:* Courtesy of Grayson Doss, Madison, WI.

into the ventricle at an approximately 45° angle. The syringe often fills slowly with each heartbeat. Avoid excess negative pressure on the plunger [4]. Upon needle withdrawal, maintain digital pressure on the site. Blood collected from the heart has a low chance of lymphatic contamination [10].

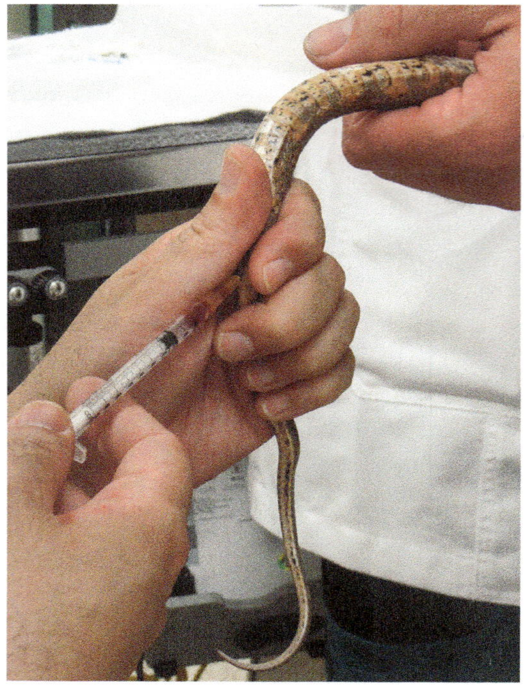

Figure 42.7 Caudal vein venipuncture in a corn snake (*Pantherophis guttatus*). A secure grip of the tail helps maintain the midline approach as the snake tries to twist away.

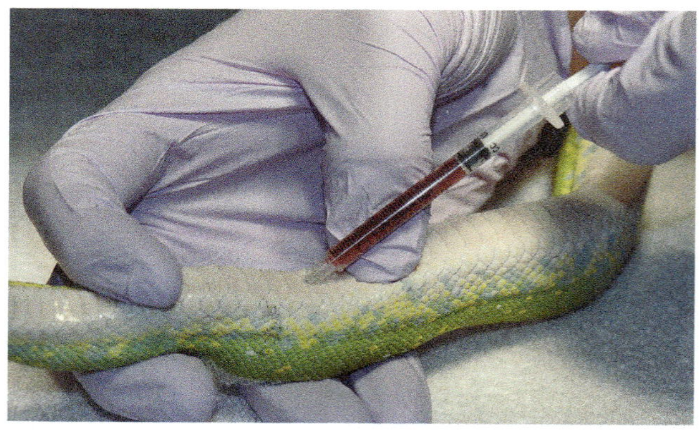

Figure 42.8 Cardiocentesis in an anesthetized green tree python (*Morelia viridis*). *Source:* Photo courtesy of Christoph Mans.

Jugular Vein

The jugular vein is not commonly utilized for venipuncture in snakes. The jugular vein cannot be visualized externally, necessitating a blind attempt to access the vessel. Begin by locating the heart and counting 4–9 ventral scutes craniad [14, 15]. Insert the needle at a shallow angle in a cranial direction both lateral to the ventral scute and medial to the ribs.

Lizards

Caudal Vein

In lizards, the caudal or ventral tail vein is the primary vessel utilized for venipuncture. This vessel runs ventral to the coccygeal vertebral bodies. It can be accessed with a ventral

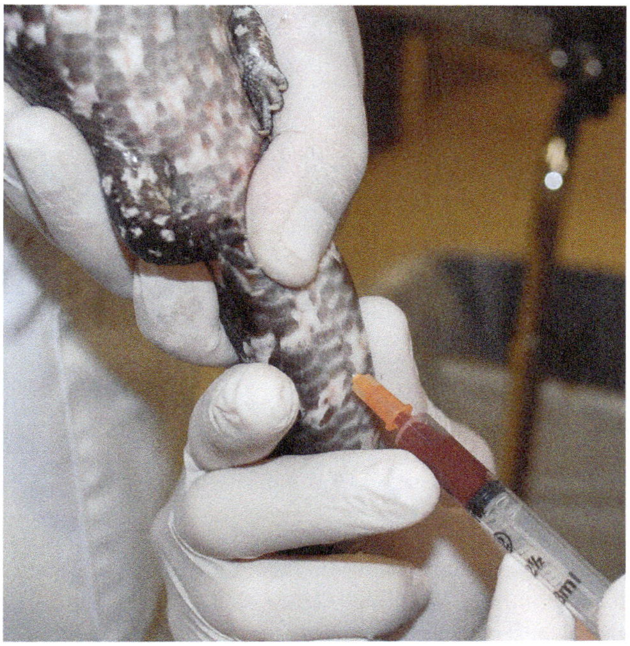

Figure 42.9 Caudal vein venipuncture in a blue-tongue skink (*Tiliqua scincoides*).

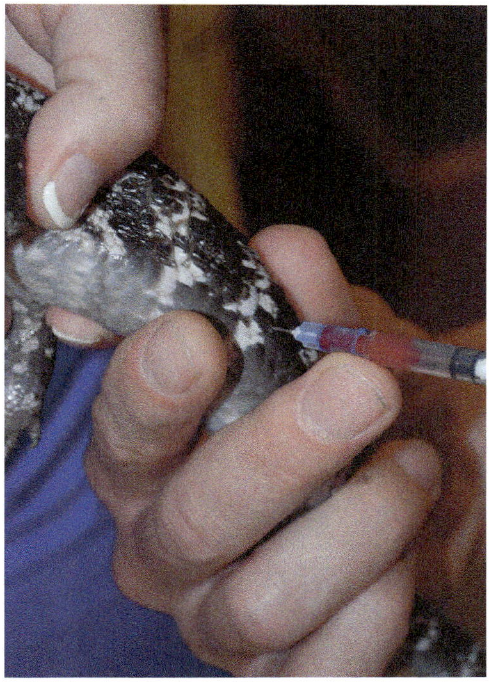

Figure 42.10 A lateral approach to caudal vein venipuncture in a blue-tongue skink (*Tiliqua scincoides*).

midline approach as in snakes or chelonians (Figure 42.9). Negative plunger pressure should be minimized to avoid collapsing the vessel. Male lizards have paired hemipenes immediately caudal to the vent which should be avoided by inserting the needle caudal to the hemipenile bulge or by using the distal 80% of the tail for venipuncture. The vein reduces in size as it progresses caudally.

The ventral tail vein can also be accessed from a lateral approach (Figure 42.10). Insert the needle into the lateral midline. The target area is just ventral to the transverse processes of the coccygeal vertebrae on midline. If the needle hits a transverse vertebral process, withdraw the needle slightly and redirect it ventral to the process. After redirection, slowly advance the needle toward the midline of the tail.

Many lizards have the ability to perform autotomy when the tail is grasped. Patient restraint prior to grasping the tail should minimize this risk. In species like geckos, sedation, or anesthesia for venipuncture is recommended.

Cephalic Vein

The cephalic vein is an uncommon venipuncture site in lizards. It runs along the dorsal surface of the front leg similar to mammals; however, it is neither visible, nor palpable.

Jugular Vein

The jugular vein can be a practical venipuncture site in lizards, although it cannot usually be visualized or palpated. The needle is often inserted blindly behind the tympanum in a caudal direction. In some small lizards like chameleons, the jugular vein can be visualized with trans-illumination [16]. A blind sampling technique has been described for small lizards where the animal is restrained with the head and neck stretched laterally. The needle is inserted in the caudal cervical area at an angle <45° to the skin surface in a caudoventral direction [17].

Cranial Vena Cava

The cranial vena cava may be a suitable alternative in species that readily autotomize their tails [18, 19]. However, this technique has not been fully described in reptiles. Sedation or anesthesia is recommended [19].

Other Sites

The ventral abdominal vein is not a common venipuncture site in lizards. This large vein runs along the ventral midline of the coelom [10, 15]. It is most easily accessed mid-coelom [10]. The needle is inserted at a shallow, craniad angle along the ventral midline. Because applying adequate pressure after sampling is difficult in this area, hemorrhage can occur.

Other blood collection sites occasionally discussed include the orbital sinus or a nail clip. However, utilization of these sites is considered painful and unethical, and often yields poor diagnostic samples [2, 10].

Amphibians

Lingual Vein

The lingual vein has traditionally been used in anurans and may be useful in salamanders [2, 4, 6, 20, 21]. The mouth is opened with a soft speculum and the tongue

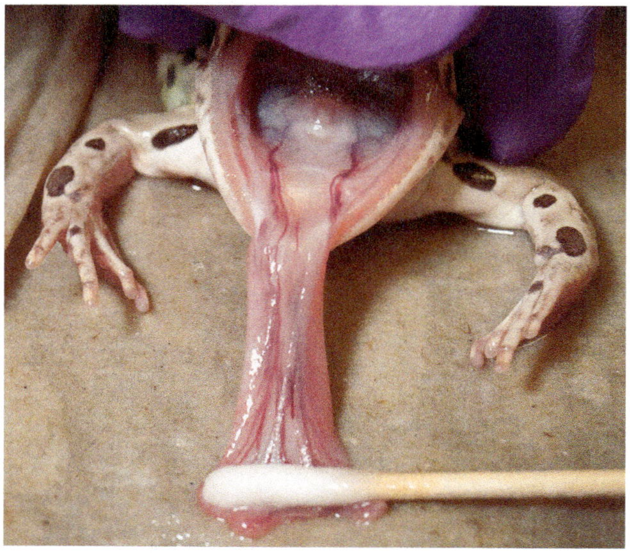

Figure 42.11 Lingual veins in a leopard frog (*Lithobates pipiens*). The vessels are typically more apparent after tongue extension. *Source:* Photo courtesy of Grayson Doss.

withdrawn with a cotton tipped applicator. Vessels located on the ventrum of the tongue or on the buccal floor can be easily visualized and are wiped clean of saliva to minimize contamination (Figure 42.11). A vessel is punctured with a small gauge needle and blood is allowed to flow from the wound and collected in a heparinized capillary tube [21]. Tongue withdrawal often provides sufficient pressure for hemostasis [21].

Ventral Abdominal Vein

The ventral abdominal vein can be used for venipuncture in amphibians. Often it is readily visible or it can be found by using a Doppler probe [2, 4, 6]. Sampling is similar to lizards. Begin midway between the sternum and pelvis [4, 21]. Blood flow is slow, and the vein can easily collapse [4]. Lymphatic contamination may occur [2].

Caudal Vein

Venipuncture of the caudal vein in salamanders is performed as in snakes and lizards. Ideally, avoid this vein in species that perform tail autotomy [2, 4, 21].

Intra-Cardiac

Cardiocentesis can be performed in amphibians. Sedation or anesthesia is recommended for this procedure as trauma to the heart or great vessels can occur [2, 4, 6, 9, 21]. The heart is located by visualizing the heart beat on the ventrum, with the aid of a Doppler probe, or with esophageal transillumination [2, 4, 21]. A small gauge needle is inserted along the ventrum toward the heart and advanced craniodorsally into the ventricle (Figure 42.12). Pericardial fluid may be observed and appears clear or cloudy-yellow [4].

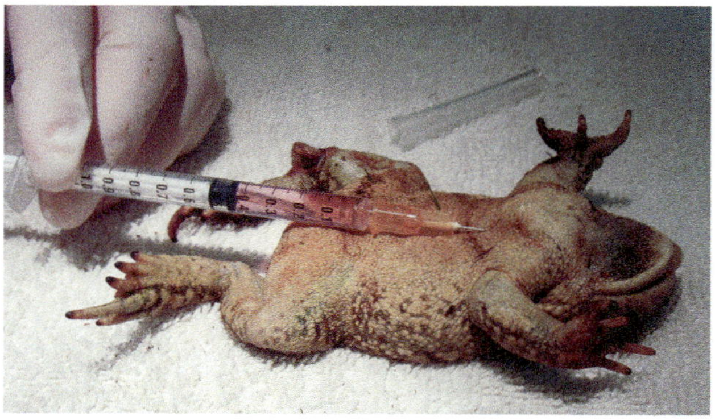

Figure 42.12 Cardiocentesis for euthanasia in a Woodhouse's toad (*Anaxyrus woodhousii*). The heart can be located by visualizing the heart beat on the ventrum, with the aid of a Doppler, or with esophageal trans-illumination.

Femoral Vein

The femoral vein has been suggested for venipuncture in anurans [9, 20]. This vein can be visualized on the medial aspect of the hind leg and blood collected with a small gauge needle [9].

Arterial Sampling

Arterial sampling is not routinely performed in reptiles and amphibians due to the small peripheral arteries and necessity of an invasive approach to access large enough vessels for sample collection.

Collection from Blood Donors

Donor Testing/Typing

Blood transfusion reactions have been anecdotally reported in reptiles, although there are no studies investigating blood types or groups in either reptiles or amphibians. It is recommended to use donors of the same species who are free of disease, and to perform major and minor crossmatching whenever possible [1, 22, 23]. However, guidelines have not been well-defined in reptiles and amphibians and a full crossmatch may not be practical in patients with small blood volumes. Mammalian major and minor crossmatching protocols in two sea turtle species demonstrated a high rate of both intraspecific and interspecific incompatibility [23]. Because even an initial blood transfusion could result in a reaction, a simplified crossmatch should be performed, at a minimum, if full major and minor crossmatching is not possible. At room temperature, mix two drops of plasma from either the recipient or donor animal on a slide along with one drop of whole blood from the opposite individual; evidence of microagglutination in <1 minute suggests incompatibility [24]. Heterologous blood transfusions should be considered a viable option in emergencies when an ideal donor (i.e. same species) is not readily available, although the risk of reaction may be increased and donor blood cells may have a reduced lifespan.

Technique and Storage

Sedation or anesthesia of the donor is performed prior to collection to minimize stress. This is especially important for jugular venipuncture in large tortoises and cardiocentesis in snakes, where donors must remain still during collection. Immobilization utilizing alpha$_2$-agonists may make collection from peripheral sites more challenging. Blood volumes of up to 1 mL/100 g body weight can be collected from a healthy donor animal. See Chapter 46: Nutrition and Fluid Therapy for specifics regarding administering blood transfusions to reptiles and amphibians.

There is little information on storage of reptilian or amphibian blood, and the ideal anticoagulant choice may be group- or species-specific. Both acid-citrate-dextrose (ACD) and citrate-phosphate-dextrose-adenine (CPDA-1) successfully preserved American alligator (*Alligator mississippiensis*) packed red blood cells for at least 35 days [25]. In Loggerhead sea turtles (*Caretta caretta*), sodium heparin was the preferred anticoagulant for short-term storage (24 hours) of whole blood [26].

Catheterization

Intravenous

Intravenous (IV) catheters are most commonly used in anesthetized or moribund reptiles, as their placement typically requires a surgical procedure and they are easily dislodged in the awake patient.

The jugular vein is one of the most common sites used for IV catheterization in reptiles. The right jugular is often larger but both can be used [27, 28]. The cephalic and caudal veins may also be used in lizards. Venous sinuses are not recommended for catheter placement [29]. For jugular or cephalic catheterization, a surgical cut down procedure aids vein visualization (Figure 42.13). For this invasive procedure, local anesthesia in addition to heavy sedation or general anesthesia is required [27, 29]. In chelonians, a central venous catheter can permit continued patency when the head is retracted [28]. In desert tortoises (*Gopherus agassizii*), jugular vein catheters were easily dislodged during manipulation or following animal movement [30].

A surgical cut down is not used for the caudal vein in lizards. The catheter is inserted ventral to the transverse vertebral processes of the coccygeal vertebrae in a cranial direction, aiming toward the midline of the tail. Bending the tail laterally may improve access to this vessel. Because there is little deflection of this vessel due to surrounding tissue, the catheter is advanced immediately after penetration to avoid passing completely through the vein [31]. It is important to remember that drugs injected in this vessel may pass through the renal or hepatic portal systems prior to reaching systemic circulation, depending on species [1, 31].

Intravenous catheterization has not been well described in amphibians. In larger amphibians, the ventral abdominal or femoral veins may be used for attempted catheterization. In tailed species, the caudal vein may be attempted as is described for lizards.

Arterial

Because unique anatomy necessitates an invasive surgical approach to suitably sized arteries, arterial catheterization is rarely performed in reptiles and amphibians other than in a research setting [28]. Arterial catheterization has been described for the carotid and femoral arteries in iguanas and the vertebral arteries of rattlesnakes [28].

Intraosseous

Because intravenous access requires a surgical approach in most reptiles, intraosseous (IO) access is an attractive alternative, although fluid administration rates may be

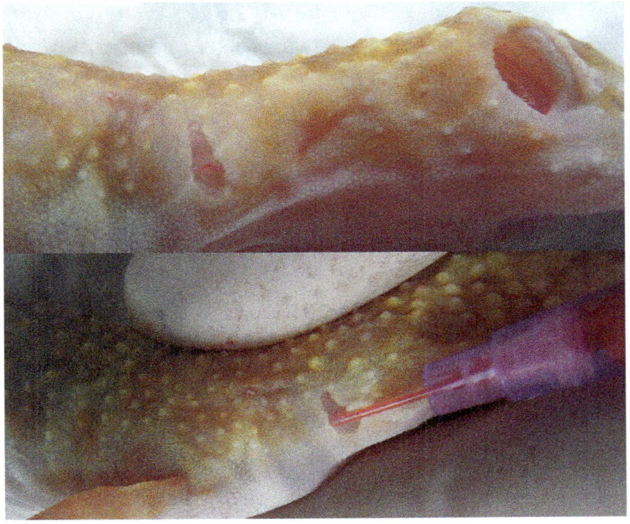

Figure 42.13 Intravenous catheterization of the right jugular vein in a leopard gecko (*Eublepharis macularius*). A cut down procedure was utilized for visualization and a 26-gauge catheter inserted.

less than with IV catheters. There are no available sites for IO catheterization in legless reptiles or amphibians and IO catheters may cause iatrogenic fractures in animals with metabolic bone disease. The potential for permanent disability, osteomyelitis and/or pain should be also considered when determining whether IO catheters are the best choice for the patient [28]. IO catheter placement should be confirmed with orthogonal radiographs and catheters should not be left in place longer than 72 hours [27].

Sites for IO catheterization in reptiles include the femur, humerus, and tibia [27, 28]. In turtles, the junction or "bridge" between the carapace and plastron has been suggested for catheterization; however, placement can be difficult and inadvertent coelomic cavity communication can occur [27, 28, 32]. In desert tortoises, the efficacy of various IO sites (humerus, femur, bridge, and plastron gular region) were compared to jugular vein catheterization using scintigraphy [30]. Results demonstrated that the humerus and femur were the best IO sites for vascular access, although they resulted in less rapid systemic circulation distribution compared with IV. When placed in the legs of chelonians, IO catheters are commonly damaged by limb movement.

IO catheter placement in the hind limb begins with flexion of the stifle joint. The skin should be aseptically prepared and heavy sedation or general anesthesia along with local anesthesia at the periosteal insertion site are recommended [27]. A spinal needle is inserted and seated firmly against the proximal tibial crest, or at the distal end of the diaphysis of the femur; the needle is rotated under gentle forward pressure to drill through the cortex of the bone (Figure 42.14). Spinal needles are preferred as they utilize a stylet, which prevents the catheter lumen plugging with a bone fragment during insertion; however, in small patients, hypodermic needles may be necessary. If proximal femoral IO catheter placement is preferred, insert the needle through the greater trochanter, which can be highlighted by adducting the leg. The greater tubercle of the proximal humerus can be exposed in a similar manner. Loss of resistance during needle insertion occurs after cortex penetration and the needle can then be advanced further into the medullary cavity. Bone marrow may be observed with negative pressure on an attached syringe and the external portion of the catheter will move simultaneously with the bone as the leg is moved. The needle tip may also grind against the medullary cavity when manipulated, helping to confirm proper placement. The catheter should flush easily. Orthogonal radiographs should always be used to confirm proper placement. Sterile antibiotic ointment can be placed on the insertion site to prevent infection and the catheter secured with tape. The leg is typically immobilized by bandaging or splinting to protect the catheter and avoid any additional trauma from limb movement (Figure 42.15).

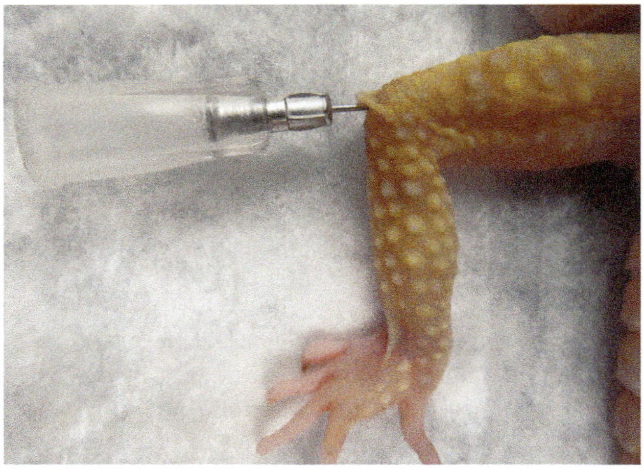

Figure 42.14 Intraosseous catheterization of the distal femur in a leopard gecko (*Eublepharis macularius*). A 25-gauge hypodermic needle was chosen due to the small size of the patient. Antibiotic cream can be put on the insertion site and the catheter secured to the leg with tape.

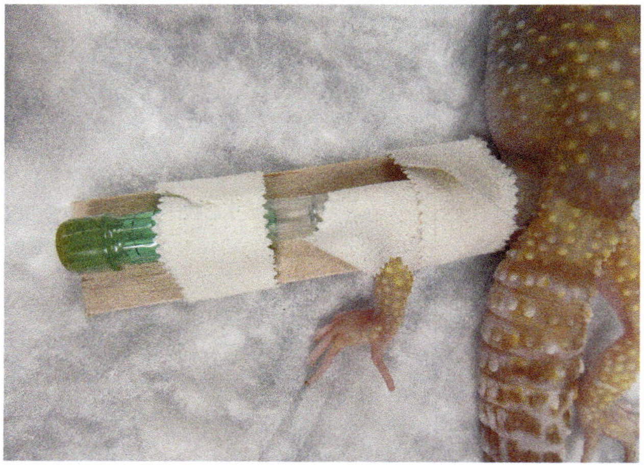

Figure 42.15 Splinting of an intraosseous catheter in a leopard gecko (*Eublepharis macularius*). In small lizards the weight of the catheter and injection cap is significant and a splint is used to prevent torque related trauma to the bone.

Urinary

Urinary catheterization is not routinely performed in reptiles or amphibians. Catheterization of the urinary bladder can be used for monitoring long-term fluid therapy or for collecting diagnostic urine samples from chelonians and lizard species that possess a urinary bladder [10]. Catheterization is ideally done under endoscopic guidance to minimize the risk of iatrogenic damage to the thin bladder wall.

References

1 Divers, S.J. and Stahl, S.J. (eds.) (2019). *Mader's Reptile Medicine and Surgery*. St. Louis: Elsevier Inc.

2 Campbell, T.W. (2015). *Exotic Animal Hematology and Cytology*. Wiley.

3 Dessauer, H.C. (1970). Blood chemistry of reptiles: physiological and evolutionary aspects. *Biol. Reptilia.* 3: 1–72.

4 Dyer, S.M. and Cervasio, E.L. (2008). An overview of restraint and blood collection techniques in exotic pet practice. *Vet. Clin. North Am. Exot. Anim. Pract.* 11: 423–443.

5 Harr, K.E., Raskin, R.E., and Heard, D.J. (2005). Temporal effects of 3 commonly used anticoagulants on hematologic and biochemical variables in blood samples from macaws and Burmese pythons. *Vet. Clin. Fathol.* 34: 383–388.

6 Wright, K. (2001). *Amphibian Hematology. Amphibian Medicine and Captive Husbandry. KM Wright and BR Whitaker (eds). Krieger Publ. Co.*, 129–146. Florida: Malabar.

7 Lyman, R.A. (1945). The anti-haemolytic function of calcium in the blood of the snapping turtle, *Chelydra serpentina*. *J. Cell. Comp. Physiol.* 25: 65–73.

8 Johnson, J.G., Nevarez, J.G., and Beaufrère, H. (2014). Effect of manually Preheparinized syringes on packed cell volume and Total solids in blood samples collected from American alligators (*Alligator mississippiensis*). *J. Exot. Pet Med.* 23: 142–146.

9 Allender, M.C. and Fry, M.M. (2008). Amphibian hematology. *Vet. Clin. North Am. Exot. Anim. Pract.* 11: 463–480.

10 Divers, S.J. (2019). Diagnostic techniques and sample collection. In: *Mader's Reptile Medicine and Surgery* (eds. S.J. Divers and S.J. Stahl), 405–421. St. Louis: Elsevier Inc.

11 Norton, T.M. (2005. Elsevier,). Chelonian emergency and critical care. *Semi. Avian Exot. Pet Med.* 14 (2): 106–130.

12 Heatley, J.J. and Russell, K.E. (2010). Box turtle (*Terrapene* spp.) hematology. *J. Exot. Pet Med.* 19: 160–164.

13 Mans, C. (2008). Venipuncture techniques in chelonian species. *Lab. Anim.* 37: 303.

14 Brown, C. (2010). Cardiac blood sample collection from snakes. *Lab Anim.* 39: 208.

15 Mosley, C.A. (2006). Intravascular access options in reptiles: what's reasonable. *Proc. NAVC*: 1654–1655.

16 Eshar, D., Lapid, R., and Head, V. (2018). Transilluminated jugular blood sampling in the common chameleon (*Chamaeleo chamaeleon*). *J. Herpetol. Med. Surg.* 28: 19–22.

17 di Giuseppe, M., Morici, M., Martinez Silvestre, A., and Spadola, F. (2017). Jugular vein venipuncture technique in small lizard species. *J. Small Anim. Pract.* 58: 249.

18 Mayer, J., Knoll, J., Wrubel, K., and Mitchell, M. (2011). Characterizing the hematologic and plasma chemistry profiles of captive crested geckos (*Rhacodactylus ciliatus*). *J. Herpetol. Med. Surg.* 21: 68–75.

19 Music, M.K. and Strunk, A. (2016). Reptile critical care and common emergencies. *Vet. Clin. North Am. Exot. Anim. Pract.* 19: 591–612.

20 Sykes, J.M. and Greenacre, C.B. (2006). Techniques for drug delivery in reptiles and amphibians. *J. Exot. Pet Med.* 15: 210–217.

21 Whitaker, B.R. and Wright, K.M. (2019). Amphibian medicine. In: *Mader's Reptile Medicine and Surgery* (eds. S.J. Divers and S.J. Stahl), 992–1013. Elsevier Inc: St. Louis.

22 Cital, S. and Goodnight, A. (2016). *Reptile and amphibian transfusion medicine* (eds. K. Yagi and M.K. Holowaychuk), 358–365. Hoboken: Wiley.

23 Donnelly, K.A., Norton, T.M., Zirkelbach, B., and Stacy, N.I. (2019). Advancing transfusion medicine in sea turtles: optimization of a cross-matching protocol. *J. Zoo Wildl. Med.* 50: 315–321.

24 Lichtenberger, M. (2004). Transfusion medicine in exotic pets. *Clin. Tech. Small Anim. Pract.* 19: 88–95.

25 Emerson, J.A., Stacy, N.I., Coverdill, C.C. et al. (2014). Preservation of red blood cells in the American alligator (*Alligator mississippiensis*) over time and in two different anticoagulants. *J. Herpetol. Med. Surg.* 24: 82–94.

26 Phillips, B.E., Stoskopf, M.K., Beasley, J.F., and Harms, C.A. (2017). Evaluation of three anticoagulants used for short-term storage of loggerhead sea turtle (*Caretta caretta*) whole blood. *J. Herpetol. Med. Surg.* 27: 97–103.

27 Briscoe, J.A. and Syring, R. (2004). Techniques for emergency airway and vascular access in special species. *Semi. Avian Exot. Pet Med.* 13: 118–131.

28 Pardo, M.A. and Divers, S.J. (2019). Catheter placement. In: *Mader's Reptile Medicine and Surgery* (eds. S.J. Divers and S.J. Stahl), 422–428. Elsevier Inc: St. Louis.

29 Mosley, C.A. (2005). Anesthesia and analgesia in reptiles. *Semi. Avian Exot. Pet Med.*, 14: 243–262. Elsevier.

30 Young, B.D., Stegeman, N., Norby, B., and Heatley, J.J. (2012). Comparison of intraosseous and peripheral venous fluid dynamics in the desert tortoise (*Gopherus agassizii*). *J. Zoo Wildl. Med.* 43: 59–66.

31 Wellehan, F., Lafortune, M., and Gunkel, C. (2004). Coccygeal vascular catheterization in lizards and crocodilians. *J. Herpetol. Med. Surg.* 14 (2): 26–28.

32 Calzada, R., Mattioli, M., De abreu, A.D., and Monteiro, R.V. (2015). Criticism over the intraosseus route for Testudines: a test with the yellow-footed tortoise (*Chelonoidis denticulata*). *J. Herpetol. Med. Surg.* 25: 45–47.

43

Wound Care and Bandaging Techniques

Anna Martel and Christoph Mans

Department of Surgical Sciences, School of Veterinary Medicine, University of Wisconsin–Madison, Madison, Wisconsin, USA

CONTENTS

Introduction

Trauma, burns, and other injuries are frequent reasons for reptiles and occasionally amphibians to be present as emergencies. Turtles and tortoises can present with shearing trauma of the shell from lawn mowers, as well as shell fractures due to predator attacks, motor vehicle impact, or from falls. Snakes, lizards, and amphibians may present with bite wounds from live prey or predators. These wounds can be profound and should be treated in a similar fashion as bite wounds in other species. Snakes, and less frequently lizards, can present with burns from inappropriate heat sources in the enclosure. When treating reptiles and amphibian wounds, management of the animal in its preferred optimal temperature zone (POTZ) during treatment is essential to optimize healing and immune system function. This temperature varies significantly by species. Similar considerations as in mammals guide wound management decisions in reptile patients; however, wound healing is much slower in reptiles.

Wound Care

Wound Healing Considerations

Stages/Factors in Wound Healing

Wound healing in most reptiles is a considerably longer process than in mammalian or avian species. Healing can take weeks to months which usually necessitates multiple follow-up visits for prolonged wound care. This should be discussed with owners prior to proceeding with treatment. If poor, the husbandry should be improved at the time therapy is initiated as healing can be delayed or incomplete with an increased risk of complications if care (e.g. improper diet, environmental temperatures) is suboptimal.

Wound Assessment/Classification

Initial wound assessment usually can be performed with manual restraint, in most species. However, sedation or anesthesia will most likely be necessary to perform interventions (e.g. lavage, debridement), particularly in cases of shell

Exotic Animal Emergency and Critical Care Medicine, First Edition. Edited by Jennifer E. Graham, Grayson A. Doss and Hugues Beaufrère.

fractures in turtles and tortoises. Gross debris should be removed manually. Lavage is the most effective way to reduce bacteria. However, it can be contraindicated in cases where the wound communicates with the coelom, particularly if the lungs are involved. If the wound penetrates into the coelomic cavity, endoscopic examination can be useful to evaluate the extent of internal tissue damage and degree of contamination. Debridement of non-vital tissue should be performed as indicated, in a manner similar to mammalian patients.

If the wound is fresh, has not been caused by a predator (e.g. dog, cat) bite, and there is limited contamination, the wound may be closed with sutures or surgical glue as appropriate, following thorough cleaning. Because reptiles have relatively poor skin elasticity compared with other animals, large wounds may have to be partially closed if skin tension becomes an issue. Delayed closure, and more commonly second intention healing, should be considered for cases with extensive tissue damage and necrosis. Reptile wounds tend to heal well by second intention (Figure 43.1). This is often the most feasible method, but may not be suitable for all wounds (e.g. extremities) or for aquatic and semiaquatic species. An open technique is recommended for management of contaminated wounds in reptiles, in particular for shell wounds and shell fractures.

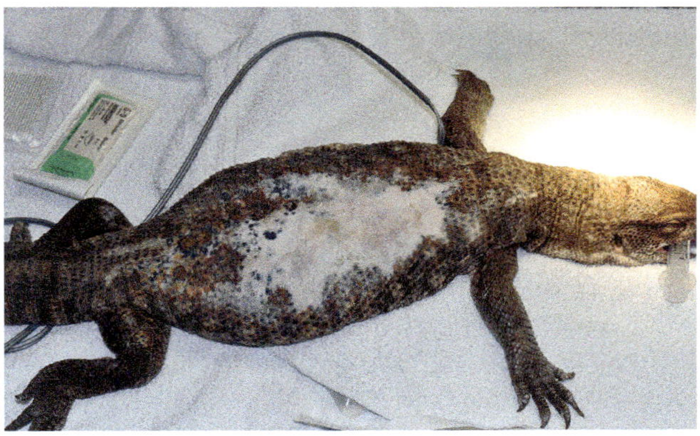

Figure 43.1 Healed, extensive burn wounds over the dorsum of a savannah monitor (*Varanus exanthematicus*).

If infection is present or highly suspected, treatment with systemic antibiotics in addition to local wound management is recommended. Antimicrobial therapy should be based on the etiology of the wound (e.g. bite wounds) in addition to bacterial culture and sensitivity. See Table 43.1 for a list of commonly used medications. Fungal infections are an important differential to rule out, as they are common in reptiles. Cytology and/or histopathology are more suitable than fungal cultures for this purpose, since many fungi isolated from reptiles do not grow under standard laboratory incubation protocols.

Wound Management

Special Considerations by Species

Turtles and Tortoises

Turtles and tortoises have an extensive shell consisting of the carapace (upper shell) and plastron (lower shell) which are connected laterally by bridges. The shell is composed of bone and covered by keratin scutes. Common causes for traumatic shell wounds and fractures include predator attacks (usually dogs or raccoons), hit-by-car, falls, being stepped on, or being hit by lawn mowers. The slower wound healing rate in reptiles should be considered when giving the client a prognosis, as bone involvement is common in traumatic shell lesions. Shell fractures associated with open coelomic wounds carry a guarded to poor prognosis. Shell wounds and fractures secondary to predator attack should be considered infected wounds and are often associated with penetration into the coelom (Figure 43.2). In these cases, intracoelomic trauma is possible, including damage to viscera (e.g. liver, lung), hemorrhage, and bacterial contamination of the coelomic cavity. Wound assessment and treatment should be staged, since tissue viability will only be assessable over several days' duration. Aggressive debridement should be avoided initially in order to preserve as much healthy tissue as possible. Shell

Table 43.1 Dosages of common medications used for wound management in reptiles.

Drug	Dosage	Frequency	Comment
Ceftazidime	30 mg/kg SC, IM	q48–72h	
Ceftiofur crystalline-free acid	30 mg/kg SC	Plasma levels >1 μg/ml for 12 d after single injection in bearded dragons	Not effective against *Pseudomonas* spp.
Enrofloxacin	5–10 mg/kg IM or PO	q24–48h	Injectable not recommended due to alkalinity, caustic to tissues
Meloxicam	0.2 mg/kg SC, IM	q24h	Parenteral preferred due to potential for poor PO bioavailability

Herptiles

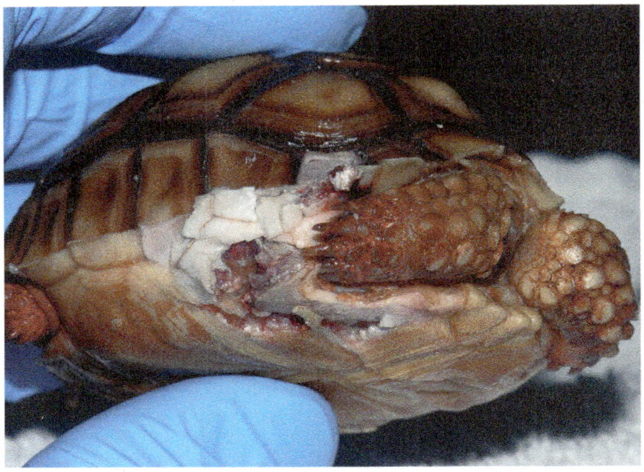

Figure 43.2 A sulcata tortoise (*Centrochelys sulcata*) with extensive shell fractures and wound communication with the coelomic cavity following a dog attack. Note the multiple shell fractures involving the cranial plastron and right cranial bridge.

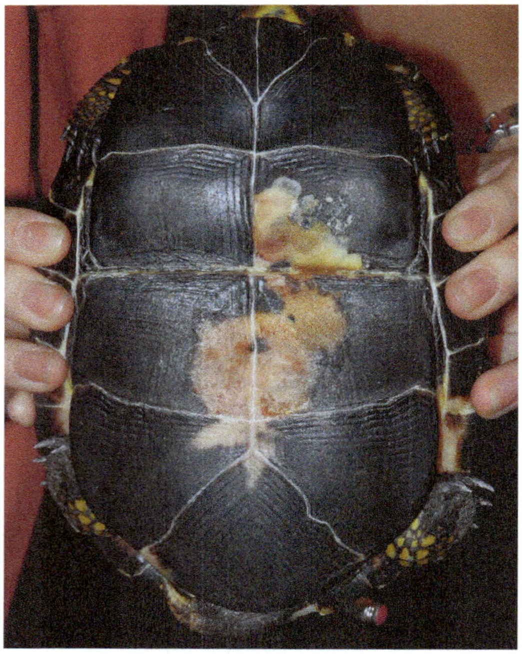

Figure 43.3 Asian box turtle (*Cuora* sp.) with necrotic bone lesions of the plastron. These lesions are often caused by bacterial emboli in septic animals. Following analgesia administration, the shell should be debrided and systemic and local antimicrobial treatment initiated. Fungal infection should be ruled out by cytology and/or histopathology.

debridement should be performed under sedation and following provision of effective analgesia.

Sepsis and bacterial emboli can lead to petechiae, fluid accumulation, and loss of keratin scutes exposing the underlying bone of the shell, often affecting the plastron (Figure 43.3). Following analgesia administration, these

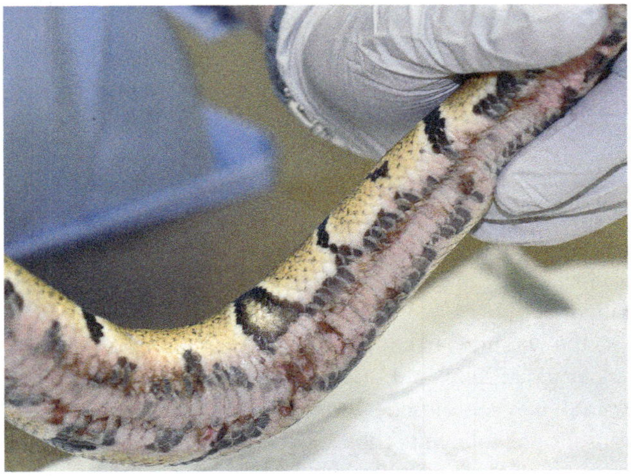

Figure 43.4 Extensive burns on the ventrum of a ball python (*Python regius*).

lesions should be opened, debrided, and managed with topical treatment and systemic antimicrobials. Fungal infection should be ruled out by cytology and/or histopathology. Blood cultures are recommended to rule out sepsis.

Aquatic turtles must often be dry-docked during treatment, which may result in anorexia. If the wound precludes the animal from being placed in water for feedings, consider placement of an esophagostomy tube for continued nutritional support (see Chapter 46: Nutrition and Fluid Therapy).

Snakes and Lizards

Burns to either the ventral body wall (Figure 43.4) or dorsum (Figure 43.1) are commonly encountered wounds in snakes and less frequently in lizards. The use of heat rocks in the enclosure, insufficient protection of heat bulbs, or insufficient distance between the heat source and the animal can lead to burns. Burn lesions are usually extensive.

Snakes that are fed live rodent prey are at risk of attack by the rodent unless the prey is removed from the enclosure quickly if not consumed. Prey bites can also occur in constrictors after the prey item has been captured. Therefore, frozen-thawed rodents should be fed or live rodents that are offered (under direct supervision) should be removed immediately if uneaten. Less frequently, feeder insects like crickets offered to ground-dwelling lizards (e.g. bearded dragons) can also cause bite wounds. Lizards and other small reptiles and amphibians attacked by insect prey may have occult illness. Prey bite wounds in snakes can be extensive and deep, involving skin, muscle, bone and the coelomic cavity. The prognosis is guarded to poor, depending on the extent of the lesions and concurrent disease processes. For most cases, long-term, open wound management is required, which is challenging in snakes, due to the difficulty in maintaining bandages on their bodies.

Amphibians

Amphibians possess a remarkable ability to heal even extensive wounds in a short period of time, as long as substantial infection does not impede the healing process. Amphibian skin is very permeable and therefore topical wound disinfectants should be avoided or used cautiously in order to avoid systemic effects. Dressing and bandages are not suitable for amphibians and wounds usually require very little management following debridement (if necrotic tissue is present). Providing excellent husbandry, including maintaining water quality, will facilitate wound healing.

Wound Prep

Most wounds should be lavaged with isotonic solution, as in other species. In cases with extensive communication with the coelomic cavity, lavage should be performed cautiously. Care must be taken not to flush bacteria and debris from the shell surface or contaminated wounds into the coelomic cavity. If the coelomic membrane is no longer intact, the patient should be positioned in a manner to facilitate immediate drainage of lavage fluid away from the coelomic cavity. Wounds may also be cleaned with antiseptics (i.e. dilute chlorhexidine) prior to treatment or bandaging.

Wound Debridement

Debridement should be performed under sedation or anesthesia with analgesia provided. With many reptile wounds, debridement may need to be performed weekly for several months.

Wound Closure Techniques

If the wound occurred fairly recently and is minimally contaminated, primary closure with everting sutures (horizontal or vertical mattress patterns) can be performed, in particular for areas that cannot be bandaged (e.g. extremities, neck of turtles, and tortoises). Care should be taken to avoid compressing tissues excessively, as focal areas of necrosis can develop. Tissue glue can be used on the exposed ends of skin to help provide an additional barrier to contamination.

Topical Medications

A topical antimicrobial medication may be applied to superficial wounds and burns as well as wounds following debridement. Antimicrobial medications should include Gram-negative bacterial coverage, especially in aquatic turtle species and for bite wounds. Silver sulfadiazine is a frequently used topical antimicrobial cream in reptiles. Ointments should not be used for exudative wounds.

Wound Dressings

Superficial wounds may be dressed with a simple, non-adherent pad (e.g. Telfa; Covidien LLC, Mansfield, MA) overlaid with an adhesive film (e.g. Tegaderm; 3M Health Care, St. Paul, MN) or bandage (Figure 43.5). Larger wounds require more extensive bandaging and more frequent bandage changes. Any fistulated or deep wounds should be packed with hydrogel material or hydrocolloid. Honey and sugar can be used for infected and exudative wounds.

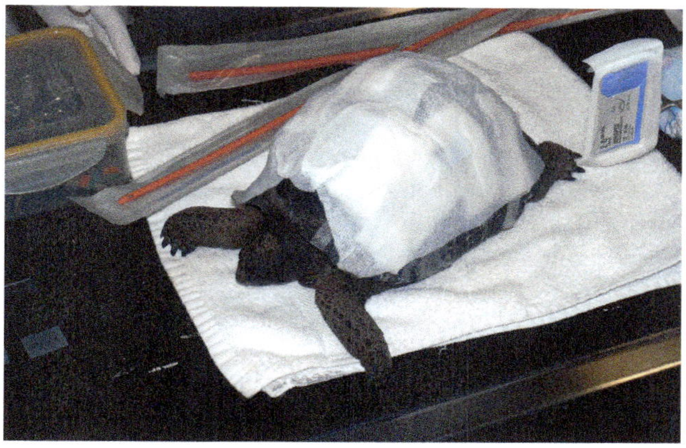

Figure 43.5 Bandaged shell lesions in a tortoise. Gauze was used as the primary layer and an adhesive permeable bandage applied as the outer layer.

Negative Pressure Wound Therapy

Negative pressure wound therapy has been used to manage shell wounds in chelonians. Reports in other reptiles are limited but negative pressure wound therapy can promote faster healing if the wound is located in an area amenable to vacuum closure placement and the patient can tolerate prolonged connection to a suction source.

Bandaging Techniques

Types of Bandages

Bandaging should involve consideration of the specific anatomy and environment of the patient. In general, bandages are challenging to maintain in snakes, and body parts other than the shell of turtles and tortoises. If a water-resistant bandage can be provided for an aquatic turtle, the time spent in water can be increased and may also eliminate the need for esophagostomy tube placement. Ventral wounds (especially burns) in snakes, turtles, and tortoises can present a challenge to bandaging and its maintenance and therefore these wounds may be better managed as open wounds with reptiles kept on newspaper as bedding.

As stated previously, superficial wounds may be managed as open wounds and a topical antimicrobial ointment or a spray-on or liquid bandage can be applied. However, deeper wounds require bandaging appropriate to the wound. Hydrogels are frequently used in wounds in reptile species. These dressings provide moisture as well as antimicrobial effects to healing wounds. Since these species produce caseous material in response to infection, heavily exudative wounds are not common.

Adhesive films or bandages (Figure 43.5) are often used as the outer, securing layer. These films can be temporarily supplemented with other dressings or wraps to allow swim time, especially if needed for feedings (e.g. aquatic turtles).

Wet-to-Dry

Wet-to-dry bandages are typically used for mechanical debridement of necrotic or exudative wounds but are uncommonly used in reptiles and amphibians due to the minimally exudative nature of wounds in these species.

Dry/Soft Padded

Soft padded bandages are most commonly used on the trunk and extremities, making them potentially useful in lizard and turtle and tortoise species but not snakes. They can be used to protect a healing wound from environmental contamination or self-trauma and may be combined with splints for external coaptation.

Tie-on

Tie-on or tie-over bandages are a useful approach in reptiles, particularly snakes, given the anatomic challenges with using traditional bandages. A major benefit of tie-over bandages is that skin suture loops are used to keep the dressings in place, permitting bandaging of challenging anatomical locations. This also permits relatively fast bandage changes.

Stabilization/External Coaptation

External Coaptation-Indications and Contraindications

The majority of principles that guide treatment of fractures in reptiles are the same as in other animals. Unstable fractures must be stabilized. External coaptation can be used for anatomic sites where fractures will stay reduced with minimal support. Contraindications to external coaptation include spiral or comminuted fractures and the presence of open wounds. External coaptation should be utilized initially for all fractures in order to prevent further tissue damage and reduce pain while definitive fracture treatment is planned.

Materials

Bandaging materials used for external coaptation include various splinting material (e.g. modified wooden tongue depressors, moldable splint material) and self-adhesive dressings. Soft padded bandages can be used to ensure proper splint placement and for protection of adjacent tissue.

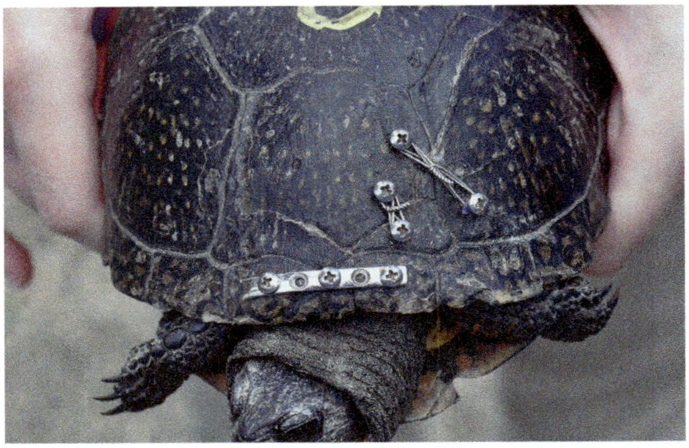

Figure 43.6 Shell fracture repair in a Blanding's turtle (*Emydoidea blandingii*) using stainless steel screws, cerclage wire and a surgical plate. These methods usually result in good fracture reduction and compression and are more durable than other techniques, while still permitting shell wound monitoring and treatment.

Species-Specific Issues

Shell fractures can be challenging to stabilize. Sterile, stainless steel screws combined with cerclage wire or (surgical) plates are recommended for stabilization of most shell fractures (Figure 43.6). These methods allow for appropriate wound care and monitoring during healing of the fracture. Shell fractures should never be covered with compounds such as epoxy, polymethacrylate or similar products, since it does not allow for continued wound monitoring and increases the risk of infection. Wounds should be lavaged and the area aseptically prepared prior to placement of surgical hardware. Guide holes should be predrilled into the shell with sterilized drill bits, taking care not to penetrate into the coelom. The shell fracture should be reduced and surgical plates ideally secured with at least two screws on either side of the fracture site. With large areas of the shell damaged, segments may slough due to loss of vascular supply. These areas often heal with fibrotic tissue if the shell is lost. Bridge fractures can be especially challenging to stabilize. Marginal scute fractures will often not heal due to the lack of underlying soft tissue.

External Coaptation

The joints proximal and distal to the fracture must be immobilized. For lizards, limbs are externally coapted in a fashion similar to other species (Figure 43.7). Stabilizing limb fractures in turtles and tortoises is challenging. Fractured limbs may be restricted in flexion inside the shell if the fracture can be maintained in an appropriate reduction (Figure 43.8). Radiographs should be performed to assess the position of the limb fracture when coapted within the shell.

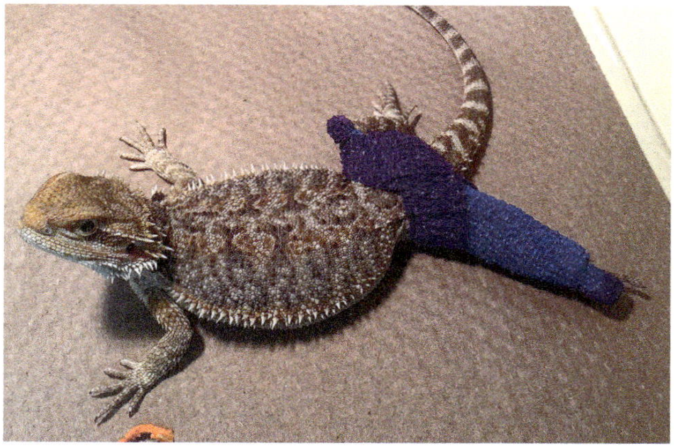

Figure 43.7 External coaptation of a left femoral fracture in a juvenile bearded dragon (*Pogona vitticeps*). Note that the coxofemoral joint has been immobilized by extending the splint dorsally over the hip to the other hindlimb. A tongue depressor has been used to provide rigidity. Care should be taken to avoid covering the vent.

Bandaging by Location

Head/Neck

Placement of bandages on the neck of reptiles and amphibians, in particular snakes, turtles, and tortoises, can be challenging to impossible due to anatomical limitations. The cervical area is more easily bandaged in lizards. Due to constant movement or poor tolerance, head bandages are not commonly utilized in reptiles and amphibians. Primary closure, tie-over bandages or second intention healing may be options for head or cervical wounds in snakes and turtles and tortoises.

Body

Body bandages are typically successful in lizard species. Stockinette can be used to assist with bandage retention. Tie-over bandages may be the most practical approach to bandaging the body of snakes. Bandages on the carapace of turtles and tortoises are fairly straight forward and can be placed as described above (Figure 43.5). However, plastron bandages can be challenging to maintain due to friction and contamination. These should be secured around the bridge or the plastron padded to reduce frictional forces on the bandage. Medical tape or duct tape usually adheres well to the shell and should be used to secure bandage edges.

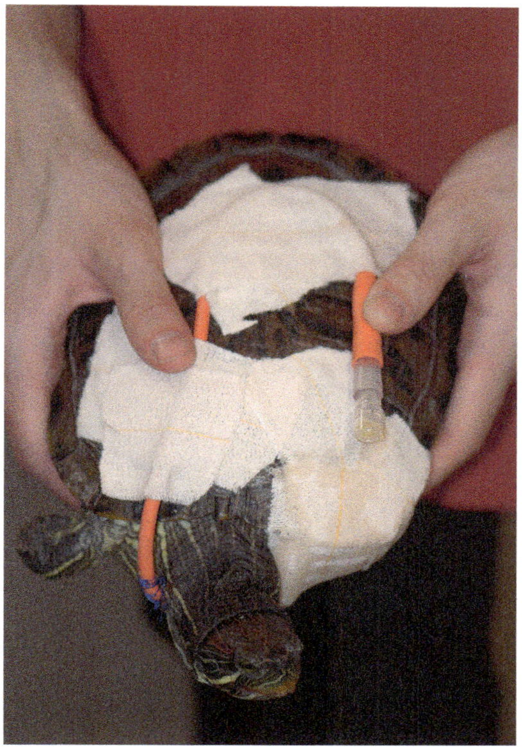

Figure 43.8 External coaptation of a left humeral fracture in a red-eared slider (*Trachemys scripta elegans*). Note that the left forelimb has been immobilized by securing it in a flexed position within the shell. A feeding tube has been placed, since this bandage does not permit water access and the turtle needs to be dry-docked until the fracture has healed.

Extremities (Legs, Tail)

Soft tissue wounds of the limbs are challenging to bandage in turtles and tortoises. The majority of these wounds may need to be left open to heal by second intention along with appropriate changes to the environment to reduce wound contamination (e.g. frequent cleaning or removal of substrate). With limb injuries in other reptile species, bandaging should be light weight and not bulky. If wounds of the lower extremities are severe and the prognosis for healing is poor, amputation of the limb should be considered. Wounds of the tail are approached similar to other extremity wounds. If the wound is located close to the vent, care should be taken during bandage application to reduce the risk of contamination.

Further Reading

Divers, S.J. and Stahl, S.J. (eds.) (2019). *Mader's Reptile and Amphibian Medicine and Surgery*, 3e. St. Louis: Elsevier, Inc.

Mader, D.R. and Divers, S.J. (eds.) (2014). *Current Therapy in Reptile Medicine and Surgery*. St. Louis: Elsevier.

Mickelson, M., Mans, C., and Colopy, S. (2016). Principles of wound management and wound healing in exotic pets. *Vet. Clin. North Am. Exot. Anim. Pract.* 19: 33–53.

Herptiles

44

CPR and Euthanasia

Grayson A. Doss and Kurt K. Sladky

Department of Surgical Sciences, School of Veterinary Medicine, University of Wisconsin-Madison, Madison, Wisconsin, USA

CONTENTS

Cardiopulmonary Cerebral Resuscitation

Cardiopulmonary cerebral resuscitation (CPCR) is comprised of basic and advanced life support, associated monitoring, and post-resuscitation care [1]. Unfortunately, there is little published information regarding CPCR in reptile and amphibian species, and most guidelines are based on recommendations for dogs and cats.

Basic life support consists of the "*ABC*s" or "*a*irway," "*b*reathing," and "*c*irculation." This approach entails securing an airway and simultaneously performing chest compressions and positive pressure ventilation. Advanced life support refers to the patient monitoring used to both evaluate the effectiveness of basic life support and to watch for the return of spontaneous breathing and heart activity; the process of establishing direct access to the circulatory system; and the administration of emergency medications by various routes [1, 2]. Post-resuscitation care involves intensive monitoring and treatment of the patient after return of spontaneous breathing and circulation, due to the high risk of complications. For CPCR in cats and dogs, the chance of survival to discharge is poor, even after return of spontaneous circulation, with rates as low as 2% [2]. Owners should be aware of the overall low success rate so as not to have unrealistic expectations about outcomes. All critically ill patients undergoing heavy sedation or anesthesia should be assigned a code status at admittance in order to avoid ambiguity during a crisis.

Performing CPCR in Reptiles and Amphibians

In reptiles, unique cardiorespiratory anatomy and physiology make the approach to CPCR a challenge. While quickly, but efficiently, examining the emergent patient, determine if the animal has a heartbeat and is breathing. Use of an ultrasonic Doppler flow detector is invaluable, as auscultation in most reptiles and amphibians is frequently challenging or impossible. To determine if the heart is beating, use transducer gel or another suitable transduction medium and place the Doppler probe over the area of the heart or a large vessel. In small amphibians, the probe can be placed over the pectoral girdle either dorsally or ventrally to obtain a reading (Figure 44.1). In chelonians, the Doppler probe can be placed on the lateral neck over the jugular vein/carotid artery or within the fossa between the forelimb and the head, adjacent to the base of the neck. Elongated or pencil-style probes (Figure 44.1) are useful for taking readings within this fossa. In lizards, the flow of blood can be detected over the jugular vein/carotid artery or heart (Figure 44.2), although a thick bony pectoral girdle can make using this latter site difficult in some species. In snakes, the Doppler probe can be placed directly over the heart (which may be localized using scale movements), caudal (ventral coccygeal) vein, or on the dorsal buccal or palatine veins in the roof of the mouth in large animals. If a pulse cannot be appreciated in the aforementioned sites, placing the probe over the spectacle may result in blood flow sounds. If a Doppler unit is not

Exotic Animal Emergency and Critical Care Medicine, First Edition. Edited by Jennifer E. Graham, Grayson A. Doss and Hugues Beaufrère.

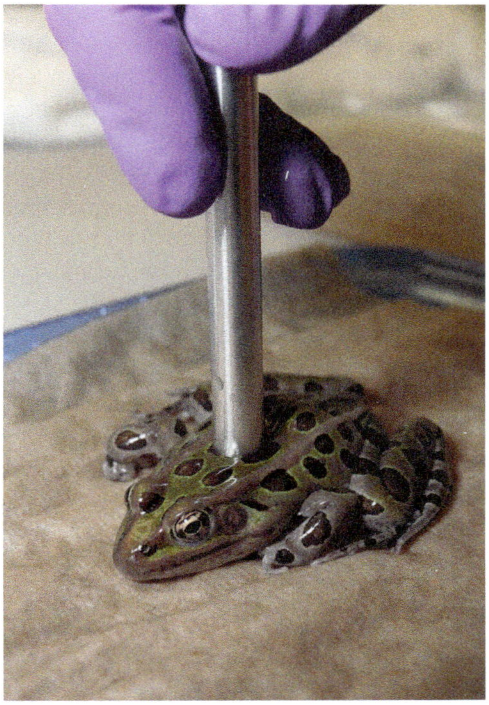

Figure 44.1 Use of an aluminum pencil-style probe for Doppler measurement of heart rate in a sedated leopard frog (*Rana pipiens*); the probe is placed over the pectoral girdle.

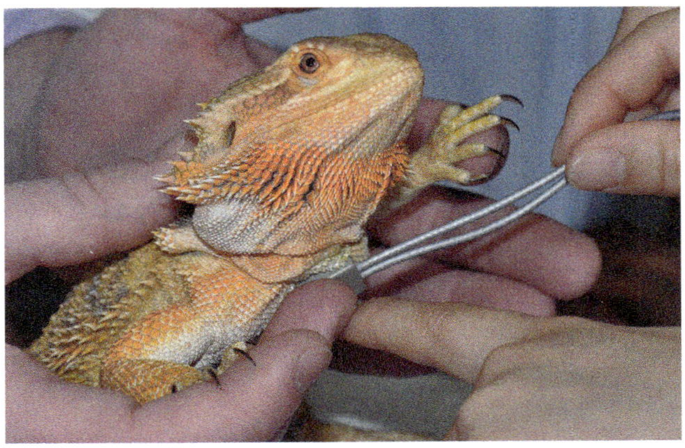

Figure 44.2 Doppler measurement of heart rate via placement of the crystal over the pectoral girdle in a bearded dragon (*Pogona vitticeps*).

available, an electronic stethoscope or placing a wet gauze pad or paper-towel between the patient and the stethoscope diaphragm may result in successful auscultation.

Because of the slow respiratory rates in some species, determining whether or not the patient is breathing normally can be a challenge in reptiles, especially if they are bradypneic. In frogs, toads, and small lizards, examine the throat area, since gular respirations are often more frequent and readily visible when compared to coelomic respirations. Do not mistake agonal breathing for normal respirations. Agonal breaths may be exaggerated, with the mouth opening in a gasping motion, or these respiratory patterns may give the impression that the animal is retching. In chelonians, monitor the limbs for forward and backward movements, as this indicates normal respiration. In snakes, watch the cranial half of the animal for intermittent inflation or swelling as the lungs fill with air.

Basic Life Support

If the patient is in cardiopulmonary arrest, initiate cardiopulmonary resuscitation measures. If only one person is available to help, initiate cardiac compressions first. Supplemental heat should be provided to mimic the preferred optimum temperature zone of the species to ensure an adequate response to CPCR, but exercise caution as higher environmental temperatures can result in an increased tissue oxygen demand [3, 4]. While CPCR is underway have an available person apprise the owner of the current status of the animal as soon as possible.

If the patient is in cardiac arrest, chest compressions may be attempted, but can be difficult due to the location of the heart within the pectoral girdle in many amphibian and lizard species, or impossible due to the presence of the plastron in chelonians. In snakes, cardiac massage is more easily performed.

Establish an airway as quickly and as safely as possible. The glottis lies caudal to the tongue in the rostral oral cavity (Figure 44.3) in most species. For species with sharp teeth, wear protective gloves or use gauze or tape strips to

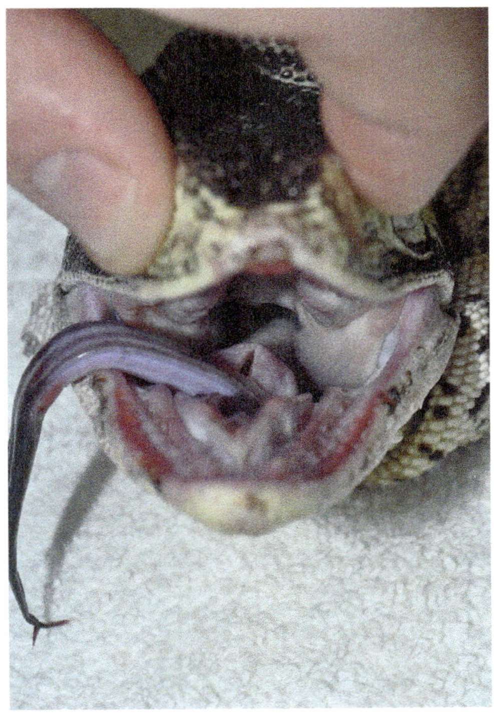

Figure 44.3 Visualization of the glottis in a sedated Argus monitor (*Varanus panoptes horni*); note its position at the base of the tongue.

open the mouth for access to the glottis. In crocodilians, the gular or palatine fold (velum palatinum) (Figure 44.4) will have to be displaced rostroventrally in order to access the glottis. In chelonians, the glottis also lies at the base of the tongue (Figure 44.5). The glottis is located cranially in snakes making intubation fairly easy.

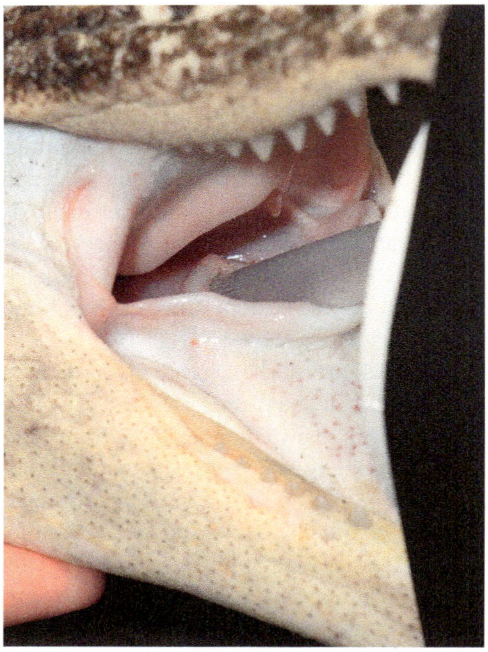

Figure 44.4 An intubated crocodilian; observe that the ventral displacement of the gular fold is required in order to visualize and access the glottis.

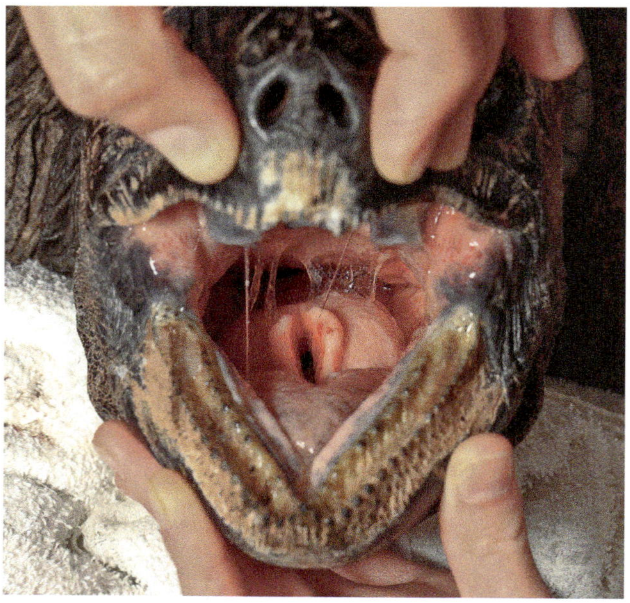

Figure 44.5 Visualization of the glottis in an anesthetized Aldabra tortoise (*Aldabrachelys gigantea*).

Once intubated, initiate positive pressure ventilation using an ambu-bag with 100% oxygen or room air. Alternatively, an anesthesia circuit with an appropriately sized reservoir bag can also be used and offers the advantage of a pressure gauge for monitoring the force of administered breaths.

Because of the distinctive respiratory physiology of reptiles, determining proper oxygen supplementation can be subjective. Both the partial pressure of oxygen and ambient temperature play a role in a reptile's drive to breathe [3, 4].

Because of the effect of inspired O_2 on respiration, recommendations regarding oxygen supplementation during ventilation under anesthesia vary [3, 5, 6]. For the emergent reptile patient, it is advocated to initially ventilate with 100% inspired O_2, transitioning to room air once the patient has a return of spontaneous circulation [3].

Recommendations for frequency and pressure of positive pressure ventilations during CPCR in reptile species are scarce. In the absence of specific guidelines the authors recommend conforming to general guidelines for reptilian anesthesia and maintaining the total pressure below 12 cm H_2O and breath rate between 2 and 6 per minute. [6–9] In one study, a rate of 1–2 breaths per minute was recommended for South American rattlesnakes (*Crotalus durissus terrificus*) to help prevent negative changes to acid–base status [10].

Advanced Life Support

Success of cardiac massage can be assessed using a Doppler flow probe placed over a peripheral vein/artery or by assessing an electrocardiogram, although electrical activity may be present long after brain activity has ceased [9]. Electrocardiogram leads can be attached using specifically designed adhesive pads or clamped to hypodermic needles inserted through the skin (Figure 44.6); lead placement has been described in detail elsewhere [8, 9].

Pulse oximetry and capnography are useful tools in canine and feline CPCR, but their use is poorly described in reptile and amphibian emergencies. Because of differences in physiology and lack of validation studies in herptiles, interpretation of individual readings can be challenging, but monitoring trends may be useful during CPCR. It is suggested to maintain the end-tidal CO_2 between 15 and 25 mmHg for anesthetized reptile species [11].

Cardiovascular access should be obtained during CPCR for fluid support and administration of emergency therapeutics. In small patients, intraosseous catheterization may be the only feasible route. See Chapter 42 for information on how to obtain intravenous or intraosseous access in reptiles and amphibians. Once access is obtained, administer any sedative/anesthetic drug reversal agents as appropriate (e.g. atipamezole, naloxone, and flumazenil).

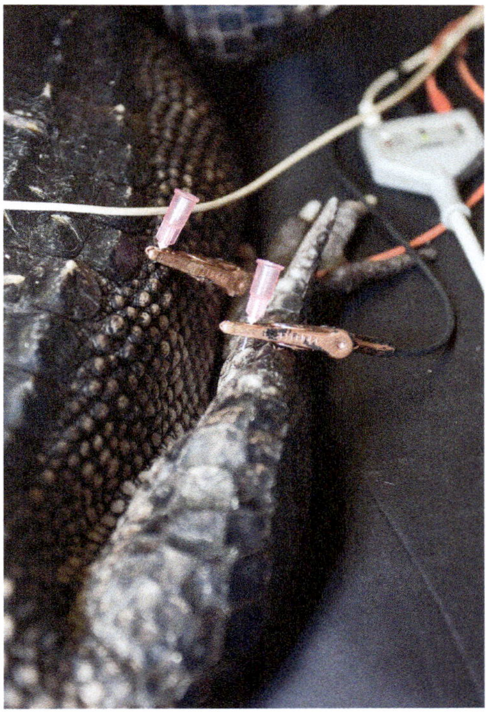

Figure 44.6 Use of hypodermic needles for electrocardiogram lead placement in a crocodilian.

Box 44.1 Commonly used medications in reptile and amphibian CPCR

Atropine	**Reptiles:** 0.01–0.04 mg/kg IV, IO, IM [9] 0.01–0.02 mg/kg IV, IM [12] 0.2 mg/kg IM [9] 0.5 m/kg IV, IO, IT, IM [3, 13] **Amphibians:** 0.03 mg/kg IM [14]
Epinephrine (1 : 1000; 1 mg/ml)	**Reptiles:** 0.1 mg/kg IV, IO, IT [3, 12] 0.5–1.0 mg/kg IV, IO, IT [13] **Amphibians:** 0.2–0.5 ml IV, IO, IT, ICe, IC [14]
Doxapram	**Reptiles:** 5 mg/kg IV, IO, IM [3, 9, 12] 20 mg/kg IV, IO, IM [13] **Amphibians:** 5 mg/kg IV, IM [14]

Abbreviations: IC, intracardiac; ICe, intracoelomic; IM, intramuscular; IO, intraosseous; IT, intratracheal; IV, intravenous.

If hypovolemia or dehydration is suspected, begin appropriate fluid therapy; see Chapter 46: Nutrition and Fluid Therapy for guidelines for fluid therapy in reptiles and amphibians.

Drugs may also be administered intratracheally through the endotracheal tube if other routes are not possible. The volume administered into the trachea will need to be large enough to push the drug to vascularized areas of the respiratory tract. This is accomplished by doubling the volume of calculated drug and diluting it in sterile saline at 1 ml/100 g of body weight [9]; a catheter passed through the endotracheal tube is used to deliver the drug.

Antagonist drugs used for anesthetic reversal, such as flumazenil for benzodiazepines, atipamezole for alpha$_2$-agonists, and naloxone for opioids, should be administered, if applicable.

Systematic studies investigating the use of common emergency medications during CPCR, including epinephrine, atropine, vasopressin, amiodarone, and sodium bicarbonate, do not exist in reptiles and amphibians. Dosages for common emergency medications are extrapolated from small mammals or birds, or are anecdotal in nature and are listed in Box 44.1.

Doxapram has been described as a respiratory stimulant for use in reptile and amphibian emergency medicine [7, 9, 12, 14]. However, its use in small animal medicine is controversial, as doxapram may increase the cerebral oxygen requirement, while decreasing cerebral blood flow [15]. Doxapram is not listed as a routine drug in current canine and feline resuscitation guidelines [2].

Ventricular defibrillation is poorly described in herptiles and may not be practical. Smaller units are often needed for most reptile and amphibian patients and the lowest possible energy setting needed to convert the abnormal rhythm should be utilized [3].

Postarrest Care

Specific guidelines for postarrest care do not exist for reptiles and amphibians. However, monitoring basic physiologic parameters with noninvasive blood pressure, pulse oximetry, electrocardiography, and capnography is recommended. Serial venous blood gas analysis and electrolyte evaluation can be useful for identifying abnormalities in the post-resuscitation patient. Frequently, herptiles may require intensive ventilatory support after successful CPCR to prevent hypoxia, and close monitoring of mental status, as well as heart rate and rhythm, is crucial [3]. Fluid therapy is warranted in order to maintain appropriate perfusion and hydration. Because of the potential for intestinal epithelial compromise from decreased blood flow, systemic antimicrobials are often warranted to prevent septicemia.

Euthanasia

Euthanasia is a method by which clinicians can prevent further discomfort or suffering in terminally ill or severely debilitated patients. By definition, the goal of euthanasia is to produce a rapid, painless death with as little associated stress as possible. The clinician must always strive for this goal and approach euthanasia in a compassionate manner. Scavenger exposure to euthanasia drugs should also be considered when selecting the euthanasia method if the owner wishes to bury their pet.

Methods by Species

The main euthanasia methods in herptiles include the use of injectable or inhalant agents, the application of topical agents in many amphibian species, and physical means. The American Veterinary Medical Association routinely publishes guidelines for euthanasia which provides a detailed framework for performing euthanasia in most animal groups encountered in veterinary medicine; the reader is referred to the latest version of these guidelines for a comprehensive list of approved and non-approved methods by animal groups or species.

An overview of approved and non-approved euthanasia methods for reptiles and amphibians is listed in Table 44.1. In herptiles, the heart may continue to beat for long periods after brain death has occurred. **Because confirmation of death in reptiles and amphibians is difficult, it is generally recommended to perform at least two approved methods to ensure successful euthanasia** [16]. This usually entails utilizing a physical method of euthanasia as the final procedure.

Reptiles

Injectable agents are commonly utilized for euthanasia of reptiles. Approved routes include intravenous (Figure 44.7) and intracoelomic [16]. Injection into the brain through the parietal eye has also been described in anesthetized lizards [16]. Intravascular routes are preferred for euthanasia, if available, and injections should be performed in the cranial portion of the body in species where this is possible [17]. Intracardiac administration of euthanasia agents is approved for unconscious or nonresponsive herptiles (Figure 44.8); however, euthanasia agents may be administered into the heart of conscious snakes, if deemed necessary (e.g. inabilty to access other vascular sites) [16].

Commercial compounds containing barbiturates, such as pentobarbital sodium, are readily available and approved for euthanasia via recommended routes. Anesthetic agents like ketamine, tiletamine-zolazepam, alfaxalone

Table 44.1 Methods of euthanasia in reptiles and amphibians.

Reptiles	*Amphibians*
Acceptable	Acceptable
Sodium pentobarbital IV, ICe	Sodium pentobarbital IV, ICe, injected into lymph spaces or sacs
Overdose of dissociative agents or intravenously-administered anesthetics	Overdose of dissociative agents or intravenously administered anesthetics
Tricaine methanesulfonate (buffered) ICe	Tricaine methanesulfonate (buffered) via immersion[a] or ICe (not *Xenopus* species)
	Benzocaine hydrochloride via immersion or topically as gel
Acceptable *with conditions*	Acceptable *with conditions*
Overdose of inhalant anesthetics	Overdose of inhalant anesthetics
Captive bolt or firearm for large species	
Blunt force trauma to head	Blunt force trauma to head
Rapid freezing	Rapid freezing
Intracardiac or intraosseous (IO) administration of approved drugs in unconscious, unresponsive, or deeply anesthetized animals	Intracardiac or intraosseous (IO) administration of approved drugs in unconscious, unresponsive, or deeply anesthetized animals
Carbon dioxide inhalation[b]	Carbon dioxide inhalation[b]
Adjunctive methods	Adjunctive methods
Pithing	Pithing
Decapitation	Decapitation
Unacceptable	Unacceptable
Hypothermia	Hypothermia
Intracardiac or IO injections of agents in conscious animals[c]	Intracardiac or IO injections of agents in conscious animals
Magnesium sulfate, potassium chloride, and neuromuscular blocking agents as sole means of euthanasia in conscious animals	Magnesium sulfate, potassium chloride, and neuromuscular blocking agents as sole means of euthanasia in conscious animals

Source: Based on Leary et al. [16].

[a] A secondary method is recommended following immersion in amphibians.

[b] Other methods are preferable.

[c] While other methods are preferable, approved euthanasia agents may be injected directly into the heart of conscious snakes if necessary (e.g. small species).

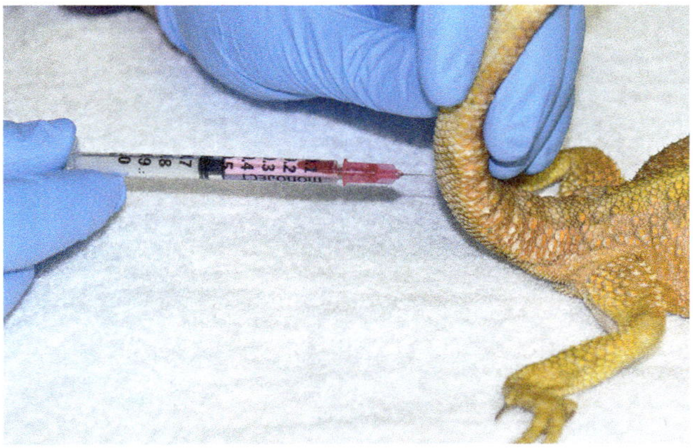

Figure 44.7 Use of the caudal (ventral coccygeal) vein for intravascular administration of a commercial sodium pentobarbital solution in a bearded dragon (*Pogona vitticeps*).

and propofol, may be used to induce rapid anesthesia and subsequent euthanasia, although a secondary method is recommended to ensure death [16].

Buffered tricaine-methanesulfonate (MS-222) may be used via the intracoelomic route for euthanasia of herptiles [16, 18]. One benefit of this method is the lack of histological artifacts observed with other injectable agents, such as pentobarbital sodium.

Inhaled agents can result in prolonged periods of breath holding in herptiles (especially chelonians), resulting in significant patient stress, therefore their use has been recommended only when other acceptable methods are not available [16]. During prolonged exposure, death must be ensured or a secondary means of euthanasia performed prior to termination of the inhalant [16].

Physical methods include use of captive bolts or firearms, rapid freezing, or blunt force trauma to the head. Because of the potential for incorrect application or risk to personnel, only trained individuals should perform euthanasia using these methods in appropriate environments. Very small reptiles and amphibians (less than 4 g) may be euthanatized by submersion in liquid nitrogen; however, this technique is not approved for species that are cold-tolerant or for animals equal to or greater than 4 g in body weight [16]. Application of blunt force trauma to the head as a means of euthanasia should be reserved as the last resort in animals of appropriate size, and should be immediately followed with an adjunctive method to confirm death [16].

In large reptile species, such as monitors or crocodilians, euthanasia may be performed using a captive bolt or gunshot targeting the brain. In American alligators (*Alligator mississippiensis*), use of penetrating and non-penetrating captive bolts resulted in rapid cessation of electroencephalogram activity [19].

Adjunctive or secondary methods to ensure death in deeply anesthetized or unconscious animals include pithing and decapitation. Only trained individuals who are familiar with the anatomy of the subject species should perform pithing in order to ensure rapid death.

Decapitation is only performed as part of a three-step euthanasia protocol [16] using specialized equipment such as heavy, sharp, metal shears, or a guillotine; because of the potential for continued central nervous system activity following cessation of blood flow, decapitation *must* be followed by pithing [16, 17]. Severance of the spinal cord alone was insufficient for eliminating electroencephalogram activity in American alligators and subsequent pithing was required for death [19].

Amphibians

Euthanasia in amphibian species is similar to described methods for reptiles; however, given their unique skin, euthanasia may also be performed by means of immersion or topical application of various compounds and injectable agents can also be administered into lymph sacs and spaces [16]. Inhalant agents are not typically recommended for euthanasia of terrestrial amphibians [20].

Dosages required for various euthanasia agents can vary by species. For example, one study examining euthanasia methods in African clawed frogs (*Xenopus laevis*) found that very high levels of topical MS-222 and injectable pentobarbital and phenytoin were required for successful euthanasia; intracoelomic injection of high concentrations of MS-222 did not result in euthanasia [21].

Tricaine methanesulfonate is commonly used to euthanatize amphibians via the immersion route; this compound requires buffering prior to administration via immersion or injection to limit distress to the animal. As demonstrated in African clawed [21] and smoky jungle frogs (*Leptodactylus pentadactylus*) [22], extremely high dosages or prolonged contact times may be required for euthanasia of some amphibians with MS-222, making follow-up with a secondary method of euthanasia desirable when using this compound. Further research is needed to determine if MS-222 is suitable as a sole euthanasia agent for many amphibian species.

Benzocaine hydrochloride can be administered via immersion or topically as a gel for euthanasia of amphibians [16, 20, 21].

Eggs and Fetuses

Recently oviposited reptile and amphibian eggs may be destroyed via freezing or through methods of maceration resulting in rapid death; later development stages should be euthanatized using adult methods [16].

(a) (b)

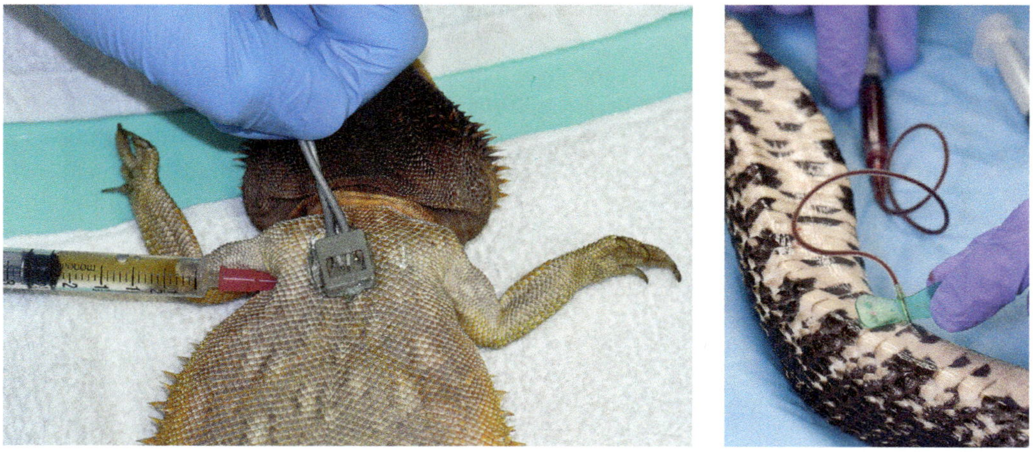

Figure 44.8 Intracardiac administration of potassium chloride solution in a deeply anesthetized bearded dragon (*Pogona vitticeps*) (a) and bullsnake (*Pituophis catenifer sayi*) (b).

Unacceptable Methods of Euthanasia

Many methods unacceptable as sole agents are approved when used as part of a two-stage process. For example, potassium chloride may be used as a conditional injectable agent once an animal is under a deep plane of anesthesia or unconscious, but it cannot be used in conscious animals; similarly, neuromuscular blocking agents and magnesium sulfate are also unacceptable as euthanasia agents in conscious vertebrates [16, 17].

Hypothermia is an unacceptable means of euthanasia in all reptiles and amphibians due to induced stress and pain [16, 17, 20].

Necropsy

If a postmortem examination is planned, use of certain euthanasia agents, such as pentobarbital, should be carefully utilized in order to prevent significant tissue artifact. Proper equipment needed to perform a postmortem examination, and collect and save appropriate tissues, should be available prior to starting the procedure. The reader is directed to texts providing detailed overviews of performing necropsies in herptiles [23] for more information on utilizing the postmortem examination in clinical practice.

Conclusion

Performing CPCR in reptiles and amphibians can be challenging when compared to other species, due to their unique anatomy and physiology. Understanding the approach to basic and advanced life support in herptiles enables the clinician to act quickly and provide emergent support for the critical patient. Reptiles and amphibians are frequently presented to the clinician for euthanasia, and choosing an appropriate method and route is important when providing the best possible care for these unique animals.

References

1 Boysen, S. (2014). Zoo and wildlife CPR. In: Zoo Animal and Wildlife Immobilization and Anesthesia, 2e (eds. G. West, D. Heard and N. Caulkett), 125–138. Ames: Wiley.

2 Fletcher, D.J., Boller, M., Brainard, B.M. et al. (2012). RECOVER evidence and knowledge gap analysis on veterinary CPR. Part 7: clinical guidelines. *J. Vet. Emerg. Crit. Care* 22 (S1): S102–S131.

3 Costello, M.F. (2004). Principles of cardiopulmonary cerebral resuscitation in special species. *Semin. Avian. Exot. Pet. Med.* 13 (3): 132–141.

4 Schumacher, J. (2011). Respiratory medicine of reptiles. *Vet. Clin. North Am. Exot. Anim. Pract.* 14 (2): 207–224.

5 Long, S.Y. (2016). Approach to reptile emergency medicine. *Vet. Clin. North Am. Exot. Anim. Pract.* 19 (2): 567–590.

6 Sladky, K. and Mans, C. (2012). Clinical anesthesia in reptiles. *J. Exot. Pet. Med.* 21: 17–31.

7 Bennett, R.A. (1998). Reptile anesthesia. *Semin. Avian. Exot. Pet. Med.* 7 (1): 30–40.

8 Mans, C., Sladky, K.K., and Schumacher, J. (2019). General anesthesia. In: Mader's Reptile Medicine and Surgery, 3e (eds. S.J. Divers and S.J. Stahl), 447–464. St. Louis: Elsevier Inc.

9 Martinez-Jimenez, D. and Hernandez-Divers, S.J. (2007). Emergency care of reptiles. *Vet. Clin. North Am. Exot. Anim. Pract.* 10 (2): 557–585.

10 Bertelsen, M.F., Buchanan, R., Jensen, H.M. et al. (2015). Assessing the influence of mechanical ventilation on blood gases and blood pressure in rattlesnakes. *Vet. Anaesth. Analg.* 42 (4): 386–393.

11 Divers, S.J. (2010). Reptile diagnostic endoscopy and endosurgery. *Vet. Clin. North Am. Exot. Anim. Pract.* 13 (2): 217–242.

12 Norton, T.M. (2005). Chelonian emergency and critical care. *Semin. Avian. Exot. Pet. Med.* 14 (2): 106–130.

13 Mitchell, M.A. (2010). Managing the reptile patient in the veterinary hospital: establishing a standards of care model for nontraditional species. *J. Exot. Pet. Med.* 19 (1): 56–72.

14 Clayton, L.A. and Gore, S.R. (2007). Amphibian emergency medicine. *Vet. Clin. North Am. Exot. Anim. Pract.* 10 (2): 587–620.

15 Plunkett, S.J. and McMichael, M. (2008). Cardiopulmonary resuscitation in small animal medicine: an update. *J. Vet. Intern. Med.* 22 (1): 9–25.

16 Leary S, Underwood W, Anthony R, et al. (2020). AVMA guidelines for the euthanasia of animals: 2020 edition. pp. 1–121. https://www.avma.org/sites/default/files/2020-01/2020-Euthanasia-Final-1-17-20.pdf.

17 Baier, J. (2006). Reptiles. In: Guidelines for Euthanasia of Nondomestic Animals (ed. C. Baer), 42–45. Yulee: American Association of Zoo Veterinarians.

18 Conroy, C.J., Papenfuss, T., Parker, J., and Hahn, N.E. (2009). Use of tricaine methanesulfonate (MS222) for euthanasia of reptiles. *J. Am. Assoc. Lab. Anim. Sci.* 48 (1): 28–32.

19 Nevarez, J.G., Strain, G.M., da Cunha, A.F., and Beaufrère, H. (2014). Evaluation of four methods for inducing death during slaughter of American alligators (*Alligator mississippiensis*). *Am. J. Vet. Res.* 75 (6): 536–543.

20 Baier, J. (2006). Amphibians. In: Guidelines for Euthanasia of Nondomestic Animals (ed. C. Baer), 39–41. Yulee: American Association of Zoo Veterinarians.

21 Torreilles, S.L., McClure, D.E., and Green, S.L. (2009). Evaluation and refinement of euthanasia methods for *Xenopus laevis*. *J. Am. Assoc. Lab. Anim. Sci.* 48 (5): 512–516.

22 Balko, J.A., Posner, L.P., and Chinnadurai, S.K. (2019). Immersion in tricaine methanesulfonate (MS-222) is not sufficient for euthanasia of smokey jungle frogs (*Leptodactylus pentadactylus*). *J. Zoo Wildl. Med.* 50 (1): 89–95.

23 Gottdenker, N. and Yau, W. (2019). Necropsy. In: Mader's Reptile Medicine and Surgery, 3e (eds. S.J. Divers and S.J. Stahl), 368–375. St. Louis: Elsevier Inc.

45

Analgesia, Anesthesia, and Monitoring

Grayson A. Doss, Christoph Mans, and Kurt K. Sladky

Department of Surgical Sciences, School of Veterinary Medicine, University of Wisconsin-Madison, Madison, Wisconsin, USA

CONTENTS

Introduction

Historically, managing anesthesia in reptiles and amphibians has been problematic due to their diversity and the lack of systematic research dedicated to advancing our understanding of effective anesthetic/analgesic induction and maintenance drugs, dose-dependent effects, duration of drug efficacy, interspecies differences, and potentially fatal drug-related adverse effects, such as cardiopulmonary depression. Therefore, the reptile and amphibian literature is rife with anecdotal information, which has persisted and, in many cases, has grown to be widely accepted dogma for clinicians. The diversity of reptiles and amphibians in terms of natural history, size, anatomy, and physiology presents a unique clinical challenge to the veterinarian. However, as with all nondomestic species, the application of safe and effective anesthetic and analgesic techniques is essential for those veterinarians dealing with reptile and amphibian patients, and effective anesthetic application will facilitate performing complete physical examinations, collecting appropriate and high-quality diagnostic samples, and performing successful surgical procedures.

Importance of Anatomy and Physiology

Cardiac shunting can play a role in inhaled anesthetic uptake and elimination, potentially causing delayed induction, and delayed or an unexpectedly rapid recovery. In addition, cardiac shunts may affect systemic blood pressure and arterial/venous oxygen concentration, which, in turn, will impact anesthetic monitoring (e.g. indirect blood pressure, pulse oximetry, and expired gases).

The **respiratory system** of reptiles and amphibians differs substantially from other animals. As a broad generalization, the reptilian lung is considered fragile, composed of a simple, endothelial-lined sac in most reptile species. Lizards and chelonians have paired, sac-like lungs. Most snakes have a vestigial left lung and a functional right lung, which ends distally as an air sac. Boid snake species tend to have functional right and left lungs, although the left tends to be smaller. In non-crocodilian reptiles, the lung is typically septate, unlike the alveolar lungs of mammals. Reptiles lack a muscular diaphragm separating the thoracic and abdominal cavities, so a variety of skeletal and smooth muscles facilitate breathing. Chelonians use their pelvic and

Exotic Animal Emergency and Critical Care Medicine, First Edition. Edited by Jennifer E. Graham, Grayson A. Doss and Hugues Beaufrère.

pectoral muscles, which are functionally analogous to a mammalian diaphragm. Snakes use a combination of smooth muscle in the lung walls as well as intercostal muscles, while lizards use lung smooth muscle, intercostal, pectoral, and abdominal muscles for respiration. In amphibians, respiratory gas exchange can occur by different modes, including cutaneous, buccopharyngeal, and pulmonic or through gills. Cutaneous respiration occurs to some degree in most amphibians, while some species lack lungs. Physiologically, because reptiles and amphibians have a low metabolic rate, rate of respiration is slower, and reptiles also have a lower rate of oxygen consumption than mammals. Respiration in reptiles is controlled by oxygen and carbon dioxide concentrations in the blood as well as environmental temperatures. Reptiles tolerate hypoxic conditions, whether it is natural hypoxia or induced breath holding during anesthesia, as they are capable of metabolically converting to a state of anaerobic metabolism. This tolerance to hypoxia seems to depend on cardiovascular shunts, environmental temperature, and ability to buffer lactic acid.

Reptiles and amphibians are poikilothermic, meaning that their body temperature is directly dependent on environmental temperature. Changes in body temperature significantly affect metabolic rate and many physiologic processes. Therefore, the temperature at which one maintains a patient is an important factor, due to the fact that the metabolism and excretion of drugs is directly related to environmental temperature. [1–3] Consequently, **it is important to maintain the reptile and amphibian patient at its preferred optimal body temperature (POBT) in order to be able to better predict the physiologic effects of anesthetic drugs, as well as drug metabolism and excretion**. POBT is generally considered to be 20–25 °C (68–77 °F) in temperate and aquatic species, and 25–35 °C (77–95 °F) in tropical species. [4] Anesthetics and sedatives administered to reptiles maintained below the POBT will result in delayed onset of effects or lack of effects, all together. Duration of drug effects and recovery is prolonged in animals maintained below their POBT. In contrast, animals maintained at higher temperatures will show faster onset times of anesthesia or sedation, shorter duration of effects, and shorter recovery times.

Drug Administration Techniques

A **hepatic first-pass effect** occurs if drugs are administered in the caudal body half of reptiles, particularly if administered in the pelvic limb musculature. Blood from the pelvic limbs in reptiles drains directly into ventral abdominal vein(s) and then into the liver, before reaching the systemic circulation. This first-pass effect can substantially lower drug plasma levels and/or reduce the clinical efficacy of anesthetic or analgesic drugs that undergo hepatic metabolism and/or excretion, when administered in the pelvic limbs or caudal body half [5, 6]. Therefore, **it is strongly recommended to administer anesthetic and analgesic drugs in the cranial body half**. An exception is the intravenous (IV) administration of anesthetic induction agents (e.g. propofol, alfaxalone) in the caudal (tail) vein. This route of administration results in reliable anesthetic induction, since the caudal vein drains predominately into the caudal vena cava, mostly or completely avoiding the hepatic first-pass effect.

Routes of Administration

Subcutaneous (SC), Intramuscular (IM)

Both the SC and IM routes are commonly used to deliver anesthetics or analgesic drugs in reptiles and amphibians. Historically, it was recommended to avoid the SC route for injections due to the potential for delayed absorption. However, more recent studies in several reptile and amphibian species have demonstrated that the SC route results in rapid drug uptake [7–10]. Additionally, the SC route permits larger injection volumes when compared to IM injections, which are often limited by the size of available muscle bellies in small patients. Large patients (e.g. sulcata tortoises) may require use of multiple injection sites or concentrated drugs.

Intracoelomic (ICe)

While the intracoelomic (ICe) route may be an option for very small patients where other administration routes may be challenging, the risk of inadvertent bladder, gastrointestinal tract, respiratory tract, or follicular puncture and the potential impedance upon normal lung or air sac expansion make this route less desirable than SC or IM in most situations.

Topical

Due to their capability for transcutaneous absorption, various anesthetic and analgesic drugs can be administered topically in amphibians via an immersion bath or other techniques.

Intravenous (IV), Intraosseous (IO) Injections

The IV route may be used for anesthetic induction using agents like alfaxalone or propofol. Similar to IV catheters, IO catheters may be used for administration of injectable anesthetics or analgesics. The caudal (tail) vein is a common vascular access point for IV injections in reptiles.

Locoregional

Locoregional anesthesia and analgesia are currently underutilized in reptile and amphibian medicine, but offer significant benefits, like the ability to reduce injectable, inhalant anesthetic, and sedative drug requirements, and to produce preemptive analgesia in the perioperative period without deleterious side effects, such as respiratory depression. Common indications for the use of local anesthetics as part of an anesthetic protocol in reptiles include: distal limb surgery, cloacal procedures (e.g. prolapse), phallectomy, and coeliotomy. Local anesthetics can be administered as part of topical or incisional (infiltration) anesthesia, peripheral or cranial nerve blocks, or neuraxial (intrathecal, spinal) anesthesia.

Constant Rate Infusions (CRIs)

Currently, there is limited information regarding constant rate infusions (CRIs) of anesthetics or analgesics in reptiles and amphibians.

Analgesia

Indications

Analgesia should be provided for any painful condition in reptiles and amphibians. Preemptive analgesia (prior to onset of a painful procedure) should be administered in order to prevent central sensitization.

Pain Assessment/Scoring

Pain assessment is challenging in reptiles and amphibians. Because species-specific ethograms and pain scales in reptiles and amphibians are scarce to nonexistent, pain assessment is typically based upon subjective evaluations and information extrapolated from other animal groups, like mammals and birds. Alterations in body position, activity level and food intake may occur secondary to pain in reptiles and amphibians. However, since these changes are nonspecific they should be interpreted only as part of a multifactorial approach to assessing pain in these species.

Principles of Analgesia

Taking a multimodal approach to analgesia in reptiles and amphibian is imperative in order to provide the best possible care for critical and traumatized patients. As prey species, uncontrolled pain can result in a significant increase in patient morbidity and mortality.

Due to the marked variation in analgesic efficacy of drugs amongst groups of reptiles (i.e. snakes vs. lizards vs. chelonians) general recommendations on analgesic protocols are challenging to make and there is very little published data with respect to the clinical efficacy of analgesic drugs in any amphibian species. The bulk of the amphibian analgesia literature is research in Northern leopard frogs (*Lithobates pipiens*) administered opioid analgesics, other anesthetics and nonsteroidal anti-inflammatory drugs (NSAIDs), and an acetic acid wipe test used to measure efficacy.

Drug Classes

Commonly used drugs that have been shown to provide analgesia in reptiles and amphibians are listed in Tables 45.1 and 45.2, respectively.

Opioids

Mu-opioid receptor agonists are currently considered the most effective analgesic drugs in lizards and turtles and tortoises. **Buprenorphine and butorphanol do not provide analgesia in any of the reptile species tested to date, and therefore should not be administered to reptiles**.

In general, most of the amphibian analgesia research highlights mu-opioid receptor agonists (e.g. morphine) as the most effective analgesics in the species studied.

NSAIDs

While NSAIDs are commonly used in reptiles and amphibians, there is very little data regarding their analgesic efficacy or safety. While they appear safe to use in reptiles and amphibians, clinicians should remain mindful of the adverse (e.g. renal, gastrointestinal) effects documented with NSAID use in other animal species and use these drugs with appropriate caution. Meloxicam is currently the most frequently administered NSAID in reptiles and amphibians.

Local Anesthetics

Lidocaine (2–4 mg/kg) and bupivacaine (1 mg/kg) are most commonly used for regional anesthesia in reptiles. Neuraxial anesthesia with preservative-free lidocaine produced loss of motor function in the pelvic limbs and cloacal relaxation in bearded dragons (*Pogona vitticeps*) [17]. Only preservative-free drugs should be utilized for intrathecal injections.

Other Drugs

There is very little information regarding the analgesic efficacy of non-opioid drugs in reptiles and amphibians. Subcutaneous dexmedetomidine resulted in antinociception and respiratory depression in ball pythons (*Python regius*) [18]. While ketamine is often administered in combination with midazolam and/or alpha$_2$-agonist drugs for its sedative effects, there is no evidence regarding its analgesic efficacy in reptiles.

Table 45.1 Analgesic drugs commonly used in reptiles [11].

Opioids			
Hydromorphone	SC, IM	0.5–1.0 mg/kg q24h	Efficacy in red-eared slider turtles
Fentanyl	TC	12 µg/h	Clinical efficacy in lizards and chelonians; pharmacokinetics in ball pythons and prehensile-tailed skinks
Morphine	SC, IM	1.0–5.0 mg/kg q24h	Efficacy in lizards, and chelonians. Respiratory depression
Tramadol	PO, SC, IM	5.0–10.0 mg/kg q24–72h	Efficacy and pharmacokinetics in chelonians; clinical efficacy in lizards
NSAIDs			
Carprofen	SC, IM	1.0–4.0 mg/kg	Extrapolated from mammals; no efficacy data
Meloxicam	PO, SC, IM	0.2–0.5 mg/kg q12–24h	Extrapolated from mammals; no efficacy data. Avoid oral route in turtles (poor bioavailability)

Abbreviations: NSAIDs, nonsteroidal anti-inflammatory drugs; TC, transcutaneously.

Table 45.2 Analgesic drugs commonly used in amphibians.

Opioids			
Buprenorphine	ICe	50 mg/kg	Experimental: Eastern red-spotted newts showed slightly faster return to normal behavior compared to controls after limb amputation [12]. No analgesic effect at this dosage and route in axolotls [13]
	SC	14 mg/kg	Experimental: antinociception in Northern leopard frogs for at least 5 h [14]
Butorphanol	Immersion/TC	0.5 mg/l	Experimental: Eastern red-spotted newts showed slightly faster return to normal behavior compared to controls after limb amputation [12]
Morphine	SC	10–100 mg/kg	Experimental: antinociception in Northern leopard frogs [15]
	SC	40 mg/kg	African clawed frogs; unknown efficacy [16]
NSAIDS			
Flunixin meglumine	SC	25 mg/kg	African clawed frogs; possible efficacy with noxious thermal stimulus; caution, may cause renal toxicity at this dosage [16]
Meloxicam	SC	0.2 mg/kg	African clawed frogs; unknown efficacy [16]

ICe, intracoelomic; TC, transcutaneous.

Sedation

Indications

Major indications for sedation in reptile and amphibians include facilitation of basic procedures like physical examination, diagnostic sample collection (e.g. venipuncture) or diagnostic imaging. When combined with analgesia, more invasive procedures (e.g. wound management, minor surgeries) can be performed under sedation. Sedation can also enable safe handling of aggressive animals.

Risks and Benefits

Sedation is often sufficient for chemical restraint of most reptile and amphibian emergencies. Since many reptiles and amphibians are chronically diseased by the time of presentation, avoiding general anesthesia by using sedation will reduce potential anesthesia-related complications, such as delayed recovery and death. A variety of injectable drugs are effective for sedation in reptiles and are preferably administered in combination, in order to reduce the need for high drug dosages. Partially or completely reversible sedative combinations

Table 45.3 Sedation and anesthesia protocols commonly used in reptiles [19, 20]

Drug	Route	Dosage (mg/kg)	Comment
Turtles and tortoises			
Alfaxalone	IV	5–9	Induction of anesthesia
	SC, IM	10	Sedation
	SC, IM	20	Deep sedation to light anesthesia
Dexmedetomidine + midazolam	SC, IM	0.1 (D) + 0.5–1 (M)	Mild to moderate sedation
Dexmedetomidine + midazolam + ketamine	SC, IM	0.1 (D) + 1(M) + 2.5 mg/kg (K)	Heavy sedation
Dexmedetomidine + ketamine	SC, IM	0.05–0.1 (D) + 10 (K)	Light to surgical anesthesia
Propofol	IV	2–10	Induction of light to surgical anesthesia
Lizards			
Alfaxalone	IV	5–10	Induction of anesthesia
	SC, IM	10–20	Sedation, species-dependent
	SC, IM	30	Anesthesia, long recovery
Alfaxalone + midazolam	SC, IM	15 (A) + 1 (M)	Sedation
Dexmedetomidine + midazolam	SC, IM	0.075–0.1 (D) + 0.5–1(M)	Sedation, fast recovery after reversal
Dexmedetomidine + midazolam + ketamine	SC, IM	0.075–0.1 (D) + 0.5–1(M) + 5 mg/kg (K)	Heavy sedation
Dexmedetomidine + ketamine	SC, IM	0.1 (D) + 10 (K)	Sedation
Propofol	IV	5–10	Induction agent
Snakes			
Alfaxalone	IV	10	Induction agent, light anesthesia
	SC	5–10	Sedation
Alfaxalone + midazolam	SC	5 (A) + 0.5 (M)	Sedation
Dexmedetomidine + midazolam	SC	0.05 (D) + 0.5 (M)	Sedation
Propofol	IV	3–10	Induction agent
Tiletamine-zolazepam (Telazol)	SC, IM	2–10	Dose-dependent prolonged recovery

Dexmedetomidine and medetomidine should always be reversed with atipamezole. Reversal of midazolam with flumazenil is recommended in most cases.

Herptiles

are preferred, in order to avoid prolonged or unpredictable recoveries. The sedative combination used should be chosen based on the desired level of sedation, the general condition of the patient, and the diagnostic and/or therapeutic procedure to be performed. In reptiles, the authors prefer a combination of midazolam and dexmedetomidine, to which either ketamine at a low dose, or an opioid, can be added for deeper sedation and/or improved analgesia. Alternatively, alfaxalone can be administered SC or IM, either alone or combined with midazolam for deeper sedation. Commonly used sedative protocols in reptiles and amphibians are summarized in Tables 45.3 and 45.4, respectively. Sedated animals should be able to maintain spontaneous breathing, and should be responsive to overtly painful stimulation. The combination of procedural sedation with either local or spinal anesthesia offers the possibility of performing surgical or invasive procedures that would otherwise only be possible under general anesthesia. Additionally, by combining sedation with local or spinal anesthesia, the dose of general anesthetic drugs can be reduced, which will lead to reduced cardiovascular depression, more rapid recoveries, and potentially fewer anesthetic complications compared to general anesthesia.

Table 45.4 Sedation and anesthesia protocols commonly used in amphibians.

Drug	Route	Dosage	Comment
MS-222 (Tricaine-methanesulfonate)	Immersion/TC	200–5000 mg/l	Lower concentrations for gilled amphibians; higher concentrations for terrestrial amphibians
Eugenol (84–100%)	Immersion/TC	200–500 mg/l	Rapid induction and prolonged recovery. Caution: medullary collapse and death can occur quickly if not monitored; no evidence of analgesic efficacy, so cannot be recommended for invasive procedures. Histopathologic evidence of hepatic necrosis, pulmonary and renal changes, and fat body hemorrhage
Isoeugenol (Aqui-S)	Immersion/TC	50 mg/l	Brown tree frog tadpoles; no evidence of analgesic efficacy, so cannot be recommended for invasive procedures
Isoflurane	TC	0.01–0.06 ml/g	Liquid anesthetic mixed with sterile lubricating gel and water; mild to moderate sedation
	TC	2.1%	Gas administered in mask or chamber to effect (approximately 4 min) in cane toads [21]
Sevoflurane	TC	37.5 μl/g	Liquid sevoflurane mixed with sterile lubricating gel and water; moderate sedation in cane toads [22]
	TC	2.6%	Gas administered in mask or chamber to effect (approximately 5 min) in cane toads [21]
Alfaxalone	Immersion/TC	200 mg/l	Mild sedation, fire-bellied toads
		2000 mg/l	Minimal sedation, bullfrogs [23]
Alfaxalone–butorphanol	Immersion/TC	3.0 (A) + 2.5 mg/100 ml (B)	Fire-bellied toads; marked sedation, respiratory depression, no analgesic efficacy [25]
Alfaxalone–morphine	Immersion/TC	3.0 (A) + 5.0 mg/100 ml (M)	Fire-bellied toads; marked sedation, respiratory depression, evidence of analgesic efficacy [25]

TC, transcutaneous.

Anesthesia

Indications

The primary indication for general anesthesia in reptiles and amphibians is for major surgical procedures (e.g. coeliotomy) where complete immobilization is needed.

Preanesthetic Assessment

Systemic disease processes may preclude general anesthesia, and instead sedation with or without regional anesthesia, may be more suitable. If general anesthesia is required, the procedure may need to be delayed until the patient has received supportive care and is stabilized. With the exception of elective procedures or acute disease (e.g. trauma), most reptile and amphibian patients present with a history of chronic problems, frequently associated with inappropriate husbandry. Therefore, a thorough history and review of husbandry is critical prior to the physical examination and any diagnostic sample collection. Hydration and cardiopulmonary status of the patient should be assessed during the physical exam. Additionally, a complete blood count, plasma biochemical profile, and diagnostic imaging should be considered, if indicated and feasible based on patient size and species. Anemia, dehydration, and underlying organ dysfunction can cause significant complications during anesthesia, and may lead to delayed or non-recovery from general anesthesia. Dehydrated patients should be adequately rehydrated (see Chapter 46: Nutrition and Fluid Therapy) and any underlying disease processes identified and treated prior to an anesthetic procedure.

Premedication

Injectable sedation agents are routinely administered for premedication prior to anesthetic induction to decrease stress and lower the dose of induction agent required to reach the desired anesthetic depth. Injectable analgesic agents are also administered prior to induction when the planned procedure may be painful. Anticholinergics are rarely used as premedicants in reptiles and amphibians.

Induction

Reptiles and amphibians can be induced with injectable or inhalant anesthetic agents. Amphibians can also be anesthetized with topical administration of certain drugs. Commonly used anesthetic protocols in reptiles and amphibians are summarized in Tables 45.3 and 45.4, respectively.

Subcutaneous (SC), Intramuscular (IM)

Reptiles and amphibians are commonly anesthetized using higher dosages of injectable drugs often used for sedation/premedication.

Intravenous (IV)

Intravenous administration of propofol or alfaxalone can be performed in certain species of sufficient size. The administration of intravenous anesthetics should not be performed in the subcarapacial sinus or dorsal tail vein in turtles and tortoises, due to the risk of accidental administration in the subdural space (which communicates with the central nervous system [CNS]) which can lead to fatal complications.

Chamber

Inhalant anesthetics are preferred in snakes and lizards, and lead to rapid induction and recovery times. Induction is performed using isoflurane or sevoflurane via a chamber or facemask (Figure 45.1). In turtles and tortoises, the use of inhalant anesthetics is often associated with very prolonged or lack of anesthetic induction, due to the cardiopulmonary shunting of blood. Therefore, injectable protocols are often preferred over inhalant anesthesia in these species. In amphibians, inhalant anesthetic agents can be administered as a gas (Figure 45.2) or applied topically (Figure 45.3).

Topical

The most efficient method for anesthetic delivery in most amphibian species is by an immersion bath, which can be applied for short-term procedures using an induction container (Figure 45.4), or longer-term procedures using a recirculating bath anesthesia delivery apparatus, as is commonly used in fish anesthesia (Figure 45.5). Bath anesthetic methods require application of the anesthetic chemical, such as tricaine methanesulfonate (MS-222), eugenol, isoeugenol or alfaxalone (Table 45.4), mixed with **non-chlorinated** water. Anesthetic induction of amphibians using a water-filled container can provide short-term chemical immobilization, permitting physical examination, common diagnostic procedures (e.g. gill biopsies, skin

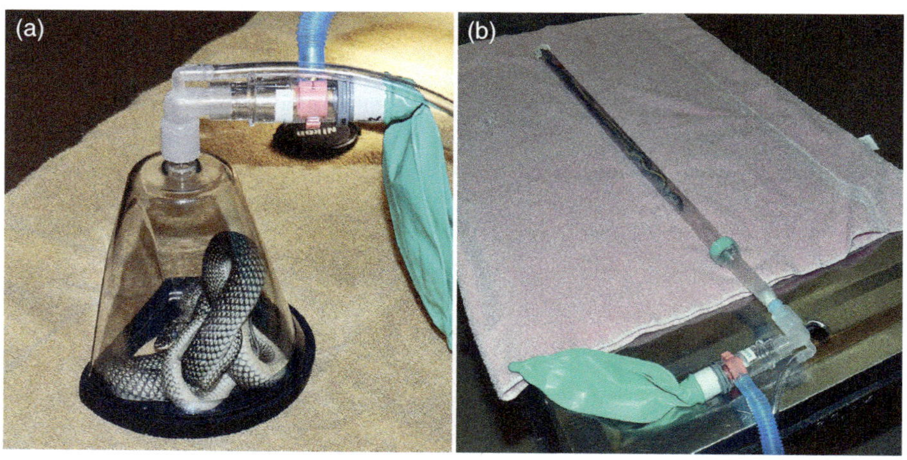

Figure 45.1 Induction of snakes with inhalant anesthetics. (a) Canine face mask is used as an induction chamber. (b) A snake restraint tube has been connected to a modified syringe case and used as an induction chamber. Snake tubes are particularly useful for aggressive or venomous snakes.

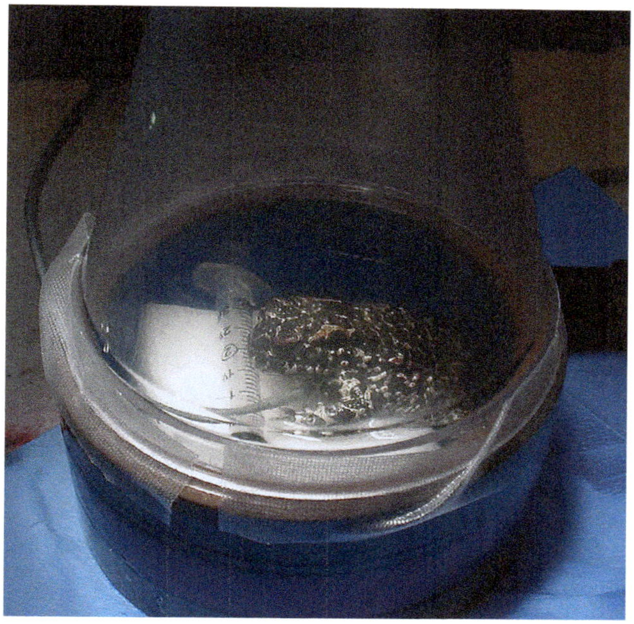

Figure 45.2 Gas anesthesia used for induction of a toad placed in a facemask.

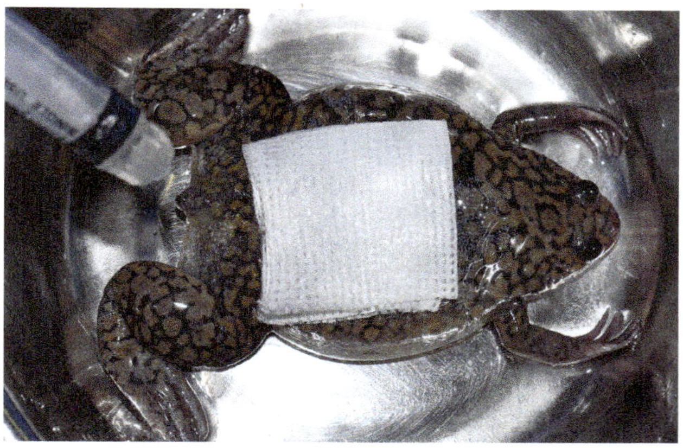

Figure 45.3 Topical application of isoflurane (dripped onto a gauze) in a frog.

scrapes), blood sample collection, and diagnostic imaging. For longer anesthetic procedures and surgery, either the recirculating anesthesia delivery apparatus with the anesthetic applied directly to the skin of the amphibian, or a gas anesthetic, is essential.

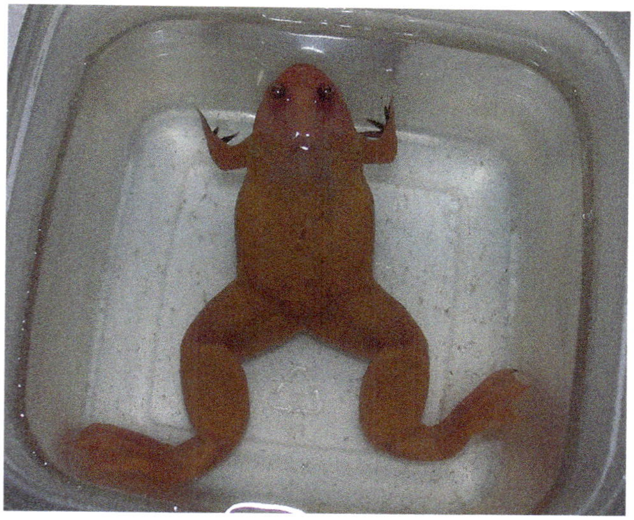

Figure 45.4 A frog placed in an immersion bath with MS-222 for anesthetic induction.

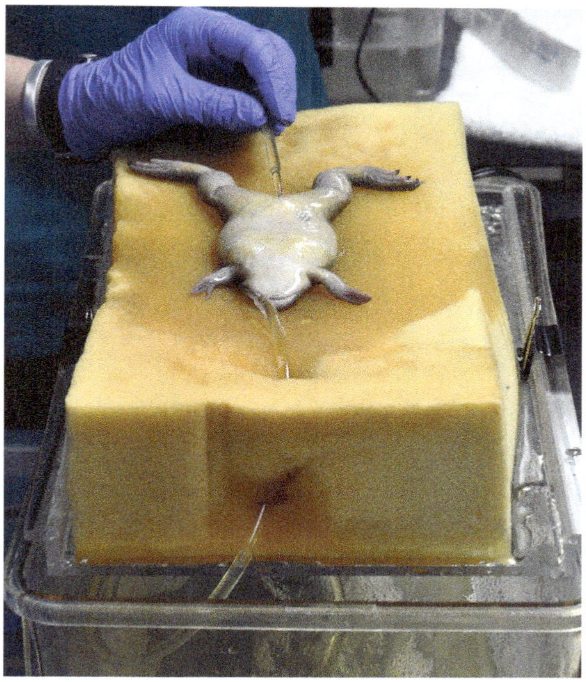

Figure 45.5 A recirculating bath anesthesia delivery apparatus is used to maintain general anesthesia in a frog.

Intubation

Following induction, endotracheal intubation should be performed using uncuffed (e.g. Cole) endotracheal tubes (Figure 45.6). Intubation is usually straightforward, but can be more challenging in chameleons due to the location of the glottis (Figure 45.7). Amphibian species with lungs can be intubated with an appropriately sized, uncuffed, endotracheal tube (Figure 45.8). The glottis is at the base of the tongue, much like reptiles, but the trachea is extremely short, so care must be taken so as not to advance the tube too far, causing intubation of a primary bronchus or doing damage to the trachea. Cole tubes (Figure 45.6) are particularly useful as they provide a limited length of the tube entering the short trachea.

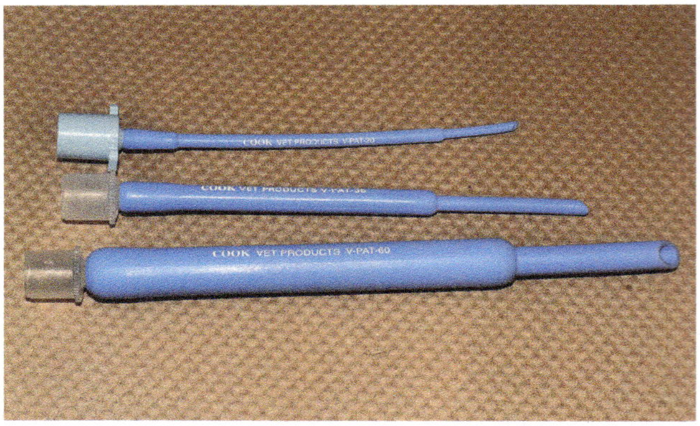

Figure 45.6 Uncuffed Cole endotracheal tubes, suitable for use in reptiles and amphibians.

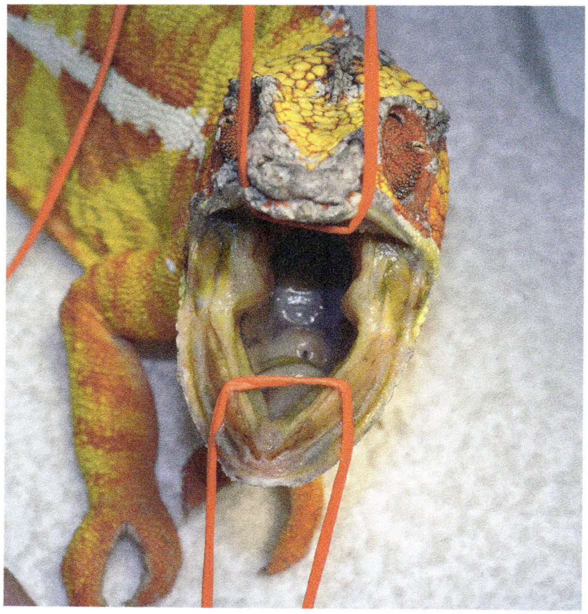

Figure 45.7 Oral cavity and glottis of a panther chameleon. Note the location of the glottis deep in the oral cavity at the base of the tongue, making intubation in chameleons more challenging.

Maintenance

Injectable

Supplemental injections (SC, IM, IV, and IO) of anesthetic agents (e.g. alfaxalone, midazolam, and ketamine) can be administered intermittently during long procedures to prolong anesthetic duration. Currently, total intravenous anesthesia (TIVA) is not readily used in reptile and amphibian anesthesia due to limited research and the relative difficulty obtaining vascular access.

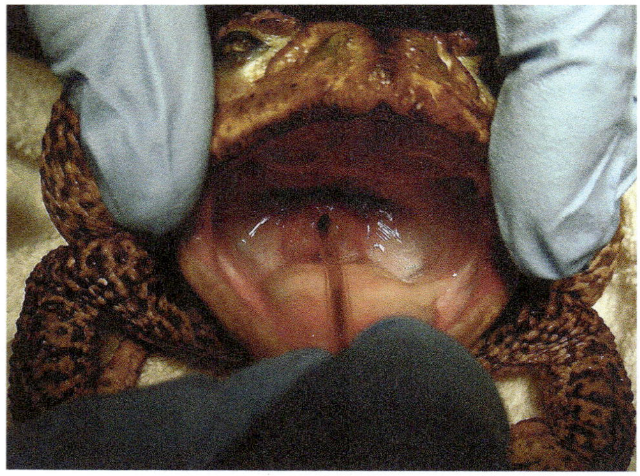

Figure 45.8 Endotracheal intubation in a toad.

Inhalant

In general, isoflurane or sevoflurane levels should be administered at the minimum required levels. The MAC of isoflurane and sevoflurane has been reported in only a handful of snake and lizard species [19].

Monitoring and Supportive Care

Anesthetic monitoring in reptiles and amphibians is challenging, due to the wide variety of anatomic and physiologic adaptations as well as the lack of validation of commonly used monitoring equipment.

Clinical Assessments

Depth of Anesthesia Reflexes

Reflex monitoring is considered one of the best methods to determine and repeatedly evaluate anesthetic depth. Multiple reflexes can be assessed, depending on the reptile or amphibian species. The corneal and palpebral reflex cannot be used in reptiles with spectacles (i.e. snakes, most geckos). Righting reflex and limb/tail withdrawal are simple reflexes to monitor and should be absent in amphibians, snakes and lizards under surgical anesthesia. Head and neck withdrawal as well as limb tap reflex can be reliably assessed in most turtles and tortoises. Jaw tone and cloacal tone can be assessed in most species.

Auscultation

In general, auscultation and palpation of pulses are challenging in reptiles and amphibians due to their unique anatomy (e.g. presence of scales). Using electronic

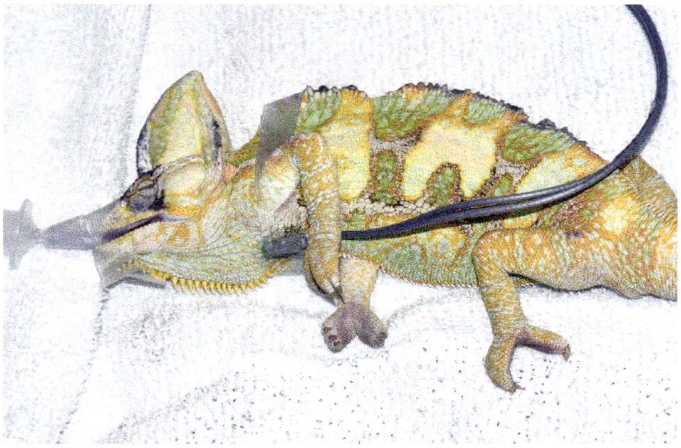

Figure 45.9 Veiled chameleon under general anesthesia. Note the placement of the Doppler probe in the area of the pectoral girdle between the forelimbs.

stethoscopes or placing a moistened gauze in between the stethoscope diaphragm and the patient can improve sound conduction.

Cardiovascular

Doppler

An ultrasonic Doppler can be used to determine heart rates in most reptile and amphibian species (Figure 45.9) and is often the most reliable and robust method of monitoring cardiovascular function. Doppler probes should be placed over the heart in amphibians, snakes, and lizards and over the thoracic inlet in turtles and tortoises.

Blood Pressure, ECG

Indirect blood pressure measurement in reptiles does not correlate with direct blood pressure, and therefore its use is not recommended. Electrocardiography (ECG) can be performed in reptiles, but interpretation is often challenging. In addition, persistent baseline ECG recordings may be present in reptiles and amphibians following CNS death.

CV Support

Intravenous or IO fluid therapy is recommended for anesthetic events. Fluid choice (e.g. crystalloids, colloids) depends on patient status. When intravascular access cannot be obtained, SC fluids should be administered. There is no published information regarding pressor use in reptiles and amphibians. Intramuscular epinephrine (0.1 mg/kg) significantly increased heart rate in anesthetized American alligators (*Alligator mississippiensis*) and common snapping turtles (*Chelydra serpentina*) but not in loggerhead sea turtles (*Caretta caretta*) [26–28]. However, the effect of IM epinephrine on cardiac output was not evaluated in these studies.

Respiratory

Pulse-oximetry, Capnography

Pulse oximetry and capnography readings in reptiles should be interpreted cautiously due to difference in respiratory physiology and the lack of validation in most species, but can be used to monitor trends. In green iguanas (*Iguana iguana*), oxygen saturation calculated by pulse oximetry was lower than SaO_2 determined by arterial blood gas analysis. [29] Reflectance probes are recommended and can be placed in the oral cavity or cloaca.

Respiratory Support

Intermittent positive pressure ventilation (IPPV) is performed for intubated reptiles and amphibians at a surgical plane of anesthesia. When ventilating reptiles and amphibians, pressures should be kept much lower than those used in mammals to prevent trauma due to their sac-like lungs.

Temperature

Monitoring, Support

As poikilotherms, the body temperature of reptiles and amphibians will correspond with environmental temperature. Patient size permitting, esophageal, and cloacal temperatures may be monitored in anesthetized reptiles and amphibians. [30] Infrared thermometers permit rapid measurement of the immediate environment but patient surface temperatures may underestimate core temperatures. [30] Many of the thermal support devices commonly used for anesthesia of other species (e.g. recirculating water blankets, forced air warmers, and conductive thermal blankets) can be used in reptiles and amphibians. When providing thermal support to amphibians, care must be taken to prevent skin desiccation. Aquarium water heaters can be used to maintain immersion and recovery anesthetic solutions at appropriate temperatures.

Post-anesthesia

Recovery times in reptiles and amphibians are dependent on the drugs used, body temperature and underlying morbidity. In general, the use of completely reversible injectable drugs (e.g. dexmedetomidine, midazolam) results in faster recovery, following administration of the respective reversal agents (e.g. atipamezole, flumazenil). Nonreversible drugs (e.g. ketamine, alfaxalone, and propofol) have to be metabolized and excreted, which is dependent on organ function and body temperature. Increased body temperature will result in reduced recovery times. Administration of high doses of nonreversible drugs should be avoided, since increased doses result in prolonged recovery times. Administration of 0.1 mg/kg epinephrine IM resulted in faster inhalant anesthetic recovery times in American alligators, common snapping turtles and loggerhead sea turtles [26–28]. In common snapping turtles, electrical stimulation of the Governing Vessel 26 (GV-26) acupuncture point resulted in faster recovery from isoflurane anesthesia [27].

Animals should be placed in a temperature-controlled environment (e.g. incubator for reptiles) and ventilated intermittently until spontaneous breathing has returned, which is a reliable indicator of anesthetic recovery. Routine anesthetic monitoring (e.g. Doppler, reflex evaluation) should continue until the patient is fully recovered.

References

1. Preston, D.L., Mosley, C.A.E., and Mason, R.T. (2010). Sources of variability in recovery time from methohexital sodium anesthesia in snakes. *Copeia* 2010 (3): 496–501.
2. Carregaro, A.B., Cruz, M.L., Cherubini, A.L., and Luna, S.P.L. (2009). Influence of body temperature on rattlesnakes (*Crotalus durissus*) anesthetized with ketamine. *Pesqui. Vet. Bras.* 29 (12): 969–973.
3. Stirl, R. and Bonath, K.H. (1998). Anesthesia of tropical boids (*Boa constrictor*) – influences of the ambient temperature? *Kleintierpraxis* 43 (11): 839–845.
4. Varga, M. (2004). Captive maintenance and welfare. In: *BSAVA Manual of Reptiles*, 2e (ed. G.S.J. RP), 6–17. Gloucester, UK.
5. Fink, D.M., Doss, G.A., Sladky, K.K., and Mans, C. (2018). Effect of injection site on dexmedetomidine-ketamine induced sedation in leopard geckos (*Eublepharis macularius*). *J. Am. Vet. Med. Assoc.* 253 (9): 1146–1150.
6. Yaw, T.J., Mans, C., Johnson, S.M. et al. (2018). Effect of injection site on alfaxalone-induced sedation in ball pythons (*Python regius*). *J. Small Anim. Pract.* 59 (12): 747–751.
7. Yaw, T.J., Mans, C., Martinelli, L., and Sladky, K.K. (2020). Comparison of subcutaneous administration of alfaxalone–midazolam–dexmedetomidine with ketamine–midazolam–dexmedetomidine for chemical restraint in juvenile blue poison dart frogs (*Dendrobates tinctorius azureus*). *J. Zoo Wildl. Med.* 50 (4): 868–873.
8. Doss, G., Fink, D., Sladky, K., and Mans, C. (2017). Comparison of subcutaneous dexmedetomidine–midazolam versus alfaxalone–midazolam sedation in leopard geckos (*Eublepharis macularius*). *Vet. Anaesth. Analg.* 44 (5): 1175–1183.
9. Yaw, T.J., Mans, C., Johnson, S. et al. (2020). Evaluation of subcutaneous administration of alfaxalone–midazolam and dexmedetomidine–midazolam for sedation of ball pythons (*Python regius*). *J. Am. Vet. Med. Assoc.* 256 (4): 573–579.
10. Hawkins, S.J., Cox, S., Yaw, T.J., and Sladky, K. (2019). Pharmacokinetics of subcutaneously administered hydromorphone in bearded dragons (*Pogona vitticeps*) and red-eared slider turtles (*Trachemys scripta elegans*). *Vet. Anaesth. Analg.* 46 (3): 352–359.
11. Sladky, K.K. and Mans, C. (2012). Clinical analgesia in reptiles. *J. Exot. Pet. Med.* 21 (2): 158–167.
12. Koeller, C.A. (2009). Comparison of buprenorphine and butorphanol analgesia in the eastern red-spotted newt (*Notophthalmus viridescens*). *J. Am. Assoc. Lab. Anim. Sci.* 48 (2): 171–175.
13. Llaniguez, J.T., Szczepaniak, M.A., Rickman, B.H. et al. (2020). Quantitative and qualitative behavioral measurements to assess pain in axolotls (*Ambystoma mexicanum*). *J. Am. Assoc. Lab. Anim. Sci.* 59 (2): 186–196.
14. Stevens, C.W., Maciver, D.N., and Newman, L.C. (2001). Testing and comparison of non-opioid analgesics in amphibians. *Contemp. Top. Lab. Anim. Sci.* 40 (4): 23–27.
15. Pezalla, P.D. (1983). Morphine-induced analgesia and explosive motor behavior in an amphibian. *Brain Res.* 273 (2): 297–305.
16. Coble, D.J., Taylor, D.K., and Mook, D.M. (2011). Analgesic effects of meloxicam, morphine sulfate, flunixin meglumine, and xylazine hydrochloride in African-clawed frogs (*Xenopus laevis*). *J. Am. Assoc. Lab. Anim. Sci.* 50 (3): 355–360.
17. Ferreira, T.H. and Mans, C. (2019). Evaluation of neuraxial anesthesia in bearded dragons (*Pogona vitticeps*). *Vet. Anaesth. Analg.* 46 (1): 126–134.
18. Bunke, L.G., Sladky, K.K., and Johnson, S.M. (2018). Antinociceptive efficacy and respiratory effects of dexmedetomidine in ball pythons (*Python regius*). *Am. J. Vet. Res.* 79 (7): 718–726.
19. Mans, C., Sladky, K., and Schumacher, J. (2019). General anesthesia. In: *Mader's Reptile and Amphibian Medicine and Surgery*, 3e (eds. S. Divers and S. Stahl), 447–464. St. Louis, MO: Elsevier.

20 Sladky, K. and Mans, C. (2012). Clinical anesthesia in reptiles. *J. Exot. Pet. Med.* 21 (1): 17–31.

21 Morrison, K.E., Strahl-Heldreth, D., and Clark-Price, S.C. (2016). Isoflurane, sevoflurane and desflurane use in cane toads (*Rhinella marina*). *Vet. Rec. Open.* 3 (1) https://pubmed.ncbi.nlm.nih.gov/27651914/.

22 Stone, S.M., Clark-Price, S.C., Boesch, J.M., and Mitchell, M.A. (2013). Evaluation of righting reflex in cane toads (*Bufo marinus*) after topical application of sevoflurane jelly. *Am. J. Vet. Res.* 74 (6): 823–827.

23 Posner, L.P., Bailey, K.M., Richardson, E.Y. et al. (2013). Alfaxalone anesthesia in bullfrogs (*Lithobates catesbeiana*) by injection or immersion. *J. Zoo. Wildl. Med.* 44 (4): 965–971.

24 Adami, C., Spadavecchia, C., Angeli, G., and D'Ovidio, D. (2015). Alfaxalone anesthesia by immersion in oriental fire-bellied toads (*Bombina orientalis*). *Vet. Anaesth. Analg.* 42 (5): 547–551.

25 Adami, C., D'Ovidio, D., and Casoni, D. (2016). Alfaxalone–butorphanol versus alfaxalone–morphine combination for immersion anaesthesia in oriental fire-bellied toads (*Bombina orientalis*). *Lab. Anim.* 50 (3): 204–211.

26 Gatson, B.J., Goe, A., Granone, T.D., and Wellehan, J.F.X. (2017). Intramuscular epinephrine results in reduced anesthetic recovery time in American alligators (*Alligator mississippiensis*) undergoing isoflurane anesthesia. *J. Zoo Wildl. Med.* 48 (1): 55–61.

27 Goe, A., Shmalberg, J., Gatson, B. et al. (2016). Epinephrine or GV-26 electrical stimulation reduces inhalant anesthestic recovery time in common snapping turtles (*Chelydra serpentina*). *J. Zoo Wildl. Med.* 47 (2): 501–507.

28 Balko, J.A., Gatson, B.J., Cohen, E.B. et al. (2018). Inhalant anesthetic recovery following intramuscular epinephrine in the loggerhead sea turtle (*Caretta caretta*). *J. Zoo Wildl. Med.* 49 (3): 680–688.

29 Hernandez, S.M., Schumacher, J., Lewis, S.J. et al. (2011). Selected cardiopulmonary values and baroreceptor reflex in conscious green iguanas (*Iguana iguana*). *Am. J. Vet. Res.* 72 (11): 1519–1526.

30 Cremer, J., Perry, S.M., Liu, C.C., and Nevarez, J.G. (2019). Comparison of surface, esophageal, and cloacal temperatures in different reptile species. *J. Zoo Wildl. Med.* 50 (2): 308–314.

46

Nutrition and Fluid Therapy

Ian Kanda and João Brandão

Department of Veterinary Clinical Sciences, College of Veterinary Medicine, Oklahoma State University, Stillwater, Oklahoma, USA

CONTENTS

Nutrition

Indications

Nutritional therapy is used to manage cachexia in patients that are unable or unwilling to eat voluntarily. Nutritional support promotes organ and immune system function, as well as healing [1]. Nutrition-related disorders are a common cause for presentation of the reptile or amphibian patient.

Based on mammalian information, nutritional intervention is recommended in cases of acute loss of 10% body weight (BW), or chronic loss of 20%. Assistance is also required if patient condition prevents ingestion of 85% of caloric requirements [2]. History and body condition scoring are used to determine the nutritional status. Vertebral processes, ribs, and pelvic girdle should be palpable but not readily visible. The tail should be full, and musculature should fill and cover the temporal fenestra of the head; these appear sunken in emaciated animals. In lizards, skin folds should be minimal with one lateral fold in most species. Hind-gut fermenting species (e.g. green iguanas) should have rounded, full-feeling coelomic cavities.

Prior to instituting nutritional therapy, the patient should be in stable condition at its optimal temperature and euhydrated. For patients in good body condition, feed 75–100% of their daily energy needs in their first 24–48 hours [2]. To avoid digestive and metabolic upset, debilitated animals should be fed slower, administering approximately 40–75% of their requirements over this period [2].

Nutritional Requirements

Species-Specific Dietary Requirements

There are thousands of reptile and amphibian species, many of which are common in the pet trade. Among this group is a diverse variety of feeding strategies and dietary niches (Figure 46.1). Smaller reptiles typically eat daily, with young, growing animals needing to be fed multiple times daily. Larger adults can be fed daily or much less often, depending on species, size of the animal, and food type. The variety of nutritional specialization makes the

Exotic Animal Emergency and Critical Care Medicine, First Edition. Edited by Jennifer E. Graham, Grayson A. Doss and Hugues Beaufrère.

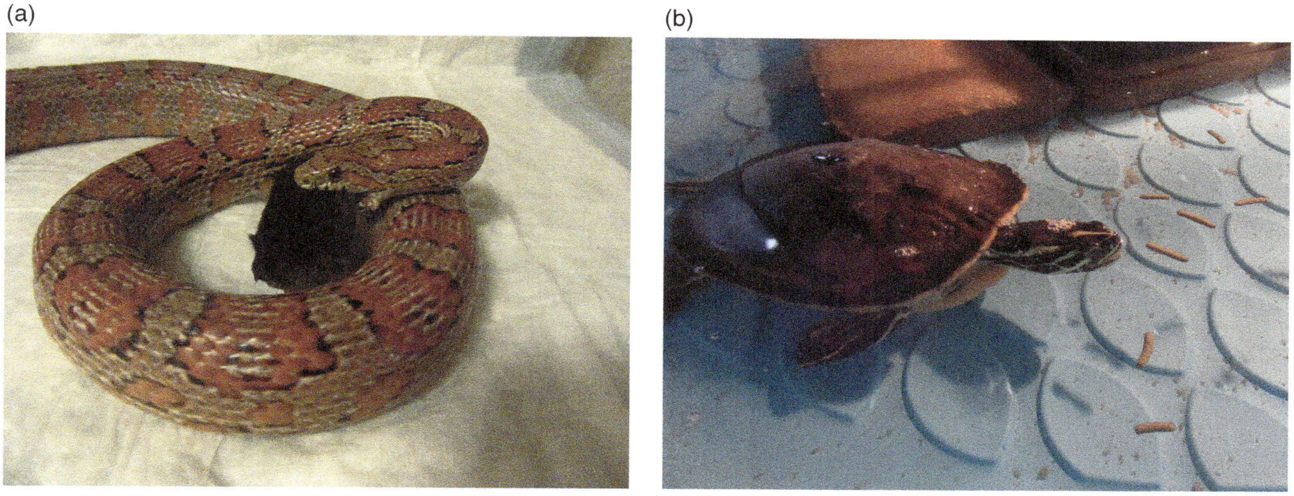

Figure 46.1 A corn snake (*Pantherophis guttatus*) eating a mouse (a). Carnivores that eat whole body vertebrate prey are less likely to be subjected to nutritional imbalances. Many aquatic turtles like the Florida red-bellied cooter (*Pseudemys nelsoni*) will only eat while in water (b).

categories of carnivore, herbivore, and omnivore insufficient to select a diet that will entice spontaneous food intake in all species. Many aquatic turtles are primarily carnivorous as juveniles, but begin ingesting more vegetation with age. All adult amphibians are carnivorous; however, many tadpoles are herbivorous [3]. For the dietary classification of some common pet reptile and amphibian species see Table 46.1.

Metabolic Rates and Caloric Requirements

The standard metabolic rate (SMR) for reptiles is calculated using SMR (kcal/d) = $32(\text{BW in kg})^{0.75}$ [2]. Daily caloric intake is SMR multiplied by factors that raise metabolic rate like activity (×1.25); reproduction (×1.5); stress or growth (×2–2.5); or wound healing (×1.5) [2]. Amphibians are not only ectotherms, but they also prefer temperatures typically much cooler than reptiles. For simplicity, calculations for amphibian SMR at 20 °C have been provided. For anurans, SMR(kcal/d) = $0.012(\text{BW in g})^{0.82}$. Multiply SMR by 2 if animals are kept at 25 °C, and halve it if environmental temperature is 5 °C [4].

Due to the subjective nature of calculating caloric needs in reptiles and amphibians, it is important to individually tailor nutritional support based on patient response.

Nutritional Diets/Feeding Formulas

Critical Care Diets

Although specific nutrient requirements for reptiles and amphibians are largely unknown, commercial critical care diets are available (see Table 46.2). Also known as elemental diets, these products are formulated to be calorically dense and easily digestible for debilitated patients and are typically formulated for different diet strategies. Recommended daily feeding volumes are product specific and frequency is based on estimated caloric needs and the patient's normal feeding habits.

Carnivores can also be fed critical care diets formulated for cats and dogs [5]. However, the purine and vitamin A content may be too high making it contraindicated in renal disease patients [5]. While hydration status should be corrected prior to nutritional therapy, these diets are typically diluted with water or can be mixed with electrolyte solutions [5].

Another alternative is to make a puree of typical prey items. This method likely does not offer the same digestibility of a critical care diet, and is more likely to clog the feeding tube. Powdered and gel diets formulated for reptiles can be made in to a slurry that can be syringe fed. Alfalfa pellets or powder can be mixed with water for herbivores. Meat, vegetable, or fruit human baby foods can be used to add palatability to diets while enticing a patient to eat voluntarily.

Routes

Syringe Feeding

Syringe feeding can begin by placing a drop of the diet on to the rostral lip margin to try and instigate licking and a feeding response (Figure 46.2). If this does not work, an atraumatic speculum can be pressed and/or rotated into the commissure of the mouth to open. In small patients, a soft-rubber baking spatula or plastic bank card can serve as an atraumatic speculum (Figure 46.3). In some lizards, gentle downward traction on the gular skin may work. Once the mouth is open, food can be deposited into the oral cavity. Avoid bolusing large amounts into the oral cavity at one time, which could increase the risk of aspiration into the adjacent glottis.

Table 46.1 Specific dietary preferences of common pet reptile and amphibian species.

Common name	Species	Dietary category
Box turtle	*Terrapene carolina*	Omnivorous
Desert tortoise	*Gopherus agassizii*	Herbivorous
Greek tortoise	*Testudo graeca*	Herbivorous
Painted turtle	*Chrysemys picta*	Omnivorous
Red-eared slider	*Trachemys scripta elegans*	Omnivorous
Russian tortoise	*Agrionemys horsfieldii*	Herbivorous
African spurred tortoise	*Centrochelys sulcata*	Herbivorous
Australian water dragon	*Intellagama lesueurii*	Omnivorous
Crested gecko	*Correlophus ciliatus*	Omnivorous
Jackson's chameleon	*Trioceros jacksonii*	Carnivorous
Veiled chameleon	*Chamaeleo calyptratus*	Carnivorous
Green iguana	*Iguana iguana*	Herbivorous
Green anole	*Anolis carolinensis*	Carnivorous
Bearded dragon	*Pogona vitticeps*	Omnivorous
Sand boa	*Eryx colubrinus*	Carnivorous
King snake	*Lampropeltis getulus*	Carnivorous
Garter snake	*Thamnophis sirtalis*	Carnivorous
Boa constrictor	*Boa constrictor*	Carnivorous
Ball python	*Python regius*	Carnivorous
Corn snake	*Pantherophis guttatus*	Carnivorous
Pacman frog	*Ceratophrys* spp.	Carnivorous
Tiger salamander	*Ambystoma mavortium*	Carnivorous
Oriental fire-bellied toad	*Bombina orientalis*	Carnivorous

Table 46.2 Critical care diets for reptiles and amphibians.

Product	Manufacturer	Patient group	Notes
Carnivore Critical Care	Oxbow	Carnivores, insectivores	Can mix with Herbivore Critical Care for omnivores
Herbivore Critical Care	Oxbow	Herbivores	Can mix with Carnivore Care for omnivores
Omnivore Critical Care	Oxbow	Omnivores	
Emeraid Carnivore	Lafeber	Carnivores, insectivores	
Emeraid Herbivore	Lafeber	Herbivores	
Emeraid Omnivore	Lafeber	Omnivores	
Emeraid Piscivore	Lafeber	Piscivores	Designed for fish-eating birds
Clinicare Canine	Zoetis	Omnivores, herbivores	
Clinicare Feline	Zoetis	Carnivores, insectivores	
Prescription Diet a/d	Hill's	Carnivores, insectivores	

Nasogastric

Most pet reptile species do not have a hard palate and the airway enters into the oral cavity from the choana, making use of nasogastric tubes impractical.

Esophagostomy Tube

Esophagostomy tubes are indicated when the mouth is difficult or painful to open. Additionally, feedings through an esophagostomy tube are likely less stressful than repeated

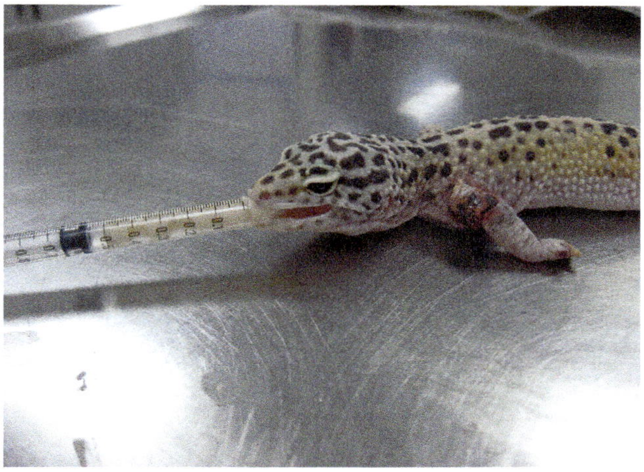

Figure 46.2 This leopard gecko (*Eublepharis macularius*) was enticed to eat by first placing a drop of a critical care formula on the rostral lip margin.

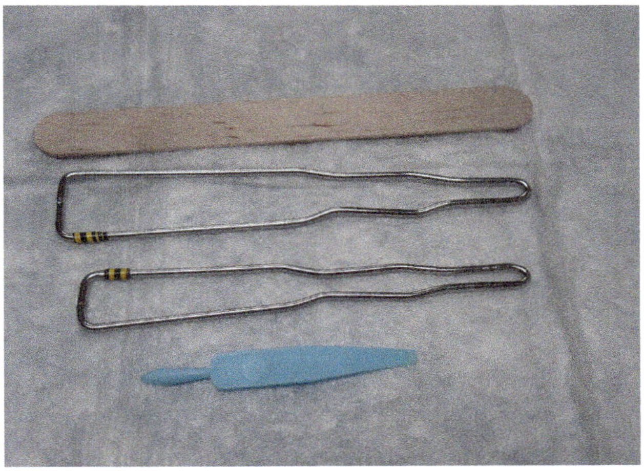

Figure 46.3 An assortment of items used as oral speculums. Softer materials are less likely to damage teeth and tissue, while the metal oral speculums allow for easy visualization and manipulation around a feeding or endotracheal tube.

restraint for passage of an orogastric tube. This method of providing nutritional support is commonly utilized in chelonians, as it is very difficult or impossible to gain oral access in a conscious turtle or tortoise, especially when the head is withdrawn. Esophagostomy tubes are less commonly utilized in snakes due to the relative ease of performing intermittent orogastric tube feedings.

Large red rubber catheter tubes are commonly used, which can usually accommodate most slurries and enteral diets. Tube-fed meals should always be followed with water to flush the tube lumen and prevent clogging. Provided it remains patent, and the stoma site is free from cellulitis, abscessation, ulceration, or other potential side effects, tubes can be left in for months until the animal is eating voluntarily [1, 6].

Heavy sedation or general anesthesia is needed for esophagostomy tube placement. The tube is premeasured from the lateral cervical region where the tube will exit the neck to the area of the stomach and the point marked with a permanent marker. In chelonians, measuring to the junction of the pectoral and abdominal scutes of the plastron is a good approximation of stomach location. In chelonians, place the cervical area exit point for the tube as caudal as possible to limit the patient's ability to pull the tube out. Tube placement can be on either side of the neck; however, the right jugular vein is typically larger in most species so left-sided placement is more common. See Figure 46.4 for a step-by-step approach to esophagostomy tube placement in chelonians.

Orogastric Tubes

Intermittent gavage or orogastric tube feedings are commonly used in reptile and amphibian critical care. The oral cavity can be accessed for tube passage in some turtles as they open their mouth to defensively bite. In most species, red rubber urinary catheters can be used; however, in chelonians, which possess strong jaw power and have sharp oral cavity edges, straight metal gavage tubes (Figure 46.5) with an atraumatic tip are typically used.

The tube is premeasured to reach the patient's distal esophagus or stomach. In snakes, this is approximately at the mid-body point (Figure 46.6a). If the patient is too long, a tube that passes the heart should suffice. For lizards and turtles, measuring to the midpoint of the coelomic cavity is adequate. Amphibians have a short esophagus and measuring to the cranial 1/3 point of the snout-to-vent length may be more appropriate [4].

The mouth is opened with a speculum and the glottis visualized and avoided (Figure 46.6b). The feeding tube is advanced down the esophagus (Figure 46.6c) with the syringe containing liquid nutrition attached. The feeding tube should be prefilled with food or water to avoid adding unnecessary air into the stomach and lightly coated with lubricant prior to insertion. For larger patients, care must be taken to avoid bites to the handler, and a mouth gag is often used to protect the tube. Use of sedation should be considered in awake patients to help alleviate potential induced stress of the procedure. Indwelling orogastric tubes are rarely used as a means of nutritional support in reptiles.

Parenteral

Information pertaining to parenteral support in reptiles is derived from mammalian species. Due to the difficulty of venous access in most reptile species, this route of

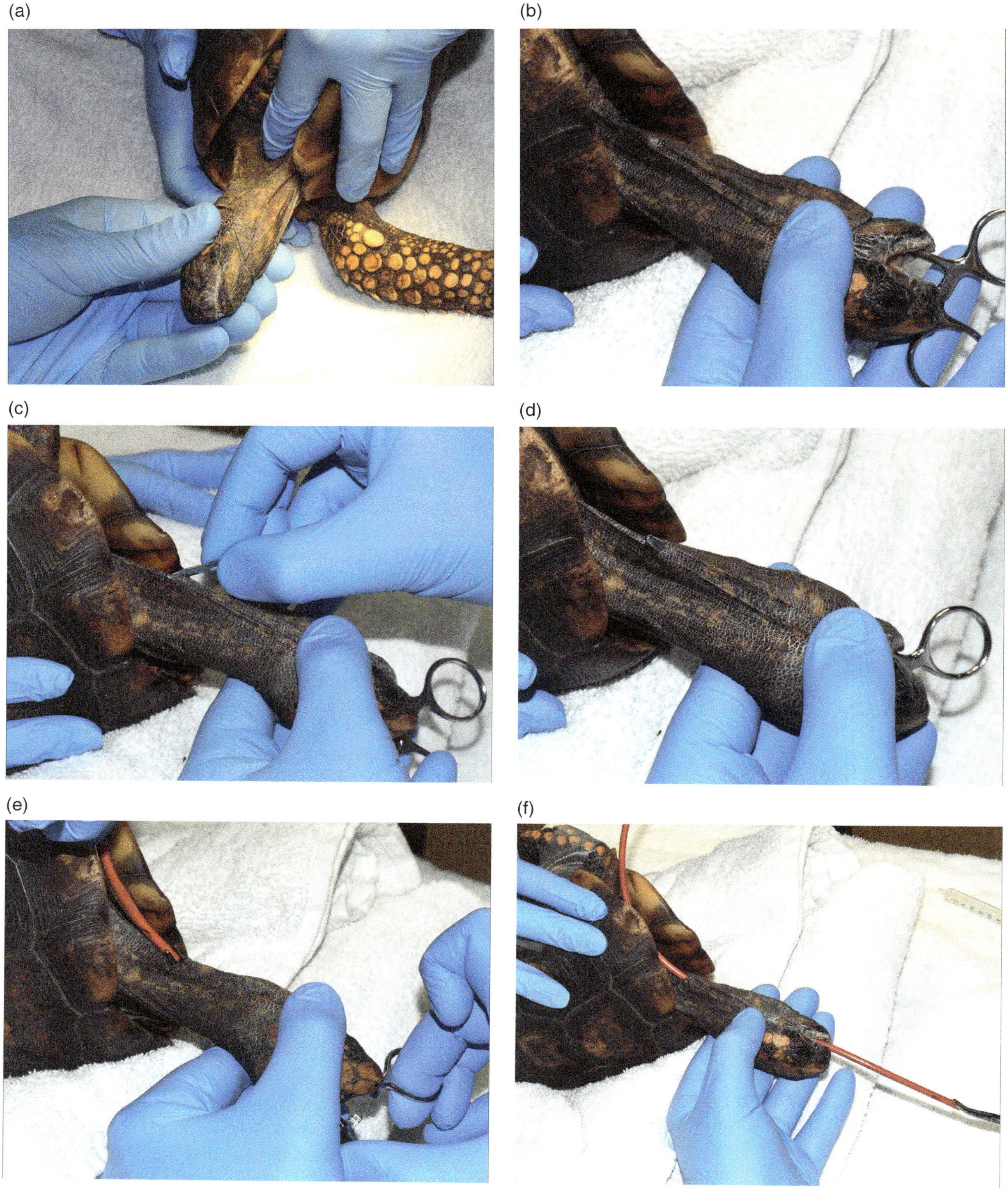

Figure 46.4 Esophagostomy tube placement in a heavily sedated red-footed tortoise (*Chelonoidis carbonaria*). The tortoise is placed in lateral recumbency to facilitate tube placement and an assistant tucks the adjacent limb out of the way (a). Long-handled hemostatic forceps are inserted into the oral cavity and down the esophagus to the selected entry point (b) and the skin and esophagus are tented. An incision is made over the tip of the hemostats (c) and the tip of the hemostats is exposed after the full-thickness skin and esophagus incision (d). The incision is made large enough to allow the hemostats to open enough to grab the end of the feeding tube and pull it back cranially out of the mouth (e, f). The tube is then redirected back down the esophagus into the stomach. Note how once the tube is successfully inserted aborad into the gastrointestinal tract, it reorients with the proximal, external end of the tube pointing cranially rather than caudally (g). The tube is moved until the premeasured depth mark is level with the skin (g) and a finger-trap pattern is used to secure the tube to the skin with nonabsorbable suture (h). The esophagostomy tube has been capped and secured to the carapace using adhesive medical tape in the awake patient (i). *Source:* Images courtesy of Grayson Doss, Madison, WI.

(g)

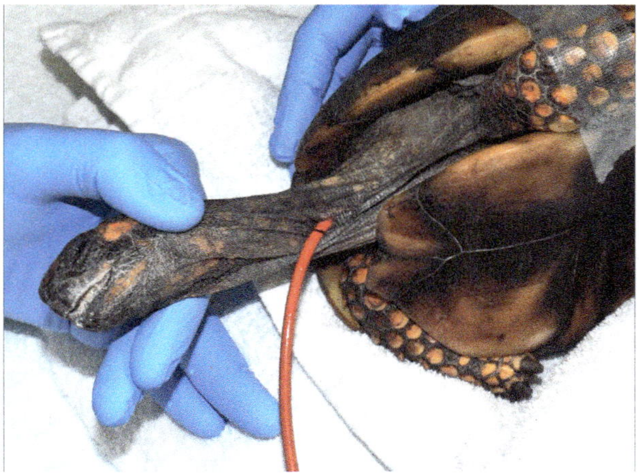

(h)

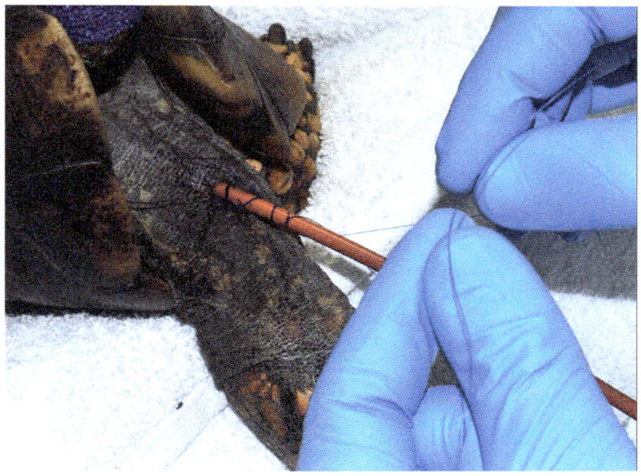

(i)

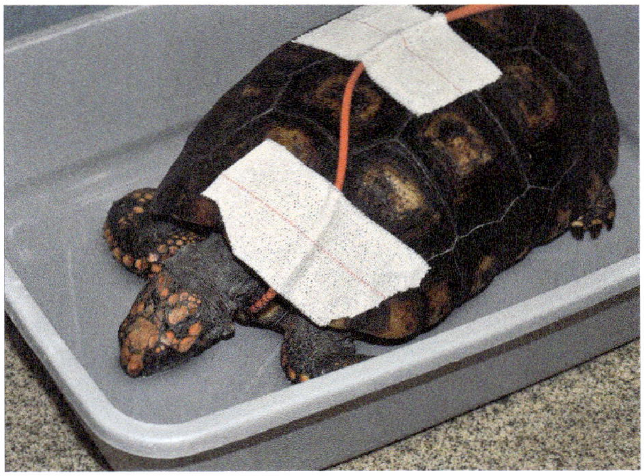

Figure 46.4 (Continued)

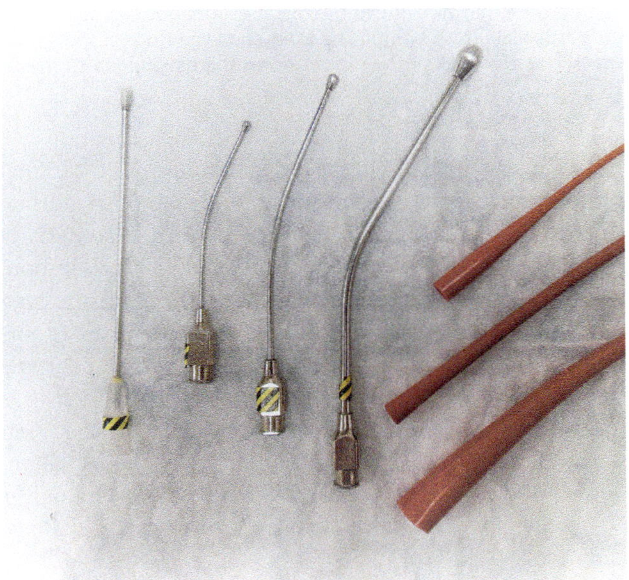

Figure 46.5 Metal ball tipped syringes, red rubber urinary catheters and feeding tubes can all be used to deliver a food bolus of critical care diet.

nutritional support is rarely utilized. Central venous access is necessary for the administration of amino acids and dextrose while lipids can be given into a peripheral vein. Sepsis, phlebitis, thrombosis, fatty liver, hyperglycemia, and hypokalemia are all potential complications of parenteral nutrition therapy and enterocytes are starved without gastrointestinal food consumption [1, 2]. Regular bloodwork should be performed to monitor patient status and recovery with a plan to transition to oral caloric intake.

Monitoring

Although poorly documented in reptiles and amphibians, a concern associated with nutritional therapy is refeeding syndrome [2, 7]. This can be avoided by beginning hydration and electrolyte corrections prior to nutritional supplementation, and feeding nutritionally balanced diets [7]. Feed 50% of estimated energy needs over a 24-hour period and repeat for several days, with incremental increases as

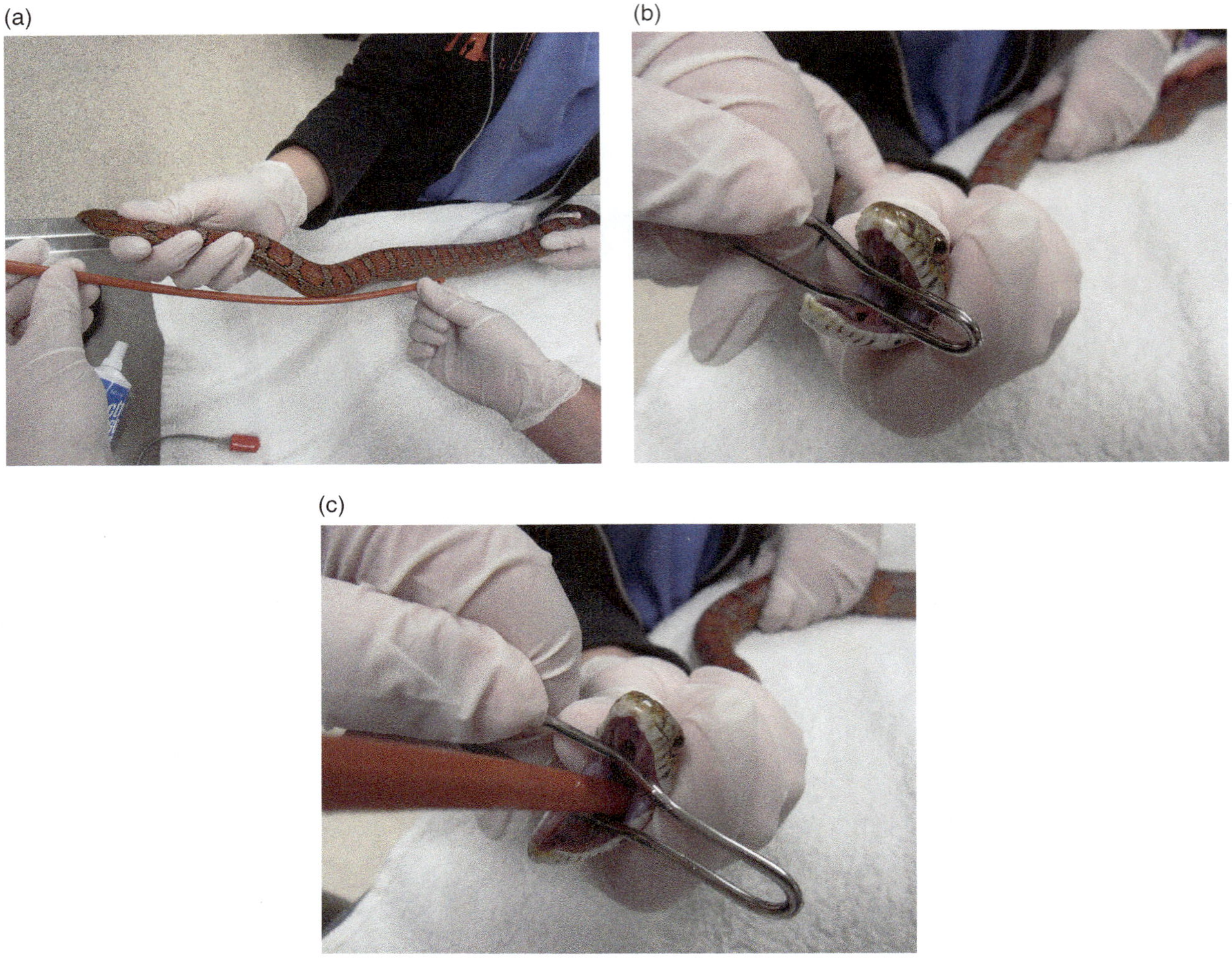

Figure 46.6 Orogastric tube passage in a corn snake (*Pantherophis guttatus*). First, premeasure the feeding tube to enter the stomach, approximately at the midpoint of the body (a). For snakes that are too long, a tube that extends to the distal esophagus can be sufficient. With a mouth speculum holding the mouth open, the glottis is easily visualized behind the tongue on the floor of the mouth (b). Avoiding the glottis, a lubricated feeding tube can easily be passed to the back of the mouth, down the esophagus, to the stomach (c).

the patient clinically improves [2]. Monitoring of patients undergoing nutritional therapy should include serum phosphorus, potassium, and glucose levels [2]. The patient should be evaluated daily for signs of fluid overload or congestive heart failure [7].

Fluid Therapy

Indications

Dehydrated reptiles often have sunken eyes, thick, ropey oral cavity mucus and tacky mucous membranes. Decreased skin turgor may also be noted [2, 6–9]. Dehydrated animals may exhibit a slow or difficult to find heartbeat [6]. Increased packed cell volume (PCV), total protein, and plasma sodium and chloride may also indicate dehydration. A history or the presence of dysecdysis is often an initial sign of hypohydration or dehydration, resulting from a lack of available lymph to fill the area between the new and old skin layers. Reptile urine is normally hyposthenuric and specific gravity does not surpass that of plasma in dehydrated reptiles [10].

Assessment of dehydration in amphibians utilizes skin tackiness, increased presence of skin folds, discoloration, and sunken eyes [11]. Some amphibians can tolerate over 30% water loss but permanent excretory system damage can occur [11].

If a patient is estimated to be less than 5% dehydrated, oral fluid replacement can be considered. If greater than

5% dehydrated, the majority of fluid therapy should be provided parenterally. Both the patient and fluids need to be warmed to the preferred temperature for the species.

Fluid Requirements

Shock Fluids

Shock is a poorly defined condition in reptiles and amphibians. As such, mammalian-based shock fluid rates have not been described for and may be contraindicated in reptiles and amphibians as they possess smaller vascular capacity and are more easily overloaded with intravenous (IV) fluids when compared with mammals. Intravascular fluid boluses of crystalloids at 5–10 ml/kg or colloids at 3–5 ml/kg can be administered to treat perfusion deficits [12]. Hypertonic saline solutions may also be useful for treatment of hypovolemic shock.

Replacement/Losses

Fluid deficits can be replenished over 48–96 hours for chronic dehydration and over 12–36 hours in acute volume loss [12]. Different from birds and mammals, reptiles have an equal fluid distribution between the intracellular and extracellular compartments [12]. Daily fluid rates should include maintenance fluid plus 25–33% of the estimated deficit [13]. To reduce the risk of fluid overload, do not exceed a 40 ml/kg/d total and reassess hydration and fluid losses frequently [6, 8, 9].

Maintenance

Maintenance fluid rates are based on the relative volume of plasma in a typical reptile [13] and blood volume is estimated to be 4–8% of total body weight in reptiles [12]. Daily maintenance fluid recommendations are typically 5–15 ml/kg/d [12, 14].

Fluid Types

Crystalloids

Isotonic crystalloid solutions seem to be acceptable for use in reptiles and commonly include 0.9% NaCl, lactated Ringer's solution, Plasma-Lyte A (Abbott Laboratories, Abbott Park, Ill 60064) or Normosol-R (Hospira, Lake Forest, Ill 60045) [6, 9]. Because 0.9% is not a physiologically buffered solution it is less commonly recommended for fluid therapy when compared with other isotonic crystalloid fluids. Plasma osmolality or osmolarity has been reported for multiple species (see Table 46.3). While use of lactated crystalloids has historically been controversial, there is little evidence that the level of lactate administered during fluid therapy is significant, as reptiles have a remarkable tolerance for high lactate levels. In dehydrated inland bearded dragons (*Pogona vitticeps*), rehydration with lactated Ringer's solution did not result in a significant change in blood lactate levels [20].

Hypotonic solutions such as 5% dextrose in water or 0.45% saline can be used cautiously to replace free water deficits in reptiles [14]. However, they should not be administered IV or intraosseous (IO) for intravascular volume expansion as they are ineffective for this purpose and may also cause cranial swelling [14, 16]. However, hypotonic solutions may be useful for patients with a decreased ability to excrete excess sodium or tolerate expansions of the intravascular volume [14]. Use of a hypotonic "reptile Ringer's" solution in dehydrated

Table 46.3 Reported osmolality and osmolarity in reptiles.

Common name	Species	Osmolality (mOsm/kg)	Osmolarity (mOsm/l)	References
American alligator	*Alligator mississippiensis*	269.3 (267.7–270.9)[a]		[15]
Corn snake	*Pantherophis guttatus*	344.5 (304.5–373.0)[b]		[16]
Bearded dragon	*Pogona vitticeps*	295.4 ± 9.35[c]		[17]
Green iguana	*Iguana iguana*	327 ± 3.3[d]		[18]
Dwarf caiman	*Paleosuchus palpebrosus*		303 (301–304)[b]	[5]
Savannah monitor	*Varanus exanthematicus*		332 (319–345)[b]	[5]
Prehensile tailed skink	*Corucia zebrata*		361 (335–373)[b]	[19]
Boa constrictor	*Boa constrictor*		306[e]	[5]

[a] Mean (95% confidence interval).
[b] Mean (range).
[c] Mean ± standard deviation.
[d] Mean ± standard error.
[e] Single value.

Herptiles

bearded dragons resulted in a persistent hyperglycemia as well as significant decreases in plasma osmolarity, phosphorus, and sodium [20].

The use of hypertonic solutions has not been well-documented in reptiles but they can potentially be used for hypovolemic resuscitation.

Colloids

Colloids are isotonic fluids that contain large molecular weight molecules which contribute to an increased osmotic pressure. They are used in patients with hypoalbuminemia, hypovolemic perfusion deficits, or with brain, heart or lung disease that precludes use of larger fluid volumes. Colloids can be given as a slow, IV or IO, 3–5 ml/kg bolus; crystalloids are given concomitantly [5, 8]. Due to documented adverse effects from use of hydroxyethyl starch solutions (a commonly utilized synthetic colloid) in mammals, use of this product in veterinary medicine is currently controversial although there is little information regarding safety in reptile and amphibian species.

Blood Products

Blood transfusion medicine is poorly described in reptiles. Whole blood transfusions are used to correct life threatening conditions of anemia or acute hemorrhage [6]. Amazingly, reptiles with a PCV >5% can sometimes be successfully managed with fluids and supportive care, without blood transfusion [6]. Reptilian blood transfusions are ideally done with a healthy conspecific donor. Heterologous blood transfusions have shown some success in birds and should be considered when a conspecific is unavailable [21]. A second heterologous blood transfusion may be contraindicated [22]. Blood should ideally be administered within a few hours of collection and warmed prior to administration. In an emergency, whole blood collected from a donor can be administered directly to the recipient as an IV or IO bolus of up to 1–2 ml/kg of body weight [23]; use of an in-line micron filter during administration is recommended. Filtration using an 18-μm filter did not result in significant hemolysis of whole American alligator blood [24]. See Chapter 42: Catheterization and Venipuncture for specifics regarding donor identification as well as blood collection, typing, and storing for transfusions in reptiles and amphibians.

Routes

Oral

Oral fluid administration should be reserved for mildly dehydrated reptiles and amphibians that have a functioning gastrointestinal tract. Oral fluid administration is contraindicated for patients that are vomiting or have ileus. Do not exceed 2–3% of the animal's body weight as a single fluid bolus in order to avoid gastric atony or regurgitation/vomiting [25]. If the patient is compliant, oral fluids can be given slowly with a syringe. However, this may increase the risk of aspiration if fluids are administered too quickly.

Subcutaneous/Intracoelomic

Fluids can be administered subcutaneously (SC) or intracoelomically (ICe) in reptiles or amphibians. The subcutaneous space in reptiles is relatively small and poorly vascularized which may lead to variable absorption rates. Because of this, the SC route should be reserved for reptiles and amphibians that are not severely dehydrated and are hemodynamically stable. In snakes and lizards, SC fluid is given over the lateral body wall (Figure 46.7a). Multiple sites can be used to obtain the desired volume, if needed. In chelonians, SC fluids can be administered in the cervicobrachial (Figure 46.7b) or prefemoral fossae (Figure 46.8). Hyperosmotic fluids should not be administered SC, as surrounding tissue fluid may be drawn into the site, causing an electrolyte imbalance. It can also result in delayed absorption and sterile abscess formation.

In addition to the abundant, vascular serosal surfaces present in the coelomic cavity, the coelomic membrane is also highly absorptive, which can permit rapid absorption of fluids. However, considering that there is no research regarding efficacy of this route for fluid therapy in debilitated animals, the ICe route should be reserved for reptiles and amphibians that are not severely dehydrated and are hemodynamically stable. Additionally, this route may be best reserved as a last resort since ICe injection carries the risk for inadvertent puncture of lung, bowel, bladder, follicles, or vasculature and large administration volumes can prevent normal lung expansion. Intracoelomic fluids are administered in the caudoventral coelom. In chelonians, a preferred site is in the prefemoral fossa where the skin meets the bridge of the shell (Figure 46.8). In snakes and lizards, avoid the ventral abdominal vein by injecting paramedian. Place the patient in dorsolateral recumbency to let the viscera fall away from the injection site. Disinfect the skin and insert a 22–25 g needle at a shallow angle below the skin, and into the coelom. Prior to injection, assert negative pressure to ascertain that the needle has not been placed into a luminal organ, follicle, or vasculature.

Submersion

Rehydration of amphibians is often performed with submersion in oxygenated, dechlorinated water. Typical amphibian plasma is approximately 230 mOsm/l [11]. An electrolyte-balanced "amphibian Ringer's" fluid solution which is isotonic to amphibian plasma can be used or, if not available, a 0.6% saline solution substituted [11].

(a) (b)

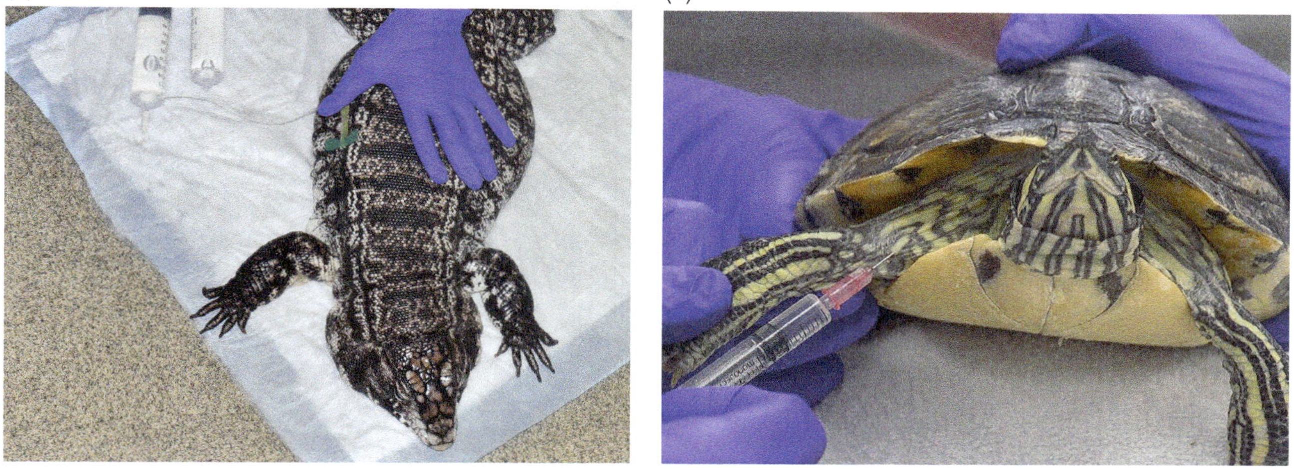

Figure 46.7 Subcutaneous fluids administered along the lateral body wall of a sedated Argentine black and white tegu (*Salvator merianae*) (a) and in the cervicobrachial fossa in a river cooter (*Pseudemys concinna*) (b). *Source:* Images courtesy of Grayson Doss, Madison, WI.

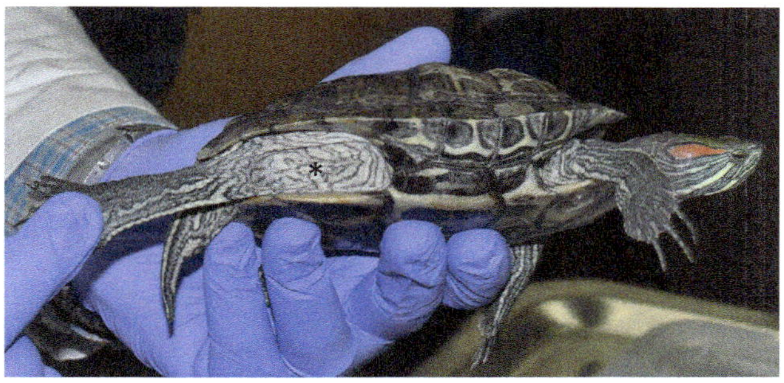

Figure 46.8 Abducting the right pelvic limb caudally reveals the right prefemoral fossa (asterisk) in this male red-eared slider (*Trachemys scripta elegans*), an area where subcutaneous or intracoelomic fluids can be administered. *Source:* Image courtesy of Grayson Doss, Madison, WI.

Intravenous/Intraosseous

For critically ill animals, fluids should be administered via IV or IO routes. IO boluses can be difficult (and potentially painful) to administer into small medullary cavities quickly; delivering the bolus over several minutes by hand or with an infusion pump is recommended. IV access is difficult and typically requires a cut-down procedure for catheter placement. See Chapter 42: Catheterization and Venipuncture for specifics regarding IV and IO catheter placement.

Monitoring

In mammals, hypovolemia leads to tachycardia. Tachycardia may also occur with hypovolemia in reptiles and amphibians but may require a warm environment to manifest. While the reptile is maintained at its preferred environmental temperature heart rate is monitored and tachycardia, if present, should resolve as blood pressure improves. Skin turgor, saliva viscosity, eye position, body weight, and mentation can also be helpful for monitoring and making sure fluid therapy goals are being met. PCV and total solids can be used for monitoring but be aware of the possibility of concurrent anemia and hypoproteinemia. Sodium and chloride levels can also be monitored to assess the patient's hydration status.

References

1 Whittington, J.K. (2013). Esophagostomy feeding tube use and placement in exotic pets. *J. Exot. Pet. Med.* 22: 178–191.

2 Donoghue, S. (2006). Nutrition. In: Reptile Medicine and Surgery, 2e (ed. D.R. Mader), 992–1013. Elsevier Inc: St. Louis.

3 Vitt, L.J. and Caldwell, J.P. (2013). Herpetology: An Introductory Biology of Amphibians and Reptiles. Academic Press.

4 Wright, K.M. and Whitaker, B.R. (2001). Amphibian Medicine and Captive Husbandry. Krieger Publishing Company.

5 Klaphake, E., Gibbons, P.M., Sladky, K.K., and Carpenter, J.W. (2018). Reptiles. In: Exotic Animal Formulary, 5e (ed. J.W. Carpenter), 81–166. Elsevier Health Sciences.

6 Norton, T.M. (2005). Chelonian emergency and critical care. *Semin. Avian Exot. Pet Med.* 14: 106–130.

7 Orosz, S.E. (2013). Critical care nutrition for exotic animals. *J. Exot. Pet. Med.* 22: 163–177.

8 Gibbons, P.M. (2002). Critical care nutrition and fluid therapy in reptiles. *Proceedings of the 15th Annual International Veterinary Emergency & Critical Care Symposium*.

9 Music, M.K. and Strunk, A. (2016). Reptile critical care and common emergencies. *Vet. Clin. North Am. Exot. Anim. Pract.* 19: 591–612.

10 Divers, S.J. and Innis, C.J. (2019). Urology. In: Mader's Reptile Medicine and Surgery (eds. S.J. Divers and S.J. Stahl), 251–298. St. Louis: Elsevier Inc.

11 Whitaker, B.R. and Wright, K.M. (2019). Amphibian medicine. In: Mader's Reptile Medicine and Surgery, 3e (eds. S.J. Divers and S.J. Stahl), 992–1013. St. Louis: Elsevier Inc.

12 Martinez-Jimenez, D. and Hernandez-Divers, S.J. (2007). Emergency care of reptiles. *Vet. Clin. North Am. Exot. Anim. Pract.* 10: 557–585.

13 Mitchell, M.A. (2006). Therapeutics. In: Reptile Medicine and Surgery, 2e (eds. S.J. Divers and S.J. Stahl), 631–664. Elsevier Inc: St. Louis.

14 Petritz, O.A. and Son, T.T. (2019). Emergency and critical care. In: Mader's Reptile Medicine and Surgery, 3e (eds. S.J. Divers and S.J. Stahl), 967–976. St. Louis: Elsevier Inc.

15 Nevarez, J.G., Acierno, M.J., Angel, M., and Beaufrere, H. (2012). Determination of agreement between measured and calculated plasma osmolality values in captive-reared American alligators (*Alligator mississippiensis*). *J. Herpetol. Med. Surg.* 22: 36–41.

16 Guzman, D.S.-M., Mitchell, M.A., and Acierno, M. (2011). Determination of plasma osmolality and agreement between measured and calculated values in captive male corn snakes (*Pantherophis* [*Elaphe*] *guttatus guttatus*). *J. Herpetol. Med. Surg.* 21: 16–19.

17 Dallwig, R.K., Mitchell, M.A., and Acierno, M.J. (2010). Determination of plasma osmolality and agreement between measured and calculated values in healthy adult bearded dragons (*Pogona vitticeps*). *J. Herpetol. Med. Surg.* 20: 69–73.

18 Fitzsimons, J. and Kaufman, S. (1977). Cellular and extracellular dehydration, and angiotensin as stimuli to drinking in the common iguana *Iguana iguana*. *J. Physiol.* 265: 443.

19 Gibbons, P.M., Klaphake, E., and Carpenter, J.W. (2013). Reptiles. In: Exotic Animal Formulary, 4e (ed. J.W. Carpenter), 83–182. Elsevier Health Sciences.

20 Parkinson, L. and Mans, C. (2020). Evaluation of subcutaneously administered electrolyte solutions in experimentally dehydrated inland bearded dragons (*Pogona vitticeps*). *Am. J. Vet. Res.* 81: 437–441.

21 Degernes, L.A., Harrison, L.D., Smith, D.W. et al. (1999). Autologous, homologous, and heterologous red blood cell transfusions in conures of the genus *Aratinga*. *J. Avian Med. Surg.* 13: 10–14.

22 Degernes, L.A., Crosier, M.L., Harrison, L.D. et al. (1999). Autologous, homologous, and heterologous red blood cell transfusions in cockatiels (*Nymphicus hollandicus*). *J. Avian Med. Surg.* 13: 2–9.

23 Pees, M. and Girling, S. (2019). Emergency care. In: BSAVA Manual of Reptiles (eds. S.J. Girling and P. Raiti), 101–114. Gloucester, UK: British Small Animal Veterinary Associaton.

24 Nevarez, J.G., Cockburn, J., Kearney, M.T., and Mayer, J. (2011). Evaluation of an 18-micron filter for use in reptile blood transfusions using blood from American alligators (*Alligator mississippiensis*). *J. Zoo Wildl. Med.* 42: 236–240.

25 Perry, S.M. and Mitchell, M.A. (2019). Routes of administration. In: Mader's Reptile Medicine and Surgery (eds. S.J. Divers and S.J. Stahl), 1130–1138. St. Louis: Elsevier Inc.

Section 2

Diagnostics

47

STAT Diagnostics

Peter M. DiGeronimo[1] *and Nicola Di Girolamo*[2]

[1] *Adventure Aquarium, Camden, New Jersey, USA*
[2] *Department of Veterinary Clinical Sciences, College of Veterinary Medicine, Oklahoma State University, Stillwater, Oklahoma, USA*

CONTENTS

Point-of-Care Blood Sampling

Bedside analysis of blood samples can help identify emergent problems and narrow lists of differential diagnoses. Ever-advancing technology allows for an increasing amount of diagnostic information to be gleaned from even very small blood samples.

PCV/TS

Capillary tubes can be used to collect small volumes of blood for a manual packed cell volume (PCV), qualitative evaluation of plasma, and estimation of total solids (TS) by refractometry. Hematocrit tubes can be filled with less than 50 μl of blood. Microhematocrit tubes can be filled with less than half this volume (~18 μl). With these smaller tubes, even the blood in the hub of an insulin syringe can be of diagnostic value. Following blood collection, results are obtained by centrifugation and manual evaluation of the sample in less than five minutes (Figure 47.1).

Manual PCV

Hematocrit tubes give the PCV, that is the percent of whole blood comprised of red blood cells. For small volume samples and microhematocrit tubes that may not fit standard hematocrit reader charts, the PCV can be determined by measuring the tube with a millimeter ruler.

Exotic Animal Emergency and Critical Care Medicine, First Edition. Edited by Jennifer E. Graham, Grayson A. Doss and Hugues Beaufrère.

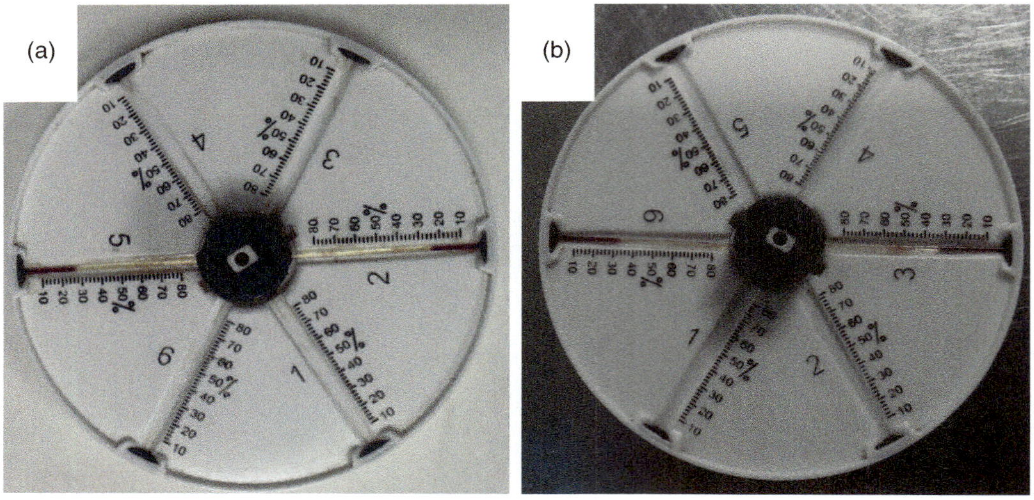

Figure 47.1 Following centrifugation, microhematocrit tubes allow for the evaluation of packed cell volume ([a]: 24–26%, [b]: 33%), gross appearance of plasma, and estimation of total solids by refractometry with less than 50 μl of whole blood.

Like all diagnostic tests, PCV must be interpreted in light of physical examination, clinical assessment of the patient, sample quality (e.g. lymph contamination) and the results of other diagnostics. Clinical signs attributed to anemia will be associated with compromised oxygen carrying capacity of blood and hypovolemia [1]. Because such small volumes are required, the PCV can be monitored serially to assess response to emergency treatment.

Refractometer TS

Hematocrit tubes can be broken to remove the packed erythrocytes from the sample so that the plasma can be used for refractometry. This will give the estimated TS content of the plasma sample. Refractometry measurements are preferred over point-of-care analyzers because their methodology (i.e. bromocresol green dye-binding method) yields inaccurate results in reptiles [2].

Plasma Appearance

Gross plasma evaluation in the capillary tube may provide some information. Plasma should be translucent and clear to straw-colored. Plasma may be ruddy or reddish secondary to acute hemolysis [1] or greenish secondary to hyperbiliverdinemia or, for some snake species, hyperbilirubinemia due to hepatic or cholestatic disease [3]. Carotenoids may result in a normally yellow-orange or green-yellow plasma in certain herbivores and snake species, respectively.

Glucose

Glucometers

Handheld glucose meters used in veterinary practice are either calibrated specifically for dogs and cats or for humans. The advantage of handheld glucose meters is that they require as little as 0.3 μl of whole blood and provide rapid results. However, due to the lack of calibration for reptiles, the absolute value provided should not be considered. Extremely elevated or decreased values may be clinically significant and should be verified with a biochemistry profile employing a hexokinase reaction. Blood glucose level extremes can result in profound clinical signs. Hyperglycemia can be paraneoplastic, secondary to stress, or seen with pancreatic disease, such as pancreatitis or glucagonoma [4, 5]. Hypoglycemia is often consistent with sepsis, but may also occur following seizure activity.

Lactate

Lactate Meters

Blood lactate can be measured by handheld point-of-care lactate meters that require ≤25 μl of whole blood and give results in seconds. Elevated lactate can be a consequence of prolonged hypoxia, ventilation–perfusion mismatch, reduced oxygen carrying capacity of blood, or inadequate tissue perfusion as in patients during shock. An elevated lactate measurement is not necessarily pathologic in reptiles, as they readily utilize anaerobic metabolism, making interpretation difficult. Lactate may also increase in states of dehydration or hibernation.

Blood Smear-Quick Assessment

WBC/Platelet Estimates

A blood smear can be made with a single drop of blood using bevel edge-to-slide or coverslip-to-slide techniques (Figure 47.2) [6]. A Wright–Giemsa stain may allow the best differentiation between leukocytes although rapid stains like Diff-Quick may be used as well. Blood smear evaluation can be used to determine a leukocyte differential and an

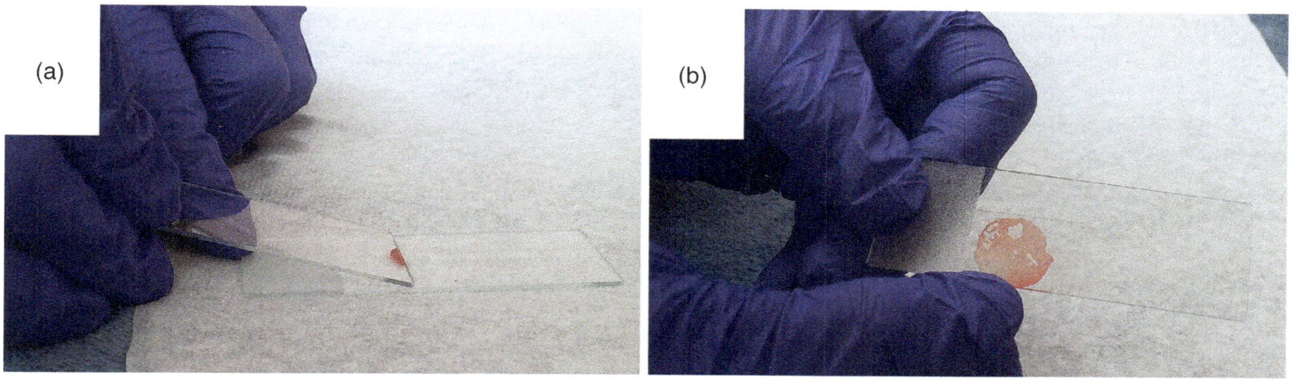

Figure 47.2 Diagnostic blood smears require a single drop of blood and can be made using (a) bevel edge-to-slide or (b) coverslip-to-slide techniques.

estimated leukocyte count, to evaluate erythrocyte and leukocyte morphology, to estimate thrombocytes, and to screen for bacteria, hemoparasites, and viral inclusions.

Coagulation Testing

Currently there are no validated diagnostic tools to evaluate coagulation in reptiles. Evaluation of coagulopathy in reptiles currently relies on physical examination, thrombocyte estimates, and the subjective evaluation of venipuncture sites for unexpected or prolonged bleeding or of whole blood samples for prolonged clotting. Commercially available assays, such as prothrombin time (PT) and activated partial thromboplastin time (aPTT) are mammalian-based, making interpretation subjective [7]. Values for PT and aPTT in clinically healthy green iguanas ranged from 453 to 831 seconds and from 170 to 242 seconds, respectively [8]. Due to the variability in results in the study, PT and aPTT were determined to be of limited diagnostic value. Buccal mucosal bleeding time (BMBT) has been suggested for use in reptiles [7]. However, there are currently no published reference intervals for BMBT in reptiles. Given that BMBT varies with the device used, requires sedation or anesthesia, and can be difficult to apply in a standardized method due to the anatomic diversity of reptiles, it is not recommended for use.

Blood Gas + Acid–Base Evaluation

Indications

Various point-of-care blood gas analyzers are available for veterinary use. Portable clinical analyzers require between 60 and 95 μl of whole blood and, depending on the unit used, can yield electrolyte (Na^+, Cl^-, K^+), urea nitrogen, lactate, glucose, hematocrit, hemoglobin, ionized calcium, pH, pO_2, pCO_2, and bicarbonate values in about 90 seconds. Blood gas evaluation in reptiles has similar indications as in mammals. It should be performed in reptile patients suspected to have metabolic disturbances and for serial monitoring during anesthesia. However, interpretation of blood gases is greatly limited by the lack of knowledge regarding reptile physiology and clinical pathology.

The pH of reptile blood is most easily interpreted when the patient is at their preferred optimal temperature zone (POTZ). Many point-of-care units auto-correct analyte values based on patient core temperature so a valid temperature measurement must be obtained at the time of venipuncture [9]. Blood at homeostasis should have a higher pH at colder temperatures and a lower pH at warmer temperatures [10]. This is necessary when interpreting acid–base values in reptiles, as a pH of 7.4 may be neutral for a reptile within their POTZ, but could indicate a severe metabolic acidosis for a hypothermic animal.

Respiratory and Non-respiratory

Acid–base balance of the blood is regulated by the respiratory and urinary systems. Respiration regulates the exchange of CO_2 in the blood. Excesses or deficiencies of CO_2 in the blood result in respiratory acidosis or alkalosis, respectively. Excesses or deficiencies of bicarbonate (HCO_3^-) in the blood result in metabolic alkalosis or acidosis, respectively. Identifying the cause and type of acid–base abnormality can elucidate the pathologic process experienced by the patient and direct treatment options. The lungs regulate carbon dioxide homeostasis. Tachypnea may be the result of the patient increasing exhalation of CO_2 to compensate for a blood pH below normal (acidosis). Acidotic patients produce more acidic urine as the kidneys remove hydrogen from circulation. Conversely, the kidneys excrete bicarbonate and produce alkaline urine in response to abnormal elevations in blood pH (alkalosis).

Acidemia and Alkalemia (SID, AG, BE)

Acid–base balance can be measured, calculated, and defined in several ways including anion gap (AG), base excess (BE), and strong ion difference (SID). Anion gap is the difference in measured cations and anions in the blood and is defined in mEq/l as $(Na^+ + K^+) - (Cl^- + HCO_3^-)$. Anion gap will increase as unmeasured cations such as Ca^{2+}, Mg^+, and globulins decrease or as unmeasured anions such as lactic acid or ketones increase. Anion gap is approximately 15–25 mEq/l in small animals, but can be more variable in reptiles; a range of 15–40 mEq/l was noted in green iguanas [11]. Increased anion gap suggests acidosis while decreased anion gap suggests alkalosis. Base excess (BE) is defined as the amount of acid required to return blood pH to 7.4 and ranges between −2 and +2 mEq/l in mammals. Elevated BE indicates a metabolic alkalosis while decreased BE indicates a metabolic acidosis. SID is simply the difference between the sums of concentrations of cations and anions and is defined in mEq/l as $(Na^+ + K^+ + Ca^{2+} + Mg^{2+}) - (Cl^-)$ − other anions (lactates, urates, sulfates, and ketones).

Respiratory acidosis suggests primary respiratory compromise or hypoventilation and the inability to exhale excess CO_2 [12]. Respiratory acidosis may coincide with metabolic acidosis with the accumulation of lactic acid secondary to anaerobic metabolism during periods of hypoxia or apnea. Metabolic acidosis may result from lactic acid accumulation due to muscle exertion or from ketoacidemia secondary to a negative energy balance or catabolic state. In critical reptile patients, marked hypocalcemia and hypomagnesemia should also be considered. Metabolic alkalosis may be a compensatory response to respiratory acidosis. It may result from hypochloremia secondary to vomiting or, in crocodilians and potentially other reptiles, be postprandial due to the mobilization of chloride ions in gastric acid secretions for digestion. Excessive excretion of bicarbonate in diarrhea or in chronic renal failure can cause a metabolic acidosis. Toxic overdoses of unmeasured anions such as methanol, ethylene glycol, or salicylates (e.g. aspirin) can also lead to an increase in anion gap and a metabolic acidosis.

Electrolytes (Na/Cl, K, Ca, Phos)

Point-of-care monitoring of electrolytes may be helpful from a diagnostic, therapeutic (e.g. choosing appropriate crystalloids for fluid resuscitation) and prognostic point of view [13]. A major advantage of point-of-care testing of electrolytes in reptiles is measurement of ionized calcium (iCa^{2+}). Evaluation of calcium homeostasis is critical in poorly managed reptiles and in females with reproductive disorders. Ionized calcium is currently regarded as the best indicator of calcium homeostasis [14]. However, it is a highly variable proportion (18–57%) of total calcium in reptiles [15], preventing accurate estimation of iCa^{2+} from total calcium. Using point-of-care instruments limits post-sampling variables known to invalidate iCa^{2+} analysis (e.g. exposure to room air, anticoagulants) [14]. Currently published values for iCa^{2+} in reptiles are listed in Table 47.1.

Biochemistry

Abnormalities in biochemistry analytes may be of diagnostic value for the critical reptile patient. Currently, cost-effective point-of-care biochemistry analyzers are either portable (e.g. i-STAT, Abbott) or bench-top (e.g. VetScan, Abbott). Such biochemistry units require as little as 100 µl of whole blood and can yield a full biochemistry profile in less than 15 minutes. Interpretation of results of units not validated for the species of interest should be performed cautiously as significant analytic discrepancies are expected [23]. When analyzing blood with multiple machines, it is recommended to exercise caution when comparing results between units since significant differences between analyte values can be found [25, 26]. All analyte values must be interpreted with caution because significant differences can be found between sex, age, reproductive status, season, and diet, even within species [27]. Some abnormalities may not be specific, but when combined with other diagnostics and physical examination can help to narrow the list of differential diagnoses and direct treatment.

Evaluation of Droppings

General by Species

Reptile droppings have three components: urine, urates, and feces (Figure 47.3). Urine is the only liquid component and is produced by the kidneys. Urates are pasty, semisolid, and opaque white or off-white in color. They are salts of uric acid, the end product of protein catabolism in most terrestrial reptiles. Feces are the end product of digestion and are excreted from the gastrointestinal tract. Aquatic species will produce few urates as most of their nitrogenous waste is excreted as urea nitrogen in urine.

Evaluation of Urine

Volume/Appearance

Gross evaluation of the urine is entirely subjective and may be of limited diagnostic value in the critical reptile patient. Volume of urine is related to the patient's habitat, anatomy, and hydration status. Aquatic reptiles may produce more voluminous urine to compensate for relatively high fluid intakes. This may be especially pronounced in species with urinary bladders such as chelonians due to their ability to store urine or even water retrofluxed from their cloaca in

Table 47.1 Summary of currently published values for ionized calcium (iCa^{2+}) in reptile species.

Species	Ionized calcium (iCa^{2+}) in mmol/l	References
Green iguana (*Iguana iguana*)	*Mean ± SD; range*	
	1.38 ± 0.1; 1.21–1.60	[16]
	1.47 ± 0.12; 1.22–1.62	[17]
	Mean ± 2 SD; range	
	Males: 1.32 ± 0.04; 1.28–1.36	[18]
	Gravid females: 1.21 ± 0.2; 1.01–1.41	
Bearded dragon (*Pogona vitticeps*)	*Mean ± SEM*	
	With UVB: 1.3 ± 0.1	[19]
	Without UVB for 83 d: 1.48 ± 0.04	
Gila monster (*Heloderma suspectum*)	*Median (range)*	
	1.23 (1.09–1.50)	[20]
Ball python (*Python regius*)	*Median (range)*	
	With UVB: 1.8 (1.71–1.92)	[21]
	With UVB for 70 d: 1.81 (1.67–1.85)	
	Without UVB for 70 d: 1.8 (1.73–1.89)	
Testudo tortoise spp.	*Median (range)*	
	1.32 (1.03–1.63)	[22]
	Portable analyzer: 1.6 (1.13–1.84)	[23]
	Benchtop analyzer: 1.45 (1.09–1.69)	
Green sea turtle (*Chelonia mydras*)	*Median (10th–90th percentiles)*	
	Rehabilitated juveniles: 0.63 (0.55–0.72)	[24]
	Wild: 1.05 (0.87–1.23)	

SD, standard deviation; SEM, standard error of the mean; UVB, ultraviolet B.

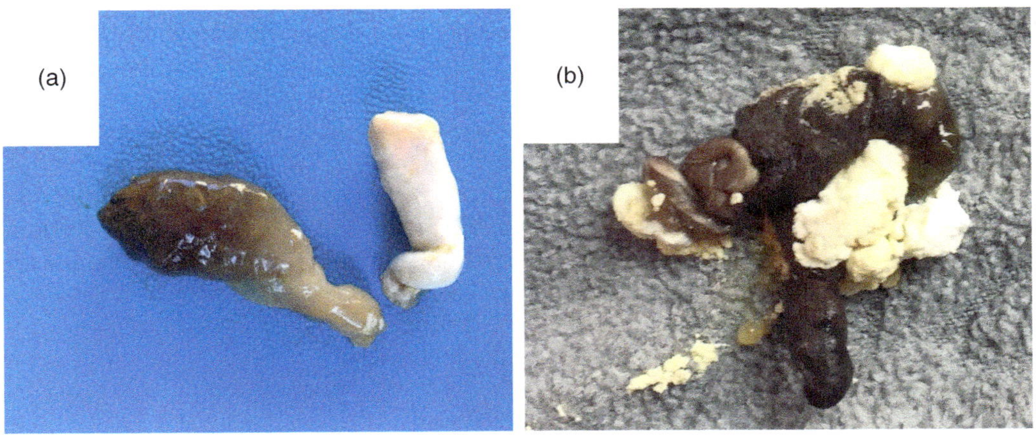

Figure 47.3 Grossly normal droppings from (a) a bearded dragon (*Pogona vitticeps*) and (b) a corn snake (*Pantherophis guttatus*). Droppings include formed to loosely formed fecal components, semisolid white urates, and liquid urine which is often absorbed by bedding or substrate.

the urinary bladder. Species adapted to more arid environments can be expected to produce smaller volumes of urine. Although urine is expected to be contaminated by urates and feces, it is generally clear and not viscous. Discolored, opaque, or viscous urine may be indicative of disease of the cloaca, urinary bladder (in species in which a bladder is present), kidneys, reproductive tract, or distal gastrointestinal tract.

Urates that are red or pink suggest hemorrhage associated with the cloaca, hemipenes or phallus, or distal gastrointestinal or urogenital tracts. Green urates may be the result of biliverdinuria secondary to hepatic disease.

Urine-Specific Gravity

Reptilian nephrons lack a loop of Henle and therefore reptiles cannot concentrate urine greater than plasma osmolality. Reptile urine is isosthenuric (urine specific gravity [USG] 1.005–1.010) [28]. USG is currently not considered an indicator of renal function in reptiles as it is in mammalian patients.

Urinalysis

Contamination of urine by the gastrointestinal and reproductive tracts can confound interpretation of urinalysis. Protein should be expected in reptile urine samples as it binds to excreted uric acid to keep it in suspension and may also be present secondary to fecal contamination [29]. Dipstick findings should be verified by sediment examination. Cellular or protein casts suggest renal tubular disease. Urine should also be microscopically evaluated for parasites, including nematodes, cestodes and coccidia and other protozoa.

Evaluation of Feces

Volume/Appearance

Evaluation of fecal samples can be of diagnostic value for a reptile emergency. While some animals may defecate prior to or during an examination, others may be encouraged to do so by placing them in a warm, shallow water bath. While defecation cannot rule out mechanical obstruction of the gastrointestinal tract, it makes a distally located obstruction less likely. Since most reptiles do not defecate daily, absence of defecation does not necessarily suggest mechanical or functional ileus. Feces should be soft but formed. Unformed or liquid feces suggests gastrointestinal infection or inflammation. Fecal concretions or fecoliths, suggest chronic dehydration, functional ileus, and secondary disease such as mechanical obstruction, gastrointestinal inflammation, and associated pain. Feces should be grossly evaluated for the presence of substrate as gastrointestinal impactions from inappropriate substrate such as sand, coconut byproducts, or crushed walnut shells are relatively common presentations. Undigested food material may indicate decreased gastrointestinal transit time and hypermotility and suggest maldigestion or malabsorption.

Cytology-Fecal Gram Stain (FGS), Direct/Float, Occult Blood

Fecal examination in reptiles requires a direct saline solution smear as well as flotation. Direct saline smears should be evaluated for the presence of moving flagellates. Fecal flotation allows for the evaluation of coccidia, and nematode, trematode, and cestode ova. Gram stains of fecal smears can confirm and define bacterial populations. The normal flora of most reptile gastrointestinal tracts should be comprised of Gram-negative rods. A preponderance of cocci or Gram-positive organisms may suggest a dysbiosis or localize disease to the gastrointestinal tract. Although not highly sensitive, acid-fast stains of abnormal feces or of regurgitated food should be considered to screen for infectious diseases such as cryptosporidiosis and mycobacteriosis. Fecal occult blood tests require a scant volume of feces and give results in <1 minute. Confirmation of occult blood in feces can potentially localize disease to the gastrointestinal tract. However, the significance of this test should be interpreted in the light of diet (will be positive in reptiles consuming meat protein), clinical signs, physical examination findings, and the other diagnostics including PCV and TS.

Cardiovascular Assessment

Clinical Assessment

Cardiovascular assessment of the reptile patient, like assessment of all organ systems, starts with the physical examination. Mucous membrane color and capillary refill time are indicators of perfusion. The patient should be examined for signs of hypovolemia (consistent with signs of dehydration) and for signs of hypoxia secondary to decreased oxygen carrying capacity of the blood, including exercise intolerance and inappropriate mentation. Snakes with cardiac disease often present with cardiomegaly, evident as a swelling toward the end of the cranial third length of their body, and they may also display swelling of the gular area. Chelonians with cardiac disease may present with generalized edema. Because no currently available diagnostics specific to the cardiovascular system have been validated for reptile species, it is important to interpret all diagnostic results in light of the clinical evaluation of the patient. In squamates, electronic stethoscopes may facilitate cardiac auscultation.

Doppler

Dopplers are a necessity in reptile practice due to the difficulty of cardiac auscultation. Dopplers convert the detection of blood flow to an audible sound by applying a crystal probe to a site with coupling gel, allowing for constant and real-time monitoring of a patient's heart rate, rhythm, and peripheral pulses. The Doppler can be used to determine heart rate and rhythm as auscultation with a stethoscope in

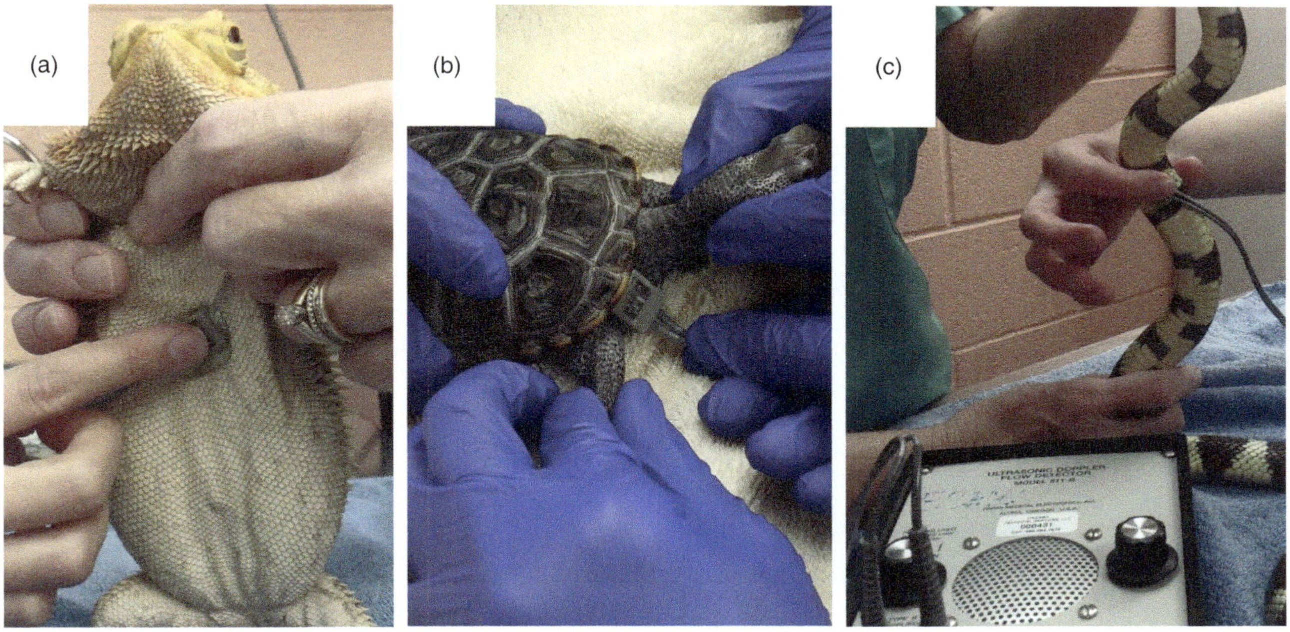

Figure 47.4 Doppler is used to monitor heart rate and rhythm in reptile patients. The probe should be placed cranially on the ventral midline of lizards as in this bearded dragon (*Pogona vitticeps*) (a), between the neck and forelimb of chelonians as in this diamondback terrapin (*Malaclemys terrapin*) (b), and at the end of the cranial third of the length of snakes as in this California kingsnake (*Lampropeltis getula californiae*) (c).

reptiles is typically unrewarding. In larger patients, Doppler can be used to detect peripheral blood flow and may be used, along with clinical signs, to identify sites of compromised perfusion. Doppler probes should be placed over the presumptive site of the heart, which is ventral cranial midline in lizards, ventral midline in the cranial third of snakes, and in between the neck and the forelimb in chelonians (Figure 47.4).

Blood Pressure

Blood pressure (BP) can be measured with automated digital oscillometric units or manually with a Doppler probe and sphygmomanometer. In chelonians and most lizards, cuffs should be applied to the highest point of the forelimb and the probe applied to the brachial artery at the palmar aspect of the antebrachium [28]. In snakes and larger chelonians, the cuff may be applied to the proximal tail distal to the vent and the probe placed over the caudal coccygeal artery or vein [28]. Manual BP readings provide systolic pressures. While oscillometric units also yield diastolic and mean arterial pressures, manual BP readings are considered more accurate especially for patients with arrhythmias. However, neither have been validated for any reptile species and therefore BP monitoring in reptile patients is used to monitor trends and response to treatments rather than to diagnose hypertension or hypotension based on absolute values.

ECG

Electrocardiogram (ECG) can be used to identify and monitor electrical activity of the heart, heart rate, and rhythm (Figure 47.5) [28]. This may be useful to monitor during prolonged resuscitation efforts, as reptiles can survive even long periods of hypoxia, apnea, and unresponsiveness. ECG waves can be less clear in reptiles that are not within their POTZ [28]. Caution is warranted, however, as cardiac electrical activity can continue for hours after the reptile has died.

Respiratory Assessment

Clinical Assessment

Assessment of patients with suspected respiratory disorders requires knowledge of species-specific anatomy as reptiles and amphibians lack a distinct thoracic cavity. Chelonians with increased respiratory effort may demonstrate increased movements of the fore limbs to expand the lungs. Snakes with increased respiratory effort usually perform deeper inspirations than usual. Any reptile that exhibits open-mouth breathing or gaping, audible wheezes, or discharge from the nares or trachea needs proper evaluation of the respiratory system. Ideally, a brief oral exam should be performed to assess for swelling, discharge, or obstruction of the trachea.

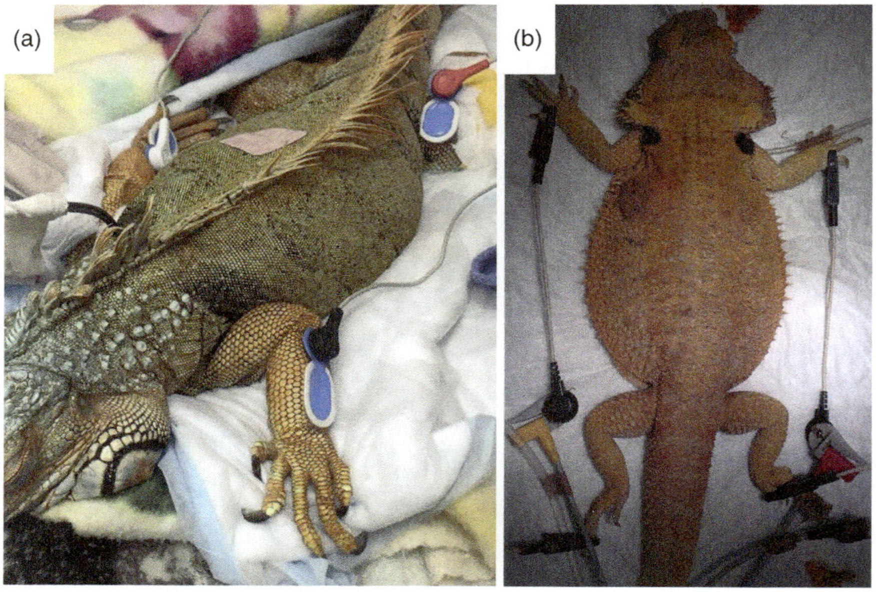

Figure 47.5 Electrocardiogram use in lizards. (a) Heart rate and rhythm are monitored in a green iguana (*Iguana iguana*) using electrocardiography in Lead II connected to the patient using adhesive pads. *Source*: Photo courtesy of La'Toya Latney. (b) In an anesthetized bearded dragon (*Pogona vitticeps*), the electrocardiogram is obtained with metal clips.

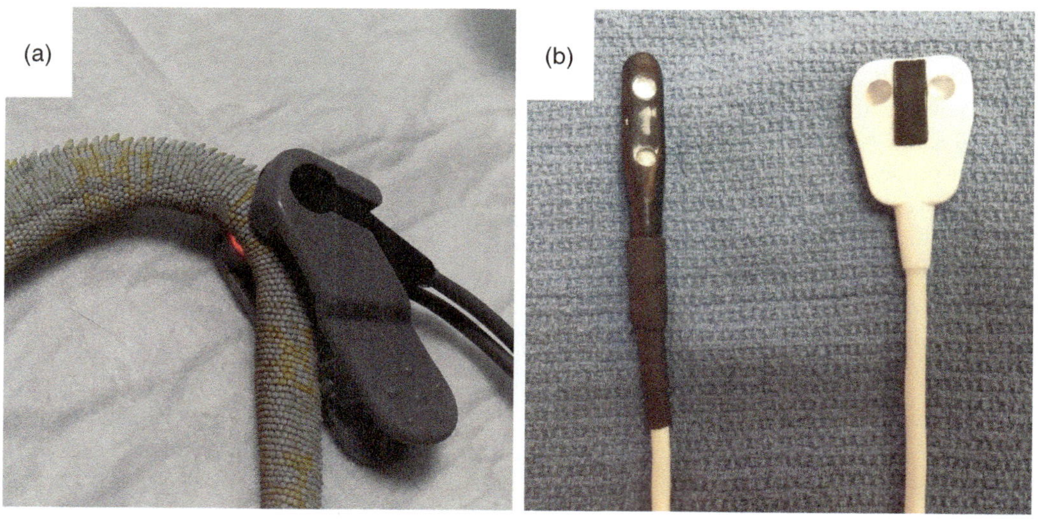

Figure 47.6 Pulse oximetry sensors. (a) A clip sensor can be used on thin part of the patient as in the tail of this veiled chameleon (*Chamaeleo calyptratus*). (b) Linear, reflectance sensors can be applied directly to mucosal surfaces such as the cloaca to avoid interference from thick or pigmented scales.

Pulse-Oximeter

Pulse oximetry is a noninvasive method of determining the oxygen saturation of hemoglobin in arterial blood. A sensor is clipped to a thin part of the patient's body such as a digit, tail, or tongue. Due to the pigmented nature of reptile skin, clip sensors often do not provide a reading. An alternative is to use reflectance probes (Figure 47.6) designed for use on vascularized surfaces. They can be placed against the reptile's oral or cloacal mucosa. SpO_2 is determined based on mammalian oxyhemoglobin dissociation curves and therefore is often inaccurate in reptile patients [28, 30]. Therefore, pulse oximetry should not be used to assess absolute hemoglobin oxygenation, but rather to monitor trends. As such, pulse oximetry can be used to assess response to treatment (e.g. oxygen therapy, fluid resuscitation), although results must always be interpreted cautiously.

Herptiles

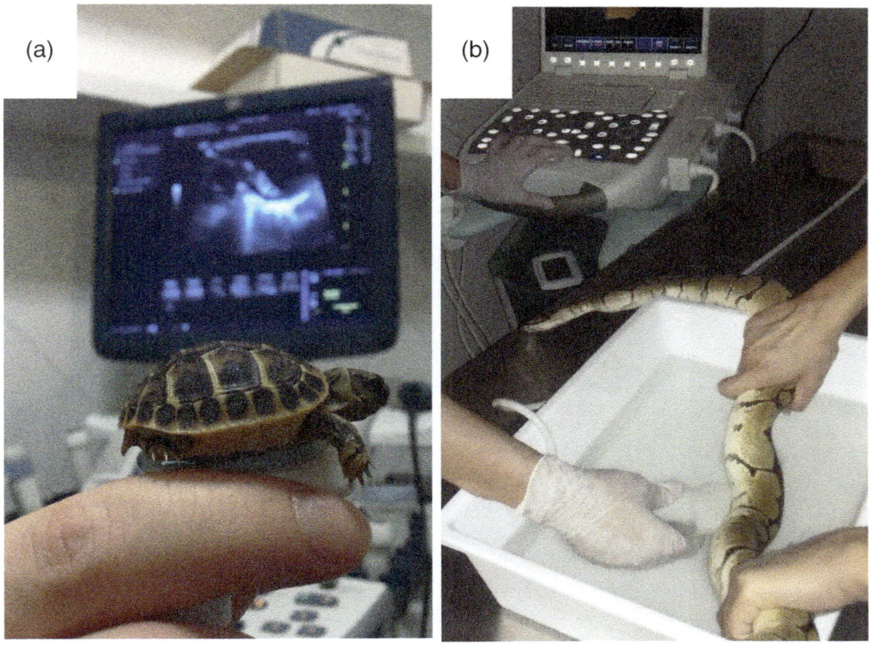

Figure 47.7 Image acquisition is improved with the use of coupling gel for transplastronal ultrasonography of a hatchling Hermann's tortoise (*Testudo hermanni*) (a) or with the use of a warm water bath for coelomic ultrasonography of an adult ball python (*Python regius*) (b).

Capnograph

Capnography monitors expired or end-tidal partial pressure carbon dioxide ($ETCO_2$). In reptiles, respiratory rate is driven by hypoxia rather than by hypercapnia as in mammals. Because reptiles can efficiently utilize anaerobic metabolism during periods of hypoxia, $ETCO_2$ may not be an accurate reflection of adequate ventilation, but can be useful to monitor trends. Capnography may also be useful to monitor respiratory rates for patients such as chelonians for which visual assessment of breathing can be difficult due to unique anatomy.

Point-of-Care Ultrasound (POCUS)

Indications

Point-of-care ultrasound (POCUS) is a quick and noninvasive diagnostic tool for the evaluation of the critical patient. POCUS may provide valuable information for any emergent patient but is particularly useful for reptiles presented following blunt force trauma, for chelonians with generalized edema in order to differentiate cardiac from renal or hepatic disorders, and for snakes with focal coelomic swelling. Even brief ultrasonographic examination of the heart and coelom can be used for cursory evaluation of cardiac function, gastrointestinal motility, organ size and appearance, and reproductive status [31]. A 7.5–10.0 MHz focused-phased array sector transducer with a small footprint is appropriate for most patients although a 5.0 MHz transducer may be used in larger animals [32]. In smaller reptiles (e.g. bearded dragons, chameleons), higher frequency transducers (10–18 MHz) provide more detailed images. Image quality is optimized by using coupling gel or submerging the portion of the patient to be examined in warm water (Figure 47.7). Direct contact with the patient can be avoided by placing the patient in a plastic box filled with warm water and positioning the transducer on the outside and is especially indicated for amphibians (Figure 47.8). Organs should be evaluated in sagittal and transverse planes and knowledge of specific reptile echo-anatomy is needed [33, 34]. When stable enough for handling, patients should be examined in both right and left lateral recumbencies and from a ventral midline approach, either in sternal or dorsal recumbency [35]. POCUS has not been validated in any reptile species and its diagnostic ability is limited by the technical skill and experience of the operator [32].

Abdominal/Coelomic (AFAST)

POCUS of the coelomic cavity, analogous to AFAST (Abdominal Focused Assessment using Sonography for Triage) in small animal medicine, is a quick, noninvasive, portable, and repeatable procedure. POCUS of the coelomic cavity is used in emergencies to screen for hemorrhage following trauma. It can also be used to identify, sample, and

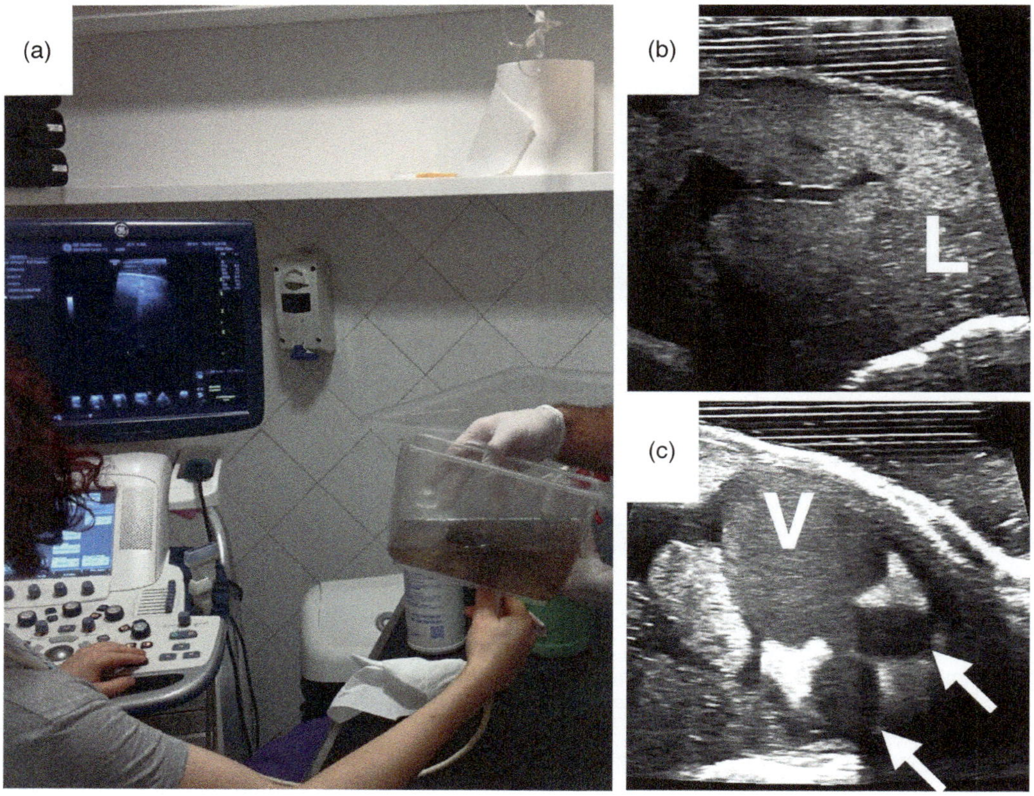

Figure 47.8 Ultrasonographic examination of a Colorado River toad (*Incilius alvarius*). Image acquisition in amphibians can be performed without directly contacting their skin by placing the patient in water in a plastic container and applying coupling gel to the outside (a). In the ultrasonographic images (b, c), the liver (L) and the heart with the single ventricle (V) and two atria (arrows) are identified.

characterize other coelomic effusions, to diagnose reproductive disease [36], to differentiate between cystic and solid masses, and to identify calculi in the urinary bladder, gastrointestinal tract, or cloaca [32]. It is especially useful in lizards (Figure 47.9), and in post-hatchling chelonians (Figure 47.7) that do not have a mineralized plastron, where the ventral coelom (including liver, gastrointestinal tract, yolk sac, and urinary bladder) is easily visualized through transplastronal ultrasonography. Coelomic evaluation should be systematic, starting with evaluation of the cranial coelom and moving caudally toward the vent.

Cardiovascular (TFAST)

In small animal emergency medicine, point-of-care thoracic ultrasound thoracic focused assessment with sonography for trauma (TFAST) is employed in cases of blunt trauma and is used to identify pneumothorax, pericardial and pleural effusion, damage to the chest wall (e.g. rib fractures), cardiac tamponade, and pulmonary edema or hemorrhage [35]. Unique anatomy limits the translation of TFAST to reptile emergency medicine. The shells of chelonians and air sacs of some squamates will preclude ultrasonographic evaluation of the pulmonary parenchyma. However, POCUS can help distinguish primary respiratory versus cardiogenic causes of dyspnea in critical patients, to differentiate cardiogenic edema versus dysproteinemic edema, and to confirm cardiomegaly in snakes with cranial third swelling [37]. Ultrasonographic evaluation of the heart may reveal congenital abnormalities, cardiomyopathy, thrombosis, carditis, or neoplasia [38] and can be used to screen for heart failure secondary to valvular insufficiency [39]. Application of Doppler increases the diagnostic information of POCUS by allowing evaluation of blood flow.

Water Quality Testing

Water quality assessment can provide information about potential sources of illness in amphibians and aquatic reptiles but is not routinely performed on an emergency basis due to logistical reasons. Major parameters to assess include pH, ammonia, chlorine, nitrates, and nitrites. Thorough reviews of water quality evaluation for amphibians have been published elsewhere [40, 41].

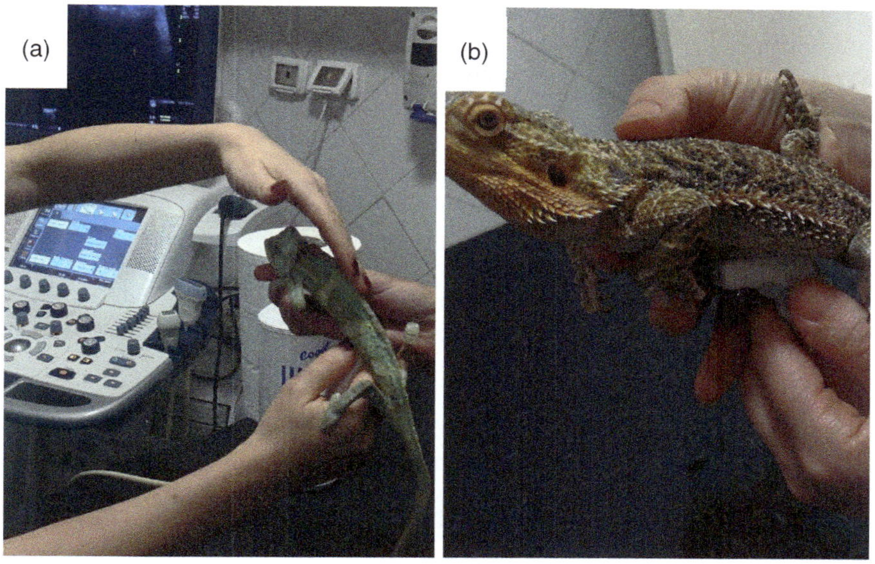

Figure 47.9 Positioning of ultrasonography probe on (a) a veiled chameleon (*Chamaeleo calyptratus*) and (b) a bearded dragon (*Pogona vitticeps*). POCUS in lizards usually allows a prompt evaluation of the heart, liver, intestines, and testes or ovaries.

References

1 Saggese, M.D. (2009). Clinical approach to the anemic reptile. *J. Exot. Pet Med.* 18 (2): 98–111.

2 Muller, K. and Brunnberg, L. (2010). Determination of plasma albumin concentration in healthy and diseased turtles: a comparison of protein electrophoresis and the bromcresol green dye-binding method. *Vet. Clin. Pathol.* 39 (1): 79–82.

3 Nardini, G., Leopardi, S., and Bielli, M. (2013). Clinical hematology in reptilian species. *Vet. Clin. Exot. Anim.* 16: 1–30.

4 Stahl, S.J. (2003). Diseases of the reptile pancreas. *Vet. Clin. Exot. Anim.* 6: 191–212.

5 Hidaldo-Vila, J., Martinez-Silvestre, A., Ribas, A. et al. (2011). Pancreatitis associated with the helminth *Serpinema microcephalus* (Nematod: Camallandiae) in exotic red-eared slider turtles (*Trachemys scripta elegans*). *J. Wildl. Dis.* 47 (1): 201–205.

6 Perpiñan, D., Hernandez-Divers, S.M., McBride, M., and Hernandez-Divers, S.J. (2006). Comparison of three different techniques to produce blood smears from green iguanas, *Iguana iguana*. *J. Herpetol. Med. Surg.* 16 (3): 99–101.

7 Fitzgerald, K.T. and Newquist, K.L. (2008). Poisonings in reptiles. *Vet. Clin. Exot. Anim.* 11: 327–357.

8 Kubalek, S., Mischke, R., and Fehr, M. (2002). Investigations on blood coagulation in the green iguana (*Iguana iguana*). *J. Vet. Med. A* 49: 210–216.

9 Lewbart, G.A., Hirschfeld, M., Denkinger, J. et al. (2014). Blood gases, biochemistry, and hematology of Galapagos green turtles (*Chelonia mydas*). *PLoS One* 9 (5): e96487.

10 Howell, B.J. and Rahn, H. (1976). Regulation of acid–base balance in reptiles. In: *Biology of the Reptilia*, vol. 5 (eds. C. Gans and W.R. Dawson). New York, NY: Academic Press.

11 Harr, K.E., Alleman, R., Dennis, P.M. et al. (2001). Morphologic and cytochemical characteristics of blood cells and hematologic and plasma biochemical reference ranges in green iguanas. *J. Am. Vet. Med. Assoc.* 218 (6): 915–921.

12 Deem, S.L., Norton, T.M., Mitchell, M. et al. (2009). Comparison of blood values in foraging, nesting, and stranded Loggerhead turtles (*Caretta caretta*) along the coast of Georgia, USA. *J. Wildl. Dis.* 45: 41–56.

13 Keller, K.A., Innis, C.J., Tlusty, M.F. et al. (2012). Metabolic and respiratory derangements associated with death in cold-stunned Kemp's ridley turtles (*Lepidochelys kempii*): 32 cases (2005–2009). *J. Am. Vet. Med. Assoc.* 240 (3): 317–323.

14 Baird, G.S. (2011). Ionized calcium. *Clin. Chim. Acta* 412 (9–10): 696–701.

15 Eatwell, K. (2009). Comparison of total calcium, ionized calcium and albumin concentrations in the plasma of captive tortoises (*Testudo* species). *Vet. Rec.* 165: 466–468.

16 Hernandez-Divers, S.J., Stahl, S.J., Stedman, N.L. et al. (2005). Renal evaluation in the healthy green iguana (*Iguana iguana*): assessment of plasma biochemistry, glomerular filtration rate, and endoscopic biopsy. *J. Zoo Wildl. Med.* 36 (2): 155–168.

17 Dennis, P.M., Bennett, R.A., Harr, K.E., and Lock, B.A. (2001). Plasma concentration of ionized calcium in healthy iguanas. *J. Am. Vet. Med. Assoc.* 219 (3): 326–328.

18 Nevarez, J.G., Mitchell, M.A., Le Blanc, C., and Graham, P. (2002). Determination of plasma biochemistries, ionized calcium, vitamin D3, and hematocrit values in captive green iguanas (*Iguana iguana*) from El Salvador. In: *Proceedings of the Association of Reptilian and Amphibian Veterinarians*, 87–93.

19 Oonincx, D.G., Van De Wal, M.D., Bosch, G. et al. (2013). Blood vitamin D3 metabolite concentrations of adult female bearded dragons (*Pogona vitticeps*) remain stable after ceasing UVb exposure. *Comp. Biochem. Physiol. B: Biochem. Mol. Biol.* 165 (3): 196–200.

20 Cooper-Bailey, K., Smith, S.A., Zimmerman, K. et al. (2011). Hematology, leukocyte cytochemical analysis, plasma biochemistry, and plasma electrophoresis of wild-caught and captive-bred Gila monsters (*Heloderma suspectum*). *Vet. Clin. Pathol.* 40 (3): 316–323.

21 Hedley, J. and Eatwell, K. (2013). The effects of UV light on calcium metabolism in ball pythons (*Python regius*). *Vet. Rec.*

22 Eatwell, K. (2010). Calcium and phosphorus values and their derivatives in captive tortoises (*Testudo* species). *J. Small Anim. Pract.* 51 (9): 472–475.

23 Di Girolamo, N., Ferlizza, E., Selleri, P. et al. (2018). Evaluation of point-of-care analysers for blood gas and clinical chemistry in Hermann's tortoises (*Testudo hermanni*). *J. Small Anim. Pract.* 59: 704–713.

24 Stringer, E.M., Harms, C.A., Beasley, J.F., and Anderson, E.T. (2010). Comparison of ionized calcium, parathyroid hormone, and 25-hydroxyvitamin D in rehabilitating and healthy wild green sea turtles (*Chelonia mydas*). *J. Herpetol. Med. Surg.* 20 (4): 122–127.

25 McCain, S.L., Flatland, B., Schumacher, J.P. et al. (2010). Comparison of chemistry analytes between two portable, commercially available analyzers and a conventional laboratory analyzer in reptiles. *Vet. Clin. Pathol.* 39 (4): 474–479.

26 Wolf, K.N., Harms, C.A., and Beasley, J.F. (2008). Evaluation of five clinical chemistry analyzers for use in health assessment in sea turtles. *J. Am. Vet. Med. Assoc.* 233: 470–475.

27 Scope, A., Schwendenwein, I., and Schauberger, G. (2013). Characterization and quantification of the influence of season and gender on plasma chemistries of Hermann's tortoises (*Testudo hermanni*, Gmelin 1789). *Res. Vet. Sci.* 95: 59–68.

28 Martinez-Jimenez, D. and Hernandez-Divers, S.J. (2007). Emergency care of reptiles. *Vet. Clin. Exot. Anim.* 10: 557–585.

29 Braun, E.J. (1998). Comparative renal function in reptiles, birds, and mammals. *Semin. Avian Exot. Pet Med.* 7 (2): 62–71.

30 Costello, M.F. (2004). Principles of cardiopulmonary cerebral resuscitation in special species. *Semin. Avian Exot. Pet Med.* 13 (2): 132–141.

31 Mitchell, M.A. (2010). Managing the reptile patient in the veterinary hospital: establishing a standards of care model for nontraditional species. *J. Exot. Pet Med.* 19 (1): 56–72.

32 Schumacher, J. and Toal, R.L. (2001). Advanced radiography and ultrasonography in reptiles. *Sem. Avian Exot. Pet Med.* 10 (4): 162–168.

33 Banzato, T., Russo, E., Finotti, L. et al. (2012). Ultrasonographic anatomy of the coelomic organs of boid snakes (*Boa constrictor imperator, Python regius, Python molurus molurus,* and *Python curtus*). *Am. J. Vet. Res.* 73 (5): 634–645.

34 Bucy, D.S., Guzman, D.S., and Zwingenberger, A.L. (2015). Ultrasonographic anatomy of bearded dragons (*Pogona vitticeps*). *J. Am. Vet. Med. Assoc.* 246 (8): 868–876.

35 Boysen, S.R. and Lisciandro, G.R. (2013). The use of ultrasound for dogs and cats in the emergency room: AFAST and TFAST. *Vet. Clin. Small Anim.* 43: 773–797.

36 Music, M.K. and Strunk, A. (2016). Reptile critical care and common emergencies. *Vet. Clin. Exot. Anim.* 19: 591–612.

37 Schilliger, L., Rossfelder, A., Bonwitt, J. et al. (2014). Antemortem diagnosis of multicentric lymphoblastic lymphoma, lymphoid leukemia, and inclusion body disease in a boa constrictor (*Boa constrictor imperator*). *J. Herpetol. Med. Surg.* 24: 11–19.

38 Snyder, P.S., Shaw, N.G., and Heard, D.J. (1999). Two-dimensional echocardiographic anatomy of the snake heart (*Python molurus bivittatus*). *Vet. Radiol. Ultrasound* 40 (1): 66–72.

39 Rishniw, M. and Carmel, B.P. (1999). Atrioventricular valvular insufficiency and congestive heart failure in a carpet python. *Aust. Vet. J.* 77: 580–583.

40 Whitaker, B.R. (2001). Water quality. In: *Amphibian Medicine and Captive Husbandry* (eds. K.M. Wright and B.R. Whitaker), 147–158. Malabar, FL: Krieger Publishing Company.

41 Odum, R.A. and Zippel, K.C. (2008). Amphibian water quality: approaches to an essential environmental parameter. *Int. Zoo Yearb.* 42: 40–52.

48

Diagnostic Imaging

Constance Fazio

Department of Small Animal Clinical Sciences, College of Veterinary Medicine, University of Tennessee, Knoxville, Tennessee, USA

CONTENTS

Image Acquisition and Normal Anatomy

Reptiles and amphibians represent a broad range of body conformation and size, along with several unique anatomical variations. This diversity among lizards, turtles, tortoises, snakes, and amphibians can create unique challenges for diagnostic imaging. While radiography remains the most common imaging modality, ultrasound (US), computed tomography (CT), and even magnetic resonance imaging (MRI) are being utilized more often. When acquiring and interpreting images with any modality, it is essential to keep species-specific considerations in mind.

Radiographs

The technical aspects of radiography are similar to those used for small animals. A key equipment capability is a portable X-ray tube permitting horizontal beam projections, in which the X-ray beam is oriented in the horizontal direction across the table toward the image receptor panel/plate (Figure 48.1). These projections allow for natural patient positioning, resulting in less coelomic organ displacement, as well as requiring less restraint. Especially small patients or extremity radiographs may require a table-top exposure without a grid.

Positioning

Patient and radiographer safety should always be the primary consideration. A clinically unstable patient should be stabilized prior to imaging. Unless necessary, manual restraint is not recommended due to radiation safety concerns and potential obscuring of the image. Depending on patient compliance, heavy sedation or anesthesia may be required. Radiography of the head requires heavy sedation or general anesthesia to accomplish proper positioning.

Turtles and Tortoises Three standard projections are used in chelonians: dorsoventral (DV), lateral, and craniocaudal (Figure 48.2). The lateral and craniocaudal views are best accomplished using a horizontal beam technique. Patients are positioned on top of a radiolucent bowl/cup or foam block. This allows for limited patient movement and encourages the limbs to hang outside the shell, reducing superimposition with the coelomic cavity. A radiolucent box can also be used to confine the patient or the patient may be positioned with cloth tape. Chemical restraint is rarely needed for proper radiographic positioning in chelonians.

Exotic Animal Emergency and Critical Care Medicine, First Edition. Edited by Jennifer E. Graham, Grayson A. Doss and Hugues Beaufrère.

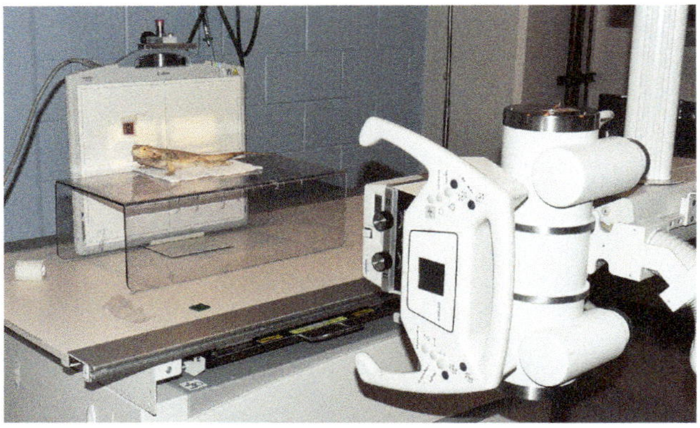

Figure 48.1 Horizontal beam X-ray tube and image receptor panel configuration for a cross-table lateral projection of a bearded dragon (*Pogona vitticeps*). The patient is positioned on top of an acrylic trough and the X-ray beam is matched to the patient elevation. The lamp light reflects the collimation of the primary X-ray beam.

Snakes Lateral and DV projections are standard for radiographic evaluation of snakes. Thin, radiolucent, acrylic restraint tubes are helpful for positioning (Figure 48.3). If a snake restraint tube is not available, chemical restraint is typically required for adequate radiographic positioning (especially lateral views). Metallic markers can mark positions on longer snakes radiographed with sequential images. The cardiac apex can be used for localization. A coiled snake position results in superimposition artifacts on lateral views and body asymmetry on a DV view, and is therefore not recommended.

Lizards Lizards are radiographed in two standard projections: lateral and DV (Figure 48.4). As in turtles, tortoises, or snakes, additional oblique projections may be helpful in further evaluation of the head. The lateral view is best accomplished using a horizontal beam with the patient positioned on an acrylic box or foam block. Certain species like chameleons are more naturally positioned on a stick-like support (Figure 48.5). A radiolucent box may also be used to confine the patient, though straight positioning for the lateral view may be challenging. When obtaining lateral views of lizards without using a horizontal beam projection, chemical immobilization, or use of the vasovagal reflex is required. For extremity evaluation, the limb should be extended from the body. Cloth tape may be used for patient positioning, though the tail should not be tied or taped. In lizards, use of cotton-balls applied to the eyes and wrapped in self-adhesive bandage material may induce a sufficient vasovagal reflex to keep the patient still for the duration of the radiographic study.

Amphibians DV projections of amphibians are readily accomplished. However, lateral projections are often limited by significant summation artifact due to the relatively short and wide body conformation of frogs and toads. Given the unique properties of their skin, tape should not be used for restraint.

Complications/Contraindications

The risks of radiography include the inherent radiation safety concerns, as well as the potential complications of patient restraint and chemical immobilization. Studies in venomous species should be considered carefully for both radiographer and patient safety.

Contrast Studies

Indications for gastrointestinal contrast studies include evidence of obstruction, to assess for gastrointestinal wall integrity, history of foreign body ingestion, an unexplained organ displacement or mass effect, or to confirm feeding tube placement (Figure 48.6).

Among reptiles, there is a great variation in gastrointestinal transit times, which are longer compared to mammals and influenced by many factors (Box 48.1). This hinders the diagnostic utility of gastrointestinal contrast studies in reptiles. Gastrointestinal contrast studies have been reported for several species, including a range of recommended dosages for either barium sulfate (25–35% w/v barium sulfate given at 8–25 ml/kg) or iodinated contrast medium [1–10]. For gastrointestinal studies in reptiles, nonionic iodinated contrast medium is recommended, as transit times are faster compared to barium sulfate. In addition, barium sulfate may solidify in the gastrointestinal tract with longer passage times.

The most common complication of upper gastrointestinal (GI) contrast studies in reptiles is regurgitation, which can be minimized with slower contrast administration. The danger of contrast medium aspiration is higher with iodinated contrast medium as it can result in pulmonary edema [11]. Therefore, it should always be administered via a gastric or esophageal tube. Barium sulfate may be administered orally. Barium should never be used if gastrointestinal perforation is suspected or if endoscopy is planned. However, the hyperosmolar nature of iodinated contrast pulls water into the GI tract, which can lead to dehydration and dilutes the contrast in more distal intestinal segments. Double contrast studies may also be used for both upper and lower GI studies. Cloacography has also been described.

Normals

Radiographic projections of clinically healthy reptiles and amphibians are included in Figures 48.7–48.10. Significant differences may exist due to species, age, size, sex, and individual variation.

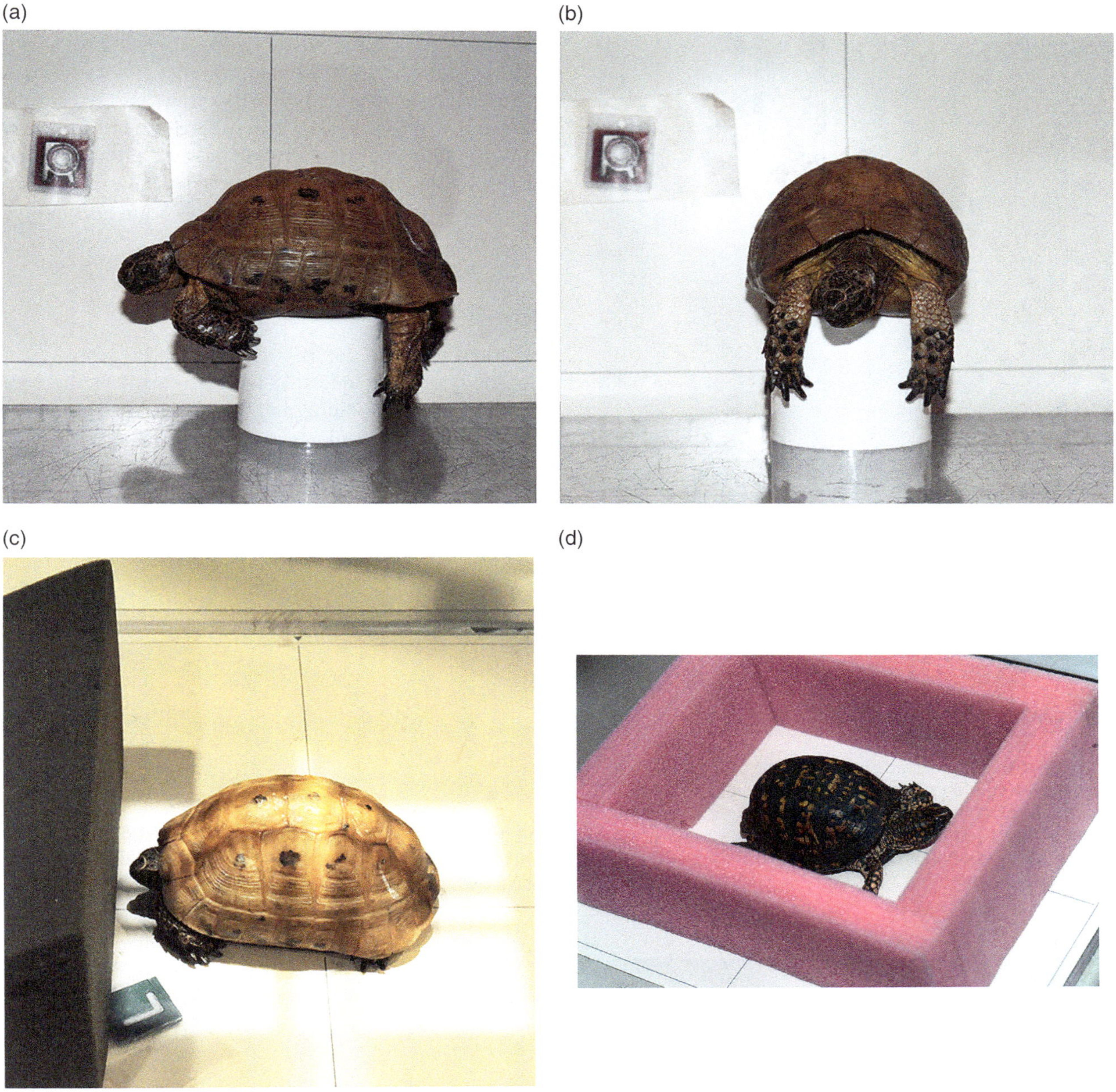

Figure 48.2 Three standard radiographic projections for tortoises and turtles. Horizontal beam lateral projection (a), horizontal beam craniocaudal projection (b), and dorsoventral projection (c, d). This Greek tortoise (*Testudo graeca*) is placed on top of a radiolucent cup (a, b), which allows the limbs to hang away from the body, rather than tucked in the shell. For this DV view, a foam wedge is used as barrier to discourage patient motion (c). Use of a radiolucent foam square to restrict a box turtle (*Terrapene carolina*) to the surface of the image receptor panel for a DV projection (d).

There are several system-based considerations when interpreting radiographs of reptiles. First, the lungs of reptiles vary greatly by species. Most lizards and snakes have sac-like lungs, while the lungs of chelonians have thin septations. The snake lung is quite elongated, and some species have a reduced or absent left lung. These differences limit the use of classical pulmonary radiographic pattern terminology (i.e. alveolar, bronchial, and interstitial).

Second, the coelomic soft tissues are often obscured due to superimposition and silhouetting in the coelomic cavity. For this reason, orthogonal projections are recommended whenever possible and a lateral projection alone is often less helpful. The heart is located in the cranial coelom in

(a) (b)

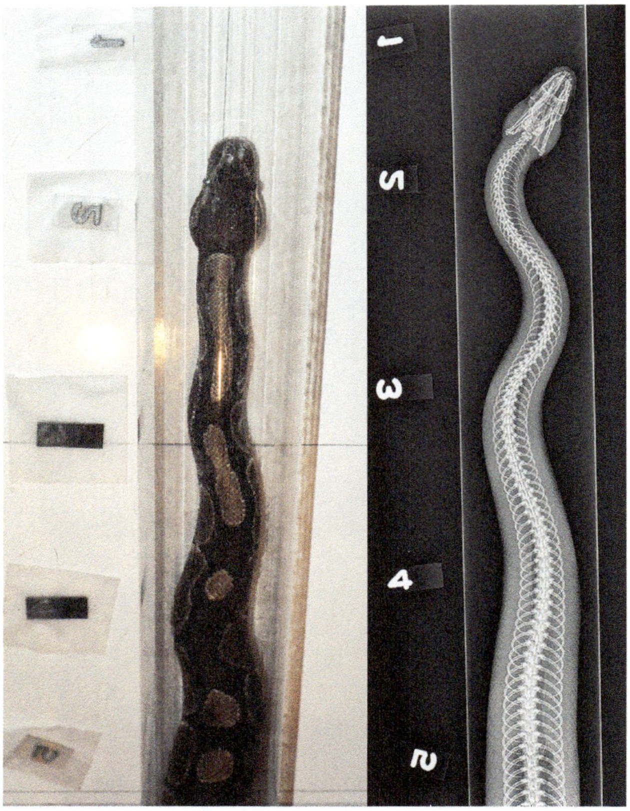

Figure 48.3 Use of a thin, radiolucent, acrylic tube for positioning of a normal ball python (Python regius) for a dorsoventral projection (a). Numerical lead markers are placed along the patient's left side to indicate position. In the corresponding DV radiograph (b), the patient has extended further cranially in the tube.

most lizards and chelonians, making it challenging to evaluate.

Third, the reproductive tract of reptiles is not routinely identified radiographically when inactive. However, when active, follicles, or eggs may occupy a large portion of the coelomic cavity, displacing and obscuring the intracoelomic organs (Figure 48.11). Non-mineralized follicles may be difficult to differentiate from non-mineralized eggs.

Ultrasound

Indications

Ultrasonography is indicated for assessment of the coelomic soft tissue structures and can be used to distinguish structures of indeterminate origin seen radiographically. Indications in the emergency setting include clinical signs or suspicion of gastrointestinal stasis or obstruction,

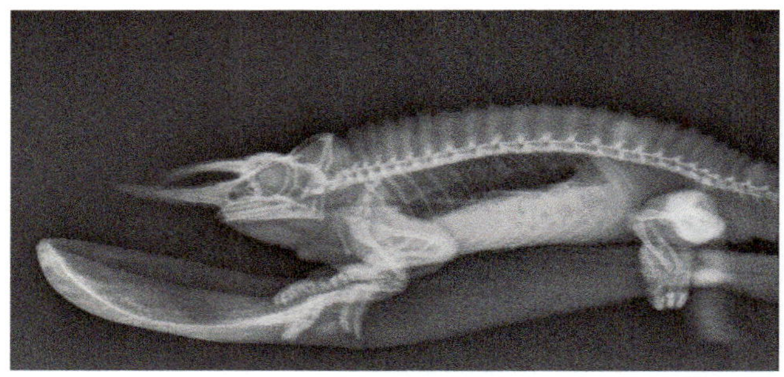

Figure 48.5 Use of a wooden spoon for supporting a Jackson's chameleon (*Trioceros jacksonii*) for a horizontal beam lateral radiograph.

(a) (b)

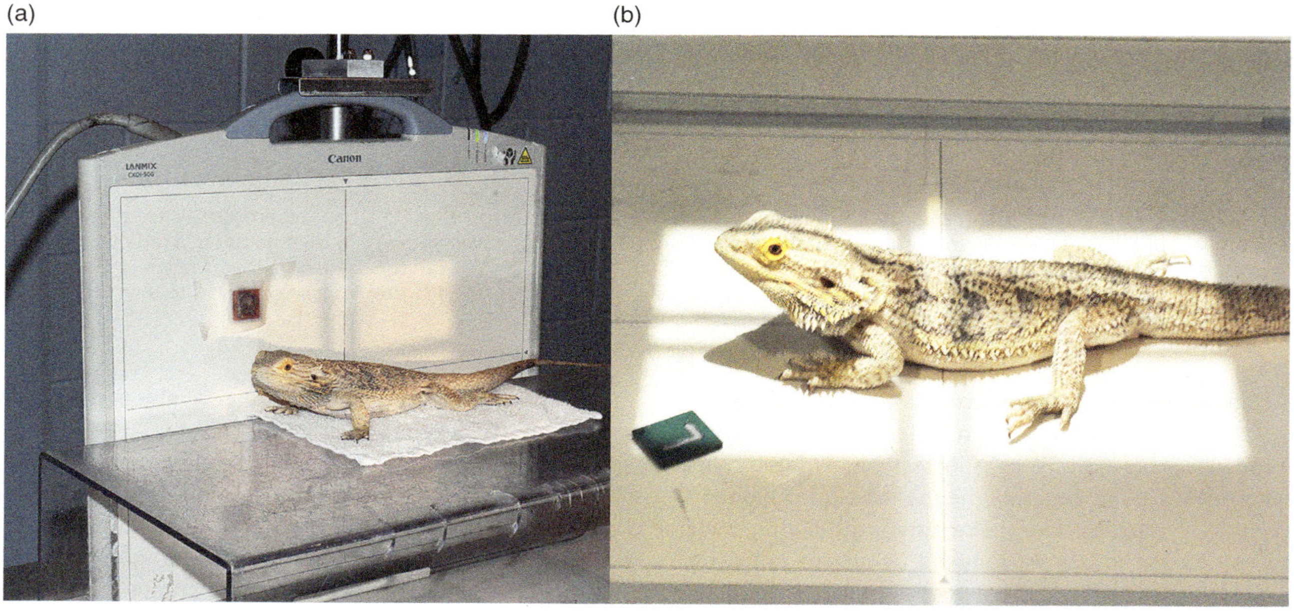

Figure 48.4 Two standard radiographic projections for lizards. Horizontal beam lateral projection (a) and dorsoventral projection (b) of a bearded dragon (*Pogona vitticeps*). Note the acrylic sheet used to protect the image receptor panel (b).

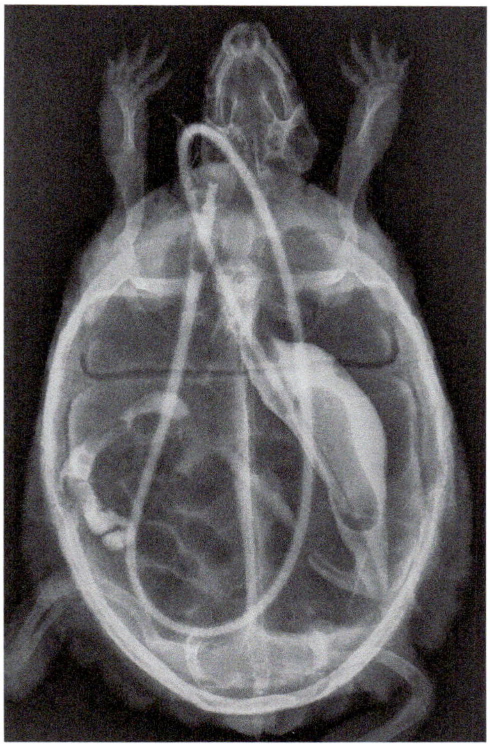

Figure 48.6 Positive contrast study using iohexol for confirmation of esophagostomy feeding tube placement in an adult box turtle (*Terrapene carolina*). The external portion of the tube is superimposed with the patient on this DV radiograph.

Box 48.1 Factors Influencing Gastrointestinal Transit Times in Reptiles

Temperature
Fasted or postprandial status
Diet strategy (e.g. herbivore, omnivore, carnivore)
Anatomy
Species
Season
Individual variation

reduced renal function, hepatic disease, disturbance in egg development or oviposition, coelomic distension, and masses. Ultrasound-guided fine needle aspiration or biopsy may also be performed.

General Information

The ideal ultrasound transducer frequency depends on patient size and structure of interest. Higher frequencies are recommended for smaller structures, at a trade-off with penetration depth. Recommended ultrasound frequencies for reptiles range from 5 to 18 MHz. When available, high frequency linear transducers are ideal for thorough evaluation. Transducers with a smaller footprint, such as microconvex or a "hockey stick" transducer are well-suited for small acoustic windows. The availability of a color Doppler function may aid investigation of organ perfusion.

Manual restraint is typically sufficient for sonographic evaluation, while sedation or anesthesia may be required for larger or more aggressive patients.

A few key factors influence the success of reptile coelomic sonography. The main factor is an appropriate acoustic window. Acoustic coupling gel can be applied in most instances. Alternatively, the patient may be partially submerged in a water bath. A stand-off may be helpful for superficial structures. In general, the presence of gas in the lungs and gastrointestinal tract causes reverberation artifact, limiting evaluation of deeper structures. The presence of ingesta may create a similar effect. Thus, not all coelomic structures will be visible sonographically in all reptiles. Organs typically identified on ultrasound in reptiles are listed in Box 48.2.

Species-Specific Information

Turtles and Tortoises

The obvious sonographic obstacle is a hard shell. Two main sonographic windows are available, the prefemoral fossa cranial to the hindlimb and the cervicobrachial fossa lateral to the neck (Figure 48.12). Both require a transducer with a small footprint and ample transducer coupling material, such as gel or a water bath. The majority of the coelomic organs visible in chelonians are visualized using the prefemoral window, including the reproductive tract, intestines, liver, kidneys, and allantois. The heart, esophagus, portions of the liver, and potentially the thyroid gland can be imaged from the cervicobrachial window.

Snakes Ventral and lateral approaches can be utilized in snakes. Shadow artifact from the numerous ribs and gas reverberation artifact from the long lung may interfere with lateral window images. It may be advantageous to hold only the area of interest in dorsal recumbency while the remainder of the snake remains in ventral recumbency. Ultrasonography of actively shedding snakes should be delayed due to artifact from air trapped between skin layers.

Lizards The majority of organs can be assessed using a ventral approach in lizards (Figure 48.13). The coelomic fat bodies are quite attenuating to the ultrasound beam, so a dorsal approach is recommended for evaluation of the kidneys in some species. Air trapped between scales or particularly thick or mineralized scales may prevent sonographic evaluation of the coelom. A water bath prior to or during sonographic evaluation may help resolve trapped air.

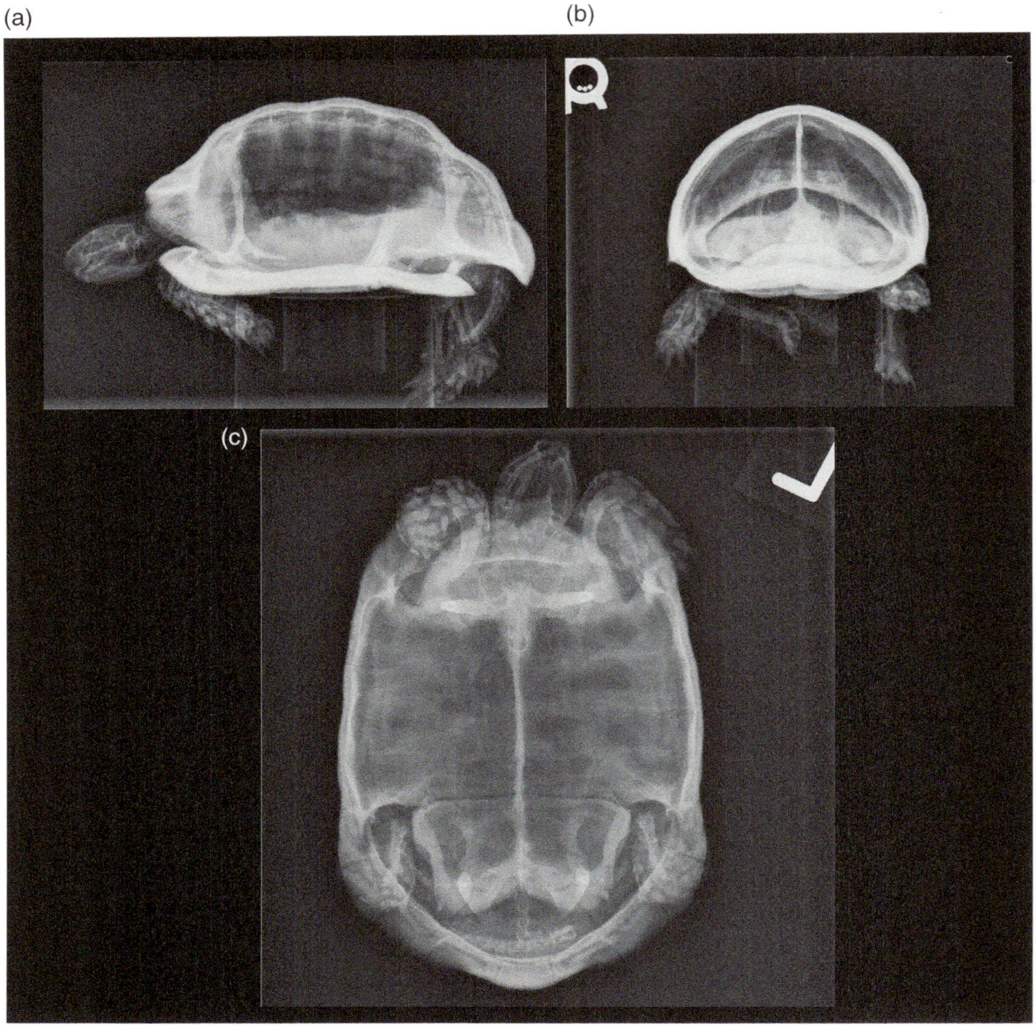

Figure 48.7 Normal radiographic study of the same Greek tortoise (*Testudo graeca*) shown in Figure 48.2. Lateral (a), craniocaudal (b), and dorsoventral (c) radiographic projections. Note the radiolucent cup used for positioning.

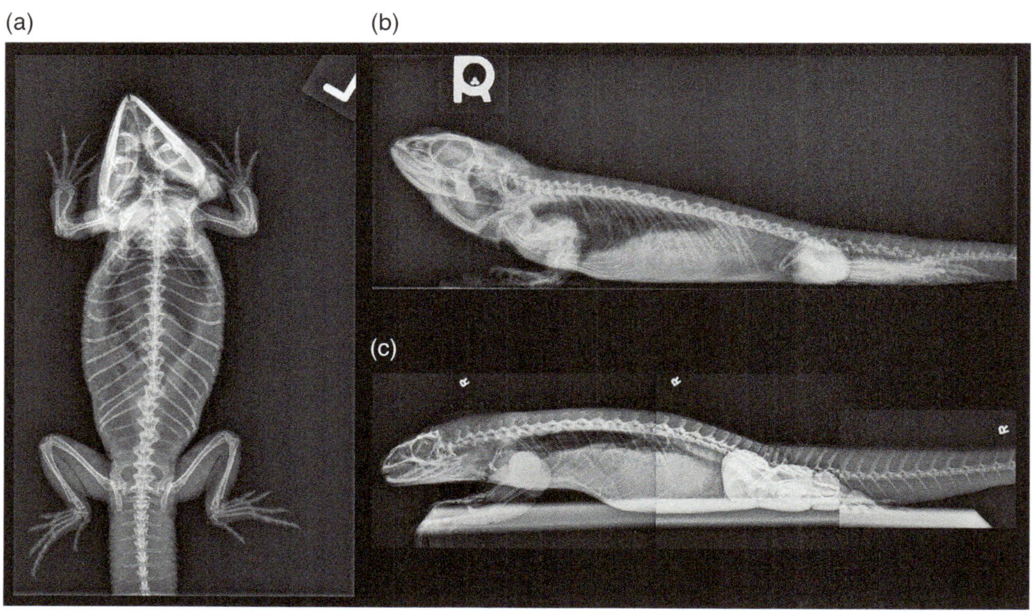

Figure 48.8 Normal adult bearded dragon (*Pogona vitticeps*), dorsoventral (a) and lateral (b) radiographic projections. Larger patients may require sequential radiographic images. Composite image of three horizontal beam lateral radiographs of a 10-year-old green iguana (*Iguana iguana*) with incidental spondylosis deformans (c).

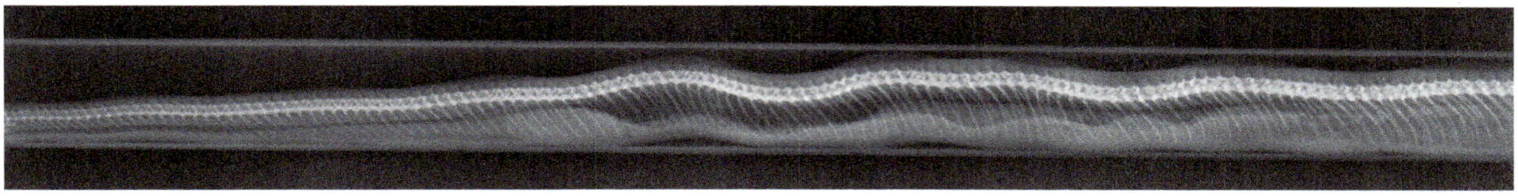

Figure 48.9 Normal two-year-old corn snake (*Pantherophis guttatus*) lateral radiograph. Cranial is to the left of the image. A normal ball python (*Python regius*) DV radiograph is shown in Figure 48.3. Note the radiolucent tube used for positioning.

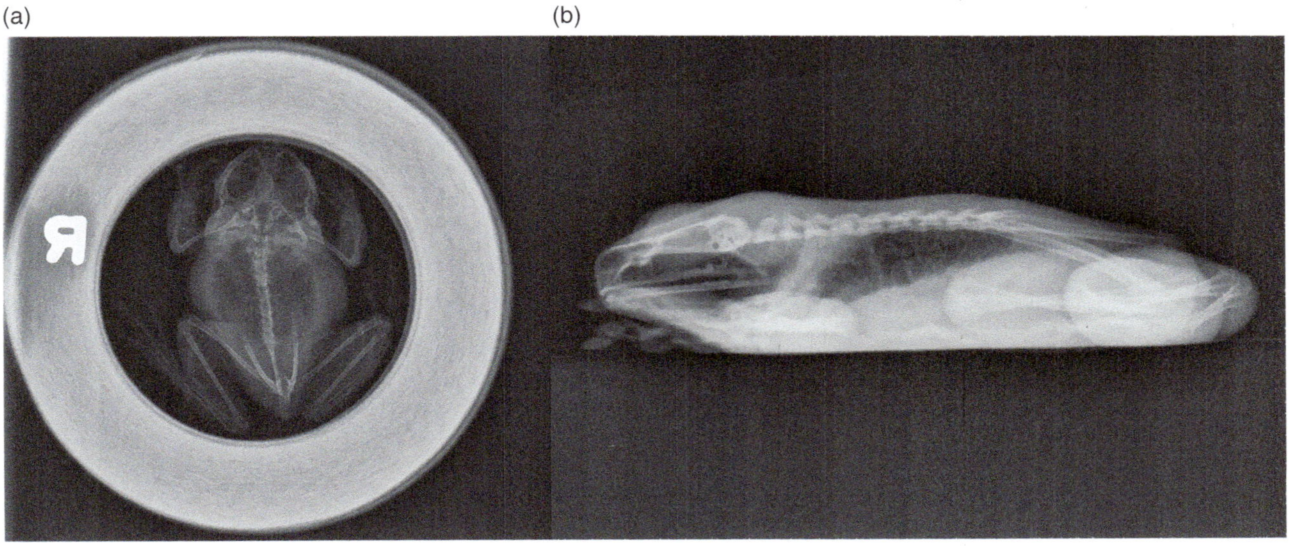

Figure 48.10 Normal radiographic study of an adult male White's tree frog (*Ranoidea caerulea*). Dorsoventral (a) and lateral (b) projections. A surrounding roll of tape limits patient motion on the DV view.

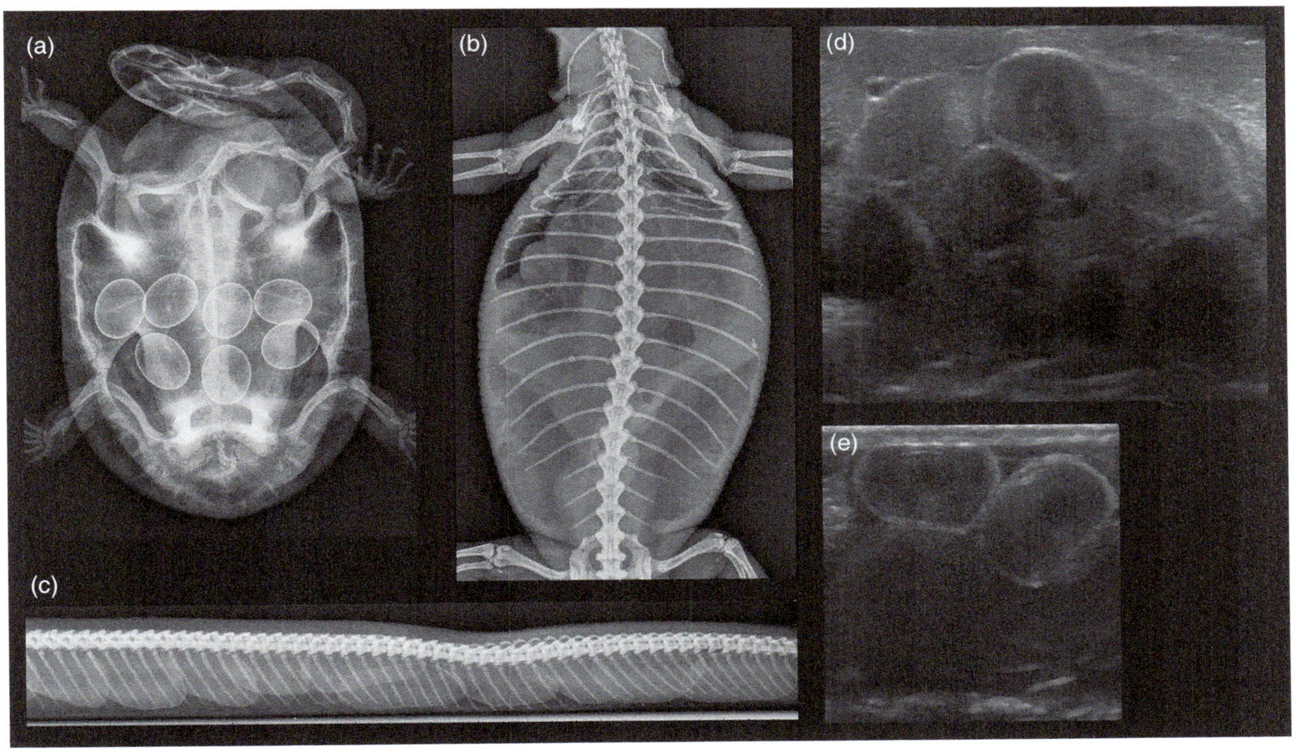

Figure 48.11 Radiographs (a–c) and ultrasound images (d, e) of female reptiles with various stages of follicles or eggs. Dorsoventral radiograph of a gravid snake-necked turtle with mineralized eggs (a). Dorsoventral radiograph of a Savannah monitor (*Varanus exanthematicus*) with suspected follicle resorption (b). Note the space-occupying effect in the coelom. Lateral radiograph of a gravid rat snake with several faintly mineralized eggs (c). Ultrasound image of several normal preovulatory partially vitellogenic follicles (d). Ultrasound image of a few postovulatory follicles in the oviduct (e).

Normals Sonographic images of clinically healthy reptiles are included in Figure 48.14. Significant differences may exist between species as well as due to individual variation. The liver should be hypoechoic to the fat bodies in lizards and snakes. The presence of echogenic gallbladder sediment has been reported in some lizards and snakes [12–14]. In some species, a small amount of free coelomic fluid is a normal finding. While portions of the gastrointestinal tract are visible, a wide range in wall layer identification has been described. Depending on the reproductive cycle in females, follicles, or eggs may occupy a large volume of the coelom (Figure 48.11).

Box 48.2 Coelomic Structures Commonly Identified with Ultrasound in Reptiles

More common

- Heart
- Liver
- Gallbladder
- Stomach
- Large intestine
- Kidneys
- Gonads (when reproductively active)

Less common

- Small intestine
- Pancreas
- Spleen
- Gonads (not reproductively active)

Advanced Diagnostic Imaging

Echocardiography

Echocardiography has been reported in some species of awake, sedated, or anesthetized reptiles and amphibians [15–18]. The reptilian heart, except for crocodilians, consists of two atria and one ventricle. A small amount of pericardial effusion may be a normal variation in chelonians [18]. While cardiac disease is rare in reptiles, echocardiography may be useful in the emergency setting for identification of pericardial effusion (Figure 48.15).

Fluoroscopy

Fluoroscopy may be useful for feeding tube placement or intraoperative imaging. Given the lengthy gastrointestinal transit times in reptiles, standard radiography is typically sufficient for routine gastrointestinal contrast studies.

Computed Tomography (CT)

CT is becoming increasingly available, leading to more routine evaluation of reptiles [1–3, 19–22]. CT cross-sectional imaging removes the limitations of superimposition

(a) (b)

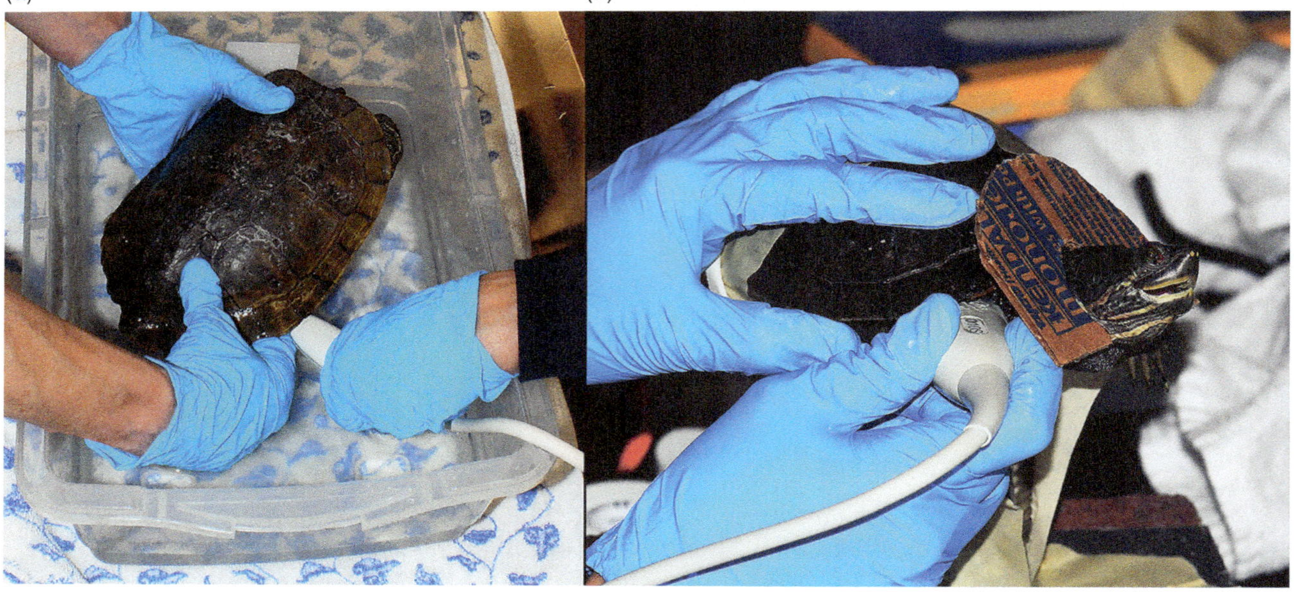

Figure 48.12 Prefemoral ultrasound transducer window in a red-eared slider (*Trachemys scripta elegans*), illustrating use of a water bath (a). Cervicobrachial ultrasound transducer window in a red-eared slider (b). Cardboard is used to protect the sonographer's hand during the examination. Source: Photographs courtesy of Christoph Mans.

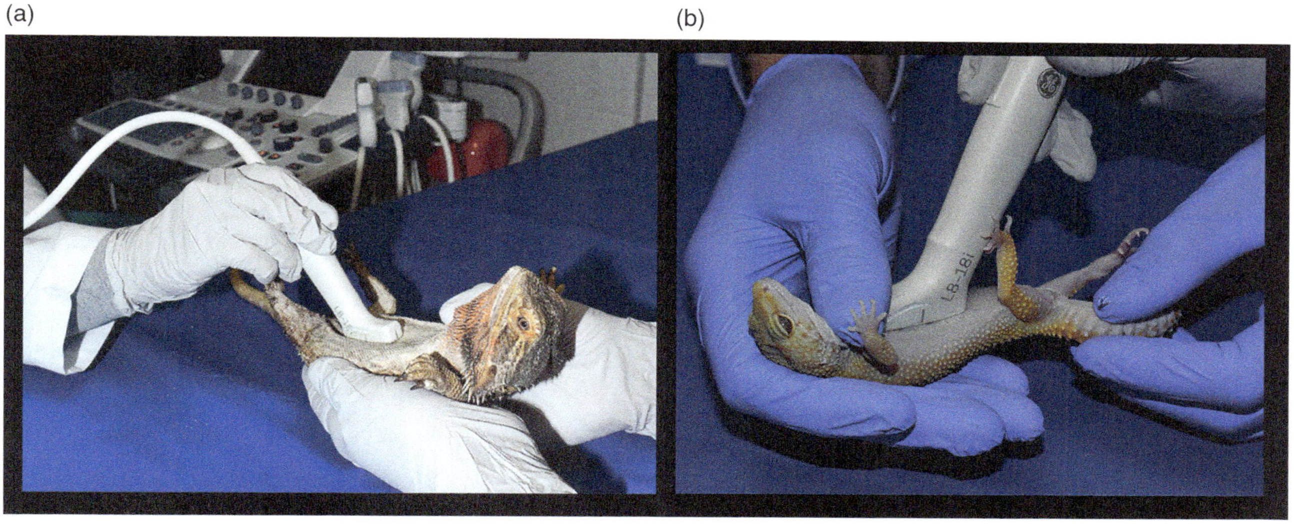

Figure 48.13 Ventral approach for ultrasound examination in a bearded dragon (*Pogona vitticeps*) (a) and leopard gecko (*Eublepharis macularius*) (b). Note use of a high frequency linear transducer with a small footprint.

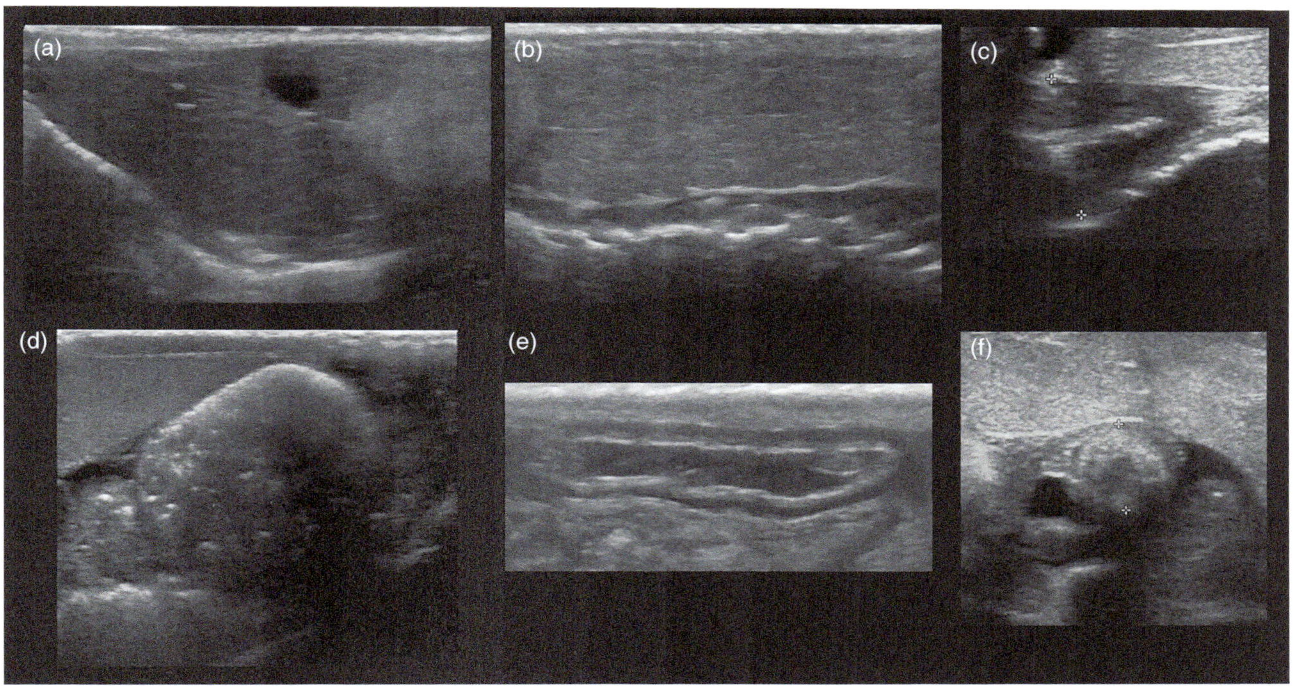

Figure 48.14 Normal coelomic ultrasound of the liver and gallbladder (a), fat body (b), kidney (c), stomach (d), small intestine containing a small amount of luminal fluid (e), and colon (f). Images are of a healthy leopard gecko (*Eublepharis macularius*) (a, b, e) and a healthy bearded dragon (*Pogona vitticeps*) (c, d, f).

of radiography and offers improved distinction of the coelomic organs. CT can offer additional information regarding the liver, kidneys, gastrointestinal tract, and reproductive status and is ideally suited for evaluation of the lungs and skeleton. As such, CT may be indicated in cases of dyspnea or in cases of trauma to the head, spine, shell, or pelvis. Patients should be positioned as straight as possible to maximize symmetry. Radiolucent tubes or boxes may be used for patient confinement. Use of the vasovagal reflex, sedation, or general anesthesia may be required for certain patients or studies. Multidetector CT allows for faster scans with thinner slice thicknesses and multiplanar reconstruction capabilities. Technique settings vary with species and

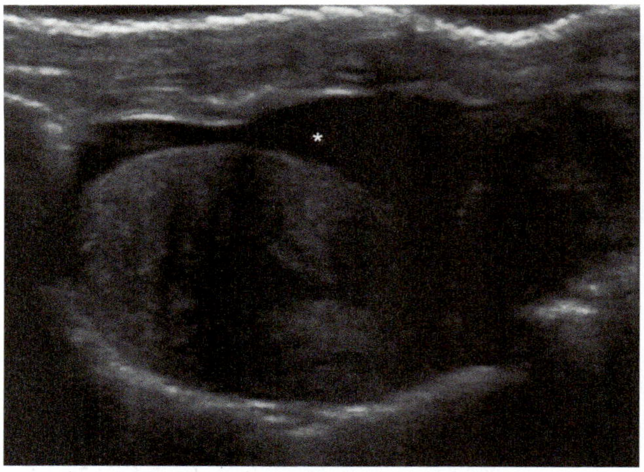

Figure 48.15 Echocardiogram of a seven-year-old bearded dragon (*Pogona vitticeps*) with pericardial effusion (asterisk) of unknown origin. This is a transverse image at the level of the ventricle.

patient size. High frequency algorithms are recommended for bone and lung, while medium frequency algorithms are recommended for soft tissues. When accessible, intravenous iodinated contrast may augment diagnostic capability.

Magnetic Resonance Imaging (MRI)

Indications for MRI include neurologic dysfunction or trauma [1–3, 23]. MRI offers improved soft tissue imaging compared to CT and may be used to evaluate the coelomic organs as well as potential masses. Prior to MRI, patients should be radiographically screened for metal that may potentially dislodge during the MRI scan becoming a safety concern, or otherwise interfere with MRI image acquisition. MRI requires longer scan times than CT, necessitating the use of general anesthesia to prevent significant motion artifact.

Clinical Presentations Requiring Emergent Imaging

Investigations

GI Disease

Radiographs are routinely utilized to assess cases of gastrointestinal disease. Localization of gastrointestinal structures is often easier on DV views compared to lateral views hindered by superimposition. The intestines should be evaluated for gas or fluid distention, though reptiles may not always display an obstructive pattern. Ingested material may accumulate in a particular intestinal segment and remain there, causing partial or complete mechanical obstruction

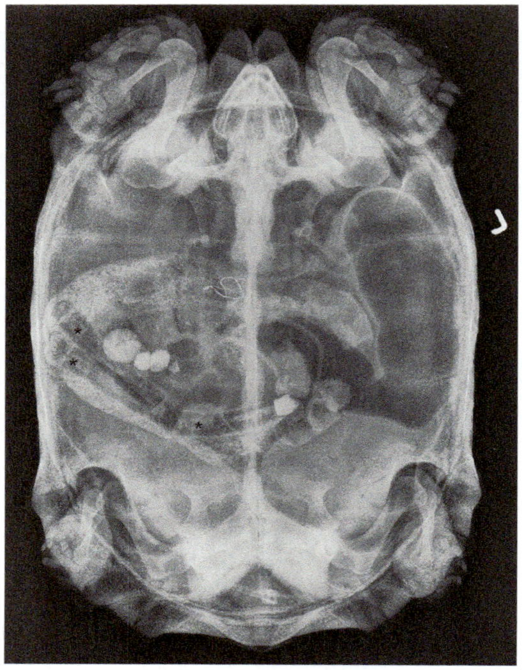

Figure 48.16 Intestinal mechanical obstruction due to foreign bodies in a five-year-old sulcata tortoise (*Centrochelys sulcata*). Note the gas distention of the gastrointestinal tract and the partially radiolucent, tubular foreign bodies. Three foam darts (asterisks) were removed via an enterotomy.

(Figure 48.16). Radiographs can screen for radiopaque foreign bodies, including metal in patients with signs of heavy metal toxicity (Figure 48.17). Foreign bodies can also be found incidentally on imaging. Images should be evaluated for the presence of coelomic effusion or free gas representing potential secondary coelomitis or perforation. Gastrointestinal contrast studies may be helpful to identify radiolucent foreign bodies, such as fishing line or plastic bags. Ingestion of food or substrate material, such as woodchips, gravel, sand, litter, bark, or towels may accumulate in the intestines and cause an impaction. Constipation/obstipation is often a diagnosis made radiographically and correlated with clinical findings (Figure 48.18). Sonographically, intussusception appears similar to that in mammals (Figure 48.19).

Dyspnea

Radiography or CT with minimal restraint should be considered for dyspneic patients. An increase in lung opacity may represent an infectious pneumonia (Figure 48.20), atelectasis due to coelomic effusion or mass effect, contusion or hemorrhage, airway collapse due to obstruction, near drowning, or pneumonitis. While radiographically focal or diffuse, CT or MRI may be required to further characterize the pulmonary changes. A radiographic diagnosis of pneumonia should

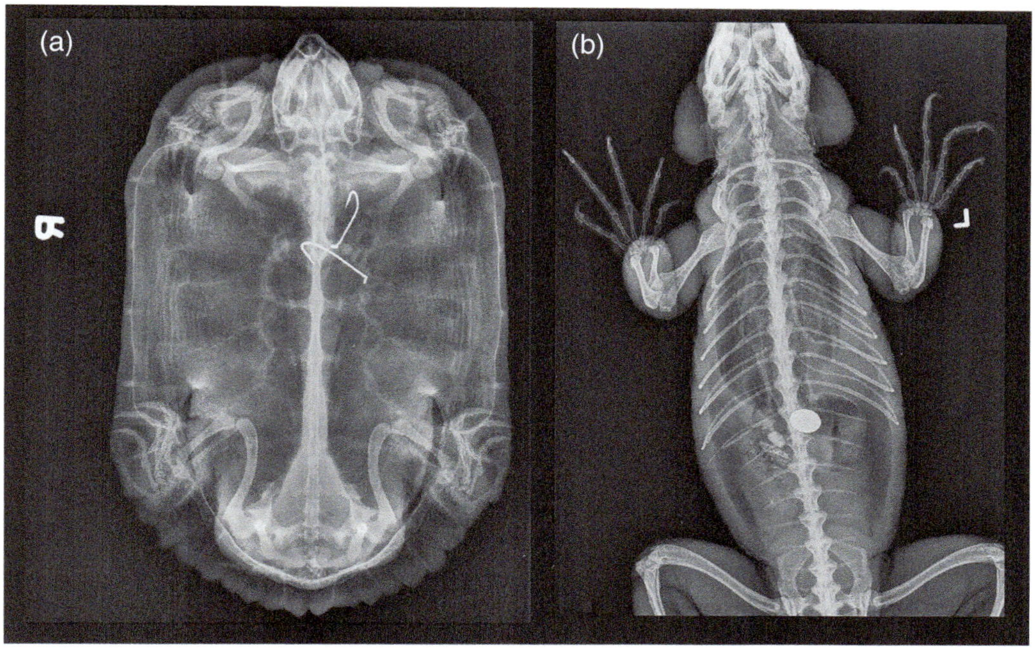

Figure 48.17 Radiographs clearly identify ingested metallic foreign bodies. Two ingested fishhooks in a three-year-old yellow-bellied slider (*Trachemys scripta scripta*), confirmed to be in the esophagus with endoscopy (a). A coin ingested by an eight-year-old male green iguana (*Iguana iguana*) with clinical signs of heavy metal toxicity (b).

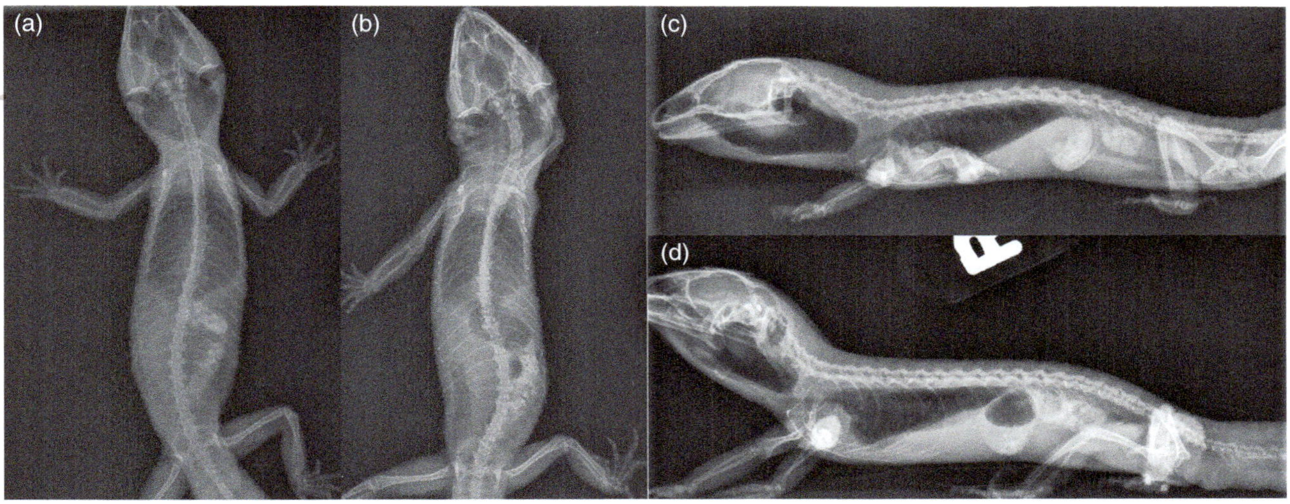

Figure 48.18 Constipation in a one-year-old male leopard gecko (*Eublepharis macularius*). Survey DV and lateral radiographs showing granular mineral material in the region of the colon (a, c). A pneumocolonogram is performed, outlining the material with gas and confirming its presence in the colon (b, d).

be correlated with clinical findings. Dyspnea may result from a coelomic space-occupying mass effect. If coelomic effusion, organomegaly, or an unknown mass effect is concurrently identified, ultrasound, CT, or MRI may be required for further investigation.

Pulmonary hyperinflation may occur secondary to upper respiratory obstructions, such as foreign bodies or soft tissue swellings (Figure 48.21).

Trauma

In cases of trauma, the skeletal structures should be thoroughly assessed for fractures, considering open or closed fracture status, comminution, and articular or physeal involvement. Rib fractures are common in snakes. Complex head or shell fractures may be challenging to fully define radiographically, hence CT is recommended (Figures 48.22 and 48.23). Pulmonary contusions or hemorrhage are seen

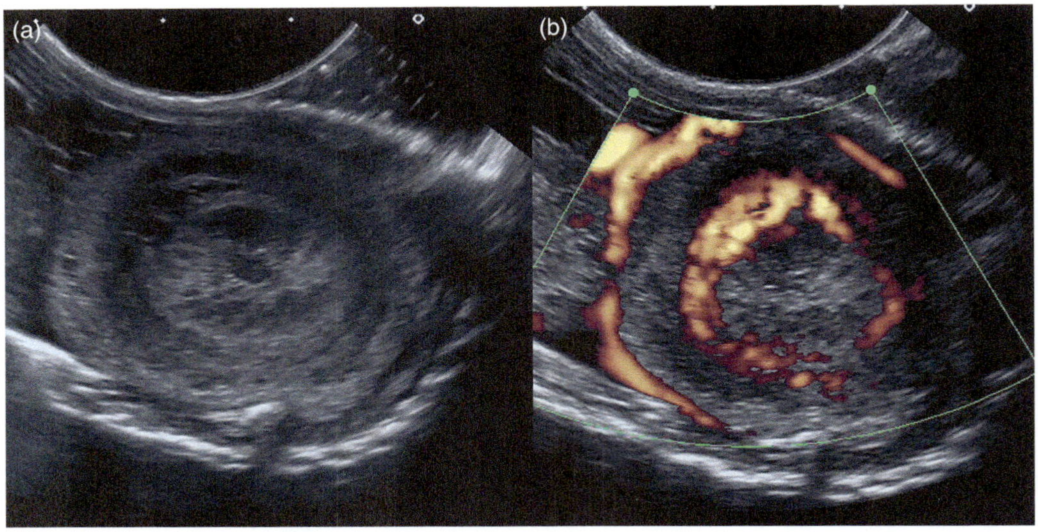

Figure 48.19 Transverse ultrasound images of an intussusception in an adult Savannah monitor (*Varanus exanthematicus*). Concentric hyperechoic and hypoechoic layering of the intestinal segments is seen with B-mode imaging (a) and Doppler confirms a concentric pattern of vascularity (b). Source: Images courtesy of Eric Norman Carmel, DMV, DACVR.

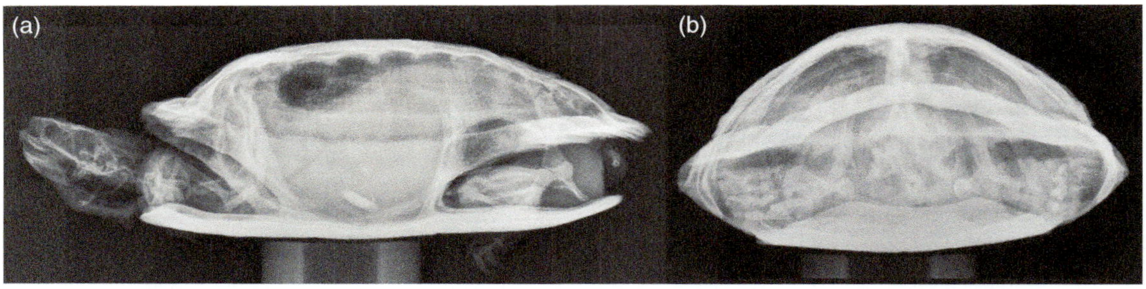

Figure 48.20 Bilateral pneumonia in a six-year-old female red-eared slider turtle (*Trachemys scripta elegans*), lateral (a) and craniocaudal (b) radiographs. There is also an incidental rock gastrointestinal foreign body.

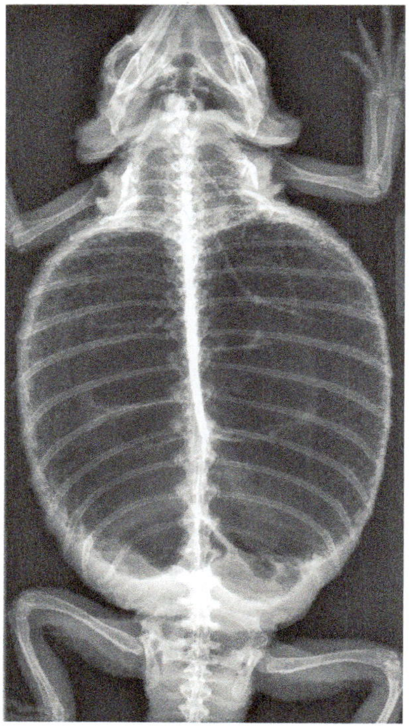

Figure 48.21 Marked pulmonary hyperinflation in a five-year-old female bearded dragon (*Pogona vitticeps*) secondary to a bronchial plug. There is marked hyperlucency and expansion of the lungs bilaterally.

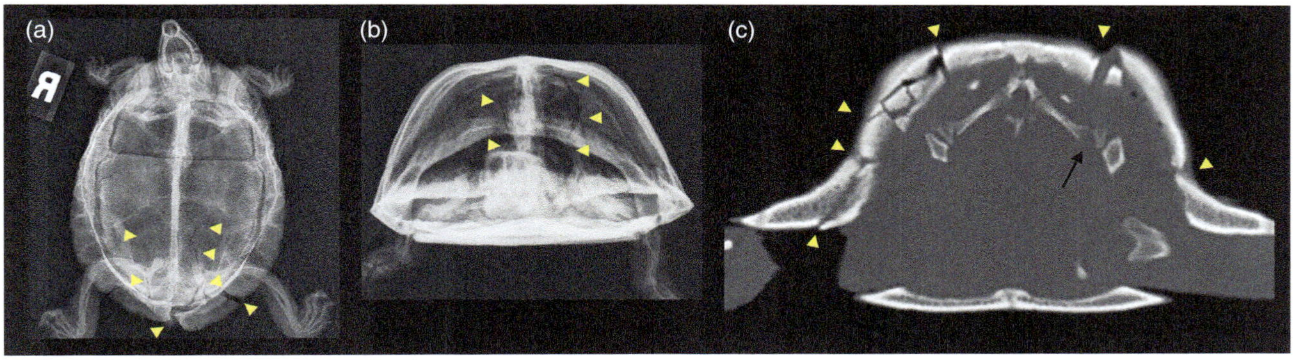

Figure 48.22 Caudal carapace and pelvic fractures (arrowheads) in a box turtle (*Terrapene carolina*) identified on DV (a) and craniocaudal radiographs (b). A transverse CT image (c) permits further characterization of the marked carapace fracture comminution (arrowheads), as well as a left pelvic fracture (arrow).

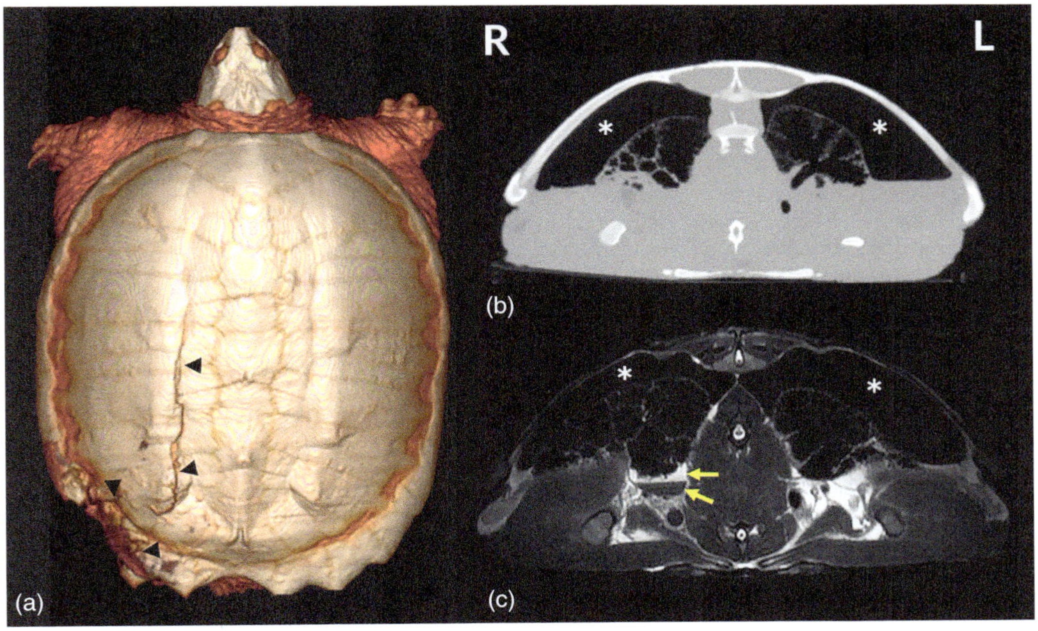

Figure 48.23 Shell fractures in chelonians may result in pulmonary contusions, pneumocoelom, or coelomic hemorrhage, as shown in this common snapping turtle (*Chelydra serpentina*) as the result of vehicular trauma. The fracture is shown on a computed tomographic 3D surface rendering (a, arrowheads). Free gas in the coelom (asterisks) is identified peripheral to the lungs on CT (b) and MRI (c) T2 transverse images at the same level. Note the hyperattenuation (b) and hyperintensity (c) in the retracted lung lobes. Horizontal fluid lines or a "double layer sign" (arrows) indicate coelomic hemorrhage on the MRI (c). Source: Images courtesy of Eric Norman Carmel, DMV, DACVR.

as increased opacity or hyperattenuation in the lungs, and should always be considered with trauma to the carapace in chelonians. Trauma involving the coelomic cavity may result in free fluid or free gas. Large volumes of coelomic effusion or hemorrhage may be evident radiographically, while ultrasound, CT, or MRI may be necessary to identify smaller amounts.

Lameness

Traumatic or pathologic fractures may cause lameness. Evidence of pathologic fracture include decreased mineral density of the bone, osteolysis, or irregular periosteal proliferation. Metabolic bone disease and osteomyelitis represent two underlying etiologies for pathologic fractures (Figures 48.24 and 48.25). Radiographic signs of metabolic bone disease are listed in Box 48.3. Imaging findings should always be correlated with patient clinical signs. The radiographic appearance of osteolysis associated with osteomyelitis or septic arthritis may lag behind clinical signs. Similarly, a radiographic bone lesion may remain visible beyond the resolution of clinical lameness. Fracture healing in reptiles shows less osseous proliferation than mammals, producing more sclerosis, thickening, blunted margins, and endosteal callus. Other chronic causes of

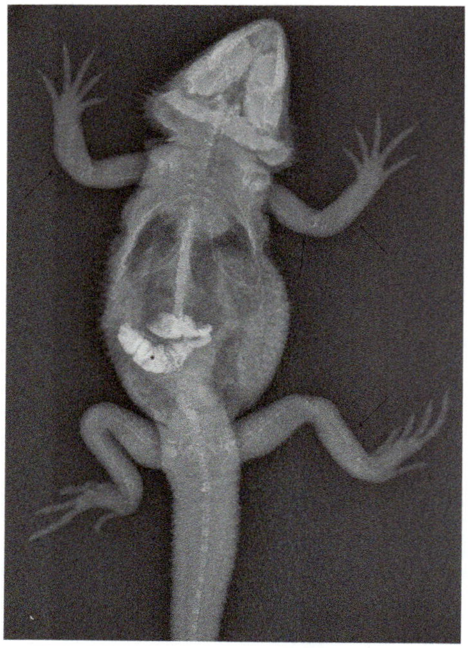

Figure 48.24 Metabolic bone disease and multiple folding pathologic fractures (arrows) in a bearded dragon (*Pogona vitticeps*). The skeleton is markedly decreased in bone opacity, less opaque even than the mineralized gastrointestinal content (asterisk).

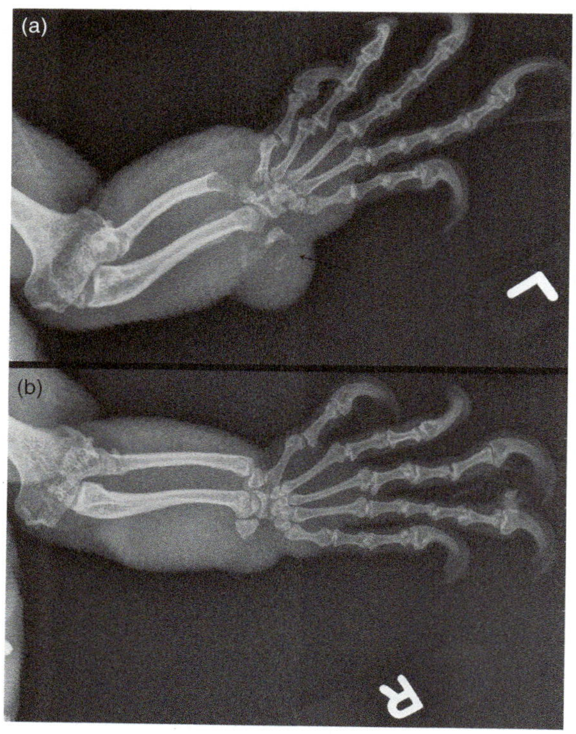

Figure 48.25 Left carpus of a seven-year-old male green iguana (*Iguana iguana*) with marked osteomyelitis of the accessory carpal bone (arrows) and associated soft tissue swelling and abscess formation (a). The normal right carpus is included for comparison (b).

Box 48.3 Radiographic Signs of Metabolic Bone Disease

- Decreased bone opacity/poor corticomedullary distinction
- Thin cortices
- Bowed or undulant long bones
- Folding fractures
- Vertebral deviation or collapse
- Mandible softening
- Angular limb deformities
- Soft tissue swelling

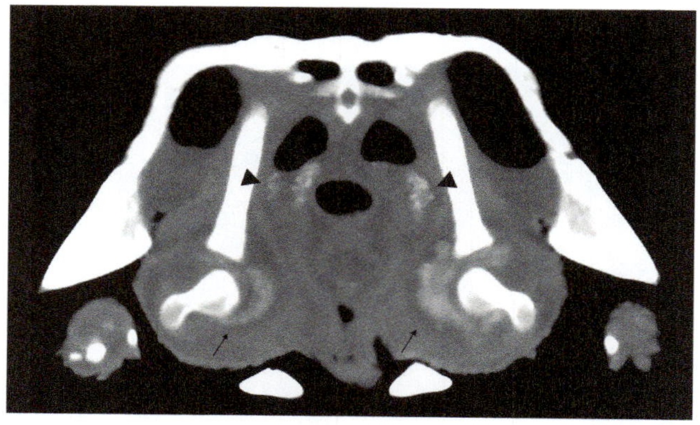

Figure 48.26 Transverse CT image of a seven-year-old female sulcata tortoise (*Centrochelys sulcata*) with gout. There is marked periarticular mineralization at the coxofemoral joints (arrows), as well as bilateral renal mineralization (arrowheads).

lameness include degenerative joint disease affecting the limbs or spine as well as gout. Spinal osteoarthrosis in snakes can limit mobility. Gout may appear as periarticular mineralization at multiple joints (Figure 48.26).

Prolapses

Cloacal prolapse in reptiles may involve the gastrointestinal, reproductive, or urinary tracts. As prolapses are predominantly soft tissue opaque radiographically, contrast studies, ultrasound, CT, MRI, and/or cloacoscopy are often required to identify which structure is prolapsed (Figure 48.27). Images should be thoroughly evaluated for potential underlying causes, such as an intracoelomic mass effect, egg retention, or gastrointestinal ileus.

Reproductive Complications

Radiographically, follicles or eggs are identified as round or ovoid soft tissue opaque structures in the caudal coelom (Figure 48.11). In gravid female lizards and snakes, eggs may be only faintly mineralized, compared to the well-defined, mineral shelled eggs seen in chelonians. Gravid females should be evaluated for egg number, size, shape, position, and overall skeletal bone density. Egg counts are often easier to accomplish on DV views of chelonians and lizards compared to lateral views. Dystocia or egg retention may be obstructive, such as secondary to pelvic fractures, or may be functional (Figure 48.28). Radiographic signs of egg retention include misshapen eggs, collapsed eggs, irregular egg margins, misplaced eggs, and incomplete or excessive egg mineralization. Depending on the stage of development, follicles or egg contents should be homogeneous to concentrically organized (Figure 48.11). Horizontal layering of liquid egg content may indicate latency or lack of viability. Egg rupture can result in egg yolk coelomitis, represented as coelomic effusion (Figure 48.29). Using ultrasound, CT, or MRI, the ruptured eggs may contain disorganized material and gas foci. For viviparous species, fetuses can be identified radiographically if skeletal mineralization has occurred or potentially earlier in development using ultrasound.

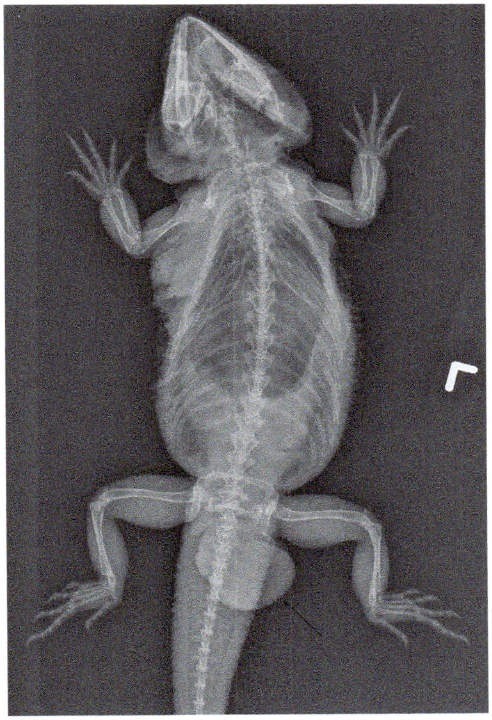

Figure 48.27 Cloacal prolapse (arrow) in a two-year-old female bearded dragon (*Pogona vitticeps*) with reported oviposition three days prior. Surgery confirmed prolapse of the colon.

Urinary Tract

Calculus formation is common in chelonians and to a lesser extent in lizards; however, calculi may or may not result in clinical signs. Though calculi are often mineral opaque, calculi may be radiolucent. Localization may require US, CT, or even MRI (Figure 48.30).

Reptile kidneys are not visible radiographically unless enlarged and/or increased in opacity. These radiographic signs may indicate infection, nephrocalcinosis, gout (Figure 48.26), degeneration, or rarely neoplasia. Ultrasonographic or advanced imaging may help characterize the kidneys.

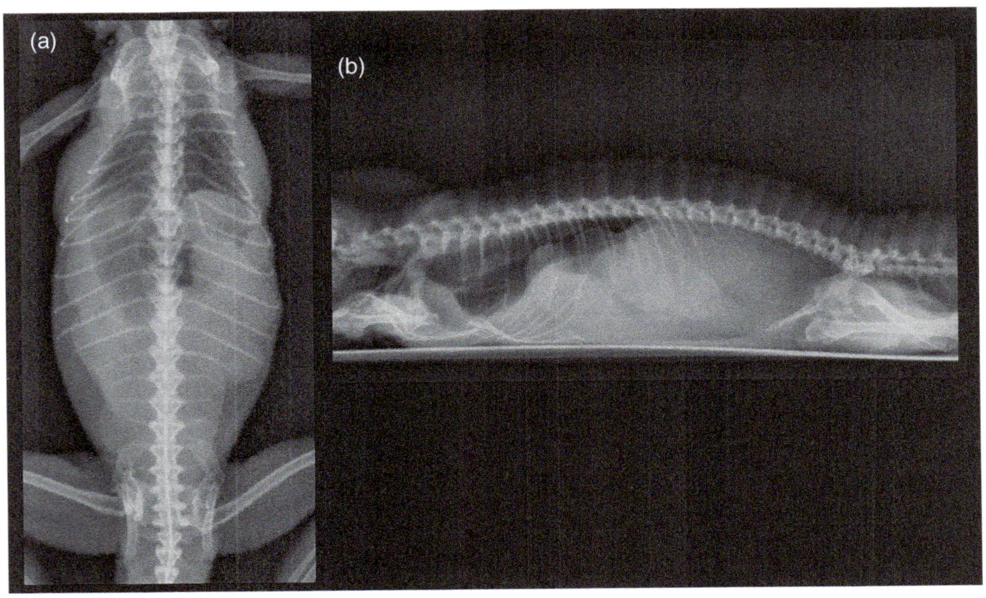

Figure 48.28 Dystocia in a five-year-old female Chinese water dragon (*Physignathus cocincinus*), dorsoventral (a) and lateral (b) radiographs. There are large, partially mineralized eggs with mild variation in shape, one of which is positioned at the cranial aspect of the pelvic canal.

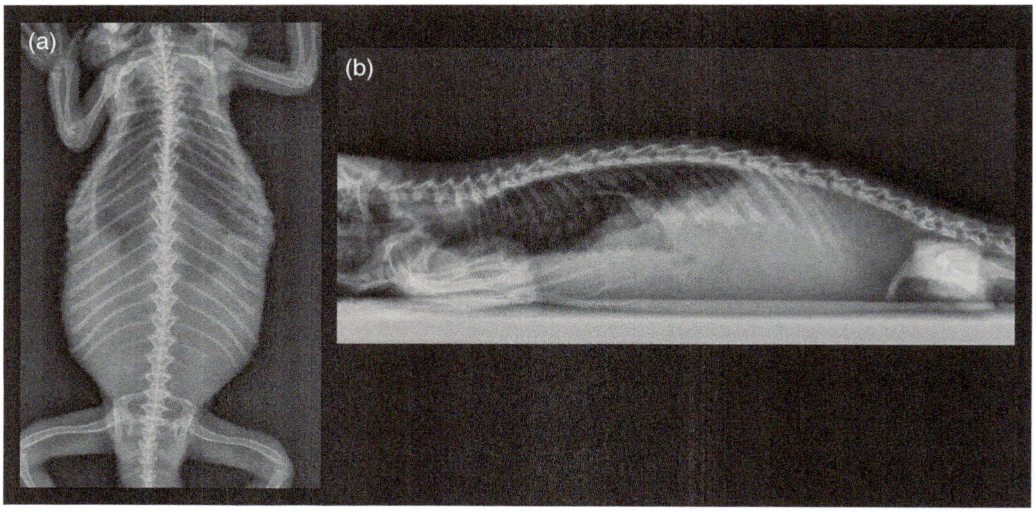

Figure 48.29 Egg yolk coelomitis in a two-year-old female bearded dragon (*Pogona vitticeps*). The caudal coelomic structures are obscured by the coelomic effusion on dorsoventral (a) and lateral (b) radiographs.

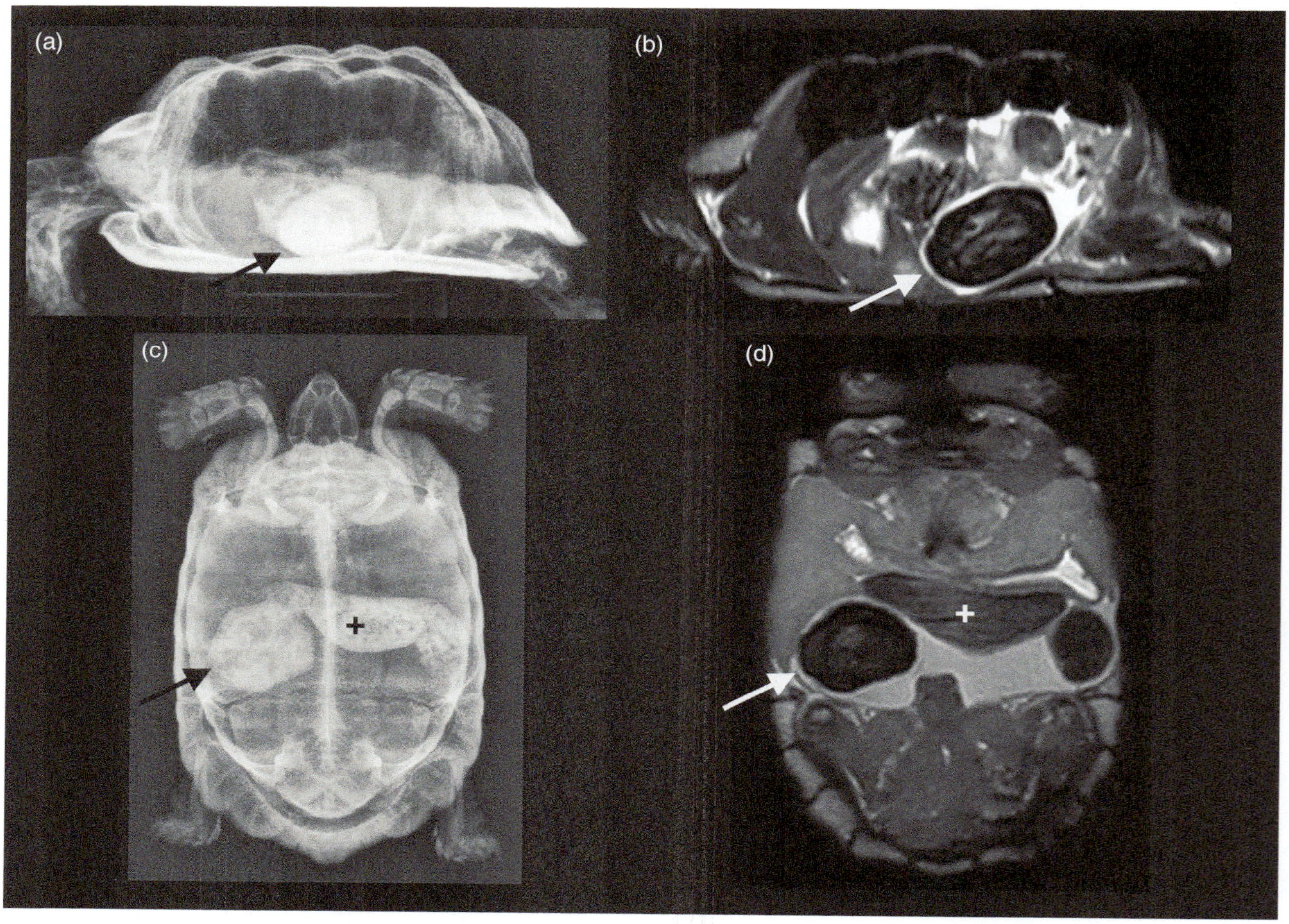

Figure 48.30 Large calculus in the allantois of a six-year-old male Egyptian tortoise (*Testudo kleinmanni*). Lateral (a) and dorsoventral (c) radiographs showing the calculus in the mid ventral abdomen (arrow), caudal and to the right of granular mineral gastrointestinal material (+). Sagittal plane T2 (b) and dorsal plane proton density (d) MRI. The calculus is surrounded by T2 hyperintense fluid in the allantois and is separate from the gastrointestinal tract content (+).

References

1 Pees, M., Kiefer, I., Ludewig, E. et al. (2011). Reptiles. In: *Diagnostic Imaging of Exotic Pets*, 1e (eds. M.E. Krautwald-Junghanns, M. Pees, S. Reese and T. Tully), 309–439. Hannover: Schlutersche.

2 Divers, S.J. and Stahl, S.J. (eds.) (2019). Diagnostic imaging. In: *Mader's Reptile and Amphibian Medicine and Surgery*, 486–588. St. Louis: Elsevier Inc.

3 Banzato, T., Hellebuyck, T., Van Caelenberg, A. et al. (2013). A review of diagnostic imaging of snakes and lizards. *Vet. Rec.* 173: 43–49.

4 Grosset, C., Daniarux, L., Guzman, D.S. et al. (2014). Radiographic anatomy and barium sulfate contrast transit time of the gastrointestinal tract of bearded dragons (*Pogona vitticeps*). *Vet. Radiol. Ultrasound* 55 (3): 241–250.

5 Banzato, T., Russo, E., Finotti, L. et al. (2012). *Am. J. Vet. Res.* 73: 996–1001.

6 Long, C.T., Page, R.B., Howard, A.M. et al. (2010). Comparison of Gastrografin to barium sulfate as a gastrointestinal contrast agent in red-eared slider turtles (*Trachemys scripta elegans*). *Vet. Radiol. Ultrasound* 51 (1): 42–47.

7 DiBello, A., Valastro, C., Staffieri, F., and Crovace, A. (2006). Contrast radiography of the gastrointestinal tract in sea turtles. *Vet. Radiol. Ultrasound* 47 (4): 351–354.

8 Smith, D., Dobson, H., and Spence, E. (2001). Gastrointestinal studies in the green iguana: technique and reference values. *Vet. Radiol. Ultrasound* 42 (6): 515–520.

9 Meyer, J. (1998). Gastrografin as a gastrointestinal contrast agent in the Greek tortoise (*Testudo hermanni*). *J. Zoo Wildl. Med.* 29 (2): 183–189.

10 Taylor, S.K., Citino, S.B., Zdziarski, J.M., and Bush, R.M. (1996). Radiographic anatomy and barium sulfate transit time of the gastrointestinal tract of the leopard tortoise (*Testudo pardalis*). *J. Zoo Wildl. Med.* 27 (2): 180–186.

11 Wallack, S.T. (2003). *The Handbook of Veterinary Contrast Radiography*, 1e, 1–25. Solana Beach: Seth T Wallack, 74–75, 89.

12 Banzato, T., Russo, E., Finotti, L. et al. (2012). Ultrasonographic anatomy of the coelomic organs of boid snakes (*Boa constrictor imperator, Python regius, Python molurus molurus, and Python curtus*). *Am. J. Vet. Res.* 73: 634–645.

13 Bucy, D.S., Guzman, D.S., and Zwingenberger, A. (2015). Ultrasonographic anatomy of bearded dragons (*Pogona vitticeps*). *J. Am. Vet. Med. Assoc.* 246: 868–876.

14 Holland, M.F., Hernandez-Divers, S., and Frank, P.M. (2008). Ultrasonographic appearance of the coelomic cavity in healthy green iguanas. *J. Am. Vet. Med. Assoc.* 233: 590–596.

15 Schroff, S., Starck, J.M., and Krautwald-Junghanns, P.M. (2012). Echocardiography in boid snakes: demonstration and blood flow measurements. *Tierarztl Prax Ausg K Kleintiere Heimtiere* 3: 180–190.

16 Bartlett, H.L., Escalera, R.B., Patel, S.S. et al. (2010). Echocardiographic assessment of cardiac morphology and function in *Xenopus*. *Comp. Med.* 60 (2): 107–113.

17 Gustavsen, K.A., Saunders, A.B., Young, B.D. et al. (2014). Echocardiographic and radiographic findings in a cohort of healthy adult green iguanas (*Iguana iguana*). *J. Vet. Cardiol.* 16: 186–196.

18 Poser, H., Russello, G., Zanella, A. et al. (2011). Two-dimensional and Doppler echocardiographic findings in healthy non-sedated red-eared slider terrapins (*Trachemys scripta elegans*). *Vet. Res. Commun.* 35: 511–520.

19 Gumpenberger, M. (2011). Chelonians. In: *Veterinary Computed Tomography*, 1e (eds. T. Schwarz and J. Saunders), 533–544. West Sussex: Wiley-Blackwell.

20 Banzato, T., Selleri, P., Veladiano, I.A. et al. (2012). Comparative evaluation of the cadaveric, radiographic and computed tomographic anatomy of the heads of green iguana (*Iguana iguana*), common tegu (*Tupinambis merianae*) and bearded dragon (*Pogona vitticeps*). *BMC Vet. Res.* 8: 53.

21 Valente, A.L., Cuenca, R., Zamora, M. et al. (2007). Computed tomography of the vertebral column and coelomic structures in the normal loggerhead sea turtle (*Caretta caretta*). *Vet. J.* 174: 362–370.

22 Pees, M., Kiefer, I., Thielebein, J. et al. (2009). Computed tomography of the lung of healthy snakes of the species *Python regius, Boa constrictor, Python reticulatus, Morelia viridis, Epicrates cenchria,* and *Morelia spilota*. *Vet. Radiol. Ultrasound* 50 (5): 487–491.

23 Anderson, C.L., Kabalka, G.W., Layne, D.G. et al. (2000). Noninvasive high field MRI brain imaging of the garter snake (*Thamnophis sirtalis*). *Copeia* (1): 265–269.

49

Clinical Pathology

Nicola Di Girolamo

Exotic pet and Zoological Medicine, Oklahoma State University, Stillwater, OK, United States

CONTENTS

The emergency veterinarian is often required to interpret analyses of blood, urine, and other body fluids. Clinical pathology is as fundamental in reptiles as in other species. However, most clinical pathology techniques are extrapolated from small mammal medicine, and are therefore limited in reptiles. The clinician should always consider the results of any analyses critically, as (i) there are large interspecific and intraspecific (e.g. sexual and seasonal) differences that may lead to inaccurate or erroneous clinical conclusions [1–3], and (ii) minimal research has been conducted to correlate mere analytical results to patient-relevant outcomes.

Although reference intervals for hematology, biochemistry, and urine analyses are published for several species, cutoff values are more often determined based only on presumed healthy individuals. Therefore, sensitivity and specificity of upper and lower reference intervals are unknown [4]. Until more definitive cutoffs are determined using populations that include healthy and diseased individuals, reference intervals should be used only as a rough guideline. The results of the analysis should be considered in combination with clinical signs and results of ancillary diagnostic techniques, instead of using them alone to make a definitive diagnosis of the condition of the reptile patient.

Hematology

Cell Blood Count (CBC)

Routine hematology may be performed on very small reptiles as only a few drops of blood are needed. The packed cell volume (PCV) may be determined through microhematocrit, while the total and differential leukocyte count, as well as the examination of blood cell morphology may be performed on a stained blood film (Figure 49.1). Hematocrit in reptiles is usually determined on blood samples collected in lithium heparin tubes as other anticoagulants (e.g. sodium citrate and K3-EDTA) may result in hemolysis [5, 6]. Manual methods for obtaining a WBC include estimated

Exotic Animal Emergency and Critical Care Medicine, First Edition. Edited by Jennifer E. Graham, Grayson A. Doss, and Hugues Beaufrère.

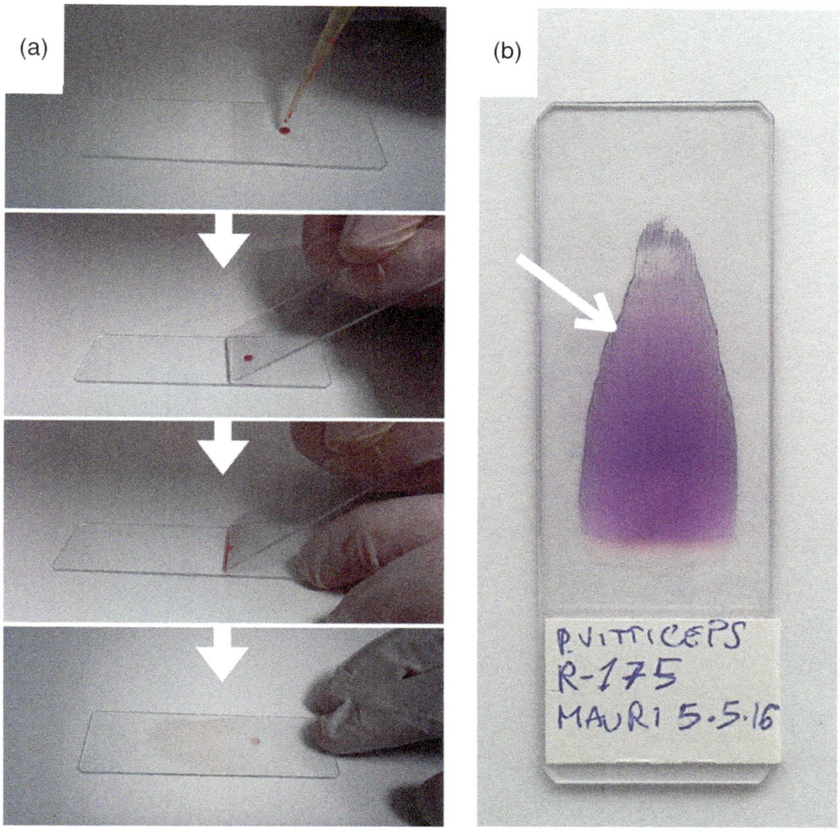

Figure 49.1 Preparation of a blood smear with the slide-to-slide method (a). After staining, the ideal counting site is where a monolayer of cells is present (arrow) (b).

counts from blood smears, semidirect methods translated from mammal hematology (e.g. erythrocyte Unopette system, Phloxine B method), and direct methods including the Natt and Herrick solution that has been developed specifically for avian and reptile blood cell counts. The estimated count method is probably the more common WBC counting method used in an emergency setting. The average number of leukocytes per field on at least 10 fields (at 400×) is multiplied by 150–200 to determine an estimated WBC [7]. Some intrinsic error is expected due to the uneven distribution of cells on the smear.

RBC Assessment

Reptilian erythrocytes are ellipsoidal cells with permanent nuclei. Their size ranges in length from 14 to 23 mm and in width from 8 to 14 mm and may adapt to external environment (e.g. latitudes) [8]. The nucleus is central, oval to round, and contains dense purple chromatin. The cytoplasm may contain rounded basophilic inclusions. These inclusions may be an artifact caused during smear preparation or may be pathologic, as in case of boids' inclusion body disease and iridovirus in bearded dragons (Figure 49.2) [9]. The reptile erythrocyte life span is much longer than that of mammals and birds, lasting over 500 days [10].

Immature erythrocytes in reptiles are rounder than mature ones, with a larger nucleus and polychromatophilic when Romanowsky-stained (Figure 49.3). They have a distinct ring of aggregated reticulum around the nucleus. The normal number of immature erythrocytes in reptiles is unknown; however, values around 2–5% of the total are considered normal [11, 12]. Old erythrocytes have swollen cytoplasm and nuclei with dark chromatin [13]. A small number of anucleated erythrocytes (erythroplastids) are found in clinically healthy animals.

WBC Assessment

In order to perform a complete leukocyte evaluation, a total leukocyte count, differential, and morphologic assessment are required.

Heterophils

Heterophils are the most common granulocytes and are analogous to neutrophils in mammals. In chelonians and snakes, they have a peripheral, round, or oval nucleus characterized by clumped blue chromatin (Figure 49.4a–d). In

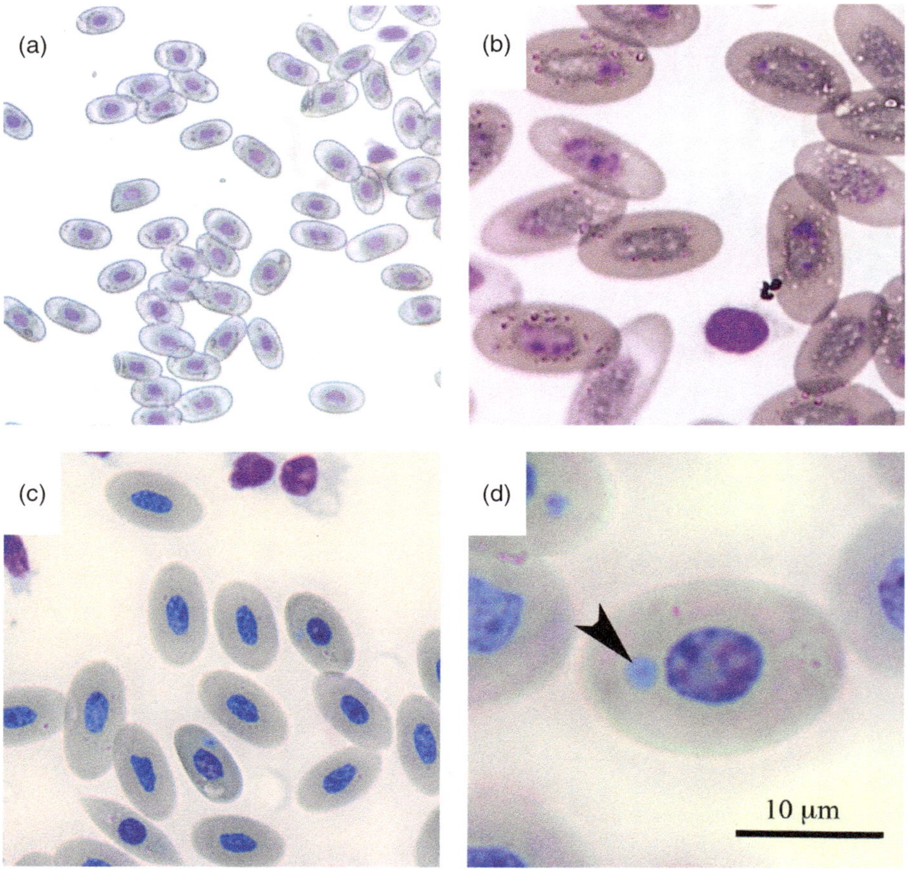

Figure 49.2 Differentiation of artifacts and inclusion bodies in reptilian erythrocytes. Smear preparation artifacts, including presence of vacuoles and improper staining of erythrocyte cytoplasm (a, b). Intraerythrocytic cytoplasmic inclusions in bearded dragons affected by iridovirus (arrowhead) (c, d). Diff-Quik stain. Magnification is approximately 400× (a) and 1000× (b–d). *Source:* (b) Photo courtesy of Alessandro Bellese; (c,d) Photos courtesy of Claire Grosset.

lizards, the nucleus is generally multilobed (Figure 49.4e,f). The cytoplasm contains variable numbers of oval, spindle-shaped granules that may be transparent, eosinophilic, or bright orange depending on the staining [1, 13–15]. The size of heterophils varies but they are generally slightly larger than erythrocytes. Toxic heterophils may be observed as a response to systemic inflammation or presence of infectious agents. They are typically larger, with an altered nuclear shape, and increased basophilia of the cytoplasm with vacuolization and toxic granulation (Figure 49.5).

Basophils

Basophils are characterized by large, extremely chromophilic granules that often obscure the nucleus (Figure 49.6) [1, 13]. The granules are deep purple-to-blue with common staining. When visible, the nucleus is slightly eccentric and rounded. Basophils are oval in some reptiles [13].

Eosinophils

Eosinophils (Figure 49.7) have an eccentric purple nucleus and a cytoplasm with chromophilic granules that are darker and rounder than in heterophils (Figure 49.8) [13]. In some species (e.g. green iguanas and tegus), granules stain blue-green with Romanowsky-type stains [15].

Monocytes and Azurophils

Currently, there is still some uncertainty on the differentiation of monocytes and azurophils and their role in different taxa. Monocytes may be the largest leukocytes, however they are variably sized and can be half the size of an erythrocyte [15]. Their nucleus is variable in shape and often oval and indented (bean-shaped); azurophilic granules may or may not be present in non-squamate reptiles (Figure 49.9) [15, 16]. Azurophils are a different cell type with similar function as neutrophils. They are typical of snakes but can be also found in other reptile groups. When colored with Wright–Giemsa stain, azurophils have blue cytoplasm and azurophilic (pink-purple) cytoplasmic granules that typically occupy the peripheral areas of the cytoplasm. The nucleus is dark pink with dense chromatin [14, 16, 17].

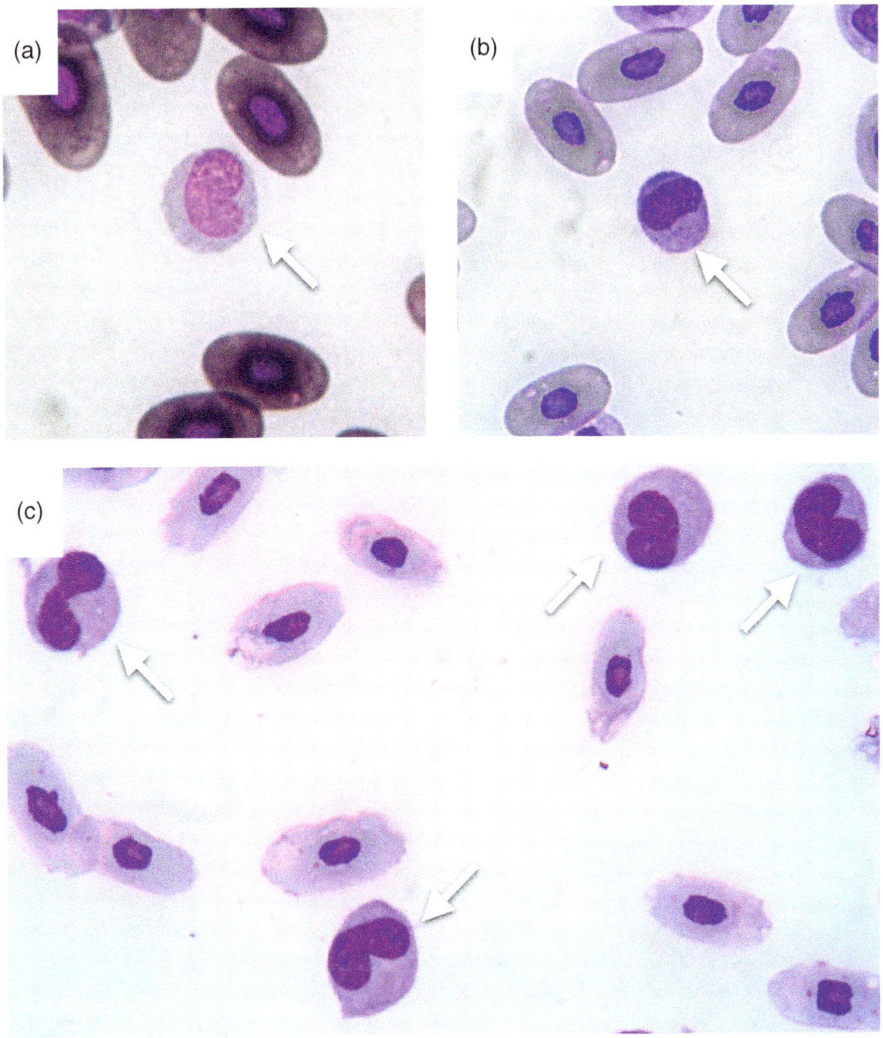

Figure 49.9 Monocytes in reptiles (arrows). Mature monocyte in a Hermann's tortoise (*Testudo hermanni*) (a). Mature monocyte in a marginated tortoise (*Testudo marginata*) (b). Marked monocytosis in a Hermann's tortoise with an active herpesviral infection (c). Diff-Quik stain. Approximately 1000×. *Source:* a: Photo courtesy of Alessandro Bellese.

nor sensitive for diagnosing liver disease in reptiles [41, 42]. ALT activity is higher in reptilian liver, kidney, and cardiac muscle, but occurs in many tissues [41, 43]. ALT activity increases with acute hepatocellular necrosis [44], but did not increase in green iguanas with acute hepatic insufficiency [45]. Also, increases in plasma LDH and AST activities are not specific for liver damage, as levels are highest in cardiac and skeletal muscles and they are present in other tissues [43]. Increased plasma ALP in reptiles, has been associated with hyperparathyroidism and bone diseases, such as Paget's disease, rather than being seen with hepatobiliary pathology [46].

CK

Creatine kinase (CK) has high activity in skeletal and cardiac muscle in iguanas [42], while in turtles it also has moderate activity in the central nervous system and gastrointestinal tissue [41] as well as the kidneys in snakes [47]. High CK values do not always indicate overt muscle disease [42].

GGT

Gamma-glutamyltransferase (GGT) is of limited clinical usefulness in squamates because of little to no activity in most tissue [42, 47]. GGT is active in the kidneys of chelonians [41, 43], but a change in levels with kidney disorders is unclear due to possible elimination through the urine rather than the blood [28].

Bile Acids

Bile acids (3α-hydroxy bile acids) are probably the most reliable biochemical indicator of hepatic function, with a

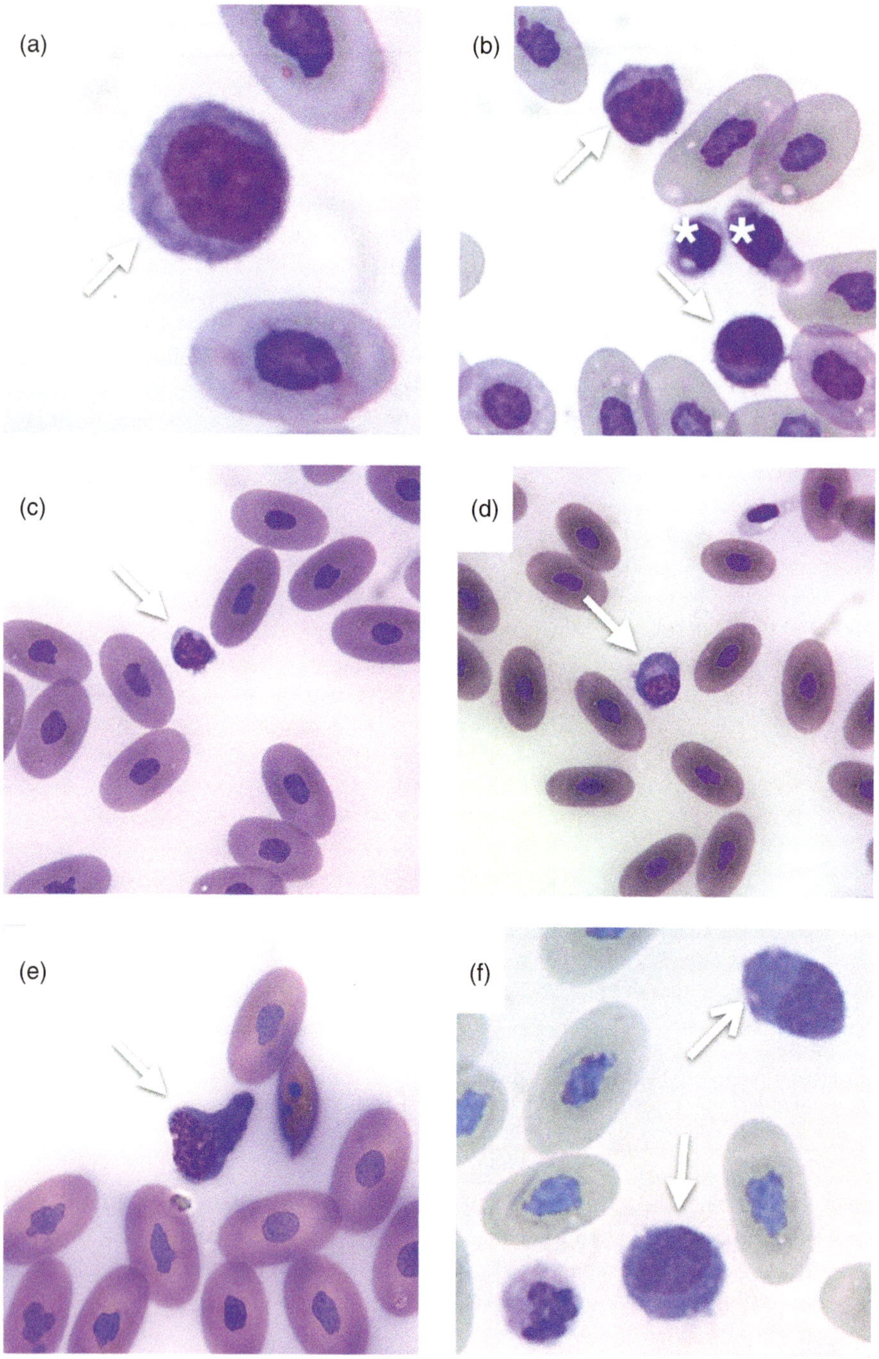

Figure 49.10 Lymphocytes in reptiles (arrows). Mature lymphocytes in marginated tortoises (*Testudo marginata*) (a, b); lymphocytes differ with thrombocytes (asterisks) in shape and size. Mature lymphocytes in a boa (*Boa constrictor*) (c). Reactive lymphocytes in a boa (d, e); notice the pseudopodal extension. Mature lymphocyte and plasmacytoid lymphocyte (empty arrow) in a veiled chameleon (*Chameleo calyptratus*) (f). Diff-Quik stain. Approximately 1000×. *Source:* (c–e): Photos courtesy of Alessandro Bellese.

transient increase following acute hepatic insult [45]. Fasting should be considered in selected species. Fasting bile acid concentrations are significantly lower than postprandial levels in the green iguana but not for red-eared sliders [48, 49].

Chol/TG

Cholesterol and triglycerides are synthetized by the liver and decreases are expected with liver failure [50]. However, plasma cholesterol and triglyceride concentrations in reptiles may vary secondary to nonhepatic disorders, or with

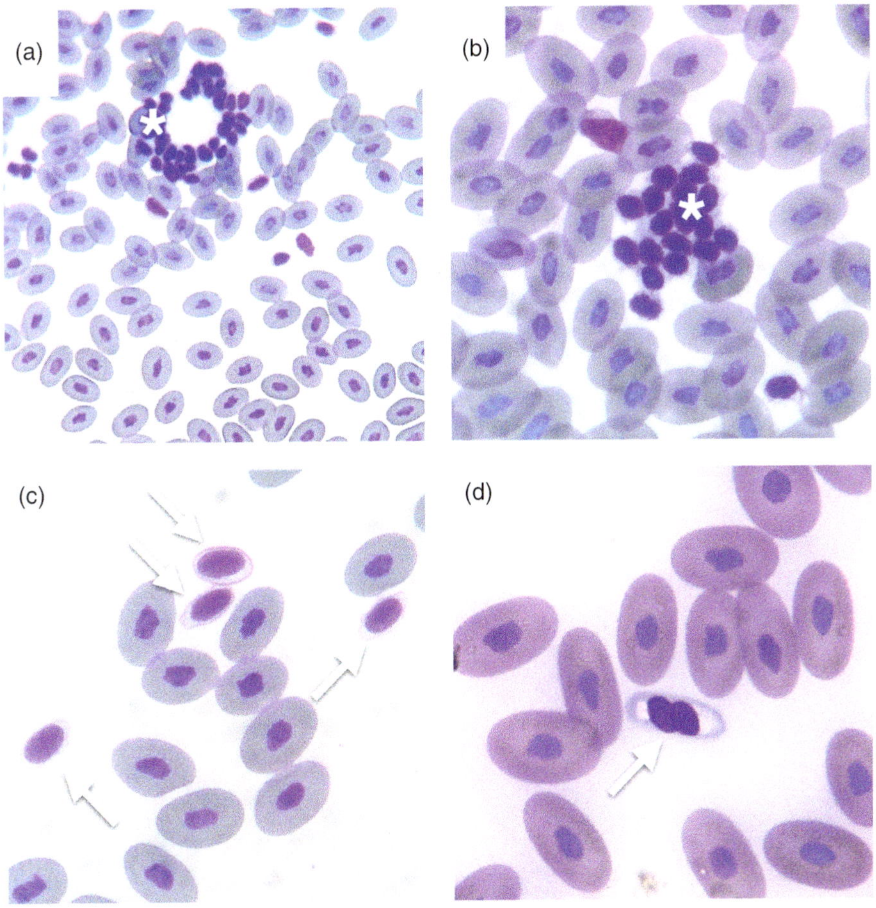

Figure 49.11 Thrombocytes in reptiles (arrows). Clumps of thrombocytes (asterisks) in bearded dragons (*Pogona vitticeps*) (a, b); these aggregations are common and explain the lack of thrombocytes in other areas of the smear. Mature thrombocytes in a bearded dragon (c). Thrombocyte at the end of mitosis in a red-eared slider turtle (*Trachemys scripta*) (d). Diff-Quik stain. Approximately 1000×. *Source:* (d): Photo courtesy of Alessandro Bellese.

season and sex [3, 28]. Hypercholesterolemia has been associated with development of xanthomatosis in mammals [51, 52], but a link has not been documented in reptiles [53].

Glucose

Blood glucose concentration in reptiles generally range between 60 and 100 mg/dl (3.33–5.55 mmol/l) [28]. Glucose concentration in whole blood decreases with sample storage time and prompt analysis is suggested [6].

Hypoglycemia may occur with hepatobiliary disease, septicemia or pancreatic islet cell tumors [54]. Although it is suggested that hypoglycemia can occur with starvation, this is not well-documented. A tortoise trapped for several months without food or water had a normal blood glucose value (70 mg/dl) [55]. This suggests that due to peculiar adaptability of reptiles, protein catabolism may be sufficient to maintain glucose concentration in the absence of any food intake for prolonged periods.

Hyperglycemia is an unspecific finding in reptiles. Physiological increases in glucose are expected during midsummer [3]. Persistent hyperglycemia has been associated with diabetes and pancreatitis in turtles, somatostatinomas (i.e. gastric neuroendocrine carcinoma) in bearded dragons, and a renal adenocarcinoma in a Chinese water dragon [56–59]. Hyperglycemia may also be a sequela of systemic disorders and stress.

Amylase/Lipase

In reptiles, amylase and lipase are the enzymes with greatest tissue specificity, with activity found only in pancreatic samples [41–43]. However, the wide range of plasma activity of amylase limits its diagnostic usefulness [42]. Further studies on amylase and lipase including reptiles with confirmed pancreatitis are required in order to ascertain the diagnostic accuracy of these enzymes.

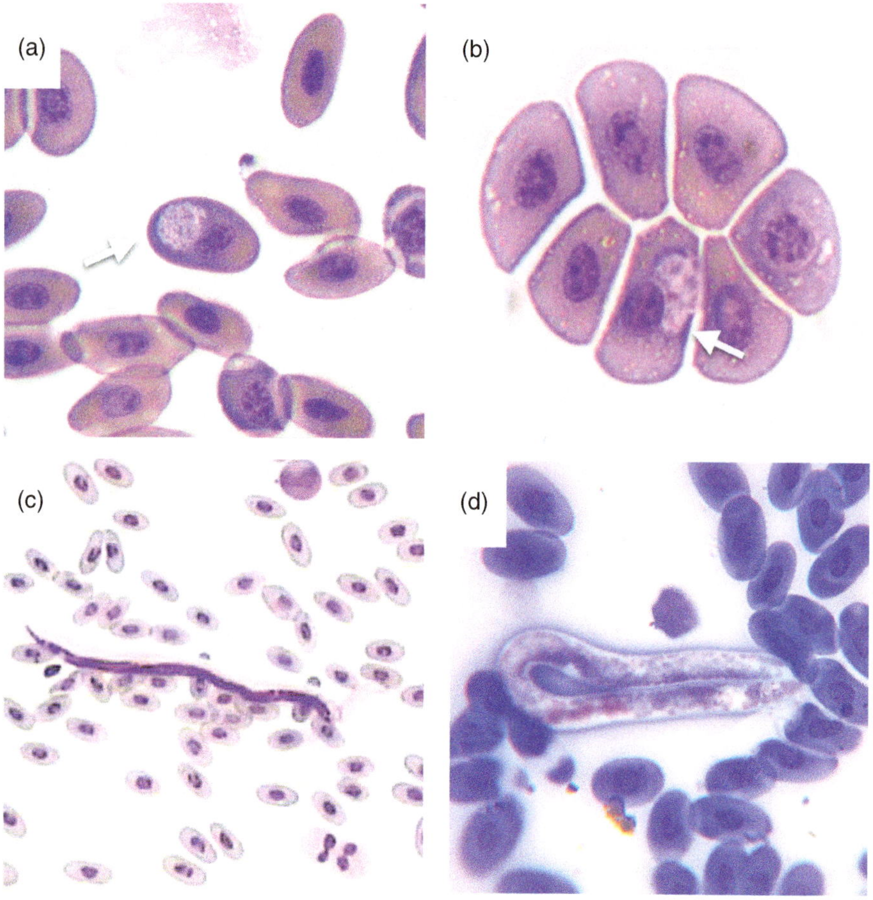

Figure 49.12 Hemoparasites in reptiles. Microgametocytes of *Plasmodium* spp. (arrows) in a Mwanza flat-headed rock agama (*Agama mwanzae*) (a, b). Circulating microfilaria (*Foleyella* spp.) in panther chameleons (*Furcifer pardalis*) (c, d). Hemacolor stain. Approximately 1000× (a, b, d) and 400× (c). *Source:* Photos courtesy of Mattia Bielli.

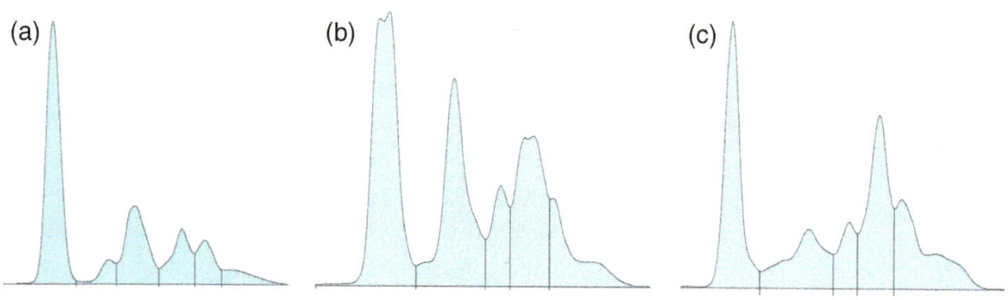

Figure 49.13 Protein electrophoresis in bearded dragons (*Pogona vitticeps*). Representative protein electrophoresis in a clinically healthy bearded dragon (a). Bisalbuminemia and increase of alpha and beta fractions (b). Bisalbuminemia is a common finding with unclear clinical significance. Increase of beta fraction (c). *Source:* Photos courtesy of Gloria Isani and Nicola Di Girolamo.

Urine Evaluation

Sample Collection

Manual/Voided Samples

Obtaining urine samples from reptiles presents some difficulties. Soaking reptiles often results in urination and defecation but makes obtaining appropriate urine samples impossible. Many chelonians will urinate and defecate as soon as they are manipulated [60]. Therefore, materials for urine collection should be prepared before removing the reptile from its kennel or its enclosure.

Manual voiding of the urinary bladder is difficult to impossible in most reptiles. In chelonians, the urinary bladder may be gently compressed with digital pressure from the prefemoral fossae. In lizards with urinary bladders (e.g. iguanas), compression of the urinary bladder is performed similar to mammals. Collecting urine samples

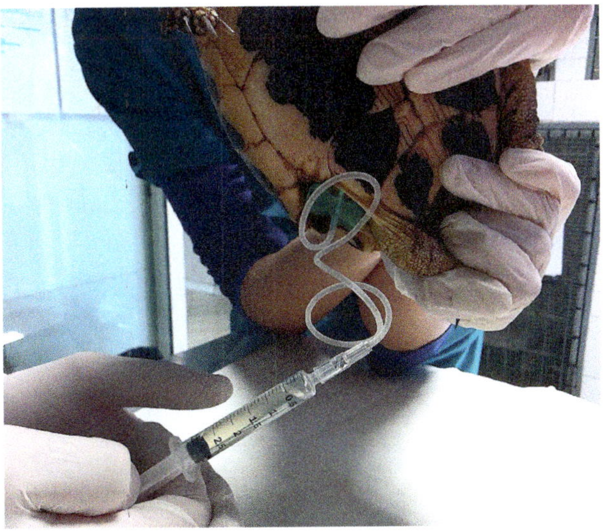

Figure 49.14 Cystocentesis in a Hermann's tortoise (*Testudo hermanni*). Urinary bladder distension was verified by ultrasonography before the procedure was performed.

in snakes and in lizards lacking a urinary bladder is complicated. Use of appropriate designed cages (i.e. with a mesh and no substrate) permit collection of urine samples but may require several days.

Cystocentesis Samples

Cystocentesis is best performed under ultrasonographic guidance or at least after visualization of urine in the urinary bladder. In lizards that have urinary bladders (e.g. iguanas) cystocentesis is performed via coelomic puncture. Puncture is not performed on ventral midline in order to avoid the ventral abdominal vein. In chelonians with distended urinary bladders, cystocentesis is performed via the prefemoral fossae (Figure 49.14).

Catheter Samples

Urinary catheter placement in reptiles is difficult and requires specific instrumentation. In chelonians, endoscopic assistance is mandatory (Figure 49.15). In anesthetized lizards, the urinary bladder can be catheterized

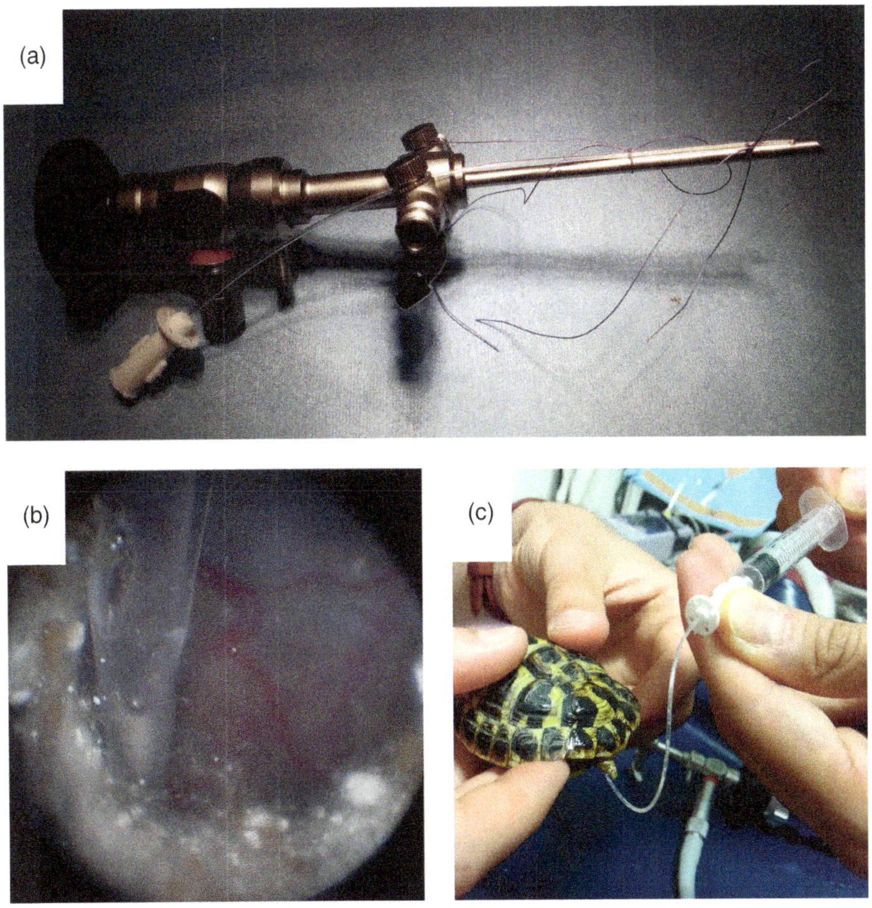

Figure 49.15 Endoscopic-assisted urinary bladder catheterization in a juvenile Hermann's tortoise (*Testudo hermanni*). A 1-mm urinary catheter is fastened to the endoscope with two stay ligatures (a long tail is left on each ligature). Once the endoscope accesses the urinary bladder, the long tails of the ligatures are pulled releasing the catheter from the endoscope (a). Endoscopic view of the catheter in the urinary bladder (b). Obtaining urine samples from the catheter. Notice the presence of thick urates (c).

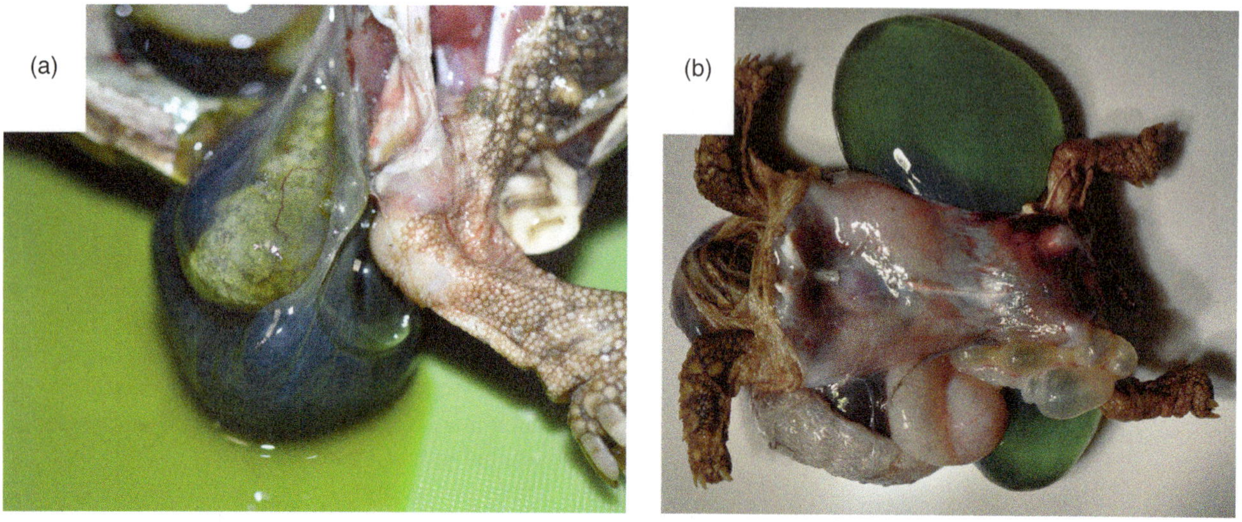

Figure 49.16 Presence of green urine during postmortem of an African spurred tortoise (*Centrochelys sulcata*) (a) and a leopard tortoise (*Stigmochelys pardalis*) (b). Although green urine has been anecdotally linked to hepatic failure, its significance remains unclear.

without endoscopy [61]. The vent is opened with a vaginal speculum and a Foley catheter inserted through the cloaca and directed dorsally into the colon. The catheter cuff is inflated and proper catheter placement verified by observing fecal matter with application of gentle negative pressure. The catheter is retracted gently to partially evert the cloaca. This permits visualization of the urethral opening and subsequent urinary bladder catheterization.

Volume/Appearance

Urine appearance varies widely, depending on the species and their environmental adaptation. Tortoise and lizard urine is composed by a liquid portion along with small to moderate amounts of white urates. The liquid portion varies from colorless to yellow. Biliverdinuria may be observed, and has been anecdotally associated with liver disease (Figure 49.16) [62]. Snakes also produce a liquid portion of urine along with large amounts of white to yellow, solid urates.

Urinalysis

Urinalysis has been the focus of little research in reptile medicine, and using mammalian parameters to evaluate reptile samples may be inappropriate or clinically unhelpful [60, 62]. Reptiles demonstrate great variation in glomerular filtration rate and tubular absorptive and secretory processes. The final urine is affected by the species' ability to modify composition and volume of the urine through the cloaca or the bladders (urinary and accessory), and to excrete ions extrarenally [63]. As with blood, urine must be collected and processed properly. The urine sample should be cooled to 4 °C (39 °F) as soon as possible. Specific gravity may be measured with a refractometer. In clinically healthy Mediterranean tortoises, specific gravity ranged from 1.003 to 1.014 (average: 1.008), while tortoises with suspected renal disease had an average specific gravity of 1.013 and values up to 1.034 [62]. In healthy and diseased box turtles (*Terrapene* sp.), urine specific gravity ranged from 1.001 to 1.019 [60]. In European tortoises with renal disease, urinary AST, urea, calcium, CK, creatinine, glucose, LDH, ammonia, and phosphorus were higher than in clinically healthy conspecifics [64].

Dipstick

There are no dipsticks currently validated for urinalysis in reptiles. Commercial urine dipsticks (Multistix7, Bayer Co., Elkhart, IN, USA) have been used for evaluation of glucose, bilirubin, ketones, occult blood, pH, and protein in reptile urine [60]. Bilirubin, ketones and large quantities of protein are not expected. Traces of blood may be found in normal chelonians.

Urine Sediment Exam

The urine sediment exam is performed as in mammals, after centrifugation and removal of the supernatant fraction. Bacteria and epithelial cells are expected to be present in almost all samples obtained with spontaneous urination, due to the passage through the cloaca. Bacteria may also be present when samples are obtained through cystocentesis [64]. Urate crystals and uric acid crystals may be found in clinically healthy reptiles (Figure 49.17). The number of epithelial cells and renal casts are increased in tortoises with renal disease [64]. Calcium oxalate, cholesterol, cystine, hippuric acid, leucine, sodium urate, tyrosine, bilirubin, triple phosphate, and uric acid crystals are

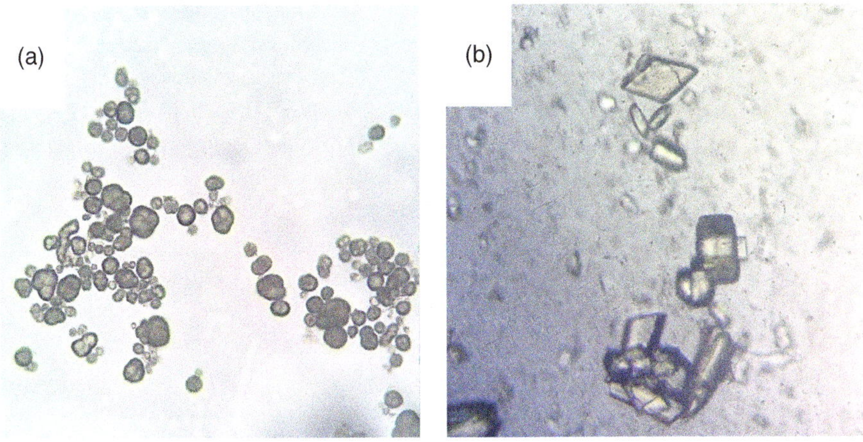

Figure 49.17 Crystals detected during sediment exam of reptile urine. Urate crystals from an eastern indigo snake (*Drymarchon couperi*) (a). Uric acid crystals from a veiled chameleon (*Chameleo calyptratus*) (b).

also increased in tortoises with renal disease [64]. Parasites, including flagellated protozoa, *Hexamita* sp., or pentastomids may be found in urine [64]. Spermatozoa are a normal finding in the urine of male chelonians and in female chelonians that have been in contact with males [60, 64].

Acknowledgments

I would like to thank Dr. Diana Binanti, DVM, DECVP for reviewing the images and Dr. Alessandro Bellese, DVM for providing many of the images used in this chapter.

References

1 Andreani, G., Carpenè, E., Cannavacciuolo, A. et al. (2014). Reference values for hematology and plasma biochemistry variables, and protein electrophoresis of healthy Hermann's tortoises (*Testudo hermanni* ssp.). *Vet. Clin. Pathol.* 43: 573–583.

2 Musilová, A., Knotková, Z., Pinterová, K., and Knotek, Z. (2015). Variations of plasma protein electrophoresis in healthy captive green iguanas (*Iguana iguana*). *Vet. Clin. Pathol.* 44: 243–248.

3 Scope, A., Schwendenwein, I., and Schauberger, G. (2013). Characterization and quantification of the influence of season and gender on plasma chemistries of Hermann's tortoises (*Testudo hermanni*, Gmelin 1789). *Res. Vet. Sci.* 95: 59–68.

4 Marshall, W.J. and Bangert, S.K. (2008). *Clinical Chemistry*, 6e. Oxford, UK: Mosby Elsevier.

5 Muro, J., Cuenca, R., Pastor, J. et al. (1998). Effects of lithium heparin and tripotassium EDTA on hematologic values of Hermann's tortoises (*Testudo hermanni*). *J. Zoo Wildl. Med.* 29: 40–44.

6 Harr, K.E., Raskin, R.E., and Heard, D.J. (2005). Temporal effects of 3 commonly used anticoagulants on hematologic and biochemical variables in blood samples from macaws and Burmese pythons. *Vet. Clin. Pathol.* 34: 383–388.

7 Sykes, J.M. 4th and Klaphake, E. (2015). Reptile hematology. *Vet. Clin. North Am. Exot. Anim. Pract.* 18: 63–82.

8 Goodman, R.M. and Heah, T.P. (2010). Temperature-induced plasticity in an ectotherm: the 'temperature size rule' examined at cellular and organismal levels. *Integr. Zool.* 5: 208–217.

9 Grosset, C., Wellehan, J.F. Jr., Owens, S.D. et al. (2014). Intraerythrocytic iridovirus in central bearded dragons (*Pogona vitticeps*). *J. Vet. Diagn. Invest.* 26: 354–364.

10 Brace, K.C. and Altland, P.D. (1955). Red cell survival in the turtle. *Am. J. Physiol.* 183: 91–94.

11 Campbell, T.W. (2006). Clinical pathology of reptiles. In: *Reptile Medicine and Surgery*, 2e (ed. D.R. Mader), 453–470. St Louis, MO: Saunders.

12 Heard, D., Harr, K., and Wellehan, J. (2004). Diagnostic sampling and laboratory tests. In: *BSAVA Manual of Reptiles*, 2e (eds. S.J. Girling and P. Raiti), 78–79. UK: Blackwell Publishing.

13 Saint Girons, M.C. (1970). Morphology of the circulating blood cell. In: *Biology of the Reptilia*, vol. 3 (eds. C. Gans and T.C. Parsons), 73–91. New York: Academic Press.

14 Salakij, C., Salakij, J., Apibal, S. et al. (2002). Hematology, morphology, cytochemical staining, and ultrastuctural

characteristics of blood cells in king cobras (*Ophiophagus hannah*). *Vet. Clin. Pathol.* 31: 116–126.
15 Harr, K.E., Alleman, A.R., Dennis, P.M. et al. (2001). Morphologic and cytochemical characteristics of blood cells and hematologic and plasma biochemical reference ranges in green iguanas. *J. Am. Vet. Med. Assoc.* 218: 915–921.
16 Alleman, A.R., Jacobson, E.R., and Raskin, R.E. (1999). Morphological, cytochemical staining, and ultrastructural characteristics of blood cells from eastern diamondback rattlesnakes (*Crotalus adamaneus*). *Am. J. Vet. Res.* 60: 507–514.
17 Bell, K.A. and Gregory, P.T. (2014). White blood cells in Northwestern Gartersnakes (*Thamnophis ordinoides*). *Herpetol. Notes* 7: 535–541.
18 Bielli, M., Nardini, G., Di Girolamo, N., and Savarino, P. (2015). Hematological values for adult eastern Hermann's tortoise (*Testudo hermanni boettgeri*) in semi-natural conditions. *J. Vet. Diagn. Invest.* 27: 68–73.
19 Schilliger, L., Rossfelder, A., Bonwitt, J. et al. (2014). Antemortem diagnosis of multicentric lymphoblastic lymphoma, lymphoid leukemia, and inclusion body disease in a boa constrictor (*Boa constrictor imperator*). *J. Herpetol. Med. Surg.* 24: 11–19.
20 Houwen, B. (2002). Blood film preparation and staining procedures. *Clin. Lab. Med.* 22: 1–7.
21 Nardini, G., Leopardi, S., and Bielli, M. (2013). Clinical hematology in reptilian species. *Vet. Clin. North Am. Exot. Anim. Pract.* 16: 1–30.
22 Chansue, N., Sailasuta, A., Tangtrongpiros, J. et al. (2011). Hematology and clinical chemistry of adult yellow-headed temple turtles (*Hieremys annandalii*) in Thailand. *Vet. Clin. Pathol.* 40: 174–184.
23 Halla, U., Korbel, R., Mutschmann, F., and Rinder, M. (2014). Blood parasites in reptiles imported to Germany. *Parasitol. Res.* 113: 4587–4599.
24 Miyamoto, M. and Mello, M.L. (2007). Chromatin supraorganization, DNA fragmentation, and cell death in erythrocytes of the rattlesnake, *Crotalus durissus terrificus* (Serpentes, Viperidae), infected with the protozoan, *Hepatozoon* spp. (Apicomplexa, Hepatozoidae). *Cell Biol. Int.* 31: 494–499.
25 Telford, S.R. (2016). *Hemoparasites of the Reptilia: Color Atlas and Text.* Boca Raton, FL: CRC Press.
26 Müller, K. and Brunnberg, L. (2010). Determination of plasma albumin concentration in healthy and diseased turtles: a comparison of protein electrophoresis and the bromcresol green dye-binding method. *Vet. Clin. Pathol.* 39: 79–82.
27 Di Girolamo, N., Ferlizza, E., Selleri, P. et al. (2018). Evaluation of point-of-care analysers for blood gas and clinical chemistry in Hermann's tortoises (*Testudo hermanni*). *J. Small Anim. Pract.* 59: 704–713.
28 Campbell, T.W. (2014). Clinical pathology. In: *Current Therapy in Reptile Medicine and Surgery* (eds. D.R. Mader and S.J. Divers), 70–92. St Louis, MO: Elsevier Saunders.
29 Moore, A.R., Allender, M.C., Mitchell, M.A., and MacNeill, A.L. (2015). Evaluation of plasma fibrinogen concentration as a diagnostic indicator of inflammation in red-eared sliders (*Trachemys scripta elegans*). *J. Am. Vet. Med. Assoc.* 246: 245–253.
30 Zhou, X., Wang, L., Feng, H. et al. (2011). Acute phase response in Chinese soft-shelled turtle (*Trionyx sinensis*) with Aeromonas hydrophila infection. *Dev. Comp. Immunol.* 35: 441–451.
31 Dantzler, W.H. and Braun, E.J. (1980). Comparative nephron function in reptiles, birds, and mammals. *Am. J. Physiol.* 239: R197–R213.
32 Knotek, Z., Hauptman, K., Knotková, Z. et al. (2002). Renal disease haemogram and plasma biochemistry in green iguana. *Acta Vet. Brno* 71: 333–340.
33 Hernandez-Divers, S.J., Martinez-Jimenez, D., Bush, S. et al. (2008). Effects of allopurinol on plasma uric acid levels in normouricaemic and hyperuricaemic green iguanas (*Iguana iguana*). *Vet. Rec.* 162: 112–115.
34 Hernandez-Divers, S.J., Stahl, S.J., Stedman, N.L. et al. (2005). Renal evaluation in the healthy green iguana (*Iguana iguana*): assessment of plasma biochemistry, glomerular filtration rate, and endoscopic biopsy. *J. Zoo Wildl. Med.* 36: 155–168.
35 Boyer TH, Getzy D, Vap L, Innis C (1996). Clinicopathologic findings of twelve cases of renal failure in *Iguana iguana*. *Proceedings of Association Reptilian and Amphibian Veterinarians*; 113.
36 Baird, G.S. (2011). Ionized calcium. *Clin. Chim. Acta* 412: 696–701.
37 Eatwell, K. (2009). Comparison of total calcium, ionised calcium and albumin concentrations in the plasma of captive tortoises (*Testudo* species). *Vet. Rec.* 165: 466–468.
38 Brischoux, F. and Kornilev, Y.V. (2014). Hypernatremia in dice snakes (*Natrix tessellata*) from a coastal population: implications for osmoregulation in marine snake prototypes. *PLoS One* 9: e92617.
39 Abou-Madi, N. and Jacobson, E.R. (2003). Effects of blood processing techniques on sodium and potassium values: a comparison between Aldabra tortoises (*Geochelone gigantea*) and Burmese mountain tortoises (*Manouria emys*). *Vet. Clin. Pathol.* 32: 61–66.
40 Innis, C.J., Ravich, J.B., Tlusty, M.F. et al. (2009). Hematologic and plasma biochemical findings in cold-stunned Kemp's ridley turtles: 176 cases (2001–2005). *J. Am. Vet. Med. Assoc.* 235: 426–432.
41 Anderson, E.T., Socha, V.L., Gardner, J. et al. (2013). Tissue enzyme activities in the loggerhead sea turtle (*Caretta caretta*). *J. Zoo Wildl. Med.* 44: 62–69.

42 Wagner, R.A. and Wetzel, R. (1999). Tissue and plasma enzyme activities in juvenile green iguanas. *Am. J. Vet. Res.* 60: 201–203.

43 Petrosky, K.Y., Knoll, J.S., and Innis, C. (2015). Tissue enzyme activities in kemp's ridley turtles (*Lepidochelys kempii*). *J. Zoo Wildl. Med.* 46: 637–640.

44 Wozniak, E.J., Kazacos, K.R., Telford, S.R. Jr., and McLaughlin, G.L. (1996). Characterization of the clinical and anatomical pathological changes associated with Hepatozoon mocassini infections in unnatural reptilian hosts. *Int. J. Parasitol.* 26: 141–146.

45 Girling, S.J. and Fraser, M.A. (2011). Cannabis intoxication in three green iguanas (*Iguana iguana*). *J. Small Anim. Pract.* 52: 113–116.

46 Preziosi, R., Diana, A., Florio, D. et al. (2007). Osteitis deformans (Paget's disease) in a Burmese python (*Python molurus bivittatus*) - a case report. *Vet. J.* 174: 669–672.

47 Ramsay, E.C. and Dotson, T.K. (1995). Tissue and serum enzyme activities in the yellow rat snake (*Elaphe obsoleta quadrivitatta*). *Am. J. Vet. Res.* 56: 423–428.

48 Knotkova, Z., Dorrestein, G.M., Jekl, V. et al. (2008). Fasting and postprandial serum bile acid concentrations in 10 healthy female red-eared terrapins (*Trachemys scripta elegans*). *Vet. Rec.* 163: 510–514.

49 McBride, M., Hernandez-Divers, S.M., Koch, T. et al. (2006). Preliminary evaluation of pre- and post-prandial 3α-hydroxy bile acids in the green iguana, *Iguana iguana*. *J. Herpetol. Med. Surg.* 16: 129–134.

50 Ghadir, M.R., Riahin, A.A., Avazpour, A. et al. (2011). The relationship between lipid profile and severity of liver damage in cirrhotic patients. *Hepat. Mon.* 10: 285–288.

51 Leonard, J.C. (1956). Hereditary hypercholesterolaemic xanthomatosis. *Lancet* 271 (6955): 1239–1242.

52 Sladky, K.K., Dalldorf, F.G., Steinberg, H. et al. (2000). Cholesterol granulomas in three meerkats (*Suricata suricatta*). *Vet. Pathol.* 37: 684–686.

53 Kummrow, M.S., Berkvens, C.N., Paré, J.A., and Smith, D.A. (2010). Cerebral xanthomatosis in three green water dragons (*Physignathus cocincinus*). *J. Zoo Wildl. Med.* 41: 128–132.

54 Naples, L.M., Langan, J.N., Mylniczenko, N.D. et al. (2009). Islet cell tumor in a Savannah monitor *(Varanus exanthematicus*). *J. Herpetol. Med. Surg.* 19: 97–105.

55 Christopher, M.M. (1999). Physical and biochemical abnormalities associated with prolonged entrapment in a desert tortoise. *J. Wildl. Dis.* 35: 361–366.

56 Frye, F.L., Dutra, F.R., Carney, J.D., and Johnson, B. (1976). Spontaneous diabetes mellitus in a turtle. *Vet. Med. Small Anim. Clin.* 71: 935–939.

57 Ritter, J.M., Garner, M.M., Chilton, J.A. et al. (2009). Gastric neuroendocrine carcinomas in bearded dragons (*Pogona vitticeps*). *Vet. Pathol.* 46: 1109–1116.

58 Hidalgo-Vila, J., Martínez-Silvestre, A., Ribas, A. et al. (2011). Pancreatitis associated with the helminth *Serpinema microcephalus* (Nematoda: Camallanidae) in exotic red-eared slider turtles (*Trachemys scripta elegans*). *J. Wildl. Dis.* 47: 201–205.

59 Hannon D, Garner M (2015). Hyperglycemia associated with renal adenocarcinoma in a Chinese water dragon. *Proceedings of Association Reptilian and Amphibian Veterinarians*; 503.

60 Gibbons PM, Horton SJ, Brandl SR (2000). Urinalysis in box turtles, *Terrapene* spp. *Proceedings of Association Reptilian and Amphibian Veterinarians*, 161–168.

61 Davis, J.R. and DeNardo, D.F. (2007). The urinary bladder as a physiological reservoir that moderates dehydration in a large desert lizard, the Gila monster *Heloderma suspectum*. *J. Exp. Biol.* 210: 1472–1480.

62 Koelle, P. (2000). Urinalysis in tortoises. In: *Proceedings of Association Reptilian and Amphibian Veterinarians*, 111–113.

63 Dantzler, W.H. (1976). Renal function (with special emphasis on nitrogen excretion). In: *Biology of the Reptilia, Physiology A* (eds. C. Gans and W.R. Dawson), 447–503. New York: Academic Press.

64 Koelle, P. and Hoffmann, R. (2002). Urinalysis in European tortoises—part II. In: *Proceedings of Association Reptilian and Amphibian Veterinarians*, 115–117.

50

Cytology

Ruth A. Houseright

Yahara Veterinary Research and Diagnostics, LLC, Madison, Wisconsin, USA

CONTENTS

As patients commonly present with subtle and nonspecific clinical signs, cytologic evaluation of blood, lesions, or body fluids is a valuable diagnostic tool for the herptile practitioner. Although it requires a degree of skill in microscopy, cytology is rapid, inexpensive, and can provide diagnostic information at the point of care. This chapter provides information on obtaining cytologic specimens from reptiles and amphibians and interpreting common cytologic findings.

Sample Collection

FNA/Impression Smears

Fine needle aspiration (FNA) is indicated to obtain samples from a variety of sites. In most species, a 20- or 22-gauge, 1- to 1½-inch needle attached to a 6 cc syringe is recommended [1]. In fractious patients, a butterfly catheter may be used to accommodate patient movement during the procedure. To obtain the specimen, air is introduced into the syringe chamber. The tip of the needle is then inserted into the tissue and redirected several times as the plunger is gently retracted. The plunger is released, the needle is withdrawn, and the specimen is expressed onto a glass slide or into an ethylenediamine tetraacetic acid (EDTA)-containing tube. Once the specimen has been applied, a second glass slide is glided along the surface of the specimen to produce a thin, even smear (Figure 50.1). The slide may then be air-dried and stained using quick stains or submitted to a cytopathologist for review.

For superficial or ulcerated skin lesions or for rapid evaluation of biopsy specimens, impression smears are useful. The lesion or cut surface of the biopsy specimen should first be blotted with a paper towel to remove blood and exuded fluid. The tissue is then touched firmly to the slide several times. The slide may be air-dried and stained as for fine needle aspirates.

GI Sampling

Specialized techniques exist for sampling the gastrointestinal tract. In most species, the oral cavity may be sampled using dry or saline-moistened cotton swabs, which are then gently applied to a glass slide by rolling. Such sampling is limited to superficial lesions; infectious organisms or neoplastic cells deeper in the tissues may be missed. Contamination of specimens obtained in this manner with oral microflora is unavoidable and may complicate interpretation. Samples of the esophagus and stomach may be obtained using swabs or by gastric lavage or endoscopy [2].

Exotic Animal Emergency and Critical Care Medicine, First Edition. Edited by Jennifer E. Graham, Grayson A. Doss and Hugues Beaufrère.

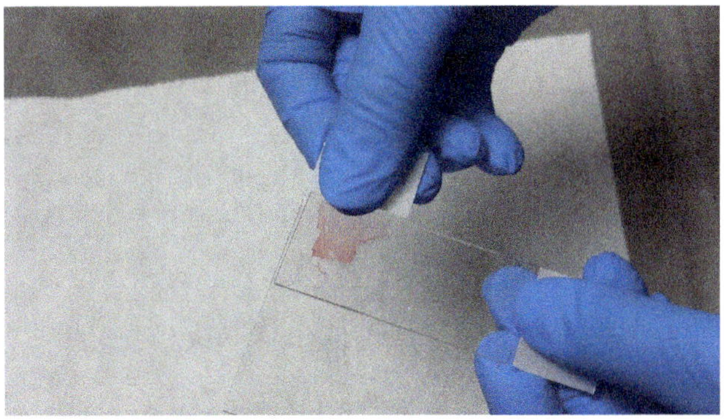

Figure 50.1 Smear preparations of specimens obtained by fine needle aspiration are prepared by expressing aspirated material onto a glass slide. A second slide is used to gently spread the aspirated material into a thin layer before the slides are air-dried and stained. Care must be taken to avoid rupturing fragile cells; the weight of the spreader slide is sufficient to distribute the specimen.

Cloacal swabs and washings and fecal evaluation are useful when parasitic or protozoal diseases are suspected. As many species defecate infrequently, collection of a fresh specimen is paramount for diagnostic utility [2]. Fecal flotations, direct stained smears, or unstained preparations of feces mixed with a drop of saline may be performed.

Respiratory Sampling

When nasal or upper respiratory disease is suspected, specimens of discharge from the oral or nasal cavities may be obtained using cotton swabs or by nasal flushing. Samples from the lower respiratory tract are obtained by lung or tracheal wash. This technique is described in detail elsewhere [3]. All fluid specimens for cytology, regardless of source, should be submitted promptly in EDTA. Preparation of direct smears at the time of fluid collection is prudent, as cells degenerate within 24 hours following sample collection. Fluid specimens for bacterial or fungal culture should be submitted in additive-free sterile tubes.

Dermatologic Sampling

While aspiration of vesicular or mass-like skin lesions may yield diagnostic specimens, for ulcerative skin lesions or evaluation of dysecdysis, other methods are recommended. Impression smears may be made by pressing a clean glass slide against the lesion, or purulent material may be collected using a cotton swab. Skin scrapings may be helpful in evaluating deeper parts of the lesion. Acetate tape impressions are useful for the diagnosis of external parasites, including mites (Figure 50.2). Shed fragments of the skin may be collected, stained, and evaluated for the presence of pathogenic microorganisms.

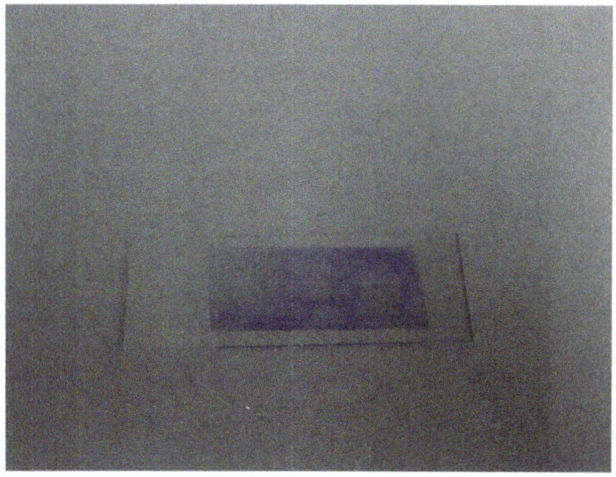

Figure 50.2 Acetate tape preparations of dry skin lesions that do not readily stick to slides are made by pressing the sticky side of the tape directly to the lesion. A drop of the third quick stain solution (dark blue) is placed on a glass slide, and the tape is placed directly onto the stain. Once air-dried, the preparation is ready to be examined by light microscopy. *Source:* Photograph courtesy of Elizabeth Layne, DVM.

Centesis

In healthy adult reptiles and amphibians, a small amount of fluid, insufficient for collection, is present in the pleuroperitoneum and pericardium to lubricate organs. In pathologic conditions, accumulated fluid may be collected by centesis. In most herptiles, centesis is performed by inserting a needle through the skin and body wall of the animal's ventrum, just lateral to the midline abdominal vein [4]. In chelonians, the peritoneal cavity may be accessed through the inguinal body wall cranial to the rear leg [4]. While most herptiles have a single pleuroperitoneal cavity, monitor lizards, chelonians, and crocodilians have a fibrous postplural or posthepatic septum separating cranial and caudal coelomic compartments, and cytologic findings may differ among compartments [5]. Fluids should be collected in an aseptic manner and submitted in EDTA tubes for cytologic evaluation. Specimens for bacterial or fungal culture should be submitted in sterile tubes. As with all fluid specimens, direct smears should be made immediately.

Although challenging in small species, fluid may also be obtained from the joints of larger reptiles by arthrocentesis. Synovial fluid should be collected in an aseptic manner and handled as with other fluid cytology specimens.

Hematology

The erythrocytes of healthy herptiles are oval and nucleated. Pinpoint to 2 μm basophilic cytoplasmic inclusions are a normal finding (Figure 50.3) [6]. In cases of regenerative anemia, immature erythrocytes, which have polychromatophilic cytoplasm and a rounded cell and nuclear shape, may be seen (Figure 50.4).

Due to the presence of nucleated erythrocytes, rapid visual evaluation at low power (10–20× objective) to estimate leukocyte counts may be misleading. In general, at high power (40–60× objective), at least one leukocyte should be present in almost every field in the monolayer area of an evenly distributed, well-made smear to be confident that leukocyte numbers are adequate. If many leukocytes are present in most fields, a leukocytosis is suspected.

Granulocyte morphology varies among herptile species. Heterophils usually have angular pink granules, while eosinophils have round, red-orange granules (Figure 50.5). However, many species have unique eosinophil granules; for example, the eosinophils of the green iguana have turquoise blue granules [7]. In inflammatory conditions, band heterophils may be noted. If toxic change is present, heterophil granules may be sparse (Figure 50.6). Basophils have a round nucleus and abundant, dark purple granules

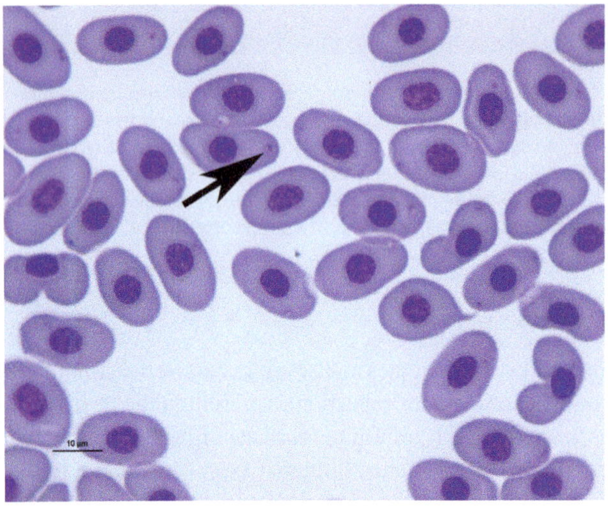

Figure 50.3 Blood film from a blue-tongued skink. Basophilic cytoplasmic inclusions (arrow) are a normal finding within the erythrocytes of reptiles. Diff-Quick stain.

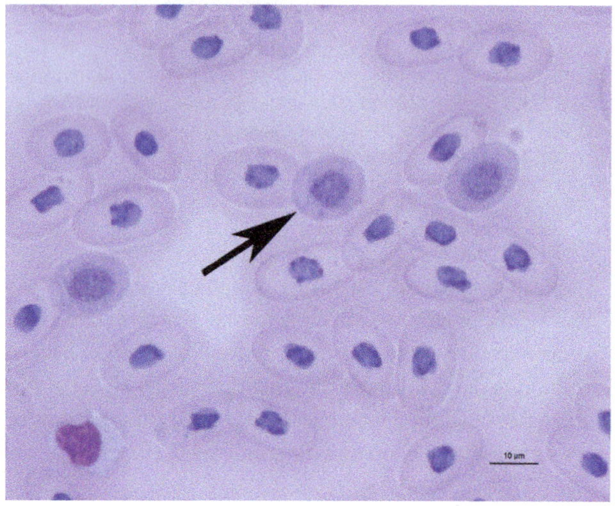

Figure 50.4 Blood film from a veiled chameleon. Immature, polychromatophilic erythrocytes, or reticulocytes (arrow), are identifiable by their round cellular and nuclear shape. The cytoplasm stains blue-gray due to the presence of residual ribonucleic acid (RNA). Increased numbers of these cells are associated with regenerative anemias. Wright's–Giemsa stain.

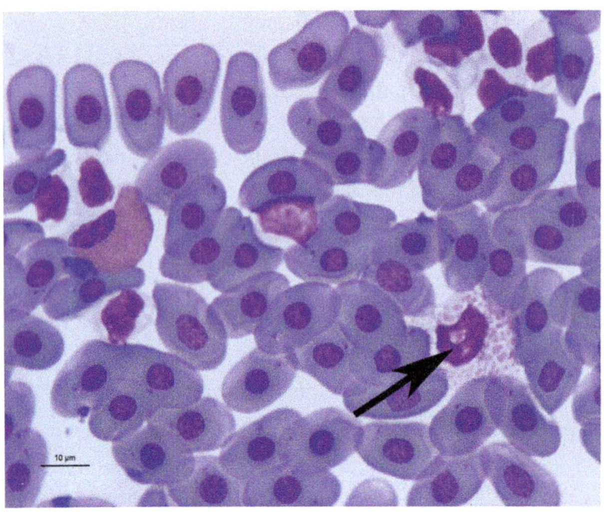

Figure 50.5 Blood film from a painted turtle. Heterophils (left) usually have elongated or angular, pink granules, while eosinophils (arrow) have round, red-orange granules. However, the appearance of eosinophil granules varies among species. Diff-Quick stain.

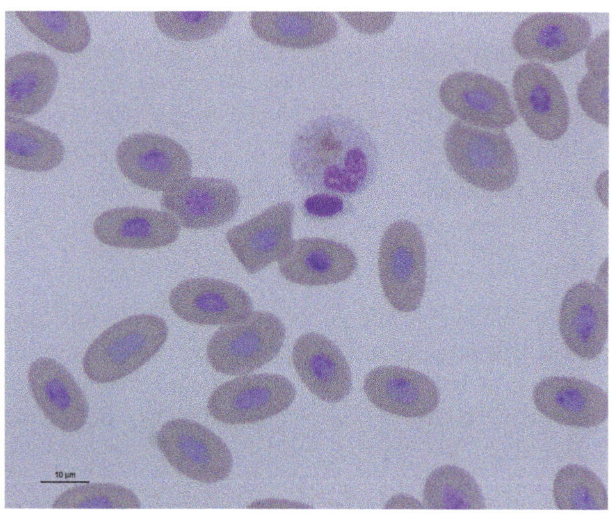

Figure 50.6 Blood film from a blue-tongued skink. Immature heterophils, or bands, have hypolobulated, c-shaped nuclei. Toxic change is also evident in this band heterophil; the cytoplasm is foamy and blue-gray, and the granules are sparse and rounded. Wright's–Giemsa stain.

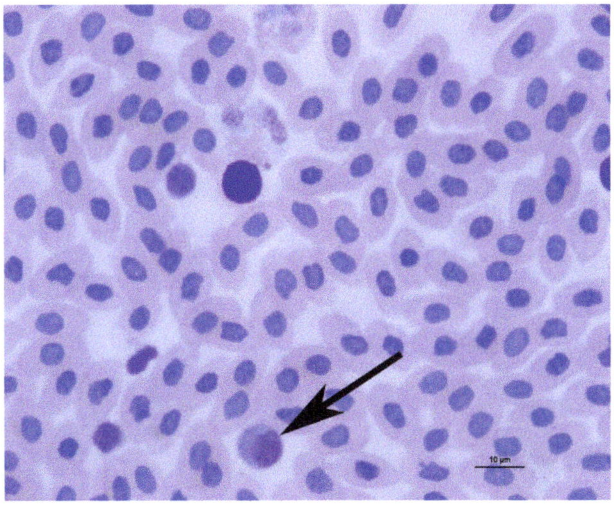

Figure 50.7 Blood film from a green iguana. Reptilian basophils have round nuclei that are often obscured by dense, purple granules. Eosinophils (arrow) of iguanas have pale blue granules. Wright's–Giemsa stain.

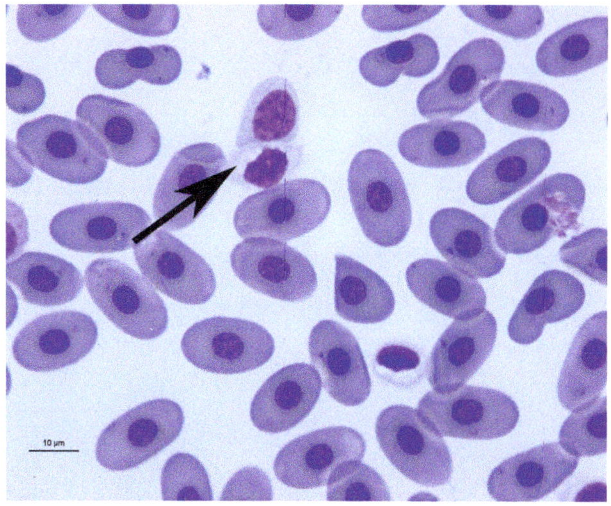

Figure 50.8 Blood film from a painted turtle. Differentiation of lymphocytes (top) from thrombocytes (bottom) can be challenging. The lymphocyte in this image is larger than the thrombocyte and has more basophilic cytoplasm. The nucleus of the thrombocyte is more condensed, and thrombocyte cytoplasm often contains clear vacuoles (arrow). Diff-Quick stain.

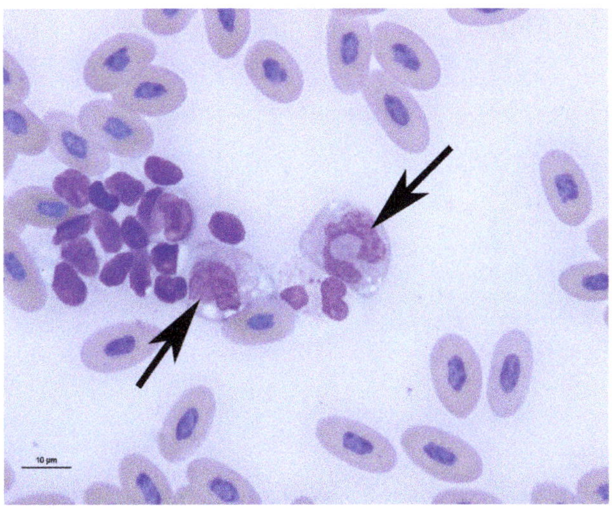

Figure 50.9 Blood film from a blue-tongued skink. In this image, two monocytes (arrows) are separated by an eosinophil and are identifiable by their large size, basophilic cytoplasm, and discrete cytoplasmic vacuoles resembling bullet holes. Monocyte nuclei may be round, ameboid (left), or horseshoe-shaped (right). The cells are accompanied by a large clump of thrombocytes. Wright's–Giemsa stain.

(Figure 50.7). High numbers of basophils are a normal finding in chelonians and some species of skinks and newborn snakes [6].

Lymphocytes are round cells, with scant basophilic cytoplasm and a round nucleus. Both large and small lymphocytes may be observed. Circulating lymphocytosis occurs with inflammation, parasitism, wound healing, and viral infection; however, in many species, lymphocytes are the most numerous leukocyte in health [6].

Differentiation of lymphocytes from thrombocytes, which are also nucleated, requires careful examination of the cells (Figure 50.8). Lymphocytes are slightly larger and much less numerous than thrombocytes, and should not form clumps, while thrombocytes tend to form large clumps, particularly at the feathered edge of the smear. Thrombocytes may contain fine vacuoles in the cytoplasm.

Monocytes are the largest of the leukocytes and have deeply basophilic cytoplasm that often contains discrete vacuoles (Figure 50.9). The nucleus may be round, horseshoe-shaped, or ameboid. In reptiles, a subset of monocytes may contain dust-like azurophilic granules and are thus named azurophils (Figure 50.10). Azurophils are a nonspecific finding.

Hemogregarines are commonly noted in the erythrocytes of both healthy and compromised herptiles, especially wild-caught specimens. Morphology is variable but generally consists of a basophilic nucleus and pale blue cytoplasm (Figure 50.11). The erythrocyte nucleus may be displaced. Microfilaria may also be noted in high numbers and are usually nonpathogenic (Figure 50.12) [8].

Diagnosis of inclusion body disease in boids relies upon careful examination of the blood smear. Pathognomonic intracytoplasmic inclusions may be found in erythrocytes, lymphocytes, or heterophils, and appear as homogenous, lightly basophilic structures that vary in shape and size (Figure 50.13) [9].

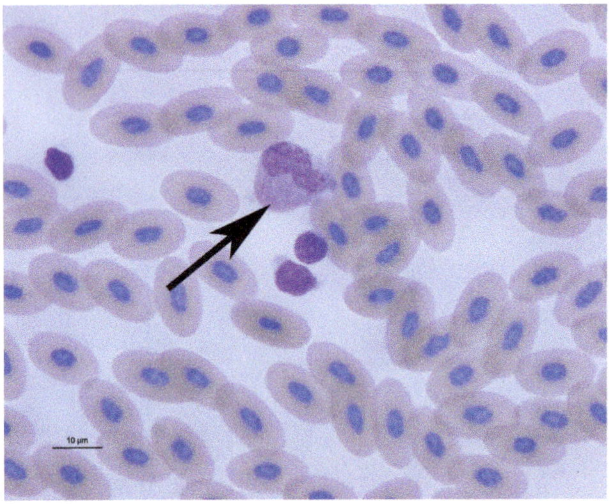

Figure 50.10 Blood film from a rainbow boa constrictor. Azurophils (arrow) resemble monocytes, except that they contain fine, dust-like azurophilic granules. Wright's–Giemsa stain.

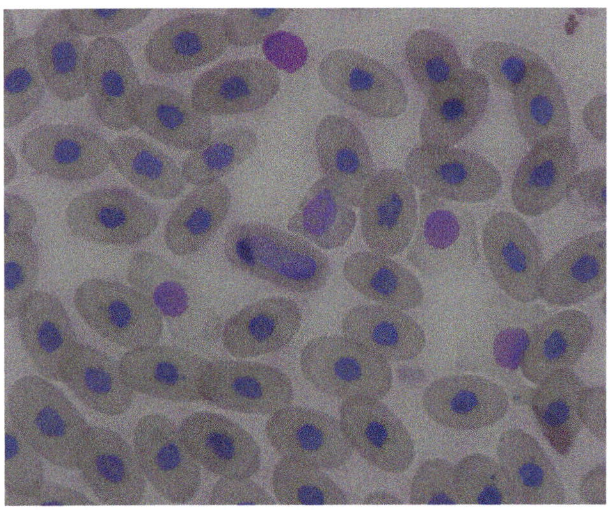

Figure 50.11 Blood film from a map turtle. Hemogregarines are found within the cytoplasm of erythrocytes, and may displace the erythrocyte nucleus. While many species exist, these protozoa are usually round to cigar-shaped, consisting of a purple nucleus and pale blue cytoplasm. Wright's–Giemsa stain, 1000× magnification.

Case reports of acute leukemia in reptiles are rare. Acute leukemia should be suspected when leukocyte counts are markedly increased and when the leukocyte population is dominated by large mononuclear cells with visible nucleoli (blasts). Determining whether the cells are of lymphoid or myeloid origin requires advanced diagnostic testing and is often unrewarding. Chronic lymphocytic leukemia is more common and is characterized by the presence of severely increased numbers of mature, morphologically unremarkable small lymphocytes (Figure 50.14).

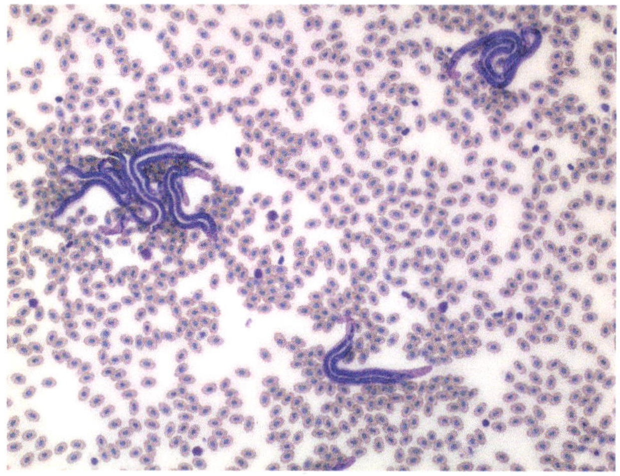

Figure 50.12 Blood film from a Jackson's chameleon. Microfilaria vary in size among species but are usually about 5–7 μm wide and 200–300 μm long, with a visible, basophilic internal structure comprising the parasite's gastrointestinal and reproductive tracts. Microfilaria are often found in pairs and groups. Wright's–Giemsa stain, 400× magnification.

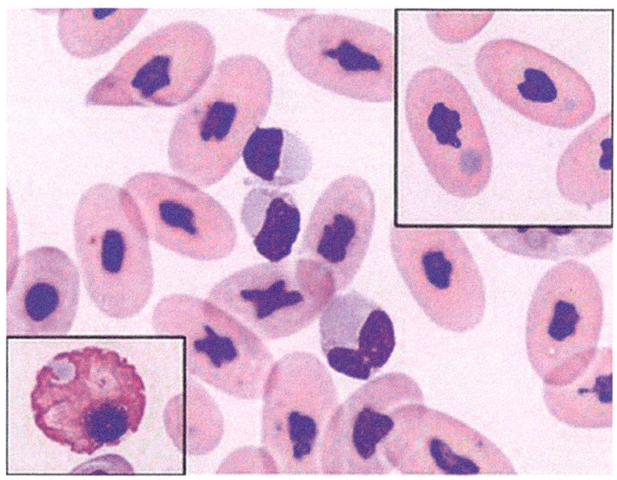

Figure 50.13 Blood film from a common northern boa constrictor. Lymphocytes, erythrocytes, and heterophils contain a single, homogenous, round, basophilic intracytoplasmic inclusion measuring 2–6 μm in diameter, which is pathognomonic for inclusion body disease. Wright's–Giemsa stain. *Source:* Reproduced with permission from Banajee et al. [9]. Copyright 2012 John Wiley & Sons, Inc.

Fluid Cytology

Sample Preparation and Analysis

Coelomic effusions are categorized based on the total nucleated cell count and total protein concentration of the fluid. Total leukocyte counts may be estimated based on visual evaluation of a stained smear; otherwise, they may be obtained by the same manual methods used to determine white blood cell counts in peripheral blood.

Coelomic effusions may be grouped as follows:

Transudates

The leukocyte count and total protein concentration of transudates (Figure 50.15) are expected to be low, fewer than 1000–3000 cells/μl and less than 2.5 g of protein/μl. Transudates are colorless to straw-colored and transparent. Macrophages predominate and may be accompanied by low numbers of lymphocytes and mesothelial cells. Heterophils are limited to those contributed by peripheral blood contamination. Causes of transudates include congestive heart failure and profound peripheral hypoalbuminemia [5].

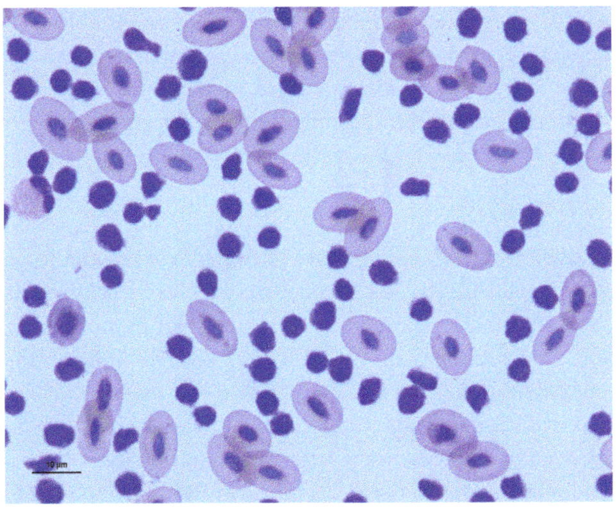

Figure 50.14 Chronic lymphoid leukemia, bearded dragon. Mature small lymphocytes, which are otherwise morphologically normal, are present in extreme numbers and outnumber erythrocytes. Wright's–Giemsa stain.

High Protein Transudates

High protein transudates are grossly hazy and have cell counts less than 1000–3000/μl. Total protein concentrations exceed 2.5 g/dl. The cytologic appearance is variable. Typically, macrophages predominate and may be accompanied by low numbers of lymphocytes and reactive mesothelial cells. However, if inflammation is contributing to the formation of the effusion, increased numbers of heterophils and plasmacytoid lymphocytes may be seen. Causes include heart failure, liver failure, and compression or torsion of internal organs [5].

Exudates

Exudates are characterized by increases in both the leukocyte count (>3000 cells/μl) and total protein concentration of the fluid (>2.5 g/dl) and often appear grossly cloudy, brown, or green [5]. A predominance of degenerate heterophils is suggestive of bacterial infection (Figure 50.15). Exudative effusions in herptiles are often granulomatous to pyogranulomatous, characterized by variable numbers of macrophages and degenerate or nondegenerate heterophils. Granulomatous exudates have been reported in cases of systemic mycobacteriosis and egg yolk coelomitis. Egg yolk coelomitis should be considered when clear lipid vacuoles and amorphous, basophilic material consistent with yolk contents is observed (Figure 50.16) [4]. Melanomacrophages (Figure 50.17), inflammatory cells that may function best at colder body temperatures, may also be observed [10].

(a) (b)

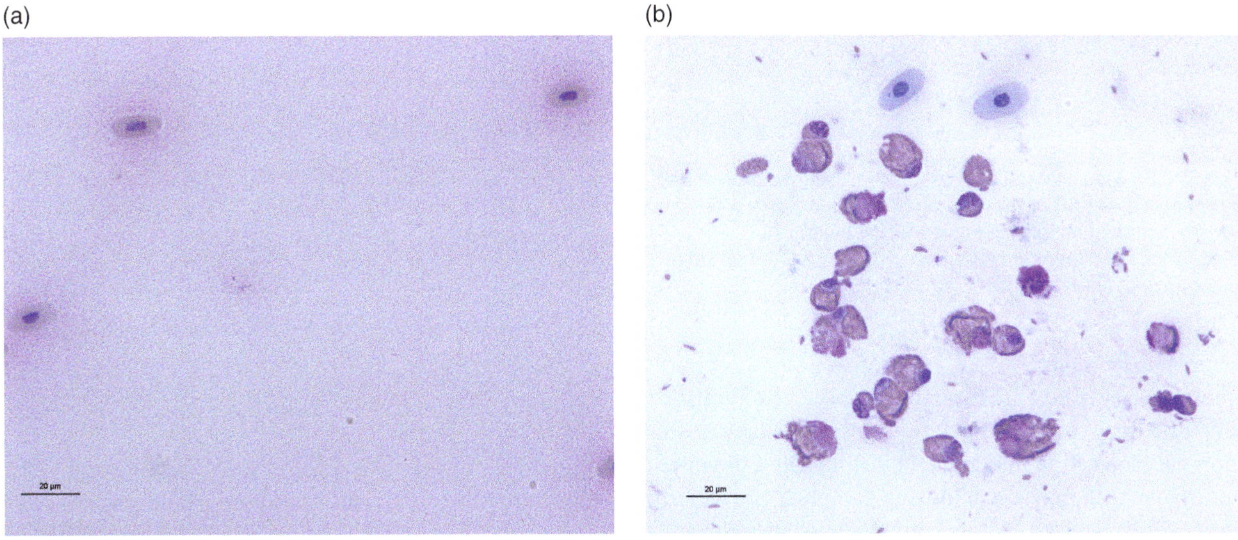

Figure 50.15 Transudative effusions (a) contain few leukocytes. This coelomic effusion from a box turtle contains a small amount of peripheral blood contamination. The total protein concentration is increased, evidenced by the eosinophilic, granular background. Exudative effusions (b) are characterized by high leukocyte counts. Heterophils predominate in this coelomic effusion from a painted turtle with pneumonia following a near-drowning incident.

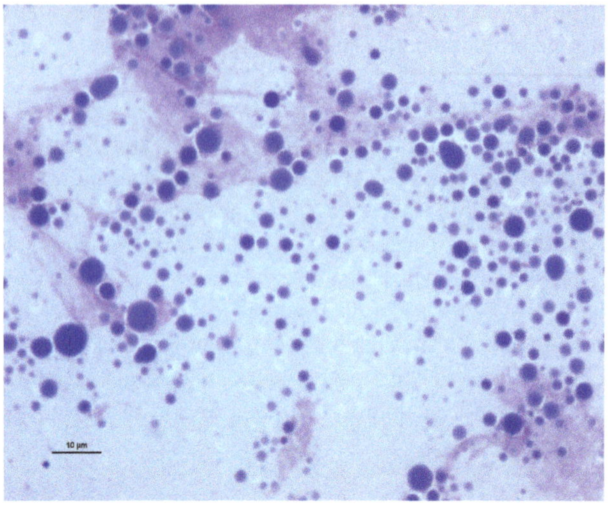

Figure 50.16 Egg yolk material appears as deeply basophilic droplets of varying sizes. Although this yolk was aspirated within the oviduct and no inflammation is observed, macrophagic inflammation is commonly associated with egg yolk coelomitis. Wright's–Giemsa stain.

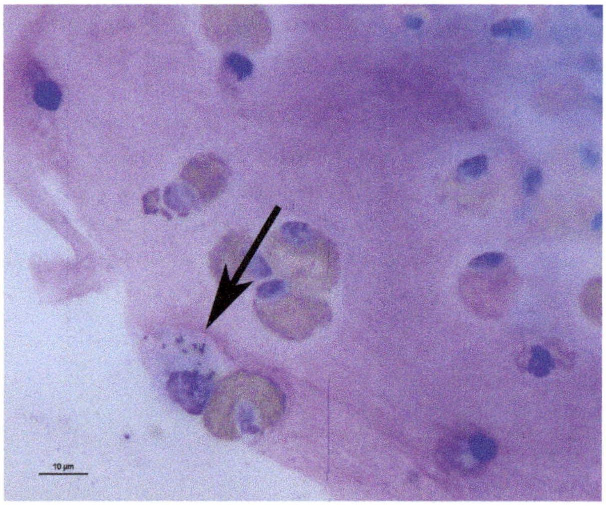

Figure 50.17 Melanomacrophages (arrow) resemble ordinary macrophages except that they contain fine, golden-brown to black, seed-shaped melanin granules, which must be distinguished from intracellular bacteria. They are often found in inflammatory lesions. Wright's–Giemsa stain.

Hemorrhagic Effusions

Hemorrhagic effusions are commonly caused by trauma or injury and may be identified by their resemblance to peripheral blood. It is important to distinguish iatrogenic hemorrhage that may occur during sampling, in which thrombocytes may be present, from clinically relevant pathologic hemorrhage, which is characterized by the presence of products of hemoglobin metabolism (hemosiderin and hematoidin) within macrophages.

Neoplastic Effusions

Neoplastic effusions are characterized by the presence of neoplastic cells in the fluid. These are most commonly of epithelial or round cell origin, for example, carcinomas or lymphomas. Multiple features of malignancy, including anisocytosis, anisokaryosis, the presence of mitotic figures, increased nuclear to cytoplasmic ratios, prominent nucleoli, and bi- or multinucleation, are often observed. An inflammatory cell population may or may not accompany the neoplastic cells.

Chylous Effusions

Chylous effusions are uncommon in herptile species but may be caused by lymphatic obstruction by granulomas, neoplasms, or distended viscera and are characterized by high numbers of small lymphocytes. Incidental aspiration of lymph may mimic the appearance of chylous effusions [5].

Synovial Fluid

Synovial fluids, in health, have leukocyte counts and total protein concentrations <3000 cells/μl and <2.5 g protein/μl. The nucleated cell population is made up of mononuclear cells (macrophages or synoviocytes) and small lymphocytes. Heterophils are rare.

In reptiles, gout causes an inflammatory arthropathy characterized by the presence of uric acid crystals in the synovial fluid specimen. Uric acid crystals are needle-shaped and birefringent under polarized light (Figure 50.18). Pseudogout can be differentiated cytologically from gout by the presence

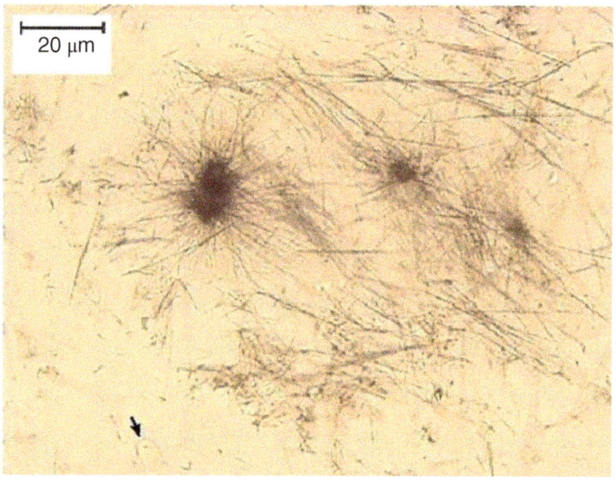

Figure 50.18 Synovial fluid from an African spur-thighed tortoise. Uric acid crystals appear in synovial fluid specimens as brown, needle-like crystals that are arranged in a starburst pattern. A peripheral blood erythrocyte (arrow) demonstrates comparative size of the crystals. Unstained direct smear. *Source:* Casimire-Etzioni et al. 2004 [11], Figure 2. Reproduced with permission of Wiley.

Herptiles

of calcium phosphate crystals, which are round and not birefringent under polarized light [11].

Increases in heterophil numbers and the presence of degenerate heterophils often indicate acute inflammation or bacterial infection, while increased numbers of large mononuclear cells are seen in mycobacterial and fungal infections and with chronic inflammation. Mixed cell inflammation is commonly observed. Infectious arthritis may occur secondary to trauma or may be due to systemic infection or septicemia.

Cytology of Body Systems

Gastrointestinal Cytology

Oral Cavity Cytology

Swabs of the normal oral cavity often contain squamous epithelial cells, bacterial microflora, and few (if any) inflammatory cells. Regardless of the inciting cause, cytologic preparations of lesions of infectious stomatitis or cheilitis are characterized by increased numbers of degenerate or nondegenerate heterophils and macrophages in varying proportions. Bacterial stomatitis is most commonly caused by Gram-negative rod-shaped bacteria in both reptiles and amphibians, which usually represent overgrowth of oral microflora [12]. Bacteria must be found intracellularly within heterophils to determine that they are pathogens. Chronic granulomatous stomatitis that is poorly responsive to antimicrobial therapy may be caused by mycobacteriosis (Figure 50.19) [13]. Granulomatous or mixed cell inflammation may also be observed in cases of fungal stomatitis. Mixed bacterial and fungal infections are common.

Neoplasia of the oral cavity may appear as proliferative masses or ulcerative lesions. In reptiles, the most commonly reported neoplasms include squamous cell carcinoma, fibroma, fibrosarcoma, and melanoma [12]. In amphibians, fibroma, lymphoma, and olfactory neuroblastoma have been reported in the oral cavity [14].

Gastric Lavage Cytology

Gastric lavage specimens from healthy reptiles contain gastric epithelial cells, heterogeneous normal bacterial flora, mucus, and ingesta. The presence of a monotonous population of bacteria with a single morphology, most commonly Gram-negative rods, is consistent with bacterial overgrowth (Figure 50.20). High numbers of macrophages, heterophils, or a combination of the two suggests infectious gastritis, and a careful examination of the slide for a causative bacterial, protozoal, or fungal organism is warranted.

Cryptosporidium spp. infection, particularly common in snakes, is diagnosed based on the finding of ~6 μm, pale, basophilic protozoal oocysts (Figure 50.21). The oocysts may be accompanied by increased numbers of hyperplastic gastric epithelial cells. The organism stains positively with acid-fast stains [15].

Neoplasia of the gastrointestinal tract occurs most commonly in snakes. Gastric adenocarcinomas often exfoliate poorly; endoscopy may be required to obtain a diagnostic specimen. Hepatomas and hepatocellular carcinomas have also been reported in snakes and may be diagnosed by aspiration of coelomic masses [12].

(a) (b)

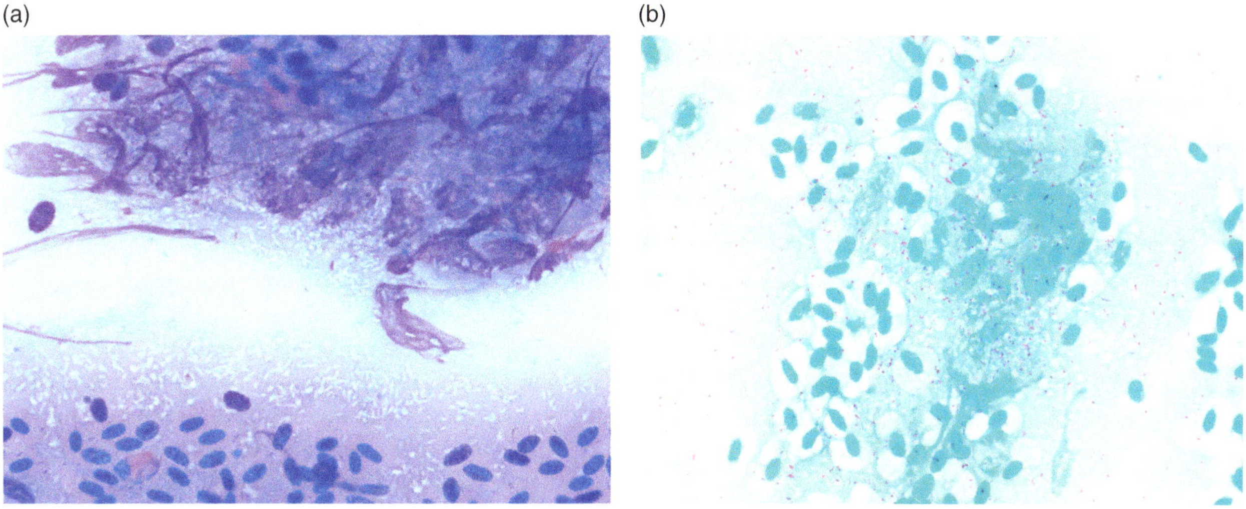

Figure 50.19 When stained with Wright's–Giemsa (a) or other routine stains, Mycobacteria appear as non-staining bacterial rods and may be found both within macrophages (top) and free in the background of the slide (bottom). When stained with Ziehl–Neelsen (b) or other acid-fast stains, Mycobacteria appear bright pink against the green counterstain. 1000× magnification. *Source:* Courtesy of Karen Young.

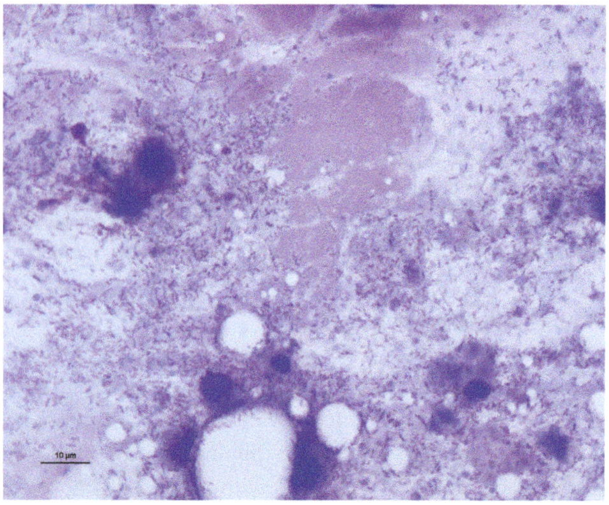

Figure 50.20 Bacterial overgrowth is characterized by an abundance of bacteria of a single morphology, usually Gram negative rods. High numbers of bacterial rods are observed in this gastric lavage smear in the absence of an appreciable inflammatory response. Wright's–Giemsa stain.

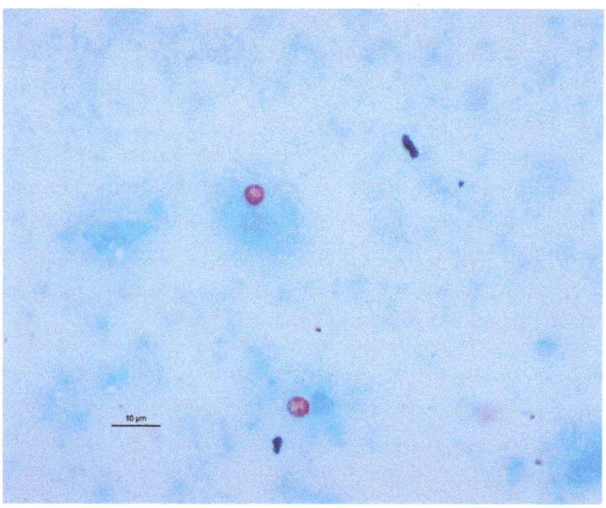

Figure 50.21 *Cryptosporidium* spp. in fecal smears are difficult to visualize with routine stains due to their blue-gray color and small size (~6 μm) but stain bright pink against the green counterstain with acid-fast stains. Ziehl–Neelsen stain. *Source:* Courtesy of Faye Hartmann.

Fecal Cytology

Most parasitic and protozoal diseases of the herptile gastrointestinal tract may be readily diagnosed by cytologic evaluation of unstained fresh feces or by fecal flotation. For some organisms, such as *Cryptosporidium* spp., stained smears are more useful.

Herptile gastrointestinal protozoal populations vary among species, and most are nonpathogenic. *Cryptosporidium* spp. and coccidia may generally be assumed to be pathogenic [12]. Coccidia are most common in lizards and are usually host-specific (Figure 50.22).

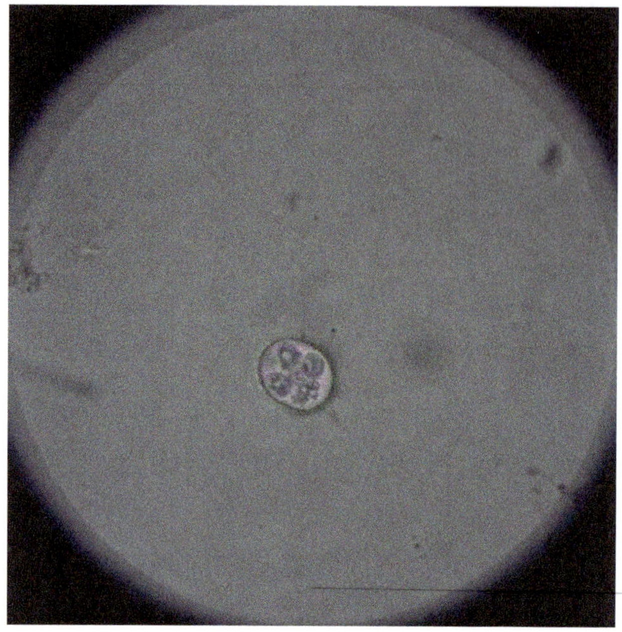

Figure 50.22 Fecal flotation from a box turtle, sporulated *Eimeria* oocyst. This coccidian parasite measures approximately 18 × 16 μm in diameter and can be identified by its small size and thin wall. This oocyst contains four sporocysts; unsporulated oocysts and oocysts with two sporocysts may also be observed. 400× magnification. *Source:* Courtesy of Linda Sullivan.

Cestode and trematode infections are most common in wild-caught specimens and rarely cause clinical disease. Thick-walled, operculated eggs of trematodes and smaller, round eggs of cestodes may be noted on fecal flotation from apparently healthy herptiles (Figure 50.23).

Oxyurids and other pinworms are commonly encountered nematode infections and are generally considered nonpathogenic but have been associated with disease in heavy infestations (Figure 50.24). Other strongyloid nematodes and ascarids are also common in reptiles and are associated with more significant pathology, including intestinal ulceration, impaction, and perforation [5].

Respiratory Cytology

Infectious respiratory disease is common in captive reptiles. Evaluation of nasal flushes is useful for diagnosing upper respiratory disease, while for lower respiratory disease, lung washes may have more diagnostic utility. Nasal flushes may contain squamous epithelial cells, respiratory epithelial cells, heterogeneous bacterial microflora, and fragments of ingesta from the nasopharynx and oronasal cavities, in addition to any inflammatory cells or infectious organisms.

Viral causes of upper and lower respiratory disease in reptiles are common but are often complicated by the presence of concurrent, secondary bacterial infections.

(a) (b)

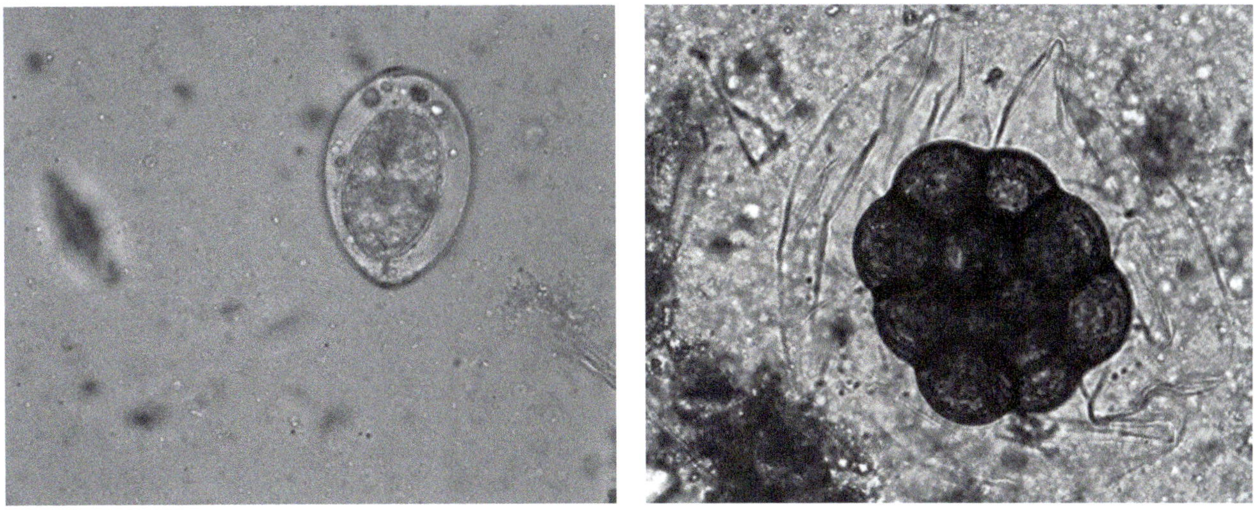

Figure 50.23 Fecal flotation from a ball python. Cestode (tapeworm) eggs may occur individually (a) or in large packets (b). 400× magnification. *Source:* Courtesy of Linda Sullivan.

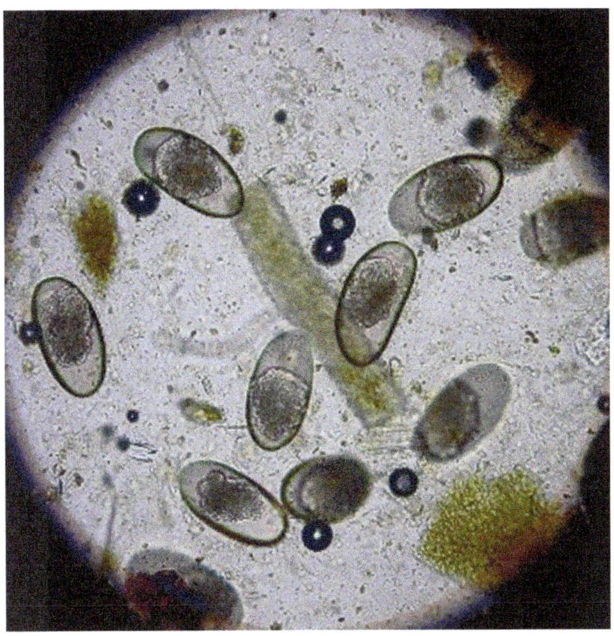

Figure 50.24 Fecal flotation from a sulcata tortoise. Oxyurid and other pinworm eggs are elongated and contain a visible morula. 400× magnification. *Source:* Courtesy of Linda Sullivan.

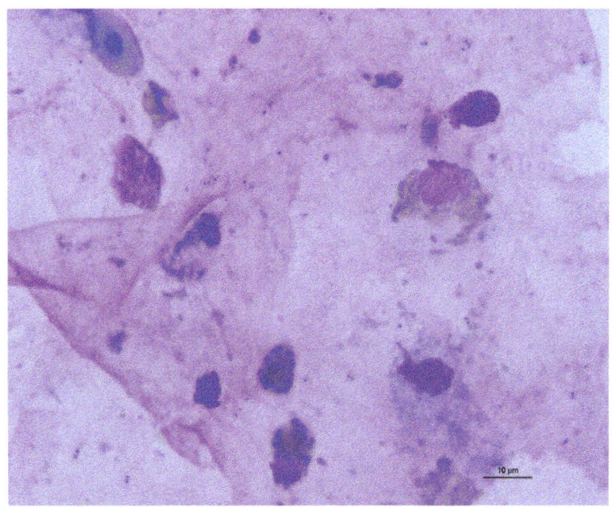

Figure 50.25 Nasal flush from a turtle, species unknown. Degenerate heterophils with swollen nuclei and abundant bacterial diplococci are consistent with septic heterophilic inflammation. Wright's–Giemsa stain.

Viral inclusions are typically not observed except in the case of inclusion body disease in boids; pale basophilic cytoplasmic inclusions similar to those found in leukocytes may be present within respiratory epithelial cells [9].

Bacterial rhinitis and pneumonia may be primary or secondary. Gram negative, aerobic rods are most common, although anaerobes and Gram positive cocci are sometimes observed [3]. Intracellular bacteria found within degenerate heterophils are particularly convincing for pneumonia (Figure 50.25).

Mycoplasmosis is characterized by the presence of 1–2 µm, pleomorphic, epicellular bacteria. Small colonies of dust-like organisms may be observed among macrophages and heterophils [16].

Fungal hyphae and spores most commonly represent systemic mycosis secondary to other causes of poor condition. Primary systemic mycosis is also reported. Lower respiratory tract specimens contain fungal elements admixed with granulomatous or mixed cell inflammation. Bacterial coinfections are common.

Parasitic pneumonia is most commonly found in snakes. Pentastomid eggs are sometimes isolated in lung wash specimens [17]. Heavy infestations of ascarids or hookworms may also cause respiratory signs and secondary bacterial pneumonia. Eosinophilic inflammation is rare in reptiles and diagnosis is usually made based on finding eggs on fecal flotation.

Primary or metastatic neoplastic disease of the respiratory tract is an infrequent finding. Sampling by lung wash is unrewarding, as neoplasms rarely communicate with the airway. Direct aspiration of the lesion yields epithelial or mesenchymal cells with many features of malignancy. Lymphoma of the lung has been reported in snakes, chelonians, and lizards [18]; it is characterized by a homogeneous population of large lymphocytes, which are larger than heterophils and have nuclei with fine chromatin and one or more prominent nucleoli (Figure 50.26). Ball pythons may develop cartilaginous granulomas that originate from the tracheal rings; these lesions are not neoplastic and aspiration yields well-differentiated cartilage [3].

Cytology of Skin and Subcutaneous Lesions

Generalized dermatitis and cellulitis are usually infectious and are often associated with poor husbandry or previous trauma. Macrophages and heterophils in varying proportions may be present. Bacterial infections are most commonly caused by Gram negative rods. Saprophytic molds are ubiquitous in habitat water and may cause dermatitis in compromised amphibians.

Some causes of dermatitis in reptiles and amphibians may be diagnosed in the absence of inflammatory cells. Dermatomycosis due to *Nannizziopsis guarroi* (yellow fungus disease), a leading cause of morbidity and mortality in bearded dragons, is characterized by rectangular arthroconidiae with little or no associated inflammation [19]. In wild-caught amphibians, chytridiomycosis, caused by *Batrachochytrium dendrobatidis*, appears as round, thick-walled zoosporangia containing multiple basophilic zoospores, which are found within the cytoplasm of amphibian keratinocytes in shed skin [20] (Figure 50.27).

Abscesses and granulomas produce mass-like lesions of the skin and subcutis. In abscesses, degenerate or nondegenerate heterophils are the dominant nucleated cell population and intracellular and extracellular bacteria are common. Granulomas consist predominantly of macrophages. Heterophils may or may not be observed. Granulomatous inflammation is associated with fungal or mycobacterial infection (Figure 50.28). Subcutaneous granulomas may be isolated or may represent systemic mycosis or mycobacteriosis.

Mass lesions may also represent neoplasia. Papillomas, squamous cell carcinomas, cutaneous lymphoma, melanoma, and sarcomas (Figure 50.29) are reported in herptiles [21]. In general, neoplastic disease should be suspected when representative cytologic preparations of the lesion lack infectious organisms and inflammatory cells and

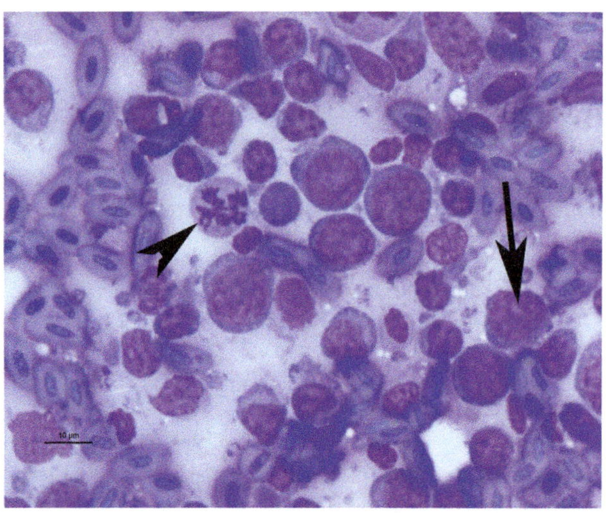

Figure 50.26 Lymphoma, bearded dragon. Large lymphocytes, which are larger than a heterophil and have high N:C ratios and basophilic cytoplasm, are the predominant cell population. Some of the lymphocytes have large, prominent, pale-staining nucleoli (arrow). Mitotic figures (arrowhead) may be seen. Round cytoplasmic fragments in the background of the smear indicate that the cells are lymphoid in origin but are not diagnostic of neoplasia. Wright's–Giemsa stain.

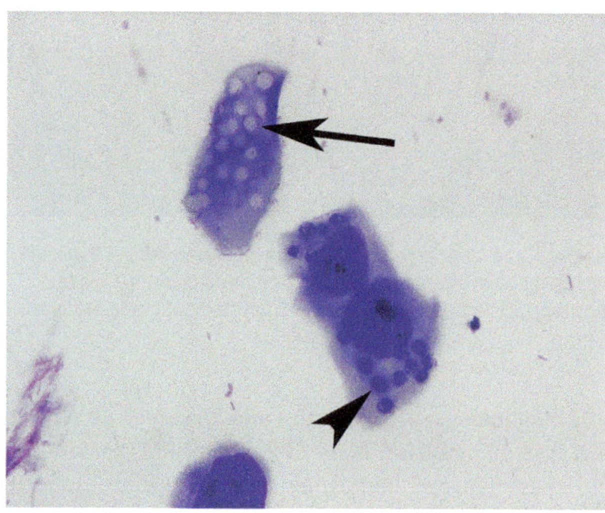

Figure 50.27 Chytridiomycosis, hellbender salamander. Empty thalli (arrow) within keratinocytes are most commonly observed; thalli containing basophilic zoospores (arrowhead) may also be seen. Inflammatory infiltrates are often absent. Wright's–Giemsa stain, 600× magnification. *Source:* Courtesy of Allison Dusick.

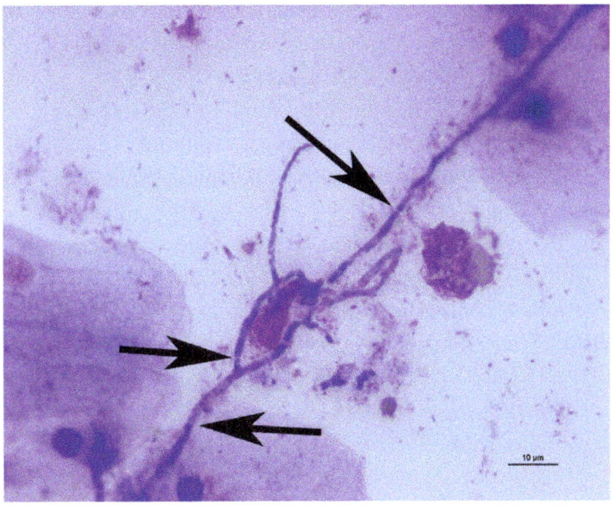

Figure 50.28 *Aspergillus* spp., painted turtle shell lesion. Fungal hyphae may be distinguished from artifact or debris by their parallel cell walls, basophilic internal structure, and septae (arrows). Acute or right-angle branching is typical of *Aspergillus* spp., but fungal culture is required for speciation. Bacteria are also present in the background of this image. Wright's–Giemsa stain.

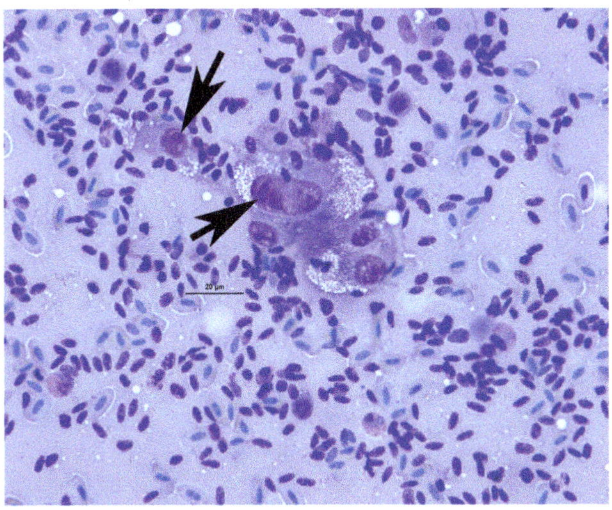

Figure 50.29 Myxosarcoma, corn snake. Neoplastic cells of sarcomas are often spindle-shaped, with oval nuclei, and may occur individually or in loose aggregates. These cells display many features of malignancy, including anisocytosis, anisokaryosis, and multiple and prominent nucleoli (arrows). Biopsy with histopathologic evaluation was needed to distinguish this sarcoma from other sarcomas. Wright's–Giemsa stain.

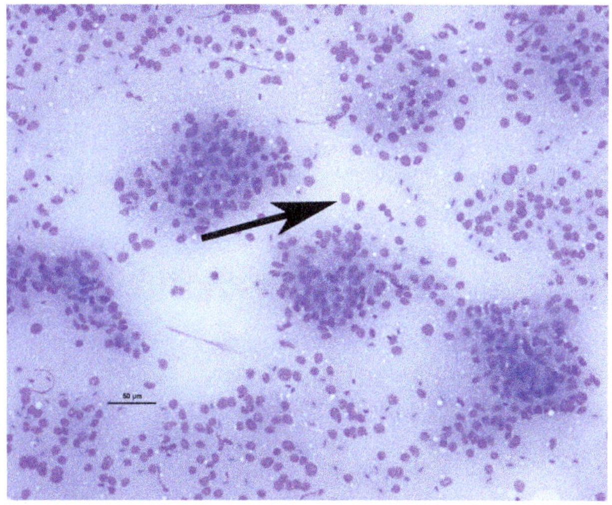

Figure 50.30 Renal adenocarcinoma, common python. Cells in this specimen are arranged in clusters, consistent with their epithelial origin, and there is a notable lack of inflammatory cells. Many bare nuclei (arrow) are scattered among clusters of cells; only intact cells should be used to evaluate features of malignancy. Wright's–Giemsa stain.

contain a homogenous population of epithelial, mesenchymal, or round cells that may display features of malignancy. Of the herptile species, neoplastic disease appears to be the most common in snakes [21].

Urogenital Cytology

Mass lesions of the urogenital tract, identified by palpation or imaging of the coelom, may represent abscesses or granulomas, which are similar in cytologic appearance to inflammatory lesions in other organs. Retained eggs within the reproductive tract may be externally palpable in some species. Neoplasia, although less common, is also reported, and as with other sites, occurs most commonly in snakes. Renal adenocarcinomas (Figure 50.30) and carcinomas and dysgerminomas of the ovary are reported, as well as leiomyomas of the oviduct. In chelonians, interstitial cell tumors of the testes are reported [21].

References

1 Raskin, R. and Meyer, D.J. (2001). *Atlas of Canine and Feline Cytology*. Philadelphia, PA: W.B. Saunders.

2 Tully, T.N. (2009). *Manual of Exotic Pet Practice*. St. Louis, MO: Saunders Elsevier

3 Schumacher, J. (2011). Respiratory medicine of reptiles. *Vet. Clin. North Am. Exot. Anim. Pract.* 14 (2): 207–224.

4 Alleman, A.R. and Kupprion, E.K. (2007). Cytologic diagnosis of diseases in reptiles. *Vet. Clin. North Am. Exot. Anim. Pract.* 10 (1): 155–186.

5 Campbell, T.W. (2015). *Exotic Animal Hematology and Cytology*, 4e. Hoboken: Wiley. Online resource (421 p).

6 Weiss, D.J. and Wardrop, K.J. (2010). *Schalm's Veterinary Hematology*, 6e. Ames, IA: Blackwell.

7 Stacy, N.I. and Raskin, R.E. (2015). Reptilian eosinophils: beauty and diversity by light microscopy. *Vet. Clin. Pathol.* 44 (2): 177–178.

8 Telford, S.R. (2009). *Hemoparasites of the Reptilia: Color Atlas and Text*. Boca Raton, FL: CRC Press.

9 Banajee, K.H., Chang, L.W., Jacobson, E.R. et al. (2012). What is your diagnosis? Blood film from a boa constrictor. *Vet. Clin. Pathol.* 41 (1): 158–159.

10 Campbell, T.W. (2007). Basics of cytology and fluid cytology. *Vet. Clin. North Am. Exot. Anim. Pract.* 10 (1): 1–24.

11 Casimire-Etzioni, A.L., Wellehan, J.F., Embury, J.E. et al. (2004). Synovial fluid from an African spur-thighed tortoise (*Geochelone sulcata*). *Vet. Clin. Pathol.* 33 (1): 43–46.

12 Mitchell, M.A. and Diaz-Figueroa, O. (2005). Clinical reptile gastroenterology. *Vet. Clin. North Am. Exot. Anim. Pract.* 8 (2): 277–298.

13 Tarigo, J., Linder, K., Neel, J. et al. (2006). Reluctant to dive: coelomic effusion in a frog. *Vet. Clin. Pathol.* 35 (3): 341–344.

14 Goodman, G. (2003). Oral biology and conditions of amphibians. *Vet. Clin. North Am. Exot. Anim. Pract.* 6 (3): 467–475.

15 Harr, K.E., Henson, K.L., Raskin, R.E. et al. (2000). Gastric lavage from a Madagascar tree boa (*Sanzinia madagascarensis*). *Vet. Clin. Pathol.* 29 (3): 93–96.

16 Jacobson, E.R., Brown, M.B., Wendland, L.D. et al. (2014). Mycoplasmosis and upper respiratory tract disease of tortoises: a review and update. *Vet. J.* 201 (3): 257–264.

17 Latney, L.V. and Wellehan, J. (2013). Selected emerging infectious diseases of squamata. *Vet. Clin. North Am. Exot. Anim. Pract.* 16 (2): 319–338.

18 Schumacher, J. (2003). Reptile respiratory medicine. *Vet. Clin. North Am. Exot. Anim. Pract.* 6 (1): 213–231.

19 Minard, H.M., Burrell, C., Delgado, J.D. et al. (2016). What's your diagnosis? Skin impression smear from a Bearded Dragon. *Vet. Clin. Pathol.* 45 (3): 505–506.

20 Baitchman, E.J. and Pessier, A.P. (2013). Pathogenesis, diagnosis, and treatment of amphibian chytridiomycosis. *Vet. Clin. North Am. Exot. Anim. Pract.* 16 (3): 669–685.

21 Hernandez-Divers, S.M. and Garner, M.M. (2003). Neoplasia of reptiles with an emphasis on lizards. *Vet. Clin. North Am. Exot. Anim. Pract.* 6 (1): 251–273.

51

Ancillary Diagnostics

Nicola Di Girolamo[1] *and Diana Binanti*[2]

[1] *Department of Veterinary Clinical Sciences, College of Veterinary Medicine, Oklahoma State University, Stillwater, Oklahoma, USA*
[2] *AbLab Veterinary Diagnostic Laboratory, Sarzana, La Spezia, Italy*

CONTENTS

The emergency veterinarian is not always involved in ancillary investigations. Nevertheless, it is important for the emergency clinician to be aware of the profound differences in terms of ancillary testing that are present between reptiles and mammals, in order to be able to refer and follow-up with the patient in the best way possible.

Infectious Disease Assessments

Once an infectious disease is suspected by the emergency clinician, the owner should be informed on the common diagnostic approaches. Pathogens of reptiles include bacteria, viruses, fungi, and parasites, including protozoan. There are several ways to establish the presence of an organism, each of those has general indication, as well as specific indications due to the pathogen in analysis (e.g. mycobacteria are slow and difficult to cultivate) or due to the clinical implications (e.g. individual patient medicine vs. population medicine) [1]. These techniques include:

- Culture and isolation, which is ideal in certain situations because they are a proof of the ability of the organism to reproduce
- Identification, which is currently usually performed via molecular diagnostic techniques
- Serology, which consists of the evaluation of the presence of antibodies directed toward such pathogen in the patient

Whichever technique will be used, the ER veterinarian should gather information on previous antibiotic use. Unfortunately, it is very common for clients, especially semi-professional reptile breeders, to attempt several antimicrobial treatments without veterinary advice.

Culture and Sensitivity Testing

The moment at which the specimen is obtained for isolation is critical. For example, viral shedding is not constant

Exotic Animal Emergency and Critical Care Medicine, First Edition. Edited by Jennifer E. Graham, Grayson A. Doss, and Hugues Beaufrère.

and obtaining samples for bacterial culture after antibiotic treatment is worthless. Characteristics of the specimen obtained are also critical. Often reptiles are small and it may not be possible to collect enough sample for bacterial, virological, and mycological investigations. Selection of the specimen depends on the organ system infected. It is mandatory for the clinician to consider the more common microorganism etiologies before referring a case for microorganism culture.

Sampling technique depends on the affected site. Common samples and sites that are cultured in reptiles are tracheobronchial lavage (Figure 51.1), urine (via cystocentesis), cloacal lavage (highly contaminated), organs (including liver and kidneys), conjunctiva, appendicular skeleton (Figure 51.2), and vertebrae. When samples are obtained percutaneously, proper positioning may need to be confirmed by diagnostic imaging techniques (e.g. ultrasound for soft tissue and radiology or computed tomography [CT] for bones) (Figure 51.3) [2]. When cultures are obtained from tissues, they should ideally be sampled from the margin of an active lesion.

The presence of a microorganism is not diagnostic of disease. Bacteria and/or fungi are normally found in the oral cavity, conjunctiva, and respiratory tract of healthy reptiles [3–6]. In order to obtain a definitive diagnosis, it is fundamental to obtain evidence of the effect of the microorganism on the tissue (e.g. with histopathology).

Sensitivity testing is indicated in bacterial and fungal infections and even parasitic infestations [7]. Currently, specific laboratories can perform sensitivity testing even on slow-growing bacteria, such as mycobacteria [8].

Bacteria

Bacteria carried by reptiles are often multidrug resistant [9, 10]. Therefore, whenever a bacterial infection is suspected sensitivity testing should precede specific antibiotic administration. As pharmacokinetics in reptiles are available for just a few antibiotics [11], the diagnostic laboratory should be contacted in advance to indicate the antibiotics to be tested for sensitivity. Specimens must be collected in a sterile container and transported to the laboratory as soon as possible. Tissue fluids, exudates, and tissue biopsies for microbial culture must be collected under aseptic conditions using sterile culture swabs or tubes. Typical media used for bacterial isolation include blood agar, brain heart infusion agar, and MacConkey agar [1].

Fungi

As for bacteria, sterile techniques are required to obtain and transport diagnostic samples for fungal culture, in order to minimize overgrowth of bacterial or fungal contaminants. Cutaneous lesions are commonly cultured for fungi. In reptiles with suspected cutaneous mycoses, skin scrapings, or small cutaneous samples can be collected under local anesthesia (Figure 51.4). In chelonians with shell mycoses, a wedge biopsy of the shell is required for culture and sensitivity testing. Histopathology is always required in order to confirm the pathogenicity. These biopsies should be collected under general anesthesia as it is difficult to understand the

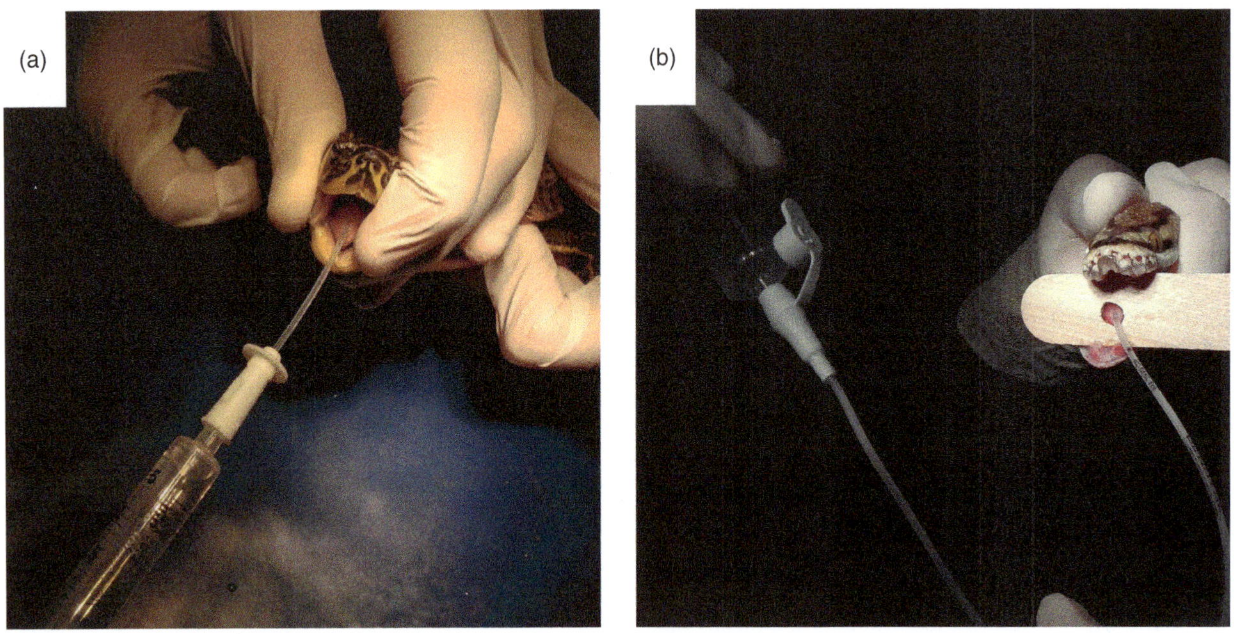

Figure 51.1 Tracheobronchial lavage in a yellow-bellied slider (*Trachemys scripta scripta*) (a) and a ball python (*Python regius*) (b). In reptiles with respiratory disorders, tracheobronchial lavage is typically performed for cytology, microbiology, and mycology (including sensitivity testing).

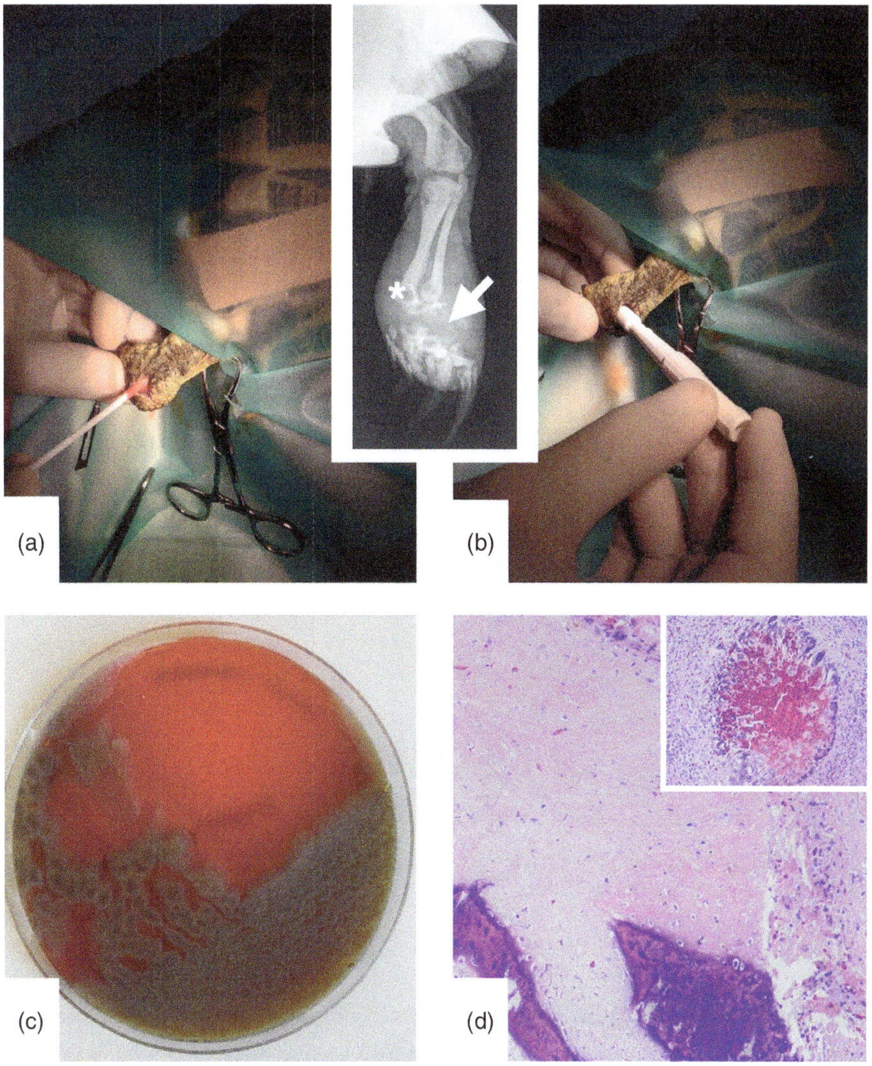

Figure 51.2 Sterile sampling of bone for microbiology in case of osteomyelitis. A Hermann's tortoise (*Testudo hermanni*) was diagnosed with osteolysis of the tarsus (inset, arrow) with involvement of both the distal tibia and ulna (asterisk). Sterile swabs (a) and tissue biopsy (b) demonstrated the presence of *Bacillus cereus* (which was also associated with *Salmonella* sp.) (c) and osteomyelitis (d), a granuloma is evident in the inset. *Source:* Photo (c) courtesy of Giorgia Matteucci.

degree of pain associated with the procedure [12]. A typical media used for mycotic isolation is Sabouraud's dextrose agar, which inhibits growth of most bacterial organisms. The owner should be informed that before being negative, fungal cultures are maintained for a minimum of two to four weeks.

Virus

Viral isolation from reptiles requires a diagnostic laboratory with specific capabilities. Viral titers decrease with storage; therefore, a prompt submission of the samples maximizes virus isolation. Samples collected for viral culture can be maintained at +4 °C for few days or at −80 °C for long-term storage. Phosphate buffered saline or saline (0.9% NaCl) can be used as media as an alternative to specific cell culture media enriched with antibiotic and antimycotic. Media such as RNAlater (Life Technologies, Grand Island, NY) can be used to preserve viability of nucleic acids. Viral isolation requires the use of live cells, e.g. cell cultures or embryonated eggs. Currently, several established cell lines have been used for culturing reptile viruses [1]. Cultures are checked daily for cytopathic effect. Cell culture medium can be collected for molecular testing. If isolation is successful, the virus can be identified and its pathogenicity determined via transmission studies [1].

PCR Screens

Polymerase chain reaction (PCR) evaluates the presence of nucleic acid, and can be used to find presence of a pathogen. Unlike culture, the pathogen need not be alive or be

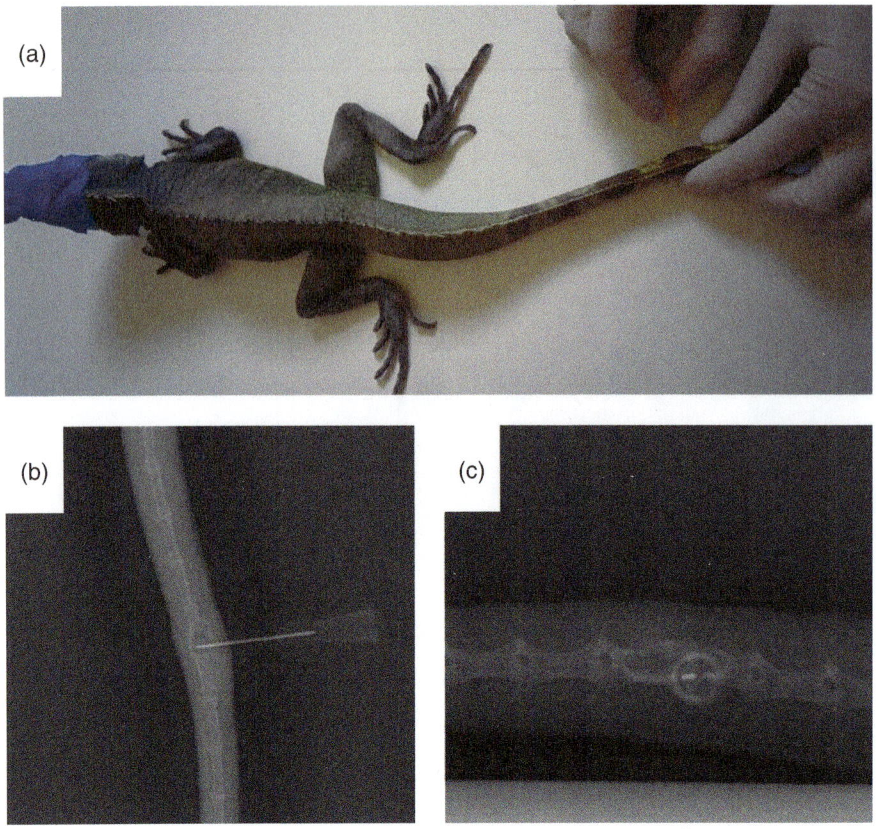

Figure 51.3 Vertebral fine-needle aspirate (a) confirmed by radiographic imaging (b, c) in a Chinese water dragon (*Physignathus cocincinus*). The proper area for sample collection may need to be confirmed by diagnostic imaging techniques, including ultrasound, radiography, CT, or MRI.

able to reproduce to be detected in PCR. Another difference from culture is that there is a need of specific primers for each pathogen, therefore a presumptive diagnosis is necessary. PCR is often a good clinical compromise to detect virus and microorganism that are difficult to cultivate (e.g. mycobacteria and *Mycoplasma*) [13]. Pathogens that are commonly screened with PCR in reptile clinical practice are listed in Table 51.1.

Correct sampling in term of timing and specimen is fundamental for isolation (Figure 51.5). A negative test does not mean that the patient does not carry the pathogen. Instead the reptile could not be shedding the pathogen in that moment of time or could not be shedding the pathogen from the site of sampling. PCR is a highly sensitive technique, and the potential for false-positive results from slight contamination anywhere in the process, from collection to laboratory, is real. As such, it is critically important that measures are taken to avoid contamination during sample collection and transport and that appropriate controls are run.

In short, the nucleic acid is extracted, then primers of pathogen DNA are added and several temperature cycles are performed to increase the amount of DNA. The PCR product must then be validated, which means that it must be determined to be the appropriate product and not an accidental binding of the primers to an unexpected site on a different DNA template. The most definitive way to determine the identity of the PCR product is to sequence it. This was once expensive, but with the rapid improvements in sequencing technology that have taken place in the past decade, costs are now minimal. Quantitative polymerase chain reaction (qPCR), also known as real-time PCR, is a PCR variant involving the use of a dye-labeled probe that binds to a sequence between the two primers. Quantitative information can be clinically useful for determining whether loads are sufficient for consideration as a disease etiology and for following trends over time for assessment of a response to therapy.

Serology

Serology refers to the diagnostic identification of antibodies in the serum, and has been used in reptiles to detect exposure to viruses, bacteria, and parasites [15]. Several techniques have been used in reptiles in order to characterize

Metabolic/Endocrine Assessments

Endocrine Panels

Gout

Gout occurs due to deposition of uric acid in the kidneys (renal gout), organ serosae (visceral gout), and /or joints (articular gout). In many reptile species, the main nitrogenous product is uric acid. Current thinking is that excess of uric acid (hyperuricemia) as a consequence of overproduction (high protein diet) or diminished excretion (kidney disorders) results in deposition of urates. In humans, however, gout may be present without hyperuricemia and vice-versa [22]. Basic diagnostic imaging including ultrasonography and radiography are useful because of the possible increase in renal radiopacity and echogenicity in advanced stages (Figure 51.6a,b). In a reptile with suspected gout, blood concentrations of uric acid should be evaluated together with a complete biochemical panel (ideally including ionized calcium, phosphorus, and protein electrophoresis). A final diagnosis is reached with cytology or biopsy showing deposition of uric acid (Figure 51.6c,d).

Hyperglycemia/Diabetes Mellitus/ Somatostatinomas

Diabetes mellitus is rare in reptiles, and may be spontaneous or iatrogenic, as a consequence of pancreas (or splenopancreas) removal [23, 24]. There is no current consensus on how to establish an antemortem diagnosis of diabetes in reptiles, however demonstration of low blood insulin concentration may be helpful. As in mammals, hyperglycemia is not pathognomonic of diabetes mellitus in reptiles [25]. In bearded dragons with persistent hyperglycemia, gastric neuroendocrine carcinomas (somatostatinomas) should be ruled out before considering diabetes [26]. Persistent hyperglycemia, glucosuria, low insulin levels, and pancreatic biopsies are all means that may support a diagnosis of diabetes, once metabolic disorders, stress, and physiological adaptation have been ruled out [25].

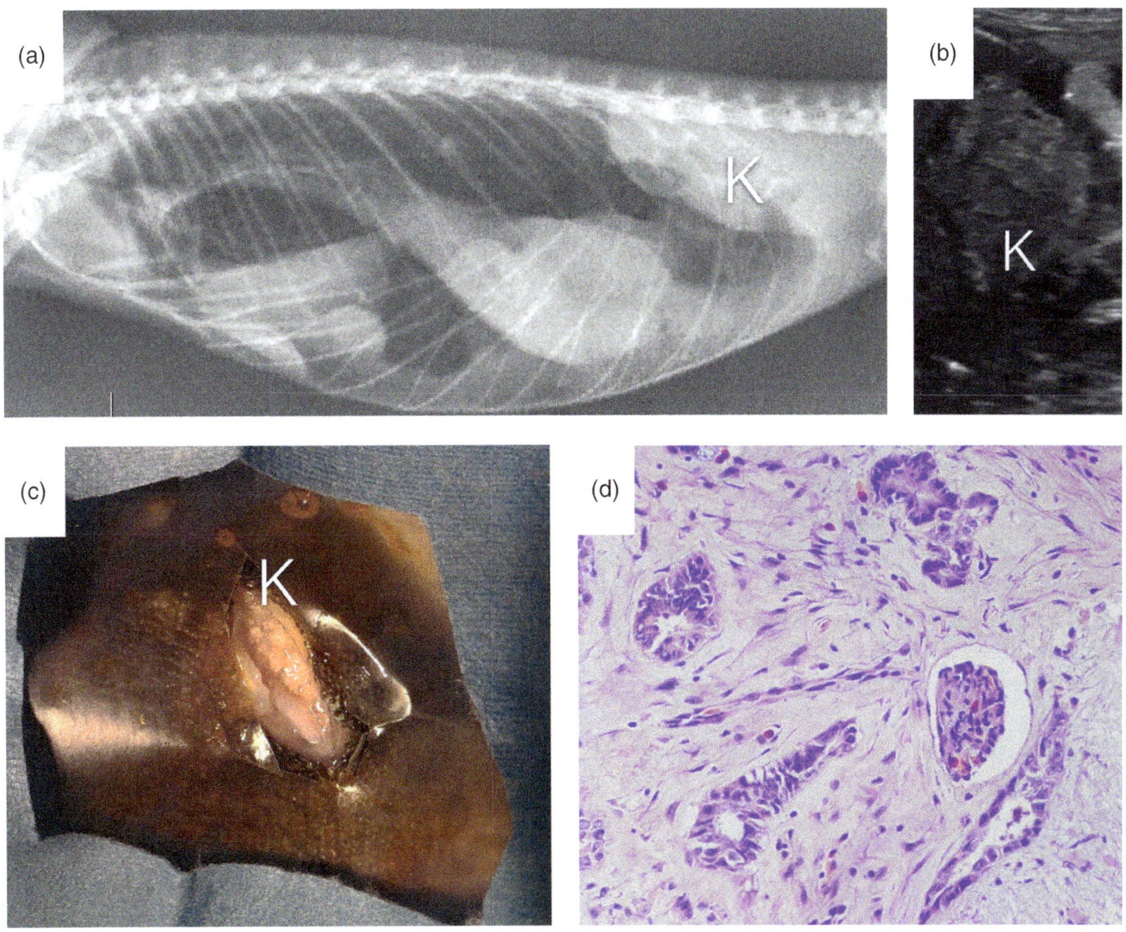

Figure 51.6 Renal gout in a veiled chameleon (*Chamaeleo calyptratus*). A dramatic increase in renal size is evident upon radiography (a). Ultrasonography shows hyperechoic renal parenchyma (b). Kidney biopsy (c) demonstrates clusters of acicular, birefringent, radiating, basophilic, or colorless structures compatible with urate crystal deposition (d). K, kidney.

Hyperthyroidism/Hypothyroidism

In reptiles, thyroid hormones maintain and stimulate metabolism, playing an important role in shedding and growth [27, 28]. Proliferative thyroid lesions and hyperthyroidism have been reported in lizards presenting with an intraoral mass, ventral throat swelling, oral bleeding, and weight loss [29, 30].

Hypothyroidism has been suspected in tortoises presenting with edema of the neck, head, and forelimbs, as well as decreased appetite and lethargy [31, 32].

When referring a reptile for a thyroid panel it should be clear that serum thyroxine levels in reptiles are sparsely reported in the literature, show important species-specific variations, and no thyroid stimulation tests have been described yet [33, 34]. The low thyroxine levels of snakes limit the validity of standard mammalian tests [35]. Therefore, a definitive clinical diagnosis of hypothyroidism and hyperthyroidism in reptiles is difficult.

Hyperparathyroidism and Hypoparathyroidism

Two forms of hyperparathyroidism are reported to be common in reptiles, secondary nutritional hyperparathyroidism, and secondary renal hyperparathyroidism.

Poor management and nutrition are still the most common causes of disease in reptiles that do not feed on whole prey items. This is typical in herbivorous reptiles (e.g. tortoises, iguanas) and omnivorous reptiles (e.g. bearded dragons) and is probably a combination between lack of sun exposure (i.e. ultraviolet light B [UVB] and temperature) and a diet containing high caloric intake and low calcium. The resulting calcium deficiency triggers an increased production of parathyroid hormone (PTH) that results in increased bone resorption. Therefore, these reptiles typically present with alterations of skeletal muscles, including curvature of long bones and softening of the jaw, or of the carapace. In order to better characterize the severity of these symptoms, radiographs, and calcium levels (total and ionized) should be measured. The reptile could also be referred for evaluation of the bone mineral content (as measured by Dual energy X-ray absorptiometry) [36] (Figure 51.7) and for measurement of vitamin D precursors and PTH.

Secondary renal hyperparathyroidism develops in patients with advanced renal disease mainly due to the lack of formation of vitamin D in the kidneys and to the increased loss of calcium through the renal tubules. Secondary renal hyperparathyroidism is suspected in reptiles with increased phosphorus, decreased calcium, and altered renal (uric acid or urea) values or evidence of renal pathology. A definitive assessment requires PTH measurement, glomerular filtration rate assessment, and renal biopsy [37].

The exact timing of decreased calcium levels, increased PTH levels, and bone resorption in reptiles with hyperparathyroidism remains unclear, despite research in this area [38]. Therefore, clinical assessment remains the main stay of diagnosis and prognosis.

Hypoparathyroidism has never been described in reptiles. However, in perfectly managed reptiles with increased phosphorus and decreased calcium and normal renal function, PTH measurement could theoretically differentiate between hypoparathyroidism and pseudohypoparathyroidism.

Bone Marrow Assessments

There are several clinical indications for bone marrow examination, including nonregenerative anemia, thrombocytopenia, lymphoproliferative disorders (e.g. leukemia), gammopathy, or suspected neoplasia. A common sampling site in small to medium lizards is the proximal femur, although the proximal tibia, proximal humerus, and the ileum can be used depending on the size of the reptile. In snakes, bone marrow biopsies are usually taken by removing a rib under general anesthesia [39]. In chelonians, suitable sites to collect specimens for histologic and cytologic evaluation of bone marrow include the pelvis, proximal portion of the humerus, femur, and thickened, peripheral portions of the cranial and caudal carapace or plastron [40]. The plastron is especially easy to access. For femoral bone marrow sampling, the reptile is anesthetized or locoregional anesthesia is performed. The area over the sampling, site is surgically prepared. A scalpel blade is used to incise the skin (or a sterile rotary tool in case of sampling from the plastron) and a spinal needle with a stylet in place is advanced into the medullary cavity by multiple gentle rotations. After removal of the stylet, negative pressure is applied with a 1-cc syringe. The sample of bone marrow is placed into ethylenediamine tetraacetic acid (EDTA) containers and slides are prepared before clotting.

Endoscopy

Due to the limits of current diagnostic capabilities in reptiles, it is more common to refer a reptile patient for endoscopy when compared to a mammal patient.

Coelioscopy

Coelioscopy involves the ingress of an endoscope (usually rigid) into the coelom. Coelioscopy permits visualization of the coelomic surface and sampling of most organs. Due to the unique unique anatomy, coelioscopy and

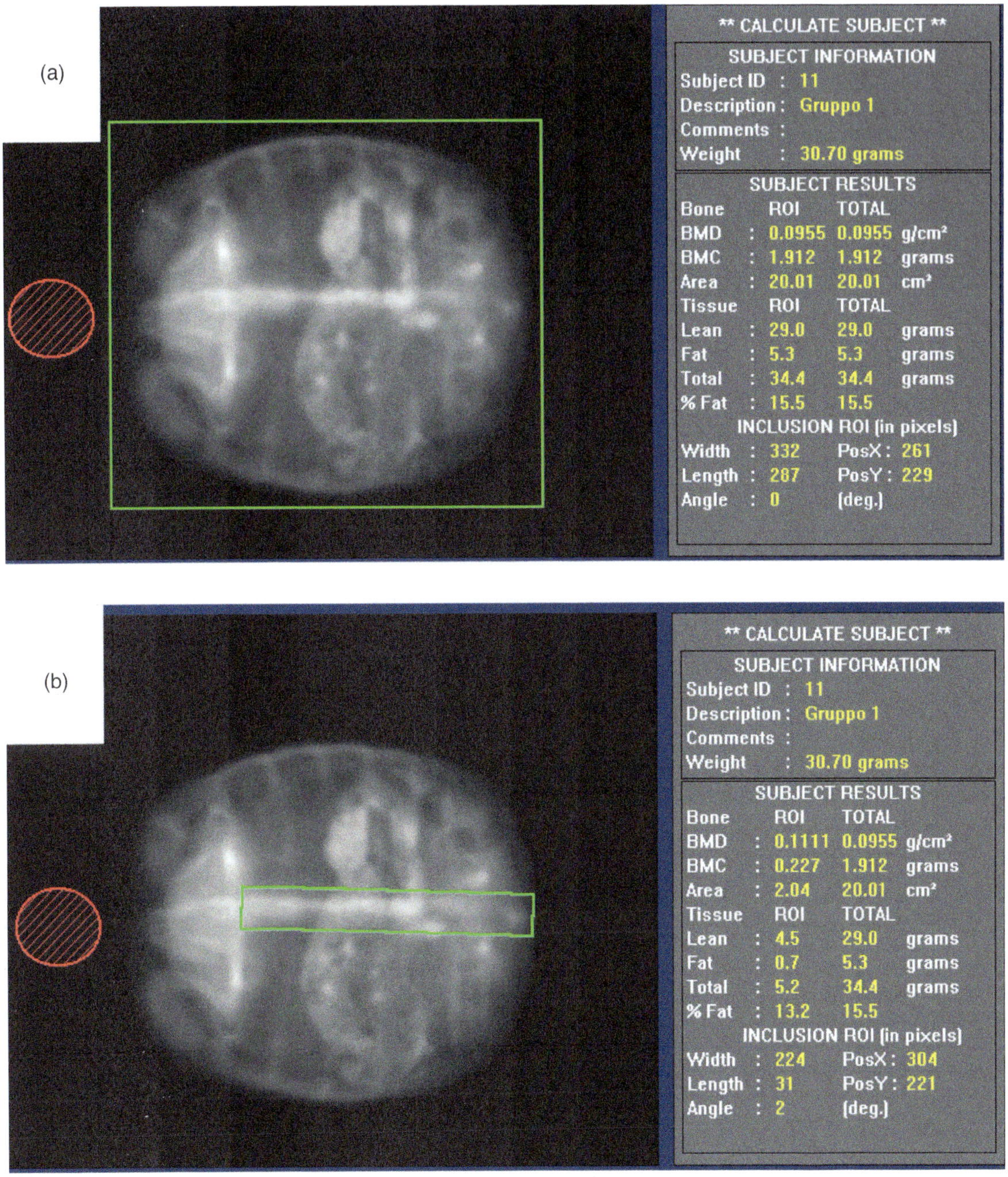

Figure 51.7 Bone mineral density measurement in a Hermann's tortoise (*Testudo hermanni*) by means of dual-energy X-ray absorptiometry. Measurements may include the entire chelonian (a), or focus on specific region of interest, e.g. the vertebral column (b).

coelioscopic surgery are most useful in chelonians [41]. In lizards, there are several indications for coelioscopy including kidney and liver biopsy [37, 42]. In snakes, diagnostic coelioscopy has fewer clinical indications, as their coelomic organs are distributed across a longer area and are not accessible through a single endoscopic breach. Additionally, most organs are easily reachable with a small incision, precluding the need for endoscopy for sampling. [43]. An alternative to coelioscopy in snakes is the examination of the coelom through percutaneous access in an air sac. This technique allows visualization of the lungs and the air sac, the bifurcation of the trachea, the external surface of the liver, the gall bladder and the spleen. In some cases, the pancreas and the surface of the stomach and colon may also be visualized [44].

Common Indications:

- Liver visualization and biopsy (Figure 51.8) [42]
- Kidney visualization and biopsy [37]
- Sexing [45]
- Diagnostic coelioscopy in case of undetermined illness

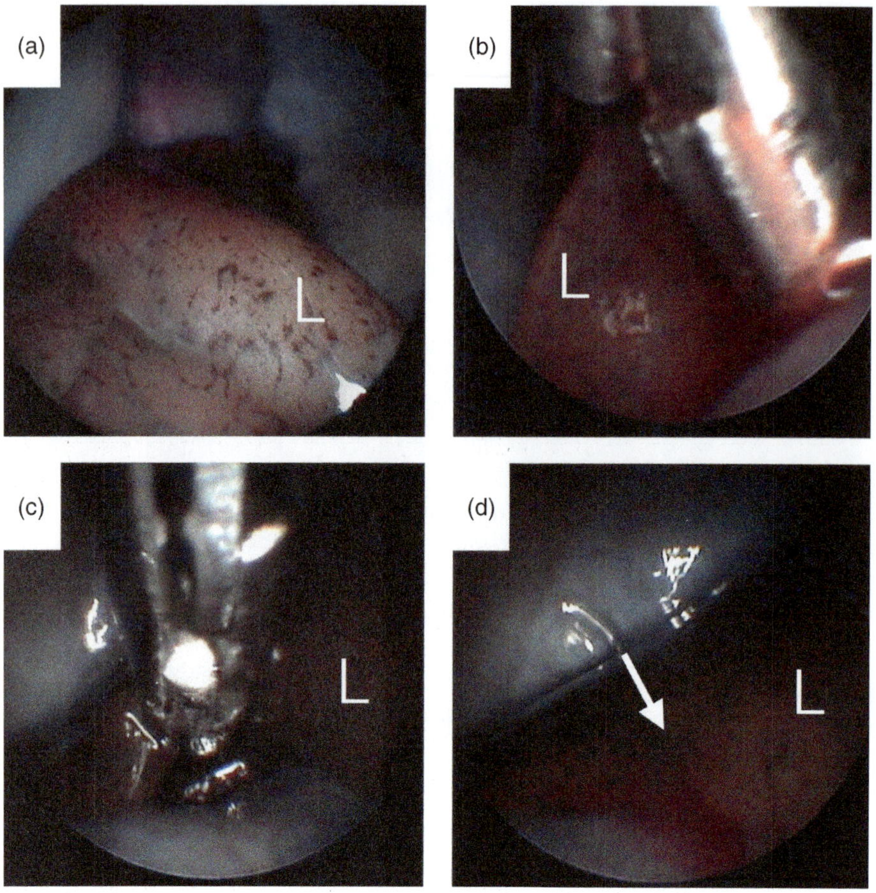

Figure 51.8 Endoscopic liver biopsy in an angulated tortoise (*Chersinia angulata*). The liver is visualized (a) and biopsy forceps are used to obtain a sample of the desired area (b, c). The liver is checked for excessive bleeding (arrow) (d). L, liver.

Technique

Coelioscopy can be performed without instillation, or with instillation of CO_2 or sterile saline. The equipment needed varies depending on the species, the size of the reptile, and on the purposes of the procedure. Coelioscopy should be performed under general anesthesia [45].

Endoscopy from Natural Openings

Endoscopic visualization of the mucosal surface of the trachea, the gastrointestinal tract and the urogenital tract are commonly indicated in clinical practice. Tracheal endoscopy permits diagnosis of intraluminal masses. Furthermore, endoscopic removal of tracheal lesions may be preferred over more invasive surgeries (i.e. tracheal resection and anastomosis) [46]. Cloacoscopy is useful to diagnose and retrieve cloacoliths or ectopic eggs [47, 48]. Foreign bodies can be retrieved with of gastrointestinal endoscopy [49]. One technique to relieve dystocia in snakes involves endoscopic visualization of the egg(s) before manual voiding [50]. Endoscopic-assisted manual voiding is advantageous over manual voiding alone because it allows endoscopic visualization and opening of the cervix, and permits instillation of fluids in the oviduct, facilitating passage of the egg(s).

Cystoscopy

Among common pet reptiles, chelonians and some lizards (e.g. green iguanas) have a urinary bladder, while snakes and other lizards (e.g. bearded dragons) lack it [51]. Many semiaquatic and semiterrestrial chelonians (typical in emydid turtles) also have accessory bladders, which typically consist of two rounded, saclike, structures dorso-lateral to the urinary bladder originating from the cloaca.

Indications

Disorders of the Urinary Bladder

Cystitis, urinary bladder stones and ectopic eggs in the urinary bladder are disorders that are ideally confirmed by cystoscopy. Urinary bladder stones and eggs may also be retrieved via cystoscopy [48], limiting the need for coelomic surgery. A common indication for cystoscopy in the emergency setting is rupture of the urinary bladder, which may occur secondary to trauma (Figure 51.9).

Cystoscopic Evaluation of the Coelom

In chelonians, cystoscopy may be used to visualize coelomic organs without surgical access to the coelom [52–54]. This is possible because the urinary bladder wall is thin and transparent when distended. Furthermore, once distended, the urinary bladder abuts most coelomic viscera, including the kidneys, gonads, adrenals, small and large intestine, stomach, pancreas, liver, lungs, and heart. This technique was developed to permit fast and minimally-invasive visualization of multiple coelomic organs and may be a useful diagnostic step to identify disease or to localize lesions in chelonians. It has particular merit for severely debilitated chelonians, where more invasive diagnostic procedures could be dangerous and for chelonians with nonspecific illness, as an initial screening technique to identify the diseased organ(s). The main limitation of cystoscopic coelomic evaluation is that it does not permit biopsy of or sample collection from the visceral organs. Therefore, histopathological, cytological, and microbiological analyses cannot be performed, and a definitive diagnosis cannot be made.

Biopsy/Histopathology Assessments

Histopathologic assessment is often thought to be a final and definitive diagnostic tool. Although this holds true for several disorders, infectious disease cannot be completely ruled out at the time of biopsy. Therefore, emergency veterinarians referring reptiles for biopsy should also request obtaining tissues for microbiology, mycology, +/− further molecular investigations. Histopathology is also required to confirm the pathogenicity of infectious agents especially when cultured from tissues that contact the external environment (Figure 51.10).

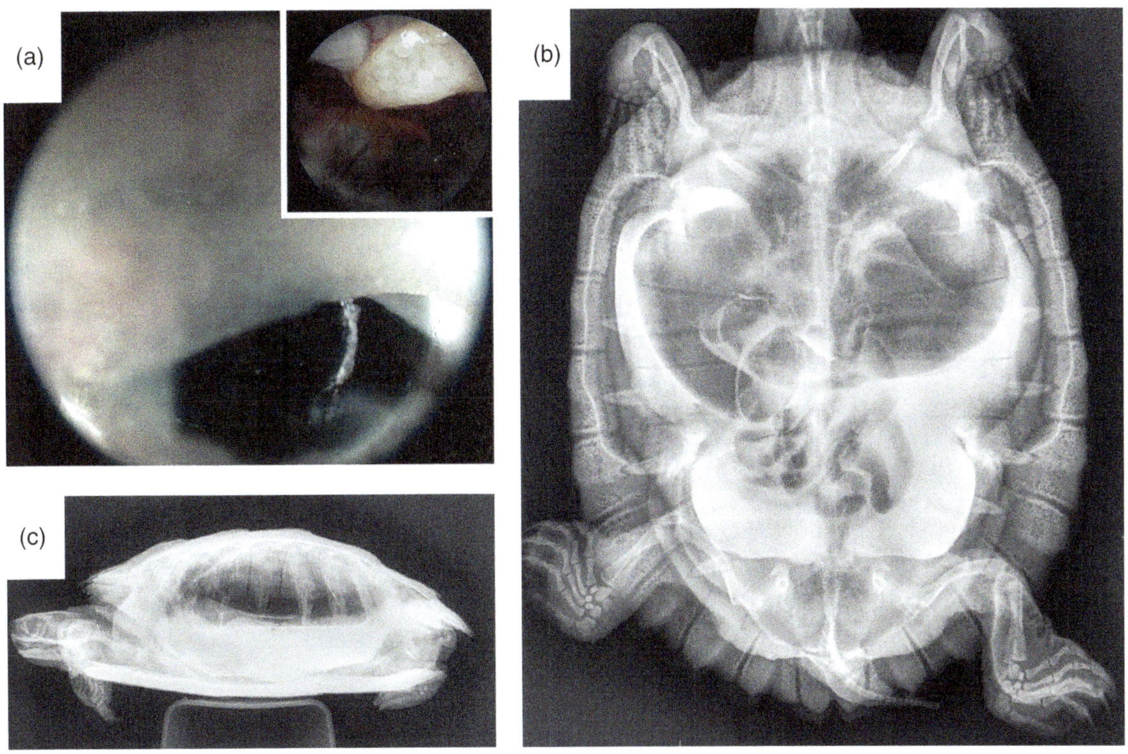

Figure 51.9 The urinary bladder may rupture in chelonians presented for trauma. Such cases should be referred for cystoscopy that may demonstrate rupture of the urinary bladder wall (a), with unhindered visualization of coelomic organs (inset). In suspect cases, contrast cystography (performed under endoscopic guidance) allows a definitive diagnosis by showing deposition of the contrast media in the entire coelom (b, c).

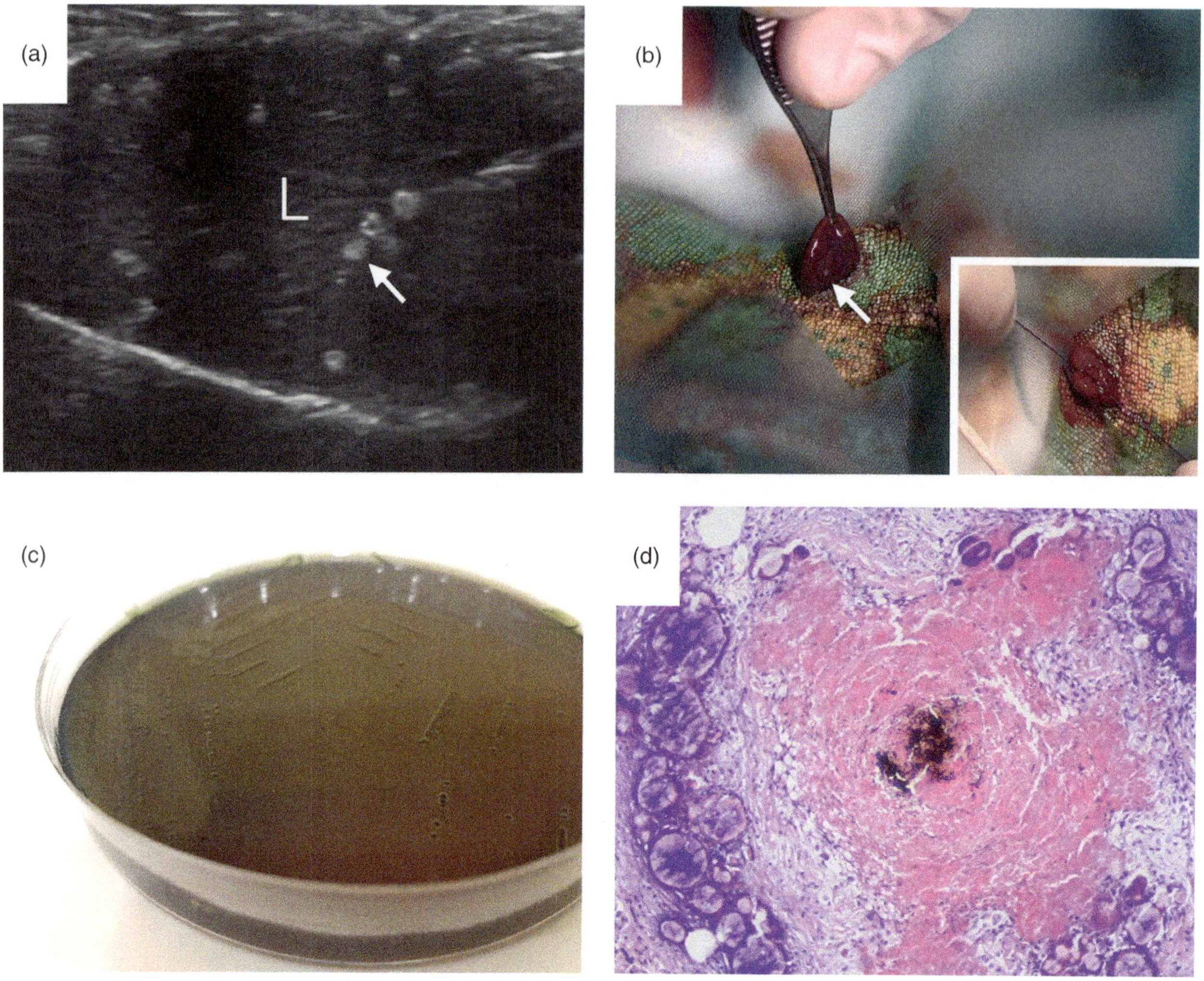

Figure 51.10 Sterile sampling of soft tissues for microbiology. A veiled chameleon (*Chamaeleo calyptratus*) was diagnosed with multiple hyperechoic lesions in the liver on ultrasound (arrow) (a). A liver biopsy was obtained (b) using a guillotine technique (inset). Culture on Hektoen Enteric Agar demonstrated growth of *Salmonella* spp. (c), and histology confirmed the presence of multiple granulomas with mineralization (d). Notice the ultrasonographic and macroscopic appearance of the granulomas (arrows). Histology and microbiology are complementary analyses in similar cases. L, liver. *Source:* Photo (c) courtesy of Giorgia Matteucci.

Invasiveness of the biopsy depends on the tissue sampled. Skin samples are easy to obtain even under local anesthesia while organ samples usually require a surgical plane of anesthesia to obtain. Biopsy of internal organs can be performed through open surgical, endoscopic, or percutaneous approaches. Although it may seem obvious that less invasive techniques (i.e. endoscopic or percutaneous) should be always elected over open surgical techniques, the preferred approach depends on the species, the tissue needed, the indications for biopsy (i.e. quantity of tissue needed), the type of lesion suspected (e.g. focal vs. multifocal vs. diffuse) and surgeon preference (Table 51.2). Plastronotomy should never be suggested for diagnostic reasons in chelonians due to its invasiveness.

Collected tissue samples must be fixed in 10% neutral phosphate buffered formalin for subsequent histopathology and special stains. Sample dimension and amount of formalin are critical for an appropriate fixation. Formalin penetrates 0.5 cm of tissue in 24 hours; therefore, thick sections can decompose despite an adequate amount of formalin.

Table 51.2 The author's favored approaches for biopsy of organs in reptiles.

Species	Organ	Preferred sampling technique	Reason	Alternative sampling technique
Liver	Chelonians	Coelioscopy	Liver is easily identifiable through endoscopic approach	—
	Lizards	Open surgical or percutaneous	The liver lies under the coastal arch and is easily accessible with a small incision	Coelioscopy
	Snakes	Open surgical or percutaneous	Liver is easily accessible with a small incision after ultrasound identification	Coelioscopy
Kidney	Chelonians	Open surgical through prefemoral fossa incision	Kidneys are retrocoelomic. In many chelonians, the kidneys are easily accessible through the dorsal aspect of the prefemoral fossa.	Coelioscopy
	Lizards	Open surgical through post-femoral incision	Kidneys are easily accessible with a small post-femoral incision	Coelioscopy
	Snakes	Open surgical or percutaneous	Kidneys are easily accessible with a small incision after ultrasound identification	Coelioscopy
Gastro intestinal	All species	Endoluminal endoscopy	Endoluminal approach avoids the need to access the coelom	Open surgical (prefemoral fossa in chelonians)
Pancreas, spleen, or splenopancreas	All species	Coelioscopy	Difficult to reach otherwise	Open surgical

These indications are for small to medium-sized reptiles. Preferred sampling techniques and procedures may differ significantly in large pet and/or captive zoological reptiles. This information is based on the personal experience of one of the authors (ND).

References

1 Origgi, F.C. and Paré, J.A. (2007). Isolation of pathogens. In: *Infectious Diseases and Pathology of Reptiles* (ed. E.R. Jacobson), 667–680. Boca Raton, FL: CRC Press.

2 Di Girolamo, N., Selleri, P., Nardini, G. et al. (2014). Computed tomography-guided bone biopsies for evaluation of proliferative vertebral lesions in two boa constrictors (*Boa constrictor imperator*). *J. Zoo Wildl. Med.* 45 (4): 973–978.

3 Plenz, B., Schmidt, V., Grosse-Herrenthey, A. et al. (2015). Characterisation of the aerobic bacterial flora of boid snakes: application of MALDI-TOF mass spectrometry. *Vet. Rec.* 176: 285.

4 Di Ianni, F., Dodi, P.L., Cabassi, C.S. et al. (2015). Conjunctival flora of clinically normal and diseased turtles and tortoises. *BMC Vet. Res.* 11: 91.

5 Taddei, S., Dodi, P.L., Di Ianni, F. et al. (2010). Conjunctival flora of clinically normal captive green iguanas (*Iguana iguana*). *Vet. Rec.* 167: 29–30.

6 Hejnar, P., Bardon, J., Sauer, P., and Kolár, M. (2007). Stenotrophomonas maltophilia as a part of normal oral bacterial flora in captive snakes and its susceptibility to antibiotics. *Vet. Microbiol.* 121: 357–362.

7 Sangster, N., Batterham, P., Chapman, H.D. et al. (2002). Resistance to antiparasitic drugs: the role of molecular diagnosis. *Int. J. Parasitol.* 32: 637–653.

8 Armas, F., Furlanello, T., Camperio, C. et al. (2016). Molecular characterization and drug susceptibility profile of a Mycobacterium avium subspecies avium isolate from a dog with disseminated infection. *J. Med. Microbiol.* 65 (4): 278–285.

9 Foti, M., Giacopello, C., Fisichella, V., and Latella, G. (2013). Multidrug-resistant *Pseudomonas aeruginosa* isolates from captive reptiles. *J. Exot. Pet. Med.* 22: 270–274.

10 Casey, C.L., Hernandez, S.M., Yabsley, M.J. et al. (2015). The carriage of antibiotic resistance by enteric bacteria from imported tokay geckos (*Gekko gecko*) destined for the pet trade. *Sci. Total Environ.* 505: 299–305.

11 Di Girolamo, N. and Selleri, P. (2015). On what evidence are reptile formularies based? *Proceedings of the Association of Reptilian and Amphibian Veterinarians, 22nd Annual Conference*, San Antonio, TX.

12 Schumacher, J. (2003). Fungal diseases of reptiles. *Vet. Clin. North Am. Exot. Anim. Pract.* 6: 327–335.

13 Ebani, V.V., Fratini, F., Bertelloni, F. et al. (2012). Isolation and identification of mycobacteria from captive reptiles. *Res. Vet. Sci.* 93 (3): 1136–1138.

14 Marschang, R.E. and Divers, S.J. (2013). Reptile viruses. In: *Current Therapy in Reptile Medicine and Surgery* (eds. D.R. Mader and S.J. Divers), 368–381. Elsevier Health Sciences.

15 Jacobson, E.R. and Origgi, F.C. (2007). Serodiagnostics. In: *Infectious Diseases and Pathology of Reptiles* (ed. E.R. Jacobson), 381–394. Boca Raton, FL: CRC Press.

16 Wellehan, J.F.X. (2013). Molecular infectious disease diagnostics. In: *Current Therapy in Reptile Medicine and Surgery* (eds. D.R. Mader and S.J. Divers), 27–31. Elsevier Health Sciences.

17 Weir, S.M., Yu, S., Knox, A. et al. (2016). Acute toxicity and risk to lizards of rodenticides and herbicides commonly used in New Zealand. *N. Z. J. Ecol.* 40 (3): 342–350.

18 Brooks, J.E., Savarie, P.J., and Johnston, J.J. (1998). The oral and dermal toxicity of selected chemicals to brown tree snakes (*Boiga irregularis*). *Wildl. Res.* 25: 427–435.

19 Sánchez-Barbudo, I.S., Camarero, P.R., and Mateo, R. (2012). Primary and secondary poisoning by anticoagulant rodenticides of non-target animals in Spain. *Sci. Total Environ.* 420: 280–288.

20 Van de Merwe, J.P., Hodge, M., Olszowy, H.A. et al. (2010). Using blood samples to estimate persistent organic pollutants and metals in green sea turtles (*Chelonia mydas*). *Mar. Pollut. Bull.* 60: 579–588.

21 Lehner, A.F., Rumbeiha, W., Shlosberg, A. et al. (2013). Diagnostic analysis of veterinary dried blood spots for toxic heavy metals exposure. *J. Anal. Toxicol.* 37: 406–422.

22 Sturrock, R.D. (2000). Gout: Easy to misdiagnose. *BMJ* 320: 132–133.

23 Stern, A.W., Velguth, K.E., and D'Agostino, J. (2010). Metastatic ductal adenocarcinoma in a Western hognose snake (*Heterodon nasicus*). *J. Zoo Wildl. Med.* 41: 320–324.

24 Frye, F.L., Dutra, F.R., Carney, J.D., and Johnson, B. (1976). Spontaneous diabetes mellitus in a turtle. *Vet. Med. Small Anim. Clin.* 71: 935–939.

25 Stahl, S. (2006). Hyperglycemia in reptiles. In: *Reptile Medicine and Surgery*, 2e (ed. D.R. Mader), 822–830. St Louis: Elsevier.

26 Ritter, J.M., Garner, M.M., Chilton, J.A. et al. (2009). Gastric neuroendocrine carcinomas in bearded dragons (*Pogona vitticeps*). *Vet. Pathol.* 46: 1109–1116.

27 Rivera, S. and Lock, B. (2008). The reptilian thyroid and parathyroid glands. *Vet. Clin. North Am. Exot. Anim. Pract.* 11: 163–175.

28 Denver, R.J. and Licht, P. (1991). Dependence of body growth on thyroid-activity in turtles. *J. Exp. Zool.* 258: 48–59.

29 Hernandez-Divers, S.J., Knott, C.D., and MacDonald, J. (2001). Diagnosis and surgical treatment of thyroid adenoma-induced hyperthyroidism in a green iguana (*Iguana iguana*). *J. Zoo Wildl. Med.* 32: 465–475.

30 Hadfield, C.A., Clayton, L.A., Clancy, M.M. et al. (2012). Proliferative thyroid lesions in three diplodactylid geckos: *Nephrurus amyae*, *Nephrurus levis*, and *Oedura marmorata*. *J. Zoo Wildl. Med.* 43: 131–140.

31 Norton, T.M., Jacobson, E.R., Caligiuri, R. et al. (1989). Medical management of a Galapagos tortoise (*Geochelone elephantopus*) with hypothyroidism. *J. Zoo Wildl. Med.* 20: 212–216.

32 Franco, K.H. and Hoover, J.P. (2009). Levothyroxine as a treatment for presumed hypothyroidism in an adult male African spurred tortoise (*Centrochelys* [formerly *Geochelone*] *sulcata*). *J. Herpetol. Med. Surg.* 19: 42–44.

33 Franco, K.H., Famini, D.J., Hoover, J.P. et al. (2009). Serum thyroid hormone values for African spurred tortoises (*Centrochelys* [formerly Geochelone] sulcata). *J. Herpetol. Med. Surg.* 19: 47–49.

34 Kohel, K.A., MacKenzie, D.S., Rostal, D.C. et al. (2001). Seasonality in plasma thyroxine in the desert tortoise, *Gopherus agassizii*. *Gen. Comp. Endocrinol.* 121: 214–222.

35 Greenacre, C.B., Young, D.W., Behrend, E.N. et al. (2001). Validation of a novel high-sensitivity radioimmunoassay procedure for measurement of total thyroxine concentration in psittacine birds and snakes. *Am. J. Vet. Res.* 62: 1750–1754.

36 Gramanzini, M., Di Girolamo, N., Gargiulo, S. et al. (2013). Assessment of dual-energy X-ray absorptiometry for use in evaluating the effects of dietary and environmental management on Hermann's tortoises (*Testudo hermanni*). *Am. J. Vet. Res.* 74: 918–924.

37 Hernandez-Divers, S.J., Stahl, S.J., Stedman, N.L. et al. (2005). Renal evaluation in the healthy green iguana (*Iguana iguana*): assessment of plasma biochemistry, glomerular filtration rate, and endoscopic biopsy. *J. Zoo Wildl. Med.* 36: 155–168.

38 Hoby, S., Wenker, C., Robert, N. et al. (2010). Nutritional metabolic bone disease in juvenile veiled chameleons (*Chamaeleo calyptratus*) and its prevention. *J. Nutr.* 140: 1923–1931.

39 Hernandez-Divers, S.J. (2006). Diagnostic techniques. In: *Reptile Medicine and Surgery* (ed. D.R. Mader), 490–532. St Louis, MI: Saunders Elsevier.

40 Garner, M.M., Homer, B.L., Jacobson, E.R. et al. (1996). Staining and morphologic features of bone marrow hematopoietic cells in desert tortoises (*Gopherus agassizii*). *Am. J. Vet. Res.* 57: 1608–1615.

41 Divers, S.J., Stahl, S.J., and Camus, A. (2010). Evaluation of diagnostic coelioscopy including liver and kidney biopsy in freshwater turtles (*Trachemys scripta*). *J. Zoo Wildl. Med.* 41: 677–687.

42 Hernandez-Divers, S.J., Stahl, S.J., McBride, M., and Stedman, N.L. (2007). Evaluation of an endoscopic liver biopsy technique in green iguanas. *J. Am. Vet. Med. Assoc.* 230: 1849–1853.

43 Di Girolamo, N. and Mans, C. (2016). Reptile soft tissue surgery. *Vet. Clin. North Am. Exot. Anim. Pract.* 19: 97–131.

44 Jekl, V. and Knotek, Z. (2006). Endoscopic examination of snakes by access through an air sac. *Vet. Rec.* 158: 407.

45 Hernandez-Divers, S.J., Stahl, S.J., and Farrell, R. (2009). An endoscopic method for identifying sex of hatchling Chinese box turtles and comparison of general versus local anesthesia for coelioscopy. *J. Am. Vet. Med. Assoc.* 234: 800–804.

46 Drew, M.L., Phalen, D.N., Berridge, B.R. et al. (1999). Partial tracheal obstruction due to chondromas in ball pythons (*Python regius*). *J. Zoo Wildl. Med.* 30: 151–157.

47 Mans, C. and Sladky, K.K. (2012). Endoscopically guided removal of cloacal calculi in three African spurred tortoises (*Geochelone sulcata*). *J. Am. Vet. Med. Assoc.* 240: 869–875.

48 Minter, L.J., Wood, M.W., Hill, T.L., and Lewbart, G.A. (2010). Cystoscopic guided removal of ectopic eggs from the urinary bladder of the Florida cooter turtle (*Pseudemys floridana floridana*). *J. Zoo Wildl. Med.* 41: 503–509.

49 Mans, C. and Braun, J. (2014). Update on common nutritional disorders of captive reptiles. *Vet. Clin. North Am. Exot. Anim. Pract.* 17: 369–395.

50 Di Girolamo, N. and Selleri, P. (2017). Diseases of the reproductive tract in snakes. *Vet. Clin. North Am. Exot. Anim. Pract.* 20 (2): 391–409.

51 Beuchat, C.A. (1986). Phylogenetic distribution of the urinary bladder in lizards. *Copeia* 1986: 512–517.

52 Selleri, P., Di Girolamo, N., and Melidone, R. (2013). Cystoscopic sex identification of posthatchling chelonians. *J. Am. Vet. Med. Assoc.* 242: 1744–1750.

53 Di Girolamo, N., Melidone, R., Catania, S. et al. (2016). Use of cystoscopy to visualize morphological alteration of the liver in a posthatchling turtle (*Cuora trifasciata*). *J. Am. Anim. Hosp. Assoc.* 52: 170–174.

54 Di Girolamo, N. and Selleri, P. (2015). Clinical applications of cystoscopy in chelonians. *Vet. Clin. North Am. Exot. Anim. Pract.* 18: 507–526.

Section 3

Emergency Presentations and Management by Species

52

Turtles and Tortoises

Krista A. Keller

Department of Veterinary Clinical Medicine Codirector, Wildlife Epidemiology Laboratory College of Veterinary Medicine University of Illinois Urbana, Illinois, USA

CONTENTS

Unique Species Considerations

- Although most species of chelonians are hard shelled, there are a few species that are not expected to have a rigid shell, most notably in the pet trade is the pancake tortoise (*Malacochersus tornieri*). The flexibility of this species' shell should not be confused with pathology
- Many species of chelonians have a hinged plastron, which should not be confused with fractures and may help in identification of a particular species. This includes the North American (*Terrapene* spp.) and Asian (*Cuora* spp.) box turtles, some mud turtles (*Kinosternon* spp.) and the Blanding's turtle (*Emys (Emydoidea) blandingii*)
- The reader is directed to Chapter 45: Analgesia, Anesthesia and Monitoring for current recommendations regarding anti-inflammatory and analgesic drug use in chelonians, as well as sedation and anesthetic protocols for these species

Common Presenting Signs

Anorexia

Introduction

- In general, anorexia without other abnormalities or complaints noted is not reason enough for an emergency visit, however, anorectic chelonians should be evaluated by their primary care provider as soon as possible
- Chelonians may exhibit a high incidence of hepatic lipidosis as a sequela to anorexia, especially if they are obese prior to the anorexic event [1]

Exotic Animal Emergency and Critical Care Medicine, First Edition. Edited by Jennifer E. Graham, Grayson A. Doss, and Hugues Beaufrère.

Diagnosis

History:

- Perform a full husbandry review (see Box 52.1)
- Previous history of hibernation and egg laying

Signalment:

- Adult breeding age females may go through a physiologic fast during the egg laying period
- Hatchlings may not require feeding for the first days to weeks of life as nutrition is provided by the internalized yolk

Clinical Signs:

- Dehydration (enophthalmos, sticky saliva)
- Lack of appetite

Differentials:

- Physiological causes (egg laying, neonate, hibernation/brumation)
- Pathological
  - Any underlying systemic disease can lead to anorexia
  - Inappropriate husbandry

STAT Diagnostics:

- Radiographs
- Ionized calcium
- Fecal direct mount + flotation

Complete Diagnostics:

- Cell blood count (CBC)/chemistry
- Contrast radiographic study
- Special stains on fecal cytology (acid fast)
- Molecular diagnostics
  - *Cryptosporidium* spp.
  - *Giardia* spp.
- Intranuclear coccidiosis
- Bacterial/fungal cultures
- Gastrointestinal (GI) endoscopy or coelioscopy +/− biopsies

Treatment

Stabilization:

- Fluid therapy (Chapter 46: Nutrition and Fluid Therapy)
- Anti-inflammatories
- Thermal support
- Empirical antibiotics (Table 52.1)
- Appropriate antiparasitics based on fecal analysis findings

Continued Care:

- Address and correct husbandry deficits
- Referral to specialist for advanced diagnostics (e.g. endoscopy)
- Nutritional support (Chapter 46: Nutrition and Fluid Therapy)

Neurologic Signs

Introduction

- A variety of non-neurologic illnesses may present with diffuse neurological signs including weakness and limb flaccidity.
- Neurological examination of reptiles has been described and should be utilized for neuroanatomical localization [2]

Box 52.1 Appropriate General Husbandry Review Questions When Evaluating the Sick Chelonian

- What diet items are offered? What components of the diet are eaten?
- What supplements are provided and at what frequency?
- What lighting sources are provided, especially is there a ultraviolet light B (UVB)-emitting bulb?
  - How far away from the patient is the UVB-emitting bulb?
  - Does the light from the bulb transmit through screen or glass?
  - When was the UVB bulb purchased? Has it passed the manufacturer's expiration date?
  - When are the lights and UVB bulb turned on/off?
- What heat sources are provided and for how many hours per day/night?
- Are there thermometers to provide accurate ambient air temperature readings? What are the coolest/warmest daytime/nighttime temperatures?
- What substrate is used? What is the cage cleaning schedule?
- Housed singly or with others? Are cage mates same species (conspecifics) or other species?
- Additional questions specific for the aquatic chelonian
  - What filtration system is utilized? How often/how is the filter cleaned?
  - Are water quality tests are performed routinely? Any recorded values?
  - Are there live plants within the enclosure?
  - Is there is an accessible haul-out area?
  - Are there thermometers to provide accurate water temperature readings? What are the temperatures achieved?

Herptiles

Table 52.1 Commonly used antibiotics, dosages, bacterial spectrum, and concerns for use in the sick chelonian.

Antibiotic	Dosage	Antibiotic spectrum	Concerns/notes
Amikacin	5 mg/kg IM, SC q48h	• Gram-negative spectrum better than Gram-positive spectrum • Aerobes (not anaerobes)	• Potential nephrotoxicity • Maintain hydration through treatment period
Ceftazidime	20 mg/kg IM, SC q72h	• Gram-positive, Gram-negative • Aerobes and anaerobes	• Not effective against *Mycoplasma* spp. • Third generation cephalosporins (in conjunction with fluoroquinolones) are first line of treatment for reptile-associated human salmonellosis
Enrofloxacin	5 mg/kg IM, SC q12–24h	• Gram-negative spectrum better than Gram-positive spectrum in most tissues • Aerobes (not anaerobes)	• Must use more frequent dosing for *Pseudomonas* infections • Intramuscular injections associated with discomfort, abscesses; if administering more than single injection, give diluted SC • Hyperexcitation noted in Galapagos tortoises

Diagnosis

History:

- Full husbandry review (see Box 52.1)
- Previous history of hibernation and egg laying
- Contact with other species
- Potential access to toxins

Signalment:

- Young, rapidly growing animals are likely to be suffering from hypocalcemia of nutritional/husbandry origin
- Older animals suffering from chronic renal disease may be suffering from hypocalcemia of renal origin

Clinical Signs:

- *Central/cranial nerve signs*: Circling, seizures, head tilt, nystagmus
- *Spinal signs*: Hemiparesis to tetraplegia, lack of tail movement, lack of vent tone

Differentials:

- Trauma
- Nutritional
  - Vitamin E deficiency
  - Thiamine deficiency in reptile species fed fish
  - Hypocalcemia
- Infectious (*Entamoeba invadens*)
- Toxins (e.g. heavy metals, insecticides, ivermectin, metronidazole, bromethalin, metaldehyde, nicotine, marijuana, chlorhexidine)
- Metabolic (gout)

STAT Diagnostics:

- Full neurologic examination
- Ionized calcium
- Blood glucose

Complete Diagnostics:

- CBC/chemistry
- Fecal direct mount + flotation
- Radiographs
- Heavy metal concentrations
- Advanced imaging (computed tomography [CT]/magnetic resonance imaging [MRI]) – may aid in evaluation of spinal disruption or intracranial disease

Treatment

Stabilization:

- Fluid therapy (see Chapter 46: Nutrition and Fluid Therapy)
- Anticonvulsant medications if seizures present
  - Diazepam 0.5 mg/kg IV
  - Midazolam 1 mg/kg IM/IV
- *Thermal support*: Patients should be kept in their preferred optimal temperature zone (POTZ)
- Correct hypocalcemia
- Empirical antibiotics (Table 52.1)

Continued Care:

- Correct husbandry deficits
- Chelation therapy
- Referral to a specialist for continued long term care
- Esophagostomy tube placement may be necessary

Prolapse

Introduction

The most important aspects of prolapse management and elucidating prognosis is identification of which tissue is prolapsed and whether that tissue is viable or devitalized.

Diagnosis

History:

- Full husbandry review (see Box 52.1)
- Previous egg laying history
- Recent change in droppings (e.g. diarrhea, change in urates)

Signalment:

- Young and fast-growing animals are at risk for cloacal prolapse secondary to nutritional secondary hyperparathyroidism and rectal prolapse secondary to endoparasitism
- Reproductively active females may prolapse the oviduct secondary to dystocia and egg retention and/or salpingitis
- Reproductively mature males may exhibit phallic prolapse during the breeding season

Clinical Signs:

- Straining (tail wagging, grunting, extended hind limbs, bubbling from nose)
- Tissue material coming from the vent opening (Figure 52.1)
- Healthy, viable tissue will be pink or red, moist, +/− bleeding
- Devitalized tissue can be dry, excessively swollen, discolored, not bleeding when manipulated

Differentials:

- Cloacal prolapse may represent oviductal, phallic, rectal, or bladder tissue.
- Oviductal tissue is pink, has linear striations and a lumen that feces does not originate from. Causes of oviductal prolapse include egg binding/dystocia, salpingitis (Figure 52.1a).
- Rectal tissue is pink, lacks linear striations and has a lumen where feces can pass. In cases where there is an obstruction due to tissue swelling or intussusception, no feces will be produced. Causes of rectal tissue prolapse include endoparasitism, diarrhea, and impaction/constipation (Figure 52.1b)
- Phalllic tissue is often pigmented, originates from the ventral aspect of the cloaca and lacks a lumen. Causes of phallus prolapse include trauma to phallus, excessive breeding activity, and hypocalcemia (Figure 52.1c)
- Bladder prolapse is the rarest form of cloacal prolapse. The tissue is pink, very thin, and lacks a lumen. Bladder prolapse is often secondary to urolithiasis

STAT Diagnostics:

- Cloacal examination – based upon size of the patient use either a lubricated gloved finger, cotton tipped applicator or red rubber tube to evaluate the presence or absence of a lumen and from where in the cloaca the tissue is arising
- Radiographs – rule out the presence of eggs, sand impaction, and urolithiasis
- Ionized calcium
- Fecal direct mount + flotation

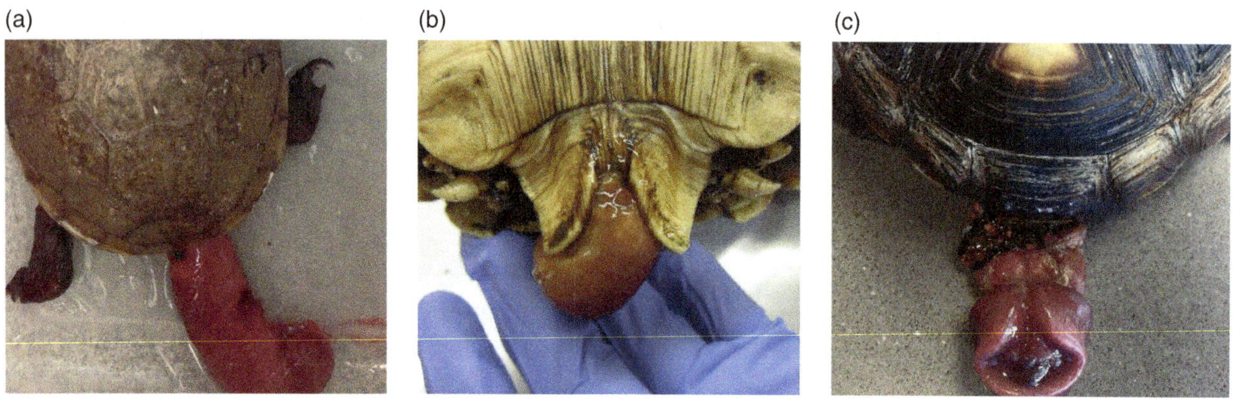

Figure 52.1 Cloacal prolapse in chelonians may represent a variety of tissues including phallic, rectal, or oviductal tissue. (a) Dorsal view of a partially devitalized oviductal prolapse in a 20 year old female three-toed box turtle (*Terrapenne carolensis triungis*). The classically described linear striations are not visible due to the large amount of edema present. (b) Ventral view of rectal prolapse without devitalization in a three year old female sulcata tortoise (*Centrochelys (Geochelone) sulcata*). (c) Dorsal view of a phallic prolapse without devitalization in a six year old male red-footed tortoise (*Chelonoidis (Geochelone) carbonaria*).

Complete Diagnostics:

- CBC/chemistry
- Cloacoscopy
- Additional fecal diagnostics – consider *Cryptosporidium* Polymerase chain reaction (PCR), intranuclear coccidia PCR

Treatment

Stabilization:

- Analgesics
- Anti-inflammatories
- Fluid administration (see Chapter 46: Nutrition and Fluid Therapy)
- Thermal support – patients should be kept in POTZ
- Prolapse reduction (if tissue is viable):
  - Most cases will be facilitated by the use of
    - Heavy sedation or general anesthesia [3]
    - Intrathecal anesthesia [4]
  - Use cooled, hypertonic (50% dextrose, 7.5% NaCl) solutions to reduce edema of tissue before utilizing lubrication and gentle pressure (digital, cotton tipped applicators) to reduce the tissue back into the cloaca
  - The vent opening should be reduced by placing lateral cloacal sutures. Ensure that feces can still pass out of the vent opening by ensuring the tip of one or two cotton tipped applicators can pass through the vent opening
- Empirical antibiotics (Table 52.1)
- Antiparasitics – based upon parasitological examination (Table 52.2)

Continued Care:

- Address husbandry deficits
- Surgical correction (devitalized tissue):
  - Phallic prolapses can be managed through amputation of the devitalized tissue. The phallus in chelonians functions only as a copulatory organ and is not required for urination
  - Oviductal prolapses can be managed with either ovari-osalpingectomy or external resection and anastomosis of the tissue. The former has the benefit of reducing incidence of recurrence and should be performed by a specialist
  - Devitalized rectal prolapses carry a poor prognosis, but management can be attempted through resection and anastomosis of the tissue

Respiratory Signs

Introduction

- Chelonians with respiratory signs can present in critical condition and require immediate attention
- Although many animals will exhibit upper respiratory signs, it is important to investigate for lower respiratory tract involvement which is often occult

Diagnosis

History:

- Full husbandry review (see Box 52.1)
- Contact with other species
- Recent hibernation/brumation

Signalment:

- *Gopherus* spp. tortoises (desert tortoise, gopher tortoise) and other species that may come into contact with these species are commonly affected with *Mycoplasma* infections [5]
- Many species are known to harbor different strains of testudid herpesvirus (e.g. Russian tortoises [*Agrioneyms horsfieldii*] may carry but not be clinically affected with Testudinid herpesvirus-1) [6]

Table 52.2 Commonly used antiparasitic agents, dosages, parasitic spectrum, and concerns for use in chelonians.

Agent	Dosage	Parasitic spectrum	Concerns/notes
Emodepside + praziquantel (Profender, Bayer)	1.12 ml/kg topical	• Nematodes • Cestodes	• Must keep aquatic turtles dry for 48 h after application
Fenbendazole	100 mg/kg PO once	• Nematodes • Protozoans (*Giardia* spp.)	• Shedding of ova may occur for 30+ d • Use with caution; can cause toxicosis (leukopenia)
Ivermectin	—	—	• Contraindicated for use in chelonians
Levamisole	5 mg/kg SC, ICe	• Nematodes	• Narrow safety margin
Metronidazole	25 mg/kg PO q24d for 5 d 50 mg/kg PO q14d	• Protozoans • Amoeba	• May cause neurological signs if overdosed or concurrent hepatopathy • May stimulate appetite

Herptiles

Clinical Signs:

- Bubbling from nares or nasal discharge
- Open mouth breathing
- Audible respiratory sounds
- Oral discharge
- Tachypnea
- Increased respiratory excursions
- Extension of the head and neck
- Buoyancy issues (aquatic species)
- Cyanotic mucous membranes

Differentials:

- Infectious (Bacterial: *Pasteurella testudinis*, *Mycoplasma* spp., other agents; viral: Testudinid herpesvirus, ranavirus; rarely fungal infections)
- Trauma
- Foreign body/material
- Vitamin A deficiency with squamous metaplasia
- Near drowning
- Smoke inhalation

STAT Diagnostics:

- Radiographs
- Pulse oximetry

Complete Diagnostics:

- CBC, chemistry
- Serology (Testudinid herpesvirus, *Mycoplasma agassizii*)
- PCR (*Mycoplasma* spp., Testudinid herpesvirus, ranavirus)
- Nasal flush or endotracheal wash for cytology and culture
- Advanced imaging (computed tomography/MRI)
- Tracheoscopy and transcarapacial/prefemoral pulmonoscopy

Treatment

Stabilization:

- O_2 therapy (Chapter 41: Oxygen Therapy)
- Fluid therapy (Chapter 46: Nutrition and Fluid Therapy)
- Empirical antibiotics (Table 52.1)
- Anti-inflammatories
- Use of bronchodilators (aminophylline 2–4 mg/kg IM)

Continued Care:

- Treat underlying cause (e.g. antibiotics, antifungals)
- Transcarapacial therapeutic catheterization for local lung therapy
- Vitamin A supplementation
  - Appropriate diet/supplementation is preferred
    - 5000 IU/kg PO or in food
  - Parenteral supplementation is likely to cause toxicity (epidermal sloughing), especially in herbivorous species
- Nutritional support (Chapter 46: Nutrition and Fluid Therapy)

Trauma

Introduction

- Inciting cause of trauma may be from conspecifics, predators, or from interaction with the enclosure or a moving vehicle
- As in mammals, the traumatized chelonian should have their neurologic, musculoskeletal, and respiratory systems evaluated
- The gregarious nature and relatively small size of most species put many individuals at risk of traumatic injury

Diagnosis

History:

- Full husbandry review (see Box 52.1)
- Length of period since traumatic event

Signalment:

- Breeding age animals during the spring in North America may be more prone to wandering behaviors and resulting trauma
- Males housed with other males may exhibit territorial and aggressive behavior
- Males housed with females of breeding age may continuously harass and bite them
- Adults housed with juveniles may exhibit aggressive behavior (species dependent)

Clinical Signs:

- Based on traumatized body system and source of trauma
- Respiratory signs – lungs, trachea
- Neurologic signs – spinal, cranial
- Musculoskeletal signs – shell, soft tissue
  - Check for presence of fly-strike (maggots) in appropriate seasons
  - Shell fractures (Figure 52.2)
    - Can be markedly unstable (involvement of one or both shell bridges) or relatively unstable (crack from marginal scutes)
    - Should be characterized as partial thickness (overlying keratin fracture only without underlying bony shell involvement) or full thickness (keratin and shell fracture)
    - Full thickness fractures should be evaluated to see if there is communication with the coelomic cavity or not

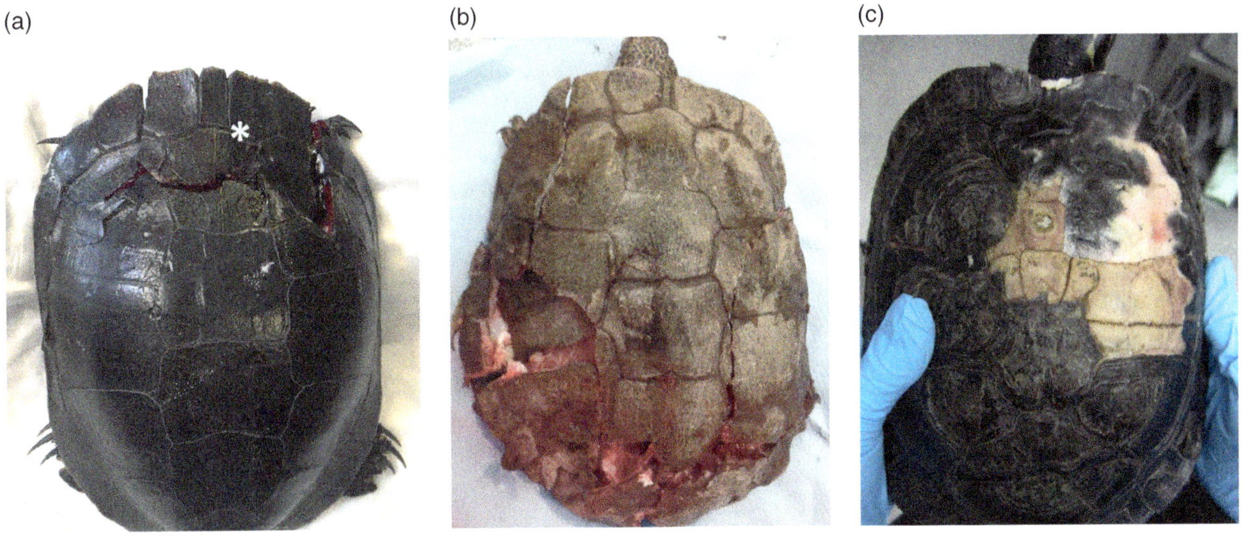

Figure 52.2 Shell fractures in chelonians can be characterized in terms of level of instability; full or partial thickness; and whether communicating with the coelomic cavity or not. (a) Full thickness carapacial fractures in a Northern red-bellied turtle (*Pseudemys rubriventris*) with an unstable fracture fragment (asterisk) that is not communicating with the coelom. (b) Multiple full thickness carapacial, bridge, and plastron fractures in a western pond turtle (*Clemmys marmorata*) with coelomic cavity involvement. This animal died shortly after presentation. (c) Partial thickness fracture with loss of keratin in a Florida cooter (*Pseudemys floridana*).

- Limb fractures
  - Patient may display weight-bearing or nonweight-bearing lameness
  - Should be characterized as an open or closed fracture
- Insidious signs – ruptured bladder or GI tract
- Wounds induced by predators
  - Distal portions of limbs, tail, and the rostral aspect of the face
  - Shell injuries
    - Gnawing lesions of the marginal scutes
    - Full thickness puncture wounds
- Falls
  - Shell and other orthopedic abnormalities common when the patient has been dropped
- Enclosure injuries
  - Appendages may be traumatized when caught by water filtration intake valves (aquatic species)
  - Shell or other orthopedic abnormalities (enclosure furniture falls)
  - Limb or digital entanglement with fibrous material can lead to lacerations or constriction injuries

STAT Diagnostics:

- Neurologic examination
- Orthopedic examination
- Radiographs (assess respiratory tract and musculoskeletal system)
- Flash coelomic ultrasound (prefemoral fossa access point) for evaluation for free fluid
- Packed cell volume (PCV)/total solids (TS) if excessive blood loss suspected
- Characterization of any wounds present

Complete Diagnostics:

- CBC/chemistry
- Computed tomography
- Wound cytology, culture, and sensitivity

Treatment

Stabilization:

- Analgesics, anti-inflammatories
- Antibiotics (Table 52.1)
- Thermal support
- Fluid therapy (Chapter 46: Nutrition and Fluid Therapy)
- Bandaging (Chapter 43: Wound Care and Bandaging Techniques)
- Removal of constricting material from digits, limbs
- Fractures
  - Irrigation with saline
    - Care must be taken if the wound is communicating with the lung (or suspected to be) so as not to cause drowning
    - Many shell fractures can be stabilized overnight using bandaging (Chapter 43: Wound Care and Bandaging Techniques)

Continued Care:

- Nutritional support (Chapter 46: Nutrition and Fluid Therapy)
- Surgical addressal of wounds (soft tissue, fractures)
- Ivermectin is contraindicated in chelonians so local therapy is required for fly-strike (flushing, manual removal, topical nitenpyram)
- For shell fractures
  - Partial thickness shell trauma
    - If the underlying bone is viable, the region can be lightly debrided under heavy sedation or general anesthesia and the area left to heal by second intention
    - If the underlying bone is nonviable, general anesthesia is needed to debride non-viable bone
      - Perform orthopedic fixation if a full thickness shell fracture is present
      - Vacuum-assisted shell repair may be useful in select cases [7]
  - Full thickness shell fractures should be surgically addressed with rigid fixation [8]. Options include
    - Cerclage wire and stainless-steel screws method
    - Stainless-steel surgical plates and stainless-steel screws method
    - Cerclage wire and hook-and-eye method
    - Nylon cable ties and mounts method

Systemic Disease

Nutritional or Renal Secondary Hyperparathyroidism and Hypocalcemia

Diagnosis

Clinical Signs:

- Acute hypocalcemia (weakness, "army-crawling," tremors, muscle fasciculation(s), seizures, cloacal prolapse)
- Chronic hypocalcemia (soft and flexible shell, kyphosis, deformed long bones, deformable jaw)
- Polyuria/polydipsia with renal secondary hyperparathyroidism
- Secondary pica can lead to GI obstruction

Differentials:

- Other causes of tremors (e.g. neurologic disease, hypoglycemia)
- Other causes of musculoskeletal abnormalities (e.g. fractures)

STAT Diagnostics:

- Ionized Ca, phosphorus, uric acid
- Radiographs (Figure 52.3a)

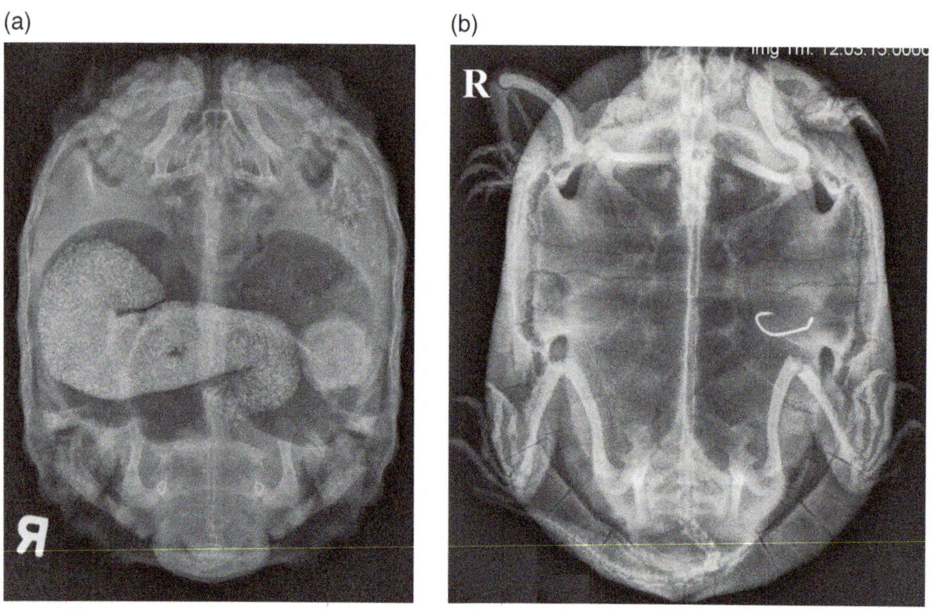

Figure 52.3 (a) Foreign material noted as gravel within the colon that was used as substrate is evident in this dorsoventral radiographic projection of a five year-old female sulcata tortoise (*Centrochelys (Geochelone) sulcata*). Poor bone density, indicative of chronic hypocalcemia, is noted based upon the lack of appropriate boney opacification of the distal limbs. A left-sided urinary bladder calculi is also evident along with mild cloacal prolapse with some radiopaque material. (b) Fish hook gastric foreign body is noted in this dorso-ventral radiographic projection of an adult male free ranging Western pond turtle (*Clemmys marmorata*).

Complete Diagnostics:

- CBC, chemistry
- Fecal direct mount + flotation
- Endoscopic renal biopsy in the case of renal secondary hyperparathyroidism
- Urinalysis (limited reference intervals available)

Treatment

Stabilization:

- Calcium therapy
  - Start parenteral supplementation if tremors are present (calcium gluconate 100 mg/kg, given diluted intramuscular [IM], subcutaneous [SC])
  - Switch to oral therapy once tremors are ameliorated (calcium glubionate or carbonate 100 mg/kg PO q12h)
- Antiseizure medications
  - Diazepam 0.5 mg/kg IV
  - Midazolam 1 mg/kg IM/IV
- Fluid therapy (see Chapter 46: Nutrition and Fluid Therapy)
- Analgesics and anti-inflammatories
- Thermal support
- Exposure to UVB radiation through unfiltered sunlight and/or through use of UVB emitting bulbs
- Empirical antibiotics (Table 52.1)

Continued Care:

- Correction of husbandry deficits
- Oral calcium supplementation until diet/UVB is corrected +/− normal radiographic bone density
- Nutritional support (Chapter 46: Nutrition and Fluid Therapy)
- Phosphate binders in the case of hyperphosphatemia
  - Aluminum hydroxide 100 mg/kg PO q12–24h

Toxins: Heavy Metals, Pesticides, Ivermectin

Diagnosis

Clinical Signs:

- Ivermectin
  - Contraindicated in chelonians
  - Neurologic (dull mentation, paralysis, coma, death)
- Pesticides
  - Organophosphates and carbamates – parasympathomimetic effects (salivation, ataxia, muscle fasciculation, meiosis, bradycardia)
  - Pyrethrins and pyrethroids – salivation, ataxia, muscle fasciculation
- Heavy metal toxicosis (zinc) – lethargy, anorexia, enteritis, pale mucous membranes, hemoglobinuria, yellow discoloration of skin and mucous membranes

STAT Diagnostics:

- Neurological examination
- Radiographs (to evaluate for metal opacities in gastrointestinal tract)
- PCV/TS

Complete Diagnostics:

- CBC, chemistry
- Blood heavy metal levels

Treatment

Stabilization:

- Pesticides, ivermectin
  - Dermal exposures should be washed with mild dishwashing liquid and large quantities of water
  - Ingestion can be treated with gastric lavage (acute ingestion) or repeated doses of activated charcoal (1% body weight (BW) q24h).
  - In cases of known or suspected carbamate/organophosphate toxicosis, atropine (0.2–0.4 mg/kg IM) should be administered
- Heavy metals
  - Chelation therapy: $CaNa_2EDTA$ 10–40 mg/kg q12h
- Anticonvulsants can be given to control seizure activity
- Fluid therapy (Chapter 46: Nutrition and Fluid Therapy)
- Thermal support

Continued Care:

- Endoscopic or surgical removal of source of intoxication (heavy metals)
- Nutritional support (Chapter 46: Nutrition and Fluid Therapy)
- Ivermectin toxicosis carries a poor prognosis and may require chronic ventilator support, although recovery has been reported

Neurological and Musculoskeletal Disease

Seizures, Muscle Tremors, or Weakness

Diagnosis

Clinical Signs:

- See Section "Toxins"

Differentials:

- Heavy metals (lead, zinc)
- Ivermectin
- Pesticide exposure
- Metronidazole

- Metaldehyde
- Marijuana ingestion
- Hypocalcemia (see Section "Nutritional or Renal Secondary Hyperparathyroidism and Hypocalcemia")

STAT Diagnostics:

- See Section "Toxins"
- Blood glucose
  - To rule out hypoglycemia as cause of clinical signs
  - However, there is no point-of-care glucometer that is validated for use in reptiles
- Ionized calcium
  - To rule out hypocalcemia as a cause of clinical signs

Complete Diagnostics:

- See Section "Toxins"

Treatment

Stabilization:

- See Section "Toxins"

Continued Care:

- See Section "Toxins"

Cardiopulmonary Disease

Upper Respiratory Tract Infection

Diagnosis

Clinical Signs, Differentials, STAT Diagnostics:

- See Section "Common Presenting Signs: Respiratory Signs"

Complete Diagnostics:

- CBC, chemistry
- Serology (Testudinid herpesvirus, *M. agassizii*)
- Sedated nasal flush
  - Cytology
  - Aerobic bacterial culture
  - PCR (*Mycoplasma* spp., Testudinid herpesvirus, ranavirus)

Treatment

Stabilization:

- O_2 therapy (Chapter 41: Oxygen Therapy)
- Fluid therapy (Chapter 46: Nutrition and Fluid Therapy)
- Empirical antibiotics (Table 52.1)
- Anti-inflammatories

Continued Care:

- Treat underlying cause (antibiotics, antifungals). Antivirals not routinely used in reptiles
- Nutritional support (Chapter 46: Nutrition and Fluid Therapy)

Lower Respiratory Tract Infection/Pneumonia

Diagnosis

Clinical Signs, Differentials, STAT Diagnostics:

- See Section "Common Presenting Signs: Respiratory Signs"

Complete Diagnostics:

- CBC, chemistry
- Advanced imaging (computed tomography)
- Serology (Testudinid herpesvirus, *M. agassizii*)
- Endotracheal lavage
  - Cytology
  - Aerobic bacterial culture
  - Fungal culture (if indicated)
- Pulmonary biopsy (if indicated)

Treatment

Stabilization:

- O_2 therapy (Chapter 41: Oxygen Therapy)
- Fluid therapy (Chapter 46: Nutrition and Fluid Therapy)
- Empirical antibiotics (Table 52.1)
- Anti-inflammatories

Continued Care:

- Treat underlying cause (antibiotics, antifungals). Antivirals not routinely used in reptiles
- Nutritional support (Chapter 46: Nutrition and Fluid Therapy)
- Transcarapacial catheterization for local pulmonary therapy

Gastrointestinal Disease

Diarrhea

Diagnosis

Clinical Signs:

- Accumulation of wet feces in the inguinal and tail regions
- Dehydration (bilateral enophthalmos, thick, ropey saliva)

- Tail wagging
- Hematochezia
- Mucoid stools
- Undigested food or visible endoparasites in stool

Differentials:

- Gastrointestinal parasitism
- Bacterial overgrowth (e.g. *Shigella*, *Salmonella*, *Proteus* spp.)
- Fungal overgrowth
- Dietary causes (inappropriate or poor quality foods fed)
- Systemic disease (hepatopathy, renal failure)
- Toxicosis (pesticides, heavy metals)
- Gastrointestinal obstruction

STAT Diagnostics

- Radiographs
- Fecal analysis
  - Direct smear
  - Flotation
  - Cytology
  - Sedimentation

Complete Diagnostics:

- CBC, chemistry
- Contrast radiographic study
- Special fecal cytology stains (e.g. acid fast)
- Molecular diagnostics
  - *Cryptosporidium*, *Giardia* spp. antigen tests
  - Intranuclear coccidiosis
- Bacterial, fungal cultures
- Gastrointestinal endoscopy or coelioscopy

Treatment

Stabilization:

- Fluid therapy (Chapter 46: Nutrition and Fluid Therapy)
- Anti-inflammatories
- Thermal support
- Empirical antibiotics (Table 52.1)
- Appropriate antiparasitics based on fecal analysis findings (Table 52.2)

Continued Care:

- Correction of underlying husbandry deficiencies
- Nutritional support (Chapter 46: Nutrition and Fluid Therapy)

Constipation

Diagnosis

Clinical Signs:

- Dehydration
- Anorexia
- Tail wagging
- Straining to defecate (grunting, extended pelvic limbs)
- Rectal prolapse
- Individuals in dystocia may also exhibit similar signs

Differentials:

- Obstructive:
  - Urolithiasis (cloacal or cystic)
  - Dystocia
  - Impaction
  - Intraluminal foreign material (e.g. substrate, phytobezoar)
  - Intestinal torsion/volvulus
  - Intussusception
  - Strictures
- Nonobstructive/functional:
  - Secondary to hypocalcemia from nutritional or renal secondary hyperparathyroidism
  - Inappropriate environmental temperatures
  - Dehydration

STAT Diagnostics:

- Radiographs
- Ionized calcium
- Plasma electrolytes

Complete Diagnostics:

- CBC, chemistry
- Contrast radiographic study
- Computed tomography
- Gastrointestinal endoscopy or coelioscopy

Treatment

Stabilization:

- Fluid therapy (Chapter 46: Nutrition and Fluid Therapy)
- Anti-inflammatories
- Thermal support
- Empirical antibiotics (Table 52.1)
- Prokinetic agents
  - Anecdotal reports only
  - Cisapride 0.5–2 mg/kg PO q24h
  - Metoclopramide 1–10 mg/kg PO q24h

- Anti-inflammatories
- Thermal support
- Empirical antibiotics (Table 52.1)

Continued Care:

- Correction of underlying husbandry deficiencies
- Nutritional support (Chapter 46: Nutrition and Fluid Therapy)
- Cystotomy for cystic calculi removal
  - Prefemoral or plastronotomy approach [11]

Reproductive (Phallus, Oviduct) or Bladder Prolapse

Diagnosis

Clinical Signs, Differentials, STAT Diagnostics, Complete Diagnostics:

- See Section "Common Presenting Signs: Prolapse"

Treatment

Stabilization, Continued Care:

- See Section "Common Presenting Signs: Prolapse"

Dystocia/"Egg-Binding"

Diagnosis

Clinical Signs:

- Straining
- Bloody discharge from vent
- Nesting behavior (digging holes, constantly walking)
- Physiologic fasting is normal in reproductively active females

Differentials:

- Obstructive
  - Enlarged or malformed eggs
  - Misshapen pelvis (previous trauma)
  - Oviductal stricture
  - Cystic or cloacal calculi
  - Pelvic mass
  - Fecal impaction
- Nonobstructive
  - Husbandry deficits (lack of appropriate nesting site, inappropriate environmental temperatures, lack of appropriate nesting area)
  - Salpingitis
  - Systemic illness
  - Malnutrition
  - Dehydration
  - Hypocalcemia

STAT Diagnostics:

- May be able to palpate egg(s) with digital cloacal exam and/or prefemoral fossa palpation
- Radiographs
  - Determine number of eggs, whether eggs are misshapen or have irregular margins (indicators of abnormally retained eggs)
  - Evaluate for comorbidities (e.g. urolithiasis)
  - Ionized calcium

Complete Diagnostics:

- CBC, chemistry
- Computed tomography to evaluate for coelomic masses
- Cloacoscopy, coelioscopy, salpingoscopy

Treatment

Stabilization:

- Fluid therapy (Chapter 46: Nutrition and Fluid Therapy)
- Anti-inflammatories
- Thermal support
- Calcium gluconate 100–200 mg/kg, diluted SC or IM
- Lubrication of the cloaca
- Once rehydrated, at POTZ and calcium supplemented, can administer increasing doses of oxytocin (1–20 IU/kg)
  - Can result in oviposition into the bladder [13]
  - Should only be used if no evidence of obstructive dystocia

Continued Care:

- Cloacoscopy +/− salpingoscopy can be used to collapse enlarged or irregularly shaped eggs and allow passage of normally-shaped eggs
- Ovariosalpingectomy to abolish further reproductive activity [14]

Neoplastic Disease

Neoplasia is not common in captive chelonians, comprising only 1.2% of necropsies in one study with no organ predilection reported [15]. The most commonly reported neoplasms of chelonians include cutaneous and visceral fibropapillomas of green sea turtles (*Chelonia mydas*) and squamous cell carcinoma in multiple species.

Herptiles

Dermatologic Disease

Aural Abscessation

Diagnosis

Clinical Signs:

- Unilateral or bilateral swellings that expand the tympanic membrane and/or pharyngeal tissues

Differentials:

- Multifactorial cause, often related to poor husbandry
- Hypovitaminosis A
  - Low vitamin A dietary levels
  - Exposure to vitamin A disrupting pesticides (organophosphates) in free-ranging animals
  - Bacterial infection (often oral cavity commensal organisms)

STAT Diagnostics:

- None

Complete Diagnostics:

- CBC, chemistry
- Radiographs to evaluate for bone involvement
- Cytology, bacterial culture of inspissated pus
- Fungal culture (if indicated)

Treatment

Stabilization:

- Fluid therapy (Chapter 46: Nutrition and Fluid Therapy)
- Anti-inflammatories
- Thermal support

Continued Care:

- Vitamin A supplementation
- Surgical debridement of abscess(es)

Developmental Shell Disorders and Secondary Complications

Diagnosis

Clinical Signs:

- "Pyramiding" of carapacial scutes
- Excessively soft shell (able to perform lateral and dorsoventral compression with digital palpation)
- Potential complications of shell abnormalities include
  - Constipation
  - Dystocia
  - Pelvic limb neurologic abnormalities

Differentials:

- Pyramiding
  - Inappropriate environmental humidity, temperature
  - High dietary protein and rapid growth
- Soft shell
  - Nutritional or renal secondary hyperparathyroidism

STAT Diagnostics, Complete Diagnostics:

- See Section "Nutritional or Renal Secondary Hyperparathyroidism and Hypocalcemia"

Treatment

Stabilization:

- Anti-inflammatories, analgesics when appropriate
- Thermal support

Continued Care:

- Correct all husbandry deficits
- See Section "Nutritional or Renal Secondary Hyperparathyroidism and Hypocalcemia"

Shell Injuries

Diagnosis

Clinical Signs, Differentials, STAT Diagnostics, Complete Diagnostics:

- See Section "Common Presenting Signs: Trauma"

Treatment

Stabilization, Continued Care:

- See Section "Common Presenting Signs: Trauma"

Ophthalmic Disease

Conjunctivitis

Diagnosis

Clinical Signs:

- Ocular discharge
- Blepharospasm
- Blepharedema

Differentials:

- Hypovitaminosis A leading to squamous metaplasia (especially prevalent in aquatic species)
- Keratoconjunctivitis sicca (KCS)

- Foreign body
- Bacterial (e.g. *Mycoplasma, Aeromonas*) [16], viral (e.g. herpesvirus), fungal infections
- Corneal ulceration, keratitis

STAT Diagnostics:

- Fluorescein staining
- Schirmer tear test or phenol red test if KCS is suspected
- Intraocular pressure using rebound tonometry

Complete Diagnostics:

- CBC, chemistry
- Conjunctival cytology
- Bacterial culture
- Fungal culture (if indicated)
- Referral to ophthalmologist and/or exotic animal medicine specialist

Treatment

Stabilization:

- Fluid therapy (Chapter 46: Nutrition and Fluid Therapy)
- Systemic, topical anti-inflammatories
- Systemic, topical antibiotics (Table 52.1)
- Flushing conjunctival sac to remove foreign material, desquamated epithelial cell debris
- Thermal support

Continued Care:

- Vitamin A supplementation

References

1 Divers, S.J. (2019). Hepatology. In: *Mader's Reptile and Amphibian Medicine and Surgery*, 3e (eds. S.J. Divers and S.J. Stahl), 649–668. St Louis: Saunders-Elsevier.

2 Mariani, C.L. (2007). The neurologic examination and neurodiagnostics techniques for reptiles. *Vet. Clin. North Am. Exot. Anim. Pract.* 10 (3): 855–891.

3 Sladky, K.K. and Mans, C. (2012). Clinical anesthesia in reptiles. *J. Exot. Pet. Med.* 21 (1): 17–31.

4 Mans, C. (2014). Clinical technique: intrathecal drug administration in turtles and tortoises. *J. Exot. Pet. Med.* 23 (1): 67–70.

5 Jacobson, E.R., Brown, M.B., Wendland, L.D. et al. (2014). Mycoplasmosis and upper respiratory tract disease of tortoises: a review and update. *Vet. J.* 201 (3): 257–264.

6 Origgi, F.C. (2012). Testudinid herpesviruses: a review. *J. Herpetol. Med. Surg.* 22 (1–2): 42–54.

7 Adkesson, M.J., Travis, E.K., Weber, M.A. et al. (2007). Vaccuum-assisted closure for treatment of a deep shell abscess and osteomyelitis in a tortoise. *J. Am. Vet. Med. Assoc.* 231 (8): 1249–1254.

8 Fleming, G.J. (2005). New techniques in chelonian shell repair. In: *Current Therapies in Reptile Medicine and Surgery* (eds. D.R. Mader et al.), 219–226. St Louis: Saunders-Elsevier.

9 Nicholas, E. and Warwick, C. (2011). Alleviation of a gastrointestinal tract impaction in a tortoise using an improvised vibrating massager. *J. Herpetol. Med. Surg.* 21 (4): 93–95.

10 Romeijer, C., Beaufrère, H., Laniesse, D. et al. (2016). Vomiting and gastrointestinal obstruction in a red-footed tortoise (*Chelonoidis carbonaria*). *J. Herpetol. Med. Surg.* 26 (1–2): 32–35.

11 Keller, K.A., Hawkins, M.G., Weber, E.P. et al. (2015). Diagnosis and treatment of urolithiasis in client-owned chelonians: 40 cases (1987–2012). *J. Am. Vet. Med. Assoc.* 247 (6): 650–658.

12 Mans, C. and Sladky, K.K. (2012). Endoscopically guided removal of cloacal calculi in three African spurred tortoises (*Geochelone sulcata*). *J. Am. Vet. Med. Assoc.* 240 (7): 869–875.

13 Minter, L.J., Wood, M.W., Hill, T.L., and Lewbart, G.A. (2010). Cystoscopic guided removal of ectopic eggs from the urinary bladder of the Florida cooter turtle (*Pseudemys floridana floridana*). *J. Zoo Wildl. Med.* 41 (3): 503–509.

14 Mans, C. and Sladky, K.K. (2012). Diagnosis and management of oviductal disease in three red-eared slider turtles (*Trachemys scripta elegans*). *J. Small Anim. Pract.* 53 (4): 234–239.

15 Sykes, J.M. and Trupkiewicz, J.G. (2006). Reptile neoplasia at the Philadelphia zological garden, 1901–2002. *J. Zoo Wildl. Med.* 37 (1): 11–19.

16 Musgrave, K.E., Diehl, K., and Mans, C. (2016). *Aeromonas* hydrophila keratitis in freshwater turtles. *J. Exot. Pet. Med.* 25 (1): 26–29.

53

Snakes

Sean Michael Perry

Mississippi Aquarium, Gulfport, Mississippi, USA

CONTENTS

Unique Species Considerations

Most snake emergency presentations are acute decompensations of a chronic disease process.

Large constrictor species require several individuals for proper restraint (i.e. one person/3 ft of snake) (Figure 53.1).

Snakes in the families *Elapidae* and *Viperidae* are venomous. Only clinicians with specialized training or experience should attend these patients. If the clinicians do not feel comfortable attending a venomous snake or do not have the appropriate training or equipment, then they should refer the case to someone who does. Exams on all venomous snakes should be performed on heavily sedated or anesthetized animals.

The reader is directed to Chapter 45: Analgesia, Anesthesia and Monitoring for an overview of current recommendations regarding anti-inflammatory and analgesic drug use in snakes, as well as sedation and anesthetic protocols for these species.

Common Presenting Signs

Abnormal Feces

Introduction

In snakes, defecation usually occurs after each meal. Intervals between defecation can be days to weeks depending on how often the snake is being fed and meal size. Feces should normally come out as a firm well defined fecal ball/pellet. If fecal material becomes too desiccated it can cause constipation/obstipation. Diarrhea can also occur in snakes. Fecal material from boids and pythons should be firm; this is in contrast to some other species like indigo snakes (*Drymarchon* spp.) which normally have a looser stool.

Exotic Animal Emergency and Critical Care Medicine, First Edition. Edited by Jennifer E. Graham, Grayson A. Doss and Hugues Beaufrère.

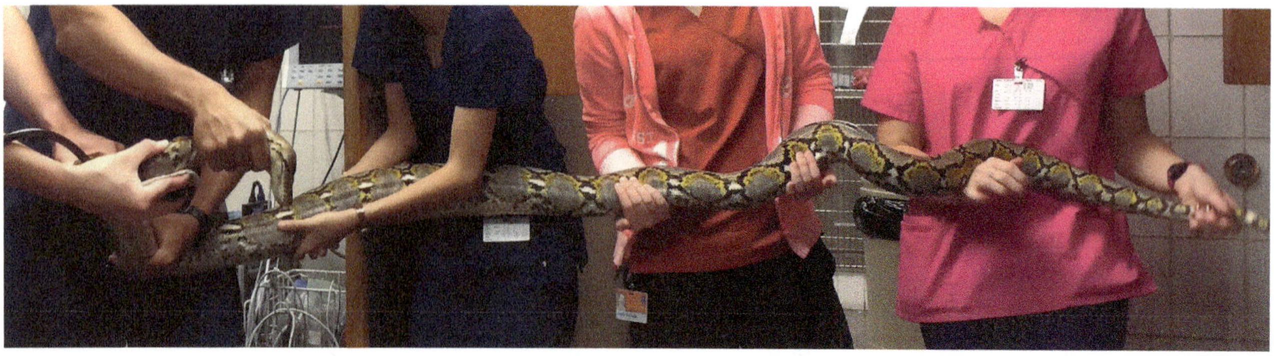

Figure 53.1 Due to their enormous strength, large snake species such as this reticulated python (*Python reticulatus*) require multiple individuals to appropriately restrain them. This animal was approximately 12 ft long.

Diagnosis

History:

- Inquire about husbandry (diet, temperatures, humidity, substrate, etc.)
- Defecation history
  - Weight loss for chronic diarrhea cases
  - Duration of abnormal feces
  - Inquire about changes to the feces (hematochezia vs. melena, increased water content, abnormal coloration, etc.)
- Cage decorations missing or history of eating substrate
- Other snakes in the household or new acquisitions
- Inquire about disinfectants in household

Clinical Signs:

- Anorexia
- Diarrhea
  - Melena can occur with proximal gastrointestinal ulcers
  - Hematochezia can occur with colon and cloacal disease
- Tenesmus
- Mid to caudal body swelling

Differentials:

- Abnormal husbandry, endoparasites (*Cryptosporidium*), bacterial/viral/fungal gastroenteritis (*Salmonella*, *Parvovirus*, *Adenovirus*), iatrogenic, dehydration, foreign body, intussusception, granuloma, neoplasia

STAT Diagnostics:

- *Physical examination*
- *Fecal flotation/direct smear*
- *Radiography*

Complete Diagnostics:

- *Cell blood count* (CBC)/*chemistry*
- *Fecal flotation/direct smear*
- *Bacterial/fungal cultures of lesions*
- *Gastric lavage*
- *Colonic lavage*
- *Radiography:* Gastrointestinal contrast series
- *Ultrasound*
- *Endoscopy*: Gastric and small intestinal biopsies
- *Exploratory surgery*: Gastric and small intestinal biopsies

Treatment

Stabilization:

- *Fluid therapy*
- *Antibiotics*: Typically not needed unless there is bacterial overgrowth
- *Antiparasitics*: Treatment should be targeted toward specific organism
- *Vitamin supplements*: Vitamin B complex 0.3 ml/kg SC, IM q24h [1]
- *Gastrointestinal protectants*: Sucralfate 500–1000 mg/kg PO q6–8h [1]
- *Deobstipation under sedation*: Warm water enemas with lubricant (1–3 ml of 50 : 50 lubricant:warm water/100 g), digital palpation and manipulation [2]

Continued Care:

- *Husbandry modifications*: Substrate, diet
- *Prokinetics*: Cisapride 0.5 mg/kg PO q24h [1]; Metoclopramide 0.06 mg/kg PO q24h × 7d [1]
- *Fecal softeners*: Lactulose: 0.5 ml/kg PO q24h [1]

Anorexia

Introduction

Anorexia is defined as a lack of appetite or the lack of feeding response. This can be quite variable in snakes. Snakes are known to go for months at a time without eating. Anorexia will be based on the owner's knowledge of their pet's feeding habits. Knowledge of the species natural history, normal behaviors, and diet is required to determine if anorexia is pathologic based on history.

Diagnosis

History:

- Inquire about husbandry (diet, temperatures, humidity, substrate, UV exposure, etc.)
- Determine the diet being offered, prey items, frequency, method of administration
- Ask if owners are actively trying to breed the animal
- Ask when the last shed was completed
- Establish if the snake is showing any other clinical signs (e.g. change in posture)
- Ask if the snake's basking behavior has changed recently
- Determine if there are any changes to the environment around the cage

Clinical Signs:

- Lack of feeding response
- No interest in a variety of prey items
- Weight loss
- Cachexia

Differentials:

- Improper husbandry (temperature, humidity, cage setup/décor)
- Prey item is too large/small or inappropriate for species
- Undergoing ecdysis (shedding skin)
- Reproductively active/seasonal anorexia
- Brumation and stress
- Gastrointestinal disease, stomatitis, gastroenteritis (bacterial, viral, parasitic)
- Respiratory disease
- Systemic disease

STAT Diagnostics:

- *Physical examination*
- *Packed cell volume* (PCV)/*total solids* (TS)

Complete Diagnostics:

- *CBC*
- *Chemistry*
- *Fecal smear/flotation*
- *Radiographs*
- *Ultrasound*
- *Infectious disease testing*: Inclusion body disease (IBD) (*Arenavirus*), paramyxovirus, Sunshine virus, protozoal

Treatment

Stabilization:

- *Fluid therapy*
- *Diet*: See Chapter 46: Nutrition and Fluid Therapy for nutritional therapy recommendations

Continued Care:

- *Dietary transition*: Entice snake with a variety of prey items based on previous feeding history and natural history. Options include frozen thawed rodents (+/− scented with other prey items), frozen thawed chicks or quail, frozen thawed lizard/snake species. Live prey items can be offered; however, risk of injury is high
- *Diet*: Continue enteral nutrition with assist feedings, if applicable

Neurologic and Musculoskeletal Disease

Opisthotonus

Introduction

In snakes, this neurologic sign is often associated with cerebral disease. Opisthotonus is a neurologic sign typically characterized by the cervical area arching backward, leaving the head pointing toward the sky or even upside down; the resulting position of the cervical area and head is also known as "stargazing." Disease localized within the cerebrum to advanced systemic disease such as septicemia can lead to this posture. Some snakes may normally adopt a "stargazing" posture intermittently (especially boid species) or this position may be a basking behavior observed when heating or UV elements are directly above the animal. It is important to differentiate the two with a thorough history and physical examination.

Diagnosis

History:

- Inquire about husbandry (diet, temperatures, humidity, substrate, UV exposure, etc.)
- Ask about other snakes in the household/collection, specifically the species
- Determine if presented animal has a history of prior illness
- For some neurologic diseases, anorexia and vomiting may precede advanced neurologic signs
- If cerebral disease presents, snakes may also display a behavior change toward humans/conspecifics
- Inquire if the snake has incurred any trauma

Clinical Signs:

- "Stargazing" posture
- Contraction of the cervical musculature
- Ataxia
- Head tilt
- Incoordination
- Loss/delay of righting reflex
- Anorexia
- Vomiting

Differentials:

- Encephalitis
  - Bacterial (*Salmonella* spp.), viral (*Arenavirus*, *Paramyxovirus*, etc.) [3–7], fungal, protozoal (*Entamoeba invadens*)
- Hepatic encephalopathy
- Renal failure
- Hepatic failure
- Electrolyte abnormalities
  - Hypocalcemia
  - Hypernatremia
- Thiamine deficiency
  - More likely in piscivorous snake species or any snake that is fed a fish-based diet
- Septicemia

STAT Diagnostics:

- *Physical examination*
- *PCV/TS*
- *Blood glucose, lactate*
- *Ionized calcium*

Complete Diagnostics:

- *CBC/chemistry*
- *Radiographs*
- *Infectious disease testing* (*IBD, paramyxovirus, protozoal*)
- *Cerebral spinal fluid* (CSF) *collection*
- *Magnetic resonance imaging* (MRI)

Treatment

Stabilization:

- *Fluid therapy*
- *Antibiotics:* Ideally, select an antibiotic that crosses the blood brain barrier. See Table 53.1
- *Antiparasitics:* Treatment should be targeted toward the specific organism
- *Antifungals* (Table 53.1)
- *Non-steroidal anti-inflammatory medications*
- *Steroidal anti-inflammatory medications*
- *Hyperosmotic fluids* (e.g. mannitol, hypertonic saline)
  - If clinical signs are suspected to be secondary to head trauma
  - Use cautiously – must extrapolate from other species since little information on use in reptiles

Continued Care:

- Treatment based on clinical signs
- *Fluid therapy*
- *Diet*: Enteral nutrition
- Continued therapy as indicated above
- *Anti-convulsant therapy*: If needed. See Section "Seizures/Convulsions/Muscle Twitching".

Seizures/Convulsions/Muscle Twitching

Introduction

Muscle tremors or muscle fasciculations are a common presenting sign in reptiles. It is difficult to determine between true seizure activity and muscle twitching in snakes. Clinical judgment, a thorough history, and experience will assist in differentiation.

Diagnosis

History

- Determine husbandry (temperature, humidity, light exposure, UV exposure, etc.)
- Obtain a thorough diet history
- Inquire about any pesticides that may have been sprayed around the exposure recently or if the owner has applied any topical medications to the snake
- Determine if any other animals are sick in the house or if there have been any new additions

Clinical Signs:

- Convulsions
- Muscle fasciculation
- Spastic muscle contractions
- Loss of righting reflex
- Ataxia
- Incoordination
- Anorexia
- Vomiting

Differentials:

- Toxicosis (permethrin, ivermectin, organophosphates)
- Septicemia
- Electrolyte abnormalities (hypocalcemia, hypernatremia)
- Encephalitis
- Renal failure
- Liver failure
- Thiamine deficiency (piscivores)

STAT Diagnostics:

- *Physical examination*
- *PCV/TS*
- *Blood glucose, lactate*
- *Ionized calcium*

Complete Diagnostics:

- *CBC/chemistry*
- *Radiographs*
- *Thiamine levels*

Table 53.1 Common systemic antibiotics and antifungals used in snakes.

Drug	Dose (mg/kg)	Route	Frequency
Antibiotics			
Amikacin[1]	5 once, then 2.5	IM	q72h
Azithromycin[8]	10	PO	q2–7d
Carbenicillin[9, 10]	200–400	IM	q24h
Ceftazidime[11]	20	SC, IM, IV	q72h
Ceftiofur crystalline-free acid[12]	15	IM, SC	q24–120h
Ceftiour sodium[1]	2.2	IM	q48h
Chloramphenicol[1, 13]	40–50	PO, SC	q12–72h
Ciprofloxacin[1]	11	PO	q48–72h
Enrofloxacin [1]	10	SC (diluted), IM	q48h; can cause significant tissue necrosis
Gentamicin[14]	2.5–3 once then 1.5	IM	q96h
Marbofloxacin[15]	10	PO	q48h
Metronidazole[16]	20	PO	q48h
Piperacillin[17]	100	IM	q48h
Antifungals			
Amphotericin B[1]	0.5	IV	q48–72h
	5 mg/150 ml saline	Nebulization for 1 h	q12h
Fluconazole[1]	5	PO	q24h
Itraconazole[1]	10	PO	q24h
Ketoconazole[1]	25	PO	q24h

SC, subcutaneous; IM, intramuscular; IV, intravenous; IT, intratracheal; PO, per os.

- *Blood cultures*: Septicemic animals
- *Infectious disease testing*: IBD (*Arenavirus*), paramyxovirus, Sunshine virus, protozoal (*E. invadens*)
- *Ultrasound*
- *MRI of the central nervous system*
- *Cerebrospinal fluid sampling*: Difficult to impossible to perform in snakes

Treatment

Stabilization:

- *Anti-convulsants*: Midazolam 0.5–2 mg/kg IM, IV [1]; diazepam 0.5–2 mg/kg IM, IV [1]
- *Muscle relaxants*: Methocarbamol (use cautiously – would require extrapolation from other species since little information on use in reptiles)
- *Hyperosmotic fluids* (e.g. mannitol, hypertonic saline)
  - If clinical signs are suspected to be secondary to head trauma
  - Use cautiously – must extrapolate from other species since little information on use in reptiles
- *Consider soaking/washing snake to remove topical toxins*
- *Vitamin supplements*: Vitamin B complex 0.3 ml/kg SC, IM q24h [1]; Thiamine 50–100 mg/kg daily [1]
- *Fluid therapy*
- *Intravenous (IV) lipid therapy for suspected toxicosis*: 0.5 ml/kg IV over 20 minutes then increase to 1.5 ml/kg IV over 30–60 minutes
  - Use cautiously; little information on use in reptiles

Continued Care:

- Treatment based on clinical signs
- *Long term anticonvulsant therapy*
  - Has been evaluated in reptiles
  - Phenobarbital, levetiracetam, potassium bromide, zonisamide

Spinal Osteopathies

Introduction

As for other species, spinal disease in snakes has significant implications, as abnormalities of the vertebral column can alter locomotion. Snakes can often compensate for decreased mobility. It is important to identify the underlying disease process. Reptiles have pronounced spinal reflexes, making it difficult to stage the severity of spinal cord involvement based on the traditional methods used in small animal medicine. In addition, snakes lack limbs, eliminating the ability to evaluate myotatic reflexes.

Diagnosis

History:

- Inquire about husbandry (temperature, humidity, enclosure environment, etc.)
- Ask about recent history of trauma
- Determine the activity level of the snake and the duration of clinical signs
- Decide if the snake has difficulty moving
- Determine when was the last time the animal defecated or passed urates
- Determine if the owners have observed any behavioral changes

Clinical Signs:

- Nodular swellings near spinal column
- Vertebral column stiffness
- Decreased mobility
- Kyphosis
- Scoliosis
- Pathologic fractures
- Muscle atrophy/decreased muscle tone caudal to the spinal column lesion
- Paresis/paralysis caudal to the lesion
- Corkscrew posture
- Loss of pain sensation
- Decreased to absent vent tone

Differentials:

- Traumatic: Fractures/luxations/bite wounds
- Infectious: Osteomyelitis/discospondylitis (*Salmonella* spp. common)
- Degenerative: Spondylosis deformans
- Nutritional: Hypovitaminosis D, hypervitaminosis A
- Neoplasia: Osteosarcoma, chondrosarcoma, fibrosarcoma

STAT Diagnostics:

- *Physical examination*
- *Spinal radiographs*: Ensure proper support of the spine to prevent further damage

Complete Diagnostics:

- *CBC/chemistry*
- *Blood cultures*
- *Computed tomography*: Evaluate the bony structures around the spinal cord, evaluate the degree of lysis and bony abnormalities
- *Magnetic resonance imaging*: Evaluate the integrity of the spinal cord and determine the degree of compression or inflammation within the cord
- *Surgical bone biopsy/culture of the affected area(s)*

Treatment

Stabilization:

- *Immobilization (for fractures)*: Prevention of any further significant movement from the spine
- *Analgesics*: Opioids, nonsteroidal anti-inflammatory drugs (NSAIDs)
- *Antibiotics*: See Table 53.1
- *Surgery*: Debridement of affected areas

Continued Care:

- Activity restriction
- Continue analgesics/NSAIDs
- Continue antibiotic therapy

Trauma/Wounds/Burns

Introduction

Snakes can present with many different types of trauma. Forms of trauma that may present on an emergency basis in snakes include: conspecific aggression; bite wounds from live prey items; degloving injuries; adherence to adhesive substances, such as tape; burns from heating elements or high levels of UVB light; and vehicular trauma. The degree and severity can vary just as in other species; therefore, a full evaluation of the patient should be performed.

Diagnosis

History:

- History of acute trauma, repeated chronic traumatic event, or exposure to heating element that is unregulated or malfunctioned. Excessive exposure to UVB light (e.g. being left out in direct sun for prolonged periods of time)

Clinical Signs:

- Lacerations or punctures present on the dorsum or along body
- Ulcerative lesions on the skin, dorsally, or ventrally
- Focal areas of erythema and petechiation, ventrally or dorsally
- Sloughed skin
- Prolapsed organs

Differentials:

- Conspecific aggression, bite wounds from prey, degloving injuries, wounds from falling cage furniture, burns from heating elements or UV bulbs, vehicular trauma

STAT diagnostics:

- *Physical examination*
- *PCV/TS*
- *Blood glucose, lactate*

Herptiles

- *Radiographs*
- *Pulse oximetry*
- *Focused Assessment using Sonography for Triage* (FAST) *ultrasound of the coelomic cavity* (see Chapter 47: STAT Diagnostics)

Complete Diagnostics:

- *Wound cytology*: If warranted
- *Bacterial and/or fungal culture*: Collect samples from area following copious saline lavage
- *CBC/chemistry*
- *Advanced imaging* (*CT, MRI*)

Treatment

Stabilization:

- *Wound management*: Promptly aseptically cover wounds to prevent further contamination
- *Fluid therapy*
- *Analgesics*: Opioids, NSAIDs; see Chapter 45: Analgesia, Anesthesia and Monitoring
- *Sedation for wound management*: See Chapter 45: Analgesia, Anesthesia and Monitoring
- *Antibiotics*: Administer broad-spectrum antibiotics; ensure both Gram-positive and Gram-negative coverage

Continued Care:

- *Wound management*
  - See Chapter 43: Wound Care and Bandaging Techniques
  - Maintaining bandages on snakes may be challenging; non-lubricated, latex condoms can be used to maintain a bandage on some snakes. Repeat surgical debridement and partial closure may be needed. Snakes should be kept in a bare cage lined with newspaper or paper towels, avoiding particulate substrate/bedding. Large wounds may take months to years to heal by second intention. Scars may interrupt the normal scale pattern
- *Rib fractures*: Most will heal without further stabilization
- *Spinal fractures*: Difficult to stabilize with external coaptation; may require surgical stabilization
- *Discontinue feeding live prey items or remove source of burn*

Vomiting/Regurgitation

Introduction

Without directly observing the event (e.g. noting the anatomic location of the food bolus) it is difficult to differentiate between vomiting and true regurgitation in snakes due to their unique anatomy and morphology. The esophagus is very long in snakes, often ending near the middle of the snake. If the food bolus is brought back up from the area of the stomach (approximately mid-body) it is usually considered vomiting. It should be considered regurgitation if the food bolus was cranial to the stomach (i.e. in the esophagus) before it was brought back up. Level of digestion (e.g. prey item grossly intact vs. partially digested) may also assist localization.

Diagnosis

History:

- Determine husbandry conditions (temperature, humidity, UV exposure, substrate, housing, etc.)
- Ask if the owners observed or recorded the regurgitation/vomiting event
- Owners usually find uneaten prey item(s) at varying levels of digestion in the snake's enclosure
  - May be found minutes to hours after ingestion or several days later
- Determine the size of prey item, the type of prey item and how often prey is offered
- Determine frequency and whether it is an acute or a chronic problem
- Determine source of the animal (wild-caught vs. captive bred)
- Has the client recently changed food items or suppliers?
- Determine, if any, previous treatments administered
- Obtain the snake's fecal and defecation habits

Clinical Signs:

- Enlarged stomach (mid-body swelling) for more than two to three days after feeding
- Weight loss
- Putrid odor emanating from snake
- Physical examination may be normal

Differentials:

- Husbandry deficiencies
- Excessive handling of the snake after meal ingestion
  - Regurgitates/vomits due to stress
- Inappropriate prey item
  - Improperly thawed before fed to snake
  - Excessively large
- Gastrointestinal tract pathology
  - Foreign body, obstruction (Figure 53.2)
  - Intussusception
  - *Cryptosporidium serpentis*
  - Enteric parasites (nematodes, ascarids, tapeworms, coccidia)
  - Neoplasia
  - Granuloma
  - Congenital abnormalities
- Extra-gastrointestinal pathology resulting in mechanical obstruction of gastrointestinal tract
  - Neoplasia or other space-occupying coelomic lesions (Figure 53.3)

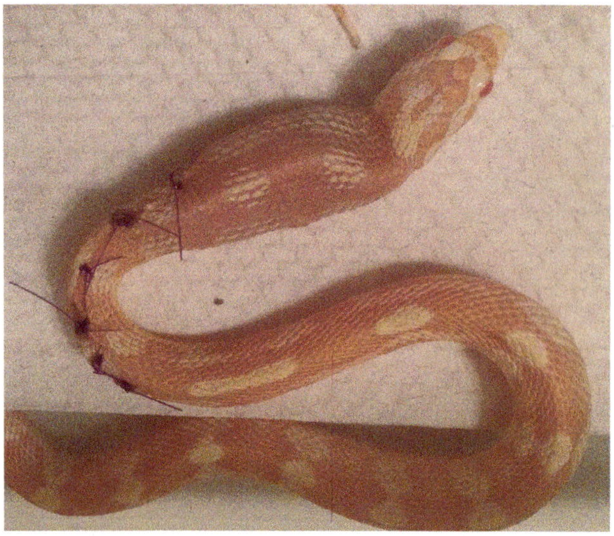

Figure 53.2 Corn snake (*Pantherophis guttatus*) with an iatrogenic esophageal stricture that occurred after surgical repair of a wound. The snake regurgitated even the smallest of meals.

- Inclusion body disease (IBD)
- *Chlamydia* spp.

Diagnostics:

STAT diagnostics:

- *PCV/TS*
- *FAST ultrasound of the coelomic cavity* (see Chapter 47: STAT Diagnostics)
- *Fecal flotation/direct smear*

Complete diagnostics:

- *CBC/chemistry*
- *Cryptosporidium diagnostics*
  - Gastric biopsy
  - Polymerase chain reaction (PCR) on gastric lavage/gastric swab sample
  - Acid fast stain on gastric lavage/swab sample (screening tool; not confirmatory) or regurgitated food item
- *Inclusion body disease diagnostics*: Liver, esophageal tonsil, renal biopsy for immunohistochemistry; PCR
- *Diagnostic imaging*
  - Radiographs
  - Gastrointestinal contrast series
  - Ultrasound
  - Endoscopy
- *Exploratory surgery*: Multiple organ biopsies

Treatment

Stabilization:

- *Fluid therapy*
- *Antibiotics*: Table 53.1
- *Antiparasitics*:
  - e.g. fenbendazole, trimethoprim-sulfa
- *Gastrointestinal therapeutics*: Protectants, anti-emetics. *Note*: The majority of gastrointestinal protectants and anti-emetics have not been evaluated in reptiles

Continued Care:

- *Correction of husbandry deficit(s)*

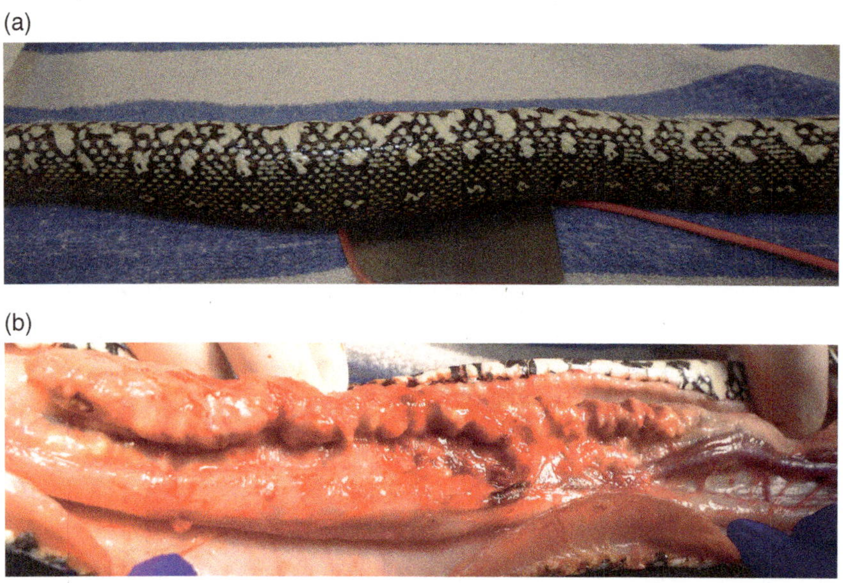

Figure 53.3 Diamond python (*Morelia spilota spilota*) presented for a mid-body swelling (a) that was preventing ingestion of food. Coelomic exploratory surgery revealed severe hepatomegaly (b) with hepatic lipidosis; blood work prior to surgery was unremarkable.

- *Diet*: Assist feeding, if necessary, once underlying etiology is corrected

Cardiopulmonary Disease

Cardiac Disease

Introduction

Cardiovascular disease in snakes is likely underreported in the literature and has received little attention clinically. Snakes have a three chambered heart with two atria and one ventricle. The ventricle has an incomplete interventricular septum which allows oxygenated and deoxygenated blood to mix [18].

Diagnosis

History:

- Inquire about husbandry (temperature, humidity, substrate, etc.)
- Ask about progression of swelling and duration of clinical signs/swelling(s)
- Determine if there is a history of any previous disease process or recent cardiocentesis

Clinical Signs:

- Cardiomegaly
  - Manifests as a swelling in the cranial 1/3 of the snake's body length
- Gular and/or cervical area swelling
- Lethargy
- Anorexia
- Tachypnea
- Dyspnea
- Tachycardia
- Ascites
- Organomegaly
- Edema

Differentials:

- Pericardial effusion
- Congestive heart failure
- Cardiomyopathy
- Endocarditis: *Salmonella enterica* subsp. *arizonae*, *Corynebacterium* spp.
- Myocarditis: *Chlamydiosis*
- Arrhythmias
- Aortic aneurysm(s)
- Enlarged thyroid gland(s)

STAT Diagnostics:

- *PCV/TS*
- *Blood glucose, lactate*
- *Diagnostic imaging*
  - FAST ultrasound of the coelomic cavity (see Chapter 47: STAT Diagnostics)
  - Coelomic radiographs
- *Pulse oximetry*

Complete Diagnostics:

- *CBC/chemistry*
- *Echocardiogram*
- *Electrocardiogram*
- *Blood cultures (if endocarditis suspected)*
- *Advanced imaging (CT, MRI)*

Treatment

Stabilization:

- *Oxygen therapy*
- *Cardiovascular drug therapy*: There are no studies examining the safety or efficacy of diuretics, positive inotropes, angiotensin-converting enzyme (ACE) inhibitors or antiarrhythmic drugs in snakes
- *Antibiotics*: See Table 53.1. Long duration of therapy for endocarditis treatment in reptiles

Continued Care:

- Long-term monitoring, dependent on underlying pathology. Monitoring to consider includes serial chemistry panels, radiographs, echocardiograms, electrocardiograms, blood cultures

Pneumonia and Upper Airway Infection

Introduction

Respiratory disease in snakes is often insidious and usually develops over a long period of time. Snakes typically compensate for a while then acutely decompensate. A typical presentation involves dyspnea with increased inspiratory effort. Dyspneic snakes often display open-mouth breathing. One must differentiate between upper airway disease and lower airway disease. Snakes are obligate nasal breathers; therefore, upper airway disease often presents as dyspnea. Nasal discharge can be seen in conjunction with lower airway disease or may be secondary to upper airway disease only. Both open-mouth breathing and/or stertor/stridor often observed with respiratory disease must be differentiated from defensive behaviors (e.g. hissing).

Diagnosis

History:

- Inquire about husbandry and identify deficiencies
- *Identify potential stressors/concurrent disease*: Recent transport, malnutrition, endoparasites, ectoparasites

- *Determine the origin of the animal*: Wild-caught vs. captive bred, specific breeder of origin
- Ask about exposure to other snakes or reptiles
- Determine the client's disinfectant protocol

Clinical Sign:

- Dyspnea; often manifests as
  - Open mouth breathing
  - Elevating cranial 1/4 to 1/3 of body length off of ground when at rest
  - Hyperinflation of lung(s)
- Nasal discharge (can manifest as bubbles from nare(s))
- Stertor/stridor
- Tachypnea

Differentials:

- Pneumonia
  - Bacterial, viral, parasitic, fungal causes
  - Secondary to infectious stomatitis (aspiration of infected oral material)
- Upper airway infection
  - Secondary to infectious stomatitis
- Respiratory clinical signs
  - Occlusion of nare(s) (e.g. retained shed)
  - Neoplasia (primary vs. metastatic)
  - Heart failure
  - Hypovitaminosis A

STAT Diagnostics:

- *PCV/TS*
- *Radiographs*: Focus on middle to cranial half of the body; the trachea ends and lung(s) begin at the level of the heart
- *Pulse oximetry*

Complete Diagnostics:

- *CBC/chemistry*
- *Tracheobronchial lavage* (see Figure 51.1)
  - Can perform cytology, microbiologic culture and infectious disease testing on fluid obtained
- *Fecal flotation for evidence of respiratory parasites* (e.g. *Rhabdias* spp., Pentastomida spp.)
- *Nasal flush*
  - Can perform cytology, microbiologic culture on fluid obtained
- *Virologic testing: Paramyxovirus, IBD (Arenavirus), Nidovirus*
- *Chlamydia testing*
- *Blood culture*
- *Computed tomography*: Improved diagnostic capability for pulmonary disease vs. radiographs
- *Pulmonoscopy*

Treatment

Stabilization:

- *Oxygen therapy*: If snake is cyanotic or apneic on presentation, consider immediate intubation. A temporary tracheostomy may be indicated if obstruction from caseous material is suspected. Tracheal obstructions may be able to be aspirated out of the trachea with gentle suction
- *Bronchodilators*: Aminophylline 2–4 mg/kg IV [1]
- *Cardiovascular therapeutics (e.g. diuretics)*: If heart disease is suspected

Continued Care:

- Correct any husbandry deficiencies
- Repeated nasal flushing and debridement of necrotic oral tissue for cases of infectious stomatitis
- *Antimicrobials* (Table 53.1): Systemic in addition to nebulized medications; based on culture and sensitivities
- *Antiparasitic medications, if needed*
- *Antifungals, if needed:* See Table 53.1
- *Nebulization therapy*
  - Amikacin or gentamicin (diluted in sterile saline)
  - Can combine an aminoglycoside with *N*-acetylcysteine and hypertonic saline
  - Can also nebulize bronchodilators or amphotericin B (1 mg/kg q24h) [1]
- *Vitamin A supplementation, if needed*: Vitamin A 2000 U/kg IM q7–10d × 4 treatments [1]

Gastrointestinal Disease

Infectious Stomatitis

Introduction

Infectious stomatitis is a very common clinical presentation in all reptiles. Infection of the oral mucosa and surrounding tissues is hallmark for this condition. This disorder can be focal or it can present diffusely throughout the oral cavity. Depending on severity, it is possible to treat it successfully; however, if not treated aggressively, snakes can develop secondary septicemia, osteomyelitis, respiratory disease, ocular disease, or die. Severe cases of infectious stomatitis with marked deformation of the oral cavity, bony involvement and the presence of one or more sequela have a poor prognosis.

Diagnosis

History:

- Owners will often present animals for "mouth rot"
- Inquire about husbandry and identify deficiencies (temperature, humidity, substrate, UV exposure, diet, etc.)

- May present for ocular disease (e.g. subspectacular abscess)

Clinical Signs (Figure 53.4):

- Oral asymmetry
  - Inability to close mouth
- Abnormal appearance of oral cavity
  - Excessive saliva or caseous exudates
  - Lingual paralysis
  - Gingivitis
  - Ecchymosis, petechiation
  - Necrotic membranes/tissue
- Anorexia
- Dysphagia

Differentials:

- Rostral trauma
- Bacterial infection (*Pseudomonas* spp., *Aeromonas* spp., *Mycoplasma* spp., *Mycobacterium* spp.)
- Fungal infection (*Candida albicans*)
- Viral infection
- Neoplasia (e.g. squamous cell carcinoma)
- Osteomyelitis
- Periodontal disease
- Gout

STAT Diagnostics:

- *PCV/TS*
- *Cytology of oral lesions*

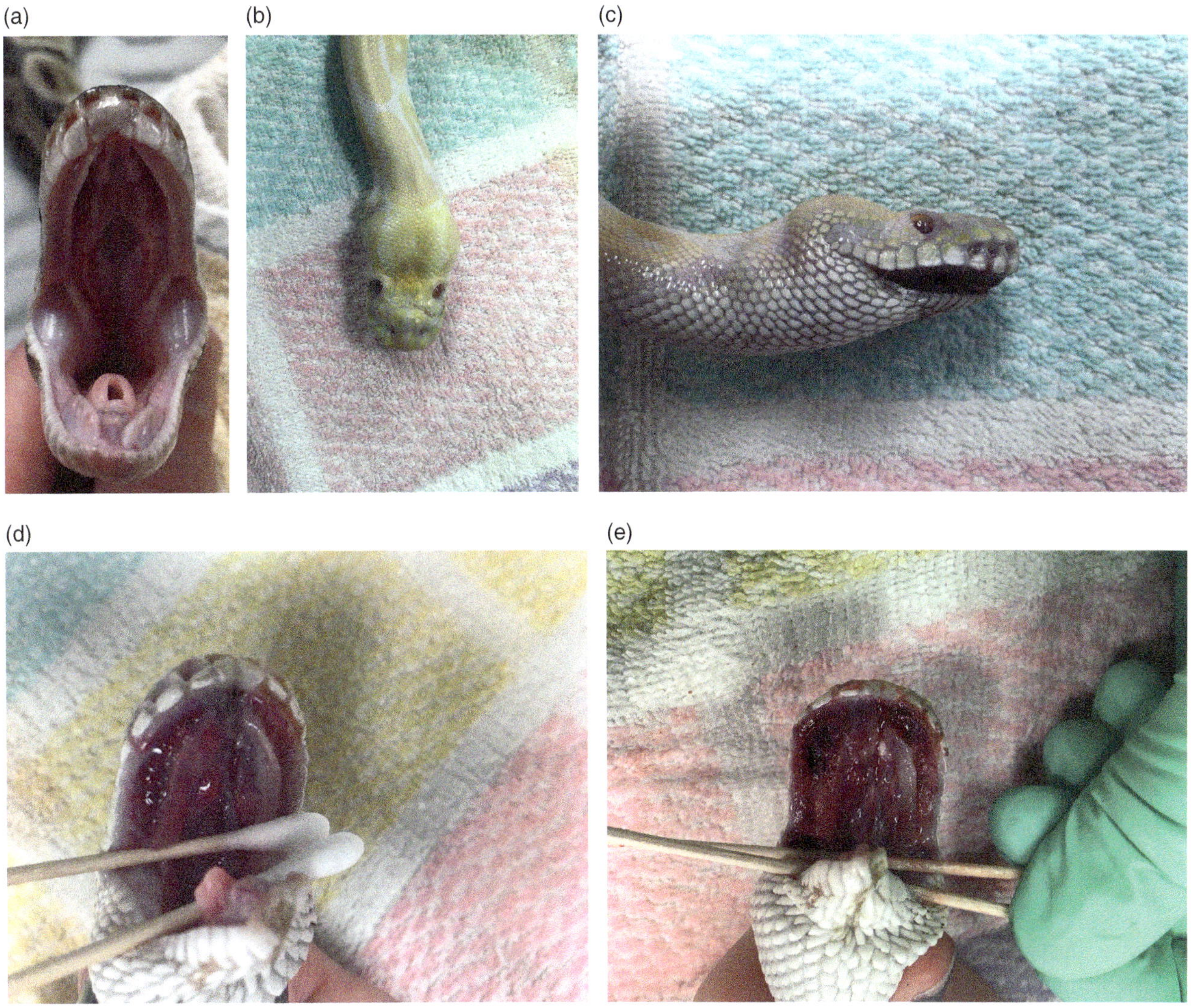

Figure 53.4 Normal oral cavity of a ball python (*Python regius*). (a) Albino ball python with a severe case of stomatitis (b–e). Notice the distortion of the rostral maxilla appreciable in this dorsal view (b) and the malocclusion between the maxilla and mandible (c). Intraoral view of the maxilla prior to (d) and after (e) flushing and debridement and flushing of caseous material from the maxilla.

Complete Diagnostics:

- *CBC*
- *Chemistry*
- *For oral lesions:* Bacterial/fungal cultures, acid fast staining, fine needle aspirates, biopsy with histopathology
- *Diagnostic imaging of skull to determine bony involvement*
  - Radiographs
  - Computed tomography

Treatment

Stabilization:

- *Fluid therapy*
- *Immobilization for surgical debridement of infected tissues and removal of necrotic debris*
- *Systemic antibiotics*: Based on culture and sensitivity results; see Table 53.1
- *Topical antibiotics*: 1% silver sulfadiazine cream; dilute povidone-iodine or chlorhexidine solution; ointments or creams containing polymyxin B sulfate, neomycin, and bacitracin
- Intralesional antibiotics: Polymethylmethacrylate (PMMA) beads with antibiotics can be utilized
- *Analgesics*: Opioids, NSAIDs
- *Antifungals*: See Table 53.1
- *Vitamin A supplementation, if needed*: See Section "Pneumonia and Upper Airway Infection".

Continued Care:

- *Diet*: Assist feeding enteral nutrition may be necessary, especially if animal has lost a significant amount of weight due to anorexia from severe stomatitis
- Repeated wound debridement of the oral cavity may be necessary
- Continued medical management

Constipation, Impaction, and Obstruction

Introduction

In snakes, feces, urates, and foreign bodies can form a full or partial obstruction of the small intestines or colon. Fecal material typically accumulates in the colon. Urate aggregates are also stored in the colon because snakes lack a urinary bladder. Dietary indiscretion can result in an intestinal obstruction. When snakes become significantly dehydrated, fecal and/or urate material can result in a colonic impaction. Foreign bodies (e.g. particulate substrate like bark, pieces of cloth) are often inadvertently ingested during a feeding period when they are located adjacent to or stuck to the prey item being consumed.

Diagnosis

History:

- Inquire about husbandry (diet, temperatures, humidity, substrate, etc.)
- Defecation/urate production history
- *Cage decorations missing*: History of eating substrate
- Availability of drinking water source
- Antiparasitic protocols and if the snake has ever been treated for endoparasites
- Determine if diet is adequate for animal and appropriate size

Clinical Signs:

- Tenesmus
- Anorexia
- Decreased to absent defecation/urate frequency
- Vomiting
- Very firm to hard structure present within the caudal 2/3's of the body

Differentials:

- Inappropriate husbandry
- Endoparasites (*Nematodes* etc., *Cryptosporidium* spp.)
- Dehydration
- Foreign body
- Granuloma
- Neoplasia

STAT Diagnostics:

- *Physical examination*
- *Fecal flotation/direct smear*
- *Radiography*: Gastrointestinal contrast series

Complete Diagnostics:

- *CBC/chemistry*
- *Fecal flotation/direct smear*
- *Bacterial/fungal cultures*
- *Gastric lavage*
- *Colonic lavage*
- *Ultrasound*
- *Cloacoscopy*

Treatment

Stabilization:

- *For constipation or fecal and/or urate impaction*
  - Fluid therapy, including enemas
  - *Vibrational stimulation*: Once rehydrated, applying a vibrating stimulus to the caudoventral coelom can assist fecal, urate passage [19]
  - *Sedated deobstipation*: Administer warm water and lubricant enemas (1–3 ml of 50:50 lubricant:warm water/100 g of body weight), gentle digital palpation and manipulation [2]

- *For foreign bodies*:
  - Ingested items large enough causing obstruction or too large to pass through the gastrointestinal tract
  - Endoscopic or surgical removal

Continued Care:

- *Diet*: Nutritional support, if needed
- *Fecal softeners*: Lactulose (0.5 ml/kg PO q24h) [1]

Urogenital and Reproductive Disease

Prolapse of Tissue from the Vent

Introduction

In reptiles, the cloaca is comprised of three compartments which include the coprodeum (terminal colon), urodeum (termination of urinary tract, reproductive system), and proctodeum (reservoir for feces and urate before excretion). Colonic and oviductal prolapses can occur in snakes and may be secondary to excessive straining (e.g. during oviposition). Snakes do not possess a urinary bladder. Prolapses of tissue from the vent may also be referred to as "cloacal prolapses."

Male snakes possess two copulatory organs (hemipenes) that are located in the base of the tail, immediately caudal to the vent. This tissue can become damaged in snakes and will prolapse from the vent. Hemipenes are for copulation only and are not required for urination to occur. Prolapse(s) can occur following breeding trauma or iatrogenic trauma during gender determination (e.g. probing).

Diagnosis

History:

- Determine if husbandry setup is appropriate for species
- For female snakes that are actively being bred
  - Inquire if the photoperiod has been altered for breeding purposes
  - Inquire about reproductive status (e.g. when the snake was bred last)
  - Ask about the animals last shed cycle, duration and time
  - Snakes often shed prior to oviposition
  - If expected to lay (i.e. is gravid), determine how long the snake has retained its eggs after the projected lay date
- For male snakes that are actively being bred
  - Determine if the male is reproductively active
  - Determine if the animal has been recently sexed and the method used
  - Ask about any recent trauma to the animal
- Inquire about defecation habit and frequency of urate production
- Evaluate if snake has adequate access to water, if the snake is dehydrated
- Assess for any signs of polytrauma
- Determine if the animal has ever been treated for parasites and the origin of the animal (private breeder, pet store, wild-caught)

Clinical signs:

- Tenesmus
- Pink-to-red tissue protruding from the vent
- Colonic prolapse
  - Tubular structure
  - May have fecal staining on surface or emanating from lumen
- Oviductal prolapse
  - Tubular structure
  - Eggs or neonates may be present within the structure
- Hemipenal prolapse (Figure 53.5)
  - Protruding tissue from the caudolateral aspect of the vent, can be either unilateral or bilateral

Differentials:

- Dystocia ("Egg-binding")
- Constipation/obstipation, impaction
- Bacterial or parasitic enteritis or cloacitis
- Renomegaly
- *Trauma*: Vehicular impact, crushing injury, polytrauma
- Hemipenal prolapse
  - Excessive copulation
  - Physical separation by owner during copulation
  - Infection
  - Damage secondary to inappropriate sexing (e.g. probing or hemipenal "popping")
  - Tenesmus/constipation
  - *Neurologic disease*: Spinal disorder
  - Severe metabolic derangement (leading to loss of smooth muscle control)
- Abscess
- Neoplasia
- Neurologic dysfunction

STAT Diagnostics:

- *PCV/TS*
- *Blood glucose*
- *FAST ultrasound of the coelomic cavity* (see Chapter 47: STAT Diagnostics)
- *Fecal float/smear*

Complete Diagnostics:

- *CBC*
- *Chemistry*

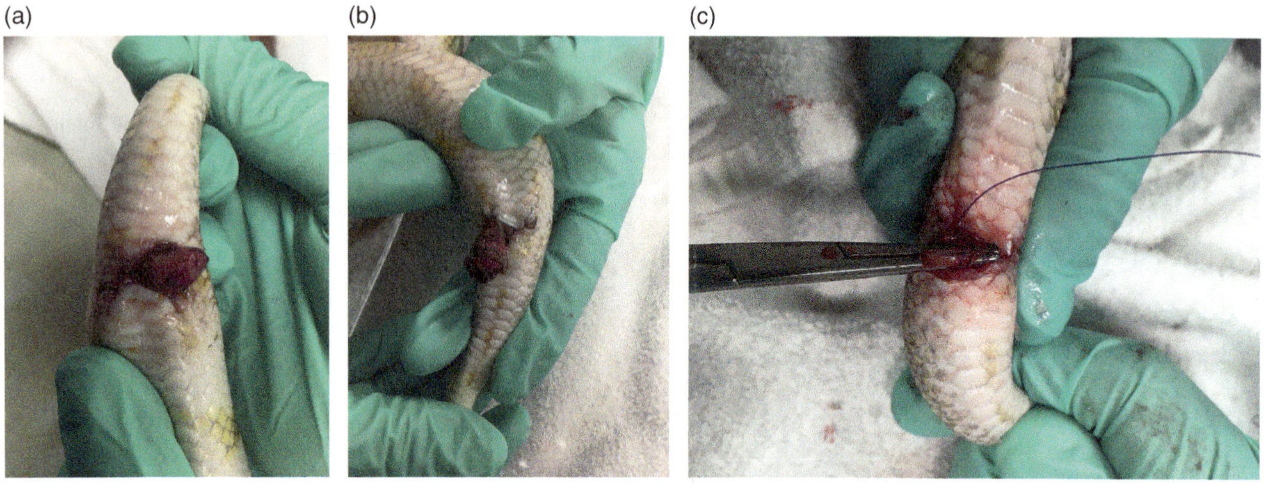

Figure 53.5 Repeated unilateral right hemipenal prolapse in a snake. Right hemipenis on initial presentation (a) and after medical management failed (b). Hemipenal amputation (c) under sedation with local analgesic. After amputation, this animal can still reproduce with the left hemipenis.

- *Radiographs*
- *Cloacal flush for cytology*
- *Biopsy, impression smear of prolapsed tissue*

Treatment

Stabilization:

- *Prolapsed tissue management*
  - Keep lubricated (to prevent desiccation) and clean until further diagnostics (e.g. cloacoscopy) and/or reduction is performed
  - Reduction (if tissue is viable)
    - Application of a hyperosmotic substance such as 50% dextrose or granulated sugar to the exposed tissue to decrease edema
    - Under chemical immobilization, attempt to reduce small prolapses with gentle pressure from moistened sterile cotton swabs; larger prolapses may require surgical reduction
    - Once reduced, place lateral cloacal sutures to reduce size of vent opening; if possible, leave enough space between the sutures to permit passage of one to two cotton swabs; remove sutures in 7–14 days
- *Analgesics:* Opioids, NSAIDs

Continued Care:

- The underlying cause of the prolapsed tissue must be fully investigated and resolution of the disease process should occur to prevent further prolapses after intervention
- Surgical reduction via coeliotomy may be needed for oviductal prolapses to prevent recurrence
- Colonic resection and anastomosis may be necessary if prolapse is large or tissue appears devitalized
- For hemipenal prolapse
  - If tissue appears necrotic or severely discolored, perform a hemipenal amputation. Discuss with owner, especially if it is a valuable breeding animal. Amputation may still affect breeding success, even if only one hemipenis needs to be surgically removed
  - Separate males from female animals (decreases reproductive activity of the male individual)

Reproductive Inertia (Follicular Stasis and Dystocia)

Introduction

Reproductive inertia refers to the cessation of progression of the normal reproductive cycle and can be caused by a variety of factors; often the etiology is unknown. The inertia can occur at different stages of development (e.g. follicle formation, parturition, or oviposition). Dystocia specifically refers to difficulty laying already-formed eggs or fetuses – termed as post-ovulatory – rather than the cessation of follicular development – termed pre-ovulatory – in snakes. However, snakes can be presented emergently for either of the two major types (pre- and post-ovulatory) of reproductive inertia events.

Pre-ovulatory inertia is characterized as the presence of static follicles rather than shelled eggs or fetuses and is also known as "follicular stasis." These follicles have stopped developing (i.e. are in stasis) for a variety of reasons. However, the simple presence of follicles in the coelomic cavity does not equal follicular stasis. Follicles may continue to develop into shelled eggs or fetuses or can even be resorbed over time, without resulting in pathology. Taking a thorough history (e.g. asking when the snake was bred and other husbandry practices [e.g. lack of nest box]) can help differentiate between normal reproduction and follicular stasis.

Post-ovulatory inertia, more specifically referred to as dystocia, is characterized by difficulty in laying shelled eggs or fetuses and is further classified into obstructive and non-obstructive patterns. The term obstructive is used when there is a mechanical reason (e.g. mass impinging upon oviduct, oviductal stricture) preventing passage of eggs or fetuses through the oviduct. Non-obstructive dystocias can occur secondary to metabolic derangements (e.g. hypocalcemia) or from oviductal abnormalities (e.g. infection) and are typically only diagnosed when an overt obstruction is ruled out. Differentiation between obstructive and non-obstructive dystocias is important as the therapeutic approach typically differs.

Diagnosis

History:

- Identify the snake species and how it reproduces; snakes are either oviparous (form shelled eggs) or ovoviviparous (neonates are birthed in membranous, non-shelled sacs)
- Determine if husbandry setup is appropriate for species as some species need nest boxes/areas to properly give birth
- Inquire if the owner is using an artificial circadian rhythm to promote laying
- Inquire about reproductive status (e.g. when the snake was last bred)
- Ask about the animal's last shed cycle (e.g. duration and time) as snakes often have a preoviposition shed
- Determine the duration of time the snake has retained its eggs after the projected lay date

Clinical Signs:

- Often clinically normal
- Anorexia
- Swollen caudal half of the snake
- Multiple movable ovoid swellings on palpation
- Increased basking
- Swelling at or around the vent
- Tenesmus (e.g. tail lifting and vent straining)
- Prolapse of tissue from vent

Differentials:

- Follicular stasis and non-obstructive dystocia
  - Poor female physical condition/malnutrition
  - *Inappropriate husbandry*: Temperature, humidity, improper/lack of nesting site
  - Dehydration
  - Salpingitis (non-obstructive dystocia)
- Obstructive dystocia:
  - Anatomic abnormality (maternal or egg/fetal)
  - Oversized egg or fetus
  - Malpositioned egg or fetus
  - Oviductal stricture
  - Renomegaly
  - Coelomic abscess
  - Coelomic neoplasia

STAT Diagnostics:

- *Ionized calcium*
- *Blood glucose*
- *Radiographs*
- *FAST ultrasound of the coelomic cavity* (see Chapter 47: STAT Diagnostics)

Complete Diagnostics:

- *CBC/chemistry*
- *Diagnostic imaging*
  - Radiographs
  - Coelomic ultrasound
- *Bacterial/fungal culture of lesions*
- *Exploratory coelomic surgery*

Treatment

Stabilization:

- Follicular stasis
  - *Correct husbandry deficits*: Offer nesting boxes in the cage that contain a suitable laying substrate
  - *Thermal support*: Increase temperature of the enclosure to ensure the preferred optimum temperature zone (POTZ) is achievable
  - *Fluid therapy*
  - *Hypocalcemic animals*: Calcium gluconate 10–100 mg/kg SC, IM, ICe q6–24h [1]
- Non-obstructive dystocia
  - *Similar stabilization suggestions for follicular stasis*
  - *Ecbolic therapy*:
    - *Oxytocin*:
    - Only after ruling out obstructive dystocia
    - Administer 1–20 U/kg IM q90min for three treatments at increasing dosages *or* administer two doses where the second dose is 1–12 hours later at 50–100% of the first dose [1]
  - *Oviparous species*:
    - *Manual removal*: After the snake is anesthetized or heavily sedated to relax the musculature, eggs can

- *Radiographs*
- *Ultrasound*
- *Computed tomography (CT)*

Treatment

Stabilization:

- *Thermal support*: Adjust the snake's immediate environment to fall within the POTZ for the specific species
  - utilize thermal support (warm enclosure, warm water blanket, warm air exchanger)
- *Fluid therapy*: Depending on patient status, may require administration of colloids in addition to crystalloids, colloids should be administered IV
- *Blood transfusion*: While a whole blood transfusion may be beneficial for both plasma and red blood cells in sepsis, the procedure is difficult to perform in snakes due to anatomic limitations (e.g. lack of readily accessible access points). See Chapter 46: Nutrition and Fluid Therapy regarding blood transfusions in reptiles
- *Antibiotics* (Table 53.1): Administer broad spectrum antibiotics initially; base further antibiotic selection on culture and sensitivity
- *Analgesics*: Opioids; NSAIDs (controversial use for septicemia in small mammals)
- *Vasoactive catecholamines*: Dobutamine, dopamine, norepinephrine, epinephrine, and phenylephrine to maintain blood pressure (little information on efficacy and safety in snakes)
- *Surgical intervention*: Indicated if an infectious nidus is identified, once patient is stabilized

Continued Care:

- Daily care and close monitoring are crucial for septic patients. Consider Kirby's rule of 20 when continuously monitoring

Herptiles

References

1 Klaphake, E., Gibbons, P.M., Sladky, K.K., and Carpenter, J.W. (2018). Reptiles. In: Exotic Animal Formulary, 5e (ed. Carpenter), 81–166. St. Louis, MO: Elsevier Saunders.

2 Anderson, N.L. and Wack, R.F. (2000). Basic husbandry and medicine of pet reptiles. In: Saunders Manual of Small Animal Practice, 2e (eds. S.J. Birchard and R.G. Sherding), 1539–1567. Philadelphia: WB Saunders Co.

3 Stenglein, M.D., Sanders, C., Kistler, A.L. et al. (2012). Identification, characterization, and in vitro; culture of highly divergent arenaviruses from boa constrictors and annulated tree boas: candidate etiological agents for snake inclusion body disease. *mBio* 3 (4): e00180-12.

4 Aqrawi, T., Stöhr, A.C., Knauf-Witzens, T. et al. (2015). Identification of snake arenaviruses in live boas and pythons in a zoo in Germany. *Tierärztliche Praxis Ausgabe K: Kleintiere/Heimtiere* 43 (4): 239–247.

5 Hyndman, T.H., Marschang, R.E., Wellehan, J.F.X., and Nicholls, P.K. (2012). Isolation and molecular identification of Sunshine virus, a novel paramyxovirus found in Australian snakes. *Infect. Genet. Evol.* 12 (7): 1436–1446.

6 Hetzel, U., Sironen, T., Laurinmaki, P. et al. (2013). Isolation, identification, and characterization of novel arenaviruses, the etiological agents of boid inclusion body disease. *J. Virol.* 87 (20): 10918–10935.

7 Hyndman, T.H., Shilton, C.M., Doneley, R.J.T., and Nicholls, P.K. (2012). Sunshine virus in Australian pythons. *Vet. Microbiol.* 161 (1–2): 77–87.

8 Coke, R.L., Hunter, R.P., Isaza, R. et al. (2003). Pharmacokinetics and tissue concentrations of azithromycin in ball pythons (*Python regius*). *Am. J. Vet. Res.* 64: 225–228.

9 Holz, P.H., Burger, J.P., Baker, R. et al. (2002). Effect of injection site on carbenicillin pharmacokinetics in the carpet python, *Morelia spilota*. *J. Herpetol. Med. Surg.* 12: 12–16.

10 Lawrence, K., Needham, J.R., Palmer, G.H. et al. (1984). A preliminary study on the use of carbenicillin in snakes. *J. Vet. Pharmacol. Ther.* 7: 119–124.

11 Lawrence, K., Muggleton, P.W., and Needham, J.R. (1984). Preliminary study on the use of ceftazidime, a broad spectrum cephalosporin antibiotic, in snakes. *Res. Vet. Sci.* 36: 16–20.

12 Adkesson, M.J., Fernandez-Varon, E., Cox, S. et al. (2011). Pharmacokinetics of a long-acting ceftiofur formulation (ceftiofur crystalline free acid) in the ball python (*Python regius*). *J. Zoo Wildl. Med.* 42: 444–450.

13 Clark, C.H., Rogers, E.D., and Milton, J.L. (1985). Plasma concentrations of chloramphenicol in snakes. *Am. J. Vet. Res.* 46: 2654–2657.

14 Hilf, M., Swanson, D., Wagner, R. et al. (1991). A new dosing schedule for gentamicin in blood pythons (*Python curtus*): a pharmacokinetic study. *Res. Vet. Sci.* 50: 127–130.

15 Coke, R.L., Isaza, R., Koch, D.E. et al. (2006). Preliminary single-dose pharmacokinetics of marbofloxacin in ball pythons (*Python regius*). *J. Zoo Wildl. Med.* 37: 6–10.

16 Bodri, M.S., Rambo, T.M., Wagner, R.A. et al. (2006). Pharmacokinetics of metronidazole administered as a

single oral bolus to red rat snakes, *Elaphe guttata*. *J. Herpetol. Med. Surg.* 16: 15–19.

17 Hilf, M., Swanson, D., Wagner, R. et al. (1991). Pharmacokinetics of piperacillin in blood pythons (*Python curtus*) and in vitro; evaluation of efficacy against aerobic Gram-negative bacteria. *J. Zoo Wildl. Med.* 22: 199–203.

18 Mitchell, M.A. (2009). Reptile cardiology. *Vet. Clin. North Am. Exot. Anim. Pract.* 12 (1): 65–79.

19 Nicholas, E. and Warwick, C. (2011). Alleviation of a gastrointestinal tract Impaciton in a tortoise using an improvised vibrating massager. *J. Herpetol. Med. Surg.* 21 (4): 93–95.

20 Hausmann, J.C., Hollingsworth, S.R., Hawkins, M.G. et al. (2013). Distribution and outcome of ocular lesions in snakes examined at a veterinary teaching hospital: 67 cases (1985–2010). *J. Am. Vet. Med. Assoc.* 243 (2): 252–260.

21 Labelle, A. (2016). Special senses: eyes. In: Current Therapy in Exotic Pet Practice, 1e (eds. M.A. Mitchell and T.N. Tully), 435–459. St. Louis, MO: Elsevier.

Further Reading

Divers, S.J. and Stahl, S.J. (eds.) (2019). Mader's Reptile Medicine and Surgery, 3e. St. Louis: Elsevier Inc.

Martinez-Jimenez, D. and Hernandez-Divers, S.J. (2007). Emergency care of reptiles. *Vet. Clin. North Am. Exot. Anim. Pract.* 10 (2): 557–585.

Music, M.K. and Strunk, A. (2016). Reptile critical care and common emergencies. *Vet. Clin. North Am. Exot. Anim. Pract.* 19 (2): 591–612.

54

Lizards

Stacey L. Wilkinson

Owner and Head Veterinarian, Avian and Exotic Animal Hospital of Georgia, Georgia, USA

CONTENTS

Unique Species Considerations

- Open mouth posturing and hissing are common in certain species and must be differentiated from dyspnea
- Lizards often have pigmented areas that are different than their mammalian or avian counterparts (tip of the tongue, oral mucosa, coelomic and intestinal serosal membranes, etc.)
- Tail autotomy is normal in some species
- The reader is directed to Chapter 45: Analgesia, Anesthesia and Monitoring for current recommendations regarding anti-inflammatory and analgesic drug use in lizards, as well as sedation and anesthetic protocols for these species

Common Presenting Signs

Abnormal Droppings

Introduction

Most lizards have commensal organisms (parasites) living in the gastrointestinal tract that can be normal in certain amounts

Exotic Animal Emergency and Critical Care Medicine, First Edition. Edited by Jennifer E. Graham, Grayson A. Doss and Hugues Beaufrère.

STAT Diagnostics:

- Physical examination, including oral cavity and nares
- Pulse oximetry not validated in reptiles, can be used to monitor trends
- Radiographs

Complete Diagnostics:

- CBC and chemistry panel
- Fecal direct and flotation
- *Trans*-oral tracheal wash
  - Can be performed on awake animal if debilitated, or with sedation
  - Cytology
  - Bacterial/fungal culture and sensitivity
- Bacterial culture and sensitivity of proximal trachea or nasal discharge if tracheal wash is not an option
  - May culture normal commensal organisms
- Echocardiogram or coelomic ultrasound based on radiographic findings
  - Aspirate and cytology of mass lesions
- Coelomocentesis and fluid analysis

Treatment

Stabilization:

- Oxygen therapy, if indicated
- Antibiotics with Gram-negative spectrum coverage
  - Ceftazidime 20 mg/kg IM, SC
  - Enrofloxacin 5–10 mg/kg SC (diluted)
  - Amikacin 5 mg/kg SC, IM: be aware of renal function
- Therapeutic coelomocentesis
- Anti-inflammatories, analgesics in trauma cases

Continued Care:

- See Sections "Respiratory Tract Infection and Trauma" for additional management details
- Congestive heart failure
  - Minimal information regarding management of cardiovascular disease in reptiles
  - Furosemide, angiotensin-converting enzyme (ACE)-inhibitors, and pimobendan have been anecdotally used
- Coelomic disease
  - Surgical management (e.g. neoplasia, abscess)
  - See Sections "Hepatic Disease, Renal Disease, and Pre-ovulatory and Post-ovulatory Stasis" for additional management details
- General supportive care (fluid therapy, nutritional, and thermal support) along with husbandry modifications

Trauma

Introduction

- Falls and drops are extremely common as many lizards are children's pets and are not held correctly, and many are flighty/nervous and may jump or run if given the opportunity
- Crickets, rodents attack lizards if left in cage and do not have food source
- Many lizards normally exhibit tail autotomy as a defense mechanism

Diagnosis

History:

- Dropped, fell, stepped on, grasped by tail
- Wire (especially chicken wire) sides of enclosure
- Unstable or improperly-sized cage furniture
- Allowed to free roam
- Low humidity, lack of water for soaking
- Improper cage materials or enclosure size
- Left outdoors unsupervised

Signalment:

- Very young animals are more likely to be dropped or have self trauma from improper caging
- Males and females in breeding season likely to traumatize nails from digging and rostrum from rubbing
- No injuries specific to gender or age

Clinical Signs:

- Open wounds
  - Bites from cagemates, predators, live prey
- Lameness, paresis, or paralysis
  - Drops, falls
  - Trapped under or in falling cage furniture
- Digit or nail loss, toe necrosis
  - Retained constricting shed
  - Fiber constriction
  - Climbing on wire caging
- Rostral trauma (Figure 54.2)
  - Rostral abrasions, abscesses, mandible/maxillary fractures
    - Rubbing rostrum on sides of cage
    - Trying to escape
    - Inappropriate husbandry
- Tail damage, necrosis
  - Constricting shed, fibers
  - Damage from bite, impact trauma

Differentials:

- Wounds, skin abnormalities

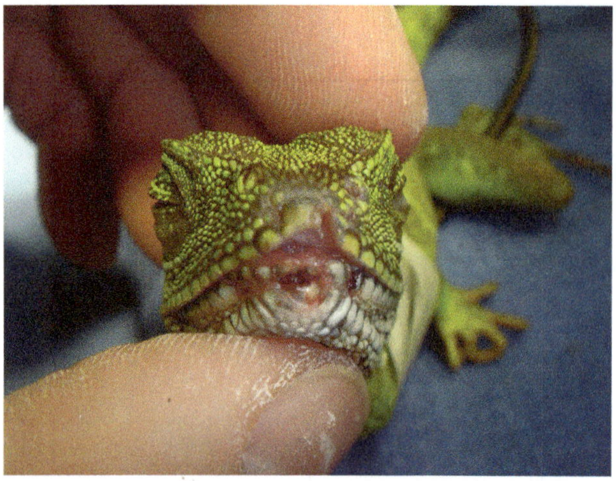

Figure 54.2 Rostral trauma in a young Chinese water dragon (*Physignathus cocincinus*). This type of trauma is common in certain nervous, young lizards. *Source:* Courtesy of Daniel Johnson.

  - Burns
  - Infectious dermatitis
- Lameness, paresis/paralysis
  - NSHP
  - Septic arthritis, osteomyelitis

STAT Diagnostics:

- Packed cell volume (PCV)/total solids (TS)
- Radiographs

Complete Diagnostics:

- Culture and sensitivity of wounds
- CBC and chemistry panel

Treatment

Stabilization:

- Control hemorrhage
- Stabilize fractures

Continued Care:

- Topical wound care, antibiotics, analgesics
- Surgical wound therapy
- Correct husbandry deficiencies
- See Sections "Abscesses, Burns, Dysecdysis, and Fractures" for further management

Systemic Disease

Septicemia

Diagnosis

History:

- Husbandry deficiencies, often inappropriately low temperatures

Signalment:

- No age or gender predilection

Clinical Signs:

- Lethargy
- Anorexia
- Stomatitis
- Petechial hemorrhages or erythema of gingiva or skin
- Episcleral injection
- Sloughing skin, blisters, abscesses
- Seizures or other neurologic signs

Differential Diagnoses:

- Burns
- Dermatitis
- See Section "Neurologic Signs"

STAT Diagnostics:

- Collect samples for culture and sensitivity before starting treatment – blood cultures, oral cavity, skin lesions, etc.

Complete Diagnostics:

- CBC and chemistry panel
- Imaging if suspicion of pneumonia, septic arthritis, osteomyelitis

Treatment

Stabilization:

- Antibiotic therapy
  - Enrofloxacin 5–10 mg/kg SC (diluted)
  - Ceftazidime 20 mg/kg SC, IM
- External wound care
  - Clean and debride
  - Topical therapy
    - Dilute chlorhexidine or povidone iodine
    - Silver sulfadiazine
- Supportive care – fluid therapy, assist feeding, thermal support

Continued Care:
- Antibiotic therapy – based on culture and sensitivity results
- Continue supportive care as needed
- Correct husbandry deficiencies

Neurologic and Musculoskeletal Disease

Nutritional or Renal Secondary Hyperparathyroidism ("Metabolic Bone Disease")

Introduction
- Due to imbalance of calcium, phosphorus, and vitamin D_3
- May be due to
  - Improper diet, lack of UVB: NSHP
  - Organ dysfunction: RSHP

Diagnosis
History:
- NSHP
  - Lack of calcium supplementation
  - Lack of exposure to UVB lighting or unfiltered sunlight
  - Recent egg laying
- RSHP
  - Lack or improper provision of water
  - High protein diets fed to herbivorous animals
  - Inappropriate humidity levels
  - Renal disease

Signalment:
- NSHP – growing animals, females developing eggs
- RSHP – most often older animals

Clinical Signs:
- Weakness
- Inability to support body weight
- Muscle fasciculations/tremors
- Seizures
- Paresis or paralysis
- Orthopedic abnormalities (Figure 54.3)
  - Bowed or soft long bones or mandible
  - Thickening of the limbs and mandible
  - Fractures
- Palpably enlarged kidneys

Differentials:
- Nutritional or renal etiologies
- See Section "Neurologic Signs"

STAT Diagnostics:
- Ionized calcium (see Chapter 47: STAT Diagnostics)
- Chemistry panel including calcium, phosphorus, uric acid

Complete Diagnostics:
- Radiographs
- CBC
- See Section "Renal Disease" for further diagnostics

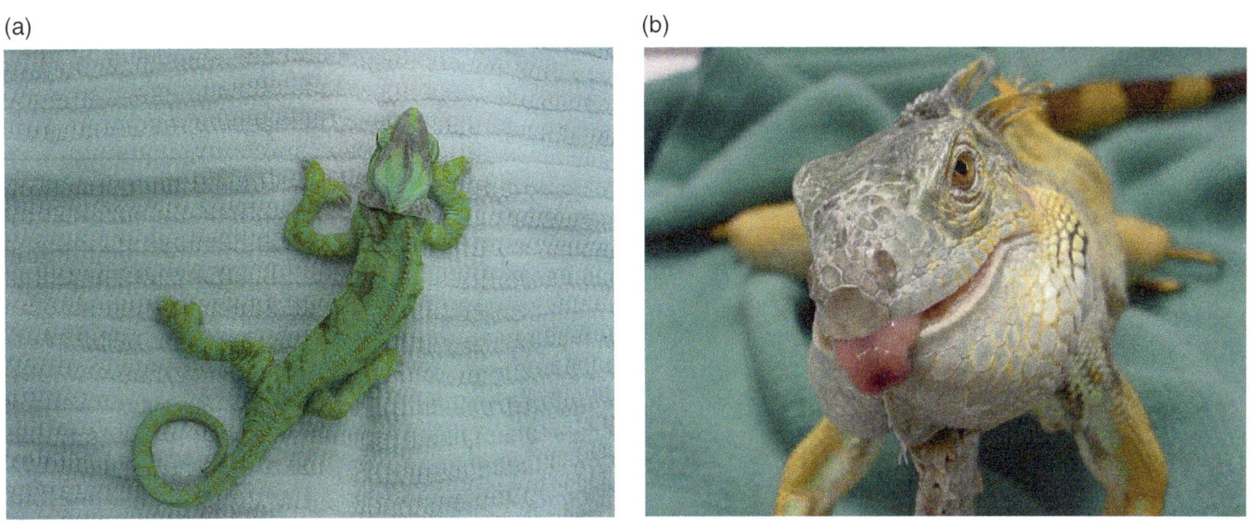

Figure 54.3 Nutritional secondary hyperparathyroidism in a veiled chameleon (*Chamaeleo calyptratus*) with flexible, bowed limbs (a) and a green iguana (*Iguana iguana*) with fibrous osteodystrophy of the mandible (b). *Source:* Courtesy of Daniel Johnson.

Treatment

Stabilization:

- Calcium gluconate 100 mg/kg (dilute) IM, SC q12h until muscle tremors or seizures stop; use caution if hyperphosphatemic
- Fluid therapy
- Thermal support, appropriate husbandry

Continued Care:

- NSHP
  - Calcium glubionate 50–100 mg/kg PO q24h × 30d
  - Husbandry corrections
    - Regular access to high quality UVB lighting, natural unfiltered sunlight
    - Temporarily remove climbing furniture
  - Vitamin D_3 – used cautiously in select cases where deficiency is documented
  - Salmon calcitonin – used cautiously in select cases; serum calcium must be within normal limits beforehand
  - Nutritional support
  - See Section "Fractures" for further management
- See Section "Pre-ovulatory and Post-ovulatory Stasis" for further management
- RSHP – see Section "Renal Disease" for further management

Toxicoses

Diagnosis

Clinical Signs:

- Muscle tremors
- Ataxia
- Weakness
- Seizures
- Paresis or paralysis
- Opisthotonus ("stargazing")
- Head tilt

Differentials:

- Inappropriate (e.g. over-the-counter) mite treatments
- Toxic substance ingestion
  - Fireflies
  - Heavy metals
  - Household chemicals, rodent baits, etc.
  - Insecticides, herbicides, etc.
- See Section "Neurologic Signs" for other differentials

STAT Diagnostics:

- Complete history and neurologic exam

Complete Diagnostics:

- CBC and chemistry panel
- Radiographs
- Heavy metal blood levels

Treatment

Stabilization:

- Bath to remove any topical chemicals, remove animal from area of exposure
- Benzodiazepines to control seizures
- Activated charcoal for acute ingestion

Continued Care:

- Endoscopic or surgical removal of toxic material
- Supportive care

Infectious

Diagnosis

Clinical Signs:

- Weakness, lethargy
- Ataxia
- Opisthotonus ("stargazing")
- Head tilt
- Circling
- Erythema or petechial hemorrhages of mouth or skin

Differentials:

- Bacterial
- Viral
  - *Atadenovirus* – bearded dragons (Figure 54.4)
- Parasitic
  - Microsporidia – bearded dragons [1]
- See Section "Neurologic Signs" for other differentials

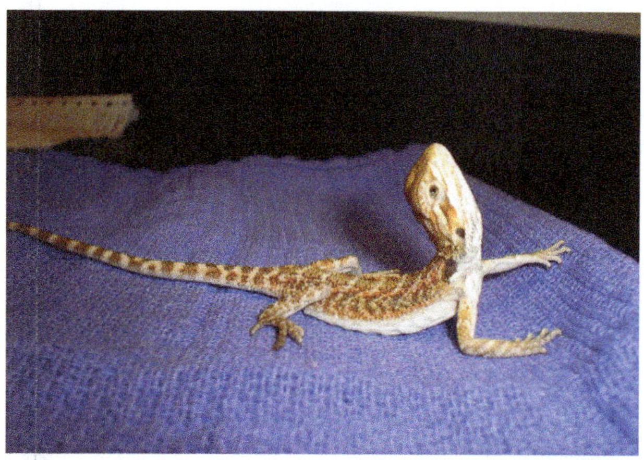

Figure 54.4 Opisthotonus ("stargazing") in a bearded dragon (*Pogona vitticeps*) infected with *Atadenovirus*.

STAT Diagnostics:

- Blood cultures

Complete Diagnostics:

- CBC and chemistry panel
- Fecal direct and flotation exam
- *Atadenovirus* PCR
- Radiographs
- CT/MRI

Treatment

Stabilization:

- Empiric antibiotics
  - Enrofloxacin 5–10 mg/kg SC (diluted)
  - Ceftazidime 20 mg/kg SC, IM
- Anti-inflammatories
  - Meloxicam 0.2 mg/kg SC, IM

Continued Care:

- Antiparasitics based on fecal exam
  - Secondary parasite overgrowth common with *Atadenovirus*
  - Fenbendazole for Microsporidia
- Supportive care

Spinal Disease

Diagnosis

Clinical Signs:

- Paresis or paralysis
- Decreased cloacal tone
- Lack of fecal production
- Muscle tremors
- Kyphosis, lordosis, scoliosis
- Deviation of or swelling around spinal column

Differentials:

- Infectious
  - Osteomyelitis
- NSHP
- Trauma
- Degenerative

STAT Diagnostics:

- Spinal radiographs
- Ionized calcium

Complete Diagnostics:

- CBC and chemistry panel
- Advanced imaging of vertebral column
- Osteomyelitis
  - Aspirate or biopsy of affected bone
  - Aerobic and anaerobic bacterial culture and sensitivity
  - Blood culture

Treatment

Stabilization:

- Calcium gluconate 100 mg/kg (dilute) IM, SC
- Fluid therapy
- Empiric antibiotics
  - Enrofloxacin 5–10 mg/kg SC (diluted)
  - Ceftazidime 20 mg/kg SC, IM
- Anti-inflammatories
  - Meloxicam 0.2 mg/kg SC, IM
- Analgesics

Continued Care:

- Cage confinement, temporarily remove cage furniture
- Nutritional support, fluid therapy
- Antibiotic therapy continued at least two to three months with spinal osteomyelitis
  - Euthanasia may become necessary
- Physical therapy after bony healing
- Warm water soaks, enemas to facilitate defecation

Limb Fractures

Introduction

Must differentiate traumatic versus pathologic etiology

Diagnosis

History:

- Improper husbandry
  - Lack of calcium supplementation or UVB lighting
  - Drops, falls
- Conspecific or predator bites

Signalment:

- Young growing animals
- Females developing eggs

Clinical Signs:

- Lameness, usually significant
- Soft-tissue swelling

Differentials:

- Trauma
- Pathologic
  - NSHP
  - Osteomyelitis
    - Bacterial (most common)
    - Fungal
    - Microsporidia

- Neoplasia (very rare)

STAT Diagnostics:

- Radiographs
- Ionized calcium

Complete Diagnostics:

- CBC and chemistry panel
- Bone aspirate, biopsy
  - Aerobic and anerobic bacterial and fungal culture and sensitivity
  - Histopathology
- Blood culture

Treatment

Stabilization:

- Splint (Figure 54.5)
  - Fractured limb pulled caudally and secured to body with tape
    - Front limb to trunk and pelvic limb to tail
- Create splint with bandage material, adding rigidity by incorporating a paper clip, tongue depressor, etc.
- Calcium gluconate for NSHP
- Empiric antibiotics for osteomyelitis
  - Ceftazidime 20 mg/kg SC, IM
  - Enrofloxacin 10 mg/kg SC (diluted) or PO + metronidazole 50 mg/kg PO

Continued Care:

- Keep splint in place at least six to eight weeks, repeat radiographs before removal
- Referral for surgical fracture fixation, depending on case
- Osteomyelitis

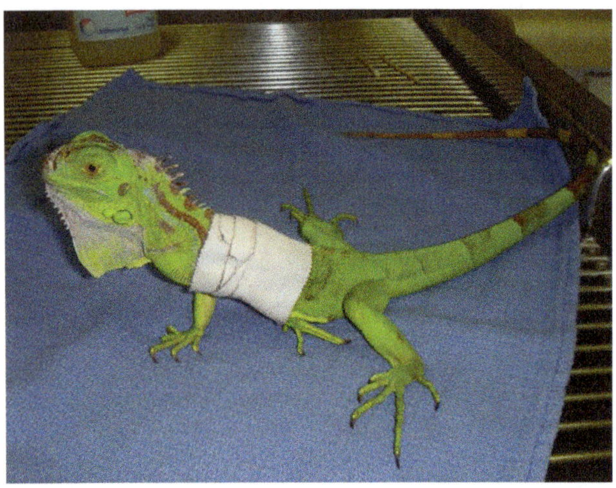

Figure 54.5 Green iguana with a fractured humerus taped to the body for stabilization. *Source:* Courtesy of Daniel Johnson.

  - Long term antibiotic therapy based on culture and sensitivity
  - Surgical debridement and/or limb amputation sometimes necessary
- See Sections "Nutritional or Renal Secondary Hyperparathyroidism ("Metabolic Bone Disease")" and "Pre-ovulatory and Post-ovulatory Stasis" for additional management details

Cardiopulmonary Disease

Respiratory Tract Infection

Diagnosis

Clinical Signs:

- See Section "Respiratory Signs"

Differentials:

- Differentiate opportunistic infection (poor husbandry) from contagious disease
- Upper respiratory tract infection
- Pneumonia
  - Bacterial – Gram-negative organisms most common
  - Parasitic
  - Viral
  - Fungal
- See Section "Respiratory Signs" for futher differentials

STAT Diagnostics:

- Physical examination, including oral cavity and nares
- Pulse oximetry not validated in reptiles, can be used to monitor trends
- Radiographs

Complete Diagnostics:

- CBC and chemistry panel
- Fecal direct and flotation
- Trans-oral tracheal wash
  - Can be performed on awake animal if debilitated, or with sedation
  - Cytology
  - Bacterial/fungal culture and sensitivity
- Bacterial culture and sensitivity of proximal trachea or nasal discharge if tracheal wash is not an option
  - May culture normal commensal organisms

Treatment

Stabilization:

- Oxygen therapy, if indicated
- Antibiotics with Gram-negative spectrum coverage

- Ceftazidime 20 mg/kg IM, SC
- Enrofloxacin 5–10 mg/kg SC (diluted)
- Amikacin 5 mg/kg SC, IM – be aware of renal function

Continued Care:

- Antibiotic therapy for at least three to four weeks based on culture and sensitivity results
  - Important to treat past when clinical signs have resolved
- Nebulization therapy
  - Antibiotics
  - Lizards can hold their breath for extended periods of time which may affect efficacy
- Increase environmental temperature, correct husbandry deficiencies
- Supportive care

Gastrointestinal Disease

Gastrointestinal Obstruction, Perforation

Diagnosis

History:

- Improper husbandry
  - Free roaming
  - Housed on particulate substrate
  - Fed excessive amount of large prey items
  - History of force-feeding

Signalment:

- Animals fed on particulate substrate predisposed

Clinical Signs:

- Anorexia
- Lack of fecal production
- Straining
- Vomiting, regurgitation
- Lethargy

Differentials:

- Obstruction
  - Ingestion of foreign material (e.g. substrate)
  - Insect prey impaction (e.g. crickets, roaches, mealworms)
  - Endoparasitism
    - Oxyurid impaction (rare)
- Perforation
  - Ingestion of cricket hydration gel
  - Iatrogenic rupture from force-feeding

STAT Diagnostics:

- Radiographs

Complete Diagnostics:

- Ultrasound
- Radiographic contrast series
- Computed tomography
- CBC and chemistry panel
- Fecal direct/flotation exam

Treatment

Stabilization:

- Fluid therapy
- Thermal support

Continued Care:

- Impaction
  - Medical therapy
    - Preferred over surgical therapy, if feasible
    - Warm water soaks, massage
    - Enemas
    - Colonoscopic removal
    - Liquid diet with supplemented canned pumpkin, mineral oil
    - Lactulose 0.5 ml/kg PO q24h
    - Continue medical therapy if lizard starts to pass feces and impacted material
  - Can take weeks to resolve
- Surgical therapy
  - Often necessary with obstructions and severe impactions
  - Lack of response to medical therapy or patient decompensation
- Obstruction, perforations
  - Surgical therapy required for perforations, many obstructions

Gastrointestinal Prolapse

See Section "Prolapse" for management

Vomiting/Regurgitation

Introduction

- Differentiating vomiting and regurgitation is difficult in lizards
- Vomiting usually indicates severe underlying illness

Diagnosis

History:

- Ingestion of foreign material, diet change, toxin exposure, etc.
- Free-roaming
- Overfed
- Low environmental temperatures

Signalment:

- No age or gender predisposition

Clinical Signs:

- Regurgitation/vomiting of food material, fluid
- Lethargy
- Anorexia
- Reduced to absent fecal output or diarrhea

Differentials:

- Inappropriately low environmental temperatures (prevents digestion)
- Inappropriately large prey item
- Infectious
  - Endoparasitism
    - *Cryptosporidium*
    - Protozoal gastritis or enteritis
  - Bacterial
  - Fungal
  - Viral
    - *Atadenovirus* in bearded dragons
- Gastrointestinal obstruction
  - Foreign body
  - Stricture
  - Torsion
  - Impaction (foreign material, prey items)
- Neoplasia
  - Gastric neuroendocrine carcinoma in bearded dragons [2]
- Metabolic (e.g. renal, hepatic) disease

STAT Diagnostics:

- Fecal direct/flotation exam
- Acid fast staining of feces or regurgitated material
- Gastric wash and cytology
- Radiographs

Complete Diagnostics:

- CBC and chemistry panel
- Gastrointestinal contrast series
- Ultrasound
- Bacterial, fungal cultures
- Specific infectious disease testing (PCR)

Treatment

Stabilization:

- Fluid therapy
- Thermal support

Continued Care:

- Surgical therapy, when indicated
  - See Section "Gastrointestinal Obstruction" for further management
- Fast temporarily, supportive feeding when appropriate
- Antibiotics, antiparasitics based on test results
- Antiemetics not typically effective
- Correct husbandry deficits

Constipation

Introduction

Extremely common presenting complaint in bearded dragons

Diagnosis

History:

- Lack of water intake or provision
- Inappropriate environmental temperatures
- Diet change or excessive ingestion of prey items

Signalment:

- No age or gender predisposition
- Bearded dragons overrepresented

Clinical Signs:

- Lack of fecal output
- Recent decrease in appetite or anorexia
  - Most lizards continue to eat normally despite lack of fecal production; appetite typically declines late in disease
- Decreased activity level

Differentials:

- Differentiate from obstruction, impaction
- Anorexia
  - Lack of fecal output due to lack of food intake
- Renal disease
  - Enlarged kidneys compress the colon, hinder passage of feces

STAT Diagnostics:

- Coelomic palpation
- Radiographs

Complete Diagnostics:

- CBC and chemistry panel
- Fecal direct exam and flotation

Herptiles

Treatment

Stabilization:

- Warm water soak
- Enema

Continued Care:

- Once feces are successfully passed, lizard typically returns to normal
- Correct underlying husbandry problems (temperature, diet, hydration, humidity)
- See Section "Renal Disease" for further management

Stomatitis

Introduction

- Also known as "mouth rot"
- Sequela of husbandry issue(s)

Diagnosis

History:

- Inappropriately low environmental temperatures
- Lack of Vitamin A supplementation for insectivores
- Rostral abrasions
- Periodontal disease
- Other husbandry deficiencies

Signalment:

- No age or gender predisposition

Clinical Signs:

- Asymmetry of oral cavity when closed
- Petechiation, erythema of oral mucosa
- Oral mucosa bleeds easily
- Caseous material in oral cavity
- Anorexia

Differentials:

- Trauma
- Periodontal disease
- *Mycobacterium* spp.
- Neoplasia

STAT Diagnostics:

- Diagnosis based on clinical signs

Complete Diagnostics:

- Cytology and bacterial +/– fungal culture and sensitivity of lesions
- Dental/skull radiographs or computed tomography of skull
- CBC and chemistry panel

Treatment

Stabilization:

- Flush oral cavity with dilute chlorhexidine
- Remove any necrotic or caseous oral material
- Empiric antibiotics
  - Enrofloxacin 5–10 mg/kg SC (diluted)
  - Ceftazidime 20 mg/kg SC, IM
- Vitamin A 2000 IU/kg SC, IM
  - Insectivores with lack of Vitamin A supplementation
  - Use caution, can overdose

Continued Care:

- Continue antimicrobial therapy based on culture results
- Correct husbandry deficits
  - Increase environmental temperature
  - Ensure preformed, active Vitamin A present in multivitamin supplementation for insectivores
- Supportive care

Cryptosporidium

Diagnosis

History:

- Chronic weight loss despite good appetite
- Exposure to new animals in recent weeks to months

Signalment:

- More common in younger animals
- Leopard geckos overrepresented [3]

Clinical Signs:

- Emaciation (Figure 54.6)
  - Lack of tail fat deposits
  - Prominent vertebral column, pelvic bones
  - Sunken eyes
- Regurgitation
- Diarrhea
- Anorexia
- Lethargy
- None (can shed the organism without clinical signs)

Differentials:

- Improper diet, amount fed
- Other internal parasites (e.g. protozoa)
- *Reovirus* – leopard geckos
- Bacterial, fungal enteritis
- Severe systemic illness (e.g. renal failure, neoplasia)

STAT Diagnostics:

- Fecal direct exam and flotation

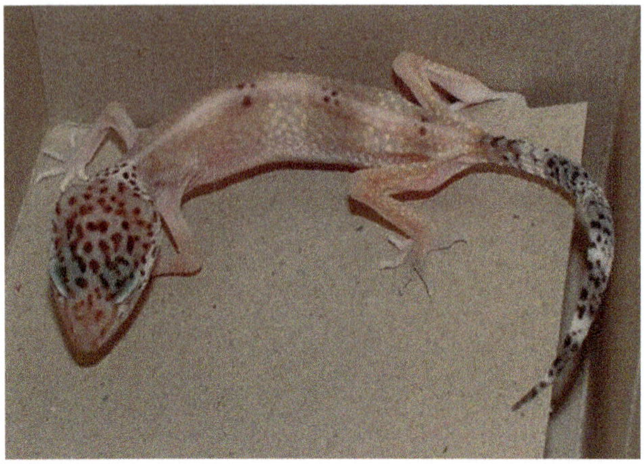

Figure 54.6 Typical emaciated appearance of a leopard gecko chronically infected with *Cryptosporidium*. *Source:* Courtesy of Daniel Johnson.

- Acid fast stain on feces, regurgitated material, cloacal, or gastric wash samples
  - Low sensitivity, specificity
    - Oocysts intermittently shed
    - Can be "pass-through" oocysts from mammalian prey

Complete Diagnostics:

- PCR on feces or regurgitated material
  - *Cryptosporidium varanii* most common species affecting lizards
- Histopathology of gastrointestinal tract

Treatment

- No effective treatment exists: prevention (e.g. proper quarantine) is paramount
- Euthanasia recommended due to poor prognosis and risk of transmission to other animals
- Theoretically a zoonotic organism
- If owner wishes to treat
  - Paramomycin 300–800 mg/kg PO q24h
    - May reduce shedding of organism
  - Supportive care
  - Initiate strict quarantine protocol
  - Oocysts very environmentally stable

Urogenital and Reproductive Disease

Renal Disease

Introduction

- Very common
- Often leads to articular or visceral gout

Diagnosis

History:

- Lack of humidity or improper provision of water
- Improper diet
  - High protein diet to herbivores
  - Excessive Vitamin D_3 supplementation
- Nutritional secondary hyperparathyroidism (NSHP)

Signalment:

- Common in older animals
- Common in green iguanas, bearded dragons, chameleons

Clinical Signs:

- Lethargy to obtundation
- Weight loss
- Anorexia
- Straining to defecate, constipation
  - Renomegaly
- Polyuria
- Swollen joints
- Fractures
- Flexible, bowed long bones, mandible
- Weakness, tremors, seizures

Differentials:

- Multiple causes
  - Dehydration
  - Improper diet
    - Excessive protein, Vitamin D_3
  - Infectious nephritis
    - Bacterial
    - Parasitic – *Hexamita* spp.
    - Fungal
  - Fibrosis
  - Dystrophic mineralization
  - Amyloidosis
  - Neoplasia
  - Toxins
- Any severe systemic illness can mimic clinical signs
  - Hepatic failure
  - Neoplasia
- Swollen joints
  - Septic arthritis
  - Trauma
- NSHP
- See Section "Constipation", page 870.

STAT Diagnostics:

- CBC and chemistry panel
  - Blood uric acid level
- Ionized calcium

Complete Diagnostics:

- Cytology from aspirate of swollen joints
- Radiographs
- Renal ultrasound
- Renal biopsy
- Calculate glomerular filtration rate [4]
- Renal scintigraphy [5]

Treatment

Stabilization:

- Fluid therapy – intravenous (IV) or intraosseous (IO) routes preferred
- Thermal support
- Calcium gluconate 100 mg/kg (dilute) IM, SC q12h for muscle tremors; use caution if hyperphosphatemic
- Phosphate binders
  - Aluminum hydroxide – 100 mg/kg PO q12–24h
- Uric acid reducers
  - Allopurinol – 10–20 mg/kg PO q24h
  - Probenecid – 250 mg/kg PO q12h

Continued Care:

- Continue uric acid reducers, phosphate binders
- Diet modification – low protein, low phosphorus
- Increase fluid intake
- Nutritional support
- Calcitriol – chronic renal disease; use cautiously
- Antibiotics, antiparasitics if indicated

Uroliths

Introduction

- Many lizards do not have urinary bladders (e.g. bearded dragons)
- Uroliths are predominantly composed of uric acid salts

Diagnosis

History:

- Chronic dehydration
- Improper environmental temperatures
- Calcium, Vitamin D, and/or Vitamin A deficiencies
- Excessive dietary protein, oxalates in diet
- Improper mineral balance of diet

Signalment:

- Green iguanas, uromastyx overrepresented
- More common in middle-aged to older animals
- No gender predisposition

Clinical Signs:

- Discomfort
- Hematuria
- Reduced appetite
- Cloacal prolapse
- Constipation
- Stranguria
- Dystocia
- Lethargy
- Stunted growth
- Rear limb paresis or paralysis
- None

Differentials:

- Gastrointestinal foreign body
- Retained or ectopic egg
- Mineralized abscess or granuloma
- Mineralized neoplasm

STAT Diagnostics:

- Radiographs

Complete Diagnostics:

- Gastrointestinal contrast series
- Coelomic ultrasound
- Cloacoscopy
- Cystoscopy
- Urinalysis
- CBC and chemistry panel
- Coelioscopy

Treatment

Stabilization:

- Supportive care
- Analgesia
- Antibiotics

Continued Care:

- Cystotomy or endoscopic removal
  - Referral to exotic or zoological medicine specialist
- Submit calculus for mineral analysis, bacterial culture and sensitivity

Preovulatory and Postovulatory Stasis

Introduction

- Preovulatory stasis
  - Production of "static" follicles: they do not progress to shelled eggs and are not resorbed
- Post-ovulatory stasis (dystocia)
  - Production of shelled eggs that are not oviposited
- Female lizards can develop follicles/eggs without a male present
- Typically lay eggs in late winter through early summer
- Can lay multiple clutches in a single season

Diagnosis

History:

- May or may not have been bred
- Decreased appetite
- May appear agitated (e.g. increased activity level, digging, pacing)

Signalment:

- Females
- Ability to reproduce is based more on animal size rather than age

Clinical Signs:

- Enlarged coelom
- Increased activity and/or digging for several weeks with no oviposition
- Normal appetite to anorexia
- Increased activity level to lethargy

Differentials:

- Ascites
- Coelomic mass
- Any underlying illness causing anorexia and lethargy

STAT Diagnostics:

- Numerous spherical structures on coelomic palpation
  - Palpate gently, follicles rupture easily
- Radiographs
  - If species produces thinly-shelled eggs, pre-ovulatory, and post-ovulatory stasis can be difficult to differentiate

Complete Diagnostics:

- Coelomic ultrasound
- CBC and chemistry panel
  - Elevated total calcium, protein seen during vitellogenesis

Treatment

Stabilization:

- Calcium gluconate 100 mg/kg (dilute) IM, SC q12h
- Fluid therapy
- Nutritional support, if needed

Continued Care:

- If patient stable, can allow time for further development/resorption of follicles and/or oviposition
  - Correct husbandry deficits, provide suitable nesting/laying environment
- If non-obstructive post-ovulatory stasis
  - Oxytocin 5–10 IU/kg IM, repeat up to three times
    - Not very effective in lizards
- Bilateral ovariectomy +/− salpingotomy/salpingectomy often needed, however, due to high recurrence rate
- Calcium supplementation
- Antibiotics, anti-inflammatories if coelomitis present
- Analgesia
- Continued fluid and nutritional support

Prolapse

See Section "Prolapse" for further management

Neoplastic Diseases

Uncommonly present as emergencies

Dermatologic Disease

Abscesses

Introduction

Reptilian pus is caseous in nature (Figure 54.7)

Diagnosis

History:

- Wound or penetrating injury (e.g. cage furniture, bites)
- Septicemia
- Low environmental temperatures

Signalment:

- No gender or age predisposition

Clinical Signs:

- Firm, raised subcutaneous (SC) swelling

Differentials:

- Granuloma
- Neoplasia
- Swollen joint

STAT Diagnostics:

- Aspirate and cytology
  - Obtaining a sample via aspirate is difficult due to caseous pus
- Radiographs of area to rule out bony involvement

Complete Diagnostics:

- Bacterial and fungal culture and sensitivity
- Biopsy and histopathology, if needed

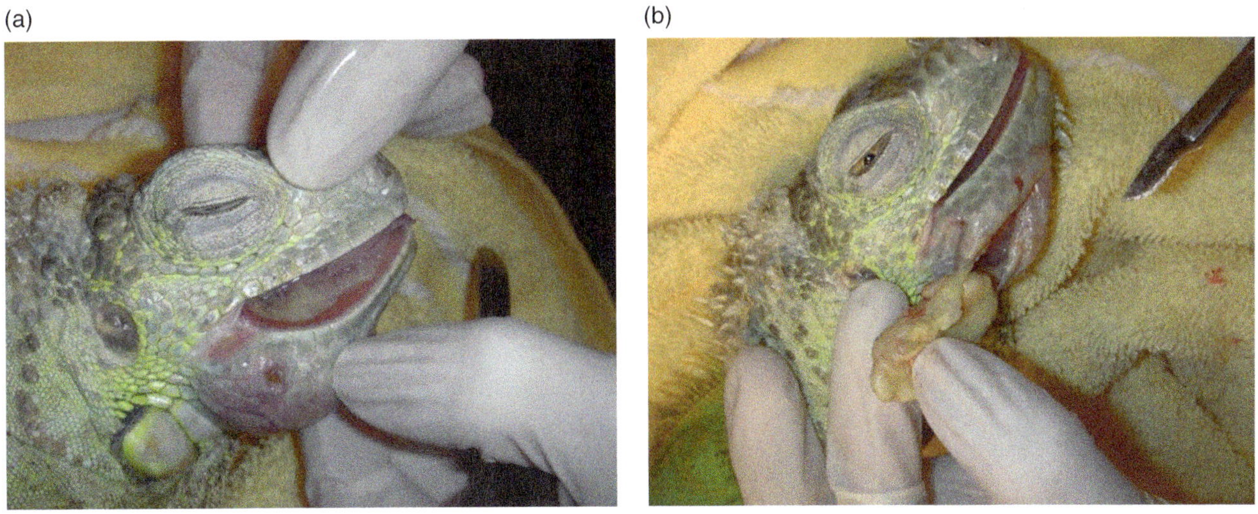

Figure 54.7 Green iguana with a mandibular abscess (a). Abscess lanced with caseous pus removed (b). *Source:* Courtesy of Daniel Johnson.

Treatment

Stabilization:

- An abscess is not an emergency
- Nutritional and fluid support, if needed

Continued Care:

- Surgical removal
- Antibiotics
- If ulcerated, topical wound care
  - Silver sulfadiazine cream
- Nutritional support
- Fluid support
- Correct husbandry deficits

Burns

Introduction

- Commonly occur with use of hot rocks, undertank heating pads adhered to glass, or heat lamps that are too close (especially with climbing species)
- Burn may have occurred weeks prior to development of clinical signs

Diagnosis

History:

- Use of certain heating equipment
  - Hot rock or undertank heater
- Heat lamp too close, unprotected, or basking spot too hot

Signalment:

- No age or gender predilection

Clinical Signs:

- Dermatologic changes
  - Erythema
  - Blisters
  - Raised crusts with serosanguinous drainage
- Lesions on ventrum or ventral aspect of limbs with hot rock or undertank heater
- Lesions on dorsum or dorsal aspect of limbs with overhead heat source
- Lethargy, anorexia if septic

Differentials:

- Bacterial or fungal dermatitis
- "Blister disease" – layman's term for dermatitis often caused by wet or dirty substrate
- Cutaneous neoplasia

STAT Diagnostics:

- Swab for bacterial culture and sensitivity

Complete Diagnostics:

- Radiographs of area to rule out underlying bone involvement
- CBC and chemistry

Treatment

Stabilization:

- Fluid therapy
- Irrigation
- Topical therapy (silver sulfadiazine) and bandaging
- Analgesia
- Antibiotics

Continued Care:

- Monitor healing – as burn progresses delineation between healthy and necrotic tissue will become clearer and surgical debridement often needed
- Continue topical therapy +/– bandaging
- Continue antibiotic therapy based on culture and sensitivity
- Provide supportive care
- Correct husbandry
- Full healing will take many shed cycles

Nannizziopsis spp. Fungal Disease

Introduction

- Nomenclature is changing [6]
  - Several pathogenic fungal organisms previously grouped together in *Chrysosporium* anamorph of *Nannizziopsis vriesii* (CANV)
  - *Nannizziopsis guarroi* – species commonly affecting bearded dragons, green iguanas [6, 7]
    - Also called "yellow fungus disease"
  - *Nannizziopsis dermatitidis* – chameleons [6]
  - Many others – any lizard species can be affected [8]
- Causes a deep, invading fungal dermatitis and can spread systemically
- End stage of chronic disease may present as emergency

Diagnosis

History:

- Lizard obtained from pet store or large-scale breeding operation
- Chronic, progressive skin lesions
- Recent stressful event (temperature drop, etc.)

Signalment:

- More common in young animals, but can occur at any age
- Bearded dragons overrepresented

Clinical Signs:

- Raised, thickened, crusty lesions that are often yellow in color initially then turn brown-black (Figure 54.8)
  - Owners often confuse with retained shed
- Ulcerations under superficial crusts
- Lethargy
- Anorexia
- Weight loss

Differentials:

- Other bacterial or fungal dermatitis
- Burns
- Retained shed
- Other systemic illness

STAT Diagnostics:

- Cytology of lesions
  - May see rectangular arthroconidia

Complete Diagnostics:

- Biopsy and histopathology
- Fungal culture of biopsy sample
- PCR for *Nannizziopsis* spp.
- Radiographs or other imaging to determine if there is underlying bony or internal organ involvement
- CBC and chemistry panel

(a) (b)

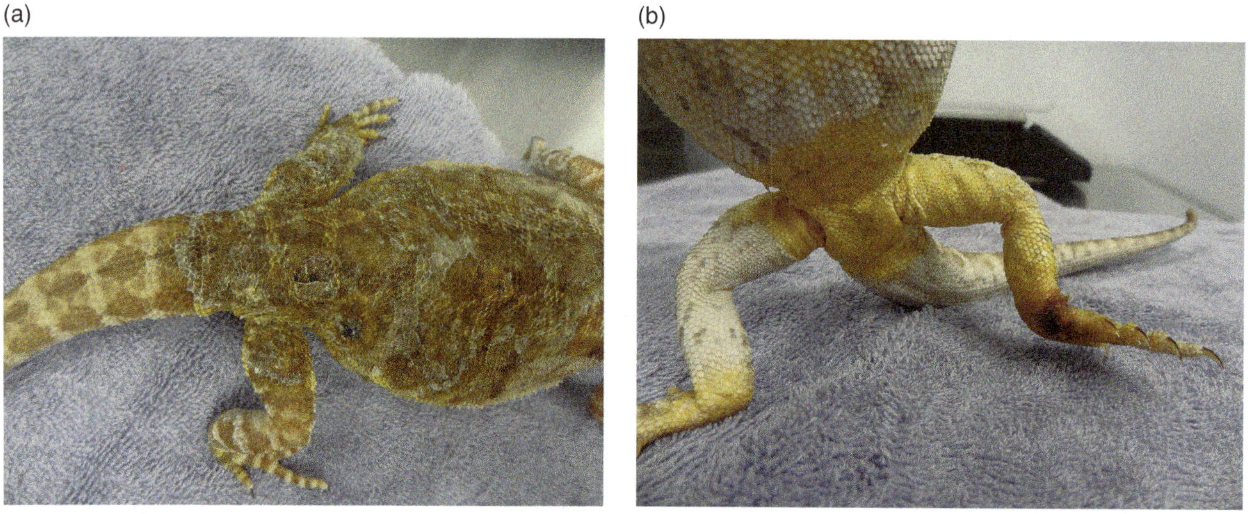

Figure 54.8 Bearded dragon with *Nannizziopsis guarroi* infection. Notes multifocal crusts on dorsum (a) and yellow skin lesions on ventrum and pelvic limbs (b).

Treatment

Stabilization:

- Debride skin lesions
- Scrub skin lesions with dilute chlorhexidine solution
- Systemic antifungals
  - Voriconazole 10 mg/kg PO q24h or itraconazole 5 mg/kg PO q24h
    - Can cause hepatocellular injury or anorexia
    - Can add in terbinafine 5 mg/kg PO q24h

Continued Care:

- Continue systemic and topical antifungal treatment, usually for months
  - Systemic
    - Voriconazole treatment of choice
      - Less hepatotoxicity than itraconazole [9]
    - Pulse therapy recommended with long term triazole therapy
      - Signs often return when medication is discontinued
  - Topical
    - Aimed at reducing spread of shed spores
    - Direct application of medications on lesions
      - Miconazole
      - Enilconazole
      - Clotrimazole
      - Terbinafine
    - Scrub body with or soak in dilute chlorhexidine to remove any spores
- If fungal lesions are confined to appendicular skeleton, amputation may be curative
- Topical antifungals
- Routine environmental decontamination to remove spores is essential
- If systemic signs present, euthanasia is recommended

Dysecdysis

Diagnosis

History:

- Low environmental humidity
- Hypovitaminosis A
- Improper environmental temperatures

Signalment:

- No age or gender predilection

Clinical Signs:

- Retained shed
  - Digits
  - Tail tip
  - Eyelids
  - Dorsal spines of iguanas
- Digit necrosis
- Nail or digit loss

Differentials:

- Bacterial or fungal dermatitis
- Trauma

STAT Diagnostics:

- Diagnosis made on physical exam

Complete Diagnostics:

- Bacterial culture and sensitivity of affected area(s) if needed

Treatment

Stabilization:

- Soak in warm water and manually remove shed
- Antibiotics in cases of tissue necrosis

Continued Care:

- Amputation of necrotic tissue
- Correct husbandry deficits (e.g. provide adequate humidity)

Ectoparasites

Introduction

- Mites, ticks
- SC cestode, filarid worms

Diagnosis

History:

- Wild-caught animal
- Recent acquisition
- Exposed to other reptiles
- Overcrowding

Signalment:

- Wild-caught and young animals predisposed
- Wild caught chameleons
  - SC filarids

Clinical Signs:

- Grossly visible mites, ticks
- Damaged dry, brown scales
- Small, soft SC swelling

Differentials:

- Abscess
- Neoplasia
- Dermatitis

STAT Diagnostics:

- Skin scrape, tape prep

- Aspirate, lance swelling

Complete Diagnostics:

- Fecal flotation and direct exam
- Parasite identification

Treatment

Stabilization:

- Mites
  - Ivermectin 0.2 mg/kg SC
  - Fipronil spray (Frontline Spray, Boehringer Ingelheim, USA) – do not apply directly to animal; spray on towel then wipe animal
- Ticks
  - Manual removal
- SC filarids and cestodes
  - Lance swelling and carefully remove it

Continued Care:

- Mites
  - Discard bedding, thoroughly clean and disinfect enclosure, discard anything with cracks/crevices
  - Repeat antiparasitic treatment every 10–14 days × 3–4 treatments
  - Completely clean cage at each treatment
- SC parasites
  - Reptile is the intermediate host, so swellings may continue to appear
  - Topical wound care, antibiotics if needed
  - Systemic treatment of *F. furcata* often results in systemic anaphylaxis due to parasite death and death of the host

Ophthalmic Disease

Conjunctivitis

Diagnosis

History:

- Low temperature, humidity
- Hypovitaminosis A – insectivores

Signalment:

- Young, rapidly growing animals are more commonly affected
- Bearded dragons – Microsporidia [1, 10]
- Chameleons and leopard geckos – hypovitaminosis A

Clinical Signs:

- Swollen, red, irritated eyelids
- Episcleral injection
- Chemosis
- Clear-to-yellow ocular discharge
- Plaques of yellow material obscuring cornea (leopard geckos, chameleons) (Figure 54.9)

Differentials:

- Bacterial
- Parasitic
  - *Trichomonas*
  - Microsporidia [1, 10]
  - SC filarids
- Hypovitaminosis A
  - Insectivores require a diet containing or supplementation of preformed, active Vitamin A, not carotenoid precursors (e.g. β carotene) alone
- Foreign body
- Trauma
- Neoplasia

STAT Diagnostics:

- Diagnosis often made based on history and physical exam

Complete Diagnostics:

- Conjunctival scraping and cytology, biopsy
- Bacterial culture and sensitivity

Treatment

Stabilization:

- Topical antibiotics

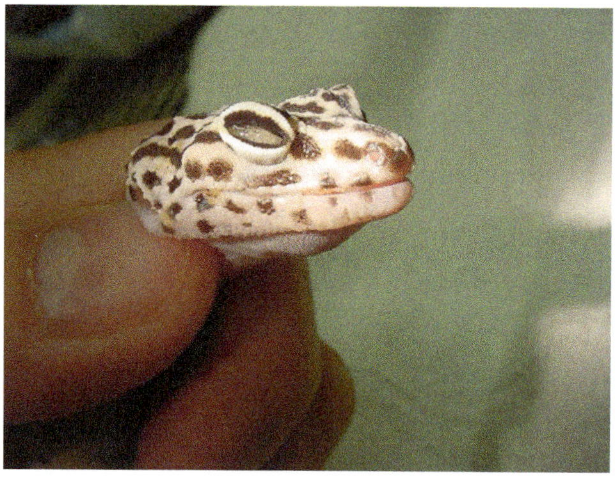

Figure 54.9 Typical presentation of a leopard gecko with ocular disease due to hypovitaminosis A with secondary infection. Note the plaque of yellow material obscuring the cornea. A similar presentation can occur in chameleons with hypovitaminosis A. *Source:* Courtesy of Daniel Johnson.

- Vitamin A supplementation
  - 2000 IU/kg SC; use caution, can overdose
  - Oral, active vitamin A safer than parenteral therapy
- Topical ophthalmic non-steroidal anti-inflammatory drugs (NSAIDs)
- Sedate or anesthetize for ocular flushing to remove foreign material and complete ophthalmic exam

Continued Care:

- Continue antibiotics and NSAIDs until resolution
- Continue Vitamin A supplementation
- Correct underlying husbandry, dietary deficiencies
- Metronidazole therapy for protozoa

Ocular Trauma

Diagnosis

History:

- Live prey left in cage
- Presence of a cagemate
- Iatrogenic trauma while attempting to remove foreign body or clean eye
- Predator attack
- Particulate substrate used in enclosure
- Other trauma

Signalment:

- No age or gender predilection
- Leopard geckos with retained shed, hypovitaminosis A overrepresented

Clinical Signs:

- Blepharospasm
- Epiphora, ocular discharge
- Chemosis
- Corneal edema
- Corneal neovascularization
- Corneal ulcer
- Hyphema
- Aqueous flare
- Visible foreign body, retained shed

Differentials:

- Corneal damage
  - Prey items
  - Foreign body
  - Cagemate
  - Predator
  - Iatrogenic
  - Hypovitaminosis A – retained shed, secondary infection
- Anterior uveitis
- Spectacle damage (ablepharine gecko species)

STAT Diagnostics:

- Diagnosis made on history and physical exam
- Fluorescein stain

Complete Diagnostics:

- Corneal scraping, cytology
- Bacterial, fungal culture and sensitivity
- CBC and chemistry panel if anterior uveitis present

Treatment

Stabilization:

- Topical antibiotics
- Proparacaine and removal of foreign body
- Vitamin A therapy, if indicated

Continued Care:

- Continue topical antibiotics until resolution
- Systemic antibiotics if indicated
- Topical and/or systemic anti-inflammatories
- Nutritional support if necessary (often do not eat if nonvisual)
- Identify underlying cause and correct husbandry

Periorbital Swelling

Diagnosis

History:

- Lack of preformed, active Vitamin A in diet
- Conjunctivitis

Signalment:

- Chameleons, leopard geckos, and bearded dragons are overrepresented
- No age or gender predilection

Clinical Signs:

- Periocular swelling
- Concurrent conjunctivitis
- Blepharospasm
- Clear to yellow ocular discharge

Differentials:

- Hypovitaminosis A
- Infectious
  - Bacterial
  - Periocular abscessation – leopard gecko

- Periocular squamous cell carcinoma in bearded dragons [11]
- Trauma
- Nasolacrimal obstruction
- Cardiovascular disease

STAT Diagnostics:

- Diagnosis made based on history, physical exam, and result of treatment

Complete Diagnostics:

- Bacterial culture and sensitivity
- Fine needle aspirate and cytology
- Biopsy and histopathology
- Radiographs
- CBC and chemistry panel

Treatment

Stabilization:

- Saline ocular flush under sedation, anesthesia
- Remove any hard debris after topical proparacaine administration

Continued Care:

- Vitamin A therapy
- Topical and systemic antibiotics
- See Section "Cardiopulmonary Disease" for further management

References

1 Jacobson, E.R., Green, D.E., Undeen, A.H. et al. (1998). Systemic microsporidiosis in inland bearded dragons (*Pogona vitticeps*). *J. Zoo Wildl. Med.* 29 (3): 315–323.

2 Ritter, J.M., Garner, M.M., Chilton, J.A. et al. (2009). Gastric neuroendocrine carcinomas in bearded dragons (*Pogona vitticeps*). *Vet. Pathol.* 46: 1109–1116.

3 Deming, C., Greiner, E., and Uhl, E. (2008). Prevalence of *Cryptosporidium* infection and characteristics of oocyst shedding in a breeding colony of leopard geckos (*Eublepharis macularius*). *J. Zoo Wildl. Med.* 39 (4): 600–607.

4 Hernandez-Divers, S.J., Stahl, S., Stedman, N.L. et al. (2005). Renal evaluation of the green iguana (*Iguana iguana*): assessment of plasma biochemistry, glomerular filtration rate, and endoscopic biopsy. *J. Zoo Wildl. Med.* 36: 155–168.

5 Greer, L.L., Daniel, G.B., Shearn-Bochsler, V.I., and Ramsay, E.C. (2005). Evaluation of the use of technetium Tc 99m diethylenetriamine pentaacetic acid and technetium Tc 99m dimerceaptosuccinic acid for scintigraphic imaging of the kidneys in green iguanas (*Iguana iguana*). *Am. J. Vet. Res.* 66: 87–92.

6 Pare, J.A. and Sigler, L. (2016). An overview of reptile fungal pathogens in the genera *Nannizziopsis*, *Paranannizziopsis*, and *Ophidiomyces*. *J. Herpetol. Med. Surg.* 26 (1–2): 46–53.

7 Abarca, M.L., Castellá, G., Martorell, J., and Cabañes, F.J. (2010). *Chrysosporium guarroi* sp. nov., a new emerging pathogen of pet green iguanas (*Iguana iguana*). *Med. Mycol.* 48 (2): 365–372.

8 Toplon, D.E., Terrell, S.P., Sigler, L., and Jacobson, E.R. (2012). Dermatitis and cellulitis in leopard geckos (*Eublepharis macularius*) caused by the *Chrysosporium* anamorph of *Nannizziopsis vriesii*. *Vet. Pathol.* 50 (4): 585–589.

9 Van Waeyenberghe, L., Baert, K., Pasmans, F. et al. (2010). Voriconazole, a safe alternative for treating infections caused by the *Chrysosporium* anamorph of *Nannizziopsis vriesii* in bearded dragons (*Pogona vitticeps*). *Med. Mycol.* 48 (6): 880–885.

10 Martel-Arquette, A., Chen, S., Hempstead, J. et al. (2017). Microsporidial keratoconjunctivitis in a pet bearded dragon (*Pogona vitticeps*). *J. Exot. Pet Med.* 26 (4): 257–262.

11 Hannon, D.E., Garner, M.M., and Reavill, D.R. (2011). Squamous cell carcinomas in inland bearded dragons (*Pogona vitticeps*). *J. Herpetol. Med. Surg.* 21 (4): 101–106.

Further Readings

Divers, S.J. (2003). Reptile critical care. *Exot. DVM* 5 (3): 81–87.

Divers, S.J. and Stahl, S.J. (eds.) (2019). *Mader's Reptile Medicine and Surgery*, 3e. St. Louis: Elsevier Inc.

Mader, D.R. and Divers, S.J. (eds.) (2014). *Current Therapy in Reptile Medicine and Surgery*. St. Louis, MO: Elsevier.

Martinez-Jimenez, D. and Hernandez-Divers, S.J. (2007). Emergency care of reptiles. *Vet. Clin. North Am. Exot. Anim. Pract.* 10 (2): 557–585.

Music, M.K. and Strunk, A. (2016). Reptile critical care and common emergencies. *Vet. Clin. North Am. Exot. Anim. Pract.* 19 (2): 591–612.

55

Amphibians

Eric Klaphake

Cheyenne Mountain Zoo, Colorado Springs, Colorado, USA

CONTENTS

Unique Species Considerations

- There are three major amphibian orders – Anura (frogs/toads), Urodela/Caudata (salamanders/newts), and Gymnophiona (caecilians)
- Most pet species seen will be frogs/toads (~5000 species); rarely salamanders (~650 species) [1]
- Caecilians are rarely encountered; consult with zoological facility familiar with these amphibians if presented
- This chapter only focuses on the adult lifestage; larval stages (i.e. tadpoles) are not addressed
- Amphibians are very sensitive to environmental changes; be cautious about water, temperature, pH, and substrate modifications
- Most amphibians tolerate cooler environmental conditions than reptiles
- Many amphibians present with chronic disease issues that are often irreversible
- The knowledge and ability to diagnose and manage disease in amphibians is primitive vs. other animals
  - This chapter will not cover organ-specific diseases, where diagnosis usually occurs at necropsy
- First, determine if presenting concern is normal or abnormal anatomy/physiology
  - White material exudes from parotoid glands on the dorsum of true toads (*Bufo* spp.) as a defense mechanism or stress response
  - Anurans can prolapse their stomach from through the oral cavity to empty undesirable contents and wipe it clean with their forelimbs; the stomach is usually replaced on its own
  - Color changes (e.g. brown to green) in the White's tree frog (*Litoria caerulea*) are normal
  - Amphibians have a varying ability to respire and to regulate electrolytes through their dermis
  - Due diligence through basic species literature search or utilizing online search engines for presenting signs/species can be helpful
- Primary differentials for amphibian illness include physiological, environmental, and nutritional causes
- Anesthesia is routinely performed using MS-222 (tricaine methanesulfonate) added to container of dechlorinated water and buffered to pH 7 with baking soda [2]

Exotic Animal Emergency and Critical Care Medicine, First Edition. Edited by Jennifer E. Graham, Grayson A. Doss and Hugues Beaufrère.

- Handle amphibians using vinyl or nitrile gloves moistened with dechlorinated water
- Zoonotic disease
  - Can harbor various Gram-negative enteric bacteria like *Salmonella* spp. as well as *Mycobacteria* spp. – both on animal and in enclosure [3]
  - Dispose of enclosure water carefully due to risk of environmental contamination with infectious organisms
- 201 species of salamanders, including from USA are prohibited to be imported/transported across state lines due to *Batrachochytrium salamandrivorans* fungus which can lead to species extinction if introduced to naïve populations [4]
- Keeping certain amphibian species banned by law because of invasiveness potential; check website of local state entity overseeing wildlife
- The reader is directed to Chapter 45: Analgesia, Anesthesia and Monitoring for an overview on current recommendations regarding anti-inflammatory and analgesic drug use in amphibians, as well as sedation and anesthetic protocols for these species

Common Presenting Signs

Anorexia

Introduction

- Normal physiologic causes or environmental, nutritional, and chronic disease-based etiologies are common
- Adult amphibians are strict carnivores, most being insectivores
- Many owners release insects into the amphibian's enclosure and are not able to quantify actual consumption vs. insect death, escape, or hiding
- Amphibians have a slower metabolism than mammals, so be careful of overfeeding as refeeding syndrome can occur
- Many owners overfeed amphibians
  - Most are opportunistic feeders normally, waiting for food to come to them
  - When owners release numerous insects directly in front of amphibians, they will gorge on prey items
  - Ideally, depending on size of the animal, anurans should eat a small number of insects that are appropriately sized, 1–2 times/wk
  - Mealworms and superworms are high in fat content; ideally feed roaches, which are more nutritious [5]

Diagnosis

History:

- Changes in ingestion pattern
- Wasted insects
- Progressive, selective eating (usually trends to high fat insects or mice)
- Perceived as inactive, lethargic
- Origin of amphibian
  - Wild caught vs. captive born
    - Wild-caught animals may have significant parasitic burdens
  - Pet store vs. private breeder sourced
    - Animals bought from pet stores may have been wild-caught or originated from facilities with poor hygiene/husbandry or exposed to infectious disease(s)
- Owner experience with amphibians in general or the specific species
- Length of ownership

Signalment:

- Period of physiologic anorexia possible for females during reproductive season
- Physiologic anorexia can occur when conditions are simulating brumation (cooler temperatures) or estivation (warmer temperatures), which are types of hibernation; changes in moisture/humidity can also induce
- Older amphibians have decreased nutritional needs and may ingest less food but maintain appropriate weight and body condition, possibly secondary to decreased activity

Clinical Signs:

- Decreased to no ingestion of food
- Prey aversion
- Weight loss, weight maintenance, or weight gain
- Decreased body condition
- Decreased fecal production
- Diarrhea
- Gastric or cloacal prolapse (Figure 55.1)
- Decreased to normal activity

Differentials:

- Environmental causes
  - Temperature, humidity, photoperiod variation
  - Ultraviolet light deficiency or excess [6]
  - Overcrowding
  - Lack of desirable hide areas
  - Wrong substrate/cage set up
  - Noise/handling stress
- Physiologic causes
  - Reproductive activity (female)
- Nutritional causes
  - Over-feeding
    - Too many prey items

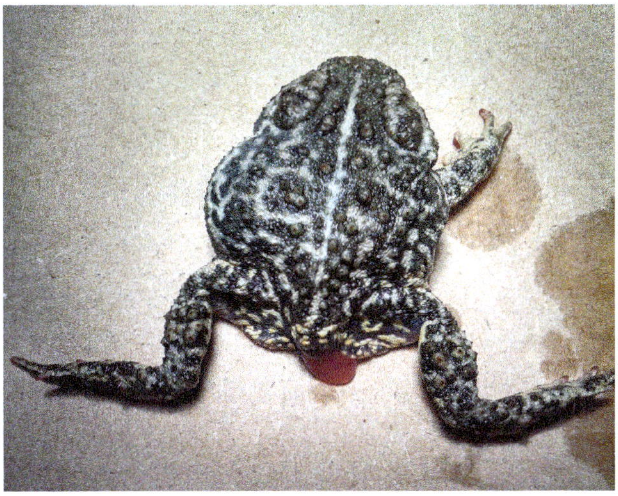

Figure 55.1 Cloacal prolapse in a Wyoming toad (*Anaxyrus baxteri*); idiopathic etiology.

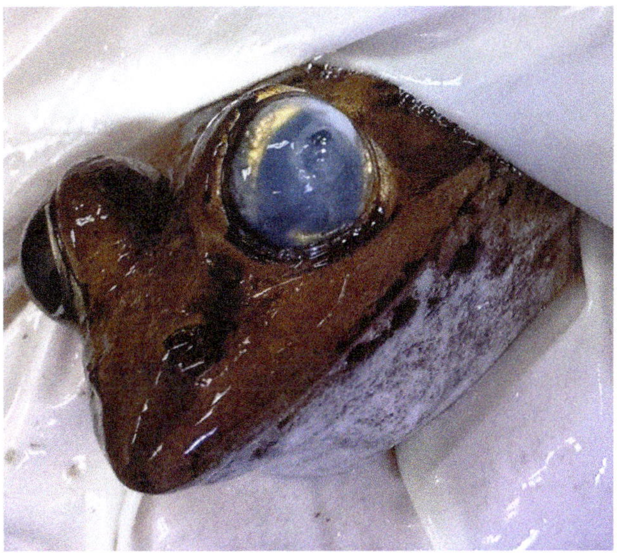

Figure 55.2 Corneal ulcer in a southern leopard frog (*Lithobates sphenocephalus*).

        - Prey items high in calories/fat leading to hepatic lipidosis
    - Underfeeding
        - Insects die before found/eaten
        - Offering unpalatable dried/canned insects
        - Outcompeted for food by cage mate
    - Food presentation
        - Wrong type, size, number, color (brightly colored prey may be interpreted as toxic)
        - Excessive calcium/vitamin powder dusting may make prey unpalatable
        - Prey attacks
            - Some prey species (e.g. crickets, mice) may attack amphibians

- Metabolic causes
    - Hepatic disease
    - Renal disease/edema syndrome [7] (Figure 55.3)
    - Nutritional secondary hyperparathyroidism [7, 8] (Figure 55.4)
    - Reproductive disease
- Mechanical
    - Hypovitaminosis A ("short-tongue syndrome") [9]
    - Gastrointestinal
        - Foreign body
            - Prey item
            - Substrate (Figure 55.5)
            - Gel water source designed for crickets [10] (Figure 55.6)
            - Fecolith
        - Intussusception, intestinal torsion
        - Ileus
        - Gastric or cloacal prolapse (Figure 55.1)
- Infectious – especially integument [11, 12]
    - Bacterial
    - Viral
    - Parasitic
    - Fungal
- Idiopathic
- Traumatic – pain
    - Musculoskeletal (Figure 55.7)
    - Ocular disease
- Neoplastic [13] (Figure 55.8)
- Toxic
    - Ammonia toxicity
    - Other water-based or aerosolized toxins in room/house
    - Contact toxins
        - Substrate – aromatic wood (e.g. cedar) chips

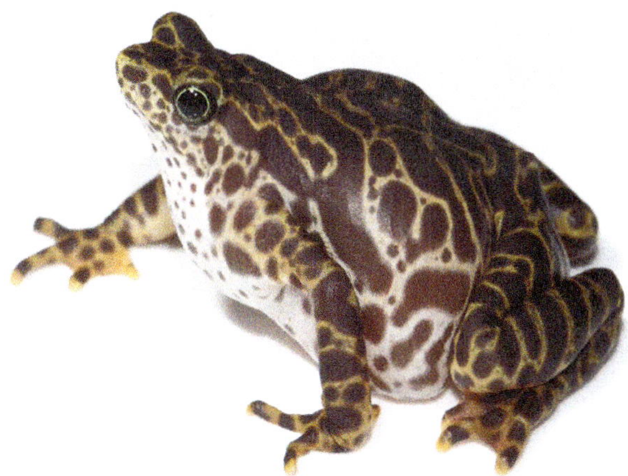

Figure 55.3 Generalized and coelomic edema in a Toad Mountain harlequin frog (*Atelopus certus*). Polycystic nephropathy was diagnosed on necropsy. *Source:* Photo courtesy of Brian Gratwicke.

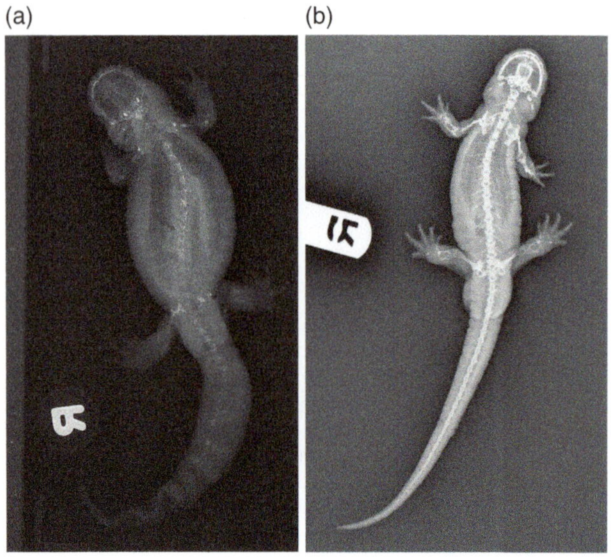

Figure 55.4 Dorsoventral radiographs demonstrating the difference in bone density of tiger salamanders (*Ambystoma tigrinum*) with (a) and without (b) nutritional secondary hyperparathyroidism (a). *Source:* (a) Photo courtesy of Erika Crook.

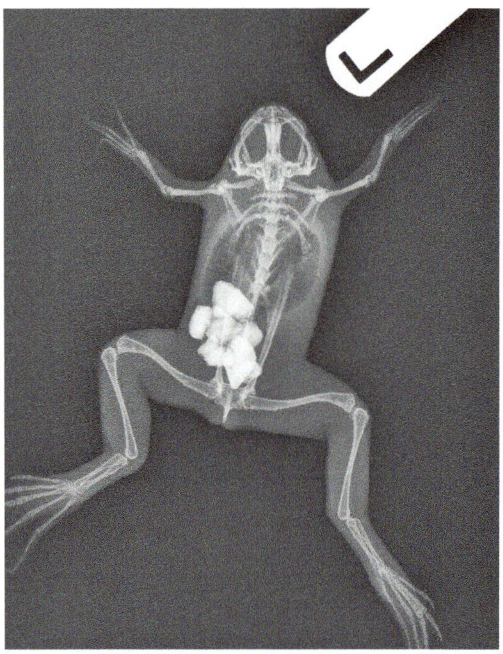

Figure 55.5 Dorsoventral radiograph of an African clawed frog (*Xenopus laevis*) found deceased with ingested intestinal rocks that had perforated the gastrointestinal tract. The pica behavior was suspected to be secondary to chronic hepatic and renal disease.

    - Cleaning products
    - Inappropriate supplements
- Ocular disease [14]
  - Pain – uveitis, corneal ulcers (Figure 55.2)

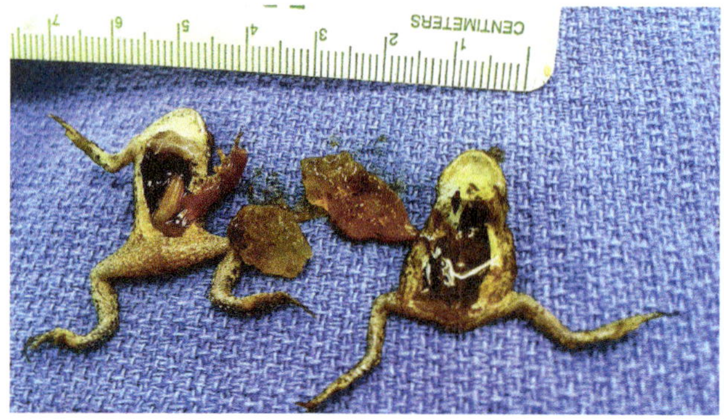

Figure 55.6 Necropsies of Wyoming toad (*Anaxyrus baxteri*) metamorphs that died following development of anorexia and coelomic swelling. Gastroliths consisting of polyacrylamide gel were found. Ingestion of numerous crickets with "water gel" in their stomachs was theorized to have caused gastrolith formation.

  - Unilateral or bilateral blindness (many species, especially those using their tongue to prehend food items, require binocular vision to successfully capture prey)
    - Cataracts
    - Retinal disease
    - Corneal lipidosis [15, 16]
- Cardiovascular
  - Vasculitis
  - Disseminated intravascular coagulation
  - Cardiac disease
  - Lymphatic heart/duct issues

STAT Diagnostics:

- Body weight
- Collect photos for body condition scoring; compare to online images of the particular species

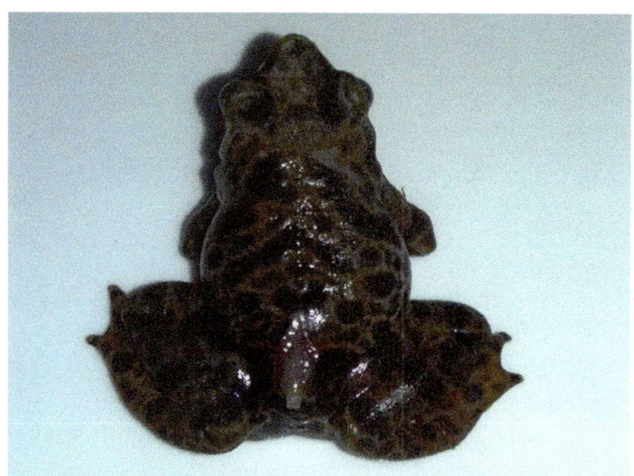

Figure 55.7 Toad Mountain harlequin frog (*Atelopus certus*) with an exposed urostyle secondary to trauma. Euthanasia was elected due to inability to surgically close the area.

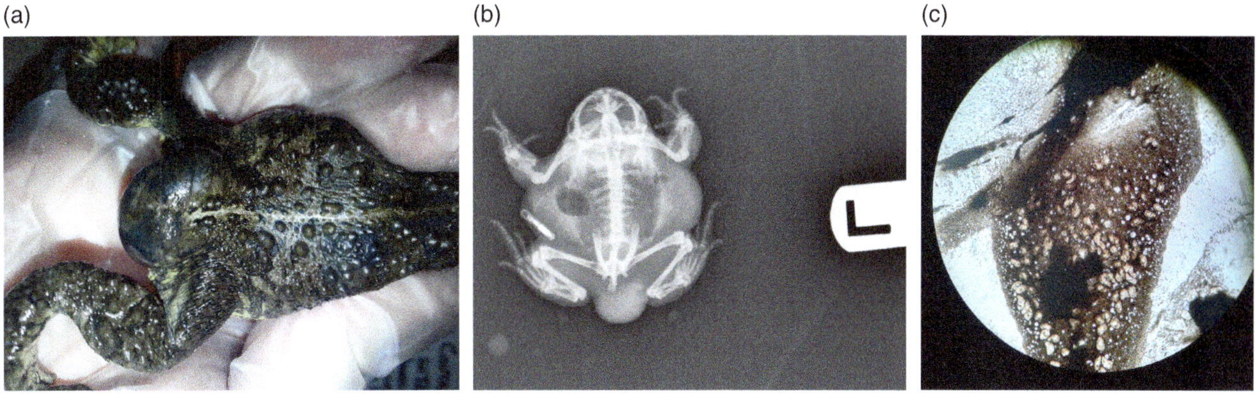

Figure 55.8 Wyoming toad (*Anaxyrus baxteri*) with a dermal, urostyle-region mass (a). Dorsoventral radiograph of the soft tissue mass (b). Unstained slide of material obtained from fine-needle aspirate of mass (c); confirmed as melanoma via histopathology. Removal was attempted, but toad euthanized following incision site dehiscence and infection.

- Physical examination
- Water quality testing – examine pH, ammonia, nitrates, nitrites, and chlorine levels [17]
- Whole body radiographs – dorsoventral and horizontal beam views (Box 55.1)

Complete Diagnostics (See Box 55.1):

- Diagnostic imaging
- Baseline blood work
- Fecal float/direct smear exam
- Complete ophthalmic examination with intraocular pressure measurement [18, 19] and fluorescein staining
- Coelomocentesis and cytology [20], if indicated
- Integument lesion cytology [20]
- *Batrachochytrium dendrobatidis* DNA polymerase chain reaction (PCR) testing [12]
- Ranavirus DNA PCR testing [12]

Treatment

Stabilization:

- Provide appropriate husbandry, fluid, and nutrition (Box 55.2)
- Maropitant citrate 1 mg/kg SC q24h
- Empiric antibiotics:
  - Trimethoprim-Sulfa 30 mg/kg PO q24h
  - Enrofloxacin 5 mg/kg PO, SC, IM, topical q24h
  - Ceftazidime 20 mg/kg SC, IM q72h
  - Ophthalmic ofloxacin 0.3% or ciprofloxacin 0.3% solution topical/eye (pH balanced): 1–2 drops q12–24h, dependent on size
- Pain management
  - If ocular in origin
    - Ophthalmic flurbiprofen 0.3% solution q12–24h or ophthalmic diclofenac 0.1% solution q12–24h
  - Meloxicam 0.2 mg/kg IM, SC, PO q24–48h
- Therapeutic coelomocentesis; see Section "Swelling (Edema Syndrome)"

Continued Care:

- Correct underlying husbandry and dietary issues
- Correct underlying etiology
- Consider continued nutritional/fluid support at home
- Refer to exotic animal medicine specialist for long term care

Unresponsive

Introduction

- It can be challenging to determine if amphibians are dead
- Place a Doppler probe directly over the heart to assess; however, the heart can continue to beat even after brain activity has ceased

Diagnosis

History:

- Progressive or acute onset
- Wild amphibians found in estivation or brumation may appear to be dead
- Temperature/hydration extremes may incur
- Found unmoving in water
- Found in dorsal recumbency

Signalment:

- No specific predilection

Clinical Signs:

- Dehydrated, normal, or overhydration
- Limp, but not in rigor mortis
- Non-responsive or limited response to noxious stimuli
- Little to no evidence of pulmonic respiration

Box 55.1 Amphibian Diagnostic Tips and Hints

- Diagnostic imaging
  - Whole body radiographs – dorsoventral and horizontal beam views
    - Can radiograph animal through small plastic containers with lids removed and placed on top of animal or with animal placed in a plastic storage bag
    - Amphibians often adopt a relaxed posture when in water which can assist in diagnosing gastrointestinal foreign bodies, lung displacement, or musculoskeletal issues
  - Gastrointestinal barium contrast series
    - Mix 1:1 with dechlorinated water
    - Remember, amphibians can evert stomach out of mouth
    - Volumes of barium contrast: <25 g body weight = 0.25 ml; 25–100 g = 1–2 ml; 100–500 g = 2–3 ml
    - Amphibians have a very simple gastrointestinal tract, but transit times are unknown and can be slower than mammals
    - Contrast study may take several days to complete
      - Increase the interval between radiographs once contrast present in the intestines
  - Ultrasound
    - Despite the small size of many amphibians, can scan them in a water bath or using a gel pad offset on the probe
- Clinical pathology
  - Phlebotomy is challenging and volumes collected are often small
    - Lymph contamination common; may skew lab results
    - Complete blood count – if scant volume obtained, prioritize packed cell volume (PCV), total solids (TS), buffy coat estimate, and blood smear evaluation [21]
    - Chemistry – remember, most amphibians excrete ammonia as nitrogenous waste
      - Normal hepatic parameters are unknown
      - Electrolyte and glucose levels may be of clinical value
  - Fecal float/direct smear
    - Dependent on sample availability
    - Parasite presence is common and **does not equal disease** [11]
      - Oxyurids are commensal in some species [11]
      - May be pass-through parasites from prey item [11]
      - Environmental contaminants (e.g. nematodes) [11]
  - Cytology of integument lesions, coelomocentesis fluid [20]
    - Bacterial/fungal culture sensitivity, if indicated
      - Many commensal/pathological organisms of amphibians grow at much lower temperature than most labs incubate plates [12]
        - Lack of growth does not necessarily mean absence of organisms
- Molecular testing for common infectious diseases
  - For positive results, need to differentiate between carriers vs. pathologic infections
  - Make sure to use the proper swabbing technique and swab materials
  - Batrachochytrium dendrobatidis ("Bd") DNA PCR testing [12]
  - Ranavirus testing [12]
    - While commonly positive, some ranaviruses are benign
- Intraocular pressure/ophthalmic examination – the Tonovet (Icare, Raleigh, NC, USA) has been used/validated on a number of amphibian species [14, 18, 19]

Differentials:

- Environmental
  - Extreme heat or cold for species
  - Dehydration
- Physiological
  - Significant dysecdysis
- Nutritional
  - Starvation
- Metabolic
  - Hepatic disease
  - Renal disease/edema syndrome [7] (Figure 55.3)
  - Nutritional secondary hyperparathyroidism [7, 8] (Figure 55.4)
  - Reproductive disease
- Mechanical
  - Gastrointestinal
    - Foreign body
      - Prey item
      - Substrate (Figure 55.5)
      - Gel water source designed for crickets [10] (Figure 55.6)
      - Fecolith
    - Perforation

Box 55.2 Husbandry, Fluid, and Nutritional Therapy Recommendations for Hospitalized Amphibians

- **Husbandry**
  - Always use dechlorinated water when cleaning and when providing a water source
    - Use a fish dechlorinating product which ideally also reduces ammonia levels
  - Rinse enclosure and cage furniture with dechlorinated water prior to use to remove contaminants; residues of commonly-used disinfectants can be toxic
  - Enclosure must be secure to prevent escape from leaping or climbing (can climb smooth plastic and glass)
  - Limit cage furniture to well-rinsed, smooth-edged, plastic hide boxes with brown paper towels soaked in dechlorinated water as substrate
  - For aquatic species – provide an adequate depth of dechlorinated water and change it frequently to manage ammonia level build-up
  - For terrestrial species – provide a shallow bowl of dechlorinated water (½ the height of the amphibian) that permits soaking; change frequently
  - For arboreal species – mist cage/animal frequently with dechlorinated water; provide sturdy, easy to clean, climbing furniture to reduce stress
  - Provide a temperature appropriate for the species; if unsure:
    - 65–70 °F (18–21 °C) for temperate species
    - 75–80 °F (24–27 °C) for tropical species
- **Fluid therapy**
  - Fluid selection is controversial and depends on health (is the amphibian edematous vs. dehydrated?) and the ideal osmolarity of the species. There is no strong evidence that amphibian Ringer's solutions are better than standard crystalloid fluids
  - The author prefers to use a standard, non-lactated, balanced crystalloid solution
  - Generally, soaking the amphibian in a shallow level of the solution is as effective as systemic routes, even when visibly dehydrated. The length of soaking time varies.
  - With some cases of edema, a hypertonic solution might be used to attempt to decrease patient edema. However, many of these amphibians have integument damage, which may result in adverse effects with hypertonic fluid use.
- **Nutritional therapy** [5, 22]
  - Offering regular or favorite prey items for self-ingestion is best
  - Nutritionally, roaches > crickets > meal/super/wax worms
  - If unwilling/unable to self-ingest (e.g. tongue issue), can try feeding with forceps
    - Use caution – some species can inflict a painful bite
    - Open mouth gently with thin plastic card (e.g. bank card) or a small rubber spatula
    - If feeding an insect, try placing it in the mouth and release the amphibian
  - If forceps feeding is unsuccessful, consider gavage feeding critical care formula
    - Prescription critical care diet formulated for carnivores (e.g. Oxbow Carnivore Critical Care, Emeraid Carnivore formulas) mixed with a small amount of a critical care diet designed for herbivores (to simulate chitin exoskeleton fiber)
    - Mix and administer via syringe when pancake batter consistency, 0.25 ml/100 g q24–48h

- Neoplastic [13]
- Infectious – especially integument [11, 12]
  - Bacterial
  - Viral – ranavirus
  - Parasitic
  - Fungal – *B. dendrobatidis*
- Idiopathic
- Trauma
- Toxic
  - Ammonia toxicity
  - Other water-based or aerosolized toxins in room/house
  - Contact toxins
    - Substrate – aromatic wood (e.g. cedar) chips
    - Cage cleaning products
    - Inappropriate supplements
- Cardiovascular
  - Vasculitis
  - Disseminated intravascular coagulation
  - Cardiac disease
  - Lymphatic heart/duct issues

STAT Diagnostics:

- Doppler to assess for presence of heartbeat
- Body weight
- Collect photos for body condition scoring; compare to online images of the particular species
- Physical examination
- Water quality testing – examine pH, ammonia, nitrates, nitrites, and chlorine levels [17]

- Whole body radiographs – dorsoventral and horizontal beam views (Box 55.1)

Complete Diagnostics (See Box 55.1):

- Ultrasound or other diagnostic imaging
  Baseline blood work
- Coelomocentesis and cytology [20], if indicated
- Integument lesion cytology [20]
- *B. dendrobatidis* DNA PCR testing [12]
- Ranavirus DNA PCR testing [12]

Treatment

Stabilization:

- Some etiologies have rapid resolution
- Slow warming or cooling if history indicates
- Provide appropriate husbandry, fluid, and nutrition (Box 55.2)
  - if providing fluid therapy by soaking, slightly tilt container to keep head from submerging
- If inappetence, try maropitant citrate 1 mg/kg SC q24h
- Empiric antibiotics:
  - Enrofloxacin 5 mg/kg PO, SC, IM, topical q24h
  - Ceftazidime 20 mg/kg SC, IM q72h
  - Ophthalmic ofloxacin 0.3% or ciprofloxacin 0.3% solution topical/eye (pH balanced): 1–2 drops q12–24h, dependent on size
- Pain management
  - Meloxicam 0.2 mg/kg IM, SC, PO q24–48h
- Therapeutic coelomocentesis; see Section "Swelling (Edema Syndrome)"

Continued Care:

- Correct underlying husbandry and dietary issues
- Correct underlying etiology
- Consider continued nutritional/fluid support at home
- Referral to exotic animal medicine specialist for long term care

Dermal Mass

Introduction

- For amphibians, skin disease is very likely to lead to systemic issues
- Amphibian skin is highly permeable to water and ions via diffusion gradients and osmosis
- Amphibians periodically undergo ecdysis of the outer epidermal layer and subsequently ingest the shed skin
- Epidermal thickenings such as warts can be seen
- Some amphibians can change the color of their skin due to the presence of chromatophores
- Amphibians' dermis is thick compared to the epidermis

Diagnosis

History:

- Recent integumentary change (e.g. mass effect, ulceration)

Signalment:

- Parasitic causes are more common in wild-caught individuals [11]

Clinical Signs:

- Integument
  - Swelling or mass
  - Ulcerated area
  - Discoloration
  - Observation of the amphibian wiping the abnormal area with its digits (i.e. wiping response), which is a sign of local discomfort in amphibians
- Need to differentiate between epidermal/dermal mass vs. coelomic mass/swelling/edema

Differentials:

- Environmental
  - Ultraviolet excess [6]
- Physiological
- Color change can be normal due to skin chromatophores
- Neoplastic [13]
  - Melanomas have been reported (Figure 55.8)
  - Benign cysts
- Infectious [11, 12]
  - Bacterial
  - Viral
    - Ranaviruses and herpesviruses may cause skin ulcers
  - Parasitic
  - If it is a wild-caught individual, filarids and cestodes are common
  - Fungal
- Idiopathic
- Traumatic
  - Hematoma
  - Seroma
  - Fracture under dermis

STAT Diagnostics:

- Body weight
- Collect photos for body condition scoring; compare to online images of the particular species
- Physical examination
- Whole body radiographs – dorsoventral and horizontal beam views (Box 55.1)

Herptiles

Complete Diagnostics:

- Baseline blood work
- Fecal float/direct smear exam
- Integument lesion cytology [20]
- *B. dendrobatidis* DNA PCR testing [12]
- Ranavirus DNA PCR testing [12]

Treatment

Stabilization:

- Provide appropriate husbandry, fluid, and nutrition (Box 55.2)
- If inappetence, try maropitant citrate 1 mg/kg SC q24h
- Empiric antibiotics:
  - Trimethoprim-Sulfa 30 mg/kg PO q24h
  - Enrofloxacin 5 mg/kg PO, SC, IM, topical q24h
  - Ceftazidime 20 mg/kg SC, IM q72h
  - Ophthalmic ofloxacin 0.3% or ciprofloxacin 0.3% solution topical/eye (pH balanced): 1–2 drops q12–24h, dependent on size
- Pain management
  - Meloxicam 0.2 mg/kg IM, SC, PO q24–48h
- If parasitic, can lance site and extract, often at multiple locations

Continued Care:

- Correct underlying husbandry and dietary issues
- Correct underlying etiology
- Consider continued nutritional/fluid support at home
- Referral to exotic animal medicine specialist for long term care
- Removal of lesion, especially neoplasia, can be challenging due to difficulty closing the surgical site and high rate of dehiscence [2]

Emaciation

Introduction

- First determine if true emaciation or species norm
- If pathologic or nutritional, usually chronic in nature
- Many owners release insects into the amphibian's enclosure and are not able to quantify actual consumption vs. insect death, escape, or hiding
- Amphibians have a slower metabolism than mammals, so be careful of overfeeding as refeeding syndrome can occur

Diagnosis

History:

- Refusal to eat
- Weight loss despite a robust appetite
- Novice owner (i.e. not feeding the amphibian appropriately)

Signalment:

- More common in older or wild-caught animals

Clinical Signs:

- Anorexia
- Robust appetite with poor body condition
- Weight loss
- Lethargy
- Hiding behavior
- Weak
- Decreased fecal production
- Cloacal prolapse (Figure 55.1)

Differentials:

- Environmental
  - Inappropriate temperature, humidity, photoperiod variation
  - Ultraviolet light deficiency or excess [6]
  - Overcrowding
  - Lack of desirable hide areas
  - Wrong substrate/cage set up
  - Noise/handling stress
- Nutritional
  - Underfeeding
    - Insects die before being found/eaten
    - Offering unpalatable dried/canned insects
    - Outcompeted for food by cage mate
  - Food presentation
    - Wrong type, size, number, color (brightly colored prey may be interpreted as toxic)
    - Excessive calcium/vitamin powder dusting may make prey unpalatable
    - Prey attacks
    - Some prey species (e.g. crickets, mice) may attack amphibians
- Metabolic
  - Hepatic disease
  - Renal disease/edema syndrome [7] (Figure 55.3)
  - Nutritional secondary hyperparathyroidism [7, 8] (Figure 55.4)
  - Reproductive disease
- Mechanical
  - Hypovitaminosis A ("short-tongue syndrome") [9]
  - Gastrointestinal
    - Foreign body
      - Prey item
      - Substrate (Figure 55.5)
      - Gel water source designed for crickets [10] (Figure 55.6)
      - Fecolith

Herptiles

    - Intussusception, intestinal torsion
    - Ileus
  - Gastric or cloacal prolapse (Figure 55.1)
- Neoplastic [13] (Figure 55.8)
- Infectious – especially integument [11, 12]
  - Bacterial
  - Viral
  - Parasitic
  - Fungal
- Idiopathic
- Traumatic – pain
  - Musculoskeletal (Figure 55.7)
  - Ocular disease [14]
- Toxic
  - Ammonia toxicity
  - Other water-based or aerosolized toxins in room/house
  - Contact toxins
    - Substrate – aromatic wood (e.g. cedar) chips
    - Cleaning products
    - Inappropriate supplements
- Ocular disease [14]
  - Pain – uveitis, corneal ulcers (Figure 55.2)
  - Unilateral or bilateral blindness (many species, especially those using their tongue to prehend food items, require binocular vision to successfully capture prey)
    - Cataracts
    - Retinal disease
    - Corneal lipidosis [15, 16]
- Cardiovascular
  - Vasculitis
  - Disseminated intravascular coagulation
  - Cardiac disease
  - Lymphatic heart/duct issues

STAT Diagnostics:

- Body weight
- Collect photos for body condition scoring; compare to online images of the particular species
- Physical examination
- Water quality testing – examine pH, ammonia, nitrates, nitrites, and chlorine levels [17]
- Whole body radiographs – dorsoventral and horizontal beam views (Box 55.1)

Complete Diagnostics (See Box 55.1):

- Diagnostic imaging
  - Gastrointestinal contrast series
  - Ultrasound
- Baseline blood work
- Coelomocentesis and cytology [20], if indicated
- Fecal float/direct smear exam
- Complete ophthalmic examination with intraocular pressure measurement [18, 19] and fluorescein staining
- *B. dendrobatidis* DNA PCR testing [12]
- Ranavirus DNA PCR testing [12]

Treatment

Stabilization:

- Provide appropriate husbandry, fluid, and nutrition (Box 55.2)
- If inappetence, try maropitant citrate 1 mg/kg SC q24h
- Empiric antibiotics
  - Trimethoprim-Sulfa 30 mg/kg PO q24h
  - Enrofloxacin 5 mg/kg PO, SC, IM, topical q24h
  - Ceftazidime 20 mg/kg SC, IM q72h
  - Ophthalmic ofloxacin 0.3% or ciprofloxacin 0.3% solution topical/eye (pH balanced): 1–2 drops q12–24h, dependent on size
- Pain management
  - If ocular in origin
    - Ophthalmic flurbiprofen 0.3% solution q12–24h or ophthalmic diclofenac 0.1% solution q12–24h
  - Meloxicam 0.2 mg/kg IM, SC, PO q24–48h
- Therapeutic coelomocentesis; see Section "Swelling (Edema Syndrome)"

Continued Care:

- Correct underlying husbandry and dietary issues
- Correct underlying etiology
- Consider continued nutritional/fluid support at home
- Refer to exotic animal medicine specialist for long term care

Limb Injury/Paresis

Introduction

- Trauma is the most common cause

Diagnosis

History:

- Sudden onset of inability to use limb
- Possible bone exposure
- Abnormal/extra limbs (more likely in wild-caught individuals)

Signalment:

- No specific predilection

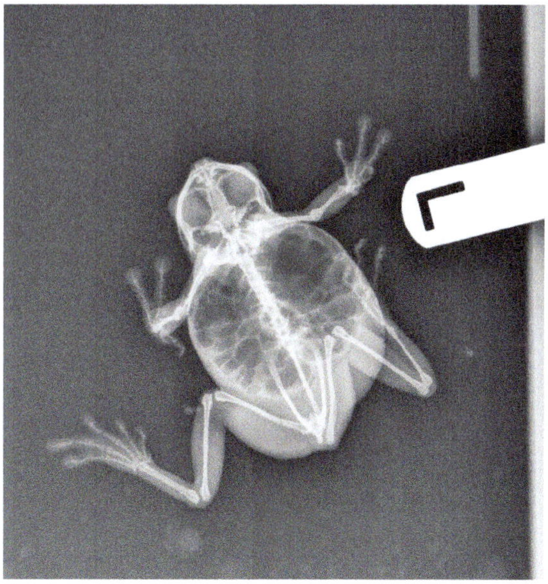

Figure 55.9 Left coxofemoral luxation identified on a dorsoventral radiograph of an inactive White's treefrog (*Litoria caerulea*), suspected to be secondary to handling injury. This frog attempted to jump from the handler's grasp and was quickly grasped by the affected leg to prevent a fall.

Clinical Signs:

- One or more limbs not being used; most noticeable when hind limb(s) are affected

Differentials:

- Developmental – "Spindly Leg Syndrome" [23]
- Environmental
  - Inappropriate cage set up
- Metabolic
  - Nutritional secondary hyperparathyroidism [7, 8] (Figure 55.4)
- Neoplastic [13] – especially nerve, muscle, or bone origin
- Idiopathic
- Infectious
  - Parasitic – trematode genus *Ribeiroia* [11, 12]
- Traumatic
  - Musculoskeletal
    - Inappropriate handling is a common cause (Figure 55.9)

STAT Diagnostics:

- Body weight
- Physical examination
- Whole body radiographs – dorsoventral and horizontal beam views (Box 55.1)

Complete Diagnostics:

- No additional diagnostics on top of STAT diagnostics readily needed

Treatment

Stabilization:

- Provide appropriate husbandry, fluid, and nutrition (Box 55.2)
- If inappetence, try maropitant citrate 1 mg/kg SC q24h
- If open fracture, prescribe empiric antibiotics
  - Trimethoprim-Sulfa 30 mg/kg PO q24h
  - Enrofloxacin 5 mg/kg PO, SC, IM, topical q24h
  - Ceftazidime 20 mg/kg SC, IM q72h
  - Ophthalmic ofloxacin 0.3% or ciprofloxacin 0.3% solution topical/eye (pH balanced): 1–2 drops q12–24h, dependent on size
- Pain management
  - Meloxicam 0.2 mg/kg IM, SC, PO q24–48h
- Consider amputation, external coaptation, or internal repair of fractures

Continued Care:

- Correct underlying husbandry and dietary issues
- Correct underlying etiology
- Consider continued nutritional/fluid support at home
- Refer to exotic animal medicine specialist for long term care

Ophthalmic Issues

Introduction

- Likely underdiagnosed
- Can be concurrent with other presentations
- Amphibians can retract their eyes into the dorsal part of the oral cavity to assist in holding or swallowing prey
  - Ocular injury or enucleation may affect ability to successfully prehend food

Diagnosis

History:

- Change in interest in food
- Attempting to eat but missing food
- Inactivity
- Hiding more frequently

Signalment:

- More common in older animals
- A wild amphibian that was unusually easy to catch

Clinical Signs:

- Anorexia
- Behavior changes
- Ophthalmic signs
  - Can be bilateral or unilateral
  - Buphthalmia, exophthalmos, and/or proptosis
  - Raised nictitans
  - Cloudy cornea
  - Hyphema
  - Mydriasis or miosis
  - Repeated wiping of ocular region with digits
  - Repeated retraction of eyeball(s) when not eating
  - Photophobia

Differentials:

- Multiple processes may manifest as ophthalmic disease [14]
- Environmental
  - Temperature variation
  - Ultraviolet light deficiency or excess [6]
  - Dehydration
- Nutritional
  - High fat diet – corneal lipidosis [15, 16]
- Mechanical
  - Foreign body
- Metabolic
  - Cataracts [14]
- Neoplastic [13, 14]
- Infectious [11, 12, 14]
  - Bacterial
  - Viral
  - Parasitic
  - Fungal
- Idiopathic
- Traumatic
- Toxic
  - Ammonia toxicity
  - Other water-based or aerosolized toxins in room/house
  - Contact toxins
    - Substrate – aromatic wood (e.g. cedar) chips
    - Cleaning products
    - Inappropriate supplements
- Ocular disease [14]
  - Corneal ulcer (Figure 55.2)
  - Cataracts
  - Non-infectious uveitis or retinal disease
- Cardiovascular
  - Vasculitis
  - Disseminated intravascular coagulation
  - Cardiac disease
  - Lymphatic heart/duct issues

STAT Diagnostics:

- Body weight
- Collect photos for body condition scoring; compare to online images of the particular species
- Physical examination
- Water quality testing – examine pH, ammonia, nitrates, nitrites, and chlorine levels [17]
- Complete ophthalmic examination with intraocular pressure measurement [18, 19] and fluorescein staining

Complete Diagnostics:

- Whole body radiographs – dorsoventral and horizontal beam views (Box 55.1)

Treatment

Stabilization:

- Provide appropriate husbandry, fluid, and nutrition (Box 55.2)
- If inappetence, try maropitant citrate 1 mg/kg SC q24h
- Empiric antibiotics
  - Trimethoprim-Sulfa 30 mg/kg PO q24h
  - Enrofloxacin 5 mg/kg PO, SC, IM, topical q24h
  - Ceftazidime 20 mg/kg SC, IM q72h
  - Ophthalmic ofloxacin 0.3% or ciprofloxacin 0.3% solution topical/eye (pH balanced): 1–2 drops q12–24h, dependent on size
- If ulcer (Figure 55.2)
  - Consider tarsorrhaphy of affected eye(s), surgical glue, topical corneal repair gel (e.g. Remend, Bayer, Janesville, WI, USA)
- Pain management
  - If ocular in origin
    - Ophthalmic flurbiprofen 0.3% solution q12–24h or ophthalmic diclofenac 0.1% solution q12–24h
  - Meloxicam 0.2 mg/kg IM, SC, PO q24–48h

Continued Care:

- Correct underlying husbandry and dietary issues
- Correct underlying etiology
- Consider continued nutritional/fluid support at home
- Consider quality of life before attempting enucleation (e.g. is animal able to eat on its own?) [24]
  - Can be challenging to surgically close; dehiscence can occur [2, 24]
- Referral to veterinary ophthalmologist ideal for long term care

Prolapse (Vent/Cloacal) (Figure 55.1)

Introduction

- Prolapse of tissue from vent/cloacal area more common than gastric prolapse
- Etiology is often idiopathic
- Stomach prolapse
  - Concerning if it stays out or becomes repetitive
  - Causes
    - Following gavage of medications/food
    - Administration of certain medications – eugenol
    - Ingested foreign body
    - Irritating or toxic insect eaten

Diagnosis

History:

- Owner notices pink-to-red structure near pelvic area (Figure 55.1)

Signalment:

- Concern for genetic component if numerous cohorts develop cloacal prolapse
- More common in metamorphs (juvenile stage following metamorphosis from tadpole)
- Females may be more predisposed during egg-laying

Clinical Signs:

- Pink to red tissue protruding from vent
- Sometimes, a small "bubble" is associated with the tissue
  - Urinary bladder prolapse
- Anorexia
- Diarrhea
- Constipation

Differentials:

- Physiological
  - Egg-laying female
- Nutritional
  - Over-feeding
    - Too many food items
  - Food presentation
    - Wrong type, size, number
- Metabolic
  - Hepatic disease
  - Renal disease/edema syndrome [7] (Figure 55.3)
  - Nutritional secondary hyperparathyroidism [7, 8] (Figure 55.4)
  - Reproductive disease
- Mechanical
  - Gastrointestinal
    - Foreign body
      - Prey item
      - Substrate (Figure 55.5)
      - Gel water source designed for crickets [10] (Figure 55.6)
      - Fecolith
    - Intussusception, intestinal torsion
    - Ileus
  - Gastric or cloacal prolapse (Figure 55.1)
- Neoplastic [13]
- Infectious [11, 12]
  - Bacterial
  - Viral
  - Parasitic
  - Fungal
- Idiopathic
- Traumatic
  - Pelvic fracture(s)
- Toxic
  - Ammonia toxicity
  - Other water-based or aerosolized toxins in room/house
  - Contact toxins
    - Substrate – aromatic wood (e.g. cedar) chips
    - Cleaning products
    - Inappropriate supplements
- Cardiovascular
  - Vasculitis
  - Disseminated intravascular coagulation

STAT Diagnostics:

- Body weight
- Collect photos for body condition scoring; compare to online images of the particular species
- Physical examination
- Water quality testing – examine pH, ammonia, nitrates, nitrites, and chlorine levels [17]
- Whole body radiographs – dorsoventral and horizontal beam views (Box 55.1)

Complete Diagnostics (See Box 55.1):

- Diagnostic imaging
  - Gastrointestinal contrast series
  - Ultrasound
- Baseline blood work
- Fecal float/direct smear exam
- Coelomocentesis and cytology [20], if indicated

Treatment

Stabilization:

- Provide appropriate husbandry, fluid, and nutrition (Box 55.2)
- Empiric antibiotics

Index

Note: Page numbers in *italic* refer to figures.
Page numbers in **bold** refer to figures.
Where subheadings "mammals", "birds" or "reptiles" are given, there may also be subheadings under the same main heading for subcategories of these, such as "poultry".

Exotic Animal Emergency and Critical Care Medicine, First Edition. Edited by Jennifer E. Graham, Grayson A. Doss and Hugues Beaufrère.

C

d

e

j

k

l

u

V

W